Diseases of

With Contributions by

WALTER BAUER
EVAN CALKINS
ABRAHAM CANTAROW
SIDNEY Q. COHLAN
GARFIELD G. DUNCAN
SAMUEL GURIN
JOSEPH M. HAYMAN, JR.
ROBERT W. HILLMAN
ABRAM KANOFF
ANCEL KEYS
BENJAMIN KRAMER
RACHMIEL LEVINE
MAX MILLER
RULON W. RAWSON
JAMES M. SALTER
MARTIN SONENBERG
TOM D. SPIES
JAMES M. STRANG
RICHARD WAGNER
CECIL J. WATSON
LOUIS G. WELT
PRISCILLA WHITE

Metabolism

DETAILED METHODS OF DIAGNOSIS AND TREATMENT

Edited by

GARFIELD G. DUNCAN, M.D.

Professor of Medicine, University of Pennsylvania; Director of Medical Divisions, Pennsylvania Hospital and The Benjamin Franklin Clinic

FOURTH EDITION — ILLUSTRATED

W. B. Saunders Company

Philadelphia and London

Reprinted, July, 1959

 Made in the United States of America. Press of W. B. Saunders Company. Library of Congress Catalog Card Number: 59-5077

Contributors

WALTER BAUER, M.D., F.A.C.P.
Jackson Professor of Clinical Medicine, Harvard Medical School. Chief of Medical Services, Massachusetts General Hospital, Boston.

EVAN CALKINS, M.D.
Assistant Professor of Medicine, Harvard Medical School. Associate Physician, Massachusetts General Hospital, Boston.

ABRAHAM CANTAROW, M.D.
Professor and Head of Department of Biochemistry, Jefferson Medical College, Philadelphia, Pennsylvania.

SIDNEY Q. COHLAN, M.D.
Associate Professor of Clinical Pediatrics, New York University-Bellevue Medical Center. Associate Attending Physician, Beth Israel Hospital, New York City.

GARFIELD G. DUNCAN, M.D., C.M., F.A.C.P.
Professor of Medicine, University of Pennsylvania. Director of Medical Divisions, Pennsylvania Hospital and the Benjamin Franklin Clinic, Philadelphia.

SAMUEL GURIN, Ph.D.
Benjamin Rush Professor of Biochemistry, University of Pennsylvania School of Medicine. Consultant: National Institute for Arthritis and Metabolic Diseases; Office of the Surgeon General, Department of the Army; National Science Foundation; United States Public Health Service; Veterans Administration Hospital, Philadelphia.

JOSEPH M. HAYMAN, JR., M.D.
Dean and Professor of Medicine, Tufts University School of Medicine. Senior Physician, New England Center Hospital, Boston, Massachusetts.

ROBERT W. HILLMAN, M.D., M.P.H., F.A.C.P.
Associate Professor, Department of Environmental Medicine and Community Health, State University of New York College of Medicine, Brooklyn. Associate Attending Physician, The Brooklyn Hospital; Physician-in-Charge, Red Hook Nutrition Clinic, Brooklyn, New York.

ABRAM KANOF, M.D., F.A.A.P.
Associate Professor of Clinical Pediatrics, State University of New York College of Medicine. Director of Pediatrics, Jewish Chronic Disease Hospital; Attending in Rehabilitation Pediatrics, Jewish Hospital of Brooklyn, New York.

ANCEL KEYS, Ph.D.
Professor, School of Public Health, University of Minnesota, Minneapolis.

BENJAMIN KRAMER, M.S., M.D., F.A.A.P.
Clinical Professor of Pediatrics, Emeritus, State University of New York Downstate Medical Center. Director of Pediatric Services, Maimonides Hospital; Consultant in Pediatrics, Jewish Hospital and Beth-El Hospital, Brooklyn, and Rockaway Beach Hospital, New York.

RACHMIEL LEVINE, M.D.
Professorial Lecturer in Physiology, University of Chicago. Chairman, Department of Medicine, and Director, Department of Metabolic and Endocrine Research, Michael Reese Hospital, Chicago.

MAX MILLER, M.D.
Associate Professor of Medicine, Western Reserve University. Associate Physician, University Hospitals of Cleveland, Cleveland, Ohio.

RULON W. RAWSON, M.D.

Professor of Medicine, Cornell University Medical College. Chief, Division of Clinical Investigation, Sloan-Kettering Institute for Cancer Research. Attending Physician and Co-Chief, Department of Medicine, Memorial Hospital; Executive Officer, Department of Medicine, Memorial Center, New York City.

JAMES MORLEY SALTER, M.A., Ph.D.

Assistant Professor, Banting and Best Department of Medical Research, University of Toronto, Toronto, Ontario, Canada.

MARTIN SONENBERG, M.D., Ph.D.

Associate Professor of Medicine, Cornell University Medical College. Associate, Sloan-Kettering Institute for Cancer Research. Assistant Attending Physician, Memorial Hospital and James Ewing Hospital, New York City.

TOM D. SPIES, M.D., F.A.C.P.

Professor and chairman of Department of Nutrition and Metabolism, Northwestern University Medical School, Chicago. Director, Nutrition Clinic, Hillman Hospital, Birmingham, Alabama.

JAMES M. STRANG, M.D., F.A.C.P.

Assistant Professor of Internal Medicine, University of Pittsburgh. Staff, Western Pennsylvania Hospital; Consultant in Disorders of Metabolism, Veterans Administration Hospital, Pittsburgh.

RICHARD WAGNER, M.D.

Professor of Pediatrics (Emeritus), Tufts University, School of Medicine. Physician, Boston Floating Hospital, Boston, Massachusetts.

CECIL J. WATSON, M.D., Ph.D., F.A.C.P.

Professor of Medicine, University of Minnesota. Chief of Medical Service, University of Minnesota Hospital, Minneapolis.

LOUIS G. WELT, M.D., F.A.C.P.

Professor of Medicine, University of North Carolina School of Medicine, Chapel Hill.

PRISCILLA WHITE, M.D., Sc.D. (Hon.), F.A.C.P.

Assistant Professor of Pediatrics, Tufts University School of Medicine. Physician, New England Deaconess and Boston Lying-In Hospitals, Boston, Massachusetts.

Preface

THE OBJECTIVE in preparing this edition has been to bring into focus progress in methods of investigation with changing concepts that have ensued and the incorporation of the modifying influences which these changes exert in the clinical field of metabolism. If this objective is fully achieved, the physician, the instructor and the student will have at hand basic considerations from which growth of clinical application has evolved. Liberal bibliographies provide opportunity for the perusal of thoughts, investigations and conclusions of those engaged in the exploratory probing of the unknown.

G. G. D.

Acknowledgements

Acknowledgement with sincere appreciation is extended to the co-authors who have brought this enterprise through its fourth edition. They have adhered to the principle of bridging the gap between the highly technical basic concepts and their clinical application. I continue to be indebted to the authors whose names appeared in previous editions but not in this one. They helped greatly in establishing the success which this work enjoys.

A cordial welcome and gratitude are extended to authors whose names appear for the first time in this undertaking. They will share some satisfaction in the successes of previous editions and they will share in maintaining and extending the standards set by their predecessors.

A special note of gratitude is due Mrs. Martha A. Hunscher who has scrutinized the dietary section of the chapter dealing with Diabetes Mellitus.

Suggestions and constructive criticisms from colleagues and reviewers have been most helpful and have been gratefully received and acted upon when it was practicable to do so. I owe much to resident physicians of the Medical Division of the Pennsylvania Hospital who helped with many details. I refer especially to Doctors Agim Leka and Guy L. Schless. Doctor Henry Ford, while he was still a medical student at the University of Pennsylvania, was of special assistance in checking references. I am indebted to him and to my former associate, Doctor Kenneth R. Knox of Hartford, Connecticut, for their tireless support in the preparation of this edition.

Also, I owe thanks to Doctor Charles L. Joiner of London, England, for his help, while a Research Fellow in Metabolism, in crystallizing our experience with oral preparations in the treatment for diabetes.

Staff members of the Pennsylvania Hospital have contributed in tangible and intangible ways through assistance, counsel and special interest in problems of a metabolic nature. I am especially indebted to Doctors Perry S. MacNeal, Charles T. Lee, John B. Alexander, Robert J. Gill, John G. Rogers, William K. Jenson and Edward A. Theurkauf, Jr.

To the Dietary and Nursing Department and to many individuals whose names do not appear but upon whose teachings and writings I have drawn in the fulfilment of our objective I am grateful, as I am for the assistant editorial services of Mrs. Lucia Carr and the secretarial help of Mrs. Catherine Danner.

My wife Dorothea continues to provide an inspiration which has lightened appreciably the burden of this undertaking.

This fourth edition extends the happy relationship of many years' standing with W. B. Saunders Company and their staff. Their patience, understanding and help are deeply appreciated.

Garfield G. Duncan

Contents

Chapter 12

Chapter 13

Chapter 14

CHAPTER 1

By JAMES M. SALTER, PH.D.

Protein Metabolism

INTRODUCTION

The word protein (derived from the Greek proteios, meaning first) was originally used by Mulder in 1839 to designate the material he described as "unquestionably the most important of all known substances in the organic kingdom." "Through its means the chief phenomena of life are produced." The term remains an appropriate one for the complex nitrogenous constituents that "stand at the center of all organic life."[1]

Attempts to elucidate the chemical structure of the proteins began early in the nineteenth century. Wollaston[2] in 1810 isolated cystine from a urinary calculus and Proust[3] in 1819 found leucine while investigating the fermentation of gluten and milk curd, but the significance of these compounds was not recognized, since they were incidental discoveries arising from work not directly concerned with protein structure. The most important early contribution was made by Braconnot, who in 1820 introduced the technique of acid hydrolysis and isolated leucine from hydrolysates of muscle and wool, and glycine from hydrolysates of gelatin. The value of Braconnot's technique was not recognized and, although Liebig[4] discovered tyrosine in 1846 by a process involving the fusion of casein with potassium hydroxide, little progress was made until 1865 when Cramer isolated serine from an acid hydrolysate of silk fibroin. Mainly through the use of acid and, to a lesser extent, alkaline hydrolysis, eleven more amino acids were isolated from proteins between 1865 and 1900. An account of the discovery of the amino acids has been written by Vickery and Schmidt.[5]

PROTEIN STRUCTURE

As the isolation and identification of the amino acids progressed, it became increasingly evident that these compounds were the structural units of proteins.

The twenty-one amino acids more commonly found in protein hydrolysates are listed in Table 1. It is apparent from these data that, with the exception of proline and hydroxyproline, which are more precisely defined as imino acids, the amino acids can be represented by the general formula.

$$\mathrm{R{-}\underset{}{\overset{NH_2}{\overset{|}{C}}}H{-}COOH}$$

The $\mathrm{{-}\overset{NH_2}{\overset{|}{C}}H{-}COOH}$ grouping is a common feature and the individuality of the acid is determined by the nature of the R-grouping.

An important chemical characteristic of the amino acids is the ability of the amino group of one molecule to react with the carboxyl group of a second, with the elimination of a molecule of water.

$$\mathrm{R{-}\overset{NH_2}{\overset{|}{C}}H{-}COOH + NH_2{-}\overset{COOH}{\overset{|}{C}}H{-}R \rightarrow}$$

$$\mathrm{R{-}\overset{NH_2}{\overset{|}{C}}H{-}CO{-}NH{-}\overset{COOH}{\overset{|}{C}}H{-}R + H_2O}$$

TABLE 1. AMINO ACIDS

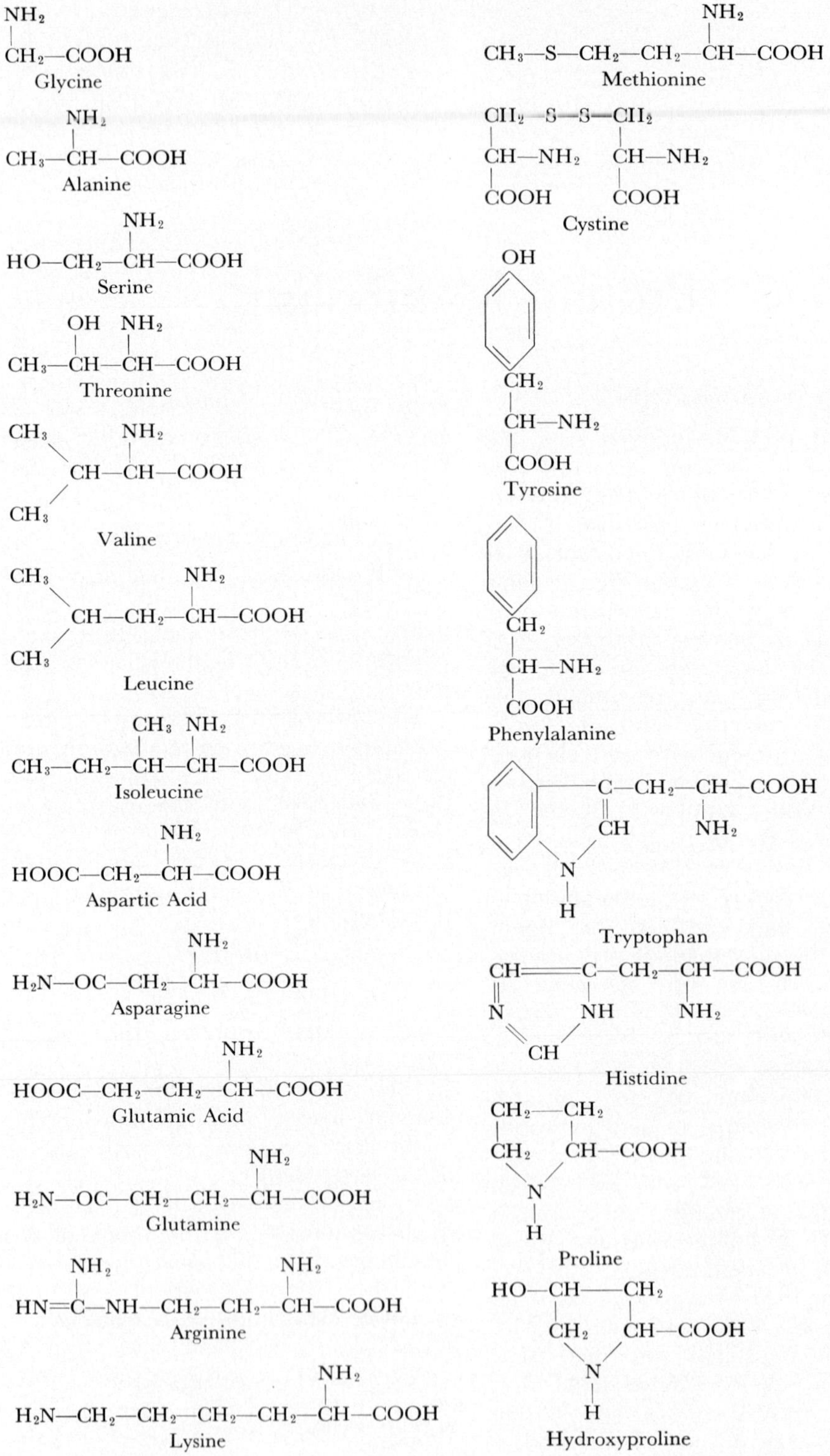

NH_2
$CH_2—COOH$
Glycine

$CH_3—CH(NH_2)—COOH$
Alanine

$HO—CH_2—CH(NH_2)—COOH$
Serine

$CH_3—CH(OH)—CH(NH_2)—COOH$
Threonine

$(CH_3)_2CH—CH(NH_2)—COOH$
Valine

$(CH_3)_2CH—CH_2—CH(NH_2)—COOH$
Leucine

$CH_3—CH_2—CH(CH_3)—CH(NH_2)—COOH$
Isoleucine

$HOOC—CH_2—CH(NH_2)—COOH$
Aspartic Acid

$H_2N—OC—CH_2—CH(NH_2)—COOH$
Asparagine

$HOOC—CH_2—CH_2—CH(NH_2)—COOH$
Glutamic Acid

$H_2N—OC—CH_2—CH_2—CH(NH_2)—COOH$
Glutamine

$HN{=}C(NH_2)—NH—CH_2—CH_2—CH(NH_2)—COOH$
Arginine

$H_2N—CH_2—CH_2—CH_2—CH_2—CH(NH_2)—COOH$
Lysine

$CH_3—S—CH_2—CH_2—CH(NH_2)—COOH$
Methionine

$CH_2—S—S—CH_2$
$CH—NH_2 \quad CH—NH_2$
$COOH \quad COOH$
Cystine

OH
(benzene ring)
CH_2
$CH—NH_2$
$COOH$
Tyrosine

(benzene ring)
CH_2
$CH—NH_2$
$COOH$
Phenylalanine

(benzene ring)—$C—CH_2—CH(NH_2)—COOH$
$\|$
CH
N
H
Tryptophan

$CH{=}C—CH_2—CH(NH_2)—COOH$
$N \quad NH$
CH
Histidine

$CH_2—CH_2$
$CH_2 \quad CH—COOH$
N
H
Proline

$HO—CH—CH_2$
$CH_2 \quad CH—COOH$
N
H
Hydroxyproline

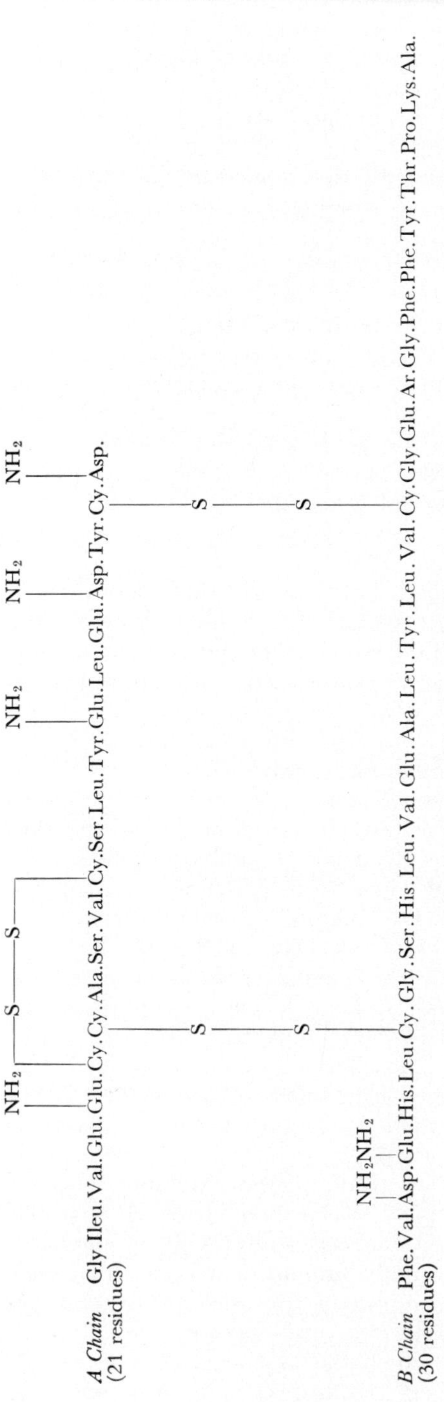

FIG. 1. The structure of beef insulin. (Sanger et al.[7]).

The link between the amino acids is called a peptide bond and the product of the reaction a dipeptide. There is adequate evidence to support the view that in this manner amino acids become linked one to the other to form long polypeptide chains which, in some instances, contain several hundred amino acid residues.

It is only within recent years that the structures of some of the simpler proteins have been determined. This was first accomplished by Sanger et al.,[6,7,8,9] who, through a series of brilliant and painstaking investigations, have determined the structures of beef, hog and sheep insulins. Sanger's work has been closely followed by the determination of the structure of hog β-corticotropin,[10] sheep α-corticotropin, and of oxytocin and vasopressin.[11] The synthesis of oxytocin by du Vigneaud and his colleagues[12] is a remarkable triumph in this field of protein chemistry. Some simple proteins such as insulin (Fig. 1) appear to be constructed of parallel polypeptide chains linked together at intervals by disulfide (or phosphate) bridges. In the case of the corticotropins, the molecule is a single polypeptide chain consisting of 39 amino acids. If the molecular weight of a protein is an index of its complexity, then insulin, which has a molecular weight of 5733, is a relatively simple structure; proteins with molecular weights of several million would appear to be formidably complex.

To obtain a picture of a protein molecule, we require not only a knowledge of the number of polypeptide chains involved and the sequences of the amino acids therein, but also a knowledge of the spatial configuration of the component parts. The reader is referred to original articles and reviews.[13,14]

AMINO ACIDS AND PROTEIN IN NUTRITION

Interest in the nutritive value of proteins was greatly stimulated by the emphasis Mulder placed on their biologic importance. Unfortunately, the view expressed by Boussingault[15] in

1851 that the nutritive value of a protein was only a function of its nitrogen content received support from Liebig and, although there was considerable evidence to the contrary, this misconception persisted for many years. Voit had observed that, despite its high nitrogen content, gelatin could not replace fresh meat in the diet, but Rubner seems to have been the first to realize that protein and nitrogen nutrition were not synonymous. In 1897 he drew attention to the fact that the nutritive value of protein depended as much upon the source of this nutrient as it did upon its nitrogen content. The first evidence indicating that the amino acids played an important role in determining the biologic value of proteins was obtained by Willcock and Hopkins in 1906, when they found that mice died when fed a diet containing zein as the only protein, and that the addition of tryptophan to the food prolonged their survival. Investigations carried out by Osborne revealed that the amino acid composition of different vegetable proteins varied remarkably, and in 1907 he wrote,[16] "What significance these differences have in respect to the nutritive value of these different proteins must be determined by future investigation, for it has only very recently been discovered that such differences exist." At this point there began an era of investigation that is not yet complete.

Before dealing with some of the current concepts of protein nutrition, a brief description is given of the principal methods used to determine their biologic value.

Methods Used to Determine the Nutritive Value of Protein

Growth of Immature Animals. One of the simplest and most popular methods of assessing the nutritive value of a specific protein, or of an amino acid mixture, consists of determining its ability to support the growth of immature animals (usually the albino rat) when it is incorporated as the chief source of nitrogen in a diet that is complete in all other respects. This method was used by Hopkins and many other early workers, but was standardized and made practicable by Osborne and Mendel, who were among the first to develop semi-synthetic diets of known composition that were capable of maintaining the health and vigor of experimental animals. The rate of growth is most frequently determined by measuring the rate of weight gain. The fact that the indispensability of many amino acids was discovered using this technique proves its value, but the method does have some shortcomings.

Weight gain is representative of true growth only when a significant part of the increase is due to a proportionate increase in the size and protein content of the various body tissues. The nutritive value, or the "protein efficiency," has been defined as the weight gain per gram of protein (or nitrogen) consumed. It is assumed that there exists a high degree of correlation between the weight gained and the amount of new protein synthesized. This assumption is not always justified, since the weight gain may be due to alterations in the content of body fat and/or water. Mitchell and associates,[17] using rats as their test animals, found that the protein efficiency of Limburger cheese and milk curd were similar when calculated by the method previously described. Subsequent analyses showed, however, that the animals fed the cheese synthesized more fat and less protein than rats fed the milk curd. Thus the ratio, weight gain to protein consumed, was not a true index of the ability of the proteins to support growth and protein synthesis.

The Rat-repletion Method. This extremely useful method, which is widely used,[18] consists essentially of depleting the body protein of a rat by placing it on a protein free diet until it has lost 25 per cent of its body weight. The rate at which the animal regains its weight when the test protein or amino acid mixture is incorporated into the diet serves as a measure of the protein's nutritive value. According to Frost and Sandy,[19] the rate at which the various tissue proteins regenerate correlates extremely well with the rate of weight gain. An attractive feature of this technique is the speed with which the assays can be carried out. Periods of 12 days for depletion and 12 days for repletion seem to be perfectly adequate. Determinations of the quality of proteins and amino acid mixtures by the growth method frequently require several months.

Nitrogen Balance. The greatest part of the nitrogen consumed is an integral part of the proteins and amino acids contained in the diet. The proteins, in the course of digestion, are degraded to amino acids before being absorbed from the intestinal tract. There is no appreciable storage of free amino acids within the body. They are either anabolized into proteins or catabolized and their nitrogenous residues excreted. Thus the determination of nitrogen balance—i.e., the difference between the amount of nitrogen ingested and the amount lost from the body in the urine, feces, perspiration, hair, dead skin, etc.—allows us to evaluate the general state of protein metabolism. When the nitrogen intake over a given period of time exceeds the nitrogen loss, the organism is in positive nitrogen balance and it is concluded that the rate of protein synthesis is greater than the rate of protein breakdown. Conversely, when the total amount of body protein is diminishing, the nitrogen loss exceeds the intake and the animal is in negative nitrogen balance. Nitrogen equilibrium is established when nitrogen intake and output are equal and thus the rates of protein anabolism and catabolism are equal.

The general practice in determining nitrogen balance is to consider only fecal and urinary nitrogen; the nitrogen lost by other routes (perspiration, hair, etc.) is small and contributes only a negligible error to the results. In many instances the changes in nitrogen balance are reflected only by changes in the urinary nitrogen excretion, fecal nitrogen remaining relatively constant. For this reason, the nitrogen balance is often estimated by determining the nitrogen content of the urine alone. Fecal nitrogen of adults, under normal conditions, averages between 1 and 2 grams daily[20] and may change little despite fairly wide variations in protein intake.[21,22] There is little justification for the assumption frequently made in metabolic studies that fecal nitrogen amounts to one-tenth of the total nitrogen ingested. Fecal nitrogen is increased by the consumption of proteins that are poorly digested[23] and by the addition to the diet of non-nitrogenous indigestible bulk.[21,24] It does not appear to be readily influenced by changes in fat or carbohydrate[25] consumption.

The amount of fecal nitrogen may, under normal conditions, remain relatively constant on a fixed dietary regimen, but it is difficult to approximate just what that amount may be. There are also many instances in which pathologic or experimental conditions alter markedly the nitrogen losses in feces. Thus, the accuracy of a nitrogen balance study can be assured only by determining the nitrogen content of both the stools and the urine.

The nitrogen content of food and of excreta can be determined with great accuracy, and balance studies afford the best means of evaluating protein quality. Unfortunately, the technique, although simple in practice, is laborious and time consuming. While the nature of the balance yields information regarding the general state of protein metabolism, it obviously cannot furnish data concerning the nitrogen metabolism in specific tissues.

The Essential Amino Acids

A major advance in the science of nutrition was made when it was discovered that health could be maintained only when the dietary protein contained adequate amounts of certain amino acids. The first intimation of the importance of amino acids was obtained by Willcock and Hopkins in 1906,[26] when they found that mice fed diets containing zein as the sole source of protein lost weight and eventually died. The addition of tryptophan to the diet did not completely remedy the situation, but it did prolong the survival time of the animals. It was later shown by Osborne and Mendel that zein was deficient in lysine as well as tryptophan, and that the growth of experimental animals could be restored only by adding both factors to the diet. Abderhalden[27] also provided convincing proof of the nutritional importance of tryptophan by feeding dogs a casein hydrolysate from which this amino acid had been removed. These animals developed a marked negative nitrogen balance and lost weight unless tryptophan was added to the diets.

It was also shown by Akroyd and Hopkins[28] that young rats lost weight when fed hydrolyzed casein from which histidine and arginine had been removed. They reported that both factors had to be replaced before normal growth could occur. Rose and Cox[29,30] were unable to confirm this observation and claimed that it was necessary to add only histidine. In a subsequent investigation, Scull and Rose[31] showed that when rats were allowed to grow on a diet that lacked arginine, their carcasses contained much more of this substance than did the carcasses of littermate controls that were killed and analyzed at a much earlier age. They correctly concluded that the rat was quite capable of synthesizing arginine. However, Rose also found that rats on an arginine deficient diet grew more slowly than controls fed diets supplemented with this amino acid. It was concluded that the rat could synthesize arginine, but not rapidly enough to sustain optimal growth. Although this amino acid has been classified as an essential dietary factor for young rats, Wolf and Corley[32] have shown that nitrogen equilibrium can be maintained in mature animals on diets free of arginine.

The early nutritional studies led inevitably to an attempt on the part of Rose to replace completely dietary protein by a mixture of amino acids. Rose found that a mixture of the 19 amino acids then known failed to maintain the weight of young rats. Since the weight gain and growth of the young animals could be restored by the addition of a little whole protein to the diet, it was assumed that the protein contained an amino acid or acids that had not yet been identified. The successful culmination of these investigations led to the isolation and identification by Rose[33,34] of threonine (α-amino-β-hydroxybutyric acid).

TABLE 2. ESSENTIAL AND NONESSENTIAL AMINO ACIDS

ESSENTIAL	NONESSENTIAL
Tryptophan	Alanine
Lysine	Glycine
Methionine	Glutamic acid
Threonine	Hydroxyglutamic acid
Phenylalanine	Aspartic acid
Leucine	Cystine
Isoleucine	Cysteine
Valine	Tyrosine
*Histidine	Proline
*Arginine	Hydroxyproline
	Serine
	Norleucine
	Citrulline

* Not required by adult man and probably not by children.

The discovery of threonine made it possible to feed a mixture of amino acids that would support the growth of rats, and greatly facilitated the study of the role of the other amino acids in nutrition. By using incomplete mixtures Rose was able to show that leucine, isoleucine, valine and phenylalanine were essential dietary factors.

It has been mentioned that arginine can be synthesized to a limited but appreciable extent by the young rat. Therefore, a dietary deficiency of arginine results only in a reduced rate of growth, whereas weight loss and death occur in the absence of any one of the remaining essential amino acids. However, some of the indispensable acids can be synthesized in adequate amounts when certain compounds that are not normally found in food are added to the rations. For example, α-keto-γ-methiolbutyrate can replace dietary methionine (see Metabolism of Methionine). It appears that Rose had such reservations in mind when he phrased his definition of an essential amino acid as "one that cannot be synthesized by the animal organism out of the materials ordinarily available, at a speed commensurate with the demands for normal growth."

Amino Acid Requirements

The amino acid requirements of various species are remarkably similar. The needs of the mouse are identical with those of the rat. Rose and Rice[35] find that the adult dog can be maintained in nitrogen balance in the absence of arginine, but the removal from the diet of any of the factors considered essential for the rat brings about an immediate loss of nitrogen and a negative balance. Almquist[36] finds that the chick needs arginine and glutamic acid as well as the rat factors. The amino acid requirements of adult man have been investigated by Holt et al.[37] and by Rose,[38,39] using the nitrogen balance technique. The results of these investigations have shown that nitrogen equilibrium can be maintained with amino acid mixtures lacking both arginine and histidine. With these exceptions, the amino acid requirements of man are the same as those of the rat.

Rose and collaborators have in recent years attempted to establish the quantitative amino acid requirements of man. The diets used in these studies supplied from 6.7 to 10.1 grams of nitrogen per day and contained, in addition to the essential amino acid supplements, glycine and urea, the latter two compounds serving as a source of nitrogen for the synthesis of the dispensable amino acids. The requirement for a given amino acid was determined by decreasing the dietary level over successsive periods until a negative nitrogen balance ensued. The diet was then supplemented with the amino acid until nitrogen equilibrium was re-established. The tentative minimal daily requirements of man for the amino acids, as determined by Rose et al.,[40,41,42] are shown in Table 3.

The Necessity for the Simultaneous Availability of Amino Acids. It appears that all of the amino acids required for protein anabolism must be simultaneously available before synthesis can proceed. Elman[43] found that dogs could be maintained in nitrogen equilibrium by the intravenous administration of casein hydrolysates that contained added tryptophan.* If an unsupplemented hydrolysate was given and the tryptophan administered a few hours later, a negative balance ensued. Cannon et al.[44] have reported that rats failed to grow if five of the essential amino acids were fed at one time and the remaining five fed one hour later. Similar results

* Tryptophan is destroyed by the acid hydrolysis of proteins.

TABLE 3. AMINO ACID REQUIREMENTS OF ADULT MAN

AMINO ACID	RANGE OF REQUIREMENTS OBSERVED	PROPOSED TENTATIVE MINIMUM	"SAFE INTAKE"
	gm. per day	gm. per day	gm. per day
L-Isoleucine	(0.65–0.70)	0.70	1.40
L-Leucine	(0.50–1.10)	1.10	2.20
L-Lysine	(0.40–0.80)	0.80	1.60
DL-Methionine[1]	(0.80–1.10)	1.10	2.20
L-Phenylalanine[2]	(0.80–1.10)	1.10	2.20
L-Threonine	(0.30–0.50)	0.50	1.00
L-Tryptophan	(0.15–0.25)	0.25	0.50
L-Valine	(0.40–0.80)	0.80	1.60

[1] L-cystine may replace up to 80 to 89 per cent of the minimal methionine needs. D-methionine is fully as active as L-methionine.

[2] L tyrosine may replace up to 70 to 75 per cent of the minimal phenylalanine requirement.

have been obtained by Geiger et al.[45] and by Henderson and Harris.[46]

Role of Nonessential Amino Acids. It must be recalled that certain of the amino acids are dispensable in the dietary sense only. All of the amino acids are essential for the maintenance and function of the body tissues. Rose[47] has reported that rats fed diets containing only essential amino acids gain 70 to 75 per cent as much weight as controls fed both the essential and nonessential acids. It seems possible that the inhibition of growth seen under these conditions may be due to a lag in the availability of the nonessential factors which must first be synthesized from the indispensable amino acids. Mention was made previously that protein synthesis can occur only when all of the precursors are simultaneously available. A delay of one hour in feeding a supplement that contains essential amino acids missing from the diet previously consumed results in a marked inhibition of protein anabolism. Although the nonessential elements can be synthesized from other amino acids, the nitrogen required for their formation can be derived from simple nitrogenous compounds. It has been shown by Frost and Sandy,[48] Lardy and Feldott,[49] and Rose[50] that essential amino acids are spared from the synthesis of nonessential amino acids by glutamic acid, glycine, diammonium citrate and ammonium acetate.

Protein Quality

Digestibility. It is apparent from the foregoing discussion that the nutritive value of protein is primarily dependent upon its amino acid composition. However, the quality of the protein is also a function of its digestibility. The biologic values of raw egg white and of soybean protein are considerably reduced by the presence of anti-tryptic factors that interfere with digestion.[51] Heating frequently improves protein utilization, in some instances by destroying anti-tryptic factors; in others the cooking may act simply by softening the material and making it more vulnerable to attack by digestive enzymes. The protein of parboiled rice is used 14.5 per cent more efficiently than that in the nonparboiled rice.[52] Dry heat often reduces protein quality, either by causing the amino acid to form new compounds that are resistant to digestion, or by destroying them.[53,54]

Supplementation of Protein with Protein. The benefits obtained from consuming high quality protein cannot be obtained simply by eating abnormally large amounts of poor quality protein, even though the latter has a relative rather than an absolute deficiency of some essential amino acids. This is well illustrated by the experimental results obtained by Bosshardt and colleagues[55] which showed that young rats fed diets containing as much as 35 per cent gluten protein did not gain weight as well as animals fed diets containing only 11 to 12 per cent of egg and milk protein. When the diet contains only a low quality protein such as gluten, its potential usefulness is lost, since only a fraction of it can be utilized for tissue synthesis, while the remainder must be catabolized. Utilization can be greatly increased either by mixing with it protein of animal origin or by combining two different low quality proteins that are capable of complementing each other's deficiencies. Sure and associates[56] have recently reported that when one half of the protein supplied by milled wheat in a diet is replaced by protein from milled rice, rat growth is enhanced 114 per cent and the total protein utilization increased by 86 per cent. Since the essential amino acids must be simultaneously available before anabolism can take place, the proteins that contain between them the full complement of essential amino acids must be consumed during the course of one meal.

Supplementation of Proteins with Amino Acids. Supplementation of poor quality proteins with the specific amino acids they lack has been given an increasing amount of consideration as a method whereby protein malnutrition can be remedied in areas of the world where cereals and vegetables serve as the main source of food. This topic, which has been the subject of many reviews[57,58,59] and original investigations, can be given only brief consideration here. Corn proteins are deficient in tryptophan and lysine, while wheat proteins are low in lysine only. The feasibility of improving the flours derived from these grains by adding lysine and tryptophan has been shown by Sure et al.,[60] Pecora and Hundley[61] and many others.

Amino Acid Imbalances. Fortification of protein can also have detrimental effects by producing what are loosely referred to as amino acid imbalances and toxicities. Elvehjem[62] demonstrated that rats fed a niacin-free diet containing 9 per cent casein supplemented with 0.2 per cent cystine gained weight at a rate of 12 grams per week. The addition of 0.078 per cent threonine to the diet reduced the growth rate to 4 grams per week, while further supplementation with tryptophan increased the rate to 20 grams per week. Elvehjem[62,63] considers this an example of an increase in the level of one amino acid (threonine) affecting the requirement of the next most limiting amino acid (tryptophan). It has been suggested that the addition of threonine potentiates protein synthesis so that the little tryptophan available is used for tissue anabolism, leaving none available for the synthesis of niacin. The animal is therefore suffering from a secondary niacin deficiency. Similarly, a severe amino acid deficiency can be precipitated and growth retarded when a diet low in histidine is supplemented with lysine,[64] and also when valine is added to a diet deficient in threonine.[60] It is evident from these and many other investigations that if supplementation of poor quality protein is to have a beneficial effect, a detailed knowledge of the protein composition is necessary. It should also be mentioned that because the amino acids are required simultaneously, the value of the supplement is reduced as the free amino acid is partially absorbed and metabolized during the time taken for digestion of the dietary protein.

Factors Affecting Protein Requirements

Caloric Intake. The relationship between dietary carbohydrate and fat and protein metabolism was the subject of some of the earliest metabolic studies. Lusk[65] in 1890, and shortly after Miura,[66] Neumann[67] and Roseman[68] reported that withdrawal of carbohydrate or fat from an adequate diet promptly increased the nitrogen excretion of their human subjects. As may be expected, the converse of this also holds true. The addition of either carbohydrate or fat to a diet that has sufficient protein, but which supplies an inadequate caloric intake, greatly improves the nitrogen balance.[69,70,71] This phenomenon has been termed the "nitrogen sparing action of carbohydrate and fat." An exception to the general rule that a reduction in caloric intake increases nitrogen excretion is found in the obese person who, when placed on a low calory diet that contains enough protein, remains in nitrogen equilibrium. It appears that the extra energy obtained from the increased rate of fat catabolism replaces that which normally would have been derived from the diet. It has also been demonstrated by Munro[72] and many others[73,74] that the addition of carbohydrate or fat to diets quite adequate in all respects produces a reduction in nitrogen excretion and enhances growth and protein synthesis. The diminution in nitrogen excretion obtained by surfeit feeding of fat or carbohydrate may be sustained for long periods in young growing animals. However, the positive nitrogen balance seen in mature animals under these circumstances must be relatively short-lived, for adults who eat excessively only grow obese.

In summary, the energy required for the maintenance of vital processes, including protein synthesis, is derived primarily from the oxidation of carbohydrate and fat. Regardless of the quantity or quality of dietary protein, nitrogen equilibrium cannot be sustained when the energy intake is less than the energy expenditure. When the caloric intake is inadequate, amino acids are

TABLE 4. RECOMMENDED* DAILY PROTEIN INTAKE

	AGE	BODY WT. KG.	CALORIES	PROTEIN GM.
Men	25	65	3200	65
	45	65	2900	65
	65	65	2600	65
Women	25	55	2300	55
	45	55	2100	55
	65	55	1800	55
Pregnancy (3rd trimester)	...	..	add 1400	80
Lactation	...	..	add 1000	100
Infants	0–1/12			
	1/12–3/12	6	Kg. × 120	3.5 gm./Kg. body weight
	4/12–9/12	9	Kg. × 110	
	10/12–1	10	Kg. × 100	
Children	1– 3	12	1200	40
	4– 6	18	1600	50
	7– 9	27	2000	60
Boys	10–12	35	2500	70
	13–15	49	3200	85
	16–20	63	3800	100
Girls	10–12	36	2300	70
	13–15	49	2500	80
	16–20	54	2400	75

* National Research Council.[75]

less efficiently utilized for protein anabolism and are more rapidly deaminated, with the subsequent oxidation of the residues filling part of the energy deficit.

Age. The protein requirement in relation to body weight is highest during infancy; the intake recommended by the National Research Council[75] is about 3.5 to 4.0 grams of protein per kilogram of body weight per day during the first three years. Specific recommendations are not given for the first month of life, since the desirable allowance is dependent upon maturation of excretory and endocrine functions. It has been pointed out[75] that although the breast-fed infant normally receives from 2 to 2.5 grams of protein per kilogram per day, an amount less than that recommended and supplied by formulas for artificial feeding, there is no convincing evidence that the breast-fed infant is lacking in protein or that the higher levels supplied by conventional formulas should be decreased.

The protein requirements drop slowly throughout childhood and adolescence and become fixed at a value of 1 gram per kilogram body weight for adults. Although the recommended absolute amount does not change with old age, the proportion in the diet increases since the total caloric intake decreases (Table 4).

Pregnancy, Lactation and Menstruation. Hyperplasia of the uterus and adnexae, as well as growth of the fetus, increases the protein requirement during pregnancy. Murlin[76] claims that on high protein diets the mother may retain, exclusive of fetal nitrogen, as much as 280 grams of nitrogen. The National Research Council[77] estimates that women who have borne and nursed six children will, between the age of puberty and 45, have synthesized twice their body weight of protein. The extent of the positive nitrogen balance during pregnancy has been variously estimated at 1.8 to 6 grams daily.[78,79] Seegers[80] reported that the proportion of ingested nitrogen retained increased steadily throughout the gestation period.

When the protein consumption drops below that required to maintain the pregnant mother's nitrogen balance, the fetus is maintained at the expense of the maternal tissues. The extent to which this can occur in some animals, and perhaps in humans, is indeed surprising. Nelson and Evans[81] found that rats given diets ranging from 10 to 25 per cent protein on the day of mating produced normal litters. The weight gained during gestation and the birth weight of the young was less on the low protein diet. Reducing the protein to 5 per cent resulted in resorption of 30 per cent of the implantations, and 17 per cent of the young were stillborn. However, doubling the amount of the vitamin B complex in this diet prevented resorption and reduced the number of stillborn to 2 per cent. On protein-free diets the mothers lost 41 grams during the gestation period, and 90 to 100 per cent of the implantations were resorbed. The remarkable feature is that a few rats were born.

It appears to be clearly established that a plentiful supply of protein confers protection against many of the complications of pregnancy. Tompkins[82] reports that raising the protein intake of pregnant women from 65 to 115 grams a day reduced the incidence of toxemia from 4.12 per cent to 0.63 per cent. Similar conclusions have been reached by Burke et al.[83] and by Leverton and McMillan.[84] Burke et al.[85] claim that a protein intake of less than 75 grams daily frequently gives rise to infants that receive low pediatric ratings. They agree that edema and toxemia are more prevalent among pregnant women on low protein diets. The high protein requirement is not reduced at parturition, since during lactation the mother must provide from 7 to 15 grams of protein each day. A considerable number of investigations[86,87,88] carried out with human subjects and with laboratory animals indicate that meat rather than vegetable protein is preferable during pregnancy and lactation. It should be recalled that utilization of the dietary protein depends upon an adequate caloric intake.

According to Kestner,[89] nitrogen losses during menstruation are from 1.5 to 3.3 grams daily. It has been estimated[77] that menstrual losses from puberty to the age of 45 require the average woman to synthesize an amount of protein equivalent to her own body weight.

Exercise. Within fairly wide limits, variations in muscular activity do not affect the nitrogen balance[90] or protein requirement. An increase in activity will increase nitrogen excretion only when the carbohydrate and fat consumption is not increased enough to cover the increased caloric expenditure.[91] However, a sudden change in living habits, with a more or less permanent increase in muscular activity, can result in a temporary increase in the amount of nitrogen retained.[92] The explanation for this would seem to lie in the hypertrophy of the body musculature. Conversely, prolonged immobilization in bed, even of healthy persons, is accompanied by a marked increase in nitrogen excretion and loss of body protein. Although there has been considerable discussion as to the cause of this, disuse atrophy of the muscles would seem to be the most obvious explanation.

Pathologic States. Disease or injury in a healthy and well nourished person invariably increases nitrogen excretion, the extent of the change paralleling the severity of the physical insult. The losses may reach enormous proportions, and the situation is aggravated by anorexia and immobilization in bed. Chronically ill or malnourished persons resist any further loss of body protein.[93] Following the fracture of a long bone or surgical procedures, the increase in nitrogen excretion is evident within 48 hours and reaches a maximum within 3 to 6 days. The azoturia gradually subsides and, as recovery commences, the nitrogen balance becomes positive. These periods are termed respectively the “catabolic” and “anabolic” phases.

The wisdom of attempting to correct the nitrogen losses and malnutrition that occur during the acute response to injury has been subjected to some debate.[94] The suggestion that the catabolic response is beneficial has been criticized by Pollack and Halpern,[94] who consider the increased catabolism of protein following trauma to be a vestigial response dating from the time a sick and wounded animal was unable to forage for himself and required an emergency supply of protein to enable him to meet the stressful situation. These authors also point out that although it is difficult to prevent the nitrogen loss during the "catabolic phase" of injury, it is hard to know where it ends and the "anabolic phase" begins. Certainly, during the latter period, the protein requirement is elevated and recovery is enhanced by the consumption of the appropriate diet.

Pollack and Halpern[94] point out that "therapeutic diets" frequently contribute to the negative nitrogen balance and are grossly inadequate. The Sippy type diets consumed by postoperative ulcer patients during the first ten days contain only half the protein recommended for normal adults. They conclude: "It is not surprising therefore, that some of these patients ingesting 'therapeutic' diets may become chronic invalids."

It is obvious that the body protein lost as a consequence of trauma or disease must be replaced and that an inadequate protein intake can delay or prevent convalescence. However, there is no convincing proof that feeding protein in amounts markedly in excess of the normal requirement accelerates recovery. In many instances, the benefits claimed for high protein diets are based on casual observation, rather than rigorously controlled investigations.

Protein Malnutrition. Symptoms attributable to the absolute lack of a single essential amino acid are rarely encountered clinically. Under experimental conditions the withdrawal from the diet of an indispensable amino acid is accompanied by the rapid onset of such symptoms as fatigue, anorexia, nervousness, irritability, weight loss and negative nitrogen balance. Severe protein malnutrition produces similar symptoms and is associated with anemia, hypoproteinemia, edema, a delay in convalescence, slow wound healing and increased susceptibility to infection. According to Lynch and Snively,[95] subacute protein deficiency is not uncommon among children and occurs because of the failure of the parents to enforce a reasonable measure of discipline with regard to the child's eating habits. The condition is difficult to diagnose because of the vague and apparently unrelated symptoms which they list as anorexia, failure to gain weight, gastrointestinal disturbances including vomiting and constipation, frequent bouts of infectious disease, dental caries and anemia. The condition responds promptly when the parents enforce the necessary discipline and realize, as the authors point out, that the child must be allowed the privilege of feeling hungry.

Malnutrition due to the inadequate consumption of good quality protein is, of course, best treated by making the appropriate adjustment in a diet comprised of natural food. It is generally agreed that meat, milk, cheese and eggs are much superior as sources of this nutrient than are vegetables, and that 60 to 75 per cent of the total dietary protein should be of animal origin.[86,58] When the patient is unable to chew properly or is anorexic, the consumption of adequate protein and other nutrients may be encouraged by the use of milk and egg concentrates that can be tube fed or flavored and made up as a pleasant drink. Where taste need not be considered (tube feeding), amino acid mixtures or protein hydrolysates may be employed if supplemented accordingly with an adequate source of calories and other dietary factors. It is important to note that when amino acid mixtures or protein hydrolysates are used either orally or intravenously the caloric requirement for the maintenance of nitrogen balance is, for an unexplained reason, higher than that needed to maintain balance when the person consumes whole protein. In recent investigations, Rose and associates[96] found that when whole casein was fed, 35 calories per kilogram of body weight resulted in a positive nitrogen balance. In contrast, when the same amount of nitrogen was given as a hydrolysate of casein the nitrogen balance remained negative until the caloric intake was raised to 45.5

per kilogram of body weight. This represents an increase of nearly 30 per cent over the basic caloric requirement and must certainly be taken into consideration when such mixtures are used clinically. The use of commercially available preparations of amino acids and protein hydrolysates for intravenous therapy in debilitated patients has become well established and little comment is required here.

Protein Digestion

Digestion in the Stomach. The digestion of protein is initiated in the stomach through the action of the enzyme pepsin which hydrolyzes the protein into short polypeptide chains called proteoses and peptones. Pepsin, like most other enzymes, shows some degree of specificity of action since it can only affect the hydrolysis of peptide bonds in which the amino group is supplied by one of the aromatic amino acids, tyrosine, or phenylalanine.[97] Its action does not appear to be limited to the nature of the amino acid supplying the carbonyl grouping. The cells of the gastric mucosa manufacture the pepsin precursor, pepsinogen, which is stable in alkaline solution but is converted to the active enzyme when the pH drops below 6. The pepsin liberated then acts on its own precursor, pepsinogen, to accelerate the formation of more pepsin. Peptic activity is optimal at about pH 2. This degree of acidity is maintained by gastric hydrochloric acid.

Gastric rennin, like other proteolytic enzymes, renders the casein of milk insoluble. The exact nature of the changes that occur during the process are not completely understood.[98] Available information indicates that the rennin, when added to milk, splits the soluble casein into soluble proteoses and a substance called paracasein. The latter material combines with calcium ions to form the insoluble curd, calcium paracasein. Rennin is especially abundant in the gastric mucosa of animals and is believed to aid in the digestion and utilization of milk. Its significance in the digestive processes of adults is unknown.

Digestion in the Small Intestine. The second phase of protein digestion occurs in the duodenum through the action of the proteolytic enzymes of the pancreatic juice, trypsin, chymotrypsin and carboxypeptidase. The activity of trypsin is limited to the hydrolysis of peptide bonds in which L-arginine or L-lysine contribute the carbonyl group.[99] Tryptic proteolysis is optimal at about pH 8. The active enzyme is formed from the inactive precursor, trypsinogen. Trypsinogen is converted to trypsin in mildly alkaline solution (pH 8) and, as in the case of pepsin, the active enzyme accelerates its own formation by attacking its inactive precursor. The formation of trypsin is also accelerated by the action of enterokinase, an enzyme secreted by the intestinal mucosa.

Trypsin, besides its digestive function, activates chymotrypsinogen to chymotrypsin. This latter proteolytic enzyme has its optimal action in a pH range similar to that of trypsin. Chymotrypsin shows some degree of specificity, attacking most rapidly peptide bonds in which the carbonyl group is supplied by L-tyrosine. It will, however, attack peptide bonds in which the carbonyl linkage is supplied by L-tryptophan, L-phenylalanine or L-methionine.

Pepsin, trypsin and chymotrypsin all possess the ability to hydrolyze peptide bonds situated in the interior of the polypeptide chain. For this reason they have been termed *endopeptidases*. Carboxypeptidase and the enzymes of the intestinal juice hydrolyze the last peptide bond in the chain and are thus called *exopeptidases*.

Carboxypeptidase is a pancreatic enzyme so named because it hydrolyzes the terminal peptide bond only when there is a free carboxyl group on the end of the chain.

$$\begin{array}{c} NH_2 \qquad\qquad\quad R \\ | \qquad\qquad\qquad | \\ R—CH—CO \,\vdots\, NH—CH—COOH \end{array}$$

Carboxypeptidase

Its precursor, procarboxypeptidase, is found in pancreatic tissue and is converted to the active enzyme by trypsin.

Digestion is completed by enzymes of the intestinal juice (succus entericus) several of which are classified as aminopeptidases because they cleave only the terminal peptide bonds adjacent to a free amino group. Many aminopeptidases appear to act on peptides of varying chain lengths; however, some act only on dipeptides or tripeptides, while another, leucine aminopeptidase, cleaves the peptide bond only when leucine supplies the adjacent free amino group. With the exception of leucine aminopeptidase, which has been highly purified by Spackman,[100] purification and characterization of the intestinal juice enzymes remains to be accomplished.

The Absorption of the Products of Protein Digestion

There is no significant absorption of amino acids from the stomach. The end products of protein digestion are most rapidly absorbed from the duodenum, and the process is more or less complete by the time the intestinal contents reach the ileocecal valve.

Fridhandler and Quastel[101] report that the amino acid can cross the intestinal wall by simple diffusion when the concentration of these substances is equal to, or greater than, 0.02 M. At concentration below 0.02 M they are actively absorbed, i.e., energy has to be expended to transport the metabolites across the intestinal wall. The exact mechanisms involved in active transport are not fully known, but the energy appears to be derived from the reactions involved in oxidative phosphorylation, since the absorption of L-amino acids is inhibited by anaerobiosis and dinitrophenol[102,103] and stimulated by adenosine triphosphate.[104]

Although the amino acids are the main products of protein digestion that are absorbed, it cannot be safely assumed that the absorption of small polypeptides is an unimportant or unphysiologic process. London and Kotchneva[105] found that in dogs polypeptides persisted throughout the length of the small intestine and could be detected in the portal blood. Mellander[106] has reported that when the milk protein casein is digested in vitro by proteolytic enzymes of the intestinal tract, there remains a considerable residue of polypeptides that are resistant to further enzymatic degradation. The resistance is apparently due to phosphorylation of the peptides, since enzymatic dephosphorylation makes them again susceptible to digestion. These peptides readily form complexes with calcium, iron or other metals. The compound formed with calcium, calcium-phosphopeptide, is highly soluble in water and can be given to rabbits by the intravenous route without producing toxic side effects or anaphylactic reactions. At least 70 per cent of the calcium of the phosphopeptide complex can be absorbed from the intestinal tract of infants. Mellander[107] suggests that large peptides may be of nutritional importance because they combine with other nutrients such as calcium and iron, thus favoring their absorption.

Unaltered protein can be absorbed from the intestinal tract of children. Gruskay and Cooke[108] recently reported that by use of the precipitin reaction 4.26 micrograms of egg albumin per milliliter of serum could be detected after this material was administered to children 5 days to 19 months of age. The mean concentration of egg albumin in the serum was increased to 22.84 micrograms per milliliter in children convalescing from diarrhea. The absorption of whole protein need not, of course, be limited to egg albumin and, since the amount of native protein absorbed may be of great importance in sensitizing the child to foreign proteins, Gruskay and Cooke favor the feeding of protein hydrolysates, rather than whole protein, to children recovering from diarrhea.

Protein Reserves

Rubner in 1911[109] postulated the existence of an unorganized storage protein that functioned to maintain nitrogen equilibrium when the food intake was intermittent. The basis for this belief was derived from experiments performed originally by Voit,[110,111] the results of which were confirmed by many investigators. Voit found that when a dog was fasted, the nitrogen excretion fell rapidly for 5 to 6 days and then became relatively constant. Similar changes were observed when the animals were fed a diet containing adequate carbohydrate and fat, but no protein. The excess urinary nitrogen excreted during the first few days was thought to originate from storage protein. It is well established that raising the level of protein in a diet that has more than an adequate amount of this nutrient produces a positive nitrogen balance that lasts for a few days. Conversely, if the protein intake is dropped, but to a level that is still perfectly adequate, the nitrogen balance turns negative for a short period. These data could easily be interpreted as indicating an increase or decrease in storage protein accompanying a corresponding change in nitrogen consumption. However, research in the intervening years has failed to reveal any depot or special form of protein that serves exclusively as a reserve supply.

The rapid fall and subsequent stabilization in urinary nitrogen excretion that occurs during the first few days of starvation can be explained by the behavior of the visceral organs, which lose their labile protein rapidly and then resist further depletion. The difference in the speed and extent of the protein loss from various tissues is evident from observations made by Addis, Poo and Lew.[112,113] They found that when rats were starved for 7 days the protein losses, when expressed as a percentage of the tissue originally present, were: liver, 40; prostate and seminal vesicles, 29; alimentary tract, pancreas and spleen, 28; kidneys, 20; drawn blood, 20; heart, 18; muscles, skin and skeleton, 8; brain, 5; eyes, testes and adrenals, 0. It was also shown that during a 48-hour fast the liver lost 20 per cent of its protein while the remaining tissues lost only 4 per cent.

The transient positive nitrogen balance observed when a completely adequate diet is supplemented with more protein is apparently due to increases in the protein content of the liver, kidney and blood. The liver shows the greatest response and the high protein intake is associated with an increase in the protein content per unit mass of tissue as well as hypertrophy and hyperplasia of the hepatic cells.[114] This protein can be easily utilized as a reserve in times of deprivation but, despite its lability, there is no evidence that it differs in any way from the protein normally found in the cell. On the contrary, the marked reduction in hepatic enzymes[18] associated with protein depletion indicates that some of the "reserve protein" is an integral part of the metabolic machinery of the cell, and its loss is accompanied by a reduction in the functional capacity of the liver.

A portion of the protein, or amino acids thereof, lost from one tissue during starvation can be utilized for the synthesis of other body proteins. This phenomenon is well illustrated by the experimental observation of Madden and Whipple[115] that, following the production of severe hypoproteinemia by repeated plasmapheresis, a normal dog can resynthesize as much as 40 to 60 per cent of its plasma proteins, even during a fast.

The increase in nitrogen (urea) excretion indicates that a large proportion of the amino acids arising from the labile proteins are deaminated and that the subsequent catabolism of these residues provides some of the energy required for vital processes.

In summary, the body tissues, particularly those of the liver, kidney and intestines, possess "labile" proteins that can be utilized during starvation to meet the caloric requirements of the organism, and also for the maintenance of other body tissues. These proteins are probably an integral part of the intracellular machinery but are not so intimately associated with the cell structure that their loss produces any permanent injury.

Specific Dynamic Action

The term specific dynamic action, originated by Rubner, applies to the increase in metabolic rate that follows the ingestion of food. When protein alone is fed to a fasting animal, in an amount possessing the heat value equivalent to the animal's basal metabolism, the heat production is raised 30 per cent above the basal level. Under the same conditions, carbohydrate and fat produce increases of approximately 4 per cent and 6 per cent respectively. The specific dynamic action of mixed food is about 10 per cent.

There is no complete explanation for the specific dynamic effect. The hypothesis that the increased metabolic rate results from the work performed in the digestion and absorption of protein is disproved by the fact that the intravenous administration of any of the amino acids provokes a specific dynamic effect equivalent to that produced by ingested protein. The reactions involved in the heat production appear to take place in the liver since the administration of glycine in vivo increases the temperature of this organ as much as 1° C., while muscle temperatures decline slightly.[116] Hepatectomy abolishes the specific dynamic action.[117] Lundsgaard[118] found that the administration of ammonium carbonate or ammonium lactate produced an increase in heat production comparable to that of glycine and alanine and felt that the energy arose from the reactions involved in urea synthesis. However, on the basis of our present knowledge, urea formation can account for only 12 to 15 per cent of the extra heat produced.

Sadhu and Brody[119] have reported that the specific dynamic action of amino acids is reduced by the administration of pyruvate. It has been suggested that the heat production centers around deamination and that the energy loss is lower when the initial step is transamination (which would be facilitated by the pyruvate), rather than oxidative deamination. Earlier claims that adrenalectomy, thyroidectomy and hypophysectomy abolish specific dynamic action have not been substantiated.[120,121] However, hormonal influences cannot be completely excluded, since Abelin and Goldstein[122] claim that the urinary excretion of the free and bound forms of epinephrine and norepinephrine is increased following the ingestion of meat. They suggest that the increased metabolic rate can be partly attributed to the action of these hormones.

Keeton and associates[123] have studied the effect of protein consumption on the energy requirements of normal adults exposed to an environmental temperature of —20° F. for 8 hours a day, 5 days a week, over a period of 5½ months. The subjects were not under stress since they were warmly clothed during the exposure to low temperatures. Keeton found that the dynamic effect over a 6 hour period following a meal of approximately 1000 calories was 116 calories for the high protein diet and 78 calories for the high carbohydrate diet. However, the subjects were resting under comfortable conditions during the period of observation. When the metabolic rate is raised through normal activity, the dynamic effect is somehow offset and the net result is that the high protein diet is more efficiently utilized than a diet low in protein. Keeton observed that body weight was maintained over the 5½ month period when the average daily intake of the high protein diet was only 2566 calories. The subjects on the high carbohydrate diet required 3025 calories to maintain their body weight. The average energy intake of the 6 subjects on the high protein diet was 162 per cent of their *basal* metabolic requirement, while the energy intake of the 6 subjects on the high carbohydrate diet was 191 per cent of their basal requirement. These results are diametrically opposed to the general beliefs that high protein diets are more effective than high carbohydrate diets in maintaining heat production in a cold environment.

THE FATES OF ABSORBED AMINO ACIDS

There are many metabolic pathways open to the amino acids once they have been absorbed from the intestinal tract. The possible fates of these metabolites may be generally classified as follows:

1. Utilization for the synthesis of purines and pyrimidines, porphyrins, creatine, proteins including plasma

proteins, structural tissue proteins, enzymes, hormones, etc.

2. Deamination. If the deaminated residue is not reaminated it becomes an intermediate in the metabolism of fats or carbohydrates and consequently can be
   (a) oxidized completely to carbon dioxide and water,
   (b) synthesized into fat,
   (c) synthesized into glucose and/or glycogen

It is quite possible for the amino acid to pass through many different reaction sequences; for example, it could be alternately incorporated and released from several different proteins before being deaminated and utilized in carbohydrate or fat metabolism. The evidence of such metabolic interchange is discussed briefly in the following section.

The Dynamic State of Body Proteins

Folin, on the basis of his experimental work, believed that creatinine was the end product of tissue or "endogenous" protein catabolism, and that urea was produced from "exogenous" or dietary protein catabolism. Since creatinine represents only a very small fraction of the urinary nitrogen and remains constant in amount, it was concluded that the tissue proteins were relatively inert in well nourished animals and that the small amount of breakdown resulting from "wear and tear" required for repair only minute amounts of the amino acids derived from the food. Folin's theory was challenged in 1935 by Borsook and Keighley[124] who, on the basis of their nutritional investigations and from the published data of other workers, suggested that tissue proteins were by no means inert and that their active metabolism utilized a large proportion of the dietary nitrogen. Proof that the body proteins were indeed labile structures was obtained in 1942 by Schoenheimer and associates[125] through the use of isotopically labelled compounds. Schoenheimer et al.[126] fed rats leucine and glycine in which the amino groups were labelled with N^{15}. If Folin's view was correct and the body proteins were more or less inert, nearly quantitative recovery of N^{15} from the urine should have been possible. This was not the case. Only part of the N^{15} could be recovered from the urine, while the remainder was found to be incorporated into the body tissues. After labelled leucine had been fed to rats for three days, it was found that the rate at which the amino acid was incorporated into different tissues varied markedly. The relative concentrations were: serum, 100; intestinal wall, 89; kidney, 82; spleen, 65; liver, 56; heart, 53; testes, 46; muscle, 18; hemoglobin, 17; skin, 11. It was also shown by Shemin and Rittenberg[127] that the tissue which incorporated the labelled amino acid most rapidly lost the isotope most rapidly when administration of the labelled metabolite was stopped. Schoenheimer[126] calculated from the data obtained with leucine labelled with N^{15} and deuterium that half of the liver protein was replaced every seven days. The results of these and many subsequent investigations indicate that tissue proteins, far from being inert, are in a constant state of change.

The rapid turnover of amino acids in various tissues has been considered by many to be due to the degradation and resynthesis of intracellular proteins and processes that involve an active interchange of amino acids between various intracellular proteins and between the cell and its external environment, as depicted in the figure below.

$$\begin{array}{ccc} & & \text{Dietary protein} \\ & & \downarrow \\ \text{Tissue protein} & \rightleftharpoons & \text{Amino acid pool} \\ & & \downarrow\uparrow \\ & & \text{Catabolic products} \end{array}$$

FIG. 2.

This view was challenged by Hogness, Cohn and Monod[128] in 1955 from the results of studies carried out with *E. coli.* They labelled the protein of *E. coli* by growing it in a medium containing S^{35} labelled ammonium sulfate. The bacteria were placed in a new medium containing unlabelled ammonium sulfate and a substance was added to induce the formation of the protein enzyme β-galactosidase. This enzyme contained no S^{35} when isolated, although the cell protein was still highly labelled. It is apparent that if a dynamic state existed between the cell proteins, some of the label should have been incorporated into the β-galactosidase. The authors conclude from these and other findings that the cell proteins, including the enzyme of *E. coli,* were relatively inert once formed, and that there was no appreciable exchange of amino acids. Cohn[129] states with regard to the experiments, "We take it as experimental fact that a given animal tissue of constant mass does synthesize and lose proteins at equal rates. We do not take as experimental fact that proteins *within a given cell* of that tissue are constantly being synthesized and degraded." It follows that what has been interpreted as intracellular turnover of protein may represent the turnover of whole cells, that is to say, the rate at which cells of the tissue are destroyed and replaced. Cohn draws attention to the fact that tissues with high protein turnover rates are those in which the mitotic rate is highest, e.g., intestinal mucosa.

There is, however, good evidence that protein turnover is not exclusively due to cellular turnover and that intracellular degradation and resynthesis do take place. Halvorson and associates[130,131,132] have reported that during the early stages of nitrogen starvation yeast cells are still able to synthesize the protein (enzyme) α-glucosidase. The same workers have also shown that when the energy supply of the yeast cells is limited, free amino acids accumulate at the expense of cell protein. Velick[133] also has obtained evidence of protein degradation and resynthesis in mammalian muscle cells.

Amino Acid Incorporation into Proteins

It is obvious that when the total amount of protein in a biologic system is increasing, protein must be synthesized de novo from amino acids. The mechanisms involved in this process will be considered in the next section. The following discussion is limited to a consideration of amino acid incorporation when the net amount of protein in the system remains constant, i.e., the rate of synthesis equals the rate of breakdown.

Schoenheimer and associates[126] in one of their early papers pointed out that the studies with isotopes gave no information concerning the intermediate processes involved in the incorporation of amino acids into proteins. They suggested that two mechanisms were possible, (1) the complete breakdown of the protein into units, followed by resynthesis, or (2) only partial replacement of units. A definite conclusion regarding the relative importance of these two processes in protein metabolism cannot yet be reached. There is, however, convincing evidence that the second process does occur and may be an extremely important one under the conditions considered here, i.e., incorporation without net increase in protein. In this situation, a given amino acid in a peptide chain is replaced without disrupting the bonds in the moieties on either side of the bonds broken and reformed in the interchange. This method of incorporation has been convincingly demonstrated by Gale and Folkes[134] who found that when *Staphylococcus aureus* was incubated with glucose and C^{14}-glutamic acid, the amino acid was incorporated into the cell protein. They reasoned that if this was a true exchange reaction then it should be possible to remove radioactive glutamic acid from the protein by incubation with unlabelled glutamic acid. Gale[135] then incubated an S. *aureus* preparation with C^{14}-glutamic acid until the radioactivity of the protein reached a constant level. The preparation was then washed free of unincorporated amino acid and incubated with unlabelled glutamic acid. It was found that in the course of 90 minutes 40 per cent of the C^{14}-glutamic acid in the protein was replaced by the unlabelled metabolite. It is important to note that under these conditions no net increase in protein could occur because only one amino acid was available. Gale[135] adds that amino acid exchange is probably limited to certain intracellular proteins, since C^{14}-glutamic acid can replace only 5 to 6 per cent of the total protein glutamate. Zamecnik et al.[136] have reported that the labelled leucine or valine incorporated into the microsome protein of cell-free rat liver preparations by a process other than exchange will subsequently not participate in exchange reactions. Evidence for the occurrence of exchange reactions in mammalian tissues has been obtained by Rabinovitz et al.[137]

It has been implied that amino acid exchange is not representative of protein synthesis, and it is difficult to determine the basic ideas underlying the many vague statements made on this subject. Certainly, amino acid incorporation need not mean a net increase in protein. Borsook[138] has given definition to this question by stating, "All amino acids are incorporated in vivo and in vitro; they are incorporated in different loci of the protein. Amino acid incorporation represents, then, breakdown and resynthesis of many, if not all, peptide bonds in the protein molecule. De facto, this is synthesis."

Protein Synthesis

The energy derived from the oxidation of carbohydrates is made available for endergonic reactions including those involved in protein synthesis by the formation of adenosine triphosphate (ATP). The ATP acts as an intermediate energy source (see chapter on Carbohydrate Metabolism). The incorporation of amino acids into proteins, either by de novo synthesis, or by exchange reactions, appears to be dependent upon energy derived from carbohydrate oxidations, since incorporation is greatly reduced or completely prevented when glucose utilization is inhibited by anaerobiosis or by enzyme poisons. The secondary participation of ATP is indicated by the fact that substances such as dinitrophenol (DNP) which interfere with the ATP formation and cause the energy liberated from glucose oxidation to be wastefully dissipated as heat prevent protein synthesis and amino acid exchange.

It should be emphasized that although there are many speculations and theories concerning the mechanisms responsible for the synthesis of proteins from amino acids, there is no conclusive proof of their validity, and opinions now held will undoubtedly undergo remarkable modifications within a few years.

The mechanisms of protein synthesis proposed by Borsook are at the moment receiving considerable experimental support. Borsook[139] suggests that there are three steps in the formation of a protein molecule. They are (1) activation of the carboxyl group of an amino acid; (2) transport of the activated amino acids to a nucleic acid template or mold, where they are arranged in a specific sequence; (3) linking together of the amino acids by peptide bond formation and subsequent peeling off of the newly formed protein molecule.

It was first suggested by Lipman in 1941 that phosphate bond energy drove the synthesis of peptide bonds. The manner in which the pyrophosphate bonds of ATP participate in the activation of amino acids for peptide synthesis has been inferred from studies of the formation of amides (glutamine), small peptides (glutathione), and quasipeptides such as hippuric acid. The reader is again referred to reviews and original articles for detailed information.[138,139]

The enzymatic synthesis of the tripeptide, glutathione, (γ-glutamylcysteinylglycine) has been shown to proceed in the manner outlined in [A] below and will serve to illustrate how ATP is believed to participate in peptide synthesis. Studies carried out with other model

---

[A]

1. Enzyme + ATP → P − Enz. + ADP (Adenosine Diphosphate)
2. $Enz._1$ − P + Glutamic Acid ⇆ $Enz._1$ − Glutamate + P
   $Enz._1$ − Glutamate + Cysteine ⇆ $Enz._1$ + γ − Glut. − Cyst.
3. $Enz._2$ − P + γ − Glut. − Cyst. ⇆ $Enz._2$ − Glut. Cyst. + P
   $Enz._2$ − Glut. − Cyst. + Glycine ⇆ γ − Glut. − Cyst. − Gly. + $Enz._2$

systems indicate that although the active form of the amino acid may differ slightly in different systems, it is always the carboxyl group that is activated and the activation occurs at the expense of ATP. The amino group of another amino acid can then combine with the activated carboxyl group to form a peptide bond. However, it is suggested that before the bonds are formed the activated amino acids are transported to a template which aligns them in the specific sequence characteristic of the protein to be synthesized. It is at this stage that the peptide bonds are forged and the protein subsequently released from the matrix of the template.

Considerable debate has arisen[139] as to whether or not polypeptides are intermediates in the synthesis of protein. The data presently available appear to support the view that the protein is formed through the simultaneous condensation of the activated residues and that peptides are not intermediates in the process.[139]

The template, if such exists, is probably a ribonucleic acid (RNA), for it has been evident for many years that RNA is intimately associated with protein synthesis. Protein synthesis can be inhibited without inhibition of RNA synthesis or turnover, but stimulation of protein synthesis is associated with an increased synthesis of RNA and, in view of this, it has been suggested that for the synthesis of protein, new RNA must be synthesized concomitantly.[140,141] The primary importance of RNA is suggested by observations that inhibition of RNA synthesis invariably inhibits the synthesis of cell proteins.

Zamecnik et al.,[136] using isotopically labelled amino acid, have recently obtained experimental results that strongly support the theory of protein anabolism proposed by Borsook and briefly outlined here. They found, in rat liver homogenate-soluble protein fractions, a mechanism for the activation of amino acids. In the presence of ATP and soluble enzymes, the amino acids are converted to aminoacyl-AMP compounds. The activated amino acids are built into proteins or large peptides in ribonucleoprotein particles located in the microsome fraction of the liver cell protoplasm. The over-all process may be represented by **A** below.

The Synthesis of Plasma Proteins

The ease and the relative lack of surgical trauma associated with the withdrawal of blood have made blood a popular tissue for the study of some aspects of protein synthesis. Studies of the effect of diet on the regeneration of plasma proteins after depletion by the plasmapheresis technique were started in 1918 by Whipple and associates.[142,115] Plasmapheresis consists of withdrawing blood, centrifuging down the erythrocytes, and, after washing with isotonic saline, returning the red cells to the animal (dog) by intravenous injection. In this way the plasma protein concentration can be markedly reduced without altering the hemoglobin level. The now classic work of Whipple et al. produced some of the earliest evidence of the dynamic state of body proteins. Convincing evidence for the synthesis of new protein from the labile body proteins was obtained when it was observed that the protein-depleted dog could regenerate 40 to 60 per cent of its circulating plasma proteins, even during a fast.

The role of dietary nitrogen in the synthesis of plasma constituents and the

---

A

Enzyme + ATP + C^{14} − Amino Acid
↓
(C^{14} − Aminoacyl ∼ AMP) Enzyme + PP — Soluble Protein
- - - - - - - - - - + - - - - - - - - - -
Ribonucleoprotein — Microsomes
↓
C^{14} Ribonucleoprotein

(Modified from Zamecnik et al.[136])

efficiency with which different proteins can be utilized in this respect has been the subject of a great deal of investigation by Whipple,[143] Melnick, Cowgill and Burack,[144] Seeley,[145] Weech et al.,[146,147] and others. Several reviews[115,148] are available to those desiring detailed knowledge of the subject. Many of the results obtained by the above workers are in accord with expectations and clearly show that high quality proteins such as beef, egg albumin and liver are extremely effective in maintaining plasma protein levels, while those of poor quality such as wheat gluten and gelatin are poor precursors of the blood components. Complete amino acid mixtures administered intravenously are well tolerated by experimental animals, and in hypoproteinemia such mixtures serve as well as dietary protein for the regeneration of the blood proteins.

The hypoproteinemia of malnutrition is primarily due to change in plasma albumin; the globulins are apparently much more stable. The reduction in plasma albumin is associated with a reduction in plasma volume; thus the concentration of albumin per unit volume may not change, while that of the globulin increases. It has been suggested[148,149] that changes in the albumin-globulin ratio in many disease states may be only the result of malnutrition.

There remains little doubt that about 90 to 95 per cent of the plasma proteins are synthesized by the liver. Knutti, Whipple and associates[150] showed in 1937 that when the products of digestion were diverted from the liver by anastomosis of the hepatic vein with the vena cava (Eck fistula), severe hypoproteinemia developed. Direct evidence for the hepatic synthesis of plasma proteins has been obtained with the aid of isotopically labelled compounds. Miller and co-workers[151] studied the problem by perfusing the isolated liver with whole blood to which had been added isotopically labelled lysine, as well as other unlabelled amino acids and glucose. They observed a synthesis of plasma protein amounting to 4.2 mg. per gram of liver protein per hour. Globulin was synthesized more rapidly than albumin, and fibrinogen showed the slowest rate of synthesis. It was also shown that the rate of incorporation of the labelled lysine fell markedly when an essential amino acid was left out of the perfusate, and that when all factors were available a decline in the rate of synthesis could be reversed by the addition of more of the amino acid mixture to the perfusate. Although the major part of the blood proteins are manufactured in the liver, it is well established that γ-globulins are also produced in lymphoid tissue.[152] In addition to maintaining the pH and osmotic pressure of the blood, the plasma proteins are a major source of protein for the maintenance of peripheral tissue. They apparently can be converted to cell protein without first being broken down to free amino acids. Yuile et al.,[153] working in Whipple's laboratory, have reported that the plasma proteins labelled with C^{14}-lysine are utilized by the dog for peripheral protein synthesis without appreciable loss of C^{14} in the urine or expired air. Babson and Winnick[154] and Gavrilova[155] found that in rats the labelled amino acids contained as an integral part of the plasma protein were incorporated into cell protein and that their concentration therein could not be reduced by the concurrent administration of the same non-labelled free amino acids. It was assumed that if the plasma protein were hydrolyzed to amino acids before being utilized, the unlabelled amino acid would mix with and dilute the labelled residue, which in turn would result in a smaller concentration of isotope in the newly synthesized protein. Since this did not occur, it is believed that the plasma protein is not broken down beyond the peptide stage before it is re-anabolized.

HORMONAL INFLUENCES ON PROTEIN METABOLISM

Anterior Pituitary Growth Hormone (Somatotrophin)

The occurrence of gigantism in humans possessing pituitary tumors and the failure of animals to grow following hypophysectomy gave rise to the theory that the pituitary gland contained a factor that exerted a marked effect on protein anabolism. The preparation of pituitary extracts that were capable of promoting growth and protein synthesis in experimental animals provided convincing support for this concept and led to the successful isolation by Li, Simpson and Evans[156] of the anterior pituitary growth hormone (somatotrophin).

Early investigation revealed that pituitary extracts had, in addition to a growth promoting effect, a marked effect on the catabolism of body fat. It was observed that these preparations increased the fat content of the liver and lowered the respiratory quotient to a value typical of that produced by the oxidation of fatty acids. The source of the liver fat was shown by Barret, Best and Ridout,[157] and Stetten and Salcedo[158] to be in the body depots. These investigators used deuterium to label the body depot fat of mice and rats, and found that the fat that accumulated in the liver following the administration of pituitary extracts was heavily deuterated. More recent work[159,160] has indicated that the factor responsible for these changes is identical with the growth hormone. It appears that because of its effect on lipid metabolism the growth promoting activity of somatotrophin is not completely dependent upon an increase in food intake. Greenbaum[161,162] found that purified growth hormone induced a rapid increase in the body weight of rats when their food intake was restricted to the amount consumed by controls whose weight remained constant. The increase in the rate of weight gain was due to an increase in the rate of protein synthesis and was maintained only until the labile fat reserves of the body were exhausted. These observations show that protein was synthesized at the expense of fat. Since the energy values of protein and fat are approximately four and nine calories per gram, the oxidation of one gram of fat could theoretically yield energy enough for the synthesis of two grams of protein. This would then allow a net increase in weight to occur despite the loss of fat. The weight increase would also be augmented by water since the deposition of one gram of protein is associated with the retention of three grams of H_2O. While there remains a distinct possibility that growth hormone may have a specific effect on the processes directly involved in peptide bond formation, the evidence presently available suggests that its protein anabolic effect is the indirect outcome of its ability to increase the catabolism of fat, thereby increasing the energy available for protein synthesis.

Insulin

The ability of insulin to normalize protein metabolism in diabetic animals is well known and clearly demonstrates its importance as an anabolic hormone. The evidence that insulin reduces the elevated nitrogen excretion characteristic of the diabetic state was reported in 1922 by Banting, Campbell and Fletcher, and a more comprehensive study of this nature was published by Allan[163] in 1924. The results of a number of early studies[164,165] indicated that insulin depressed the non-protein nitrogen level in the blood, but the most convincing demonstrations of an effect of insulin on amino acid metabolism were reported by Mirsky and co-workers[166,167] in 1938. These investigators found that in nephrectomized dogs, insulin caused a marked inhibition of urea formation, and in eviscerated-nephrectomized dogs this hormone inhibited the rise of blood amino acids and stimulated the utilization of exogenous amino acids, presumably for protein synthesis, since the eviscerated-nephrectomized animal obviously cannot excrete the amino acids or form urea. These observations have been adequately confirmed and extended by many others.[168,169]

Tracer studies indicate that protein synthesis is impaired during diabetes. Hoberman[170] measured the incorporation of labelled glycine into protein and concluded that in alloxan diabetes there is a depression in protein synthesis as well as an increase in protein catabolism.

Forker[171] has observed that S^{35} labelled methionine is incorporated into muscle protein three to five times more rapidly in the normal dog than in the diabetic animal.

The results of the few experiments carried out in vitro are in accord with those obtained from in vivo studies. Sinex, MacMullen and Hastings[172] found that the incorporation of C^{14} labelled alanine into the protein of rat diaphragm in vitro was markedly stimulated by the addition of insulin to the incubation fluid. Similarly, Krahl[173] reported that insulin enhanced the incorporation of C^{14} labelled glycine into glutathione and protein fractions of the rat diaphragm in vitro. Krahl[173] also observed that the uptake of amino acids by diaphragms and liver slices from diabetic rats was greatly reduced. This reduction in uptake is overcome in the diaphragm by the addition of glucose alone to the medium, but in the liver slice, glucose and insulin are required to restore the rate of incorporation to normal. It is of interest in this regard to note that Bollman et al.[174] claim that insulin plus glucose will suppress the rate of rise of blood amino acids in the hepatectomized-depancreatized dog, but glucose alone has no effect.

The evidence cited above clearly indicates that insulin promotes protein synthesis. However, studies of the effect of prolonged administration of insulin on protein synthesis in the absence of anterior pituitary growth factors were hindered by the extreme sensitivity of the hypophysectomized animal to the hypoglycemic action of insulin. Salter and Best[175,176,177] were able to overcome these difficulties by paying careful attention to diet and insulin dosage and, in 1953, they reported that the administration of insulin to hypophysectomized rats caused a marked increase in body weight. The increase in weight represented true growth, since it was due to an increase in protein, as well as fat and water; it was accompanied by an increase in the weight of the visceral organs and by an increase in the rate of skeletal growth. A growth promoting effect of insulin has also been obtained in vitro. Leslie and Paul[178] found that the addition of insulin to the incubation fluid stimulated the growth of chick heart explants cultured in vitro. A similar effect on chick bone cultured in vitro has been reported by Fell.[179]

Although conclusive proof is lacking, it is assumed that insulin increases lipogenesis and protein synthesis by increasing the rate of oxidation of glucose and thereby increasing the energy available for these endergonic reactions. Experimental support for this conjecture was obtained when it was found that insulin had no anabolic effect in hypophysectomized rats when their food intake was restricted to the amount consumed prior to treatment.[161] When the animals are allowed to consume more glucose, but no more protein, insulin has a pronounced protein anabolic effect. This effect of insulin was not obtained when the glucose supplement was replaced by fat. While the protein anabolic action of insulin is dependent upon the supply of carbohydrate, conversely, the protein sparing action of carbohydrate is largely dependent upon an adequate supply of insulin. There is little change in the nitrogen balance of hypophysectomized diabetic animals when they are fed extra glucose unless insulin is administered simultaneously.

The Relationship between Insulin and Growth Hormone

Reids, Cotes and Young,[180] and Campbell et al.[181] have shown that highly purified preparations of somatotrophin produce permanent diabetes in cats and dogs. It has been suggested that following the administration of this hormone the demand for insulin is increased to such an extent that the pancreatic reserves are eventually exhausted and the β-cells irreversibly damaged. Conclusive proof for this speculation has not been obtained; there is, however, convincing evidence that somatotrophin does increase insulin secretion from the pancreas and that its protein anabolic activity is dependent upon an adequate supply of insulin. Milman, DeMoor and

Lukens[182] have shown that somatotrophin has no effect on nitrogen balance in hypophysectomized-depancreatized cats. They also showed that the administration of growth hormone to pancreatectomized cats, given a constant amount of food and insulin, resulted in nitrogen retention; but the amount of nitrogen retained was only half that retained by normal animals given the same dose of somatotrophin. The impaired ability of somatotrophin to induce nitrogen retention was due to the limitation in the amount of insulin available and was corrected if the insulin dosage was increased three to five times. Additional and more direct evidence for an increased secretion of insulin following growth hormone administration has been obtained by Randle,[183] who found that the insulin content of blood from cats was elevated after injecting the pituitary hormone. In keeping with these observations are reports by Randle[184,185] that the insulin content of the blood from acromegalics is abnormally high, and very low in humans suffering from hypopituarism.

Although other possibilities must not be denied, it is probable that insulin promotes protein synthesis and lipogenesis by increasing the oxidation of carbohydrate and thereby increasing the energy available for these endergonic processes. It also seems likely that growth hormone increases the energy available for protein formation by limiting lipogenesis.

Sex Hormones

The androgens are well known for their ability to promote protein synthesis, and they have been used with limited success in the treatment of dwarfism in children of both sexes.[186] Unfortunately, their activity in this respect is only of limited duration. Kenyon[187] and McCullagh and Rossmiller[188] found that methyltestosterone increased the weight of eunuchoid subjects for forty to seventy days. The anabolic action ceased after this time, despite continued androgen therapy. In rats testosterone propionate increases nitrogen retention for about a week.[189] Kochakian[190] has shown that in dogs the anabolic activity of androgen is not dependent upon the pituitary gland. It accelerates growth for a limited time in young hypophysectomized rats and potentiates the action of somatotrophin in this preparation.[191]

Some nitrogen retention can also be obtained with estradiol preparations,[192] but large doses of this compound inhibit growth, presumably because of suppression of pituitary hormone production.[193] The estrogens stimulate ossification in both humans and laboratory animals and may induce sealing of the epiphyseal disk. The indiscreet use of estrogens during childhood or adolescence may bring about the premature closure of the epiphyses and leave the person permanently stunted.

Thyroxine

It is well known that thyroidectomy or hypothyroidism is accompanied by a cessation of growth in both humans and laboratory animals and that the administration of thyroxine causes a resumption of growth. The fact that thyroxine therapy fails to restore growth in hypophysectomized animals has led Evans and associates[194] and Eartly and Leblond[195] to conclude that in the hypothyroid state metabolic processes are disturbed in the pituitary gland, as well as in other tissues, and that thyroxine treatment restores the ability of the hypophysis to manufacture growth hormone. It was first shown by Collip[196] that in very young rats cessation of growth does not occur until several weeks after hypophysectomy. Scow[197] and Geschwind and Li[198] have shown that the administration of physiologic amounts of thyroxine increase the growth and protein synthesis during this posthypophysectomy growth period. However, once growth has stopped in a hypophysectomized animal, it cannot be initiated with thyroxine.[199] Despite its inability to act alone, the thyroid hormone potentiates the growth induced by insulin and by anterior pituitary growth hormone,[200] but the physiologic significance of this potentiating action is questionable, since thyroxine also enhances the action of growth antagonists such as cortisone.[201,202] This potentiation of catabolic hormones is not seen in the hypophysectomized animal, since the adrenal cortices are atrophic. A catabolic influence of thyroxine is also evident from the well known fact that thyroxine overdosage produces a hyperthyroid state which is accompanied by a general wasting away of the body tissues. Thyroxine, even in physiologic amounts, tends to increase the nitrogen excretion of hypophysectomized rats, but the appetite of the animal is also stimulated so that the loss is compensated by the increased food consumption. It is apparent that the net effect of thyroxine on protein synthesis depends upon dosage, food intake, hormonal balance, etc., and that its action cannot be considered primarily as either catabolic or anabolic.

Adrenal Cortical Hormones

In a now classic paper, Long, Katzin and Fry[203] in 1940 presented data showing that the adrenal cortex stimulated gluconeogenesis from protein. Subsequent work has shown that the adrenal steroids affecting protein and carbohydrate metabolism are of the cortisone or hydrocortisone type, i.e., compounds bearing an alcoholic or ketonic group at the C-11 position. These hormones are generally referred to as glucocorticoids. The increased conversion of amino acids to carbohydrate, induced by the administration of glucocorticoids, appears to be the indirect outcome of a suppression in the accumulation of body protein. It is not definitely known whether these steroids inhibit protein synthesis or accelerate its catabolism,[204,205] although current data favor the latter point of view.

Cortisone in large doses greatly increases urinary nitrogen excretion,[206] and when administration is prolonged, the azoturia is accompanied by hyperglycemia and glucosuria. It can bring about complete cessation of growth in normal animals, obliterate growth induced by insulin,[175] and antagonize the anabolic action of pituitary growth hormone.[207]

While the net effect of cortisone-like compounds is to retard peripheral protein synthesis, Clark[208] and Roberts[209] have reported that in rats it increases the liver and blood proteins. Russell[205] suggests that under the influence of excess cortical hormone increased quantities of amino acids are released from the peripheral tissues, and that the subsequent increase in the supply of amino acids to the liver enhances protein synthesis in this organ.

A growth promoting effect of adrenal cortical hormones has been inferred from the observation that adrenalectomized rats, which can be maintained in excellent health simply by limiting their potassium intake and supplying them with adequate salt in their food or drinking water, grow more slowly than intact controls. However, the reduced growth rate is due to a reduction in food intake, and when the controls are limited to the food consumed by the adrenalectomized animals, the latter grow more rapidly. In small doses, cortisone may improve the nitrogen balance of human subjects. It is, however, difficult to interpret these changes, since the appetite of the patient is often greatly enhanced and the improvement in nitrogen balance may reflect only a better state of nutrition.

Glucagon (Pancreatic Hyperglycemic-Glycogenolytic Factor)

Shortly after the discovery of insulin it was noted that the intravenous administration of preparations containing this hormone produced an initial elevation in blood sugar before the characteristic fall occurred. On the basis of this observation, Murlin[210] proposed that pancreatic extracts contained, in addition to insulin, a hyperglycemic factor. Considerable purification of the substance was accomplished by Sutherland and Cori, and it was obtained in crystalline form in 1953 by Staub and associates.[211] Sutherland and Cori[212,213,214] have shown that this substance, like epinephrine, causes rapid hepatic glycogenolysis by activation of the enzyme phosphorylase, which converts glycogen to glucose-1-phosphate. Glucose-1-phosphate is enzymatically converted through glucose-6-phosphate to glucose. It is clearly established that glucagon acts at the phosphorylase level, and many of the details have been elucidated by Sutherland and associates.[212,213,214] This substance also exerts a profound influence on amino acid metabolism. Tyberghein[215] reported that a two hour infusion of glucagon increased urea production. Salter, Davidson and Best[216] found that following the administration of glucagon, blood amino acids fell and urea excretion increased remarkably. These changes are not mediated by the adrenal gland or the hypophysis, and are of sufficient magnitude that animals chronically treated with large amounts of glucagon lose weight and eventually die. Very small amounts of this hormone have less drastic effects, but nevertheless, cause a marked inhibition of growth. The anti-anabolic action has been obtained in mice, rats, dogs, monkeys and humans.

It is apparent that under experimental conditions glucagon acts as a powerful catabolic agent. However, it is not yet known whether this substance plays an important role in normal physiologic processes. The mechanism through which it affects amino acid catabolism also requires elucidation.

THE METABOLISM OF THE AMINO ACIDS

The conversion of protein to glucose and/or ketone bodies is evident from the increase in the excretion of these substances that occurs following the ingestion of protein by animals afflicted with phlorizin or pancreatic diabetes. The conversion is a relatively rapid one since insulin-induced hypoglycemia can be relieved within 30 minutes after the ingestion of amino acids. The importance of the conversion of amino acids to carbohydrates in the maintenance of normal blood sugar levels can also be seen when partial inhibition of this transformation is accomplished by removing the adrenal glands, certain secretions of which greatly accelerate gluconeogenesis. The newly adrenalectomized animal, when fasted for a period that would produce an inconsequential change in the blood sugar level of an intact animal, will develop fatal hypoglycemia. Simple deamination of the many amino acids will produce keto acids that are intermediates in the metabolic pathways of carbohydrate. Thus, alanine is deaminated to pyruvic acid, glutamic acid to α-ketoglutaric acid, aspartic acid to oxaloacetic acid, etc. In other instances the conversion to carbohydrate or acetoacetate may be less direct, but nevertheless, deamination represents the initial step in the catabolism of most of the amino acids.

Deamination

Oxidative Deamination. D-AMINO ACID OXIDASES (DEHYDROGENASES). It was known to both Neubauer[217] and Knoop[218] that animal tissues were capable of producing α-keto acids by deaminating amino acids, but the first accurate studies of the process were carried out by Krebs.[219] Krebs found that liver or kidney preparations of most species were able oxidatively to deaminate alinine to pyruvic acid according to the equation [A] below. Since catalase is present in most crude tissue preparation, the hydrogen peroxide is de-

---

[A]

$$R\text{—}\overset{\overset{\displaystyle NH_2}{|}}{C}H\text{—}COOH + O_2 \xrightarrow{\text{enzymatic}} R\text{—}\overset{\overset{\displaystyle NH}{\|}}{C}\text{—}COOH + H_2O_2 \quad (1)$$

$$R\text{—}\overset{\overset{\displaystyle NH}{\|}}{C}\text{—}COOH + H_2O \xrightarrow{\text{spontaneous}} R\text{—}\overset{\overset{\displaystyle O}{\|}}{C}\text{—}COOH + NH_3 \quad (2)$$

$$R\text{—}\overset{\overset{\displaystyle O}{\|}}{C}\text{—}COOH + H_2O_2 \rightarrow R\text{—}COOH + CO_2 + H_2O \quad (3)$$

stroyed and reaction 3 does not take place.

The D-amino acid oxidases are easily extracted from tissues with water, but Krebs was unable to extract the enzymes with L-amino acid oxidase activity. Blanchard et al.[220] have been able to isolate an amino acid oxidase from rat kidney that is specific for the L form of the amino acids. However, the L-amino acid oxidase has not been obtained from animal tissues other than those of the rat, and it is unlikely that this enzyme plays a significant role in the catabolism of amino acids in mammals.

Since the naturally occurring amino acids are predominantly of the L form, the significance of the D-amino acid oxidases is unknown. It has been suggested that they may act to destroy D-amino acids consumed with the food or formed accidentally by the cells.

Non-oxidative Deamination. Dehydrases. A group of enzymes found in bacteria and in mammalian tissue deaminate serine, threonine and homoserine. The reaction does not require oxygen and is brought about by an initial dehydration of the substrate. The enzymes are accordingly named dehydrases. In the case of serine, the water is removed through the action of serine dehydrase. The product of the reaction, α-aminoacrylic acid, is unstable and proceeds spontaneously to α-iminopropionic acid, which in turn is hydrolyzed to ammonia and pyruvic acid (see [A] below).

Transaminases. Transamination is a reversible process through which the amino group of an amino acid is transferred to a keto acid. The enzymes mediating the reaction are accordingly called transaminases. Biologic transamination was first described by Braunstein and Kritsmann in 1937.[221] These investigators found that minced pigeon muscle preparation catalyzed the transfer of the amino group of glutamic acid to pyruvic acid with the formation of α-ketoglutaric acid and alanine (see [B] below). Oxaloacetic acid and α-ketoglutaric acid were, according to Braunstein, transaminated by most of the α-amino acids. Cohen[222,223] could confirm the presence of only two transaminating systems in swine heart. They were as shown in [C] below. However, it has since been conclusively demonstrated by Meister and Tice,[224] Cammarata and Cohen,[225] and others[226,227] that enzymatic transamination is a common reaction and that a very large number of amino acids are capable of transaminating with α-ketoglutaric acid.

The transamination reactions described above all involved glutamate, aspartate or their α-keto analogues. Studies carried out within recent years have revealed that transamination can occur without the participation of these

[A]

$$\underset{\text{Serine}}{\begin{matrix}CH_2OH\\ |\\ CH{-}NH_2\\ |\\ COOH\end{matrix}} \xrightarrow{-H_2O} \begin{matrix}CH_2\\ \|\\ C{-}NH_2\\ |\\ COOH\end{matrix} \leftrightharpoons \begin{matrix}CH_3\\ |\\ C{=}NH\\ |\\ COOH\end{matrix} \xrightarrow{+H_2O} \underset{\text{Pyruvic acid}}{\begin{matrix}CH_3\\ |\\ C{=}O\\ |\\ COOH\end{matrix}} + NH_3$$

[B]

$$\underset{\text{Glutamic acid}}{\begin{matrix}COOH\\ |\\ CH_2\\ |\\ CH_2\\ |\\ CH{-}NH_2\\ |\\ COOH\end{matrix}} + \underset{\text{Pyruvic acid}}{\begin{matrix}CH_3\\ |\\ O{=}C\\ |\\ COOH\end{matrix}} \rightarrow \underset{\alpha\text{-ketoglutaric acid}}{\begin{matrix}COOH\\ |\\ CH_2\\ |\\ CH_2\\ |\\ C{=}O\\ |\\ COOH\end{matrix}} + \underset{\text{Alanine}}{\begin{matrix}CH_3\\ |\\ CH{-}NH_2\\ |\\ COOH\end{matrix}}$$

[C]

Glutamic acid + oxaloacetic acid → α-ketoglutaric acid + aspartic acid
Glutamic acid + pyruvic acid → α-ketoglutaric acid + alanine

substances. Quastel and Witty[228] have reported that kidney and liver preparations catalyze transamination between ornithine and pyruvic acid. Meister[229] has also demonstrated that in liver preparations ornithine transaminates with several keto acids, including glyoxylate, α-ketobutyrate, and α-ketoglutarate. The general reaction scheme is represented by [A] below. Sallach[230] has recently achieved partial purification of an enzyme from dog liver that catalyzes the transamination of hydroxypyruvic acid from alanine with the production of serine. It appears, then, that what was originally thought to be a relatively limited reaction is, in reality, one that is responsible for a multitude of biochemical transformations involving a whole spectrum of enzymes.

Role of Pyridoxine in Transamination. The role of pyridoxine, vitamin B_6, in transamination reactions has received considerable attention. Snell,[230,231] in 1944, showed that pyridoxamine, when heated with α-ketoglutaric acid, reacted to yield pyridoxal and glutamic acid, and it was suggested that vitamin B_6 was involved as a co-factor in transamination reactions. Support for this concept was obtained from experiments which showed that transaminase activity was greatly reduced in the livers of vitamin B_6 deficient rats[233,234] and also in bacterial preparations grown on media lacking vitamin B_6.[235] Activity could be restored in both preparations by the addition of pyridoxal phosphate or pyridoxal and adenosine triphosphate. Direct evidence for the participation of pyridoxamine phosphate was obtained by Meister and associates,[236] who showed that the addition of this compound, or pyridoxal phosphate, activated the glutamic-oxaloacetic transaminase resolved from pig heart.

The available data indicate that the pyridoxal phosphate or pyridoxamine phosphate acts as a coenzyme in transamination and that the role played by the coenzyme is that of an amino group acceptor and donor. Meister and associates[236] believe, on the basis of their experimental work, that the pyridoxal phosphate first combines with the enzyme before taking part in the reaction. A tentative scheme for the intermediate reactions involved in transamination is as shown in [B] below.

Transamination-deamination. Liver preparation also catalyzes transamination between the amino acid amines, glutamine and aspargine, and α-keto

[A]

$$\underset{\text{Ornithine}}{CH_2(NH_2)-CH_2-CH_2-CH(NH_2)-COOH} + R-\overset{\displaystyle O}{\overset{\|}{C}}-COOH \rightleftharpoons \underset{\text{Glutamic-}\gamma\text{-semialdehyde}}{CHO-CH_2-CH_2-CH(NH_2)-COOH} + R-\underset{\displaystyle NH_2}{\underset{|}{CH}}-COOH$$

[B]

$$\underset{\alpha\text{-keto acid}}{R-C(=O)-COOH} + \underset{\text{Pyridoxamine phosphate}}{NH_2-H_2C-\text{[pyridine ring: }CH_2OPO_3H_2\text{, N, HO, }CH_3]} \underset{+H_2O}{\overset{-H_2O}{\rightleftharpoons}} R-C(COOH)=N-H_2C-\text{[pyridine ring: }CH_2OPO_3H_2\text{, N, HO, }CH_3]$$

$$\underset{\text{Amino acid}}{R-HC(NH_2)-COOH} + \underset{\text{Pyridoxal phosphate}}{OHC-\text{[pyridine ring: }CH_2OPO_3H_2\text{, N, HO, }CH_3]} \underset{+H_2O}{\overset{-H_2O}{\rightleftharpoons}} R-HC(COOH)-N=HC-\text{[pyridine ring: }CH_2OPO_3H_2\text{, N, HO, }CH_3]$$

acids, resulting in the formation of ammonia, α-ketoglutarate and another amino acid. This process has been most actively investigated by Meister et al.,[237] who now believe that the reaction proceeds in two stages: (1) transamination of the keto acid involving the α-amino group of glutamine with the formation of α-ketoglutaramic acid, (2) hydrolysis of the α-ketoglutaramic acid by a specific amidase to yield α-ketogluturate and ammonia as shown in [A] below.

The prevalence of transamination reactions is strikingly illustrated by the experiments of Schoenheimer et al.,[125,126] which have been previously described. When the amino acids were isolated from the tissues of the rat after feeding N^{15} labelled glycine and leucine, it was found that not only the glycine and leucine, but nearly all the amino acids isolated from the tissue proteins contained isotopic nitrogen. These results indicate that, in vivo, the interchange of amino groups between various amino acids occurs easily and very rapidly in most animal tissues.

Transamination is undoubtedly one of the most important metabolic reactions. By linking together the metabolism of amino acids and carbohydrates, it provides pathways through which amino acids can be catabolized or synthesized de novo through intermediates of the Krebs cycle.

Clinical Significance of Serum Transaminase. The glutamate-aspartate transaminase activity of serum has evoked considerable clinical interest within recent years because of its possible usefulness in following the course of coronary disease. After myocardial infarction the serum transaminase activity rises markedly within 48 hours and may reach a level two to ten times that normally observed.[238,239] The activity returns to normal within 5 days if additional areas of the myocardium are not affected. Coronary insufficiency without myocardial infarction produces no change in serum transaminase activity. The enzyme is widely distributed throughout body tissues and its activity in the serum is elevated by other traumas such as bowel infarction, biliary cirrhosis and abdominal surgery.[240] Thus, the estimation of serum transaminase activity may be of little diagnostic value unless used in conjunction with standard procedures.

Glycine

Glycine is the simplest of the amino acids and the only one that does not have two isomeric forms. It is actively incorporated into tissue proteins and, despite its simplicity, enters into a large number of metabolic transformations. Vertebrates, with the exception of birds and reptiles, possess the ability to conjugate benzoic acid with glycine to form hippuric acid (benzoylglycine) which

---

[A]

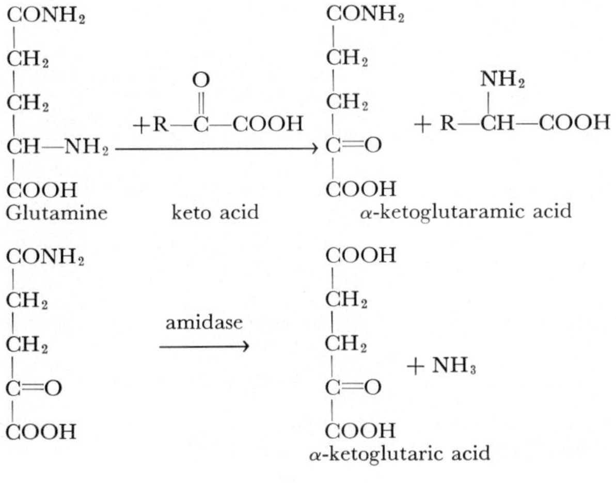

$$CONH_2{-}CH_2{-}CH_2{-}CH(NH_2){-}COOH + R{-}C({=}O){-}COOH \longrightarrow CONH_2{-}CH_2{-}CH_2{-}C({=}O){-}COOH + R{-}CH(NH_2){-}COOH$$

Glutamine + keto acid → α-ketoglutaramic acid

$$CONH_2{-}CH_2{-}CH_2{-}C({=}O){-}COOH \xrightarrow{\text{amidase}} COOH{-}CH_2{-}CH_2{-}C({=}O){-}COOH + NH_3$$

α-ketoglutaric acid

is excreted in the urine (see [A] below). Studies of factors that influence the rate of synthesis of hippuric acid and of the incorporation of isotopes into the glycine moiety have contributed a great deal to present knowledge of glycine metabolism. Reference to such studies is frequently made throughout the following discussion.

In the mammalian organism glycine is readily synthesized. It has been estimated by Quick,[241] from studies of the rate of hippuric acid synthesis, that man can mobilize 9 mg. of glycine per hour per kilo of body weight. Quick[241] has suggested that this estimation is low. Early studies carried out by Swanson[242] showed that following the administration of benzoic acid, hippuric acid excretion increased and urea excretion decreased. The results indicate that glycine was synthesized from nitrogen which would have otherwise been used for urea synthesis. Conclusive evidence of the de novo synthesis of glycine was obtained by Schoenheimer,[125] who showed that the ammonium ions of N^{15} labelled ammonium citrate can be rapidly incorporated into glycine.

Mechanisms responsible for glycine synthesis have been the subject of a great deal of investigation. The enzyme, glycine oxidase, which is present in liver and kidney tissue, catalyzes the oxidative deamination of glycine to yield glyoxylic acid (see [B] below). Ratner[243] has suggested that this reaction constitutes a catabolic pathway for glycine. However, the formation of glycine from glyoxylic or glycolic acid has been demonstrated in intact animals and in liver slices.[244,245] Thus, one mechanism of glycine synthesis appears to occur through either transamination or the reversal of oxidative deamination.

Serine appears to be a major precursor of glycine. This was conclusively demonstrated by Shemin,[246] who administered isotopically labelled serine along with benzoic acid and recovered heavily labelled glycine in the hippuric acid isolated from the urine. Shemin has suggested that the conversion takes place in the manner shown in [C] below. The reverse of this process, the synthesis of serine from glycine, has been proved to occur easily both in vivo and in vitro. Siekevitz and Greenberg[247] have found that glycine can give rise to formate, which can in turn unite with another molecule of glycine to yield serine. Since serine can also be broken down to pyruvic acid (see Serine), it represents an intermediate in the catabolism of glycine. Threonine, which is structurally similar to serine, also gives rise to glycine (see Threonine).

The conversion of sarcosine to glycine was suggested in 1935 by Gordon and Jackson,[248] who found that it increased the excretion of hippuric acid. Handler et al.[249] subsequently described a system in liver which demethylated sarcosine to formaldehyde and glycine. The conversion was attributed to the action of an enzyme termed sarcosine oxidase (see [D] below).

The relationship between these two compounds is of considerable interest since it places glycine directly in the

---

[A]

$$\underset{\text{Benzoic acid}}{C_6H_5{-}COOH} + \underset{\text{Glycine}}{NH_2{-}CH_2{-}COOH} \rightarrow \underset{\text{Hippuric acid}}{C_6H_5{-}CO{-}NH{-}CH_2{-}COOH} + H_2O$$

[B]

$$\underset{\text{Glycine}}{NH_2{-}CH_2{-}COOH} + \tfrac{1}{2}O_2 \rightarrow \underset{\text{Glyoxylic acid}}{HO{-}C{-}COOH} + NH_3$$

[C]

$$\underset{\text{Serine}}{HO{-}CH_2{-}\overset{\overset{NH_2}{|}}{CH}{-}COOH} \underset{}{\overset{-2H}{\rightleftharpoons}} \underset{\text{Formylglycine}}{O{=}\overset{\overset{H}{|}}{C}{-}\overset{\overset{NH_2}{|}}{CH}{-}COOH} \overset{+H_2O}{\rightleftharpoons} \underset{\text{Glycine}}{\overset{\overset{NH_2}{|}}{CH_2}{-}COOH} + \underset{\text{“Formate”}}{H{-}COOH}$$

[D]

$$\underset{\text{Sarcosine}}{CH_3{-}NH{-}CH_2{-}COOH} + \tfrac{1}{2}O_2 \rightarrow \underset{\text{Glycine}}{NH_2{-}CH_2{-}COOH} + \underset{\text{Formaldehyde}}{HCHO}$$

metabolic scheme involving transmethylation reactions and the resultant synthesis and catabolism of choline (see Transmethylation).

Glycine in Porphyrin Synthesis. Shemin and Rittenberg[250] in 1945 reported that after one of them had ingested a considerable amount of isotopically labelled glycine, the label appeared in the pyrrole rings of his blood hemin. The subsequent elucidation of the processes that account for this observation have, as Shemin[251] has stated, "revealed that the complicated looking molecule, protoporphyrin, is synthesized from two simple and available compounds, glycine and succinate, by relatively simple reactions." Following confirmation of their original observation, it was shown, with isotopically labelled compounds, that the four nitrogen atoms and eight of the carbon atoms of protoporphyrin were derived from glycine[251] and that the remaining twenty-six carbons came from succinate.[252,253]

The results of experiments which showed that succinate was involved in porphyrin synthesis gave rise to the postulate that "active" succinate condensed with the α-carbon of glycine to form α-amino-β-ketoadipic acid. Subsequent decarboxylation of the latter compound would give rise to δ-aminolevulinic acid, which could in turn condense to form a pyrrole ring (see A below).

The utilization of isotopically labelled glycine, succinate, and δ-aminolevulinic acid for porphyrin synthesis, by duck erythrocytes in vitro serve as convincing evidence that the synthesis of the pyrrole ring occurs in the manner depicted in the scheme above.[254,255,256,257] Shemin's elucidation of the metabolic relationship between the Krebs cycle and glycine metabolism has given rise to what is now termed the succinate-glycine cycle

A

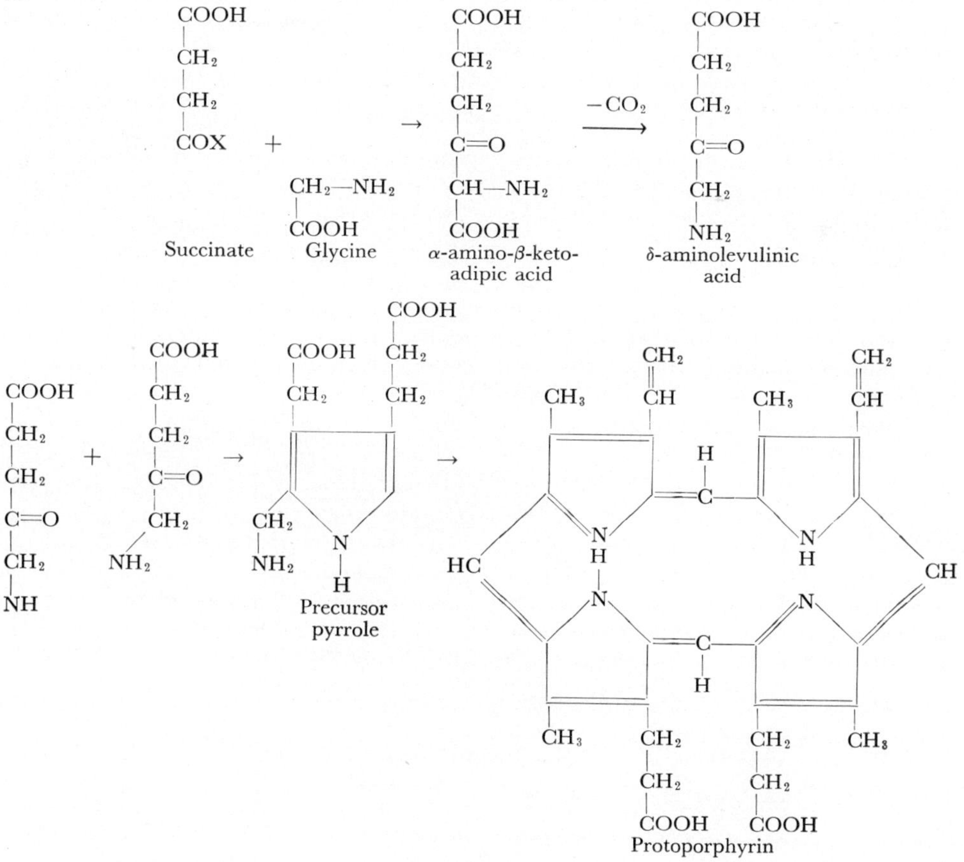

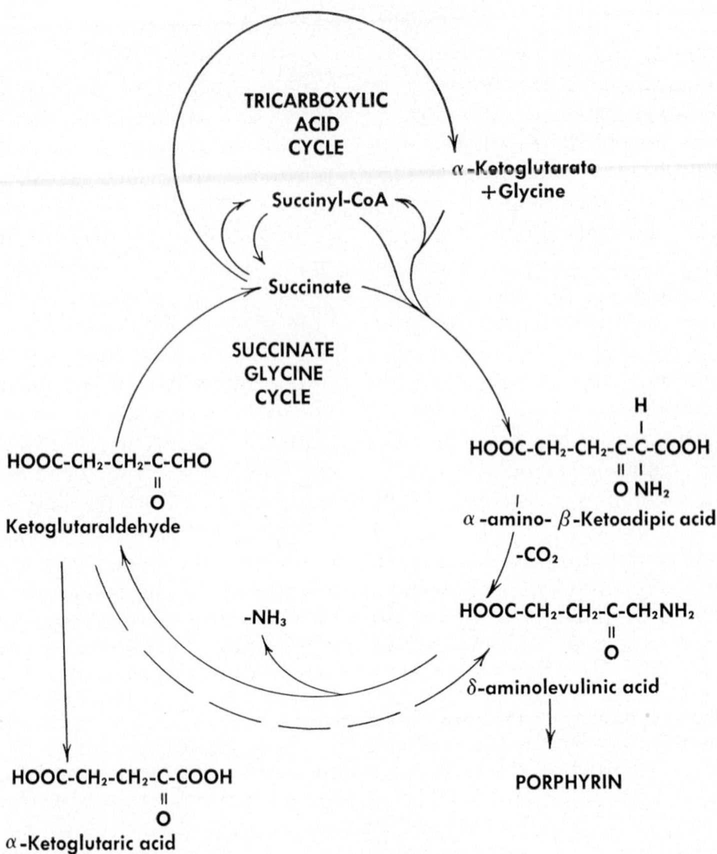

FIG. 3. The succinate-glycine cycle.

(Fig. 3). The way in which four pyrrole rings unite to form the complete porphyrin molecule has not been defined.

Serine

The synthesis of serine from glycine has been previously discussed. It was noted that the catabolism of serine also represents a pathway for the catabolism of glycine. Serine can be synthesized by the transamination of hydroxypyruvic acid from alanine.[230] The transaminase involved has a relatively high activity in liver and kidney and it has been suggested that the reaction represents a major pathway of serine metabolism in these tissues. Many animal tissues possess an enzyme, serine dehydrase, that catalyzes the degradation of serine to pyruvic acid[258] (see A below). The incorporation of N^{15} labelled glycine into ethanolamine was originally demonstrated by Stetten[259] in 1941. The hypothesis that this transformation occurred through the reduction of glycine was discarded when it was shown by Greenberg and Harris[260] that glycine in which the carboxyl group was labelled with C^{14}, failed to produce labelled ethanolamine. The suggestion that glycine was first converted to serine, which was in turn decarboxylated to form ethanolamine, was confirmed by Levine and Tarver,[261] who found that labelled ethanolamine could be recovered from the livers of animals after the adminis-

---

A

$$\underset{\text{Serine}}{\begin{matrix}CH_2OH\\|\\CH{-}NH_2\\|\\COOH\end{matrix}} \xrightarrow{-H_2O} \begin{matrix}CH_2\\\|\\C{-}NH_2\\|\\COOH\end{matrix} \rightarrow \begin{matrix}CH_3\\|\\C{=}NH\\|\\COOH\end{matrix} \xrightarrow{+H_2O} \underset{\text{Pyruvic acid}}{\begin{matrix}CH_3\\|\\C{=}O\\|\\COOH\end{matrix}} + NH_3$$

tration of serine labelled with C^{14} in the position. Since the carbon of serine does not participate in glycine formation, the ethanolamine must have arisen from the decarboxylation of serine (see A below).

Threonine

Available data suggest that vertebrates possess no ability to synthesize threonine. Apparently even simple deamination is an irreversible process, since the threonine of body tissues contains no isotope after the administration of N^{15} labelled glycine.[262]

The manner in which threonine is catabolized was first indicated by Braunstein and Valenkina,[263] when they reported that liver and kidney tissue of many species degraded threonine to glycine. Confirmation of these findings was obtained by Meltzer and Sprinson[264] and Lien and Greenberg.[265] An alternate pathway for the catabolism of threonine has been indicated by Lien and Greenberg,[266] who found that it could give rise, in vivo, to α-aminobutyric acid. The latter substance appears to be formed from the transamination of α-ketobutyric acid (see B below).

Lysine

Gortner[267] has pointed out that lysine is a prime example of the dependency of the higher animals on the plant kingdom. He exclaims that vertebrates cannot even insert an amino group on the ϵ-carbon of α-aminocaproic acid to form lysine in spite of the fact that they may be dying from a deficiency of this amino acid.

Ringer[268] in 1913 suggested that lysine might be catabolized to glutaric acid, but experimental support of this speculation was not obtained until 1948 when Borsook et al.[269,270] found that guinea pig liver homogenates converted lysine to α-aminoadipic acid. These investigators also obtained conclusive evidence, using C^{14} labelled α-aminoadipic acid, that it was converted by liver to α-ketoadipic and glutaric acids. It was originally thought that the α-aminoadipic acid arose from deamination of the ϵ-amino group of lysine. The reaction now appears to be more complex. Rothstein and Miller[271] and Schweet et al.[272] report that pipecolic acid is intermediate between lysine and α-aminoadipic acid. Cahill[273] in 1944 suggested that the

---

A

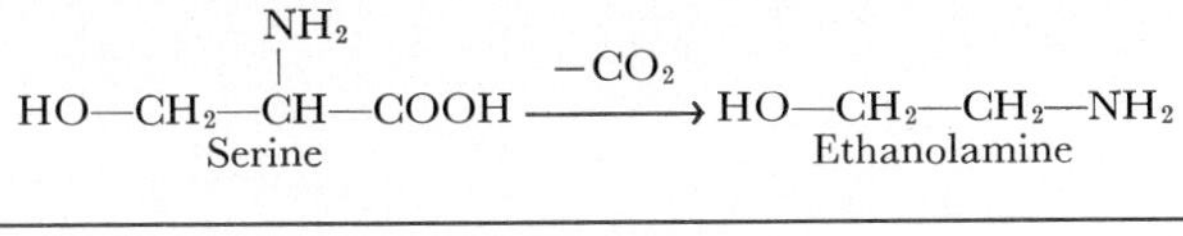

$$\underset{\text{Serine}}{HO{-}CH_2{-}\overset{\displaystyle NH_2}{\overset{|}{C}H}{-}COOH} \xrightarrow{-CO_2} \underset{\text{Ethanolamine}}{HO{-}CH_2{-}CH_2{-}NH_2}$$

B

$$\underset{\text{Threonine}}{CH_3{-}CHOH{-}CHNH_2{-}COOH} \longrightarrow \underset{\text{Glycine}}{NH_2{-}CH_2{-}COOH} + \underset{\text{Acetaldehyde}}{CH_3{-}CH{=}O}$$

$$\text{Threonine} \xrightarrow{-H_2O} CH_3{-}CH{=}C(NH_2){-}COOH \longrightarrow CH_3{-}CH_2{-}C({=}NH){-}COOH \xrightarrow[+H_2O]{NH_3} \underset{\alpha\text{-ketobutyric acid}}{CH_3{-}CH_2{-}C({=}O){-}COOH}$$

$$\alpha\text{-ketobutyric acid} \longrightarrow \underset{\text{Propionic acid}}{CH_3{-}CH_2{-}COOH}$$

$$\alpha\text{-ketobutyric acid} \longrightarrow \underset{\alpha\text{-aminobutyric acid}}{CH_3{-}CH_2{-}CHNH_2{-}COOH}$$

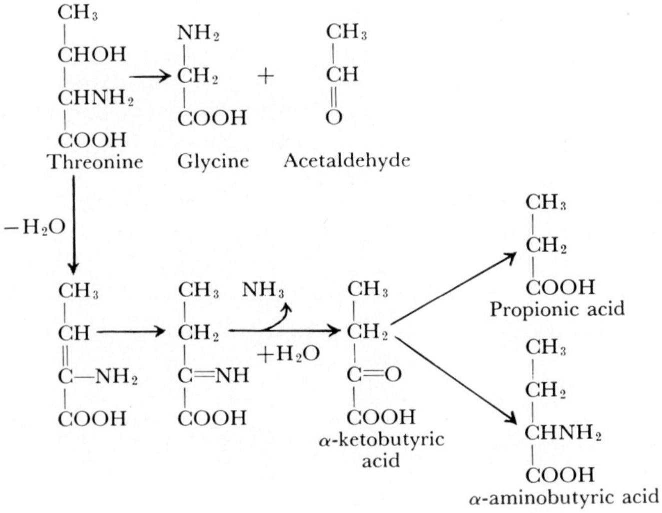

α-keto group of the oxidatively deaminated residue of lysine could react with the terminal amino group to form a substituted piperidine. The work of Rothstein et al. and of Borsook et al. indicates that the catabolism of lysine occurs according to the scheme given in A below:

Leucine

Leucine is an essential dietary factor that aroused early interest because it is the most strongly ketogenic of the amino acids. The ketogenic effect of isovaleric acid was observed in 1906 by Embden in his perfusion studies and led him to

---

A

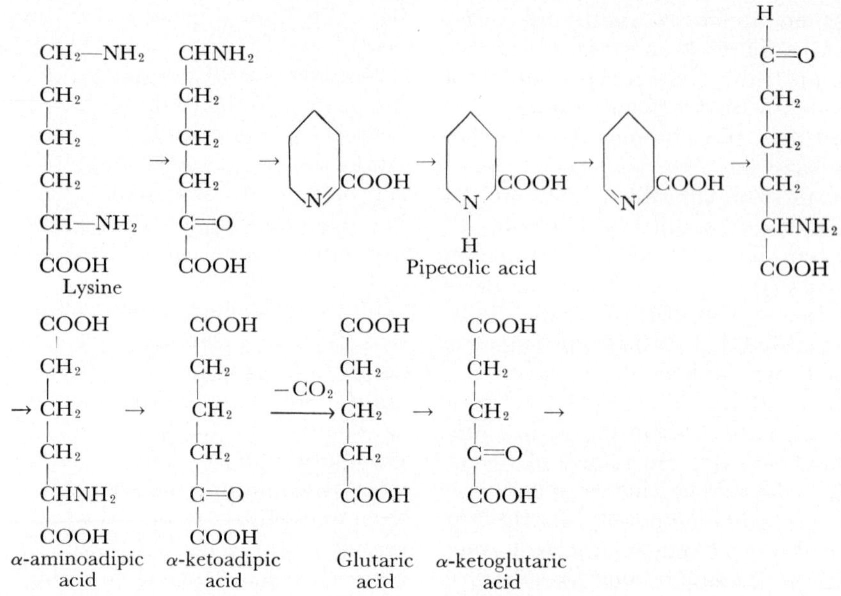

$CH_2NH_2—CH_2—CH_2—CH_2—CHNH_2—COOH$ (Lysine) → $CHNH_2—CH_2—CH_2—CH_2—C{=}O—COOH$ → [piperideine ring, N=C]—COOH → [piperidine ring, N—H]—COOH (Pipecolic acid) → [piperideine ring, N=C]—COOH → $HC{=}O—CH_2—CH_2—CH_2—CHNH_2—COOH$

→ $COOH—CH_2—CH_2—CH_2—CHNH_2—COOH$ (α-aminoadipic acid) → $COOH—CH_2—CH_2—CH_2—C{=}O—COOH$ (α-ketoadipic acid) $\xrightarrow{-CO_2}$ $COOH—CH_2—CH_2—CH_2—COOH$ (Glutaric acid) → $COOH—CH_2—CH_2—C{=}O—COOH$ (α-ketoglutaric acid) →

B

Leucine	$CH_3—CH(CH_3)—CH_2—CHNH_2—COOH$
	⇅
α-ketoisocaproic acid	$CH_3—CH(CH_3)—CH_2—CO—COOH$
	↓ CoASH
Isovaleryl-CoA	$CH_3—CH(CH_3)—CH_2—CO—S—CoA$
	⇅
Senecioyl-CoA	$CH_3—C(CH_3){=}CH—CO—S—CoA$
	⇅ H_2O
β-hydroxyisovaleryl-CoA	$CH_3—C(OH)(CH_3)—CH_2—CO—S—CoA$
	⇅ CO_2, ATP
β-hydroxy-β-methylglutaryl-CoA	$HOOC—CH_2—C(OH)(CH_3)—CH_2—CO—S—CoA$
	⇅
	$CH_3—CO—CH_2—COOH$ (Acetoacetic acid) + $CH_3—CO—S—CoA$ (Acetyl-CoA)

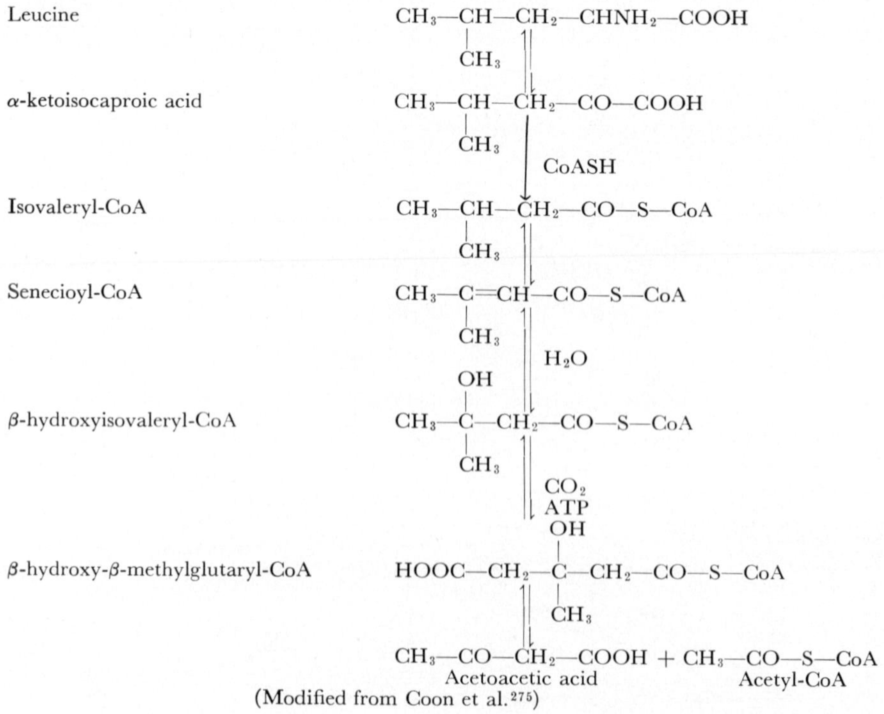

(Modified from Coon et al.[275])

suggest that this substance was an intermediate in the catabolism of leucine. However, the elucidation of the catabolic pathway proved to be a difficult task, and the problem has been resolved only within recent years.

The early suggestion that isovalerate was an intermediate in the catabolism of leucine was supported by Bloch[274] in 1944 when he observed that either leucine or isovalerate labelled with deuterium gave rise to 2-carbon compounds in vivo. Clarification of the intermediate steps shown in B on page 34 has recently been achieved by Coon et al.[275] Participation of coenzyme A (CoA) in the reaction sequence was indicated by the discovery that heart tissue extracts would catalyze the conversion of senecioyl-CoA and β-hydroxyisovaleryl-CoA to acetoacetate, while the corresponding free acids were inactive.

The hydration of senecioyl-CoA to β-hydroxyisovaleryl-CoA is catalyzed by the enzyme crotonase, which is found in both liver and heart tissue. Clarification of the reaction sequence was greatly facilitated when Coon[276] in 1950 demonstrated that acetoacetate production from leucine involved the fixation of carbon dioxide. Additional work showed that fixation occurred in the presence of ATP during the conversion of β-hydroxyisovaleryl-CoA to acetoacetate. The prediction that the fixation of carbon dioxide gave rise to the intermediate β-hydroxy-β-methylglutaryl-CoA received support from the observation that the synthetic material was rapidly converted to acetoacetate by the enzyme preparation. The second product of the reaction, acetyl-CoA, may condense with another acetyl-CoA to produce more acetoacetic acid. As Coon et al.[275] point out, this sequence of reactions fully accounts for the strongly ketogenic properties of leucine.

Isoleucine

Isoleucine, in contrast to leucine, is glycogenic and only weakly ketogenic. Meister et al.[277] have shown that preparations of pig heart transaminate isoleucine to yield α-keto-β-methylvaleric acid. It is assumed that this compound is decarboxylated to α-methylbutyric acid. Subsequent transformations have been clarified chiefly through the work

---

A

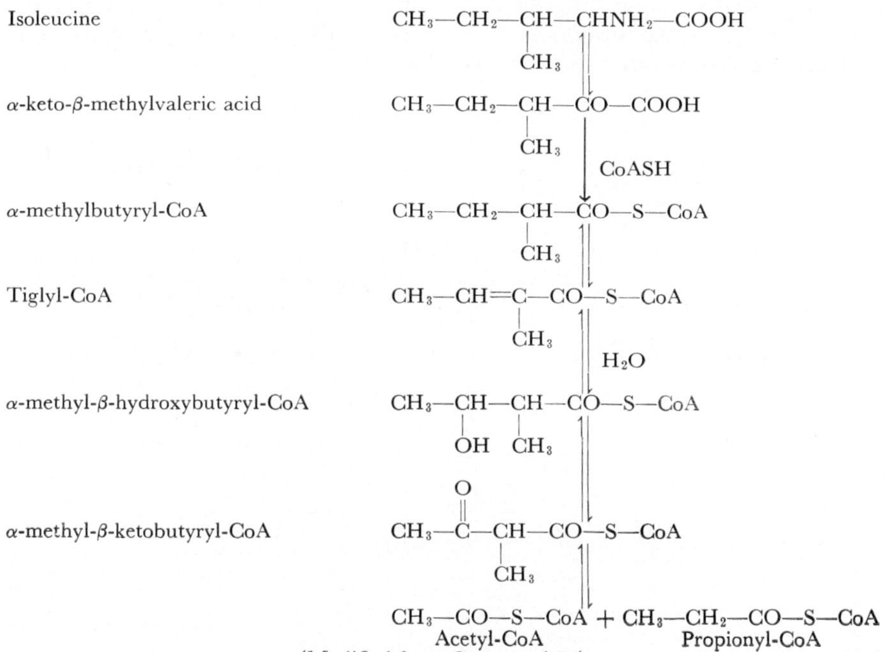

Isoleucine	$CH_3—CH_2—CH(CH_3)—CHNH_2—COOH$
	⇅
α-keto-β-methylvaleric acid	$CH_3—CH_2—CH(CH_3)—CO—COOH$
	↓ CoASH
α-methylbutyryl-CoA	$CH_3—CH_2—CH(CH_3)—CO—S—CoA$
	⇅
Tiglyl-CoA	$CH_3—CH{=}C(CH_3)—CO—S—CoA$
	⇅ H_2O
α-methyl-β-hydroxybutyryl-CoA	$CH_3—CH(OH)—CH(CH_3)—CO—S—CoA$
	⇅
α-methyl-β-ketobutyryl-CoA	$CH_3—C({=}O)—CH(CH_3)—CO—S—CoA$
	⇅
	$CH_3—CO—S—CoA$ + $CH_3—CH_2—CO—S—CoA$
	Acetyl-CoA + Propionyl-CoA

(Modified from Coon et al.[275])

of Coon et al.,[278,279] who demonstrated that C^{14} labelled α-methylbutyrate, when incubated with liver slices, gave rise to "acetate" and propionic acid. Evidence for the participation of tiglic acid as an intermediary metabolite was furnished by the observation that tiglyl-CoA was converted by liver preparations to acetyl-CoA and propionyl-CoA.[275] Chromatographic analysis also revealed the presence of α-methyl-β-hydroxybutyric acid.[275] This latter substance has been shown to arise by hydration of tiglyl-CoA through the action of crotonase (see [A] on page 35).

Valine

Several of the details in the degradation of valine are unknown. Rose and associates[280] found that three of the carbon atoms of either valine α-ketoisovaleric acid or isobutyric acid can be utilized for the synthesis of glucose, and proposed the latter two substances as the initial products of valine catabolism. The production of α-ketoisovaleric acid has been supported by Cammarata and Cohen[225] who found that valine is readily susceptible to transamination. Atchley[281] has found that kidney and liver homogenates convert isobutyric acid to propionic acid. Kinnory and Greenberg[282] proved with the aid of C^{14} labelled valine that the propionic acid arose from decarboxylation of the isobutyric acid, and not by demethylation; however, the intermediate reactions leading to propionic acid are not completely known. Coon[275] suggests on the basis of his work that isobutyryl-CoA is converted to methylacrylyl-CoA, which in turn is hydrated by the action of the enzyme crotonase to β-hydroxyisobutyryl-CoA. Flavin, Ortiz and Ochoa[283] indicate that propionyl-CoA is metabolized in animal tissues via methylmalonyl-CoA to succinyl-CoA, which is in turn converted to succinate (see [A] below).

Phenylalanine and Tyrosine

Many of the diseases classified as "inborn errors in metabolism" occur because of defects in the metabolism of phenylalanine and tyrosine and are frequently characterized by the excretion of either intermediary or abnormal metabolites of these aromatic amino acids. Studies of patients afflicted with these diseases brought early contributions to our knowledge of the metabolism of phenylalanine and tyrosine. In the condition known as alcaptonuria, homogentisic acid is excreted. Its presence is easily detected since the urine turns dark brown or black upon standing. It was noted by Abderhalden in 1907[284] that homogentisic acid excretion was increased by feeding either tyrosine

---

[A]

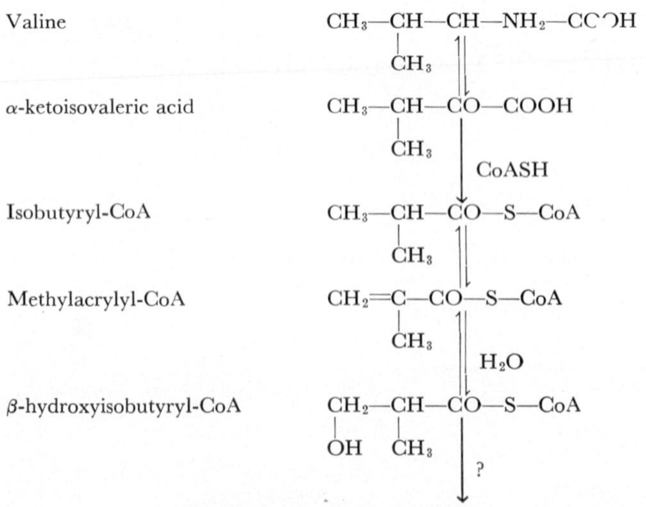

Valine	$CH_3—CH(CH_3)—CH—NH_2—COOH$
	⇅
α-ketoisovaleric acid	$CH_3—CH(CH_3)—CO—COOH$
	↓ CoASH
Isobutyryl-CoA	$CH_3—CH(CH_3)—CO—S—CoA$
	⇅
Methylacrylyl-CoA	$CH_2{=}C(CH_3)—CO—S—CoA$
	⇅ H_2O
β-hydroxyisobutyryl-CoA	$CH_2(OH)—CH(CH_3)—CO—S—CoA$
	↓ ?

(Modified from Coon et al.[275])

or phenylalanine to alcaptonurics. His suggestion that phenylalanine was converted to tyrosine received further experimental support when Embden[285] in 1913 reported that tyrosine was produced by perfusing the liver with solutions containing phenylalanine.

Phenylalanine	Tyrosine	Homogentisic Acid
C_6H_5–CH_2–$CHNH_2$–COOH	HO–C_6H_4–CH_2–$CHNH_2$–COOH	(HO)(OH)C_6H_3–CH_2–COOH

Proof that this conversion occurs in rats has been obtained by the use of isotopically labelled phenylalanine.[286]

The proposal made by Neubauer[287] in 1909 that the initial step in tyrosine catabolism was conversion to p-hydroxyphenylpyruvic acid has been verified only within recent years.[288,289] This step apparently involves transamination with α-ketoglutarate,[290] since it is accompanied by the formation of glutamic acid and no appreciable ammonia production. The manner in which the oxidation and rearrangement of the p-hydroxyphenylpyruvate to homogentisic acid is accomplished remains obscure.

Embden, during his liver perfusion experiments, observed that the addition of homogentisic acid to the perfusate resulted in the formation of acetoacetate, an observation in keeping with reports that the aromatic amino acids are ketogenic and not glucogenic. Schepartz and Gurin[291] and Weinhouse and Millington[292] with the aid of isotopically labelled phenylalanine have shown conclusively that acetoacetate is a product of tyrosine and phenylalanine catabolism. Suda and Takeda[293] and Ravdin and Crandall[294] have obtained an enzyme preparation from rabbit and rat liver that splits the ring of homogentisic acid to yield fumarylacetoacetic acid. The latter compound, according to Ravdin and Crandall, is hydrolyzed to fumaric and acetoacetic acid by another enzyme. The metabolic scheme proposed by these investigators has recently received general confirmation from experiments carried out by Dische and Rittenberg.[295]

Ascorbic Acid and Tyrosine Catabolism. A relationship between ascorbic acid and tyrosine metabolism became evident when Sealock and Silberstein[296,297] observed that scorbutic guinea pigs were alcaptonuric. The experimental alcaptonuria, which also occurred in vitamin C deficient humans, differed from the hereditary condition in that it was accompanied by the excretion of other phenolic metabolites such as p-hydroxyphenylacetic acid, p-hydroxyphenyllactic acid and p-hydroxyphenylpyruvic acid. Subsequent work by Painter and Zilva[298,299] showed that the oxidation of tyrosine by liver slices and homogenates was impaired in tissues from scorbutic guinea pigs, and that the addition of ascorbic acid in vitro improved tyrosine utilization. The study of tyrosine utilization in liver brei was greatly facilitated by Knox and associates,[300] who found that the metabolic changes were more pronounced when the tissue preparations were fortified with α-ketoglutarate, as well as ascorbic acid.[301] According to Knox,[301] ascorbic acid plays its most specific role in the oxidation of p-hydroxyphenylpyruvic acid, but the nature of its action in this process remains obscure. In view of the fact that activation of the liver brei preparation can also be obtained with isoascorbic acid, glucoascorbic acid, dichlorophenolindophenol and hydroquinone, it seems unlikely that ascorbic acid acts as a co-enzyme in the reaction.

There is some evidence indicating that folic acid and vitamin B_{12} are also involved in tyrosine metabolism. Uchida, Suzuki and Ichahara[302] have identified two enzymes from rabbit liver preparation. One enzyme converts p-hydroxyphenylpyruvic acid to 2,5-dihydroxyphenylpyruvic acid. The activity of the enzyme requires the presence of both ascorbic acid and vitamin B_{12}. The B_{12} requirement is very low. These authors suggest that the active enzyme is a B_{12} complex and that vitamin C stabilizes the

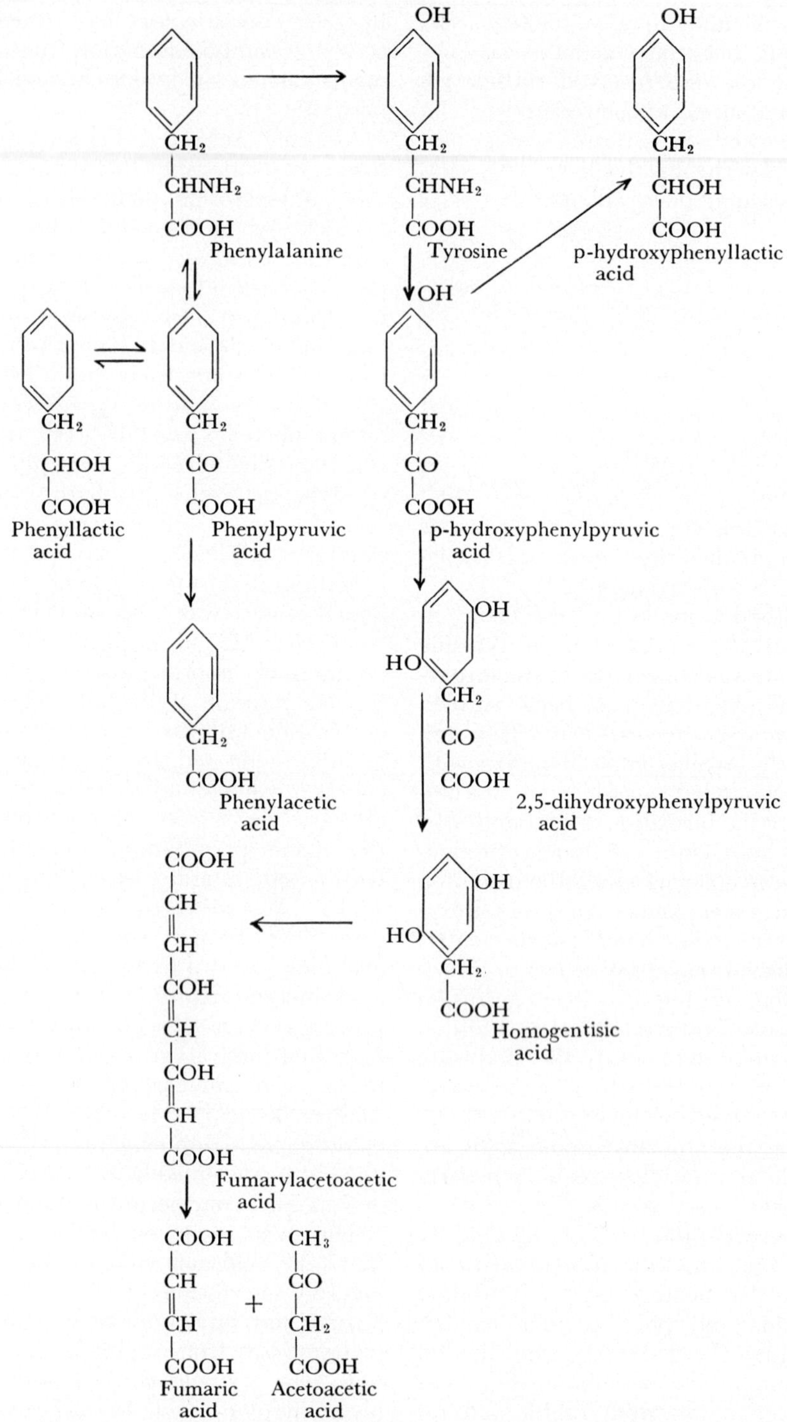

CH_2
$CHNH_2$
COOH
Phenylalanine

OH
CH_2
$CHNH_2$
COOH
Tyrosine

OH
CH_2
CHOH
COOH
p-hydroxyphenyllactic acid

CH_2
CHOH
COOH
Phenyllactic acid

CH_2
CO
COOH
Phenylpyruvic acid

OH
CH_2
CO
COOH
p-hydroxyphenylpyruvic acid

OH
HO
CH_2
CO
COOH
2,5-dihydroxyphenylpyruvic acid

CH_2
COOH
Phenylacetic acid

OH
HO
CH_2
COOH
Homogentisic acid

COOH
CH
CH
COH
CH
COH
CH
COOH
Fumarylacetoacetic acid

COOH
CH
CH
COOH
Fumaric acid

+

CH_3
CO
CH_2
COOH
Acetoacetic acid

FIG. 4. Metabolic pathways of phenylalanine and tyrosine.

reaction form of the coenzyme. The conversion of the 2,5-dihydroxyphenylpyruvic acid to homogentisic acid is catalyzed by the second enzyme,[302] but does not appear to be influenced by the vitamins under discussion. Folic acid is thought to participate in the subsequent transformation of homogentisate, but the nature of its influence remains a matter of speculation. Suda and co-workers[303] reported that the activity of homogentisicase (homogentisic acid oxidase), the enzyme responsible for the cleavage of the ring in homogentisic acid, was greatly reduced in livers from scorbutic animals. The activity could be restored by the addition of either ascorbic acid or ferrous iron; ferric iron was without effect. It has been suggested that this is a nonspecific effect of ascorbate and that by acting as a reducing agent it maintains iron in the ferrous state.[303] It has been amply demonstrated that ferrous iron is required for the enzymatic oxidation of homogentisic acid.[304,301]

It was originally observed by Levine et al.[305,306] that p-hydroxyphenylpyruvate and p-hydroxyphenyllactate were excreted by premature infants fed high protein diets, and that the excretion of these substances ceased when ascorbic acid was given. Additional investigations have shown that in some instances the hydroxyphenyluria can be decreased by the administration of folic acid.[307] Vitamin B_{12} and liver extracts, although of some value, were less effective in this respect.[308]

Biogenesis of Epinephrine and Thyroxine. Important metabolic routes of phenylalanine and tyrosine are those which give rise to the hormones epinephrine and thyroxine.

Proof of the conversion of phenylalanine to epinephrine was obtained with the use of the C^{14} labelled acid. The first step in the biogenesis of adrenaline occurs through the action of tissue tyrosinase, which converts tyrosine to 3,4-dihydroxyphenylalanine. A specific decarboxylase catalyzes the conversion of the latter compound to 3,4-dihydroxyphenylethylamine, which has been reported to be present in the adrenal gland[309] and is a normal constituent of urine.[310] The conversion of 3,4-dihydroxyphenylethylamine to norepinephrine requires the addition of a hydroxyl group to the side chain; however, the manner in which this simple transformation occurs is unknown. The formation of epinephrine from its precursor, norepinephrine, needs only the introduction of a methyl group to the side chain, a step that probably involves transmethylation from methionine.

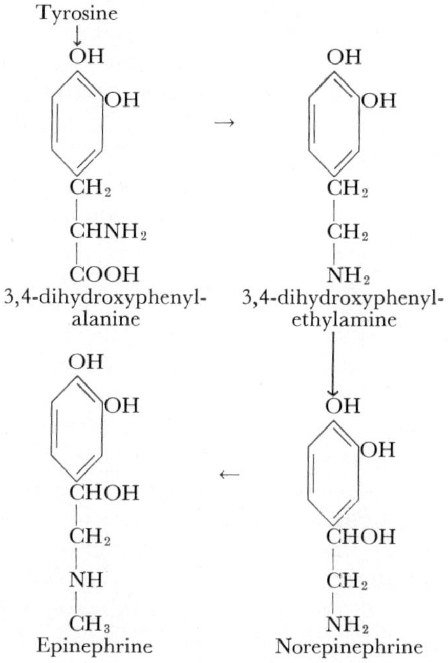

Tyrosine → OH, OH, CH_2—CHNH$_2$—COOH
3,4-dihydroxyphenylalanine
→
OH, OH, CH_2—CH_2—NH_2
3,4-dihydroxyphenylethylamine
↓
OH, OH, CHOH—CH_2—NH_2
Norepinephrine
←
OH, OH, CHOH—CH_2—NH—CH_3
Epinephrine

The details of thyroxine biogenesis are not yet known. The use of I^{131} has confirmed the earlier conclusion that in the thyroid gland tyrosine is converted to 3,5-diiodotyrosine, which in turn is converted to thyroxine. It has also been shown that incubation of diiodotyrosine in alkaline solution will give rise to small amounts of thyroxine. There has been some speculation as to the true nature of the thyroid hormone since Gross and Pitt-Rivers[311] isolated triiodothyronine from the plasma and thyroid gland. This substance is approximately five times as active as thyroxine. It has been suggested that triiodothyronine is formed either by the deiodination of thyroxine, or by the combination of one molecule of diiodotyrosine with one of monoiodotyrosine[312] (see A below).

Phenylketonuria (Phenylpyruvic Oligophrenia). Phenylketonuria, a condition first described by Folling in 1934, is biochemically characterized by the excretion in the urine of phenylalanine, phenylpyruvic acid, phenyllactic acid, phenylacetic acid and phenylacetylglutamine. The latter substance is a normal constituent of urine, but in phenylketonurics the excretion may be elevated 5 to 9 times. The disorder is inherited as a Mendelian recessive character and afflicts about 4 persons per 100,000. In addition to mental deterioration and convulsive seizures, the patients exhibit fair hair and dermatitis and have a peculiar musty smell.

Jervis,[313] in 1947, indicated that the metabolic defect in phenylketonurics lies in their inability to hydroxylate phenylalamine, thereby converting it to tyrosine. Under these conditions, phenylalanine tends to accumulate and is converted to abnormal products (see scheme). It has been suggested that the lack of pigmentation accompanying phenylketonuria may be due to a secondary lack of tyrosine and a subsequent reduction in melanin formation. The mental aberrations are thought to be due to a neurotoxic action of one or more of the abnormal metabolites but, thus far, absolute proof of this speculation has not been obtained.

Attempts to control phenylketonuria by feeding diets low in phenylalanine have produced equivocal results.[314] Some degree of improvement in mental and motor performance has been reported following the use of such diets. Since the most striking remissions appear to be obtained when treatment is started within the first year of life,[315] it has been suggested that earlier recognition and dietary therapy may be beneficial if started before permanent brain damage appears.[316]

Tyrosinosis. The only known case of tyrosinosis was described in 1932 by Medes.[317] The patient, while eating a normal diet, excreted extremely large amounts of p-hydroxyphenylpyruvic acid and, when fed supplements of tyrosine, excreted in addition to tyrosine, p-hydroxyphenyllactic acid and 3,4-dihydroxyphenylalanine. Phenylalanine supplements increased the excretion of p-hydroxyphenylpyruvate, tyrosine and p-hydroxyphenyllactate, while additional p-hydroxyphenylpyruvate was excreted either unchanged or as p-hydroxyphenyllactate. Homogentisic acid was completely utilized. Medes concluded that p-hydroxyphenylpyruvic acid was formed during the early stages of tyrosine catabolism and, since homogentisic acid was utilized while no 2,5-dihydroxy derivatives were formed, the metabolic impasse lay between p-hydroxyphenylpyruvic acid and homogentisate.

Alcaptonuria. Although alcaptonuria has been recognized for centuries, the first accurate clinical description of it was given in 1859 by Boedecker.[318] The disease is characterized by the excretion of urine that turns dark brown or black upon standing. The chromogenic material, which was called alcapton by Boedecker, was isolated by Wolkow and Baumann[319] and identified as 2,5-dihydroxyphenylacetic acid, more commonly called homogentisic acid. This substance is a reducing agent and when present in the urine produces a violet

---

A

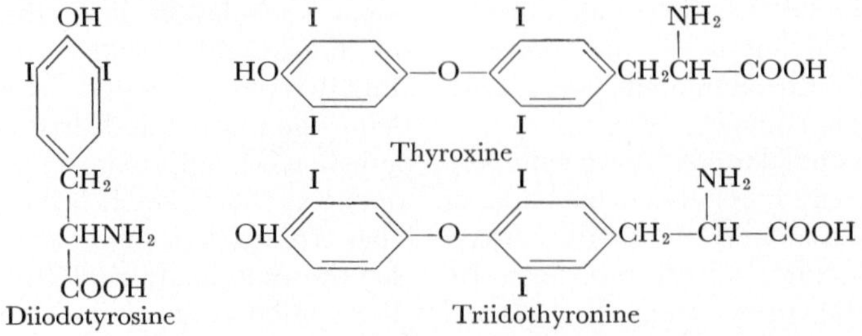

OH / I I / CH_2 / CHNH$_2$ / COOH

Diiodotyrosine

I I NH$_2$ / HO–(ring)–O–(ring)–CH_2CH—COOH / I I

Thyroxine

I I NH$_2$ / OH–(ring)–O–(ring)–CH_2—CH—COOH / I

Triidothyronine

color upon the addition of ferric chloride. Alcaptonuria is transmitted as a Mendelian recessive character but, unlike phenylketonuria, it is not accompanied by mental disease. The relatively high concentration of homogentisic acid in the body fluids leads eventually to pigmentation of the cartilaginous tissues in the body (ochronosis). It has been previously mentioned that the administration of phenylalanine and tyrosine increases the excretion of homogentisic acid. It appears, therefore, that the metabolic defect lies in the inability to utilize homogentisic acid, possibly because of the absence of the enzyme homogentisicase.

Tryptophan

Tryptophan was isolated in 1901 by Hopkins and Cole[320] and was the first amino acid shown to be nutritionally indispensable. In 1853 Liebig discovered in urine a substance he called kynurenic acid. Interest in tryptophan metabolism was stimulated when it was discovered that this amino acid increased the secretion of kynurenic acid. In 1925 Matsuoka and Yoshimatsu[321] found kynurenine in the urine of rabbits after the administration of tryptophan. Masajo[322] in 1937 isolated xanthurenic acid from rats fed a high protein diet. The relationship between tryptophan and xanthurenic acid was shown by Lepkovsky and associates.[323] They found that the excretion of xanthurenic acid by pyridoxine deficient rats ceased when tryptophan was removed from their diet. Interest in this compound was further aroused by evidence that tryptophan was involved in the synthesis of nicotinic acid, the pellagra preventative factor. Goldberger[324] in 1922 claimed that tryptophan was beneficial in the treatment of pellagra, but the significance of this was not appreciated until 1945 when Krehl and Elvehjem[325] confirmed Goldberger's observation in nicotinic acid deficient rats. The reactions through which the metabolites of tryptophan are thought to arise are represented in Figure 5.

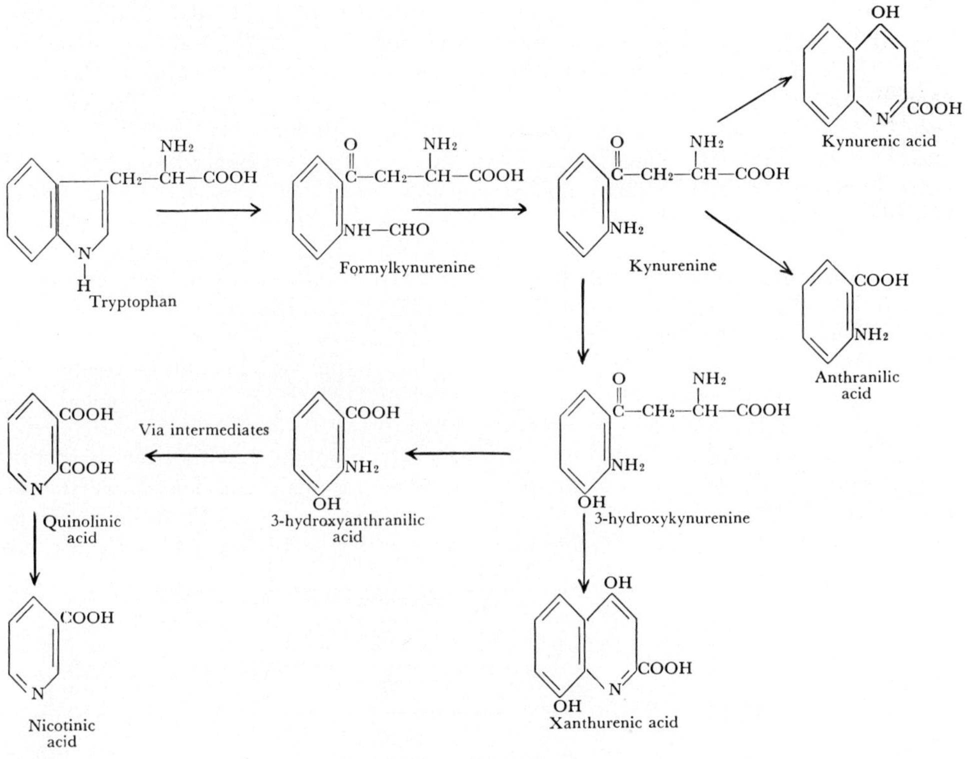

FIG. 5. Metabolic pathways of tryptophan.

The general validity of the reactions shown above has been supported by studies carried out by Heidelberger et al.[326] These investigators have reported that the administration of tryptophan labelled with C^{14} in the β position gives rise to β-labelled kynurenine in rabbit urine, and to kynurenic acid labelled in the 3-position in the urine of dogs. These observations have been substantiated by the work of Schayer.[327] The suggestion made by Albanese et al. that the indole ring of tryptophan may be utilized in the synthesis of hemoglobin has received no support from the tracer experiments of Schayer.[327] Recent work has revealed that the conversion of tryptophan to formylkynurenine is catalyzed by an enzyme system present in the liver.[328,329] This system is composed of peroxidase and an oxidase and initiates the reactions shown in A below. An enzyme, formylase, brings about the hydrolysis of formylkynurenine to kynurenine and formic acid (see B below). Kynureninase, an enzyme found in both liver and kidney tissue,[330] decomposes kynurenine to anthranilic acid and alanine. It is believed that pyridoxal phosphate is a co-factor involved in the conversions induced by kynureninase[331,332] and that in pyridoxine deficiency, removal of the alanyl side chain cannot be accomplished. The mechanism responsible for the formation of 3-hydroxykynurenine is not known and its derivation from kynurenine is largely a matter of speculation. The conversion of 3-hydroxykynurenine to 3-hydroxyanthranilic acid is also catalyzed by the enzyme kynureninase. Although the conversion of hydroxyanthranilic to nicotinic acid in the rat has been unequivocally demonstrated with the use of isotopes, the intermediates formed in the process are not known. It should be mentioned that the biosynthesis of this vitamin is not sufficient to maintain growth in experimental animals maintained on diets deficient in nicotinic acid.

Interest in xanthurenic acid has been stimulated by reports by Kotake and associates[333,334,335] that this metabolite would produce diabetes and was present in the urine of diabetics. Although the Japanese workers have reported that they have confirmed their original observations, support from other laboratories has not been obtained[336,337] and the importance of the claim cannot be evaluated at this time.

5-Hydroxytryptamine (Serotonin, Enteramine). Many investigations have been undertaken in recent years in an effort to determine the role of 5-hydroxytryptamine in normal physiologic processes.[338] This interesting substance, when given in very small doses, produces vasoconstriction, increases the frequency and amplitude of the heart beat, affects respiration, water excretion, and the activity of the intestine and some other smooth muscles. Gaddum[339] claims that there are specific cell receptors for 5-hydroxytryptamine located in various peripheral structures that are insensitive to histamine, epinephrine and acetylcholine. The detection of serotonin in the vertebrate brain has led to suggestions that it is a neurohormone, and also to the suggestion by Wooley and Shaw[340] that mental aberrations may arise from either a deficiency or excess of 5-hydroxytryptamine.

The synthesis of serotonin by mammalian tissue has been investigated by Undenfriend et al.[341] It is believed that tryptophan is first converted to 5-hydroxytryptophan, but the details of this process are unknown. The conversion of 5-hydroxytryptophan to 5-hydroxytryptamine has been shown by Undenfriend

---

A

$$\text{Tryptophan} + H_2O_2 \xrightarrow{\text{Peroxidase}} (\text{Tryptophan}) \xrightarrow[\text{Ox.}]{O_2} \text{Formylkynurenine} + H_2O_2$$

B

$$\text{Formylkynurenine} \xrightarrow{\text{Formylase}} \text{Kynurenine} + \text{Formic Acid}$$

et al.[342,344] to occur through the action of a specific decarboxylase which is found in kidney, liver, stomach, lung and blood platelets.

Serotonin is destroyed through the action of an amine oxidase found in liver and kidney tissue[343,344] which converts it to 5-hydroxyindoleacetic acid, probably by way of an aldehyde intermediate.[344] Since indoleacetic acid arising from tryptamine is known to be excreted as indoleacetic acid conjugated with glycine, it is suggested that 5-hydroxyindoleacetic acid is conjugated and excreted in a similar manner (see A below).

Histidine

Histidine is an essential amino acid for rats, mice, chicks and dogs, but is not required by the adult human and is probably not required by children. It is not known whether this amino acid is synthesized in the body tissues or whether it is formed by the intestinal flora and subsequently absorbed. Histidine, besides being an integral part of tissue protein, is found in muscle of vertebrates as a part of the compound carnosine (β-alanylhistidine) and anserine (β-alanyl-1-methylhistidine). The physiologic significance of these substances is unknown (see B below).

A number of steps in the catabolism of histidine have not yet been clarified. Experiments with C^{14} labelled histidine show that, in vivo, it is rapidly and completely degraded to carbon dioxide.[345] Information regarding some of the intermediate steps involved in its catabolism was first reported by Edlbacher[346] and Gyorgy and Rothler,[347] who found that liver preparations were capable of converting histidine to ammonia and a substance that yielded formic acid, glutamic acid and ammonia when hydrolyzed with acid or alkali. The degrada-

A

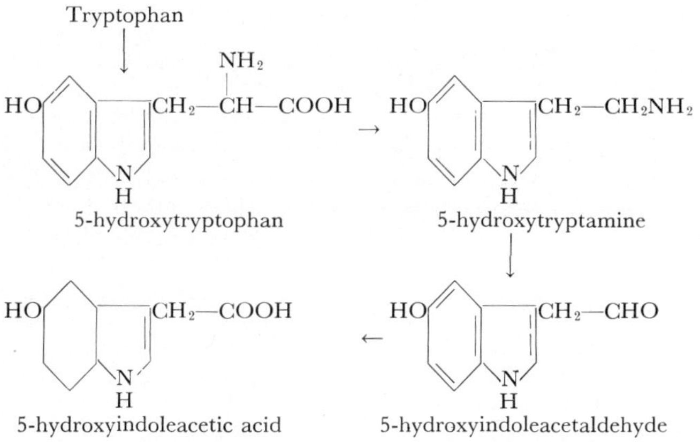

Tryptophan → 5-hydroxytryptophan → 5-hydroxytryptamine → 5-hydroxyindoleacetaldehyde → 5-hydroxyindoleacetic acid

5-hydroxytryptophan: HO–(indole)–CH_2—CH(NH_2)—COOH

5-hydroxytryptamine: HO–(indole)–CH_2—CH_2NH_2

5-hydroxyindoleacetaldehyde: HO–(indole)–CH_2—CHO

5-hydroxyindoleacetic acid: HO–(indole)–CH_2—COOH

B

Histidine: HC═C—CH_2—CH(NH_2)—COOH (imidazole ring: N, NH, CH)

Carnosine: HC═C—CH_2—CH(COOH)—NH—CO—CH_2—CH_2—NH_2 (imidazole ring: N, NH, CH)

Anserine: HC═C—CH_2—CH(COOH)—NH—CO—CH_2—CH_2—NH_2 (imidazole ring: N, NCH_3, CH)

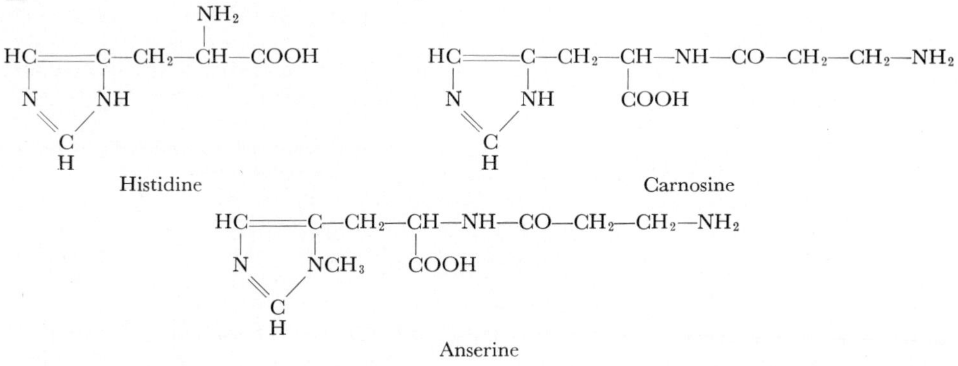

tion was originally attributed to the action of a single enzyme named histidase. The possibility that urocanic acid was an intermediate in this process was suggested by reports that it could be isolated from the urine of animals fed large amounts of histidine.[348] Additional support for this hypothesis was obtained by Sera et al.,[349,350] who found that the liver of vertebrates contained an enzyme called urocanase that broke down urocanic acid to the intermediate that yields glutamic acid, formic acid, and ammonia. It now appears that histidase is, in reality, two enzymes, urocanase and histidine deaminase. The latter enzyme converts histidine to urocanic acid.

Evidence has been obtained by Borek and Waelsch[351,352] and by Tabor and Mehler[353] that the intermediate giving rise to glutamic acid is formamido-L-glutamic acid. However, the formation of this compound is thought to involve another intermediate, imidazolone propionic acid, which arises from the addition of a molecule of water to urocanic acid. The imidazolone propionic acid then takes on another molecule of water to form formamido-L-glutamic acid. The fact that the latter substance is degraded very slowly by liver preparations, while histidine is rapidly converted to carbon dioxide in vivo, indicates the need for additional information on the factors regulating histidine catabolism (see [A] below).

Histamine. There has been considerable debate as to the origin of the histamine found in the body. According to one school, histamine is a vitamin which is either present in the food or manufactured by the intestinal flora and subsequently absorbed into the blood stream. The second group[354] believes that histamine is formed in the body tissues by the action of the enzyme histidine decarboxylase. Although both theories have been proved correct, Schayer[355] believes that most of the histamine found in the organism arises from histidine in the tissue, and not from that formed in the intestinal lumen.

The enzyme histidine decarboxylase is found in the kidney, liver, stomach and small intestine of most rodents, but its presence in the tissues of other species has not been ascertained.[354]

The enzymatic destruction of histamine was described by Eustis in 1915 and was more accurately and intensively investigated in 1929 by Best,[356] who named the enzyme responsible for the oxidative deamination of histamine, histaminase. Zellers,[357] in 1938, found that preparations which destroyed histamine also degraded other diamines and called

---

[A]

Histidine [imidazole ring: CH, N, NH; HC=C] —C—CH_2—CH(NH_2)—COOH $\xrightarrow{-NH_3}$ H—C=C—CH=CH—COOH Urocanic acid [imidazole ring: CH, N, NH]

Urocanic acid $\xrightarrow{+H_2O}$ Imidazolone propionic acid: [ring: CH, N, NH] O=C——CH—CH_2—CH_2—COOH

Imidazolone propionic acid $\xrightarrow{+H_2O}$ Formamido-L-glutamic acid: NH=CH—NH—CH(COOH)—CH_2—CH_2—COOH (HOOC—CH—CH_2—CH_2—COOH)

Formamido-L-glutamic acid $\xrightarrow{-NH_3}$ Formyl-L-glutamic acid: CHO—NH—CH; HOOC—CH—CH_2—CH_2COOH

Formyl-L-glutamic acid $\xrightarrow{+H_2O}$ HOOC—CH_2—CH_2—CH(NH_2)—COOH + HCOOH

Glutamic acid Formic acid

the enzyme diamine oxidase. Tabor[358] and Schayer[359] using radioactive histamine, have shown that the product of the deamination gives rise to imidazoleacetic acid, probably by way of imidazoleacetaldehyde. Tabor[360] has also found a second product of histamine catabolism in urine which he has tentatively identified as imidazoleacetic acid riboside. In addition to degradation initiated by histaminase, histamine may be acetylated[361] and excreted as acetylhistamine (see [A] below).

It is well established that during pregnancy the uterus and placenta of many species contain abnormally large amounts of histaminase, and that the blood level of this enzyme is elevated in pregnant women. The suggestion that histaminase protects the mother against histamine has little experimental support, since the ability of injected histamine to produce the flare of the triple response, gastric secretion, uterine motility and vasodilatation is unimpaired.[362,363,364,365,366] Despite these observations, the increased level of histaminase appears to be necessary in maintaining normal pregnancy and allowing it to terminate successfully. Roberts[367] has reported that the histaminase inhibitor, aminoguanidine, given to rats in doses that produce more than 50 per cent inhibition of the maternal placental histaminase, disturbs the normal course of pregnancy. The litters are frequently resorbed, stillborn or die shortly after delivery. The metabolism of histidine is also altered during pregnancy. Histidine appears in the urine about five weeks after conception and disappears immediately after parturition.[368,369,370,371] The observation that administered histidine is quantitatively excreted during pregnancy but completely metabolized under normal conditions[370] suggests that the formation of histamine from histidine may be impaired. However, histidinuria occurs not infrequently in healthy men;[372] thus, its significance when associated with pregnancy is difficult to interpret.

Methionine

The relationship between methionine and cystine remained obscure for many years. Osborne and Mendel[373] found, during their early investigations, that diets which contained 18 per cent casein as the sole source of protein supported vigorous growth in young rats, but any appreciable reduction in casein below the 18 per cent level resulted in a markedly diminished growth rate. The addition of cystine to the diet restored its ability to support growth; thus, cystine was considered to be an essential amino acid. This conclusion was later proved incorrect. Jackson and Block[374] reported that when the casein content of the diet had just reached the suboptimal level, the addition of either methionine or cystine restored the nutritive value of the food. It was finally demonstrated by Womack and Rose[375] that rats fed diets lacking both cystine and methionine lost weight and eventually died. The addition to the diet of methionine alone restored the health and growth of the animals, but the addition of cystine alone had no beneficial effect. Thus, methionine was the essential amino acid and

---

[A]

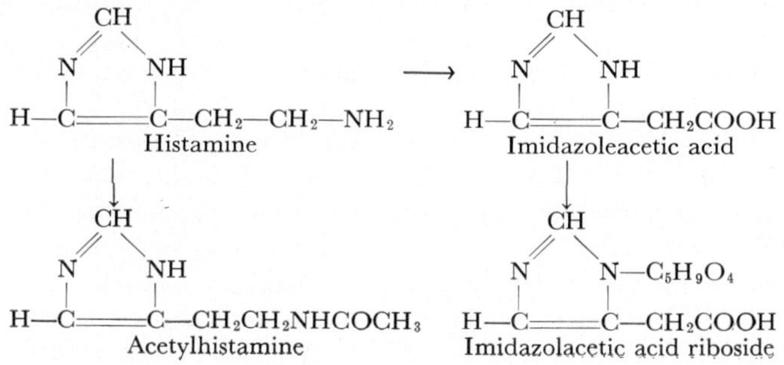

```
        CH                                       CH
      //  \                                    //  \
     N     NH                    ──→          N     NH
     |     |                                  |     |
H—C═══════C—CH2—CH2—NH2                  H—C═══════C—CH2COOH
        Histamine                            Imidazoleacetic acid
     ↓                                            ↓
        CH                                       CH
      //  \                                    //  \
     N     NH                                 N     N—C5H9O4
     |     |                                  |     |
H—C═══════C—CH2CH2NHCOCH3                H—C═══════C—CH2COOH
      Acetylhistamine                     Imidazolacetic acid riboside
```

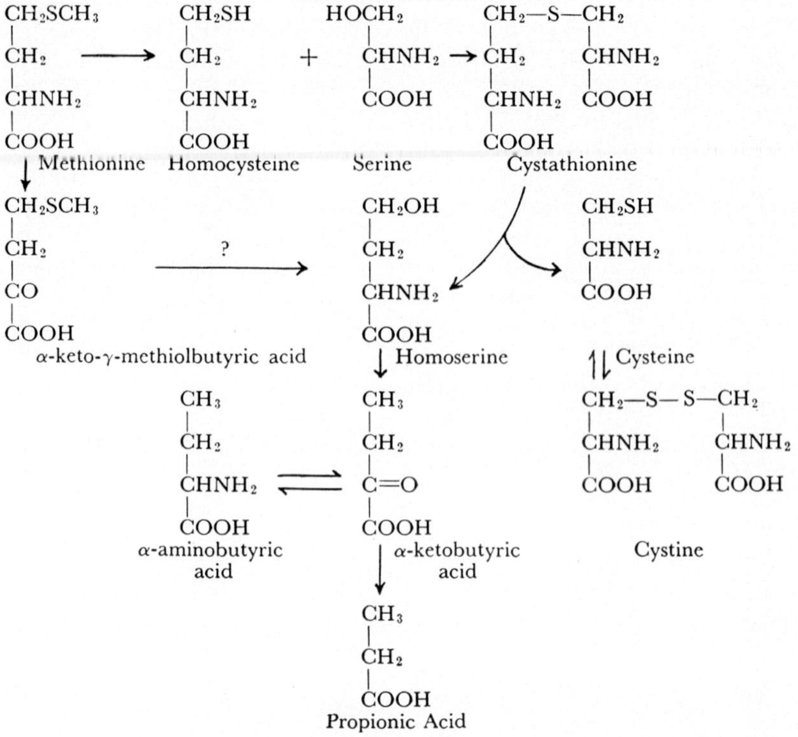

$CH_2SCH_3—CH_2—CHNH_2—COOH$ (Methionine) → $CH_2SH—CH_2—CHNH_2—COOH$ (Homocysteine) + $HOCH_2—CHNH_2—COOH$ (Serine) → $CH_2—S—CH_2$ with $CH_2—CHNH_2—COOH$ and $CHNH_2—COOH$ (Cystathionine)

Methionine ↓ $CH_2SCH_3—CH_2—CO—COOH$ (α-keto-γ-methiolbutyric acid) —?→ $CH_2OH—CH_2—CHNH_2—COOH$ (Homoserine)

Cystathionine → Homoserine + $CH_2SH—CHNH_2—COOH$ (Cysteine)

Cysteine ⇅ $CH_2—S—S—CH_2$, $CHNH_2$, $CHNH_2$, $COOH$, $COOH$ (Cystine)

Homoserine ↓ $CH_3—CH_2—C{=}O—COOH$ (α-ketobutyric acid) ⇌ $CH_3—CH_2—CHNH_2—COOH$ (α-aminobutyric acid)

α-ketobutyric acid ↓ $CH_3—CH_2—COOH$ (Propionic Acid)

FIG. 6. Metabolic interrelationships between methionine, cysteine and cystine.

cystine the dispensable factor. The confusion arose from the use of casein which has a relatively low methionine content. When the dietary level of this protein (provided that it is the sole source of protein) is reduced below 18 per cent, the biologic requirement for methionine cannot be filled. It appears that if the deficiency is not too great the metabolic requirement for methionine can just be fulfilled if some of it is spared from cystine synthesis by the addition of the latter substance to the diet.

The fact that removal of cystine from diets containing adequate methionine had no deleterious effects on experimental animals suggested that cystine could be synthesized from methionine. Conclusive proof that the sulfur of methionine could be used for cystine synthesis was obtained by Tarver and Schmidt,[376] and later by du Vigneaud and associates[377] when they isolated S^{35} labelled cystine from rats fed S^{35}-methionine. Convincing evidence had been obtained that the demethylation of methionine with the formation of homocysteine was the initial step in methionine transformation (see Transmethylation). Brand et al.,[378,379] who had noted that the administration of homocysteine increased cystine excretion in patients with cystinuria, suggested that transulfuration to serine, with the subsequent formation of cysteine, occurred through an intermediate called cystathionine. This speculation received strong support from Stetten,[380] who observed that heavily labelled cystine could be isolated from rat tissue after feeding isotopically labelled serine. Conclusive proof of cystathionine formation in vivo came when it was reported by Tabachnick and Tarver[381] that labelled cystathionine could be recovered from the liver and other internal organs of rats after the administration of S^{35} labelled methionine. The cleavage of cystathionine by rat liver preparations to cysteine and α-ketobutyric acid was demonstrated by du Vigneaud et al.[382] The fact that homoserine was also converted to α-ketobutyric acid supported speculations that it was an intermediate in cystathionine catabolism. Matsuo and Greenberg,[383] using C^{14} labelled methionine, have provided direct evidence for the formation of homoserine from cystathionine.

There is also good evidence that methionine can be degraded to homoserine without the intermediate formation of cystathionine. It was shown in 1939 by Waelsch and Borek[384] that methionine incubated with kidney slices was converted to α-keto-γ-methiolbutyric acid. There is more recent evidence that this can occur by enzymatic oxidative deamination,[385] and also by transamination.[225] The reversibility of this reaction has been indicated by the observation that the methionine in the diet of rats could be replaced by α-keto-γ-methiolbutyric acid.[386] The cleavage of α-keto-γ-methiolbutyric acid with the formation of methyl mercaptan has been recently demonstrated by Canellakis.[387] Theoretically, this should leave homoserine as the second product of the reaction.

Cystine and Cysteine

Cystine, in the presence of cytochrome oxidase and cytochrome C, is easily reduced to cysteine. The reaction is reversible.[388,389]

$$\begin{array}{lll} CH_2\!-\!S\!-\!S\!-\!CH_2 & & CH_2\!-\!SH \\ | \qquad\qquad | & & | \\ CHNH_2 \quad CHNH_2 & \rightleftharpoons & 2CHNH_2 \\ | \qquad\qquad | & & | \\ COOH \quad COOH & & COOH \\ \text{Cystine} & & \text{Cysteine} \end{array}$$

It was first shown by Fromageot et al.[390] that animal tissues converted cysteine sulfur to H_2S. Subsequently Smythe[391] discovered that this reaction was accompanied by the production of ammonia and pyruvic acid. The conversion has been attributed to the action of an enzyme termed desulfurase and is thought to proceed by way of the intermediate aminoacrylic acid[392,393] (see [A] below).

The fact that the reaction previously described did not proceed rapidly enough to account for the disappearance of cysteine indicated that it was subject to other metabolic transformations. Cammarata and Cohen[225] have shown that in heart and liver preparations, cysteine transaminates with α-ketoglutaric acid to produce β-mercaptopyruvic acid. The latter compound is, according to Meister et al.,[394] rapidly converted by most animal tissues to pyruvic acid and sulfur.

$$\begin{array}{ccccccc} & & COOH & & COOH & & CH_2SH \\ & & | & & | & & | \\ CH_2SH & & CH_2 & & CH_2 & + & C{=}O \\ | & + & | & \rightarrow & | & & | \\ CHNH_2 & & CH_2 & & CH_2 & & COOH \\ | & & | & & | & & \\ COOH & & C{=}O & & CHNH_2 & & \\ & & | & & | & & \\ & & COOH & & COOH & & \\ \text{Cysteine} & & \alpha\text{-Ketoglutaric acid} & & \text{Glutamic acid} & & \end{array}$$

$$\begin{array}{ccccc} CH_2SH & & CH_3 & & \\ | & & | & & \\ C{=}O & \rightarrow & C{=}O & + & S \\ | & & | & & \\ COOH & & COOH & & \\ \beta\text{-mercaptopyruvic acid} & & \text{Pyruvic acid} & & \end{array}$$

Besides transamination and desulfuration, cysteine is subjected to oxidation. This mode of transformation was suggested by Pirie[395] in 1934, when he observed that inorganic sulfate was formed by liver slices incubated with cystine, cysteine or methionine. Pirie theorized that cysteinesulfenic and cysteinesulfinic acids were intermediates in the oxidative process. Support for this suggestion was obtained by Medes and Floyd[389,396] who found that inorganic sulfate was rapidly formed from cysteine sulfinate in cell-free liver preparation. The ease

---

[A]

$$\begin{array}{ccccc} CH\!-\!SH & & CH_2 & & CH_3 \\ | & & \| & & | \\ CHNH_2 & \xrightarrow[\text{Desulfurase}]{H_2S\nearrow} & CHNH_2 & \xrightarrow{H_2O} & C{=}O \;+ NH_3 \\ | & & | & & | \\ COOH & & COOH & & COOH \\ \text{Cysteine} & & \text{Aminoacrylic acid} & & \text{Pyruvic acid} \end{array}$$

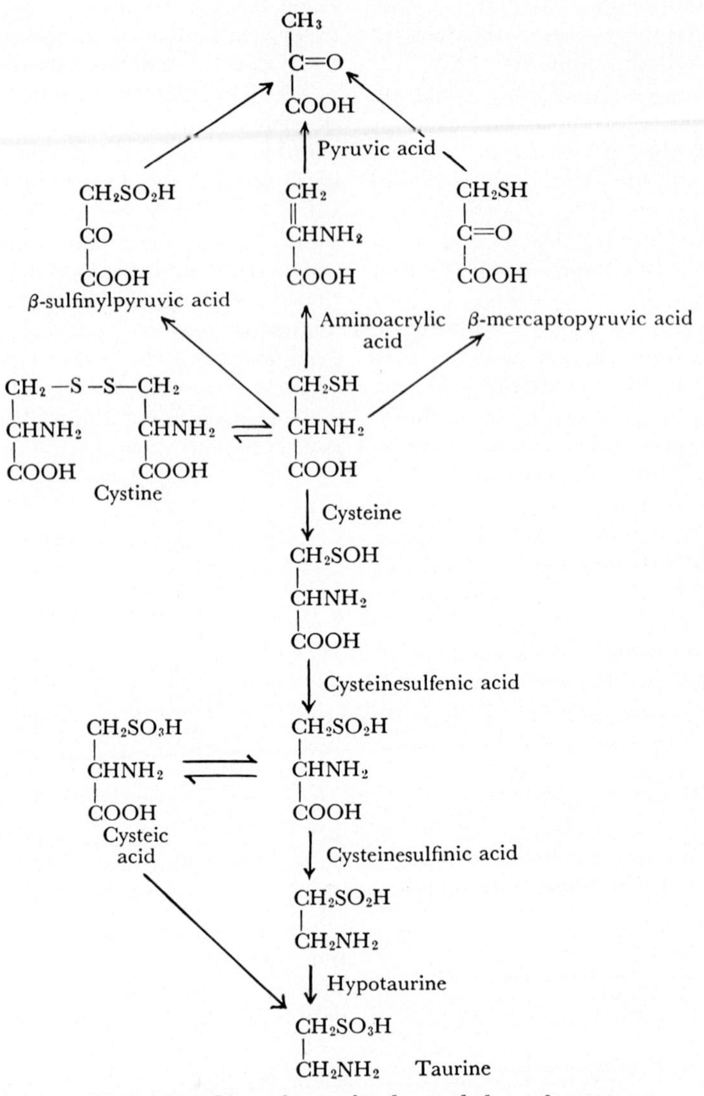

FIG. 7. Possible pathways for the catabolism of cysteine.

with which the liver preparations utilized this product suggested that it was a naturally occurring metabolite. Final proof that cysteine is converted to cysteinesulfinic acid in vivo was recently obtained by Chapeville and Fromageot,[397] who isolated the S^{35} labelled compound from rat tissue after the administration of S^{35} labelled cysteine to intact animals. Cysteinesulfinic acid can in turn suffer many fates. There is some evidence that it may be further oxidized to cysteic acid, but this appears to be an unimportant reaction.[398] Singer and Kearney[398] have shown that rat liver and beef heart preparation transaminate cysteinesulfinate with α-ketoglutarate and other keto acids to produce β-sulfinylpyruvate, which is rapidly cleaved to yield pyruvate and inorganic sulfate. This reaction has been shown to be reversible. Chapeville and Fromageot[399] found that they could recover S^{35} labelled cysteinesulfinic acid from kidney preparations which contained $S^{35}O_2$, pyruvic acid and glutamic acid.

Another important pathway in this array leads cysteinesulfinic acid through hypotaurine to taurine. Awapara and Wingo[400] reported in 1953 that cysteine injected into rats was converted to hypotaurine. Confirmation of this, with evidence of the decarboxylation of hypotaurine to taurine, has been obtained by Bergeret[401] and Cavallini et al.[402,403] A scheme summarizing the various metabolic pathways of cystine and cysteine is given in Figure 7.

Transmethylation

Methionine was discovered by Mueller[404] in 1922. In 1928 Barger and Coyne[405] showed it to be a methylated sulfur-containing amino acid. When Jackson and Block[374] in Mendel's laboratory at Yale University found in 1931 that supplements of methionine promoted the growth of animals on a diet low in cystine, doubts were raised that cystine was indeed an essential amino acid. Five years elapsed before Rose and his colleagues[375] supplied unequivocal evidence that methionine, and not cystine, is the essential sulfur-containing amino acid, but meanwhile a renewed interest had developed in sulfur compounds.

In 1932 Butz and du Vigneaud[406] discovered that hot, strong sulfuric acid converts methionine to a product giving a positive reaction like that of cystine with the reagent of Folin and Marenzi, and a year later du Vigneaud, Dyer and Harmon[407] established its structure as the disulfide form of the next higher homologue of cysteine. The metabolic importance of homocystine was indicated by the finding of Dyer and du Vigneaud[408] that both the D- and L-forms promoted the growth of rats fed a basic diet low in cystine. Several groups of workers including Brand, Cahill and Harris,[409] and Brand, Cahill and Block[378] had previously observed phenomena suggesting that methionine might be a metabolic precursor of homocystine (see [A] below). The conversion of dietary methionine to tissue cystine was finally proved in 1939 by Tarver and Schmidt.[376] They fed methionine labelled with S^{35} to a rat and subsequently isolated, from a hydrolysate of the fur and of the tissues, cystine containing radioactive sulfur.

Further studies on the conversion of methionine to cystine, and on the growth-promoting effects of homocystine on rats fed diets free from methionine and cystine, led to opposite results in the laboratories of Rose and of du Vigneaud. The rats given supplements of homocystine grew in Rose's laboratory, but in du Vigneaud's they lost weight and most of them died with fatty livers, which suggested a lack of choline in the diet.[410] The difference in results was traced to the use of 150 mg. milk-vitamin concentrate and 100 mg. tiki-tiki (rice bran extract) by Rose to supply the B vitamins, whereas du Vigneaud's colleagues used mainly crystalline vitamins with only 25 mg. of ryzamin B as a source of unrecognized factors. Choline was subsequently isolated from the crude sources of the vitamin B complex used in Rose's studies.

Proof that the amount of choline present in the crude vitamin supplement would promote growth in rats fed du Vigneaud's diet containing homocystine led to a new concept in biochemistry—transmethylation. Du Vigneaud and his colleagues suggested that the

---

[A]

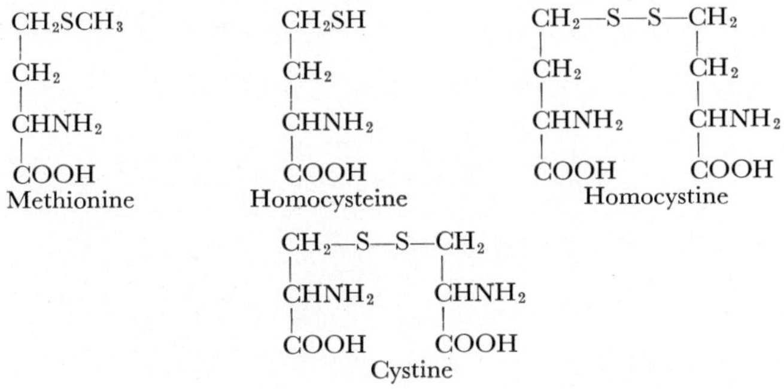

```
CH2SCH3          CH2SH            CH2—S—S—CH2
|                |                |        |
CH2              CH2              CH2      CH2
|                |                |        |
CHNH2            CHNH2            CHNH2    CHNH2
|                |                |        |
COOH             COOH             COOH     COOH
Methionine       Homocysteine        Homocystine

           CH2—S—S—CH2
           |        |
           CHNH2    CHNH2
           |        |
           COOH     COOH
              Cystine
```

rat is able to transfer methyl groups from choline to homocysteine to produce the essential amino acid, methionine (see [A] below). Betaine produced a similar growth response when added to a methyl-free synthetic diet containing homocystine in place of methionine. It was also found that rats would grow well without being fed any choline, provided sufficient methionine was in the diet. These observations could be accounted for by the hypothesis that the biologic transfer of methyl groups from choline or betaine to form methionine is reversible. This hypothesis provided an explanation for some of the observations that had been made by Best and his colleagues, by Tucker and Eckstein[411] and others that addition of choline, betaine or methionine to diets lacking these substances prevented the development of fatty livers. Homocystine is not lipotropic[412] but, as du Vigneaud has noted, this fact is not inconsistent with the hypothesis of transmethylation.

Du Vigneaud and his associates soon supplied experimental support for the new concept. Reduction of carbon monoxide with deuterium gas at high pressure, in the presence of a nickel catalyst, gave a methyl iodide in which the methyl group was labelled with heavy hydrogen. Synthetic methionine and choline made with this methylating agent contained deuteriomethyl groups that could be followed in the products of metabolism. Deuteriomethionine was fed to a rat at a dietary level of 1.4 per cent for three days. The animal was then killed; tissue choline was isolated and found to contain deuterium. In later experiments labelled methionine was fed for longer periods (three weeks in one case, ninety-four days in another). In other experiments deuteriocholine was fed. The biologic transfer of methyl groups from dietary choline or methionine to tissue choline, methionine and creatine was proved conclusively when, by chemical degradation of these metabolites, the deuterium was proved to be in the methyl groups.[413] This suggested the transfer of intact methyl groups. It was not until a few years later, however, when compounds containing doubly labelled methyl groups (i.e., with radioactive carbon and deuterium) became available, that direct proof was provided of the biologic transfer of intact methyl groups.[414] Dubnoff[415] and Muntz[416] have provided evidence that the methyl groups of choline are not labile until it has been oxidized by the enzyme choline oxidase to betaine (see [B] below).

[A]

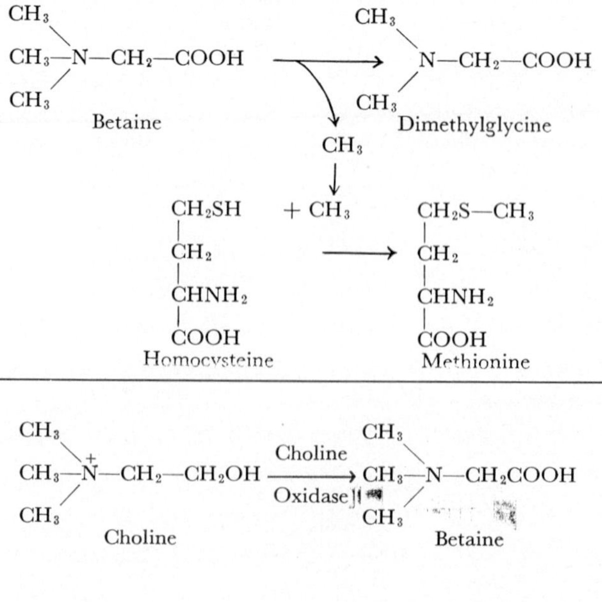

$$(CH_3)_3N\text{—}CH_2\text{—}COOH \text{ (Betaine)} \longrightarrow (CH_3)_2N\text{—}CH_2\text{—}COOH \text{ (Dimethylglycine)} + CH_3$$

$$\underset{\text{Homocysteine}}{HSCH_2\text{—}CH_2\text{—}CHNH_2\text{—}COOH} + CH_3 \longrightarrow \underset{\text{Methionine}}{CH_3\text{—}SCH_2\text{—}CH_2\text{—}CHNH_2\text{—}COOH}$$

[B]

$$\underset{\text{Choline}}{(CH_3)_3\overset{+}{N}\text{—}CH_2\text{—}CH_2OH} \xrightarrow[\text{Oxidase}]{\text{Choline}} \underset{\text{Betaine}}{(CH_3)_3N\text{—}CH_2COOH}$$

Borsook and Dubnoff[417] and Cantoni[418] have shown that the methionine methyl group is labile only after this substance has been converted to an active form by ATP, i.e., S-adenosylmethionine.

It was noted by du Vigneaud and associates[419] that occasionally an animal lost some weight and then began to grow slowly even though its choline-free diet contained homocystine in place of methionine. It will be recalled that the essential amino acid, methionine, can be synthesized from homocystine only when there is a source of labile methyl groups (choline) available. This unexpected growth on a diet lacking methyl compounds, which was also encountered by Toennies, Bennett and Medes,[420] gave rise to the speculation that the synthesis of choline or other methyl donors occurred in vivo, possibly through the action of the intestinal bacteria. To try to determine whether or not the biosynthesis of labile methyl groups does occur, du Vigneaud et al.[413] in 1945 injected D_2O into two rats fed a diet containing adequate protein (20 per cent casein) and vitamins. The deuterium content of the body water of the rats was maintained at about 3 atoms per cent for three weeks by providing D_2O in the drinking water. Tissue choline from these rats was isolated and degraded to trimethylamine. Evidence was obtained that a small but definite number of the methyl groups contained deuterium; thus, the biosynthesis of methyl groups had occurred. To determine whether the synthesis occurred in the animal body or by intestinal bacteria, the aid was sought of Professor Reyniers and his colony of germ-free rats at the Laboratory of Bacteriology, University of Notre Dame. Methyl groups were synthesized by the germ-free rats to about the same degree as in the animals reared under normal, nonsterile conditions.

Meanwhile, Welch and Sakami[421] circumvented the problem of bacterial synthesis of methyl groups by working with tissue slices in vitro. They not only in-

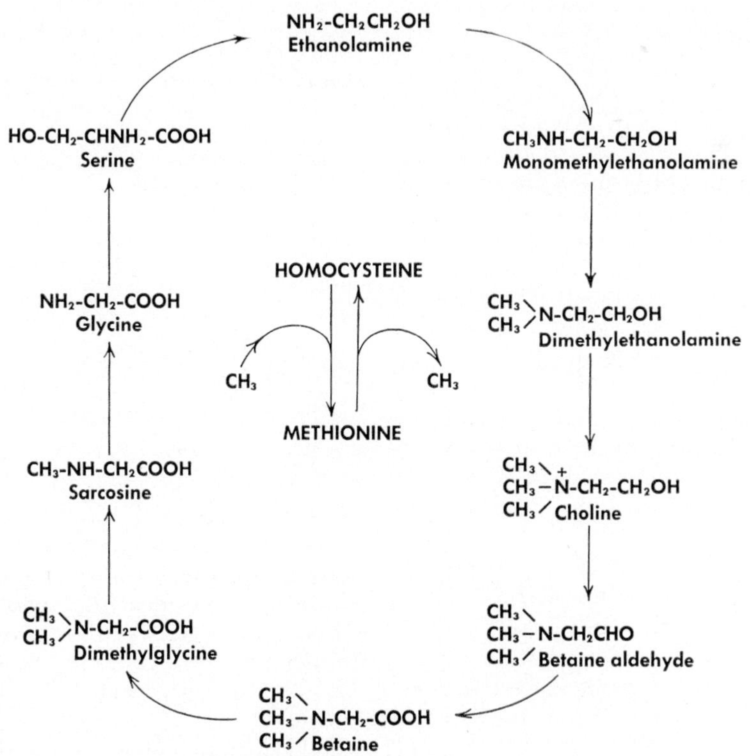

FIG. 8. Metabolic pathways in transmethylation.

jected formate labelled with C^{14} into rats, but also added it to rat liver slices. In both cases, methyl groups containing C^{14} were detected in the methionine and choline.

Although it had long been known that intact methyl groups are eliminated from the body in creatinine and creatine, it was not until 1947 that Mackenzie, du Vigneaud et al. provided evidence that the process of oxidative demethylation (which was generally assumed to occur) does actually take place. After methionine with C^{14} in the methyl group was given to a rat, expired carbon dioxide was found to be radioactive within one hour; the peak rate of excretion of radioactive carbon dioxide was at about 6 to 7 hours, but some radioactivity continued to appear in the expired air for some days. Other studies showed more than 12 to 33 per cent of the methyl groups of injected choline, betaine, dimethylthetin, and dimethyl-β-proprothetin are oxidized to carbon dioxide within 24 hours since these amounts were collected in the expired air.[422] The methyl groups of creatine and creatinine were not oxidized to any extent. The proof that biologically labile methyl groups give rise in the body of the rat to formaldehyde and formate[423] led to the suggestion that the term "one-carbon fragment" be used until the actual nature of the product of intermediate metabolism was established. Sakami[424] had shown that the carbon of labile methyl groups appeared in serine in the β-position, and earlier still, he had found that in the rat, glycine could be converted to serine by condensation with formate or some derivative of it.[425] In spite of many advances in the intervening years, the metabolism of the one-carbon fragment is not yet fully elucidated.

In 1949 three groups reported that vitamin B_{12} and folic acid were involved in the metabolism of labile methyl compounds. A large number of studies have established that vitamin B_{12} is not concerned in transmethylation, but isotope techniques have shown that it does aid in the synthesis de novo of methyl groups. Deficiency of folic acid does not reduce the transmethylation reaction (radiomethyl group from betaine into tissue methionine) in rats, mice or chicks,[426] but there is abundant evidence that folic acid is concerned in the metabolism of the one-carbon fragment. Whether by this we mean a hydroxymethyl group, formaldehyde, a formyl radical or a formate ion is less clear, although there is a growing body of evidence for the importance of the hydroxy-methyl group.

Further details of work on the synthesis and metabolic fate of biologically labile methyl groups, the so-called metabolism of the one-carbon fragment, has been reviewed by du Vigneaud.[427]

Glutamic Acid, Proline, Hydroxyproline and Ornithine

The interconversion of glutamic acid, proline, hydroxyproline and ornithine has long been suspected because of the structural similarities between these compounds.

```
CH2——CH2                  OH
|     |                   |
CH2   CH—COOH             CH——CH2
  \  /                    |   |
   N                      CH2  CH—COOH
   |                        \ /
   H                         N
                             |
                             H
    Proline               Hydroxyproline

   COOH                    CH2NH2
   |                       |
   CH2                     CH2
   |                       |
   CH2                     CH2
   |                       |
   CHNH2                   CHNH2
   |                       |
   COOH                    COOH
 Glutamic acid           Ornithine
```

Evidence for the conversion of proline to α-ketoglutaric acid by rat kidney slices was reported by Weil and Malherbe.[428] Neber[429] reported the isolation of glutamic acid from the media of tissue slices incubated with proline. Direct evidence for the formation of glutamate and of ornithine from proline was obtained by Stetten and Schoenheimer,[430] who isolated these doubly labelled compounds from rat tissues after feeding proline labelled with N^{15}

and deuterium. Stetten and Schoenheimer found in the same experiments that after feeding L Proline-N^{15}-D, hydroxyproline contained more of the isotope than any other amino acid with the exception of proline itself. It was assumed from these results that the conversion to hydroxproline was direct. It was also shown by Stetten and colleagues,[431,432] using both deutero-ornithine and N^{15} labelled ornithine that this compound could be transformed in vivo to glutamic acid, proline and hydroxyproline. Additional investigations carried out by Stetten[433] revealed that the proline-hydroxyproline conversion was irreversible and also that dietary hydroxyproline was not utilized for tissue synthesis. When labelled proline was fed, the tissue hydroxyproline was more heavily labelled than when the labelled hydroxyproline itself was administered. These results have led to the conclusion that most of the hydroxyproline in body tissues is formed from proline that is already bound, presumably in peptide linkages. The utilization of glutamic acid for the synthesis of proline and arginine has been demonstrated with the use of the C^{14} labelled material.

Although many compounds have been considered as possible intermediates of glutamic acid metabolism, relatively little is known about the transformations in mammalian tissues. Taggart and Krakaur[434] have found that rabbit kidney preparations are capable of rapidly oxidizing proline, hydroxyproline and glutamic acid. If the experimental conditions are adjusted, the utilization of proline results in the accumulation of a compound tentatively identified as glutamic semialdehyde. A proline oxidase preparation that converts L-proline to glutamic semialdehyde has been reported by Lang and Schmidt.[435] Spontaneous cyclization of the semialdehyde to a pyrroline carboxylic acid should

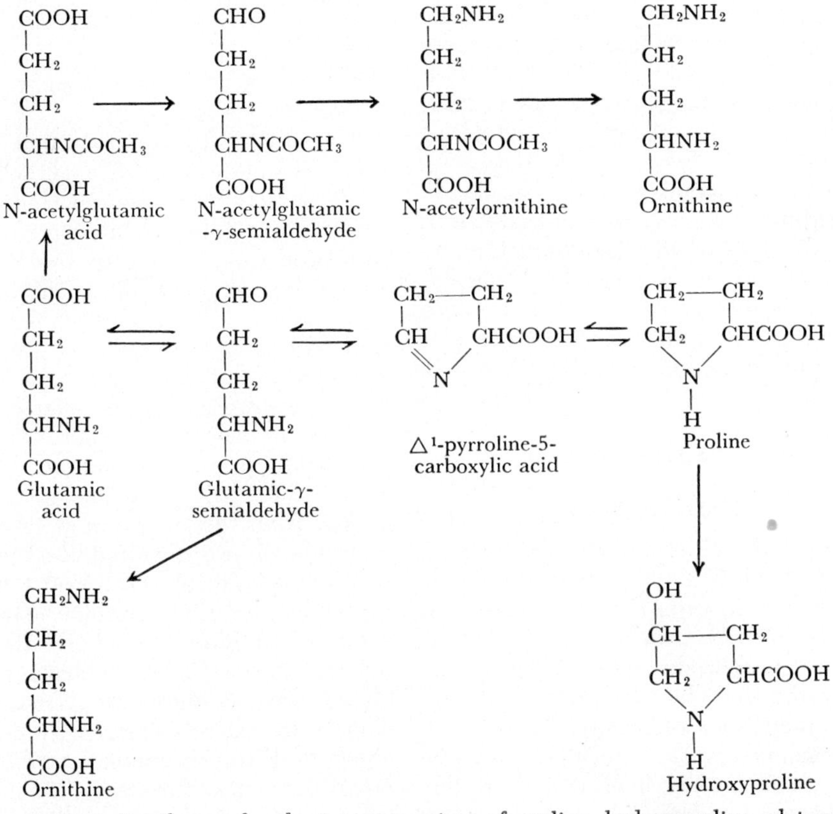

COOH–CH_2–CH_2–$CHNCOCH_3$–COOH (N-acetylglutamic acid) → CHO–CH_2–CH_2–$CHNCOCH_3$–COOH (N-acetylglutamic-γ-semialdehyde) → CH_2NH_2–CH_2–CH_2–$CHNCOCH_3$–COOH (N-acetylornithine) → CH_2NH_2–CH_2–CH_2–$CHNH_2$–COOH (Ornithine)

COOH–CH_2–CH_2–$CHNH_2$–COOH (Glutamic acid) ⇌ CHO–CH_2–CH_2–$CHNH_2$–COOH (Glutamic-γ-semialdehyde) ⇌ CH_2—CH_2, CH, CHCOOH, N (Δ¹-pyrroline-5-carboxylic acid) ⇌ CH_2—CH_2, CH_2, CHCOOH, N–H (Proline)

Glutamic acid → N-acetylglutamic acid

Glutamic-γ-semialdehyde → CH_2NH_2–CH_2–CH_2–$CHNH_2$–COOH (Ornithine)

Proline → OH–CH—CH_2, CH_2, CHCOOH, N–H (Hydroxyproline)

FIG. 9. Suggested pathways for the interconversions of proline, hydroxyproline, glutamic acid and ornithine.

proceed with ease. Reduction of this product would give rise to proline, while oxidation of the semialdehyde would produce glutamic acid. Such reactions have been shown by Vogel to account for the synthesis of proline by *E. coli* and by Neurospora. It has also been demonstrated by Vogel[436,437,438] that in *E. coli* the conversion of glutamate to ornithine proceeds by way of acetylated intermediates shown in Figure 9.

The enzymatic acetylation of glutamic acid by *E. coli* has been demonstrated by Maas et al.[439] According to Vogel,[440] a second enzyme acts in the presence of glutamate to catalyze the conversion of N-acetylglutamic-γ-semialdehyde to N-acetylornithine. The step from N-acetylornithine to ornithine is mediated by a third enzyme, acetylornithinase. However, the latter enzyme is absent from bacillus species and fungi, and ornithine degradation or synthesis is believed to proceed by transamination catalyzed by δ-transaminase.

The presence of ornithine transaminase in rat liver homogenates has been reported by Quastel and Witty.[228] It is apparent that the action of this enzyme would give rise directly to glutamic semialdehyde. The available data suggest the likelihood that the formation of ornithine in mammalian tissue proceeds by way of the transamination reaction, rather than through the acetylated intermediates found in *E. coli;* however, the validity of these speculations can be ascertained only by further studies.

END PRODUCTS

Urea Synthesis

Urea is the chief end product of protein metabolism in mammals. Although its presence in urine was discovered by Rouelle in 1773, over a century elapsed before von Schroder showed that it can be synthesized by the liver perfused with ammonium carbonate. Subsequent experimental work indicated that in higher animals the liver is indeed the only organ capable of manufacturing urea. In a now classic investigation, Bollman, Mann and Magath[441] found that following the removal of the liver from dogs, amino acids accumulated in the blood, while blood urea levels remained low and urea excretion diminished. It was also shown that the increase in blood urea that occurred in nephrectomized dogs ceased upon extirpation of the liver. Identical results were obtained with monkeys by Maddock and Svedberg.[442]

The earliest contribution to our present knowledge of urea synthesis was made by Kossel and Dakin,[443] who found that a tissue enzyme, arginase, hydrolyzed arginine to urea and ornithine in the manner shown below.

$$\underset{\text{Arginine}}{\begin{array}{l} NH_2 \\ | \\ C{=}NH \\ | \\ NH \\ | \\ (CH_2)_3 \\ | \\ CHNH_2 \\ | \\ COOH \end{array}} \xrightarrow[\text{Arginase}]{H_2O} \begin{array}{l} NH_2 \\ | \\ C{=}O \\ | \\ NH_2 \text{ Urea} \\ + \\ NH_2 \\ | \\ (CH_2)_3 \\ | \\ CHNH_2 \\ | \\ COOH \\ \text{Ornithine} \end{array}$$

The next and most important step in the elucidation of urea synthesis was made in 1932 by Krebs and Henseleit.[444] These investigators, while studying urea formation from carbon dioxide and ammonia by rat liver slices surviving in vitro, found that the addition of ornithine to the incubation fluid greatly accelerated the formation of urea. Very low concentrations were effective, and the amount of urea formed was out of proportion to the amount of ornithine added. Since the ornithine did not disappear from the system, and since each molecule of it stimulated the synthesis of 30 molecules of urea, it was inevitably concluded that ornithine acted as a catalyst. Krebs also found that the addition of either citrulline or arginine stimulated urea synthesis to a remarkable degree. In order to explain the catalytic effect of these compounds, Krebs proposed the series of reactions outlined below, which are known collectively as the "ornithine cycle." Although further research has greatly elaborated Krebs' ornithine cycle and also served to integrate it with other metabolic mechanisms, its basic form remains unaltered.

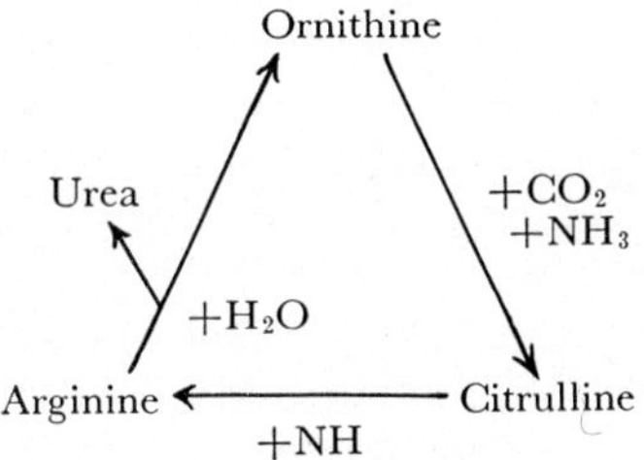

The elucidation of the details in the mechanism of urea synthesis was greatly facilitated by the development by Cohen and associates[445,446,447,448] of cell-free preparations of liver tissue that would synthesize urea, and the subsequent separation of the preparation into a mitochondrial fraction that carried out the conversion of ornithine to citrulline and a soluble protein fraction responsible for the transformation of citrulline to arginine. Cohen et al.[449,450,451] have shown that the fixation of carbon dioxide and ammonia occurs through the enzymatically mediated reaction of these substances with carbamylglutamate to form a compound of unknown structure termed "compound X."* A second enzyme then catalyzes the formation of citrulline from ornithine and compound X (see [A] below).

The steps involved in the formation of arginine from citrulline have become known chiefly through the work of Ratner, who has recently presented several excellent reviews of urea synthesis.[452,453] Ratner and associates[454,455,456,457] have shown that the conversion of citrulline to arginine occurs by two enzymatically mediated reactions. The first step in the sequence is the formation in the presence of ATP and magnesium ions of the intermediate argininosuccinic acid by the condensation of citrulline with aspartic acid. The intermediate is then split by a second enzyme to yield L-arginine and fumaric acid. The subsequent hydrolysis of arginine to urea and ornithine by the enzyme arginase completes the cycle (see [A] on page 56).

Creatine and Creatinine

The subject of creatine synthesis has been clarified largely through the work

* Recent data indicate that "Compound X" is carbamyl phosphate, $H_2N-\overset{O}{\overset{\|}{C}}-OPO_3$.[461,462,463]

[A]

$$\underset{\text{Carbamylglutamic acid}}{\begin{array}{l} COOH \\ | \\ CH_2 \\ | \\ CH_2 \\ | \\ CHNHCONH_2 \\ | \\ COOH \end{array}} + NH_3 + CO_2 \xrightarrow[Mg^{++}]{ATP} \underset{\text{Compound X*}}{\left[\begin{array}{l} COOH \\ | \\ CH_2 \\ | \\ CH_2 \\ | \\ CHNHCONH_2 \\ | \\ COOH \end{array} + NH_3 + CO_2 + P\right]}$$

$$\left[\begin{array}{l} COOH \\ | \\ CH_2 \\ | \\ CH_2 \\ | \\ CHNHCONH_2 \\ | \\ COOH \end{array} + NH_3 + CO_2 + P\right] + \underset{\text{Ornithine}}{\begin{array}{l} NH_2 \\ | \\ CH_2 \\ | \\ CH_2 \\ | \\ CH_2 \\ | \\ CHNH_2 \\ | \\ COOH \end{array}} \rightarrow \underset{\text{Citrulline}}{\begin{array}{l} NH_2 \\ | \\ CO \\ | \\ NH \\ | \\ CH_2 \\ | \\ CH_2 \\ | \\ CH_2 \\ | \\ CHNH_2 \\ | \\ COOH \end{array}} + \underset{\text{Carbamylglutamic acid}}{\begin{array}{l} COOH \\ | \\ CH_2 \\ | \\ CH_2 \\ | \\ CHNHCONH_2 \\ | \\ COOH \end{array}} + P$$

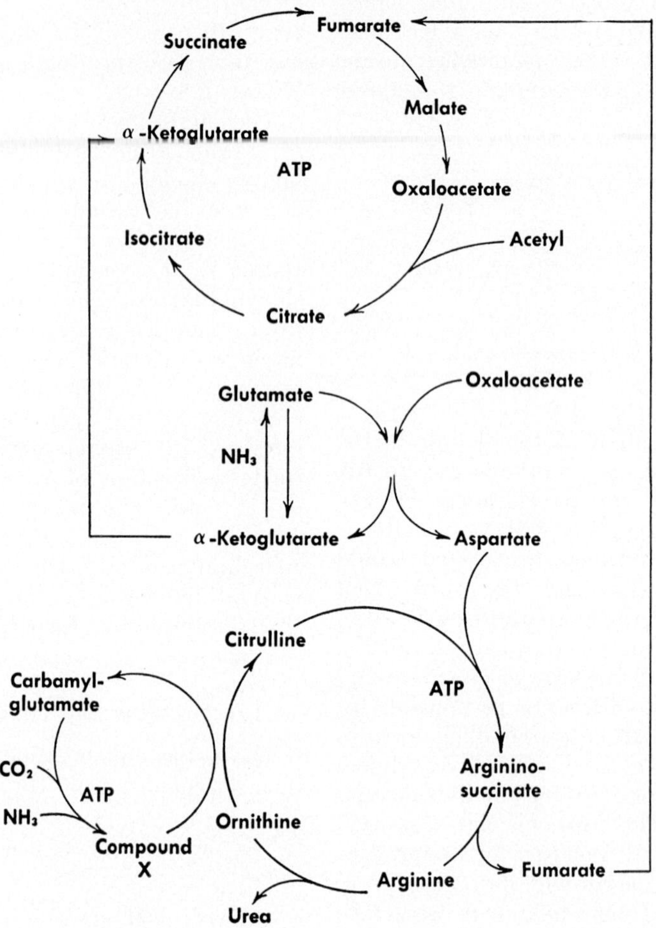

FIG. 10. Interrelationships between urea synthesis and the citric acid cycle.

of Bloch and Schoenheimer,[458,459] and of Borsook and Dubnoff.[417,460] The initial step in its formation takes place in the kidney, where arginine and glycine react through a process called transamidination to form the compound guanidinoacetic acid. This compound is then carried to the liver where it is transmethylated from methionine to creatine. Before creatine is excreted it is

---

A

Citrulline		Aspartic acid		Argininosuccinic acid			Arginine		Fumaric acid
NH_2				NH_2	COOH		NH_2		
CO		COOH		C=N—CH			C=NH		COOH
NH	+	$CHNH_2$	$\xrightarrow[Mg^{++}]{ATP}$	NH_2	CH_2	→	NH	+	CH
CH_2		CH_2		CH_2	COOH		CH_2		‖ CH
CH_2		COOH		CH_2			CH_2		COOH
CH_2				CH_2			CH_2		
$CHNH_2$				$CHNH_2$			$CHNH_2$		
COOH				COOH			COOH		

converted to its cyclic anhydride, creatinine.

$$\begin{array}{l} NH_2 \\ | \\ C{=}NH \\ | \\ NH \\ | \\ (CH_2)_3 \\ | \\ CHNH \\ | \\ COOH \end{array} + \begin{array}{l} NH_2 \\ | \\ CH_2 \\ | \\ COOH \end{array} \rightarrow \begin{array}{l} NH_2 \\ | \\ C{=}NH \\ | \\ NH \\ | \\ CH_2 \\ | \\ COOH \end{array} + \begin{array}{l} NH_2 \\ | \\ (CH_2)_3 \\ | \\ CHNH_2 \\ | \\ COOH \end{array}$$

Arginine — Glycine — Guanidino-acetic acid — Ornithine

$$\begin{array}{l} NH_2 \\ | \\ C{=}NH \\ | \\ NH \\ | \\ CH_2 \\ | \\ COOH \end{array} \xrightarrow{+CH_3} \begin{array}{l} NH_2 \\ | \\ C{=}NH \\ | \\ N{-}CH_3 \\ | \\ CH_2 \\ | \\ COOH \end{array} \xrightarrow{-H_2O} \begin{array}{l} NH{-}\!\!\!-\!\!\!-\!\!\!-\urcorner \\ | \qquad\quad | \\ C{=}NH \quad | \\ | \qquad\quad | \\ N{-}CH_3 \;\, | \\ | \qquad\quad | \\ CH_2{-}C{=}O \end{array}$$

Guanidino-acetic acid — Creatine — Creatinine

Creatine is excreted in the urine of children but disappears from the urine of the male at puberty. Adult women have intermittent creatinuria, which becomes continuous during pregnancy and is intensified for two or three weeks following parturition. Creatine is excreted by both sexes during starvation, carbohydrate deprivation, and very high protein intake. Creatinuria is also markedly intensified in disease states such as diabetes, fever, exophthalmic goiter, poliomyelitis, myasthenia gravis and progressive muscular atrophy. It appears that in most instances the increased excretion of this metabolite can be associated with the wasting away of body tissues. Since creatine phosphate plays an important physiologic role in the mechanism of muscular contraction, it cannot be considered an end or waste product of metabolism.

The amount of creatinine excreted daily by a given individual remains remarkably constant despite wide variations in activity and in food consumption. Variations between individuals range from 1.5 to 2.0 grams daily for men, and 0.8 to 1.5 grams for women. Because of the constancy of creatinine excretion, its determination during nitrogen balance studies with humans provides an excellent check on the thoroughness of the urine collection.

References

1. Verworn, M.: General Physiology. London, The Macmillan Co., 1899, p. 479.
2. Wollaston, W. H.: Trans. Roy. Soc., 223, 1810.
3. Proust: Ann. chim. phys., *10:*29, 1819.
4. Liebig, J.: Ann., *57:*127, 1846.
5. Vickery, H. B. and Schmidt, C. L. A.: Chem. Rev., *9:*169, 1931.
6. Sanger, F. and Thompson, E. O. P.: Biochem. J., *53:*353, 1953.
7. Sanger, F., Thompson, E. O. P. and Kitai, R.: Biochem. J., *59:*509, 1955.
8. Ryle, A. P., Sanger, F., Smith, L. F. and Kitai, R.: Biochem. J., *60:*541, 1955.
9. Brown, H., Sanger, F. and Kitai, R.: Biochem. J., *60:*556, 1955.
10. Bell, P. H.: J. Am. Chem. Soc., *76:*5565, 1954.
11. du Vigneaud, V., Lawler, H. C. and Popenoe, E. A.: J. Am. Chem. Soc., *75:*4880, 1953.
12. du Vigneaud, V. C., Ressler, C., Swan, J. M., Roberts, C. W. and Katsoyannis, P. G.: J. Am. Chem. Soc., *76:*3115, 1954.
13. Edsall, J. T.: J. Cell. & Comp. Physiol., *47:* Suppl. 1, 163, 1956.
14. Pauling, L., Corey, R. B. and Branson, H. R.: Proc. Nat. Acad. Sc., *37:*205, 1951.
15. Boussingault: Economie Rurale, Paris, 1851.
16. Osborne, T. B. and Clapp, S. H.: Am. J. Physiol. (B), *17:*231, 1906–07.
17. Beadles, J. R., Quisenberry, J. H., Nakamura, F. I. and Mitchell, H. H.: J. Agric. Res., *47:*947, 1933.
18. Allison, J. B.: Physiol. Rev., *35:*664, 1955.
19. Frost, D. V. and Sandy, H. R.: Proc Soc. Exper. Biol. & Med., *68:*51, 1948.
20. Peters, J. P., in Steiglitz, E. V., ed.: Geriatric Medicine. Philadelphia, W. B. Saunders Co., 1943, Ch. 41.
21. Mitchell, H. H.: Bull. Nat. Res. Council, Part I, No. 55, p. 21, 1926.
22. Smith, M.: J. Biol. Chem., *68:*15, 1926.
23. Mitchell, H. H. and Beadles, J. R.: J. Nutrition, *14:*597, 1937.
24. Mendel, L. B. and Fine, M. S.: J. Biol Chem., *11:*1, 1912.
25. Mitchell, H. H. and Beadles, J. R.: J. Biol. Chem., *105:*537, 1934.
26. Willcock, E. G. and Hopkins, F. G.: J. Physiol., *35:*88, 1906–07.
27. Abderhalden, E.: Ztschr. f. physiol. Chem., *96:*1, 1915.
28. Ackroyd, H. and Hopkins, F. G.: Biochem. J., *10:*551, 1916.
29. Rose, W. C. and Cox, G. J.: J. Biol. Chem., *61:*747, 1924.

30. Rose, W. C. and Cox, G. J.: J. Biol. Chem., *68:*217, 1926.
31. Scull, C. W. and Rose, W. C.: J. Biol. Chem., *89:*109, 1930.
32. Wolf, P. A. and Corley, R. C.: Am. J. Physiol., *127:*589, 1939.
33. McCoy, R. H., Meyer, C. E. and Rose, W. C.: J. Biol. Chem., *112:*283, 1935–36.
34. Meyer, C. E. and Rose, W. C.: J. Biol. Chem., *115:*721, 1936.
35. Rose, W. C. and Rice, E. E.: Science, *90:*186, 1939.
36. Almquist, H. J.: Fed. Proc., *1:*269, 1942.
37. Holt, L. E., Jr., Albanese, A. A., Brumback, J. E., Jr., Kajdi, C. and Wangerin, D. M.: Proc. Soc. Exper. Biol. & Med., *48:*726, 1941.
38. Rose, W. C., Haines, W. J. and Johnson, J. E.: J. Biol. Chem., *146:*683, 1942.
39. Rose, W. C., Haines, W. J. and Warner, D. T.: J. Biol. Chem., *148:*457, 1943.
40. Rose, W. C.: Fed. Proc., *8:*546, 1949.
41. Rose, W. C., Lambert, G. F. and Coon, M. J.: J. Biol. Chem., *211:*815, 1954.
42. Rose, W. C., Wixom, R. L., Lockhart, H. B. and Lambert, G. F.: J. Biol. Chem., *217:*987, 1955.
43. Elman, R.: Proc. Soc. Exper. Biol. & Med., *40:*489, 1939.
44. Cannon, P. R., Steffee, C. H., Frazier, L. J., Rowley, D. A. and Stepto, R. C.: Fed. Proc. *6:*390, 1947.
45. Geiger, E. and Geiger, L. E.: J. Nutrition, *36:*813, 1948.
46. Henderson, R. and Harris, R. S.: Fed. Proc., *8:*385, 1949.
47. Rose, W. C., Oesterling, M. J. and Womack, M.: J. Biol. Chem., *176:*753, 1948.
48. Frost, D. V. and Sandy, H. R.: J. Biol. Chem., *189:*249, 1951.
49. Lardy, H. A. and Feldott, G.: J. Biol. Chem., *179:*509, 1949.
50. Rose, W. C., Smith, L. C., Womack, M. and Shane, M.: J. Biol. Chem., *181:*307, 1949.
51. Allison, J. B., Anderson, J. A. and White, J. I.: Tr. Am. A. Cereal Chemists, *7:*24, 1949.
52. Klik, M. C.: J. Agr. Food Chem., *3:*600, 1955.
53. Clandinin, D. R. and Robblee, A. R.: J. Nutrition, *46:*525, 1952.
54. Eldred, N. R. and Rodney, G.: J. Biol. Chem., *162:*261, 1946.
55. Bosshardt, D. K., Ydse, L. C., Ayres, M. M. and Barnes, R. H.: J. Nutrition, *31:*23, 1946.
56. Sure, B., Easterling, L., Dowell, J. and Crudup, M.: J. Agr. Food. Chem., *1:*1207, 1953.
57. Nutrition Rev., *13:*272, 1955.
58. Flodin, N. W.: J. Agr. Food Chem., *1:*222, 1953.
59. Flodin, N. W.: Cereal Sc. Today, *1:*165, 1956.
60. Sure, B.: J. Agr. Food Chem., *2:*1111, 1954.
61. Pecora, L. J. and Hundley, J. M.: J. Nutrition, *44:*101, 1951.
62. Elvehjem, C. A.: Fed. Proc., *15:*965, 1956.
63. Harper, A. E.: Nutrition Rev., *14:*225, 1956.
64. Winje, M. E., Harper, A. E., Benton, D. A., Boldt, R. E. and Elvehjem, C. A.: J. Nutrition, *54:*155, 1954.
65. Lusk, G.: Ztschr. f. Biol., *27:*459, 1890.
66. Miura, K.: Beitr. z. Lehre v. Stoffwechsel d. ges. u. Krank. Menschen, *1:*1, 1892.
67. Neumann, R. O.: Arch. f. Hyg., *36:*1, 1890.
68. Rosemann, R.: Arch. f. ges. Physiol., *86:*307, 1901.
69. Jansen, W. H.: Deutsche Arch. f. klin. Med., *124:*1, 1917.
70. Zuntz, N. and Lowey, A.: Biochem. Ztschr., *90:*244, 1918.
71. Allison, J. B., Anderson, J. A. and Seeley, R. D.: Ann. New York Acad. Sc., *17:*245, 1946.
72. Cuthbertson, D. P. and Munro, H. N.: Biochem. J., *31:*694, 1937.
73. Munro, H. N.: Physiol. Rev., *31:*449, 1951.
74. Larson, P. S. and Chaikoff, I. L.: J. Nutrition, *13:*287, 1937.
75. National Research Council, Report of Food and Nutrition Board: Pub. 302, 1953.
76. Murlin, J. R.: Harvey Lectures, *12:*203, 1916.
77. National Research Council: Bull. 123, 1950.
78. Hoffstrom, K. A.: Skandinav. Arch. f. Physiol., *23:*326, 1910.
79. Wilson, K. M.: Bull. Johns Hopkins Hosp., *27:*121, 1916.
80. Seegers, W. H.: Am. J. Obst. & Gynec., *34:*1019, 1937.
81. Nelson, M. M. and Evans, H. M.: J. Nutrition, *51:*71, 1953.
82. Tompkins, W. H.: Clinical Obstetrics. Philadelphia, J. B. Lippincott Co., 1953, Ch. 9.
83. Burke, B. S. and Stuart, H. C.: J. A. M. A., *137:*118, 1948.
84. Leverton, R. M. and McMillan, T. J.: J. A. M. A., *130:*134, 1946.
85. Burke, B. S., Harding, V. V. and Stuart, H. C.: J. Pediat., *23:*506, 1943.
86. Lund, C. J.: J. A. M. A., *128:*344, 1945.
87. Turner, D. F.: J. A. M. A., *128:*590, 1945.
88. Youmans, J. B.: J. A. M. A., *128:*439, 1945.
89. Kestner, O.: Ztschr. f. physiol. Chem., *130:*208, 1923.
90. Wilson, D. W., Long, W. L., Thompson, H. C. and Thurlow, S.: J. Biol. Chem., *65:*755, 1925.

91. Shaffer, P. A.: Am. J. Physiol., *22:*445, 1908.
92. Cuthbertson, D. P., McGirr, J. L. and Munro, H. N.: Biochem. J., *31:*2293, 1937.
93. Browne, J. S. L., Hoffman, H. M., Schenker, V., Venning, E. H. and Weil, P.: Conference on Metabolic Aspects of Convalescence, Ninth Meeting, Josiah Macy, Jr., Foundation, p. 15.
94. Pollack, H. and Halpern, S. L.: Advances in Protein Chemistry, *6:*383, 1951.
95. Lynch, H. D. and Snively, W. D., Jr.: J. A. M. A., *147:*115, 1951.
96. Rose, W. C., Coon, M. J. and Lambert, G. F.: J. Biol. Chem., *210:*331, 1954.
97. Baker, L. E.: J. Biol. Chem., *193:*809, 1951.
98. Berridge, N. J.: Advances in Enzymology, *15:*423, 1954.
99. Hofmann, K. and Bergmann, M.: J. Biol. Chem., *138:*243, 1941.
100. Spackman, D. H., Smith, E. L. and Brown, D. M.: J. Biol. Chem., *212:*255, 1955.
101. Fridhandler, L. and Quastel, J. H.: Arch. Biochem., *56:*424, 1955.
102. Wiseman, G.: J. Physiol. (London), *120:*63, 1953.
103. Agar, W. T., Hird, F. J. R. and Sidhu, G. S.: Biochim. et biophys. acta, *14:*80, 1954.
104. Shishova, O. A.: Chem. Abstr., *49:*11843i, 1955.
105. London, E. S. and Kotchneva, N. P.: Arch. d. sc. biol. (USSR), *37:*3, 1935.
106. Mellander, O.: Acta Soc. med. upsalien, *52:*107, 1947.
107. Mellander, O.: Nutrition Rev., *13:*161, 1955.
108. Gruskay, F. L. and Cooke, R. E.: Pediatrics, *16:*763, 1955.
109. Rubner, M.: Arch. f. Anat. u. Physiol., physiol. Abt., *61* and *67:*1911.
110. Voit, C.: Ztschr. f. Biol., *2:*307, 1866.
111. Voit, C.: Hermann's Handbuch der Physiologie. Vol. 1, Physiologie des allgemienen Stoffwechsels. F. C. W. Vogel, Liepzig.
112. Addis, T., Poo, L. J. and Lew, W.: J. Biol. Chem., *115:*111, 1936.
113. Addis, T., Poo, L. J. and Lew, W.: J. Biol. Chem., *115:*117, 1936.
114. Luck, J. M.: J. Biol. Chem., *115:*491, 1936.
115. Madden, S. C. and Whipple, G. H.: Physiol. Rev., *20:*194, 1940.
116. Turkel, E. and Wachstein, M.: Klin. Wochschr., *15:*1435, 1936.
117. Mann, F. C., Wilhelmj, C. M. and Bollman, J. L.: Am. J. Physiol., *81:*496, 1927.
118. Lundsgaard, E.: Acta physiol. Scandinav., *4:*330, 1942.
119. Sadhu, D. P. and Brody, S.: Am. J. Physiol., *151:*130, 1947.
120. Evans, H. M., Luck, M. J., Pencharz, R. I. and Stoner, H. C.: Am. J. Physiol., *122:*533, 1938.
121. Gaebler, O. H.: J. Biol. Chem., *81:*41, 1929.
122. Abelin, I. and Goldstein, M.: Biochem. Ztschr., *327:*72, 1955.
123. Keeton, R. W., Lambert, E. H., Glickman, N., Mitchell, H. H., Last, J. H. and Fahnestock, M. K.: Am. J. Physiol., *146:*66, 1946.
124. Borsook, H. and Keighley, G.: Proc. Roy. Soc. (London), s. B., *118:*488, 1935.
125. Schoenheimer, R.: The Dynamic State of Body Constituents. Cambridge, Mass., Harvard University Press, 1942.
126. Schoenheimer, R., Ratner, S. and Rittenberg, D.: J. Biol. Chem., *130:*703, 1939.
127. Shemin, D. and Rittenberg, D.: J. Biol. Chem., *153:*401, 1944.
128. Hogness, D. S., Cohn, M. and Monod, J.: Biochim. et biophys. acta. *16:*99, 1955.
129. Cohn, M.: Enzymes: Units of Biological Structure and Function. Ed. by O. Gaebler. New York, Academic Press, Inc., 1956, p. 96.
130. Halvorson, H. O., Fry, W. and Schwemmin, D.: J. Gen. Physiol., *38:*549, 1955.
131. Halvorson, H. O. and Spiegelman, S.: J. Bact., *65:*496, 1953.
132. Halvorson, H. O. and Jackson, L.: Bacteriol. Proc., p. 125, 1955.
133. Velick, S. F.: Enzymes: Units of Biological Structure and Function. Ed. by O. Gaebler. New York, Academic Press, Inc., 1956, p. 90.
134. Gale, E. F. and Folkes, J. P.: Biochem. J., *59:*661, 1955.
135. Gale, E. F.: Symposium on Amino Acid Metabolism. Ed. by D. McElroy and B. Glass. Baltimore, Johns Hopkins Press, p. 171, 1955.
136. Zamecnik, P. C., Keller, E. B., Littlefield, J. W., Hoagland, M. B. and Loftfield, R. B.: J. Cell. & Comp. Physiol., *47:* Suppl. 1, 81, 1956.
137. Rabinovitz, M., Olson, M. E. and Greenberg, D. M.: J. Am. Chem. Soc., *77:*3109, 1955.
138. Borsook, H.: Chemical Pathways of Metabolism. Ed. by D. Greenberg. New York, Academic Press, Inc., *2:* 211, 1954.
139. Borsook, H.: J. Cell. & Comp. Physiol., *47:* Suppl. 1, 35, 1956.
140. Pardee, A. B.: Proc. Nat. Acad. Sc., *40:*263, 1954.
141. Spiegelman, S. H., Halvorson, O. and Ben-Ishai, R.: Symposium on Amino Acid Metabolism. Ed. by W. D. McElroy and B. Glass. Baltimore, Johns Hopkins Press, p. 124, 1955.
142. Kerr, W. J., Hurwitz, S. H. and Whipple, G. H.: Am. J. Physiol., *47;*356, 1918.

143. Whipple, G. H.: Hemoglobin, Plasma Protein and Cell Protein. Springfield, Ill., Charles C Thomas, 1948.
144. Melnick, D., Cowgill, G. R. and Burack, E.: J. Exper. Med., *64*:877, 1936.
145. Seeley, R. D.: Am. J. Physiol., *144*:369, 1945.
146. Weech, A. A., Gottsch, E. and Reeves, E. B.: J. Exper. Med., *61*:299, 1935.
147. Weech, A. A. and Gottsch, E.: Bull. Johns Hopkins Hosp., *53*:154, 1938.
148. Chow, B. F.: Ann. New York Acad. Sc., *47*:297, 1946.
149. Young, E. C. and Webber, R. V.: Canad. J. M. Sc., *31*:45, 1953.
150. Knutti, R. E., Erickson, C. C., Madden, S. C., Reckers, P. E. and Whipple, G. H.: J. Exper. Med., *65*:455, 1937.
151. Miller, L. L., Bly, D. G., Watson, M. L. and Bale, W. F.: J. Exper. Med., *94*:431, 1951.
152. White, A. and Dougherty, T. F.: Endocrinology, *36*:207, 1945.
153. Yuile, C. L., Lamson, B. G., Miller, L. L. and Whipple, G. H.: J. Exper. Med., *93*:539, 1951.
154. Babson, A. L. and Winnick, T.: Cancer Research, *14*:606, 1954.
155. Gavrilova, K. I.: Chem. Abstr., *49*:9799e, 1955.
156. Li, C. H., Evans, H. M. and Simpson, M. E.: J. Biol. Chem., *159*:353, 1945.
157. Barret, H. M., Best, C. H. and Ridout, J. H.: J. Physiol., *93*:367, 1938.
158. Stetten, D., Jr., and Salcedo, J.: J. Biol. Chem., *156*:27, 1944.
159. Reid, E.: J. Endocrinol., *9*:210, 1953.
160. Reid, E.: J. Endocrinol., *9*:323 and 329, 1953.
161. Greenbaum, A. L.: Biochem. J., *54*:400, 1953.
162. Greenbaum, A. L. and McLean, P.: Biochem. J., *54*:407 and 413, 1953.
163. Allan, F. N.: Am. J. Physiol., *67*:275, 1924.
164. Janney, N. W. and Shapiro, I.: Arch. Int. Med., *38*:96, 1926.
165. Daniels, A. C. and Luck, J. M.: J. Biol. Chem., *77*:151, 1928.
166. Mirsky, I. A., Swadesh, S. and Ransohoff, J.: Proc. Soc. Exper. Biol. & Med., *37*:223, 1937.
167. Mirsky, I. A.: Am. J. Physiol., *124*:569, 1938.
168. Russell, J. A. and Capiello, M.: Endocrinology, *44*:127, 1949.
169. Lotspeich, W. D.: J. Biol. Chem., *185*:22, 1950.
170. Hoberman, H. D.: Yale J. Biol. & Med., *22*:341, 1950.
171. Forker, L. L., Chaikoff, I. L., Entenman, C. and Tarver, H.: J. Biol. Chem., *188*:37, 1951.
172. Sinex, F. M., MacMullen, J. and Hastings, A. B.: J. Biol. Chem., *198*:615, 1952.
173. Krahl, M. E.: J. Biol. Chem., *200*:99, 1953.
174. Bollman, J. L., Flock, E. V., Grindlay, J. H., Mann, F. C. and Block, M. A.: Am. J. Physiol., *174*:467, 1953.
175. Salter, J. M. and Best, C. H.: Brit. M. J., *2*:353, 1953.
176. Lawrence, R. T. B., Salter, J. M. and Best, C. H.: Brit. M. J., *2*:437, 1954.
177. Salter, J. M., Davidson, I. W. F. and Best, C. H.: Canad. J. Biochem. & Physiol. In press.
178. Leslie, I. and Paul, J.: J. Endocrinol., *11*:110, 1954.
179. Fell, H. B.: International Symposium, Hypophyseal Growth Hormone, Nature and Actions. New York, Blakiston Div., McGraw-Hill, 1955.
180. Cotes, P. M., Reid, E. and Young, F. G.: Nature, *164*:209, 1949.
181. Campbell, J., Davidson, I. W. F., Snair, W. D. and Lei, H. P.: Endocrinology, *46*:273, 1950.
182. Milman, A. E., DeMoor, P. and Lukens, F. D. W.: Am. J. Physiol., *166*:354, 1951.
183. Randle, P. J. and Young, F. G.: J. Endocrinol., *13*:335, 1956.
184. Randle, P. J.: Lancet, *1*:441, 1954.
185. Randle, P. J.: Lancet, *1*:809, 1954.
186. Wilkins, L., Fleischmann, W. and Howard, J. E.: Bull. Johns Hopkins Hosp., *69*:493, 1941.
187. Kenyon, A. T.: Endocrinology, *23*:121, 1938.
188. McCullagh, E. P. and Rossmiller, H. R.: J. Clin. Endocrinol., *1*:507, 1941.
189. Kochakian, C. D.: Vitamins and Hormones, *4*:256, 1946.
190. Kochakian, C. D.: Conference on Metabolic Aspects of Convalescence Including Bone and Wound Healing. New York, Josiah Macy, Jr., Foundation, 1943, p. 125.
191. Simpson, M. E., Marx, W., Becks, H. and Evans, H. M.: Endocrinology, *35*:309, 1944.
192. Reifenstein, E. C., Jr.: The Protein Anabolic Activity of Steroid Compounds. New York, Josiah Macy, Jr., Foundation, 1942.
193. Reece, R. P. and Leonard, S. L.: Proc. Soc. Exper. Biol. & Med., *42*:200, 1939.
194. Evans, H. M., Simpson, M. E. and Pencharz, R. I.: Endocrinology, *25*:175, 1934.
195. Eartly, H. and Leblond, C. P.: Endocrinology, *45*:455, 1949.
196. Collip, J. B., Selye, H. and Thomson, D. L.: Virchows Arch. f. path Anat., *290*:23, 1933.
197. Scow, R. O.: Endocrinology, *55*:344, 1954.
198. Geschwind, I. I. and Li, C. H.: J. Clin. Endocrinol., *12*:937, 1953.

199. Smith, P. E., Greenwood, C. F. and Foster, G. L.: Am. J. Path., *3:*669, 1927.
200. Smith, P. E.: Proc. Soc. Exper. Biol. & Med., *30:*1252, 1933.
201. Wells, B. B. and Kendall, E. C.: Proc. Staff Meet. Mayo Clin., *15:*565, 1940.
202. Salter, J. M.: Unpublished data.
203. Long, C. N. H., Katzin, B. and Fry, E.: Endocrinology, *26:*309, 1940.
204. Hoberman, H. D.: Yale J. Biol. & Med., *22:*341, 1950.
205. Russell, J. A.: Fed. Proc., *14:*696, 1955.
206. Ingle, D. J.: Recent Progress in Hormone Research, *7:*375, 1952.
207. Evans, H. M., Simpson, M. E. and Li, C. H.: Endocrinology, *33:*237, 1943.
208. Clark, I.: J. Biol. Chem., *200:*69, 1953.
209. Roberts, S.: J. Biol. Chem., *200:*77, 1953.
210. Murlin, J. R., Clough, H. D., Gibbs, C. B. F. and Stokes, A. M.: J. Biol. Chem., *56:*253, 1923.
211. Staub, A., Sinn, L. and Behrens, O. K.: Science, *117:*628, 1953.
212. Sutherland, E. W. and Cori, C. F.: J. Biol. Chem., *188:*531, 1951.
213. Sutherland, E. W. and Wosilait, W. D.: J. Biol. Chem., *218:*459, 1956.
214. Sutherland, E. W. and Wosilait, W. D.: J. Biol. Chem., *218:*469, 1956.
215. Tyberghein, J.: Arch. internat. de physiol., *61:*104, 1953.
216. Salter, J. M., Davidson, I. W. F. and Best, C. H.: Diabetes, *6:*248, 1957.
217. Neubauer, O.: Deut. Arch. klin. Med., *95:*211, 1909.
218. Knoop, F.: Ztschr. f. physiol. Chem., *67:*489, 1910.
219. Krebs, H. A.: Biochem. J., *29:*1620, 1935.
220. Blanchard, M., Green, D. E., Nocito, V. and Ratner, S.: J. Biol. Chem., *155:*421, 1944.
221. Braunstein, A. E. and Kritsmann, M. G.: Enzymologia, *2:*129, 1937.
222. Cohen, P. P.: Biochem. J., *33:*1478, 1939.
223. Cohen, P. P. and Hekhius, G. L.: J. Biol. Chem., *140:*711, 1941.
224. Meister, A. and Tice, S. V.: J. Biol. Chem., *187:*173, 1950.
225. Cammarata, P. S. and Cohen, P. P.: J. Biol. Chem., *187:*439, 1950.
226. Feldman, L. I. and Gunsalus, I. C.: J. Biol. Chem., *187:*821, 1950.
227. Hird, F. J. R. and Rowsell, E. V.: Nature, *166:*517, 1950.
228. Quastel, J. H. and Witty, R.: Nature, *167:*556, 1951.
229. Meister, A.: J. Biol. Chem., *206:*587, 1954.
230. Sallach, H. J.: Symposium on Amino Acid Metabolism. Ed. by W. D. McElroy and B. Glass. Baltimore, Johns Hopkins Press, 1955, p. 782.
231. Snell, E. E.: J. Biol. Chem., *154:*313, 1944.
232. Snell, E. E.: J. Am. Chem. Soc., *67:*194, 1945.
233. Ames, S. R., Sarma, P. S. and Elvehjem, C. A.: J. Biol. Chem., *167:*135, 1947.
234. Meister, A., Morris, H. P. and Tice, S. V.: Proc. Soc. Exper. Biol. & Med., *82:*301, 1953.
235. Lichstein, H. C., Gunsalus, I. C. and Umbreit, W. W.: J. Biol. Chem., *161:*311, 1945.
236. Meister, A., Sober, H. A. and Peterson, E.: J. Biol. Chem., *206:*89, 1954.
237. Meister, A.: Symposium on Amino Acid Metabolism. Ed. by W. D. McElroy and B. Glass. Baltimore, Johns Hopkins Press, 1955, p. 3.
238. LaDue, J. S. and Wroblewski, F.: Circulation, *11:*871, 1955.
239. Rudolph, L. A. and Lyons, R. H.: Clin. Research Proc., *III(2):*113, 1955.
240. Steinberg, D. and Ostrow, B. H.: Proc. Soc. Exper. Biol. & Med., *89:*31, 1955.
241. Quick, A. J.: J. Biol. Chem., *92:*65, 193.
242. Swanson, W. W.: J. Biol. Chem., *62:*565, 1924–25.
243. Ratner, S., Nocito, V. and Green, D. E.: J. Biol. Chem., *152:*119, 1954.
244. Weinhouse, S. and Friedmann, B.: J. Biol. Chem., *191:*707, 1951.
245. Chao, F. C., Delwiche, C. C. and Greenberg, D. M.: Biochim. et biophys. acta, *10:*103, 1953.
246. Shemin, D.: J. Biol. Chem., *162:*297, 1946.
247. Siekevitz, P. and Greenberg, D. M.: J. Biol. Chem., *180:*845, 1949.
248. Gordon, W. G. and Jackson, R. W.: J. Biol. Chem., *110:*151, 1935.
249. Handler, P., Bernheim, F. and Klein, J. R.: J. Biol. Chem., *138:*211, 1941.
250. Shemin, D. and Rittenberg, D.: J. Biol. Chem., *159:*67, 1945.
251. Shemin, D.: Currents in Biochemical Research. Ed. by D. E. Green. New York, Interscience Publishers, Inc., 1956, p. 518.
252. Shemin, D. and Wittenberg, J.: J. Biol. Chem., *192:*315, 1951.
253. Shemin, D. and Kumin, S.: J. Biol. Chem., *198:*827, 1952.
254. Shemin, D., London, I. M. and Rittenberg, D.: J. Biol. Chem., *173:*799, 1948.
255. Shemin, D., London, I. M. and Rittenberg, D.: J. Biol. Chem., *183:*587, 1950.
256. Shemin, D. and Russell, C. S.: J. Am. Chem. Soc., *75:*4873, 1953.
257. Shemin, D. and Abramsky, T.: J. Biol. Chem., *215:*613, 1955.
258. Chargoff, E. and Sprinson, D. B.: J. Biol. Chem., *151:*273, 1943.
259. Stetten, D., Jr.: J. Biol. Chem., *140:*143, 1941.
260. Greenberg, D. M. and Harris, S. C.: Proc. Soc. Exper. Biol. & Med., *75:*683, 1950.

261. Levine, M. and Tarver, H.: J. Biol. Chem., *184:*427, 1950.
262. Elliot, D. F. and Neuberger, A.: Biochem. J., *46:*207, 1950.
263. Braunstein, A. E. and Valenkina, G. Y.: Doklady Akad. Nauk. S.S.S.R., *66:*243, 1949.
264. Metzler, H. L. and Sprinson, D. B.: J. Biol. Chem., *197:*461, 1952.
265. Lien, W. G., Jr., and Greenberg, D. M.: J. Biol. Chem., *151:*273, 1943.
266. Lien, W. G., Jr., and Greenberg, D. M.: J. Biol. Chem., *200:*367, 1953.
267. Gortner, R. A.: Outlines of Biochemistry. 2nd ed. New York, John Wiley & Sons, Inc., 1946.
268. Ringer, A. I.: J. Biol. Chem., *14:*539, 1913.
269. Borsook, H., Deasy, C. L., Haagen-Smit, A. J., Keighley, G. and Lowy, P. H.: J. Biol. Chem., *173:*423, 1948.
270. Borsook, H., Deasy, C. L., Haagen-Smit, A. J., Keighley, G. and Lowy, P. H.: J. Biol. Chem., *176:*1383, 1395, 1948.
271. Rothstein, M. and Miller, L. L.: J. Am. Chem. Soc. *76:*1459, 1954.
272. Schweet, R. S., Holden, J. T. and Lowy, P. H.: Fed. Proc., *13:*293, 1954.
273. Cahill, W. M.: Outline of the Amino Acids and Proteins. Ed. by M. Sahyun. New York, Reinhold Pub. Corp., 1944, p. 206.
274. Block, K.: J. Biol. Chem., *155:*255, 1944.
275. Coon, M. J., Robinson, W. G. and Bachhawat, B. K.: Symposium on Amino Acid Metabolism. Ed. by W. D. McElroy and B. Glass. Baltimore, Johns Hopkins Press, 1955, p. 431.
276. Coon, M. J.: J. Biol. Chem., *187:*71, 1950.
277. Meister, A.: J. Biol. Chem., *195:*813, 1952.
278. Coon, M. J. and Abrahamsen, N. S. B.: J. Biol. Chem., *195:*805, 1952.
279. Coon, M. J., Abrahamsen, N. S. B. and Greene, G. S.: J. Biol. Chem., *199:*75, 1954.
280. Rose, W. C., Johnston, J. F. and Hanes, W. J.: J. Biol. Chem., *145:*679, 1942.
281. Atchley, W. A.: J. Biol. Chem., *176:*123, 1948.
282. Kinnory, D. S. and Greenberg, D. M.: Fed. Proc., *12:*320, 1953.
283. Flavin, M., Ortiz, P. J. and Ochoa, S.: Nature, *176:*823, 1955.
284. Abderhalden, E., Bloch, B. and Rona, P.: Ztschr. f. physiol. Chem., *52:*435, 1907.
285. Embden, G. H. and Baldes, K.: Biochem. Ztschr., *55:*301, 1913.
286. Moss, A. R. and Schoenheimer, R.: J. Biol. Chem., *135:*415, 1940.
287. Neubauer, O.: Deut. Arch. f. klin. Med., *95:*211, 1909.
288. Le May-Knox, M. and Knox, W. E.: Biochem. J., *49:*686, 1951.
289. La Du, B. N. and Greenberg, D. M.: J. Biol. Chem., *190:*245, 1951.
290. Schepartz, B.: J. Biol. Chem., *193:*293, 1951.
291. Schepartz, B. and Gurin, S.: J. Biol. Chem., *180:*663, 1949.
292. Weinhouse, S. and Millington, R. H.: J. Biol. Chem., *175:*995, 1948.
293. Suda, M. and Takeda, Y.: J. Biochem. (Japan), *37:*381, 1950.
294. Ravdin, R. G. and Crandall, D. I.: J. Biol. Chem., *189:*137, 1951.
295. Dische, R. and Rittenberg, D.: J. Biol. Chem., *211:*199, 1954.
296. Sealock, R. R. and Silberstein, H. E.: Science, *90:*517, 1939.
297. Sealock, R. R. and Silberstein, H. E.: J. Biol. Chem., *135:*251, 1940.
298. Rienits, K. G.: J. Biol. Chem., *182:*11, 1950.
299. Painter, H. A. and Zilva, S. S.: Biochem. J., *46:*542, 1950.
300. Le May-Knox, M. and Knox, W. E.: 291st Meeting Biochem. Soc., Biochem. J., *48:*XXII, 1951.
301. Knox, W. E.: Symposium on Amino Acid Metabolism. Ed. by W. D. McElroy and B. Glass. Baltimore, Johns Hopkins Press, 1955, p. 836.
302. Uchida, M., Suzuki, S. and Ichihara, K.: J. Biochem. (Japan), *41:*41, 1954.
303. Suda, M., Takeda, Y., Sujishi, K. and Tanaka, T.: J. Biochem. (Japan), *38:* 297, 1951.
304. Schepartz, B.: J. Biol. Chem., *205:*185, 1953.
305. Levine, S. Z., Marples, E. and Gordon, H. H.: Science, *90:*620, 1939.
306. Levine, S. Z., Marples, E. and Gordon, H. H.: J. Clin. Invest., *20:*199, 209, 1941.
307. Nitowsky, H. M., Govan, C. D. and Gordon, H. H.: Am. J. Dis. Child., *85:*462. 1953.
308. Nutrition Rev., *11:*332, 1953.
309. Shepard, D. M. and West, G. B.: J. Physiol., *120:*15, 1953.
310. von Euler, U. S., Hamberg, U. and Hellner, S.: Biochem. J., *49:*655, 1951.
311. Gross, J. and Pitt-Rivers, R. V.: Lancet, *262:*439, 593, 1952.
312. Dalgliesh, C. E.: Advances in Protein Chemistry, *10:*31, 1955.
313. Jervis, G. A.: J. Biol. Chem., *169:*651, 1947.
314. Bickel, H., Gerrard, J. and Hickmans, E. M.: Acta paediat., *43:*64, 1954.
315. Armstrong, M. D. and Tyler, F. H.: J. Clin. Invest., *34:*565, 1955.
316. Nutrition Rev., *14:*42, 1956.
317. Medes, G.: Biochem. J., *26:*917, 1932.
318. Boedeker, H.: Ztschr. f. rat. Med., *7:*130, 1859.
319. Wolkow, M. M. and Baumann, E. A. G.: Ztschr. f. physiol. Chem., *15:*228, 1891.

320. Hopkins, F. G. and Cole, S. W.: J. Physiol., *27:*418, 1901.
321. Matsuoka, Z. and Yoshimatsu, S.: Ztschr. f. physiol. Chem., *143:*206, 1925.
322. Masajo, L.: Gazz. chim. ital., *67:*165, 171, 182, 1937.
323. Lepkovsky, S., Roboz, E. and Haagen-Smit, A. J.: J. Biol. Chem., *149:*195, 1943.
324. Goldberger, J. and Tanner, W. F.: Pub. Health Rep., *37:*462, 1922.
325. Krehl, W. A., Teply, L. J., Sarma, P. S. and Elvehjem, C. A.: Science, *101:* 489, 1945.
326. Heidelberger, C., Gullberg, M. E., Morgan, A. F. and Lepkovsky, S.: J. Biol. Chem., *179:*143, 151, 1949.
327. Schayer, R. W.: J. Biol. Chem., *187:*777, 1950.
328. Mehler, A. H. and Knox, E.: J. Biol. Chem., *187:*431, 1950.
329. Knox, E. and Mehler, A. H.: J. Biol. Chem., *187:*419, 1950.
330. Kotake, Y. and Nakayama, T.: Ztschr. f. physiol. Chem., *270:*76, 1941.
331. Knox, W. E.: Biochem. J., *53:*379, 1953.
332. Braunstein, A. E., Goryachenkova, E. V. and Pashkina, T. S.: Biokhimiya, *14:* 163, 1949.
333. Kotake, Y., Jr. and Inada, T.: Proc. Japan Acad., *28:*68, 1952.
334. Kotake, Y., Jr. and Kamada, J.: Proc. Japan Acad., *30:*122, 1954.
335. Kotake, Y., Kotake, Y., Jr., Hishikawa, M., Sakan, T. and Yamaguchi, M.: Proc. Japan Acad. *29:*143, 1953.
336. Weitzel, G., Buddecke, E., Strecker, F. J. and Roester, U.: Ztschr. f. physiol. Chem., *298:*169, 1954.
337. von Holt, C., Heinrich, W. D. and von Holt, L.: Ztschr. f. physiol. Chem., *297:*241, 1954.
338. Erspamer, V.: Pharmacol. Rev., *6:*425, 1954.
339. Gaddum, J. H. and Hameed, K. A.: Brit. J. Pharmacol., *9:*240, 1954.
340. Wooley, D. W. and Shaw, E.: Science, *119:*587, 1954.
341. Undenfriend, S., Clark, C. T. and Titus, E.: J. Am. Chem. Soc., *75:*501, 1953.
342. Elk, A. and Witkop, B.: J. Am. Chem. Soc., *76:*5579, 1954.
343. Pugh, E. E. M. and Quastel, J. H.: Biochem. J., *31:*2306, 1937.
344. Titus, E. and Undenfriend, S.: Fed. Proc., *13:*411, 1954.
345. Borsook, H., Deasy, C. L., Haagen-Smit, A. J., Kieghly, G. and Lowy, P. H.: J. Biol. Chem., *187:*839, 1950.
346. Eldbacher, S.: Ztschr. f. physiol. Chem., *157:*106, 1926.
347. Gyorgy, P. and Rothler, H.: Biochem. Ztschr., *173:*334, 1926.
348. Kotake, Y. and Konishi, M.: Ztschr. f. physiol. Chem., *122:*230, 1922.
349. Sera, K. and Yada, S.: J. Osaka M. Soc., *38:*1107, 1939.
350. Sera, K. and Yada, S.: J. Osaka M. Soc., *41:*745, 1942.
351. Borek, B. and Wallsch, H.: J. Am. Chem. Soc., *75:*1772, 1953.
352. Borek, B. and Wallsch, H.: J. Am. Chem. Soc., *205:*549, 1953.
353. Tabor, H.: Symposium on Amino Acid Metabolism. Ed. by W. D. McElroy and B. Glass. Baltimore, Johns Hopkins Press, 1955, p. 373.
354. Gaddum, J. H.: Ciba Foundation Symposium on Histamine. Ed. by G. E. W. Wolstenholme and C. M. O'Connor. London, J. & A. Churchill, Ltd., 1956, p. 285.
355. Schayer, R. W.: Ciba Foundation Symposium on Histamine. Ed. by G. E. W. Wolstenholme and C. M. O'Connor. London, J. & A. Churchill, Ltd., 1956, p. 298.
356. Best, C. H.: J. Physiol., *67:*256, 1929.
357. Zeller, E. A.: Helvet. chim. acta., *21:*880, 1645, 1938.
358. Tabor, H., Mehler, A. H. and Schayer, R. W.: J. Biol. Chem., *200:*605, 1953.
359. Schayer, R. W.: J. Biol. Chem., *196:*469, 1952.
360. Tabor, H. and Hayaishi, O.: J. Am. Chem. Soc., *77:*505, 1955.
361. Tabor, H. and Mosettig, E.: J. Biol. Chem., *180:*703, 1949.
362. Janowitz, H., and Grossman, M. I.: Am. J. Physiol., *157:*94, 1949.
363. Clark, D. H. and Tankel, H. I.: Lancet, *2:*886, 1954.
364. McElin, T. W. and Horton, B. T.: Am. J. M. Sc., *218:*432, 1949.
365. Kullander, S.: Acta endocrinol. (Copenhagen), *10:*135, 1952.
366. Wicksell, F.: Acta physiol. scandinav., *17:*395, 1949.
367. Roberts, M.: J. Endocrinology, *11:*338, 1954.
368. Voge, C. I. B.: Brit. M. J., *2:*829, 1929.
369. Kapeller-Adler, R.: Biochem. Ztschr., *264:*131, 1933.
370. Kapeller-Adler, R. and Haas, F.: Biochem. Ztschr., *280:*232, 1935.
371. Kapeller-Adler, R.: J. Obst. & Gynaec. Brit. Emp., *48:*141, 1941.
372. Tschopp, W. and Tschopp, H.: Biochem. Ztschr., *298:*206, 1938.
373. Osborne, T. B. and Mendel, L. B.: J. Biol. Chem., *20:*351, 1915.
374. Jackson, R. W. and Block, R. J.: J. Biol. Chem., *98:*465, 1932.
375. Womack, M., Kemmerer, K. S. and Rose, W. C.: J. Biol. Chem., *121:*403, 1937.
376. Tarver, H. and Schmidt, C. L. A.: J. Biol. Chem., *130:*67, 1939.
377. du Vigneaud, V., Kilmer, W. G., Rachele, J. R. and Cohn, M.: J. Biol. Chem., *155:*645, 1944.

378. Brand, E., Cahill, G. F. and Block, R. J.: J. Biol. Chem., *110:*399, 1935.
379. Brand, E., Block, R. J., Kassell, B. and Cahill, G. F.: Proc. Soc. Exper. Biol. & Med., *35:*501, 1936.
380. Stetten, D., Jr.: J. Biol. Chem., *144:*501, 1942.
381. Tabachnick, M. and Tarver, H.: Arch. Biochem., *56:*115, 1955.
382. Carroll, W. R., Stacy, G. W. and du Vigneaud, V.: J. Biol. Chem., *180:*375, 1949.
383. Matsuo, Y. and Greenberg, D. M.: J. Biol. Chem., *215:*547, 1955.
384. Waelsch, H. and Borek, E. J.: J. Am. Chem. Soc., *61:*2252, 1939.
385. Binder, A. E. and Krebs, H. A.: Biochem. J., *46:*210, 1950.
386. Cahill, W. M. and Rudolph, G. G.: J. Biol. Chem., *145:*201, 1942.
387. Canellakis, E. S. and Tarver, H.: Arch. Biochem., *42:*387, 1953.
388. Keilin, D.: Proc. Roy. Soc. (London), s.B., *106:*418, 1930.
389. Medes, G.: Biochem. J., *33:*1559, 1939.
390. Fromageot, C., Wookey, E. and Chaix, P.: Enzymologia, *9:*198, 1941.
391. Smythe, C. V.: J. Biol. Chem., *142:*387, 1942.
392. Smythe, C. V.: Advances in Enzymology, *5:*237, 1945.
393. Green, D. E. and Stumpf, P. K.: Ann. Rev. Biochem., *13:*18, 1944.
394. Meister, A., Fraser, P. E. and Tice, S. V.: J. Biol. Chem., *206:*561, 1954.
395. Pirie, N. W.: Biochem. J., *28:*305, 1934.
396. Medes, G. and Floyd, N.: Biochem. J., *36:*259, 1942.
397. Chapeville, F. and Fromageot, P.: Biochim. et biophys. acta, *17:*275, 1955.
398. Singer, T. P. and Kearney, E. B.: Symposium on Amino Acid Metabolism. Ed. by W. D. McElroy and B. Glass. Baltimore, Johns Hopkins Press, 1955, p. 558.
399. Chapeville, F. and Fromageot, P.: Biochim. et biophys. acta, *14:*415, 1954.
400. Awapara, J. and Wingo, W. J.: J. Biol. Chem., *203:*189, 1953.
401. Bergeret, B. and Chatagner, F.: Biochim. et biophys. acta, *14:*543, 1954.
402. Cavallini, D., Mondovi, B. and DeMarco, C.: J. Biol. Chem., *216:*577, 1955.
403. Cavallini, D., DeMarco, C., Mondovi, B. and Stirpe, F.: Biochim. et biophys. acta, *15:*301, 1954.
404. Mueller, J. H.: Proc. Soc. Exper. Biol. & Med., *19:*161, 1922.
405. Barger, G. and Coyne, F. P.: Biochem. J., *22:*1417, 1928.
406. Butz, L. W. and du Vigneaud, V.: J. Biol. Chem., *99:*135, 1932.
407. du Vigneaud, V., Dyer, H. M. and Harmon, J.: J. Biol. Chem., *101:*719, 1933.
408. Dyer, H. M. and du Vigneaud, V.: J. Biol. Chem., *109:*477, 1935.
409. Brand, E., Cahill, G. F. and Harris, M. M.: Proc. Soc. Exper. Biol. & Med., *31:*348, 1933.
410. Best, C. H. and Huntsman, M. E.: J. Physiol., *75:*405, 1932.
411. Tucker, H. F. and Eckstein, H. C.: J. Biol. Chem., *121:*479, 1937.
412. Singal, S. A. and Eckstein, H. C.: Proc. Soc. Exper. Biol. & Med., *41:*512, 1939.
413. du Vigneaud, V., Simmonds, S., Chandler, J. P. and Cohn, M.: J. Biol. Chem., *159:*755, 1945.
414. Keller, E. B., Rachele, J. R. and du Vigneaud, V.: J. Biol. Chem., *177:*733, 1949.
415. Dubnoff, J. W.: Arch. Biochem., *24:*251, 1949.
416. Muntz, J. A.: J. Biol. Chem., *182:*489, 1950.
417. Borsook, H. and Dubnoff, J. W.: J. Biol. Chem., *171:*363, 1947.
418. Cantoni, G. L.: J. Biol. Chem., *189:*745, 1951.
419. du Vigneaud, V., Chandler, J. P., Moyer, A. W. and Keppel, D. M.: J. Biol. Chem., *131:*57, 1939.
420. Toennies, G., Bennet, M. A. and Medes, G.: Growth, *7:*251, 1943.
421. Welch, A. D. and Sakami, W.: J. Biol. Chem., *187:*379, 1950.
422. Ferger, M. F. and du Vigneaud, V.: J. Biol. Chem., *185:*53, 1950.
423. MacKenzie, C. G. and du Vigneaud, V.: Fed. Proc., *8:*223, 1949.
424. Sakami, W.: J. Biol. Chem., *179:*495, 1949.
425. Sakami, W.: J. Biol. Chem., *176:*995, 1948.
426. Stekol, J. A. and Weiss, K.: J. Biol. Chem., *226:*95, 1957.
427. du Vigneaud, V.: A Trail of Research, Ithaca, N. Y., Cornell University Press, 1952.
428. Weil-Malherbe, H. and Krebs, H. A.: Biochem. J., *29:*2077, 1935.
429. Neber, M.: Ztschr. f. physiol. Chem., *217:*191, 1936.
430. Stetten, M. R. and Schoenheimer, R.: J. Biol. Chem., *153:*113, 1944.
431. Stetten, M. R.: J. Biol. Chem., *189:*499, 1951.
432. Roloff, M., Ratner, S. and Schoenheimer, R.: J. Biol. Chem., *136:*561, 1940.
433. Stetten, M. R.: J. Biol. Chem. *181:*31, 1949.
434. Taggart, J. V. and Krakaur, R. B.: J. Biol. Chem., *177:*641, 1949.
435. Lang, K. and Schmidt, G.: Biochem. Ztschr., *322:*1, 1951.
436. Abelson, P. H. and Vogel, H. J.: J. Biol. Chem., *213:*355, 1955.

437. Vogel, H. J. and Bonner, D. M.: Proc. Nat. Acad. Sc., *40:*688, 1954.
438. Scher, W. I. and Vogel, H. J.: Bacteriol. Proc., p. 123, 1955.
439. Maas, W. K., Novelli, G. D. and Lipmann, F.: Proc. Nat. Acad. Sc., *39:*1004, 1953.
440. Vogel, H. J.: Proc. Nat. Acad. Sc., *39:*578, 1953.
441. Bollman, J. L., Mann, F. C. and Magath, T. B.: Am. J. Physiol., *64:*371, 1924.
442. Maddock, S. and Svedberg, A.: Am. J. Physiol., *121:*203, 1938.
443. Kossel, A. and Dakin, H. D.: Ztschr. f. physiol. Chem., *41:*321, 1904.
444. Krebs, H. A. and Henseleit, K.: Ztschr. f. physiol. Chem., *210:*33, 1932.
445. Cohen, P. P. and Hayano, M.: J. Biol. Chem., *166:*239, 1946.
446. Cohen, P. P. and Hayano, M.: J. Biol. Chem., *166:*251, 1946.
447. Cohen, P. P. and Hayano, M.. J. Biol. Chem., *170:*687, 1947.
448. Cohen, P. P. and Hayano, M.: J. Biol. Chem., *172:*405, 1948.
449. Grisolia, S. and Cohen, P. P.: J. Biol. Chem., *191:*189, 1951.
450. Grisolia, S. and Cohen, P. P.: J. Biol. Chem., *198:*561, 1952.
451. Grisolia, S. and Cohen, P. P.: Fed. Proc., *11:*222, 1952.
452. Ratner, S.: Symposium on Amino Acid Metabolism. Ed. by W. D. McElroy and B. Glass. Baltimore, Johns Hopkins Press, 1955, p. 231.
453. Ratner, S.: Advances in Enzymology, *15:*319, 1954.
454. Ratner, S. and Pappas, A.: J. Biol. Chem., *179:*1183, 1949.
455. Ratner, S. and Pappas, A.: J. Biol. Chem., *179:*1199, 1949.
456. Ratner, S. and Petrack, B.: J. Biol. Chem., *191:*693, 1951.
457. Ratner, S. and Petrack, B.: J. Biol. Chem., *200:*175, 1953.
458. Bloch, K. and Schoenheimer, R.: J. Biol. Chem., *133:*633, 1940.
459. Bloch, K. and Schoenheimer, R.: J. Biol. Chem., *134:*785, 1940.
460. Borsook, H. and Dubnoff, J. W.: J. Biol. Chem., *169:*247, 1947.
461. Jones, M. E., Spector, L. and Lipmann, F.: J. Am. Chem. Soc., *77:*819, 1955.
462. Marshall, R. O., Hall, L. M. and Cohen, P. P.: Biochem. et biophys. Acta, *17:*279, 1955.
463. Reichard, P. and Hanshoff, G.: Acta chem. scand., *10:*548, 1956.

CHAPTER 2

By RACHMIEL LEVINE, M.D.

Carbohydrate Metabolism

Carbohydrate metabolism is a subject difficult to discuss without reference to other metabolic processes. This section is, however, limited to the metabolism of carbohydrates chiefly because this is a traditional subject division in the larger area of metabolism. It is hoped that the reader will keep in mind the necessity for relating what is here set down to the material in the sections on Protein and Lipid Metabolism.

THE CARBOHYDRATES IN FOOD

The particular carbohydrates present in the ordinary American diet, the food sources from which these carbohydrates are derived, and the quantitative importance of each carbohydrate in the total intake are indicated in Table 1.

THE DIGESTION OF CARBOHYDRATES

The digestion of carbohydrates starts in the oral cavity. Here the secretion of the parotid gland, which contains an amylase called "ptyalin," is mixed with the food and begins the conversion of starch, glycogen and the dextrins into maltose. This digestion continues in the stomach until the hydrochloric acid which is secreted there destroys the amylase activity and substitutes acid hydrolysis for enzymatic splitting. If continued long enough, the acid hydrolysis could reduce many of the digestible carbohydrates to the monosaccharide stage. However, the stomach usually empties itself before this can occur, and the digestion of carbohydrate is taken up in the enzymes of the small intestine, operating in the more alkaline medium which prevails there. The enzymes in the small intestine are: an amylase secreted by the pancreas; and an amylase, a maltase, an invertase and a lactase secreted by the wall of the small bowel. All these enzymes are capable of splitting the particular sugars which they attack to the monosaccharide stage.

We have accounted for the digestion of starch, glycogen, the dextrins and the disaccharides. Those sugars which are ingested in the form of monosaccharides do not require digestion. All the remaining carbohydrates pass through the stomach and small intestine unchanged. In the large bowel they are subjected to the enzymatic influence of the profuse bacterial flora which is normal there, and they may be broken down to monosaccharides to some extent. It is possible that minor amounts of carbohydrate are made available in this manner for absorption into the blood stream.

THE ABSORPTION OF CARBOHYDRATES

The monosaccharides, ingested as such or arising from the digestion of carbohydrates, are practically completely absorbed in the small intestine. Small amounts may be absorbed from the stomach. It is also possible to show that, when solutions of monosaccharides are introduced into the large bowel for experimental or therapeutic purposes, some sugar can be absorbed from this portion of the gastrointestinal tract.

TABLE 1. TYPES AND SOURCES OF CARBOHYDRATES IN THE AMERICAN DIETARY

CARBOHYDRATES	APPROXIMATE PERCENTAGE OF TOTAL CARBOHYDRATE INTAKE *	CHIEF FOOD SOURCES	END-PRODUCTS OF DIGESTION	REMARKS
Polysaccharides:				
a) Indigestible	3			
1. Celluloses and hemi-celluloses		Stalks and leaves of vegetables; outer covering of seeds	0	May be partially split to glucose by bacterial action in large bowel
2. Pectins		Fruits	0	Chemical hydrolysis yields galactose and arabinose
b) Partially digestible	2			
1. Inulin		Jerusalem artichokes, onions, garlic	Fructose	Digestion incomplete; further splitting by bacteria may occur in large bowel
2. Galactogens		Snails	Galactose	
3. Mannosans		Legumes	Mannose	
4. Raffinose		Sugar beets	Glucose, fructose, and galactose	
5. Pentosans		Fruits and gums	Pentoses	
c) Digestible:				
1. Starch and dextrins	50	Grains; vegetables (especially tubers and legumes)	Glucose	The most important group quantitatively. Usually accompanied by some maltose
2. Glycogen	Negligible	Meat products and sea food	Glucose	
Disaccharides:				
1. Sucrose	25	Cane and beet sugars; molasses; maple syrup	Glucose and fructose	
2. Lactose	10	Milk and milk products	Glucose and galactose	
3. Maltose	Negligible	Malt products	Glucose	
Monosaccharides:				
a) Hexoses:				
1. Glucose	5	Fruits; honey; corn syrup	Glucose	In fruits and vegetables the contents of glucose and fructose depend on species, ripeness, and state of preservation
2. Fructose	5	Fruits; honey	Fructose	
3. Galactose	0	0	Galactose	These monosaccharides do not occur in free form in foods; see under lactose and mannosans
4. Mannose	0	0	Mannose	
b) Pentoses:				
1. Ribose	0	0	Ribose	These monosaccharides do not occur in free form in foods. They are derived from pentosans of fruits and from the nucleic acids of meat products and sea food
2. Xylose	0	0	Xylose	
3. Arabinose	0	0	Arabinose	
Carbohydrate derivatives:				
1. Ethyl alcohol	Variable	Fermented liquors	Absorbed as such	These substances are the products of natural or induced carbohydrate breakdown
2. Lactic acid	Negligible	Milk and milk products		
3. Malic acid	Negligible	Fruits		
4. Citric acid	Negligible	Fruits		

* Calculated from the average dietary of the middle-income group in the United States.

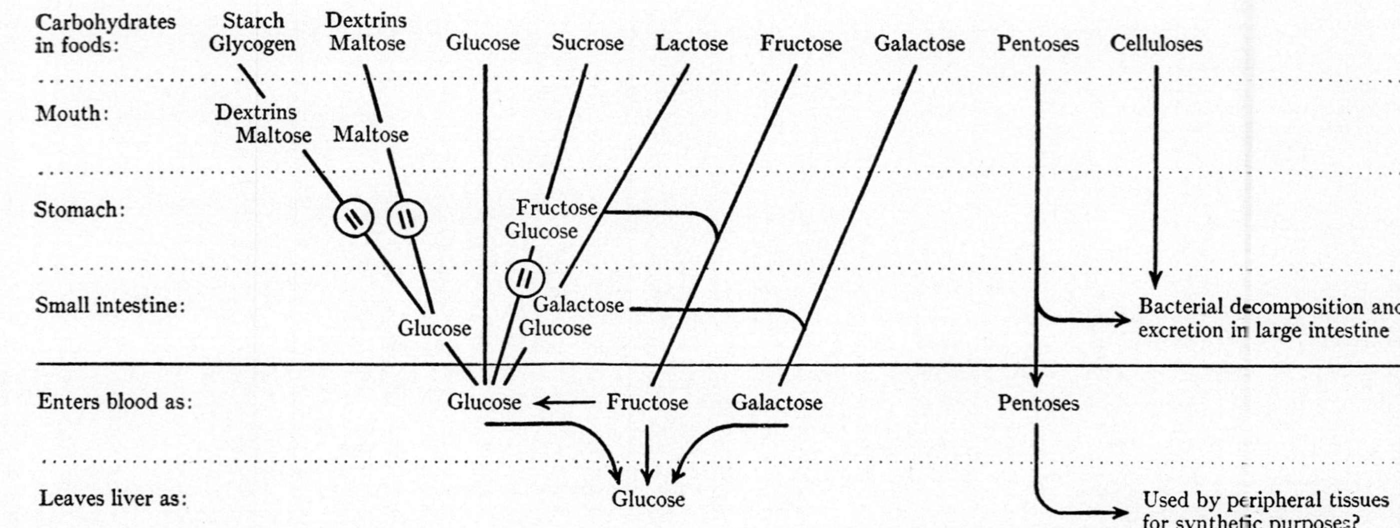

FIG. 1. Products of carbohydrate digestion at various levels of the gastrointestinal tract, and subsequent fate. ⦶ indicates that the same products as at the preceding level continue to appear. (Soskin and Levine: (Carbohydrate Metabolism, Univ. of Chicago Press.)

Two types of absorption occur in the small intestine: (a) a specific absorption of particular monosaccharides, and (b) a nonspecific absorption of all monosaccharides, by diffusion resulting from osmotic forces across the mucous membrane. Glucose, fructose and galactose are absorbed by both processes. Consequently, the absorption of these sugars differs in two respects from that of those sugars that are absorbed by diffusion alone: they are absorbed more rapidly, and their rates of absorption are largely independent of their concentrations in the intestine.[1] The mechanism of sugar transfer across the epithelial cell of the intestine is unknown. The present evidence points against a phosphorylation process. The specificity of the actively absorbed sugars differs from that of the enzyme system, hexokinase, which would be involved in phosphorylation.[2] Glucose is for the most part absorbed as such into the portal circulation, although a significant proportion may be degraded to lactic acid in the intestinal epithelium and may enter the blood in that form.[3] Fructose is transferred unchanged to the extent of about 50 per cent; some is transformed to glucose and another portion to lactic acid.[4]

The actual rates of absorption of the three monosaccharides which are phosphorylated vary rather widely, though all are much higher than the absorption rates of such monosaccharides as mannose or the pentoses, which are handled by diffusion. Thus it has been shown in rats that, if the rate for glucose is represented as 100, that for galactose would be 110, for fructose 43, and for mannose and the pentoses only 9. There are few reliable data on the absolute rates at which the various monosaccharides can be absorbed from the gastrointestinal tract of the human being under normal circumstances. The best available evidence from the work of Groen[5] indicates that the rate of absorption of glucose from a 50 cm. length of jejunum (small intestine) is about 8.0 gm. per hour; that for galactose, about 9.5 gm. per hour; and that for fructose, about 5 gm. per hour. These rates are for concentrations of sugar of 10 per cent and above. Below 10 per cent the rate of absorption varies directly with the concentration.

From the practical standpoint, the figures quoted above may have little relationship to the rate at which a monosaccharide enters the blood stream, whether eaten as such or arising from the processes of digestion under the usual conditions of feeding. Under the latter circumstances, the time which elapses before it is absorbed from the gastrointestinal tract will be governed largely by (a) the rate at which it enters the small intestine and (b) the mixture of foods in the small intestine at the time of absorption. The rate at which the sugar arrives in the small intestine depends largely on the motility of the stomach and the control of the pyloric sphincter, which can be affected by such various phenomena as hunger, emotion, local irritation (including condiments), and the composition and consistency of the food mass after mastication. The food mixture in the small intestine affects the rate of absorption by competition of the mucosa and, in the case of those monosaccharides which are specifically absorbed, by competition for the available phosphorylating capacity.

Other factors which influence the amount of carbohydrate absorbed in a given individual at a particular time are: (a) the normality of the mucous membrane of the small intestine and the length of time during which the carbohydrate is in contact with it; (b) endocrine function, particularly that of the anterior pituitary gland, the thyroid,[6] and the adrenal cortex;[7] and (c) the adequacy of vitamin intake, especially that of the B complex.[8] Since the absorption of the important end-products of carbohydrate digestion requires chemical activity by the mucous membrane, it is obvious that any abnormality of the mucosal cells might interfere with carbohydrate absorption. Enteritis (inflammation) is a not uncommon disturbance of this kind. Celiac disease may represent a more obscure disturbance of a similar nature. However, even when the mucosa is normal, an excessive rate of movement of the carbohydrate along the gastrointestinal tract, accompanying diarrheas of various origins, may hurry a portion of the ingested carbohydrate into the large bowel before it can be absorbed.

Normal absorption of carbohydrate does not occur in the presence of an anterior pituitary deficiency. This probably depends, for the most part, upon the secondary hypofunction of the thyroid gland, for the same result may be obtained after removal of the thyroid gland when the hypophysis is intact. Furthermore, the defect in absorption accompanying hypopituitarism may be relieved by the administration of thyroid extract.[6] Indeed, Althausen and coworkers[9] have attempted to make use of this phenomenon as a clinical test of the state of activity of the thyroid gland. They administer a standard amount of galactose by mouth, follow the rise of galactose concentration in the blood, and use the rate of the latter as a criterion of thyroid function.

The adrenal cortex influences carbohydrate absorption through its regulation of the sodium chloride (NaCl) exchange in the body. The absorption of carbohydrate from the intestine is subnormal in adrenal cortical deficiency but can be restored to normal without the use of adrenal cortical extracts if the NaCl of the blood is raised to normal levels by adequate salt intake.[7]

Insulin, which has such an important influence on other aspects of carbohydrate metabolism, is without apparent effect upon the absorptive capacity of the intestinal mucous membrane.

Deficiency of the B complex is associated with diminished absorption of the hexoses.[8] Recent work on this subject has been concerned with the separate effects of the various pure components of the complex. Thiamine, pantothenic acid and pyridoxine affect absorption. Riboflavin is without action.

THE DISTRIBUTION OF CARBOHYDRATE IN THE BODY

In order to understand the distribution of carbohydrate in the body and appreciate its particular functions and uses, it is necessary first to consider the relation of carbohydrate metabolism to that of the other two major foodstuffs.

Protein constitutes 75 per cent of the dry weight of the soft tissues of the body. In view of the protein nature of the tissue enzymes, it is a fair generalization to say that the proteins, with the hormones, vitamins and minerals, constitute the metabolic machinery of the body. In emergencies a certain amount of the protein machinery can be broken down and converted into fuel.* However, the amount of body protein which is available for this purpose at any one time is strictly limited, as is also the length of survival which is possible when the body has exhausted its fat stores and is forced to depend upon endogenous protein alone.

Fat differs from protein in that it can be stored in practically unlimited quantities. It is deposited chiefly within layers of connective tissue and not as an integral part of the working organs of the body. When food intake is inadequate to supply the caloric needs of the organism, sufficient fat is mobilized to make up the caloric deficit. In this way practically the entire fat stores of the body can be depleted without detriment to health. Whatever harm accompanies extreme emaciation can be explained by specific deficiencies in the protective food factors incidental to the general restriction in food intake and by the loss of certain secondary structural functions of fat having to do with heat insulation and the architectural cushioning of organs. Fat is, therefore, primarily a fuel-storage material. When food is in-

* Strictly speaking, the tissue proteins are in a constant state of flux, being continuously broken down and replaced. Therefore, "the emergency use of a portion of the protein machinery for fuel" actually means a temporary shift of the dynamic equilibrium toward the catabolic side, so that, for the duration of the emergency, synthesis no longer keeps pace with breakdown.

gested in excess of caloric expenditure (whether taken in the form of carbohydrate, protein or fat), the equivalent of the excess calories is deposited as fat in the adipose tissues.

Carbohydrate resembles fat in being a fuel material but differs from fat in that it is an indispensable one. The tissues of the body constantly require and use carbohydrate under all physiologic conditions. Even a temporary fall in the blood sugar below certain critical levels is accompanied by serious disability. Nevertheless, the amount of carbohydrate present in the body at any one time is very small. This amount, if it were not replaced as used, could sustain life for only a fraction of one day. Table 2 compares the total effective carbohydrate content of a hypothetical average normal man with his caloric requirement. Thus, unless large amounts of carbohydrate are continually ingested with the food, the needs of the body must be met by the conversion of the other foodstuffs into carbohydrate. It is, therefore, the active fuel of the body which is stored only in small quantities and which is taken in or made as required.

The carbohydrate of the body is largely present in the form of glycogen in the skeletal, cardiac and smooth muscles. In these motor tissues it serves as an emergency reserve of fuel, one which can be mobilized more rapidly than carbohydrate can reach these organs through the regular channels. Most of the remaining carbohydrate in the body is found in the manufacturing and distributing system, namely, in the liver as glycogen and in the blood and extracellular fluids as glucose. Relatively small amounts of glycogen are also found in practically all other organs and tissues of the body.

That the greater part of the body carbohydrate is present as glycogen (the polymerized storage form of glucose) depends upon the fact that all the hexoses, which result from the digestion of carbohydrate in the intestine and are absorbed into the blood stream, are converted into glucose. This occurs largely, but perhaps not entirely, in the liver.[10] Similarly, in the postabsorptive state or during fasting, when the liver must supply sugar to the blood from the body's own resources, glucose is the carbohydrate which is manufactured from protein and fat. Nevertheless, there are other forms of carbohydrate in most tissues and organs. Among these are special-purpose carbohydrates, which are presumably not used as fuel—for example, the galactose in the galactolipins of nervous tissues, the pentoses associated with the nucleoproteins, and the glucose derivatives of the widely distributed mucopolysaccharides. Under special circumstances, such as in the lactating woman, lactose is made in the breast and is present in the secreted milk. Finally, there are a number of degradiation products of glucose, such as the hexose and triose phosphates, which are caught in transit as the glucose is utilized.

Table 3 summarizes the distribution of the quantitatively important forms of carbohydrate in man and in certain laboratory animals. To some extent we must rely on the data from animals to interpret the relatively meager data available for human beings. This is because

TABLE 2. CALORIC EQUIVALENT OF CARBOHYDRATE CONTENT OF NORMAL MAN

Body weight, 70 kg.; liver weight, 1800 gm.; muscle mass, 35 kg.; volume of blood and extracellular fluids, 21 liters.

	PER CENT	GM.
Muscle glycogen	0.70	245
Liver glycogen	6.00	108
Blood and extracellular fluid sugar	0.08	17
Total body carbohydrate		370 gm.
Caloric equivalent (370 × 4.1)		1,517 cal.
Caloric requirement (sedentary occupation)		2,800 cal. per 24 hr., or 116.7 cal. per hr.
Total body carbohydrate could supply caloric needs for (1,517 ÷ 116.7)		13 hr.

TABLE 3. DISTRIBUTION OF CARBOHYDRATE IN VARIOUS TISSUES OF RAT, DOG AND MAN
(Figures Represent Ranges Found on a Mixed Diet)

TISSUE	RAT		DOG		MAN	
	Glycogen (per cent)	Glucose (mg. per cent)	Glycogen (per cent)	Glucose (mg. per cent)	Glycogen (per cent)	Glucose (mg. per cent)
Skeletal muscle	0.81–1.06	50–70	0.55	40–60	0.4–0.6	
Liver	2.5 –8.3	......	6.10	.....	1.5–6.0	
Heart	0.3 –0.6	......	0.47	.....	....	.....
Kidney	....	......	0.15	.....	0.4	
Brain	0.08	......	0.1	57		
Skin	0.07	77	0.08	71	0.08	60–82
Blood and extracellular fluids	....	90–129	....	60–80	....	60–90

both glucose and glycogen (especially the latter) are labile substances when present in the tissues, and few opportunities present themselves to obtain human tissues under the proper conditions for accurate analysis. However, the close agreement of the reliable human data which we do have with that obtained from animals increases their significance.

Glucose

Glucose is the chief, and for practical purposes the only, transport form of carbohydrate. Carbohydrates enter the blood from the gastrointestinal tract largely as glucose. In the postabsorptive state, glucose is the carbohydrate which the liver supplies to all the other tissues of the body. For these reasons the level of glucose in the blood is normally higher than in other tissues or fluids of the body.

The average normal level of glucose in the blood does not vary appreciably with the species of animal. In most animals it is very similar, ranging from 60 to 80 mg. per 100 cc. of whole blood. It has been customary to express these amounts as "60 to 80 mg. per cent." Strictly speaking, this is incorrect; for whole blood is not homogeneous, nor is it of the same specific gravity as water. Nevertheless, with the reservations noted, we shall make use of this shorthand designation of concentration for the sake of convenience.

The blood-sugar levels reported by different observers depend, to a certain extent, upon the methods employed for chemical analysis. Glucose is an aldohexose (Fig. 2) in which the aldehyde group on the first carbon atom acts as a reducing agent. Hence, the most practical and most commonly used chemical methods for determining glucose are procedures in which a metallic ion in the oxidized state (usually copper) is reduced by the sugar. Such methods were devised by Bertrand, Folin, Hagedorn, Somogyi and many others. They differ from each other chiefly as regards the means by which reducing substances other than glucose are removed from the reaction. To the extent that these means differ in efficiency, there are differences in blood-sugar values reported from various laboratories. For example, the range of normal values quoted for mammals is obtained by the Somogyi modification of the Shaffer-Hartman method. When the Folin-Wu method is used, a range of from 80 to 120 mg. per cent is obtained. Somogyi has shown[11] that his method of precipitation removes virtually all the noncarbohydrate reducing substances (chiefly glutathione); hence, the results obtained by using his method are sometimes referred to as values for "true" blood sugar. The most specific method for the estimation of glucose consists of the use of the enzyme system "glucose oxidase" to remove glucose from a sample of blood and tissue. The reducing power is estimated before and after the exposure to glucose oxidase.[12]

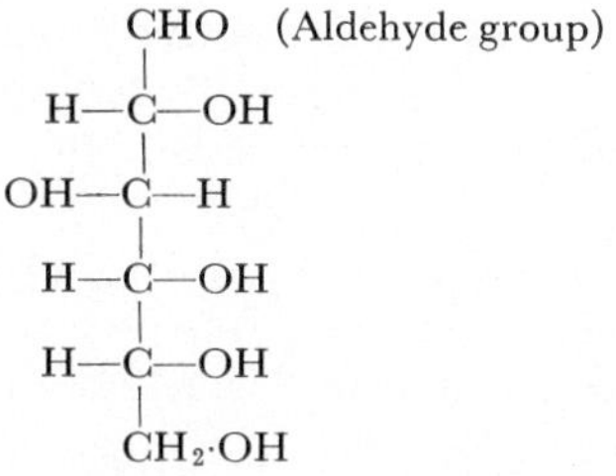

```
        CHO   (Aldehyde group)
         |
    H—C—OH
         |
  OH—C—H
         |
    H—C—OH
         |
    H—C—OH
         |
        CH₂·OH
```

FIG. 2. Glucose.

When the level of sugar in a sample of whole blood is 100 mg. per cent, the concentration of sugar in the plasma of the same blood is about 115 mg. per cent. This difference is due to the fact that the sugar is not equally distributed between the blood plasma and the red blood cells. (There is an equal distribution of glucose between the blood plasma and the water phase of the red blood cells.) The precise difference between the whole-blood sugar and the plasma sugar in a given instance will depend upon whether or not the normal number of red blood cells per unit volume of blood is present.

Because the peripheral tissues are constantly removing sugar from the blood, samples of arterial or capillary blood will show a level of sugar a few milligrams per cent higher than that of simultaneously drawn samples of venous blood. This so-called A-V difference varies with the existing rate of utilization of sugar and also depends upon the rate of blood flow through the tissues at the time of sampling. It is obvious that, if the rate of sugar utilization were constant, a doubling of the rate of blood flow would result in a diminution of the A-V difference to half its former value. Neglect of this simple consideration has given rise to some confusion in the literature.[13]

Being a crystalloid of small molecular weight, glucose diffuses readily out of the blood stream into all other body fluids. Tissues like liver or skeletal muscle are composed of at least two phases, namely, the tissue cells and the fluid filling the interstices between them (extracellular fluid). Analysis of normal whole muscle for its glucose content (using the proper precautions to prevent glycolysis) usually yields a range of values between 30 and 60 mg. per cent. Still lower values are obtained using the specific "glucose oxidase" technique. The intracellular glucose level in tissues like muscle is essentially zero under most conditions.[14] Liver cells contain appreciable quantities of free glucose. Using isotopic glucose it has been shown that it distributes in about 25 per cent of the body weight. With the exception of some tissues, free glucose is essentially an extracellular material. An estimate of the amount of glucose actually present within the tissue cells may be made by determining the amount of extracellular fluid and calculating the intracellular sugar from the sugar content of the whole tissue.

Normal urine contains a small amount of glucose. An average adult human excretes from ½ to ¾ gm. in the approximately 1500 cc. of urine voided in twenty-four hours. In clinical medicine such urine is termed "sugar-free," because the routine methods for the qualitative detection of sugar are not sufficiently sensitive to indicate its presence in this concentration. That the concentration of glucose in normal urine is far below that occurring in other body fluids is not because the membranes of the kidney are less permeable to sugar. The kidney glomerulus actually passes a filtrate containing glucose in the same concentration as is present in blood plasma. But this filtrate is then subject to the action of the cells of the kidney tubules, which reabsorb most of the sugar in it.

The process by which the kidney tubules reabsorb glucose is unknown. It probably resembles the sugar transfer system of the intestinal mucosa. The glucoside phlorhizin prevents the reabsorption of the sugar and results in so-called "phlorhizin diabetes." Abnormal amounts of sugar also appear in the urine whenever the blood-sugar level is raised to such heights that the amount of glucose filtering through the glomeruli exceeds the reabsorptive capacity of the tubules. The critical level at which this begins to occur is usually about 180 mg. per cent and is often referred to as the "kidney threshold" for glucose.[15]

Fructose

Fructose is so rapidly converted to glucose in the adult mammal that there is never any appreciable amount of free fructose present in the peripheral blood and most other tissues. However, it is produced by the seminal vesicles, presumably from glucose, and appears in the seminal fluid in high concentrations (300–700 mg. %). The amount of fructose in seminal fluid is influenced by castration and hypophysectomy and is apparently under the control of testosterone. There are other observations which link fructose with the process of reproduction. For example, the blood sugar of fetal sheep consists mainly of free fructose although some glucose is present.

Fructose has reducing properties similar to glucose and is readily fermented by yeast. Hence the usual methods for the determination of glucose, with the exception of the glucose oxidase technique, do not distinguish between these two hexoses. However, there are two practical colorimetric procedures for this purpose.[16,17]

Glycogen

Glycogen in the animal body is similar in form and function to the starch in plants. It is a polymer consisting of many glucose molecules joined to each other. The —C—O—C— linkage between adjoining glucose molecules is known as the "glucosidic linkage." It is here that the glycogen molecule splits into hexose units with the introduction of a phosphate group.

Glycogen, when isolated in the laboratory, is a stable compound. But in the presence of the tissue-enzyme systems it breaks down very easily. For this reason the glycogen content of a dead tissue gives no indication of its content during life, and accuracy of estimation is not assured even when tissue is removed from the living organism. This is especially true when any degree of anoxia is allowed to occur while the tissue is being removed for analysis or, in the case of muscle, when twitching of the muscle fibers is induced by careless handling.

The standard method for glycogen estimation in tissues depends upon the fact (discovered by Claude Bernard and put to practical use by Pflüger) that hot concentrated potassium hydroxide destroys all carbohydrates except glycogen. As described by Good, Kramer and Somogyi,[18] the method is accurate and relatively simple, once the tissue is dissolved in the alkali. The difficulty consists in removing and transferring the living tissue into the alkali before any significant amount of glycogen disappears. Fairly good and consistent results may be obtained by anesthetizing the animal with an anesthetic (such as Amytal or pentobarbital) which does not itself tend to break down glycogen. The tissue to be studied is then carefully dissected out without interfering with its blood supply. At the appropriate moment it is quickly removed and transferred to a tared vessel containing hot alkali. But the technique by which the true pre-mortem glycogen content of a tissue is most nearly determinable is the following: The animal is anesthetized, and the tissue prepared as above. The tissue is then frozen *in situ* by the use of liquid air or crushed CO_2 ice. It is removed and weighed in the frozen state and immersed in the hot alkali.

Lactic Acid

When the body is at rest and in the postabsorptive state, the lactic acid content of the blood ranges between 10 and 15 mg. per cent. The lactic acid content of other tissues is in equilibrium with that of the blood plasma, for lactic acid is freely diffusible across cell membranes. Under these circumstances, the small amount of lactic acid which is present probably arises from a few special tissues, such as the red blood cells, the intestinal mucous membrane, the retina, etc. Adult mammalian erythrocytes do not possess the enzymatic machinery for the use of oxygen but readily produce lactic acid from blood glucose. The cells of the intestinal mucosa and the retina have a high aerobic glycolysis; that is, they differ from most tissue cells, in which an adequate oxygen supply inhibits lactic acid production.

In most tissues of the body, lactic acid is not a necessary intermediate of carbohydrate metabolism. It is formed by the reduction of pyruvic acid only when the oxidative removal of the latter is relatively or absolutely deficient. A relative oxygen lack may occur during strenuous physical exercise, when the rate of oxygen supply to the muscles is temporarily inadequate in comparison with the rate of glycogenolysis, whereupon the lactic acid in the muscles increases and diffuses out into the blood. Certain organs, particularly the liver (but also the heart), will then remove the excess lactic acid from the blood and reoxidize it to pyruvic acid.

An absolute lack of oxygen, leading to high lactic acid levels even when the body is at rest, may result from pulmonary or cardiovascular diseases, which interfere with the oxygenation of the blood or tissues, respectively, and in states of shock. A similar end-result may be caused by hepatic disease, when the impairment of the oxidative systems in this organ prevent it from utilizing the oxygen available in the blood for the removal and oxidation of the blood lactic acid.

The importance of anoxia in lactic acid formation necessitates the same precautions as for glycogen when sampling tissues for chemical analysis. The addition of sodium fluoride to blood prevents further glycolysis. Lactic acid is usually estimated by the method of Friedemann, or by that of Miller and Muntz. The latter method was modified and adapted to tissue analysis by Barker and Summerson.[19]

Pyruvic Acid

Since pyruvic acid is one of the most reactive metabolic intermediates, it is not surprising that the amounts of pyruvic acid normally found in the blood and other tissues do not exceed 1.0 mg. per cent. The level rises somewhat with the increased breakdown of carbohydrate accompanying muscular work or following carbohydrate administration. The pyruvic acid content of blood and tissues also increases during thiamine deficiency, for many of the reactions which dispose of pyruvic acid require thiamine diphosphate as a coenzyme. This fact has been used as an aid in the diagnosis of this avitaminosis.[20]

It should be noted that, despite the fact that pyruvic acid is by far one of the most important substances in intermediary metabolism, its normal concentration in blood and tissues is only about one tenth to one twentieth that of lactic acid. This is because of the many mechanisms available for pyruvate removal, while lactic acid disposal is limited to one reaction—its oxidation to pyruvate. This illustrates the general rule that the concentration of a substance in blood and tissues is not necessarily an indication of its importance in the metabolic scheme. Some metabolic intermediates are never present in detectable amounts unless special methods are employed to stop the metabolic reactions at that stage.

The method commonly used for pyruvate estimation is that of Lu, or the subsequent modifications of this method.[21]

Phosphate Compounds

The phosphate compounds important in intermediary metabolism are: inorganic phosphate, phosphorylated intermediates, and phosphate-transfer substances.

Inorganic Phosphate (P_0). The P_0 in the body is largely derived from the inorganic phosphates present in foods. Under certain circumstances the P_0 of the blood may be increased by the mobilization of $Ca_3(PO_4)_2$ from the bones. The P_0 of blood and soft tissues may also rise as the result of an increased breakdown of organic phosphate compounds, owing to anoxia or the interruption of the activity of certain enzyme systems. Hence,

TABLE 4. DISTRIBUTION OF PHOSPHATE COMPOUNDS IN VARIOUS TISSUES OF MAN, RAT, RABBIT, AND DOG*

TISSUE	INORGANIC PHOSPHATE (P_0)	CREATINE PHOSPHATE (CrP)	ADENOSINE DI- AND TRI-PHOSPHATES (ADP AND ATP)	HEXOSE-6-PHOSPHATE (HMP)	PHOSPHOGLYCERATE (PGly)	DIPHOSPHOGLYCERATE (di-PGly)	TOTAL ACID-SOLUBLE PHOSPHATE (P TOTAL)
Skeletal muscle......	15–25	50–70	30–40	8–15	40–50	.....	150–200
Cardiac muscle......	23–29	5–13	18–28	14	.....	.....	80–100
Liver..............	18	0	15–25	....	.....	.....	90–100
Brain..............	7–9	9–11	16–19	4–6	0	.....	70
Blood..............	3–5	0	10–20	....	.....	30–50	50–80

* All values are in terms of mg. % P.

the sampling of tissues for the correct estimation of P_0, as well as of the other phosphate derivatives, involves the same precautions as for glycogen. With more careful handling of tissues, lower P_0 values have been reported. Table 4 summarizes the most reliable observations as to the levels of P_0 and other important phosphate compounds in various bodily tissues.

Phosphorylated Intermediates. The only phosphorylated intermediates of carbohydrate metabolism which are normally present in the tissues in significant quantities are (a) hexose-6-phosphate, (b) monophosphoglyceric acid, and (c) diphosphoglyceric acid (in red blood cells only). Table 4 lists the levels which have been reported. The other known phosphorylated intermediates, such as glucose-1-phosphate, hexose diphosphate, etc., are metabolized as rapidly as they are produced and therefore are not found except when steps have been taken to interfere with their disposal.

Phosphate-transfer Substances. This group consists of (a) adenosine diphosphate, (b) adenosine triphosphate and (c) creatine phosphate. The levels normally found in tissues appear in Table 4. The adenosine polyphosphates are present in all tissues of the body to a greater or lesser extent. However, creatine phosphate seems to be limited to contractile or conducting tissues—i.e., striated, smooth, and cardiac muscle, neurones, and the nerve fibers. It has also been found in spermatozoa. There is no creatine phosphate in blood or liver.

THE ENZYMATIC MACHINERY OF CARBOHYDRATE METABOLISM

In the process of digestion or in the liver after absorption, carbohydrates are largely converted to glucose. Hepatic gluconeogenesis leads to the same end-product. The further course of carbohydrate metabolism is therefore chiefly concerned with the chemical transformations undergone by glucose. These include the synthesis of glycogen and the formation of fat. But more basic than either of these is the breakdown of the sugar to carbon dioxide (CO_2) and water (H_2O), with the liberation of the energy that supports the various functions of living cells.

The work of Pasteur on yeast fermentation initiated a series of scientific developments, which led to our present knowledge of cell mechanisms for metabolism. The epoch-making discovery of Buchner that a cell-free extract of yeast could substitute for the living cell in the process of fermentation showed that what had been considered to be a process inseparable from life is, after all, only a special kind of chemical reaction —a reaction that is catalyzed by a complex organic substance (enzyme) in the cell. This paved the way for a rational and materialistic explanation of cell processes. Other enzymes were discovered and isolated. Evidence mounted that the chemical machinery of the living cell consists of a series of organic catalysts which operate on complex molecules, step by step, to produce simpler and more labile products. It was realized that the enzymes made possible such chemical reactions in the cell as would otherwise require high temperatures or strong reagents incompatible with life. The step-by-step catabolism controlled by the multiple enzymes also offered a reasonable basis for the regulated release of energy in small units, a process which was much more reasonable, from the point of view of the use of such energy, than the explosive type of reaction, implied in the idea of "combustion."

By the early years of this century biochemists and physiologists using biochemical methods had collected a great deal of data concerning the kinds and amounts of intermediate metabolites present in the different tissues of the body under a variety of conditions. These data guided the enzyme chemists in the isolation and study of the enzyme systems which were responsible for the various products. The last twenty-five years have witnessed a tremendous and constantly accelerating growth in the application of enzyme chemistry to metabolic problems. It has become evident that, in the process called "oxidation" in the tissues, molecular oxygen does not interact directly with the foodstuffs and that CO_2 largely arises by a splitting-off of carboxyl groups from lower metabolic intermediates. It is with these and other fundamental enzyme reactions that we shall now deal.

NATURE OF CELL ENZYMES

The enzymes in the living cell resemble the known inorganic catalysts in that they are more or less specific for a particular chemical reaction or type of reaction; also, in that they are not measurably consumed by the reaction which they accelerate. All the tissue enzymes which have thus far been isolated and sufficiently purified that their essential natures are known have turned out to be proteins. As more and more of the enzymes have been recognized and studied, it has become less possible to distinguish between purely structural proteins, constituting, as it were, the skeleton of the cell, and the enzyme proteins, representing the active organs of the cell.

Studies of the optimal conditions for the activity of various enzyme proteins have uncovered a number of other normal constituents of the living cell which must be present if a particular enzyme is to exert its fullest effect. In some instances these accessory substances are simple ions, like phosphate or magnesium, and are referred to as "cofactors" of the enzyme. When the accessory element is a complex organic but nonprotein substance, it is known as a "coenzyme." A protein enzyme (or the activating protein) together with its particular coenzyme and/or other cofactors is known as an "enzyme system."

The Enzyme Systems Involved in Carbohydrate Metabolism

The following is a list of the various types of enzymatic reactions which are known to be involved in the breakdown and synthesis of carbohydrates in mammalian tissue. The enumeration is followed by a brief description of the nature of each reaction and an important example of each type, including mention of the coenzymes and cofactors involved.

1. Oxidation (oxidoreduction)
2. Decarboxylation (oxidative and nonoxidative)
3. Carbon dioxide assimilation (addition of CO_2)
4. Phosphorylation and phosphorolysis
5. Intermolecular phosphate transfer
6. Walden inversion
7. Deamination
8. Amination
9. Transamination
10. Hydrolysis
11. Condensation

1. Oxidation. The term "oxidation" may be applied to a reaction when there is (a) the addition of oxygen atoms to a substance, (b) the removal of hydrogen atoms from a substance, or (c) the removal of electrons from a substance. The transformation of lactic to pyruvic acid is such a reaction and may be indicated as in [A] below. The hydrogen is not given off in gaseous form but rather in the form of hydrogen ions and electrons. This means that for each hydrogen ion one electron is also released. The correct chemical notation for this reaction is indicated in [B] below. Since this particular oxidation consists of the removal of hydrogen atoms, it is often referred to as a "dehydrogenation."

Lactic acid, dissolved in H_2O and with free access to oxygen at 37.5° C, will be oxidized to pyruvic acid at such a slow rate as to be hardly measurable. But when a specific protein derived from animal or plant cells is added to the solution, significant amounts of pyruvic acid appear in a matter of minutes. This influence of the activating protein or enzyme may be regarded as one which loosens the bonds joining the two hydrogen atoms to the second, or alpha C, atom of the lactic acid molecule. More accurately stated, the activating protein changes the form of the electron energy, uniting the hydrogen and carbon in such a way as to increase the tendency of the hydrogen atoms to fly off. Thus, any suitable chemical substance which can bind the hydrogen atoms (hydrogen acceptor) will remove the "loosened" hydrogen from the orbit of the lactic field, leaving pyruvic acid.

The hydrogen acceptor necessary for the above reaction is diphosphopyridine nucleotide (DPN) (Fig. 3). This, then, is the coenzyme which, with the protein, makes up the lactic acid oxidase (or dehydrogenase) system. Despite this nomenclature, however, the system is reversible and will actually reduce pyruvic acid to lactic acid under the proper conditions. The direction of the reaction depends largely on whether the DPN is present in its oxidized or reduced form (as DPN or as H_2DPN), which, in turn, depends upon whether other systems which can remove the hydrogen from H_2DPN are present. For example, the activity of the lactic acid oxidase system in the living animal is most frequently observed during relative or absolute anoxia in skeletal muscle, when the H_2DPN cannot readily be reoxidized and hence serves to convert pyruvic acid to lactic acid. In chemical notation the reaction may therefore be represented somewhat more completely, as in [C] below.

While the activating protein of the lactic acid oxidase system is completely specific for the one substrate, lactic acid, and is just as specific for the particular transformation of lactic acid which we have described, the coenzyme is less discriminating. It also serves as a hydrogen acceptor for other reactions. Each of these reactions is catalyzed by a separate activating protein in combination with DPN. Some biologic oxidations are carried on by systems consisting of proteins and TPN (Fig. 3). These two groups constitute the class of pyridinoprotein enzymes. Another group of oxidation systems are known as the "yellow

---

[A]

1 mol. lactic acid − 2 hydrogen atoms = 1 mol. pyruvic acid

[B]

$$CH_3\cdot\overset{\alpha}{C}HOH\cdot COOH - 2H^+ - 2\epsilon \rightleftarrows CH_3\cdot CO\cdot COOH$$

[C]

$$CH_3\cdot CHOH\cdot COOH + DPN \underset{\text{protein}}{\overset{\text{activating}}{\rightleftarrows}} CH_3\cdot CO\cdot COOH + H_2DPN$$

enzymes"—proteins combined with alloxazine derivatives—which are yellow in aqueous solution (Fig. 4).

The various oxidation systems that have been listed are responsible for the removal of hydrogen from all substrates and intermediate substances whose metabolic fate is known. The hydrogen removed from the original owner, while under the influence of a specific protein, is simply transferred to the coenzyme of the system, be it DPN, TPN, or an alloxazine. It will be noted that no mention has been made of the appearance of oxygen upon the scene. As a matter of fact, the hydrogen seized by the coenzyme is passed on through a series of other systems, in the manner of a bucket brigade, before it finally arrives at the point where it may com-

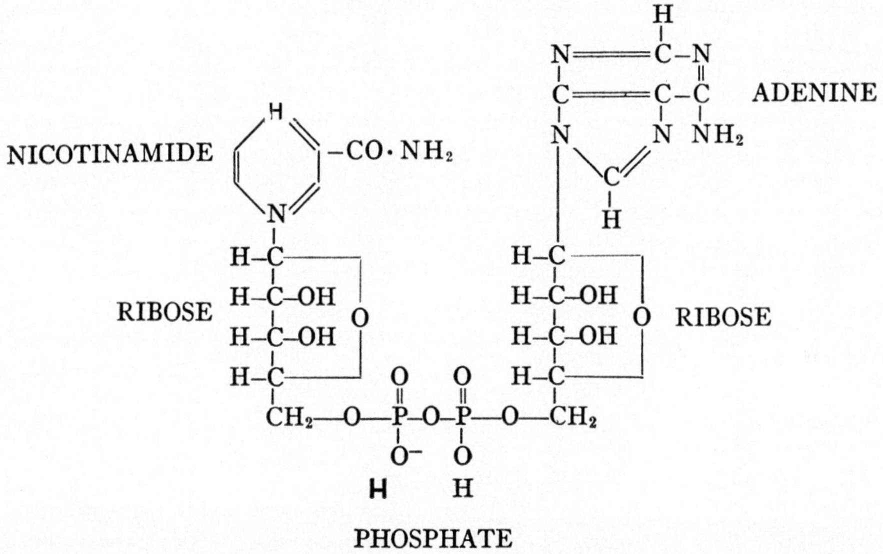

NICOTINAMIDE — ADENINE — RIBOSE — RIBOSE — PHOSPHATE

FIG. 3. Diphosphopyridine nucleotide (DPN). **H** = hydrogen atoms from substrate. (Triphosphopyridine nucleotide (TPN) differs from DPN in possessing an additional phosphate group on carbon 2 of the ribose moiety of the adenosine portion of the molecule). (Soskin and Levine: Carbohydrate Metabolism, Univ. of Chicago Press.)

PHOSPHATE — RIBOSE — RIBOSE — ALLOXAZINE — ADENINE

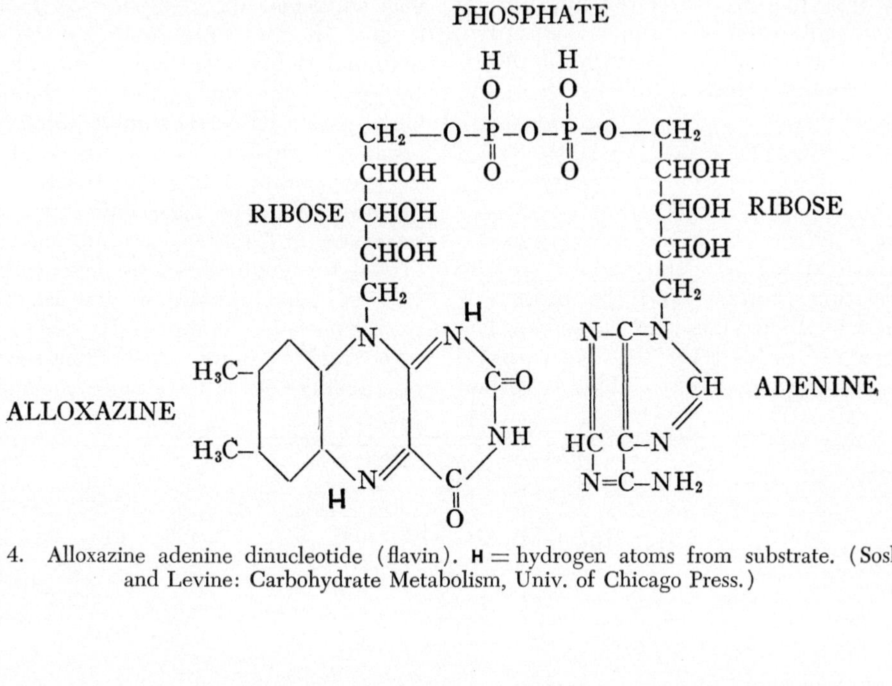

FIG. 4. Alloxazine adenine dinucleotide (flavin). **H** = hydrogen atoms from substrate. (Soskin and Levine: Carbohydrate Metabolism, Univ. of Chicago Press.)

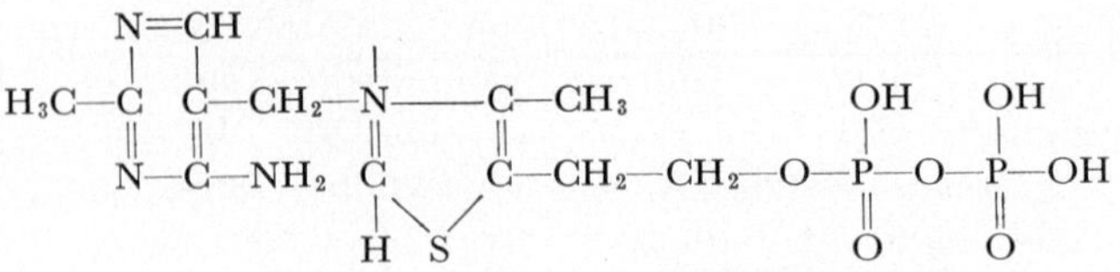

$$\begin{array}{l} \text{N=CH} \\ \text{H}_3\text{C—C}\quad\text{C—CH}_2\text{—N———C—CH}_3 \qquad \text{OH} \quad \text{OH} \\ \text{N—C—NH}_2\ \ \text{C}\qquad\text{C—CH}_2\text{—CH}_2\text{—O—P—O—P—OH} \\ \qquad\qquad\quad \text{H}\ \ \text{S} \qquad\qquad\qquad\qquad \text{O}\qquad \text{O} \end{array}$$

FIG. 5. Diphosphothiamine (cocarboxylase).

bine with oxygen to form H_2O. This will be discussed in detail later.

2. Decarboxylation. Carbon dioxide is one of the end-products of the complete breakdown of foodstuffs. It is not formed, as was formerly thought, by the direct oxidation of the carbon by molecular oxygen but arises from the splitting-off of carboxyl groups (—COOH) from intermediate organic acids which arise in the course of catabolism. The exact mechanism of decarboxylations is, at yet, obscure; but we can distinguish two types: the oxidative and the nonoxidative. In the first of these the CO_2 is split off a molecule while, at the same time, hydrogen atoms are removed from another group in the same substance. For example, pyruvic acid, $CH^3 \cdot CO \cdot$-COOH, containing three carbon atoms, is oxidized to acetic acid $CH_3 \cdot COOH$, which contains only two carbon atoms, the third having been split off as CO_2. In chemical notation this double process of oxidation plus decarboxylation can be presented as in [A] below. In the second type of decarboxylation there is no concurrent oxidation. Again using pyruvic acid as an example, this type of decarboxylation proceeds as follows:

$$\underset{\text{Pyruvic}}{CH_3\cdot CO\cdot COOH} \rightarrow \underset{\text{Acetaldehyde}}{CH_3\cdot CHO} + CO_2$$

Just as in the oxidations, the various decarboxylations are catalyzed by specific activating proteins, and the process is aided by coenzymes and cofactors. The coenzyme needed for the decarboxylation of pyruvic acid is diphosphothiamine (also called "cocarboxylase") (Fig. 5). Magnesium ion is also an essential component as a cofactor in the foregoing systems.

The oxidative decarboxylation of pyruvate has been shown recently to be more involved. Another coenzyme, called α-lipoic or thioctic acid (Fig. 6), forms a complex with diphosphothiamine. This complex, lipothiamide, in the presence of the specific proteins and of coenzyme A, leads to the formation of acetyl CoA from pyruvate.[22]

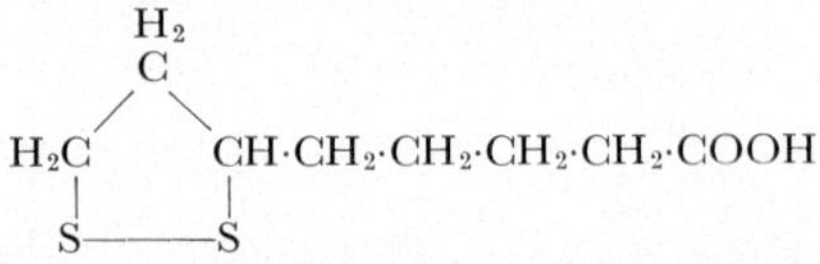

$$\begin{array}{l} \qquad\ \ H_2 \\ \qquad\ \ C \\ H_2C \qquad CH\cdot CH_2\cdot CH_2\cdot CH_2\cdot CH_2\cdot COOH \\ S \text{———} S \end{array}$$

FIG. 6. Lipoic or thioctic acid.

3. Carbon Dioxide Assimilation. It has been known for some time that CO_2 produced by the dissimilation of foodstuffs may combine with hemoglobin (carbamino compound) or may be used for the production of urea. It was supposed that by these and other means all the CO_2 produced by the mammalian organism was eventually excreted by the lungs and the kidneys. Only plants or certain autotrophic bacteria were thought to possess the ability to incorporate CO_2 into usable cell products. In 1936 this ability was first observed in bacteria; later it was confirmed for mammalian tissue (especially liver) that certain in vitro reactions undergone by compounds containing three carbon atoms (the trioses) could be speeded up if CO_2 were present in

---

[A]

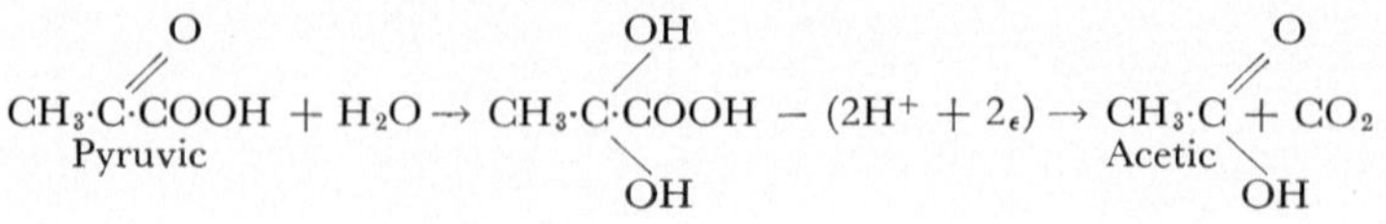

$$\underset{\text{Pyruvic}}{CH_3\cdot \overset{O}{\overset{/\!/}{C}}\cdot COOH} + H_2O \rightarrow CH_3\cdot \overset{OH}{\underset{OH}{C}}\cdot COOH - (2H^+ + 2\epsilon) \rightarrow \underset{\text{Acetic}}{CH_3\cdot \overset{O}{\underset{OH}{C}}} + CO_2$$

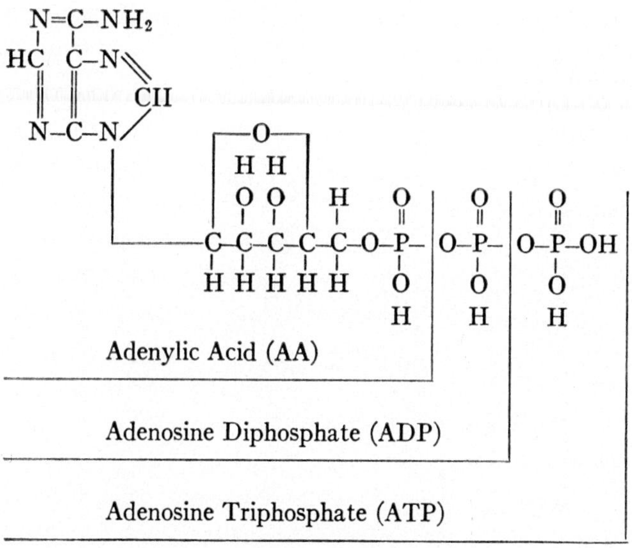

Adenylic Acid (AA)

Adenosine Diphosphate (ADP)

Adenosine Triphosphate (ATP)

FIG. 7. The coenzyme system for phosphorylations. (Soskin and Levine: Carbohydrate Metabolism, Univ. of Chicago Press.)

the medium. It was shown that this was not a consequence of the mere presence of CO_2 but that the CO_2 took part in the reactions and was incorporated into other substances.

Again pyruvic acid will serve as a good example. In the presence of the specific proteins, diphosphothiamine, inorganic phosphate and magnesium ion, pyruvic acid (a three-carbon-atom compound) and CO_2 will form oxalacetic acid (a four-carbon-atom compound) as indicated in [A] below. This is probably the first step in the series by which pyruvic acid (or lactic acid) is reconverted to sugar and glycogen.

The use of CO_2 for synthetic purposes by the mammalian cell is only now being studied in detail. But it has already taken on tremendous significance, since it completely reverses the hitherto firmly accepted view that CO_2 is merely a waste product of animal metabolism.

4. a. Phosphorylation. Early in the development of our knowledge of the enzymatic breakdown of carbohydrates it was known that the presence of phosphate was necessary for the fermentation of glucose by yeast extracts, and for the breakdown of sugar that takes place in active muscle extracts. It was later demonstrated that the phosphate is used for the formation of various intermediaries of carbohydrate breakdown which were shown to contain phosphate in their molecules. Among such metabolites are the glucose and fructose monophosphates, fructose diphosphate, glyceraldehyde phosphate, etc. The role of these phosphorylated intermediate substances in facilitating certain reactions and in the transfer of energy from one chemical reaction to another has only recently been elucidated. We shall discuss these aspects in detail in the section dealing with the utilization of metabolic energy. For the present it will suffice to present the mechanics of phosphorylation by suitable examples.

The first step in the series of reactions by which sugar enters the metabolic cycle of the cell is the addition of phosphate (P) to the sixth carbon atom of the glucose molecule. The enzyme necessary for this initial reaction in animal tissues (hexokinase) has not yet

---

[A]

$$\underset{\text{Pyruvic}}{CH_3{\cdot}CO{\cdot}COOH} + CO_2 \rightleftarrows \underset{\text{Oxalacetic}}{COOH{\cdot}CH_2{\cdot}CO{\cdot}COOH}$$

PHOSPHATE DONORS — PHOSPHATE ACCEPTORS

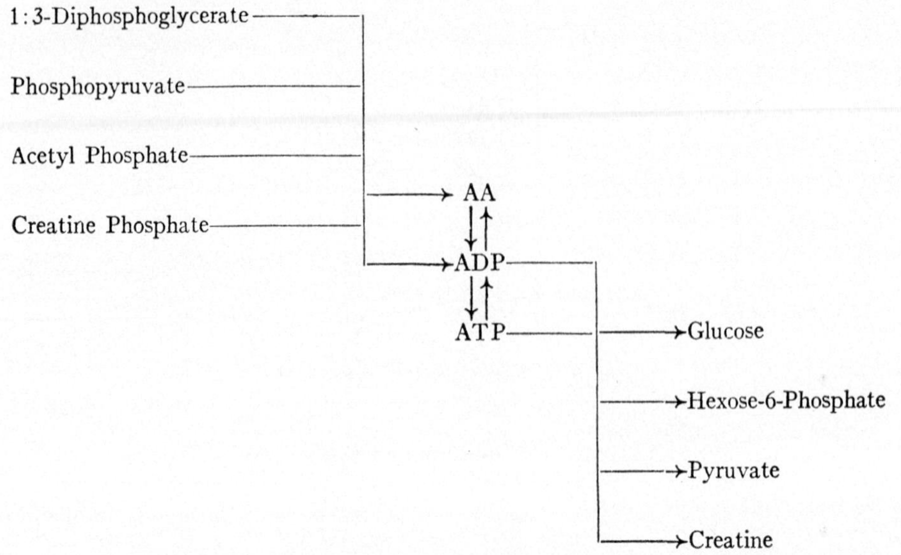

FIG. 8. Phosphate transfer by the adenylic system. (Soskin and Levine: Carbohydrate Metabolism, Univ. of Chicago Press.)

been purified, but it apparently activates the glucose molecule in such a way that it can receive a phosphate from a suitable source. The phosphate donor in this case is adenosine triphosphate (ATP) (Fig. 7), which is the coenzyme of this phosphorylation reaction. In chemical notation the reaction may be represented as in [A] below. The coenzyme ATP has two phosphate groups, which can be split off easily in the presence of the suitable enzymes:

$$\begin{array}{lll} \text{ATP} \rightarrow & \text{ADP} \rightarrow & \text{AA (adenylic acid)} \\ & + & + \\ & P_0 & P_0 \text{ (inorganic phosphate)} \end{array}$$

But the amount of ATP present in the cell at any one time is very small as compared to the amount of material to be phosphorylated. Hence ADP and AA must be continuously reconverted to ATP in order that the latter can serve as a continuous phosphate donor. The central position of this adenylic system for receiving and donating phosphate groups is illustrated in Figure 8, in which the direction of the arrows represents the direction of phosphate transfer.

4. b. Phosphorolysis. Glycogen is a complex molecule consisting of glucose units connected to one another by glucosidic (C—O—C) linkages. Two types of linkages occur, the 1:4 and the 1:6. The glycogen complex is, therefore, not a straight-chain polymer but a highly branched structure. The 1:6 linkages form the branch points of the complex

---

[A]

```
         (6) CH2OH                          CH2·O·PO3H
              |                                 |
              C——O                              C——O
       H    / |     \     H              H    / |     \     H
       |   /  H      \    |              |   /  H      \    |
       C                  C + ATP →      C                  C + ADP
       | \  OH    H    /  |              | \  OH    H    /  |
      OH  \  |    |   /  OH             OH  \  |    |   /  OH
             C————C                            C————C
             |    |                            |    |
             H    OH                           H    OH
```

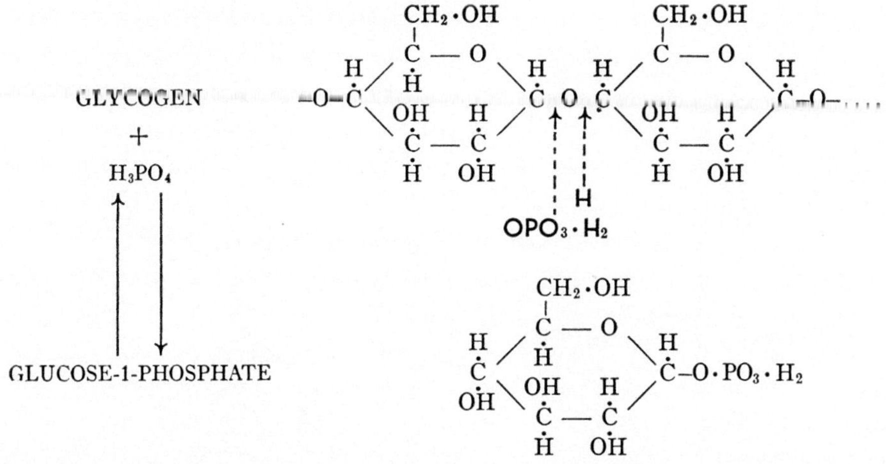

GLYCOGEN + H_3PO_4 ⇅ GLUCOSE-1-PHOSPHATE

FIG. 9. Glycogen phosphorolysis. (Soskin and Levine: Carbohydrate Metabolism, Univ. of Chicago Press.)

arboreal structure, and are present in a ratio of 1 to 10 or 18 of the 1:4 linkages. The breakdown of glycogen to hexose units is accomplished by two enzymes, each of which is specific for one of the linkages. The better studied and now purified system is the 1:4 enzyme, known as "glycogen phosphorylase." In the presence of inorganic phosphate and glycogen this enzyme catalyzes a reaction by which orthophosphoric acid (H_3PO_4) cleaves the glucosidic linkage, leaving H_2PO_4 attached to carbon atom 1 of one glucose unit and H attached to carbon atom 4 of the next glucose unit. This is analogous to a hydrolytic cleavage (H·OH) except that instead of elements of H_2O, those of the orthophosphate are added; because of this analogy the name "phosphorolysis" (compare with hydrolysis) is given to this type of reaction. The reaction is visualized in Figure 9. The 1:6 linkage is broken by the enzyme amylo-1:6-glucosidase, with the liberation of free glucose. This latter system is also known as the "debranching" enzyme.

Phosphorolysis is reversible. The direction of the reaction is determined by the relative concentrations of glucose-1-phosphate and inorganic phosphate, so that removal of inorganic phosphate favors glycogen synthesis, while addition of inorganic phosphate hastens glycogen breakdown. There is evidence that this is one of the regulating devices of glycogenolysis in the living cell. The reversal of phosphorolysis accounts only for the adddition of glucose residues in the 1:4 linkage. Branch points (the 1:6 linkage) are formed by a second enzyme, amylo-(1:4 → 1:6)-transglucosidase, which forms a 1:6 bond at the expense of a 1:4 bond.[23]

5. Intermolecular phosphate Transfer. During the degradation of glucose or glycogen certain reactions involving phosphorus occur in which a phosphate group already present in the molecule is transferred to another position in the same molecule. For example, glycogen is broken down into a glucose-phosphate compound in which the phosphate group is attached to carbon atom 1 of the glucose ring. This is therefore known as "glucose-1-phosphate" (Glucose-1-P). An enzyme protein, called "phosphoglucomutase,"[24] in the presence of a small amount of glucose-1:6-diphosphate (which acts as a coenzyme) facilitates the transfer of the phosphate group to carbon atom 6, the resulting substance being glucose-6-phosphate. The reaction (A below)

A

Glucose 1:6 di P + Glucose-1-P ⇄ Glucose-6-P + Glucose 1:6 di P

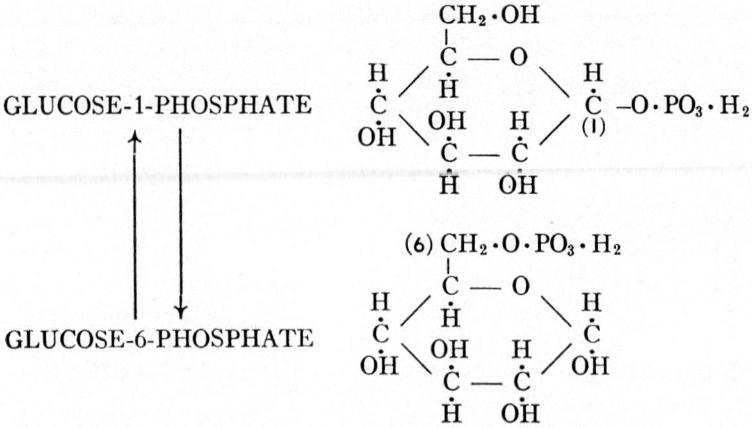

GLUCOSE-1-PHOSPHATE

$CH_2 \cdot OH$
C — O
H H H
C C $-O \cdot PO_3 \cdot H_2$
OH OH H (1)
C — C
H OH

↑↓

GLUCOSE-6-PHOSPHATE

(6) $CH_2 \cdot O \cdot PO_3 \cdot H_2$
C — O
H H H
C C
OH OH H OH
C — C
H OH

FIG. 10. Intermolecular phosphate transfer. (Soskin and Levine: Carbohydrate Metabolism, Univ. of Chicago Press.)

is reversible, as indicated; and its necessary cofactor is magnesium. These two phosphate glucose esters differ from each other in various chemical properties. See Figure 10 above. A similar intermolecular phosphate transfer occurs in the reaction:

3-phosphoglyceric acid ⇄ 2-phosphoglyceric acid

6. Walden Inversion. The conversion of galactose to glucose is known to occur readily in liver and kidney. The structural formulae of these sugars differ only in the position of the H and OH groups on carbon atom four (see [A] below). "Galactowaldenase," recently discovered and named by Leloir et al,[25] facilitates the conversion of galactose-1-phosphate to glucose-1-phosphate by "inverting" the H and OH groups. The necessary coenzyme is the substance, uridine-di-phosphoglucose, UDPG. Actually two linked reactions account for the transformation (see [B] below). In the rare metabolic disorder known as galactosemia, there is a congenital deficiency in the above systems, leading to the presence of free galactose in blood and urine, cataract formation, etc.[26]

The uridine phosphates from which the above coenzymes are derived represent a newly discovered group of compounds analogous to the adenosine phosphates. They seem important both as coenzymes and as energy transfer systems.[27]

7. Deamination. The term "deamination" refers to the removal of an NH_2 (amino) group, generally from amino acids. Since certain amino acids form glucose in the body and since the re-

---

[A]

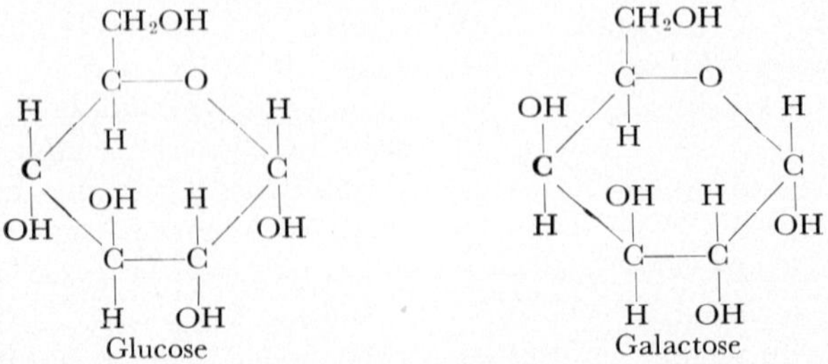

CH_2OH
C — O
H H H
C C
OH OH H OH
C — C
H OH
Glucose

CH_2OH
C — O
OH H H
C C
H OH H OH
C — C
H OH
Galactose

[B]

(1) galactose-1-phosphate + UDP-glucose ⇄ glucose-1-phosphate + UDP-galactose
(2) UDP-galactose ⇄ UDP-glucose

moval of the NH_2 group is the first step in such a transformation, the mechanism of deamination is pertinent to the general discussion of carbohydrate metabolism.

The actual loss of the NH_2 group from an amino acid is a spontaneous reaction not requiring an enzyme. However, the amino acid must first lose hydrogen before it can react with H_2O to lose the NH_2 group. Hence the whole process is called "oxidative deamination." For example, an enzyme system known as "amino acid oxidase," consisting of a protein and a coenzyme of the alloxazine group, removes two hydrogen atoms from the alpha C atom of alanine:

$$\underset{\text{Amino acid}}{CH_3\cdot\overset{\alpha}{C}HNH_2\cdot COOH} \xrightarrow{-2H} \underset{\text{Imino acid}}{CH_3\cdot C{:}NH\cdot COOH}$$

The resulting substance is known as an imino acid because of the NH or imino group. Such an acid will react with H_2O as indicated in [A] below. The final result is the formation of pyruvic acid and ammonia. The NH_3 produced may be excreted as such or transformed to urea. The pyruvic acid is either oxidized to $CO_2 + H_2O$ or built up into glucose or glycogen.

8. Amination. The synthesis of amino acids from the corresponding keto acids and ammonia has been suggested from model in vitro experiments, and one enzyme preparation has been shown to be able to form glutamate from α-keto-glutarate plus NH_3:

$$\underset{\alpha\text{-Ketoglutaric acid}}{\begin{array}{c} COOH \\ | \\ CO \\ | \\ CH_2 \\ | \\ CH_2 \\ | \\ COOH \end{array}} + NH_3 \rightleftarrows \underset{\text{Glutamic acid}}{\begin{array}{c} COOH \\ | \\ CHNH_2 \\ | \\ CH_2 \\ | \\ CH_2 \\ | \\ COOH \end{array}}$$

Although other enzymes of this kind remain to be isolated, this type of reaction must be quite general; for Schoenheimer has shown that, following the feeding of a labeled NH_4 salt (N^{15} isotope) to experimental animals, the isotopic nitrogen is found in the amino groups of all the amino acids (except lysine) of their tissue proteins.[28] That extensive amination must occur is also shown by the fact that the corresponding keto or hydroxy acids may be substituted in the diet for the essential amino acids. Thus NH_3, like CO_2, long considered to be merely a waste product, is now known to be able to re-enter the metabolic cycle and function again.

9. Transamination. Another type of reaction involving amino acids and related to carbohydrate metabolism is the mutual exchange of amino and keto groups between certain α-keto acids (derived from carbohydrate breakdown) and certain specific amino acids. For example:

$$\underset{\text{Glutamic}}{\begin{array}{c} COOH \\ | \\ CH_2 \\ | \\ CH_2 \\ | \\ CH(NH_2) \\ | \\ COOH \end{array}} + \underset{\text{Oxalacetic}}{\begin{array}{c} COOH \\ | \\ CH_2 \\ | \\ C(O) \\ | \\ COOH \end{array}} \rightleftarrows \underset{\alpha\text{-Keto Glutaric}}{\begin{array}{c} COOH \\ | \\ CH_2 \\ | \\ CH_2 \\ | \\ CO \\ | \\ COOH \end{array}} + \underset{\text{Aspartic}}{\begin{array}{c} COOH \\ | \\ CH_2 \\ | \\ CHNH_2 \\ | \\ COOH \end{array}}$$

Although the evidence is not yet complete, the coenzyme of the transamination reactions seems to be pyridoxal phosphate, derived from the vitamin, pyridoxine.[29]

This interchange is another link between carbohydrates and protein derivatives and provides a means for the transamination of one amino acid into another. It probably also represents a channel through which the amino acids contribute to the common metabolic pool formed by all the foodstuffs.

10. Hydrolysis. This type of reaction

[A]

$$CH_3{-}C{:}NH{-}COOH + H_2O \rightarrow \underset{\text{Pyruvic acid}}{CH_3\cdot CO\cdot COOH} + \underset{\text{Ammonia}}{NH_3}$$

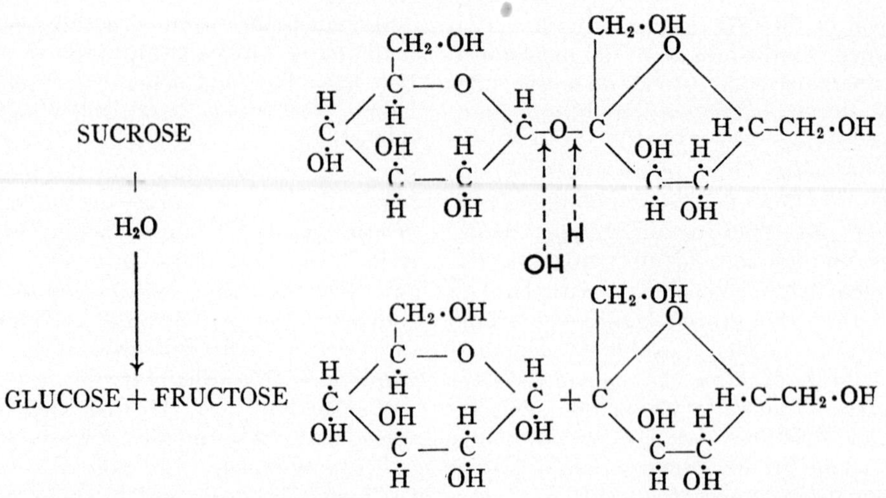

SUCROSE

H_2O

GLUCOSE + FRUCTOSE

FIG. 11. Hydrolysis of sucrose. (Soskin and Levine: Carbohydrate Metabolism, Univ. of Chicago Press.)

is very common in the processes of digestion in the gastrointestinal tract. Water is added to a molecule in such a way that the molecule is split into two portions, one receiving the H, the other the OH group, of the H_2O. Thus sucrose, a disaccharide consisting of one molecule of glucose and one of fructose, is split into its constituent hexoses by the enzyme invertase. The glucosidic linkage is opened by the entry of the elements of H_2O.

Other examples of hydrolysis are:

Lactose ⇄ Glucose + Galactose
Maltose ⇄ Glucose + Glucose

However, many reactions which formerly were thought to be examples of hydrolysis have recently been shown to be phosphorolysis, e.g., glycogen breakdown.

11. Condensation. It has become evident in recent years that all the major foodstuffs are split enzymatically to 2 and 3 carbon atom fragments which are then oxidized by way of a cycle of transformations, known as the tricarboxylic acid cycle. The manner in which a 2 carbon fragment, such as acetic acid, enters this cycle is by "condensing" with a 4-carbon acid, oxalacetic, to form a 6 carbon tricarboxylic acid:

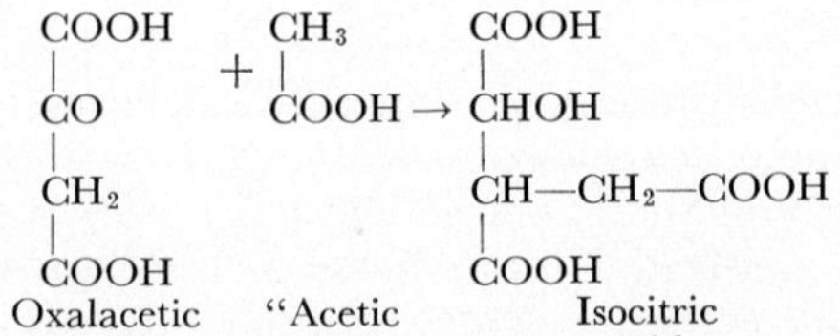

$$\begin{array}{c} COOH \\ | \\ CO \\ | \\ CH_2 \\ | \\ COOH \end{array} + \begin{array}{c} CH_3 \\ | \\ COOH \end{array} \rightarrow \begin{array}{l} COOH \\ | \\ CHOH \\ | \\ CH—CH_2—COOH \\ | \\ COOH \end{array}$$

Oxalacetic acid (4C) — "Acetic acid" (2C) — Isocitric acid (6C)

This condensation has recently been achieved with a purified enzyme system. It has been shown that the "acetic acid" is really an activated molecule acetyl CoA, and it is known that the coenzyme of this and similar addition reactions with acetate is a derivative of the vitamin, pantothenic acid.[30]

The Oxidation of the Hydrogen Removed from the Substrate

The final products of metabolism are substances which cannot be broken down further by the tissue cells. These are urea, CO_2 and H_2. Of these, urea and CO_2 are excreted via the kidneys and lungs, respectively. The problem that remains is the final fate of the H_2 removed from the foodstuffs by the coenzymes (hydrogen acceptors). The coenzymes are DPN, TPN, and flavin. Although we are not in full possession of all the details, it may safely be assumed that the reduced pyridine nucleotides are relieved of their H_2 by flavin enzymes. A final common path for H_2 is reached, and all of it exists as flavin: H_2 for an instant. The scene shifts now to a series of iron-containing proteins, the cytochromes[31] and the "respiratory ferment" known as "cytochrome oxidase." The iron in these substances is in organic combination, in a group resembling the heme of hemoglobin. The iron can oscillate between the reduced and oxidized form

$$Fe^{++} \underset{+\epsilon}{\overset{-\epsilon}{\rightleftarrows}} Fe^{+++}$$

by the addition or loss of an electron. The H_2 of the foodstuffs, having arrived at the flavin stage, reacts with the oxidized cytochrome:

$$\text{Flavin } H_2 + CyFe^{+++} \rightarrow CyFe^{++} + \text{Flavin} + H^+$$

The electron reduces $CyFe^{+++}$, while the H^+ remains in the medium. The reduced cytochrome ($CyFe^{++}$) reacts with cytochrome oxidase:

$$CyFe^{++} + OxFe^{+++} \rightarrow OxFe^{++} + CyFe^{+++}$$

This serves to restore the oxidized cytochrome and to reduce the oxidase. This oxidase is unique in that it can react with molecular oxygen dissolved in the cell:

$$OxFe^{++} + O \rightarrow OxFe^{+++} + O^-$$

The oxygen keeps the oxidase in its oxidized form and gains an electron. The free H^+ available from the flavin H_2 then reacts with O^- to form H_2O. Thus the over-all change resulting from the whole series of reversible transformations is

$$2H^+ + O^- \rightarrow H_2O$$

The series itself has been a succession of electron transfers in which every step has tended to restore the previous step to its original state.

THE INTERMEDIARY STEPS IN CARBOHYDRATE METABOLISM

Our knowledge of the intermediary steps in carbohydrate breakdown and synthesis is by no means complete. However, many lines of evidence derived from studies in vivo and in vitro in animals and in plants are converging toward a generally accepted scheme.[32] This scheme is outlined in Figures 12 and 13, which include the most thoroughly studied and, in all probability, the most important pathways. Others have been suggested and discarded from time to time. But, of these, only certain pathways for which some evidence exists will be mentioned. It should be remembered that the present scheme is subject to revision as to detail as new data appear and that it may not apply in its entirety to all organs or tissues which utilize carbohydrates. One or another of the enzyme systems may be missing in a particular tissue, thus modifying the intermediates or the end-products. The scheme, therefore, should be regarded merely as an architect's preliminary sketch, showing the general size and shape but not the final plans of the edifice to be erected.

It may be seen from Figures 12 and 13 that the orderly progression of carbohydrate breakdown can be divided conveniently into two parts: (1) down to the stage of pyruvic (or lactic) acid and (2) the reactions below pyruvic acid. The first stage is characterized by the phosphorylation of a glucose unit (as such or from glycogen) to hexose-1:6-diphosphate, which is then cleaved into a pair of phosphorylated three-carbon-atom units. At this point the first oxidative step occurs via DPN. Then the molecule is rearranged, loses its phosphate, and emerges as pyruvic acid. The over-all reaction up to this point can be expressed as shown in [A] below.

It should be noted that two molecules of ATP were used for phosphorylation but that four molecules were formed as a result of the oxidation of phosphoglyceraldehyde and the dephosphorylation of phosphopyruvic acid, respectively. This gain in ATP represents the useful energy of glycolysis, as will be discussed in detail later. Meanwhile two

---

[A]

$$C_6H_{12}O_6 + 2(\text{ATP}) + 2(\text{DPN}) \rightarrow 2(CH_3\cdot CO\cdot COOH) + 4(\text{ATP}) + 2(\text{DPN}\cdot H_2)$$

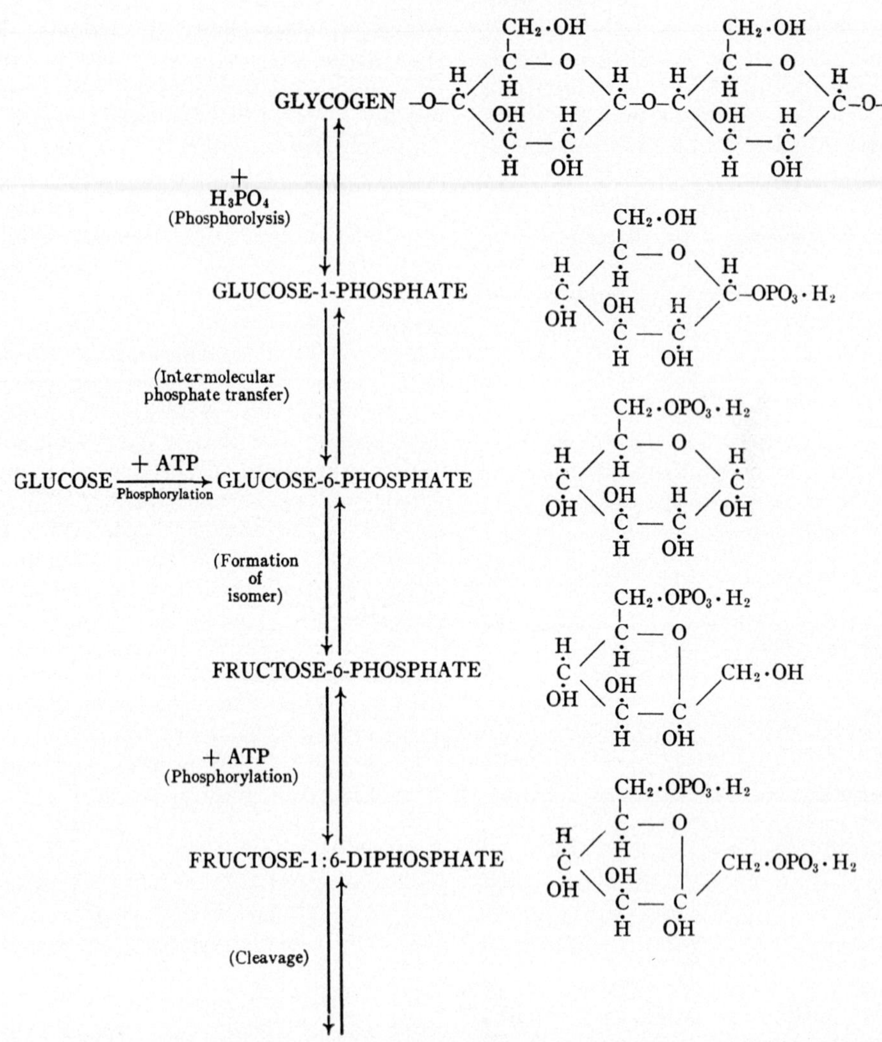

FIG. 12. Intermediary steps to pyruvic acid.

molecules of DPN have been reduced, and in order to function again these must be reoxidized. In the presence of sufficient oxygen this is probably accomplished by a flavoprotein. When oxygen is lacking, the pyruvic acid accepts the hydrogen of the DPN·H_2 and is thereby reduced to lactic acid. These two alternatives may be indicated as in [A] below. Thus it is clear that lactic acid is not an obligatory intermediate of carbohydrate metabolism. But the breakdown of hexoses to lactic acid (glycolysis) can produce useful energy and can sustain cell functions during short periods of relative or absolute anoxia.

Because of the many alternative pathways which exist below pyruvic acid, the course of its breakdown to CO_2 and H_2O is far more complex than the degradation of glucose to pyruvate. Only the more important pathways are indicated in Figure 13. The orientation toward one or another path at a particular time will be determined by the

---

[A]

(1) 2(DPN·H_2) + Flavin + Cytochrome, etc. + $O_2 \rightarrow$ 2(DPN) + $2H_2O$
(2) 2(DPN·H_2) + $2CH_3$·CO·COOH $\rightarrow$ 2(DPN) + $2CH_3$·CHOH·COOH

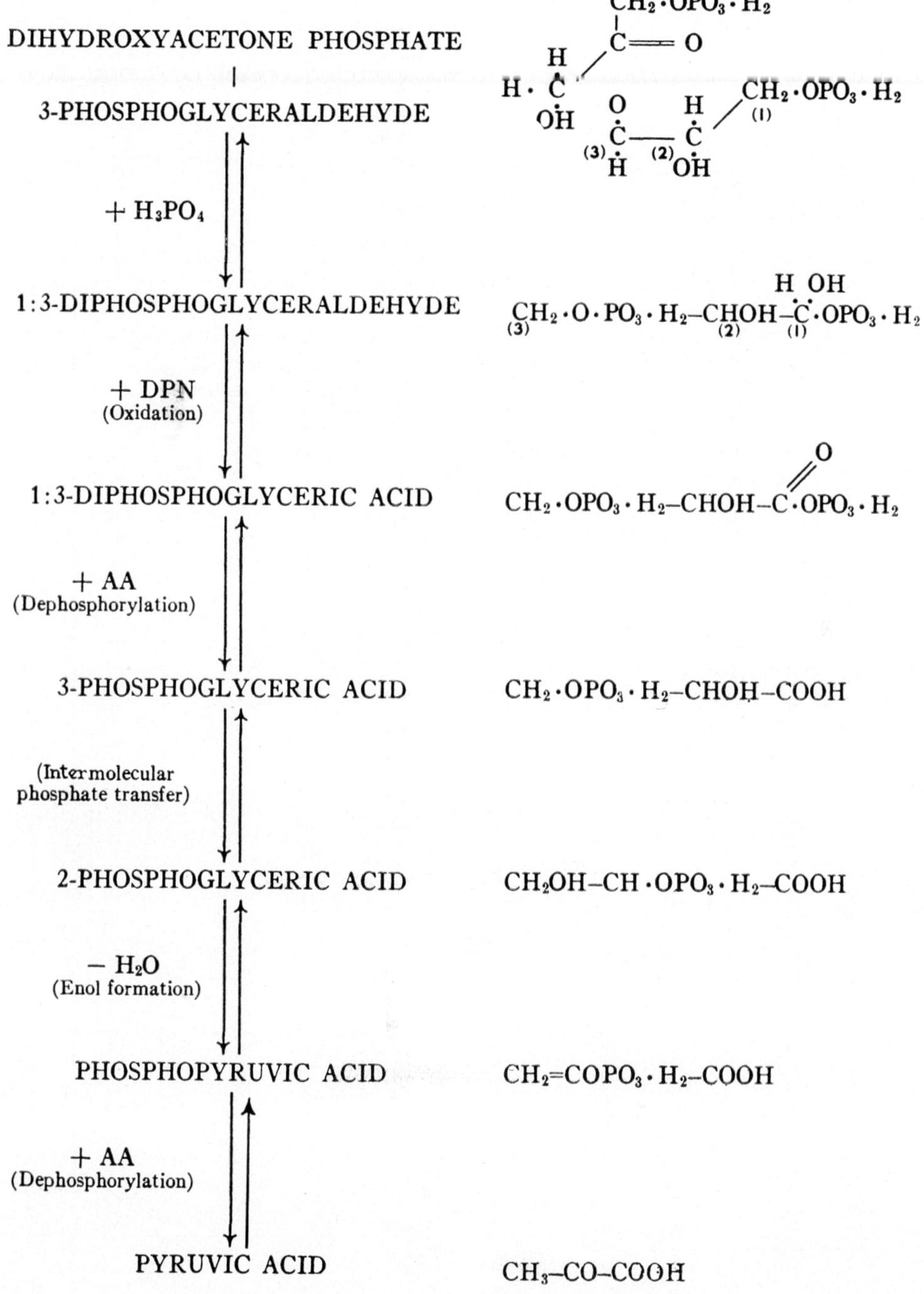

FIG. 12. Intermediary steps to pyruvic acid (*continued*). (Soskin and Levine: Carbohydrate Metabolism, Univ. of Chicago Press.)

equilibrium conditions, availability of catalysts, etc. Despite this confusing multiplicity there has emerged a principal scheme of pyruvate breakdowns to $CO_2 + H_2O$ which is logically consistent and which helps to integrate the separate metabolism of the three major foodstuffs.

This scheme, the so-called "tricarboxylic acid cycle," envisages the formation of a six-carbon-atom acid (citric) by the condensation of a two-carbon-atom frag-

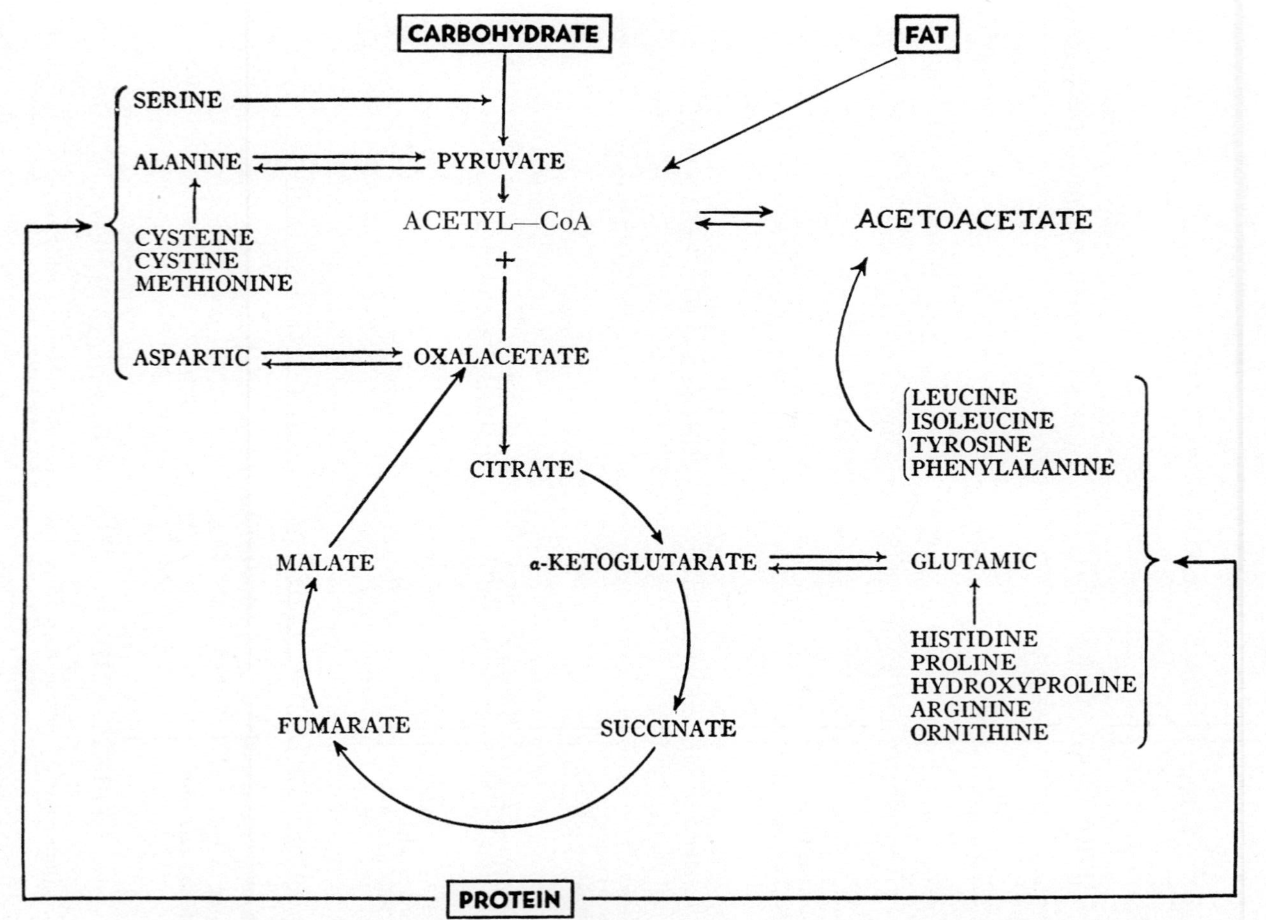

FIG. 13. The final common pathway of metabolism. (Soskin and Levine: Carbohydrate Metabolism, Univ. of Chicago Press.)

ment (acetyl CoA) derived from pyruvate with one molecule of oxalacetate. The oxalacetate is itself formed from pyruvate by the addition of CO_2 or by the deamination of aspartic acid. The citrate formed goes through a cycle of oxidations and decarboxylations until one molecule of oxalacetate is regenerated. The latter can then start the cycle off again. It will be noted that the cycle begins with one molecule of oxalacetate and one of pyruvate and ends with one molecule of oxalacetate. In other words, in one revolution of the cycle a molecule of pyruvate has been dissimilated. The exact mechanism of these steps is not completely understood, but there is evidence that many of the oxidative steps involved are coupled with phosphorylation, so that ATP is formed.

THE FINAL COMMON PATHWAY OF METABOLISM

The tricarboxylic acid cycle assumes a significance far beyond its function in carbohydrate breakdown. The catabolisms of carbohydrate, protein and fat respectively pursue more or less independent courses until they reach the stage of the alpha or beta-acids. These keto-acids (pyruvic, ketoglutaric, acetoacetic, etc.) then enter the tricarboxylic acid cycle directly, or are broken down to a two-carbon-atom fragment ("acetyl CoA") which enters the cycle by condensing with oxalacetate (Fig. 13). From this point on, the lower intermediates of all three foodstuffs are indistinguishable from each other; and from this "pool" of two-carbon and three-carbon intermediates, any of the three foodstuffs can be built up again. Hence, the cycle is probably the final common pathway for carbohydrate, protein, and fat, as well as the locus for interconversions between the three foodstuffs (Fig. 13). With this in mind, much of the older controversy as to the interconvertibility of the foodstuffs, (e.g., fat to carbohydrate) becomes pointless.

ALTERNATIVE PATHWAYS

While the overwhelming mass of evidence supports the metabolic scheme outlined above, there are strong indications that alternative pathways may exist. For example, in certain lower animal forms (fungi and bacteria), glucose may break down without the intercession of phosphorylations. Nonphosphorylative glycolysis does not seem to be significant in vertebrate tissues so far as they have been examined. On the other hand, there is evidence that glucose may be partially oxidized by a pathway which connects with the ordinary glycolytic scheme, as shown in Figure 14. This pathway would account for hexose ⇄ pentose transformations and may represent, in organs such as liver, a significant portion of hexose turnover.[33] It has been shown that com-

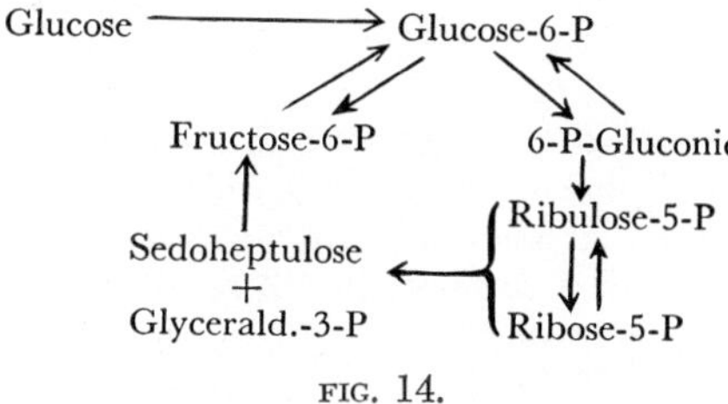

FIG. 14.

plete oxidation proceeds unhampered in the presence of special inhibitors which stop glycolysis completely. Although the alternative pathway has not been established, there is some evidence to support the theory that hexose-6-phosphate may be oxidized directly.

PATHWAYS FOR FRUCTOSE AND GALACTOSE

It has been shown for many years that the animal body can and does transform fructose and galactose to glucose and glycogen. It has also been apparent that certain organs and tissues are able to produce these hexoses from glucose or its derivatives. However, until very recently our detailed knowledge of the enzymatic mechanisms underlying the above metabolic relationships were practically unknown.

The hexokinases of certain tissues (muscle, brain) can catalyze the formation of fructose-6-phosphate from fructose. Other tissues (especially liver) contain a specific fructokinase which leads to the formation of fructose-1-phosphate which in turn is split to trioses. The trioses may be transformed to pyruvic and lactic acids or resynthesized to fructose diphosphate. This ester proceeds, by reversal of the glycolytic steps, to glycogen, or to free glucose by the action of glucose-6-phosphatase[34] (Fig. 15).

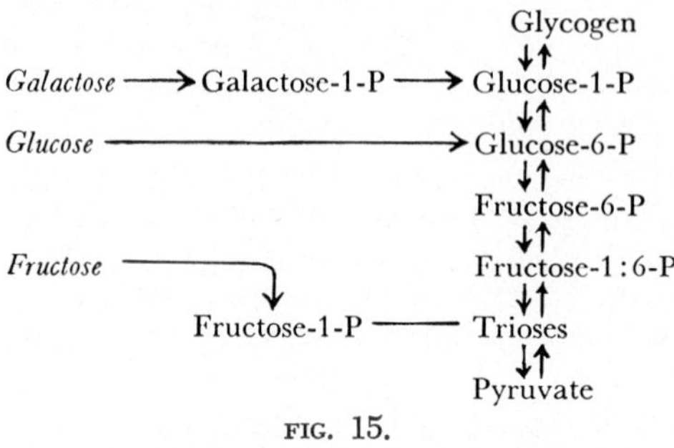

FIG. 15.

In 1938 Kosterlitz isolated galactose-1-phosphate after incubation of liver with galactose. Recently Leloir's laboratory[35] has shown that this ester is the primary phosphorylation product of galactose. They have also isolated a new enzyme system which catalyzes the conversion of galactose-1-phosphate to glucose-1-phosphate.

In the animal body galactokinase seems to be restricted to liver and kidney.

THE LIBERATION AND TRANSFER OF THE ENERGY DERIVED FROM CARBOHYDRATE BREAKDOWN

The total energy available from the complete breakdown of a molecule of a foodstuff to CO_2 and H_2O is inherent in its chemical structure. The same amount of energy would be necessary to synthesize that foodstuff from CO_2 and H_2O. Hence, the energy can be said to reside in the chemical bonds which link the atoms to form the complex molecule. Different chemical bonds vary qualitatively and quantitatively. Some bonds are more stable than others and are therefore less reactive. A substance held together largely by such bonds is one from which the energy is less available than that from substances with unstable bonds. Different chemical bonds also vary in the amounts of energy they represent. In general, the high-energy bonds tend to be the most unstable or reactive.

According to the first law of thermodynamics, no more than the total bond energy of a substance can be derived from its complete breakdown, regardless of the pathway or the number of intermediate steps through which this occurs. But common experience tells us that the form of the energy can be changed. For instance, the living organism can transform the original chemical energy of a foodstuff into mechanical energy (e.g., movement). Physiologists have long known that the body also produces electrical energy (e.g., nerve impulses). When the chemical or bond energy of a substance is released, it raises the temperature of the medium in which the chemical reaction takes place. We speak of this as a "transformation to heat." The body temperature of animals is maintained by a multitude of such reactions. There are other reactions in which the converse is true; i.e., energy has to be supplied from an outside source in order to make these reactions proceed. In the laboratory we generally supply the energy in the form of heat and call such reactions "endothermic," in contrast to the "exothermic" reactions, which give off heat. In the living organism, where temperatures are very constant, the energy necessary to make some reactions proceed is applied not as heat but as chemical or bond energy. It is therefore more precise to characterize these reactions as "endergonic" and to speak of reactions in the living organism which yield energy as being "exergonic."

It is obvious that neither the total heat produced nor the total oxygen consumed by the body during a given period of time can give any insight into the various forms through which the original energy has passed, nor can they indicate what bodily functions have been served. The situation is analogous to the measurement of the heat produced by an electric-light bulb made of opaque glass and of unspecified internal construction. From the total heat given off one could calculate the amount of electric current which must have been used by the bulb, and perhaps also the amount of coal which it must have taken to produce that much electrical energy. But one could not tell the amount of light present inside the bulb.

The Energy-transfer Function of Phosphate Groups

It is now known that the various phosphorylations which occur throughout the dissimilation of carbohydrate are the means by which the energy liberated from oxidative steps is prevented from being dissipated as heat and is held or built up for use in endergonic reactions. Different phosphorylations carry different amounts of energy and are, therefore, suitable for motivating different kinds of endergonic reactions.[36,37] According to the amount of energy transferred, we speak of high-energy or of low-energy phosphate compounds or bonds. Inorganic phosphate is, of course, at the lowest energy level. The high-energy phosphate bonds (8,000–10,000 cal/mol) are present in such compounds as adenosine triphosphate (ATP), creatine phosphate, acetyl phosphate, phosphopyruvic, etc. As an example of how a high-energy phosphate bond performs its function, let us consider the manner in which glucose is transformed into glycogen, a carbohydrate of higher potential energy than its precursor. A superficial representation of the chemical steps between glucose and glycogen might be written as indicated in [A] below. From an energetic standpoint this reaction by itself is impossible, since it requires the addition of energy to raise glucose to the energy level of glycogen, and there is no indication whence this energy is derived. These reactions can be made to proceed in vitro by adding certain protein enzymes and ATP. The energy which drives the reactions is derived from the high-energy phosphate bonds in the ATP. The latter loses its labile phosphates, becoming adenylic acid in the process.

Since the amount of ATP present in living cells is limited, the more complete story of the series of reactions in the living organism must include the manner in which adenylic acid is rephosphorylated to ATP. This may occur in more than one way, but an important means is through the energy liberated by the oxidation of 3-phosphoglyceraldehyde to 1:3 phosphoglyceric acid. The energy made available by the oxidation of the aldehyde to the acid is incorporated in a high-energy phosphate bond in the acid, in a sense, therefore, we may say that the oxidative energy has raised the inorganic phosphate involved in the reaction to a higher energy level. The ultimate use of the original oxidative energy, applied through ATP, is to raise the lower-energy foodstuff (glucose) to the higher-energy storage product (glycogen). At the latter point the phosphate group involved in the series of reactions is divorced from the substrate and may re-enter the cycle at the beginning.

The raising of glucose to the energy level of glycogen is only one of the functions which ATP performs. Indeed, the reversible systems AA $\rightleftharpoons$ ADP $\rightleftharpoons$ ATP seem to be the central mechanisms for energy transfer from exergonic to endergonic reactions in carbohydrate metabolism. Figure 16 summarizes their relationships to all the known energy cycles.

Because of its high-energy phosphate bonds, some authors have ascribed to creatine phosphate a role similar to that indicated for ATP. It now seems more likely that the latter is not the case but that creatine phosphate acts as an emergency store of high-energy phosphate bonds. This store is built up at times when the AA $\rightleftharpoons$ ATP systems are producing an excess of energy over the requirements of the moment and is broken down when the ATP mechanisms cannot supply energy as rapidly as is re-

---

[A]

Glucose $\rightarrow$ Glucose-6-phosphate $\rightleftarrows$ Glucose-1-phosphate $\rightleftarrows$ Glycogen

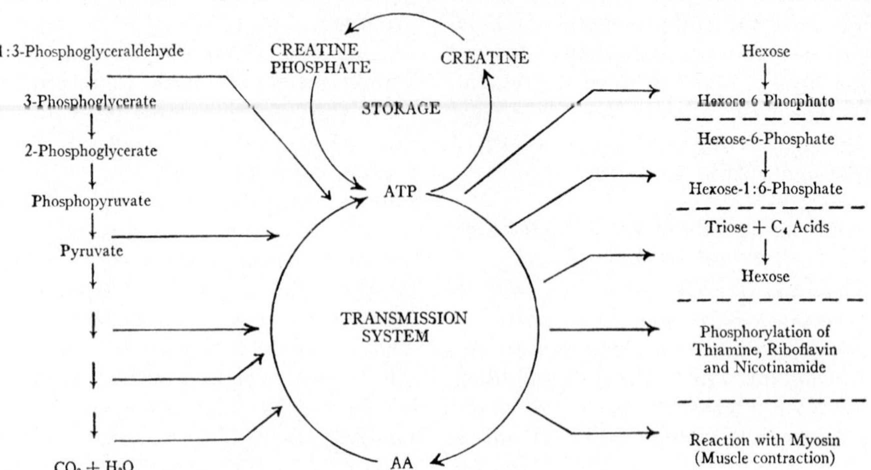

FIG. 16. Central position of the adenylic system in energy transfer. (Soskin and Levine: Carbohydrate Metabolism, Univ. of Chicago Press.)

quired. Thus, creatine phosphate stands in the same relationship to the storage of energy as glycogen stands in relation to the storage of carbohydrate substrate.

Finally, it should be noted that the transference of energy by means of phosphate bonds accounts for the ready reversibility of most of the reactions of carbohydrate metabolism. This is because the energy which is yielded by substrate remains "attached" to the product of the reaction and is therefore not lost from the system. For example, the hydrolytic splitting of glycogen by amylase produces glucose and liberates energy as heat. The analogous phosphorolytic cleavage of glycogen in the body produces glucose-1-phosphate, with the energy retained in the phosphate bond. Here, no outside energy is necessary to reverse the process.

Since we do not, as yet, possess a detailed knowledge of all or most phosphate-energy transfer reactions, the efficiency of this mechanism can be judged only approximately. It has been estimated that, during the complete dissimilation of 1 mol. of glucose to CO_2 and H_2O, about 38 high-energy phosphate bonds are formed. The energy content of these phosphate bonds is, therefore, $(38 \times 8000) = 304{,}000$ cal. Since 1 mol. of glucose going to CO_2 and H_2O yields 680,000 cal., the energy transferred by means of phosphate bonds represents about 45 per cent of the total. It is interesting to compare these figures with that of the efficiency of muscular work, which is generally considered to be about 30 per cent.

THE USE OF ENERGY FOR MUSCULAR CONTRACTION

The contractile element responsible for the shortening and elongation by which muscle performs its physiologic function is actomyosin, a complex formed by two proteins, myosin and actin. Actomyosin is present in the form of elongated, threadlike structures called "muscle fibrils." These are microscopic in size. A bundle of fibrils, composed of large numbers in parallel formation, constitutes a muscle fiber. The gross structure of a muscle is composed of aggregates of fibers. The myosin of the muscle fibrils represents approximately half of the total muscle protein.

The Chemical Events Accompanying Muscle Contraction

The first chemical changes to be related to the change in the physical state of the muscle during contraction were the breakdown of glycogen and the appearance of lactic acid. Lundsgaard's demonstration that contraction of muscle was possible in the presence of iodoacetate, which prevented lactic acid formation, forced the abandonment of this hypothesis. He further demonstrated a parallelism between the breakdown of creatine phosphate and the energy liberated by the iodoacetate-treated muscle. This led to the hypothesis that the immediate source of energy for muscular contraction was the breakdown of creatine phosphate, while the glycolytic process served to resynthesize the creatine phosphate from its split products.

The current conception of the means by which metabolic energy is applied to the muscle fibrils was initiated by the work of Lohman, who showed that adenosine triphosphate (ATP) was necessary both for glycolysis in muscle and for the synthesis of creatine phosphate. This was followed by Parnas' demonstration that the breakdown of creatine phosphate merely served to supply phosphate for the conversion of adenylic acid to ATP, without the liberation of energy, while the subsequent breakdown of the ATP actually supplied the energy for contraction and the phosphate for glycolysis. The glycolytic reactions, in turn, provided the energy for the resynthesis of both creatine phosphate and ATP.

It may be seen that, as our knowledge of the subject has developed, the breakdown of glycogen to lactic acid has been gradually relegated to a secondary process with a restorative function. As a matter of fact, the most recent evidence indicates that, under ordinary physiologic conditions, glycogen breaks down without the appearance of lactic acid at all. When the rate of oxygen supply to the muscle is adequate for the rate of glycogen breakdown, pyruvic acid is oxidized completely and none of it is reduced to lactic acid. Under these conditions, oxidative steps above and below pyruvic acid supply energy for the rephosphorylation of ATP and thus maintain the metabolic cycle in the absence of lactic acid. It is only when the oxygen supply is inadequate (as it was in most of the experiments of the earlier investigators) that lactic acid appears. This occurs because pyruvic acid partially substitutes for oxygen by becoming the hydrogen acceptor from reduced DPN and, in so doing, is itself reduced to lactic acid.

In a sense, therefore, the formation of lactic acid by muscle is merely an emergency mechanism enabling muscular contractions to occur, for a short time, despite a lack of oxygen. This may be useful at the beginning of sudden or severe muscular work, to tide the muscle over a period of circulatory adjustment, that is, while the blood supply is changing from the slow rate adequate during rest to the more rapid rate necessitated by the exertion. It also enables the muscle to exert a relatively tremendous effort for a short space of time, at a rate with which the maximal rate of oxygen supply could never cope. The lactic acid which accumulates during such an effort is reoxidized to pyruvic acid when the exertion is over. This process may be regarded as the repayment, during comparative leisure, of an energy debt contracted under stress.

Figure 17 graphically illustrates the development of our concepts concerning the sequence of chemical events which occur during muscular contraction.

The Connection between the Physical and Chemical Events in Muscle Contraction

Thus far, we have merely described the chemical events which occur coincidentally with muscular contraction. It remained for Engelhardt to demonstrate the direct causal link between the chemical reactions and the change in the physical state of the myosin.[38,39] By injecting a thin stream of purified myosin preparation into water, Engelhardt was able to make threads of myosin analogous to muscle fibrils and possessing similar elastic properties. When suitably weighted and suspended in water, these myosin threads were not affected by the presence of the various mineral and organic substances normally found in mammalian muscle. But the addition of

I

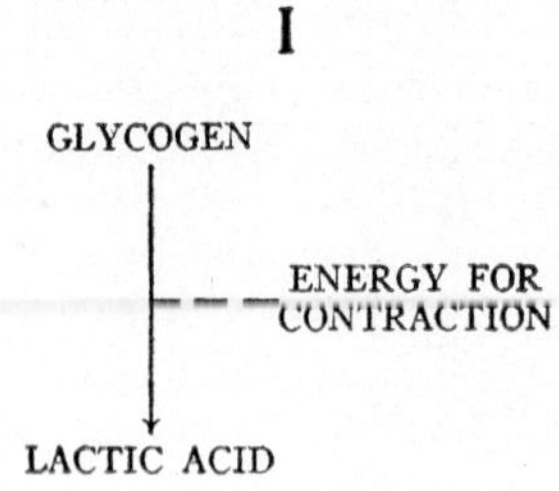

II

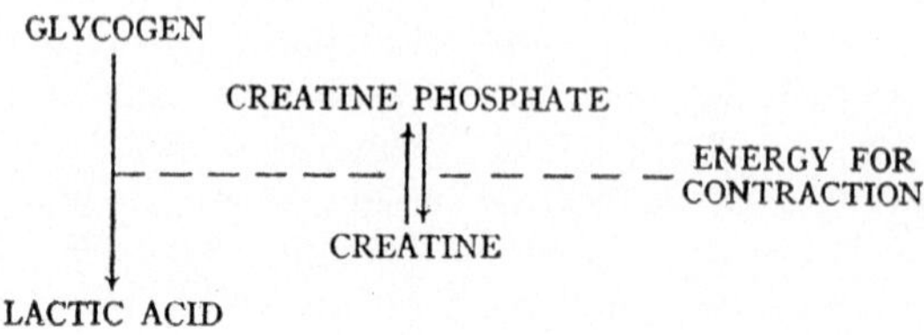

III

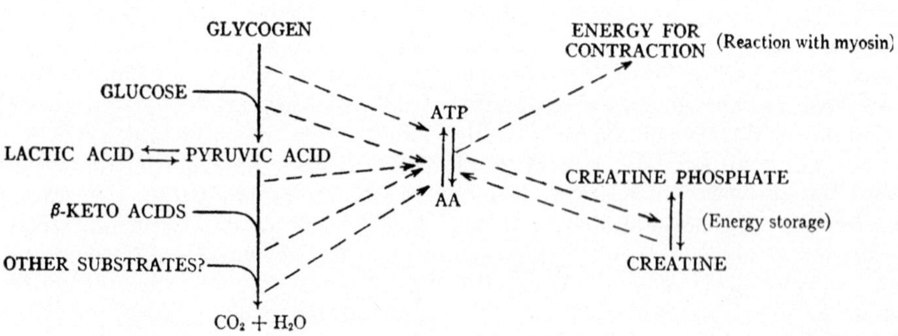

FIG. 17. Development of concepts of the chemistry of muscular contraction. *I:* Hopkins-Meyerhof hypothesis: *II:* Lundsgaard modification; *III:* current scheme indicating the secondary role of lactic acid, the central position of the adenylic system, the energy-storage function of creatine phosphate, and the use of energy in ATP by myosin. (Soskin and Levine: Carbohydrate Metabolism, Univ. of Chicago Press.)

ATP to the water was followed by a definite increase in the length of the threads, which could be reversed by flushing away the ATP.

Szent-Györgyi and his co-workers confirmed Engelhardt's work and extended it into a more complete analogy of in vivo muscular contraction. They found that a purer preparation of myosin than that used by Engelhardt would not form threads when injected into water. But when another muscle protein (which they named "actine") was added to the myosin, the compound behaved like Engelhardt's preparation. They named this complex "actomyosin" and found that threads formed from it could be made to extend or contract at will by varying the proportions of ATP, potassium, and magnesium added to the water in which they were suspended.[40]

The extremely simple conditions of Engelhardt's and Szent-Györgyi's experiments leave no doubt that ATP is the prime agent concerned in muscle contraction. The peculiar appropriateness of ATP for this purpose lies in the fact that it had previously been shown that myosin is an enzyme which can split ATP $\rightarrow$ ADP + P^o. For the time being, we may therefore accept the current scheme shown in Figure 17 as representing the cycle of events by which metabolic energy derived from the utilization of carbohydrate is transferred by ATP and applied to the contractile elements of the muscle. The train of reactions is such that both the original physical state of the muscle and the original amount of ATP are restored subsequent to contraction.

It is evident from our present conception that any metabolic intermediate which can supply the energy necessary to restore AA to ATP can serve as a fuel of muscular exercise. This applies to the alpha and beta-ketoacids derived from protein and fat as well as to carbohydrate derivatives.

The Fuel of Muscular Exercise. In his exhaustive review of the subject, Gemmill[41] has aptly reviewed the situation as regards the fuel of muscular exercise as follows:

"From the survey of the literature it is obvious that the use of carbohydrate is of primary importance as a fuel for muscular exercise in man. The evidence comes from the slight increase in efficiency on a carbohydrate diet, the prolongation of muscular effort when carbohydrate is ingested, the fall in blood sugar during long continued muscular exercise and the production of lactate at the beginning of exercise and during severe exercise. The evidence that protein is used during exercise indicates that it is of secondary importance, probably to supply carbohydrate or carbohydrate intermediates. The results of experiments on fat utilization during muscular work have demonstrated that this substance is used indirectly. There is no experimental evidence at the present time for the direct utilization of fat by mammalian muscle. However, the indirect utilization of protein or fat must be an efficient process, since the exclusive feeding of these substances to man does not have a marked effect on muscular efficiency during short periods of exercise."

However, since Gemmill's review was written some evidence has been brought forward to indicate that fatty acids can be oxidized by the liverless animals,[42] and by muscle extract in vitro. But whether this occurs in intact muscle or to what extent it occurs in relation to the total caloric expenditure has not been determined. As a matter of fact, the work on the whole animal was done under resting conditions so that the peripheral oxidation of fat observed may have no bearing as regards the fact of muscular exercise.

Hence it is still necessary to conclude that carbohydrate is the most readily useful fuel of muscular exercise, and the significance of the foregoing from the standpoint of nutrition is obvious. If carbohydrate is not available in foods, it must be made by the body from those materials which are in the diet, in order to satisfy the fuel requirements of the active tissues. The eating of adequate amounts of carbohydrate therefore spares the body the work of making it. This role of carbohydrate is naturally more important during moderate or severe muscular exertion than when the body is at rest. The great demand for fuel accompanying muscular exercise may rapidly exhaust the carbohydrate store. This is evidenced by a decrease in glycogen content of the liver and muscles and, if the exertion is sufficiently severe and prolonged, may result in an abnormal lowering of the blood-sugar level. These phenomena are accompanied by increased breakdown of body protein (which is reflected in an increased excretion of nitrogen in the urine) and by an accelerated breakdown of body fat (as evidenced by a rise of the level of ketone bodies in blood and urine). When violent exercise is preceded or accompanied by a large intake of carbohydrate, the body works somewhat more efficiently, as judged by the calories expended per unit of oxygen intake. The increased nitrogen excretion and ketone formation are also minimized. The latter two effects of carbohydrate are examples of its protein-sparing and its antiketogenic actions.

The Efficiency of Carbohydrate as a Fuel. It has been noted above that carbohydrate is a more efficient fuel for muscular exercise than either protein or fat. This does not imply that portions of the protein or fat molecules are wasted when they are used. It does mean that the protein and fat molecules, when used as fuel, yield less than their total caloric value in the form which can be used by muscle. The remainder is used for the conversion of these molecules into suitable fuel. These conversions occur largely in the liver, which supplies the other organs with fuel by way of the blood stream.

Since the amount of glycogen present in the muscle at any one time is sufficient for only short periods of work, the carbohydrate used by the muscle must eventually come from the blood sugar. The glycogen within the muscle cells may be reasonably supposed to serve best in emergencies, when the muscle is unable to draw sugar from the blood as quickly as needed. But, as a matter of fact, glycogen is more than merely a conveniently packaged form of carbohydrate lying on the pantry shelf. It is now known that more energy is derivable from a certain amount of glycogen than from an equivalent amount of blood sugar. It requires a certain amount of energy to bring the blood sugar into the metabolic system of the muscle (as hexose-6-phosphate), and therefore all the energy inherent in the glucose is not available for useful work. On the other hand, the breakdown of glycogen to the same stage does not require the addition of energy and hence makes all its inherent energy quickly available. This is not to say that one gets something for nothing from glycogen, for some energy was required to build up the glycogen in the first place. But this energy was expended during a quiescent period when plenty of it was available.

The application of these physiologic facts to clinical phenomena is exemplified by the greater stores of glycogen and of phosphate esters found in the muscles of animals which have been trained to perform prolonged work. This probably also applies to the physical abilities of manual laborers and of athletes. Conversely, the characteristically low muscle-glycogen levels found in poorly controlled diabetic patients and in hyperthyroid individuals are accompanied by muscular weakness.

SITE OF ORIGIN OF BLOOD SUGAR

It is well established that, in the fasting animal, the liver is virtually the sole source of the blood sugar. There is some recent evidence that the kidney may contribute sugar to the blood, but in amounts that are hardly significant in relation to the total carbohydrate requirements of the normal intact animal.[43] The other tissues of the body continually require and use the blood sugar for the maintenance of their metabolism and functions. Since the blood-sugar level is well maintained throughout long periods of fasting, it is evident that the sugar which the liver secretes into the blood under these conditions must be derived from stored carbohydrate or noncarbohydrate precursors.

The brilliant pioneer work of Claude Bernard was the first to indicate the predominant role of the liver in supplying blood sugar and to demonstrate the existence of liver glycogen. His early reports claimed that, in fasting animals or those fed on meat, the blood entering the liver through the portal vein contained no sugar. Repetition of these experiments by some of his contemporaries led to disagreement and controversy, for they found sugar in the portal vein blood. As it turned out, the reasons for these differences lay in the then inadequate knowledge concerning the proper handling of blood samples and the crude methods for sugar analysis. Bernard and his contemporaries eventually agreed that, while sugar was constantly present in the portal blood, there was always more sugar in the blood leaving the liver.

Claude Bernard also demonstrated that a liver flushed free of sugar by perfusion with cold water acquired a high sugar content after a few hours in the laboratory. He recognized the starch-like nature of the precursor of this sugar and called it "glycogen." He confirmed Chauveau in the finding that the sugar of arterial blood throughout the body was higher than that of venous blood.

On the basis of these essential facts and a number of other observations, Bernard arrived at the following conception, which is as valid today as when he enunciated it:

"In the liver sugar is produced, although a little is also destroyed in that organ; in the muscles sugar is destroyed. Destruction of sugar probably occurs throughout the organism, in all the organs, in all the tissues . . . The normal blood sugar level is the result of a precise equilibrium between the processes of anabolism (assimilation) and catabolism (dissimilation)."

The Evidence Derived from the Liverless Animal

The obvious crucial test for the existence of the balanced rates of production and consumption of sugar responsible for the maintenance of the normal blood-sugar level was to remove the supposed source of the sugar and to observe whether or not the blood sugar progressively diminished as it was utilized. Such observations were made by Bernard's contemporaries and by a series of investigators in later years. The results were uniform in demonstrating the development of hypoglycemia following hepatectomy or total abdominal evisceration of birds and mammals. However, there was some uncertainty as to the quantitative aspects of the results in mammals because of the technical difficulty of the operative procedures involved in total removal of the liver.

The work of Mann and collaborators finally established the liver as the prime factor for the maintenance of the normal blood-sugar level. The presence of appreciable quantities of glycogen in the muscles of their hepatectomized dogs during profound hypoglycemia led them to conclude that muscle glycogen is incapable of sufficiently rapid conversion of glucose to play a significant role in maintaining the blood-sugar level.[44] This conclusion was confirmed and extended by Soskin,[45] who demonstrated that the known hyperglycemic agents—

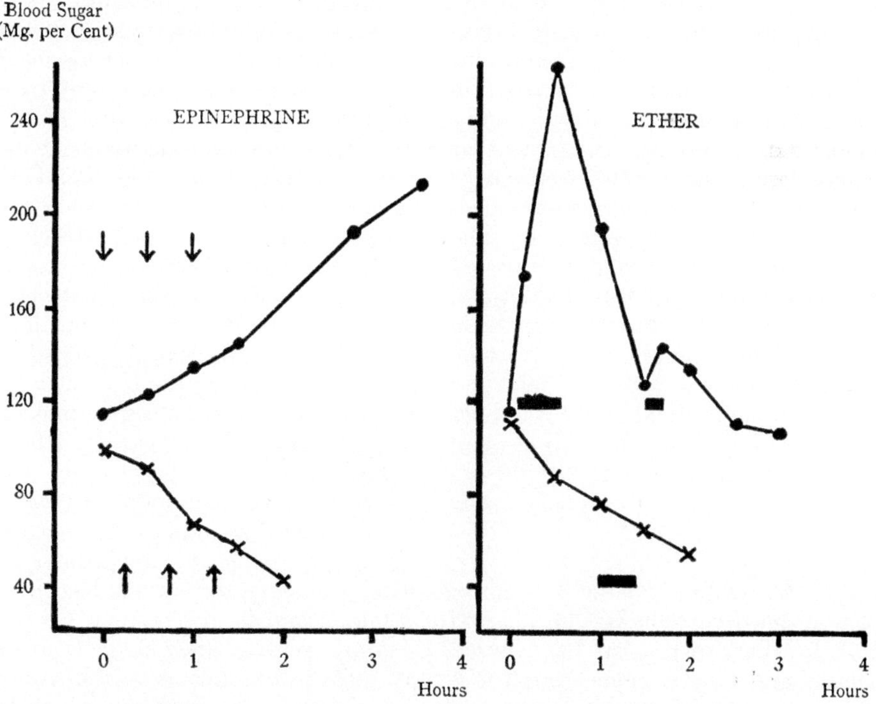

FIG. 18. The influence of epinephrine administration (↑ ↑ ↑) and of ether anesthesia (■ ■) on the blood-sugar level of normal intact dogs (·—·—·), and the lack of influence of these agents on the falling blood-sugar level of the same dogs after hepatectomy (×—×—×).

epinephrine, ether anesthesia, and asphyxia—have no influence whatever on the falling blood-sugar level of liverless dogs. More recently, Houssay and his associates have found a similar absence of the hyperglycemic action of extracts of the anterior pituitary gland in hepatectomized toads and dogs. Soskin concluded that muscle glycogen is not an available source of blood sugar in the absence of the liver and that the liver is the sole source of supply of glucose for the blood in the fasting organism. Figure 18 shows the characteristically rapid and progressive fall in the blood-sugar level of dogs after removal of the abdominal viscera, including the liver. It also shows the lack of effect of hyperglycemic agents on the rate of fall in the blood sugar, in contrast to the hyperglycemic effects of these agents on the same animals with intact livers.

Tissue enzyme chemists have since demonstrated the biochemical reasons for uniqueness of the liver (and the kidney, to some extent) in being able to liberate free glucose into the blood. All tissues are able to take glucose from the blood by converting it to glucose-6-phosphate. But under the conditions which exist in the tissues this reaction is not reversible. Hence the only pathways for the glucose are through other phosphorylative steps. However, liver and kidney contain a phosphate which can split glucose-6-phosphate to free glucose and inorganic phosphate, and this enzyme accounts for the special ability of liver and kidney.[46] It has been shown that this phosphatase is specific and is not identical with the acid and alkaline phosphatases, also found in liver and kidney and some other tissues, and which have been shown to be able to hydrolyze a variety of phosphate esters in vitro.

The Lactic Acid Cycle

The evidence which has been cited also shows that, once sugar has entered the peripheral tissues, even though it is stored rather than used, it cannot reenter the blood as glucose. This, of course, is in accord with what is known of the enzyme systems in skeletal muscle. However, under special circumstances, significant amounts of carbohydrate can leave the muscle in altered form, as when lactic acid accumulates in the muscle and diffuses into the blood stream. This occurs during a relative or absolute deficiency in the oxygen supply to the muscle. At such times the lactic acid may be carried to the liver and converted into hepatic glycogen, and thus eventually reappear as blood sugar. This so-called "lactic acid cycle" has been investigated and elaborated by Geiger, Himwich, Cori, and others. But it is fair to say that, while it constitutes a possible indirect source for some blood sugar during abnormal or emergency conditions, it is of little or no significance as regards the blood-sugar supply under normal conditions.

Special Functions of Carbohydrate in the Liver. Aside from its use as fuel in the liver, carbohydrate in this organ has protective and detoxifying actions and a regulating influence on protein and fat metabolism.

The liver of a well-fed normal animal contains a high percentage of glycogen, as compared to any other tissue. It is known that such a liver is more resistant to various types of noxious agents than one which has been deprived of its glycogen by starvation or disease. This has been shown in animals for such various types of poisons as carbon tetrachloride, alcohol or arsenic and in man for a variety of diseases accompanied by toxemias of bacterial origin. The defenses of the liver against toxic agents are of great importance to the body as a whole, for it is one of the chief functions of this organ to remove or destroy such toxins before they reach other vital tissues, which are not equipped to deal with them. From this point of view, the maintenance of a high glycogen level in the liver is an essential for the health of the whole organism.

More definite knowledge is available as regards the role of carbohydrate in specific chemical reactions which transform certain poisons into relatively innocuous substances. One such mechanism is the conjugation of glucuronic acid derived from carbohydrate with poisons which possess a hydroxyl group. Indeed, this mechanism is one of the means by which the body regulates its steroid hormone metabolism and protects itself from the harm which could result from an excess of the sex hormones. It is also possible that the carcinogenic substances of the steroid type might be disposed of in the same manner. Another hepatic mechanism is the acetylation of such substances as p-aminobenzoic acid and sulfanilamide. In this type of conjugation the acetyl groups are derived from carbohydrate and fat via pyruvate and acetyl phosphate. The rates of glucuronate formation and of acetylation have been shown to depend directly upon the concentration of carbohydrate in the liver.

The protein-sparing action of carbohydrate has already been mentioned. This action occurs partly in the liver, for it is this organ which is primarily responsible for the deamination of amino acids. Up to the point of deamination the fate of amino acids in metabolism has not been finally determined. They may be used as building blocks from which to form proteins for the repair or growth of tissues, or they may be broken down for use as fuel. Once deamination has occurred, the amino acids are divorced from protein metabolism. The amino group is converted to urea and excreted, while the non-nitrogenous fraction is either used as a source of energy or converted to carbohydrate or fat.* The rate of deamination in the liver decreases as the available carbohydrate increases. An ample supply of carbohydrate thus conserves the products of protein breakdown in a form which may be used by the body to build or maintain its own protein structure. To put it in another way, a minimal intake of protein which may be adequate for the body's needs when taken together with good amounts of carbohydrate, may become inadequate when the carbohydrate intake is deficient. It has been shown by Geiger[47] that for optimal protein sparing, carbohydrate and protein should be ingested simultaneously or within a short time of each other. Otherwise the amino acids will be largely deaminated.

The availability of carbohydrate to the liver also determines how much fat is broken down by this organ. There is no direct index of the rate of fat metabolism in the liver, for, unlike protein metabolism, fat metabolism is not accompanied by the excretion of a characteristic end-product in the urine. However, it happens that fatty acids are not completely metabolized by the liver and that the end-products of fatty-acid metabolism in this organ are the so-called "ketone bodies": beta-hydroxybutyric and acetoacetic acids. These ketone bodies must then go to the peripheral tissues for complete oxidation. Ordinarily the rate of breakdown of fat and of the formation of ketone bodies is such that the latter are promptly disposed of by the peripheral tissues, so that no significant amounts appear in the blood or urine. But when fatty-acid breakdown becomes excessively rapid and the rate of ketone formation in the liver begins to exceed the rate of disposal by the peripheral tissues, there begins to occur an accumulation of the ketone bodies in the blood and an excretion of these substances in the urine (ketosis). Under these circumstances in an otherwise normal animal the administration of carbohydrate causes a prompt disappearance of the ketone bodies (antiketogenic action). With the protein-sparing action of carbohydrate, its antiketogenic action serves to regulate the proportion of the different foodstuffs which are prepared by the liver for use as fuel by the peripheral tissues.

In discussing the special functions of carbohydrate in the liver we have referred both to its "glycogen content" and to the "availability" of carbohydrate to this organ. These terms may or may not be synonymous, for it is still not known whether sugar may be used directly by the liver cells or must first be

* Under certain circumstances the non-nitrogenous fraction may also be reaminated and restored as an amino acid.

built up to glycogen. In any case, the glycogen content of the liver is a good index of the amount of carbohydrate which is available to the hepatic cells; and from a nutritional standpoint it is important to remember that carbohydrate is the foodstuff which leads to the highest levels of liver glycogen. Fairly good glycogen stores in the liver can be obtained when protein is predominant in the diet, while a high fat diet results in a liver which is poor in glycogen. The medical uses of the high carbohydrate diet or of the intravenous administration of dextrose solution are directed toward the protection of the liver by insuring rich glycogen stores. Protein has been used with the same ultimate purpose in mind, but it is less effective, probably in proportion to its convertibility to sugar.

Carbohydrate and the Heart. The previous discussion of carbohydrate as the most efficient fuel of muscular exercise, and of the muscle glycogen as an important emergency source of contractile energy, applies in even greater measure to cardiac muscle than it does to skeletal muscle. The latter can in some measure accommodate itself to a decreased supply of carbohydrate by decreasing its work. The heart cannot stop to rest. A temporary reduction in the supply of sugar to the normal heart (as in induced attacks of hypoglycemia) has little apparent effect on the organ, although a definite change in the electrocardiogram may be noted. The apparent lack of influence of hypoglycemia on the normal heart may be due to the good glycogen stores to be found there. But, in the heart which is damaged by disease and in which the initial glycogen stores are poor, hypoglycemia may precipitate stenocardial symptoms with angina and may even result in death.

The Indispensability of Carbohydrate to the Central Nervous System. Of all the organs and tissues in the body, the central nervous system is most dependent upon the minute-by-minute supply of glucose from the blood. In connection with the discussion on the fuel of muscular exercise it was stated that carbohydrate was of primary importance, while protein and fat could be used only indirectly. As regards the central nervous system, it has been well established that only carbohydrate can be used. The need of nerve tissue for glucose is even more specific than the previous statement would indicate. It is true, when slices of brain tissue are studied in vitro regarding their ability to maintain respiration at the expense of various substrates, that a number of degradation products of glucose will serve as well or better than glucose itself. However, none of these intermediates has been shown to have any ameliorating effects upon the hypoglycemic symptoms caused by lowering the blood-sugar level in vivo. In other words, glucose as such has a specific influence and is indispensable for the maintenance of the functional integrity of the nerve tissue. This may be due to the presence of the hematoencephalic barrier which does not allow the other substrates to enter the brain readily. When the blood sugar is lowered in a living organism, those tissues which have ample stores of glycogen may use the latter to tide them over the lean period. The nervous tissue has little glycogen, and it is doubtful whether the little which is present can be mobilized for use in emergencies. The glycogen content of nervous tissue remains more or less constant under most conditions, including hyperglycemia and hypoglycemia, and may be largely an integral part of the nerve structure. The unavailability for metabolic use of the glycogen present in the nerve cells is evidenced by the dramatically rapid development of hypoglycemic symptoms when the blood sugar is lowered.

THE TRANSFORMATION OF CARBOHYDRATE INTO FAT

In the previous discussion of fat as a fuel-storage material it was pointed out that, when food in excess of caloric expenditure is ingested (whether in the form of carbohydrate, protein, or fat), the equivalent of the excess calories is deposited as fat in the adipose tissues.

With this in mind it is, strictly speaking, incorrect to label any of the foodstuffs as being particularly "fattening." Any one of them can be so if taken in sufficient quantities. But because of its proportion in the diet, its lower cost, and its use in confections, carbohydrate is quantitatively the most important precursor of fat. Lipogenesis from carbohydrate proceeds most probably via formation of acetyl CoA, which is then built up in steps of 2 C atoms to a fatty acid-CoA. This in turn is incorporated into a triglyceride by reaction of three fatty acids with glycerol. The rate of lipogenesis depends upon the availability of a factor or factors derived during the glycolytic breakdown of carbohydrates. In starvation and in diabetes lipogenesis is retarded since carbohydrate utilization is decreased. The necessary factor may play a catalytic role in the step from acetyl to butyryl-CoA.[51,52]

It has usually been thought that the transformation of carbohydrate into fat occurs exclusively in the liver. This is apparently not so; for, using C^{14} labeled glucose, Chaikoff et al.,[48] showed that the liverless animal could perform that transformation, although it occurred five times as rapidly in the presence of the liver. The exact location of the extrahepatic interconversion was not apparent from this work. One site is probably in the adipose tissue itself, as Wertheimer[49] has shown both in vivo and in vitro. According to the work of Hausberger[50] the rate of lipogenesis from carbohydrate is as high in adipose tissue as in liver.

The fat which arises from carbohydrate in the body is the so-called "hard" fat, composed, in the main, of the highly saturated palmitic and stearic acids. This is probably of more concern to stock-raisers than to human nutritionists. The former have long known that they could control the physical qualities of the fat in meats by varying the proportion of carbohydrate and of oils in the diet of their animals. Of course, carbohydrate cannot completely substitute for fat in the diet, since it does not carry with it the essential fatty acids and the fat-soluble vitamins, which cannot be manufactured by the body.

GLUCONEOGENESIS FROM PROTEIN

The literature up to the year 1930 relating to the conversion of amino acids to carbohydrate was comprehensively reviewed by Rapport.[53] The available information is derived from the following types of experiments:

In vivo:

1. Amino acids are fed to depancreatized or phlorhizinized dogs, and the urine is analyzed for the extra glucose excreted over and above the amounts excreted on previous days.
2. Amino acids are fed to starving normal animals, and the rise in liver glycogen is used as an index of transformation to carbohydrate. An increase of the ketone bodies in the blood and urine is taken as evidence of conversion of the amino acids to beta-keto acids.

Perfusion Experiments:

1. The liver is perfused with blood to which the various amino acids are added. A rise in the glucose or ketone content of the perfusing blood is taken as evidence for transformation.

In vitro:

1. Tissue slices (generally liver) are incubated in the Warburg respirometer with various amino acids; and the rise in total carbohydrate, carbohydrate intermediates, and ketone body content of the slices is measured.
2. Enzyme preparations from animal tissues are employed to follow the pathway of the intermediate metabolism of amino acids.

A critical examination of the information derived from these various kinds of investigation, reveals that few of them have any real quantitative significance. Using the glycosuria of diabetic animals as an index of gluconeogenesis from protein ignores the very considerable quantities of glucose which are utilized by the tissues and not excreted. The increase in liver glycogen which follows the feeding of protein or amino acids was not regarded as a quantitative index even by those who used this criterion. The perfusion and the in vitro experiments have yielded conflicting and contradictory results depending upon the conditions of the experiment. This is not surprising when one considers the known pathways for entry of the amino acids into the tricarboxylic acid cycle, as shown in Figure 13.

We may summarize the present knowledge by saying that, whatever its empirical usefulness, the figure of 44 to 58 per cent commonly used in metabolic and nutritional work to calculate the carbohydrate equivalent of protein is a very approximate figure. Even under the simplest conditions, using amino acids and in vitro technique, it has thus far been possible to ascertain the quantitative fate of only a few of the amino acids. Much work remains to be done in this field.

GLUCONEOGENESIS FROM FAT

The most recent work which is pertinent to the subject has involved the use of fatty acids and their derivatives, labeled with radioactive and heavy carbon (C^{13} and C^{14}) isotopes at one or more of their carbon atoms. Wood, Lorber, et al.[54,55] fed such labeled fatty acids to normal rats, then sacrificed the animals and estimated the liver glycogen. A pure glucose sample, derived from this glycogen, was then broken down in a number of ways, in order to determine the proportionate amounts of isotopic carbon at each of the six positions in the glucose molecule. They found significant amounts of isotopic carbon in the glucose, which they felt had come from the labeled fatty acid which had been fed. The distribution of the marked carbon atoms in the glucose was consistent with the hypothesis that the fatty acids broke down to two-carbon atom fragments, which entered the tricarboxylic acid cycle (TCA), and that the marked glucose was derived from constituents of the TCA cycle.

It must be recalled that with each revolution of the TCA cycle one two-carbon atom fragment enters and two CO_2 molecules are given off and that the latter are not necessarily the same carbons that entered the cycle as the two-carbon atom fragment. Hence, although the labeled carbon can be transmitted to the glucose, no net gain in carbohydrate need result from this type of conversion. For this reason Wood and Lorber[54,55] and other enzyme chemists are inclined to doubt the existence of gluconeogenesis from fat in the classic sense. However, this conclusion does not take into account other important implications of the TCA cycle.

Fatty acids represent only one source of two-carbon atom fragments for the cycle. They are also derived from protein and from carbohydrate itself. If an abundance of two-carbon atom fragments is not available from the breakdown of fatty acids, a certain amount of protein or carbohydrate or both will be broken down to CO_2 and water, to provide for the operation of the cycle, and will diminish by that amount the net gain in carbohydrate formed. Hence the breakdown of fatty acids contributes to gluconeogenesis from other precursors. This could explain the progressive fall in the urinary D:N ratios of depancreatized or phlorhizinized dogs maintained on subcaloric diets. It might also explain the impaired gluconeogenesis and low D:N ratios of hypophysectomized depancreatized dogs and equivalent preparations, which have difficulty in mobilizing fat.

From this standpoint, it is hardly correct to speak any longer of gluconeogenesis from fat or from protein. All the foodstuffs contribute lower intermediary products to the TCA cycle, and each of the foodstuffs can be regenerated in whole or in part from the cycle. When the latter occurs, it cannot be at the expense of any single other foodstuff. The situation is analogous to pouring a quantity of water into a vessel which is already brimful of water. An equivalent amount of water to that which was added will overflow, and the particular water molecules which leave the vessel need not be the molecules which were added, although the added molecules will be responsible for the overflow.

We have thus far assumed that all two-carbon atom fragments enter the TCA cycle by condensation to citrate. This is not necessarily so, since the possibility exists that two molecules of acetic acid could condense to form a C_4 acid like succinic acid. This could also account for the distribution of isotopic carbon observed by Wood and Lorber, and, under these circumstances, a net gain in carbohydrate could easily occur. A net gain of glycogen from acetate is suggested by the work of Parnes and Wertheimer,[56,57] who showed that, in the isolated rat diaphragm, acetate itself or acetate in the presence of low concentrations of glucose leads to a definite and significant rise in glycogen, while depressing the rate of glucose uptake from the medium.

Whatever the pathways by which carbon atoms originating in fatty acids can appear in glucose molecules, it should be noted that such methods of study cannot, by themselves, either prove or disprove the net conversion of one foodstuff into another. Net conversion must be shown by quantitative-balance methods which exclude the possibility that carbohydrate could have come from any other source than fatty acid. The recent work with isotopes suggests that there are at least two ways in which the formation of glucose is increased: One is the sparing of the amino acid molecules for more complete conversion into carbohydrate, and the other is most likely condensation of two-carbon atom fragments from fatty acid, which provides material for the net conversion of fat into carbohydrate.

UTILIZATION, DISSIMILATION AND OXIDATION OF CARBOHYDRATE

The use of the term "oxidation" to describe the complete breakdown of a foodstuff to CO_2 and H_2O in the tissues carries with it certain traditional physiologic connotations which are no longer acceptable in the light of present day biochemistry. Chief among these is the old conception that the original foodstuff can liberate its energy for use by the tissue by the simple addition of oxygen to its atoms. But, as previously shown, the oxidative breakdown of the energy materials in the tissues is actually a far more complicated matter, involving the processes of oxidoreduction, decarboxylation, addition of CO_2, phosphorylation, hydrolysis and transamination.

It is true that the net result of a whole series of reactions may be written as if it were a simple oxidation, as, for example:

$$C_6H_{12}O_6 + 6O_2 \rightarrow 6CO_2 + 6H_2O$$

Indeed, it was our limited knowledge of the intermediate steps in this equation which originally led to the inaccurate use of the term "oxidation." But, now that most of the intermediate steps are known, the continued use of "oxidation" for the all-over process is a source of great confusion. For example, when the biochemist speaks of the "oxidation of lactate," he means specifically the withdrawal of hydrogen from lactate with the formation of pyruvate. The physiologist uses the same words to denote the breakdown of lactic acid to CO_2 and H_2O. It would be far better for all branches of biologic science to use the term "oxidation" in its strict chemical sense, and this is the sense in which it is used here. For the complete breakdown of a substrate to CO_2 and H_2O we employ the term "complete oxidation" or "dissimilation."

There is a practical need arising out of the conditions of experimental work for another term, namely, "utilization." In working with the whole living organism or even with isolated tissue in vitro, it is often possible to follow the disappearance of a substrate from the blood or nutritive medium or from the tissues themselves without being able to ascertain the extent to which the oxygen consumed and the CO_2 evolved in the interim were actually concerned with the substrate that disappeared. Other substrates are necessarily always present under these conditions, and their participation in the reactions under observation is not necessarily ruled out by an approximate equivalence between the respiratory exchange and the disappearance of the experimental substrate. Such equivalence may be coincidental; for it also happens, not infrequently, that the disappearance of a substrate bears no discernible relationship to the respiratory exchange. Under these circumstances, when it is impossible to determine the exact chemical fate of the substrate which is disappearing, it is best to employ the term "utilization." As used here, and applied to carbohydrate, for example, it means the disappearance of sugar from the blood or nutritive medium or tissue without storage as glycogen or accumulation as hexose or lactic acid.

Utilization of Carbohydrate as Determined by the Disappearance of the Blood Sugar in Liverless Animals

The rapid disappearance of the blood sugar after removal of the liver from the normal animal has been discussed in connection with the site of formation of the blood sugar. The mere withdrawal of sugar from the blood by the extrahepatic tissues cannot, of course, be regarded as proof of its utilization by those tissues. However, it has been the universal experience that the carbohydrate content of the tissues and the accumulation of lactic acid or any other substance in the blood do not account for the sugar that disappears from the blood of the liverless animal. The rate of disappearance of blood sugar in such animals may therefore be taken as at least a rough indication of the utilization of sugar by the extrahepatic tissues.

In view of this, it is significant that the blood sugar disappears after hepatectomy or abdominal evisceration in animals which have been supposed to have ceased utilizing carbohydrate, as judged by the D:N, ketosis, and R.Q. exhibited before removal of the liver. Such evidence is available after hepatectomy of depancreatized birds, dogs, and rabbits and after evisceration of phlorhizinized dogs, of depancreatized and pituitary-diabetic dogs, and of normal dogs fasted to the point of so-called "hunger diabetes." A similar incongruity between the conclusions drawn from the classic metabolic criteria and the disappearance of the blood sugar occurs after hypophysectomy of the depancreatized dog and during prolonged injections of epinephrine in the normal dog.

Utilization of Carbohydrate as Determined by Chemical Balance Studies in Liverless Animals

The groundwork for future chemical balance studies of carbohydrate utilization was laid in the laboratory of H. H. Dale. At that time, practical methods for total abdominal evisceration in the cat were not available. The liver was left in situ, with its afferent blood supply tied off. However, the asphyxiated organ (with a high free-sugar content) could still contribute sugar to the blood by seepage into the vena cava. In their later experiments Best and Dale[58] recognized this source of error and corrected for it by including the changes in sugar content of the liver in their chemical balances.

In these experiments eviscerated spinal cats were given constant intravenous infusions of known amounts of glucose. The balance was constructed from the amounts of sugar which disappeared from the blood and from the difference in glycogen and free-sugar content between certain muscles removed at the beginning of the experiment and the corresponding muscles of the opposite leg removed at the end of the experiment. In an experiment which these workers selected as being one of those most free from technical criticism, it may be calculated that their animal utilized glucose at the rate of 392 mg. per kilogram per hour. This utilization occurred while they were maintaining a blood-sugar level of about 240 mg. per cent.

Subsequent work (except for the experiments of Wick and Drury[59] on rabbits) has shown that the rate of utilization of carbohydrate varies with the blood-sugar level and that utilization figures should be referred to sugar concentration. Soskin and Levine[60] studied the utilization of carbohydrate in totally abdominally eviscerated dogs by striking a chemical balance between the blood sugar, the blood lactic acid, and the muscle glycogen at the end of the experiment. In later work the total carbohydrate content of the muscle was determined instead of muscle glycogen, and the lactic acid content of the muscle was taken into account, as well as the blood lactic acid. The results were substantially the same by both methods.

Figure 19 summarizes the relationship between the blood-sugar level and sugar utilization in all the experiments on eviscerated normal dogs. The lower plateau of the S-shaped curve indicates that the peripheral tissues cannot accommodate themselves to a supply of blood sugar which is less than that available at normal blood-sugar levels. Under these circumstances the minimal rate of carbohydrate utilization persists, and it must be carried on at the expense of tissue stores if it is to proceed at all. The upper plateau of the curve indicates that there is a maximum capacity for the utilization of carbohydrate. Between these two plateaus carbohydrate utilization varies directly with the height of the blood-sugar level.

INFLUENCE OF HORMONES ON CARBOHYDRATE METABOLISM

Within recent years it has become increasingly evident that the internal secretions of the endocrine glands are important regulators of metabolic processes. There is not a single hormone which has not been shown to exert some influence on carbohydrate metabolism, although there is, as yet, no definite knowledge as to the precise mode and locus of action of the hormones in the intermediary steps of metabolism. However, certain general conclusions concerning the nature of the activities of the hormones are possible—conclusions that are based on their chemical nature and on the order of magnitude of their effective concentrations.

THE PANCREAS (INSULIN)

The known physiologic effects of insulin are:

1. Hypoglycemia. Since highly purified insulin has been available for experimental and clinical use, it has been administered to animals and humans under the most diverse conditions. Except for differences in the magnitude of the effect obtained with a given amount of insulin (so-called "sensitivity"), a hypoglycemic effect is invariably obtained, regardless of the state of

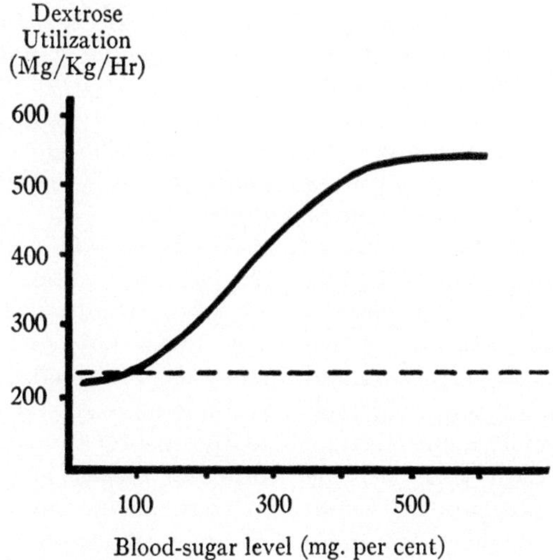

FIG. 19. The relationship between the blood-sugar level and sugar utilization in eviscerated normal dogs. (Soskin and Levine.[60])

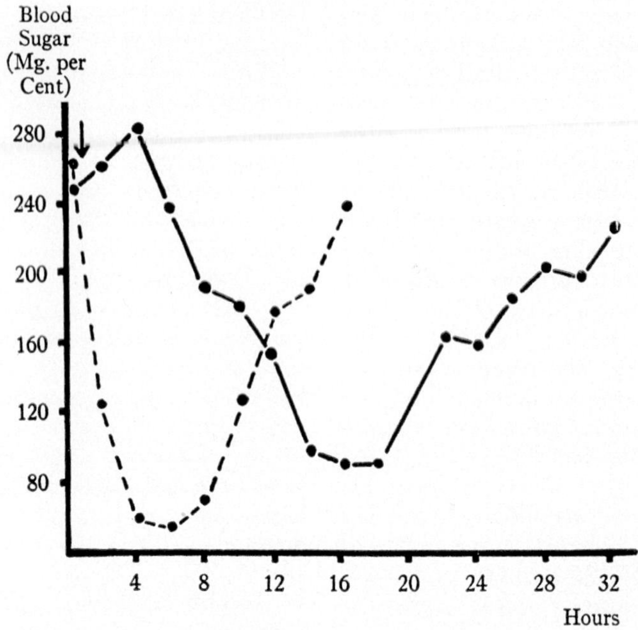

FIG. 20. The blood-sugar-lowering effects of regular and protamine insulin. The arrow indicates the administration of 80 units of regular (*broken line*) and of protamine (*continuous line*) insulin to the same diabetic patient at different times. Throughout the period of observation, in each instance, the patient was given 20 gm. of glucose (by mouth) every 2 hours.

the animal. This is true for animals at any age, in whatever state of nutrition and lacking the various endocrine glands or visceral organs. It is clear, therefore, that the hypoglycemic effect of insulin is a general one, which is not mediated by any particular organ or tissue. Figure 20 shows the typical curves of action of regular and of protamine insulin.

Numerous attempts have been made to determine whether the action of insulin might be on the blood itself. It has been impossible to demonstrate any change in blood in vitro by the addition of insulin. At one time it was claimed that insulin changed the blood glucose to a more reactive form, but this was never substantiated. It is also known that insulin has no influence on the distribution of glucose between plasma and red blood cells or on the rate of glycolysis of the blood sugar. It seems certain, therefore, that the lowering of the blood-sugar level in vivo under the influence of insulin is a result of the more rapid withdrawal of sugar from the blood by the other tissues. A decreased supply of sugar to the blood from the liver may be an additive factor.

2. Glycogen Deposition. Next to its hypoglycemic effect, the glycogenetic effect of insulin in skeletal muscle is its most thoroughly substantiated direct action. It is readily demonstrable in vitro on thin sheets of muscle (diaphragm or abdominal muscle of the young rat) in the Warburg apparatus. *This action of insulin in vivo is related to the existing blood-sugar level from moment to moment, both because of the amount of sugar available for deposition and because of the secondary counterregulations evoked by hypoglycemia.* Thus, unless the blood sugar is maintained by the administration of sugar, the hypoglycemia resulting from insulin action will evoke a secretion of epinephrine from the adrenal medulla, which, in turn, may mask the glycogenetic effect of the insulin by causing a rapid breakdown of muscle glycogen to lactic acid.

That insulin influences the deposition of liver glycogen is evident from the characteristically low glycogen levels of the diabetic liver and their return to normal with insulin treatment. But there is a paradoxical situation as regards the effects of administered insulin in normal animals, for normal animals invariably exhibit a decreased amount of hepatic glycogen after insulin administration. Part of this effect may be ascribed to the hypoglycemia-induced secretion of epinephrine and the consequent breakdown of liver glycogen to blood sugar. But this is by no means the whole explanation, for Bridge[61] has shown that insulin administered with sufficient glucose to maintain a certain blood-sugar level results in a smaller deposition of hepatic glycogen than the administration of that amount of sugar alone which will reproduce the same blood-sugar level. He also showed that this anomalous effect of insulin in normal animals could be obtained in the absence of the adrenal medulla. There is considerable uncertainty whether insulin affects the sugar uptake and glycogen deposition of the liver by any direct action on the hepatic cell. A more detailed discussion of this point will be found on p. 119.

The normal heart, like skeletal muscle, deposits increased glycogen under the influence of insulin. But cardiac glycogen is apparently more dependent upon the concentration of sugar available in the blood than is the glycogen of other organs; for the heart of the completely depancreatized animal may contain large amounts of it[62]—amounts which are reduced by restoring the blood-sugar level to normal with insulin. The finding of Junkersdorf of a high glycogen content in the cardiac muscle of phlorhizinized dogs with low blood-sugar levels also suggests the possibility of the formation of cardiac glycogen in situ from noncarbohydrate sources. Recently Russell and her coworkers[63,64] have brought forth evidence that the cardiac glycogen deposition which occurs during fasting or after phlorhizinization or pancreatectomy depends upon the hormonal activity of the anterior pituitary (most probably the growth hormone moiety).

The glycogen content of the brain and nervous tissues, on the other hand, is influenced little, if at all, by either the blood-sugar level or by the insulin content of the blood. Indeed, it seems likely that the small amount of glycogen which is found in these tissues has more structural than metabolic significance, since the amount is little affected by various nutritional, physiologic and pharmacologic factors.

3. Antiketogenesis. Ketogenesis in the liver is best correlated with a lack of glycogen. Accordingly, insulin is antiketogenic under conditions in which it increases liver glycogen (in the diabetic organism), but it may actually be ketogenic[65] under conditions in which it decreases liver glycogen (in the nondiabetic organism). Insulin has no influence whatever on the rate of disposal of ketone bodies by the extrahepatic tissues.[66]

4. Change in the R.Q. Whatever the significance of the R.Q., insulin has a definite effect upon it. But the situation with respect to the difference between the normal and the diabetic organism and the influence of the amount of carbohydrate available is somewhat similar to that which obtains for glycogen deposition in the liver. Thus, in the absence of insulin the diabetic organism fails to exhibit the rise in the R.Q. which follows the administration of sugar to the normal animal. The administration of insulin alone to the fasting diabetic organism results in an elevation of the quotient. However, insulin administration to the fasting normal organism results in variable changes of small magnitude, although insulin plus sugar does cause a more abrupt and more pronounced rise in the R.Q. than does sugar alone. Insulin either has no effect on the oxygen consumption or may actually decrease it.[67]

When insulin does affect the R.Q., the results bear no quantitative relation to the fall in the blood-sugar level. According to Bridge,[68] the R.Q. changes correlate best with the level of hepatic glycogen.

5. Decrease in Serum Inorganic Phosphate. In the absence of insulin the diabetic organism exhibits an abnormally high level of inorganic phosphate in the blood. This is corrected by treatment with insulin. The administration of insulin to the normal animal causes a diminution of serum inorganic phosphate below the normal level. There have been variable and contradictory reports concerning supposedly parallel changes in the hexosemonophosphate content of muscle, presumably due to the entrance of the blood-serum inorganic phosphate into muscle in this esterified form. But Soskin, Levine and Hechter[69] have shown that the phosphate changes in blood and muscle are not directly related to each other and that only the fall in the blood inorganic phosphate is a direct consequence of insulin action. The confusion was due to the counterregulatory reactions, whereby excessive insulin activity evokes a secretion of epinephrine, and vice versa. When the actions of the individual hormones are isolated by excision of the counterregulating gland, the unopposed action of the administered hormone can be observed.

The administration of insulin to the normal intact animal is followed by both the blood- and the muscle-phosphate effects. In the absence of the adrenal glands, the action of insulin on the blood phosphate persists, while the hexosemonophosphate in muscle is not affected. The responsibility of reflexly secreted epinephrine for the muscle-phosphate changes after insulin administration also accounts for the absence of those changes in normal animals when sufficient dextrose to prevent hypoglycemia is administered with the insulin. Conversely, epinephrine in the normal animal causes both a fall in the inorganic phosphate in the blood and a rise in the hexosemonophosphate in the muscle. But in the depancreatized animal, only the muscle effect of epinephrine occurs.

6. Decrease in Serum Potassium. A number of investigators have observed a lowering of the potassium content of the blood serum following the administration of insulin to normal animals. There has been no elucidation of the mechanism of this effect, except perhaps in so far as it may be related to the increased rate of entry of sugar into tissues under the influence of the hormone. Fenn has shown that potassium enters tissues in proportion to the amount of carbohydrate which is taken up.

7. Influence on Nitrogen Metabolism. In the absence of insulin the diabetic organism excretes abnormally large amounts of nitrogen in the urine. This indicates that insulin must act to inhibit protein catabolism at some point. The in vitro work of Bach and Holmes with liver slices showed that insulin inhibits the deamination of amino acids, as judged by the decreased rate of appearance of urea. This was accompanied by a decreased rate of appearance of carbohydrate, leading to the conclusion that insulin inhibits gluconeogenesis from amino acids and therefore from protein. Stadie and his co-workers[70] who performed similar experiments, were able to confirm this insulin effect with d-alanine but not with the naturally occurring l-alanine, as had Bach and Holmes. This nitrogen-sparing effect of insulin was further demonstrated by Gaebler[71] and Mirsky,[72] in an indirect way. They found that, whereas extracts of the anterior pituitary administered to normal animals resulted in nitrogen retention, the same treatment in diabetic animals caused an increased nitrogen excretion.

The administration of insulin to the normal animal is followed by uncertain and contradictory results. There may be either no change or an actual increase in nitrogen excretion. However, the amino acid level of the blood does decrease significantly. Like other effects of insulin under similar circumstances, this is probably due to the counterregulatory effects of other glands, particularly the adrenal medulla. Luck and his co-worker[73] have shown that in adrenal-demedullated animals insulin fails to lower the blood amino acids, while epinephrine will do so, just as it does in the normal animal. It seems reasonable to conclude, therefore, that the apparent influence of insulin on the amino acid level of the blood of the normal animal is actually due to the reflex secretion of epinephrine resulting from hypoglycemia. This same sequence of events could, of course, also account for the increased excretion of nitrogen which sometimes follows the administration of insulin to normal animals, for epinephrine has been shown to increase protein catabolism.

However, it is not at all certain that, aside from secondary effects due to epinephrine secretion, insulin does not have a direct action of its own upon the blood amino acids. Mirsky and his coworkers[74] found that in eviscerated and nephrectomized dogs maintained by a constant injection of insulin and glucose the blood amino acids rose more slowly, and injected glycine disappeared more rapidly, than in similar animals maintained on sugar alone. Since the absence of the liver and kidneys precludes a loss of the amino acids by deamination, these experiments suggest that insulin facilitates the use of amino acids in the muscles for synthetic purposes, either directly or indirectly.

*The Mode of Action of Insulin**

From a biologic standpoint, the hormones form a more uniform group of materials—that of humoral signal systems. They serve to integrate organ and cell functions in a manner which appears goal-directed in respect to the organism as a whole, especially in its adaptation to induced changes.

In the test tube the rates of enzymatic processes depend upon concentrations of substrate and catalyst, inorganic ion strengths, *p*H, substrate removal, etc. In the cell the innumerable chemical reactions are in addition controlled by structural characteristics at the submicroscopic level—the macromolecular complexes, organelles, and the resulting multitude of surfaces. More and more attention is being paid to these geometric aspects of biologic chemistry, despite the difficulties in approach. In a multicellular organism, it would seem likely that it is the role of the hormones (as it is of the peripheral nervous system) to bring about, reversibly, subtle changes in submicroscopic form and thus to trigger a change in functional direction as well as in rate of a process. This viewpoint is supported in part by the repeated observations that it becomes more and more difficult to elicit a hormonal effect as one proceeds from the whole organism to isolated organs, tissue slices, homogenates, and subcellular preparations. A certain degree of morphologic intactness seems necessary for hormonal (and drug) actions. The gun needs to be at least partially assembled for the demonstration of the action of the trigger.

During the last few years several comprehensive reviews dealing with the mechanism of action of insulin have been published,[75,76,77,78] and the reader is referred to them for detailed references and for variety of viewpoint. Sanger's elucidation of the amino acid sequence and the structure of the insulin molecule is one of the most brilliant chemical achievements of the recent era.[79] However, thus far the structure of the molecule has remained unrelated to any of its effects, and no notions as to the mode of action can be derived from it. Insulin is a simple protein of unit molecular weight of about 6000. Since the intravenous injection of 4-μg/kg body weight lowers the blood sugar of a susceptible animal about 50% from the initial level, it can be calculated that approximately 4000 molecules are available per cell of assumed average volume of 8000 μ^3, or one molecule for every 2 μ^3. The minimal effective dose of insulin is closer to one-fifth of the above amount. It is thus evident that we are dealing with a material of the type associated with active catalysis or the initiation of a chain of reactions.

In certain animal species (dog, cat, rat), complete pancreatectomy effec-

* From Levine, R.: On the Mechanisms of Action of Hormones on Cells. In Glass, B. (editor): Survey of Biological Progress, Volume III, New York, Academic Press, Inc., 1957, pages 186–201. By permission of the publisher.

tively removes all insulin-secreting cells. The syndrome of diabetes becomes established in the following sequence: the blood sugar rises; liver glycogen diminishes; liver fat content rises; the blood β-keto acid level increases as does the rate of urea formation in the liver; muscle glycogen levels fall more slowly, and that of the heart and the kidney tubules rises. The urinary findings of increased excretion of glucose, ketones, urea, water, and chlorides are all clearly secondary to internal events. It has been clearly established that kidney functions are themselves normal in experimental diabetes.

The discovery of insulin gave rise to a period of intensive investigation into the mechanism by which this hormone was able to restore to normal all the metabolic deviations of the diabetic state. Because of the sequence of events which follows pancreatectomy, it was assumed (correctly in most instances) that practically all the metabolic changes of diabetes were secondary and more remote consequences of the inability to "burn" or to "store" sugar, or both. It followed therefore that primary effect of insulin was to be sought in the areas of glucose oxidation and storage. This was the conclusion of the classic papers of Best, Dale, Hoet, and Marks in 1926.[58] Using the eviscerated spinal cat preparation, they could account for the glucose disappearing under "the action of insulin" by an increase in muscle glycogen and by oxidation (assuming that all of the O_2 consumed was used for oxidation of sugar). From their data it is apparent that the major quantitative effect of insulin in this preparation was the increase in muscle glycogen.

In view of all the effects of insulin which have been observed over the years, the fall in blood sugar and the increase of skeletal muscle glycogen (in the presence of glucose) are the effects characterized by the greatest consistency and least controversy. We shall return to a discussion of the contradictory data on the effects of insulin and glucose on liver uptake of sugar and liver storage of glycogen, as seen in the light of our present-day knowledge. At this point, however, we may take it as uncontroverted that, under the influence of insulin, skeletal muscle *in vivo* takes in more glucose from the blood and deposits more glycogen than in the absence of added insulin. The data of Bridge[48] on the intact normal rabbit and the work from Lundsgaard's laboratory[86] on perfused hind limbs demonstrate these facts.

In 1937, Soskin and Levine drew attention to the fact that the rate of uptake of sugar by the extrahepatic tissues of the dog depended upon the height of the blood sugar level maintained by the animal. This was true for the depancreatized animal (complete absence of insulin), the normal animal (endogenous insulin), and the insulinized normal animal (excess insulin). The defect exhibited by the peripheral tissues of the depancreatized animal consisted of a reduction in rate of glucose uptake at any but the highest blood sugar levels. On the other hand, a rise in blood sugar level (increased sugar pressure, so to speak) could compensate for the lack of the hormone. It was therefore concluded at that time that insulin was not absolutely essential for sugar disposal, but that it facilitated it by bringing it faster into the intermediary scheme of metabolic disposal of carbohydrate in the cell.[75] In conformity with the concepts of the enzymatic scheme, it was postulated that "insulin facilitates the formation from glucose of an intermediate substance (phosphorylated hexose?) which precedes and is necessary for both catabolism and synthesis."[75]

The relationship between the level of blood sugar and its rate of disappearance into the tissues was observed by Lundsgaard et al.[81] in the isolated hind limbs of cats and rabbits; and by Villee and Hastings[82] in rat diaphragm in vivo taken from normal as well as alloxan-diabetic animals. The significance of these observations lies in the fact that they offer a means of distinguishing between the "primary" and derivative effects of insulin. It seems entirely logical to assume that any observed effect of insulin which can be duplicated by the administration of large amounts of glucose (maintenance of a high blood glucose level) to the depancreatized animal (devoid of insulin) could be classified as a derivative effect. Such an effect is due to the forced uptake of sugar by tissues and is not a direct and immediate consequence of insulin action. Thus it was shown by Mirsky that glucose can and does lower the increased nitrogen excretion and the ketonemia of the depancreatized dog.

Soon after the discovery of insulin, it was shown that its administration is followed by a lowering of the serum and urine inorganic phosphate contents. Moderate amounts of glucose given to the depancreatized animal did not lower the P level of the serum, but did so in normal animals. However, if one gives fructose or larger amounts of glucose, there is a significant fall in blood inorganic phosphate in the complete absence of insulin.[83]

The positive effects of insulin on protein anabolism are well documented. Recently, Krahl[84] showed that in the tissues of diabetic animals there is a reduction in the rate of glutathione synthesis from glycine. This is raised to normal by insulin or by glucose. Insulin will lower the rate of amino acid accumulation which follows hepatectomy. Whether or not glucose will do so in the absence of the hormone has been both asserted[85] and denied.[86]

The review of events thus far leads plainly to the conclusion that insulin in some manner facilitates the uptake of sugar, at least by the extrahepatic tissues. The development of our knowledge of intermediary metabolism lent impetus to a search for the step or steps in the enzymatic machinery in which insulin participated, in such a manner as would lead to greater glucose utilization. The possibilities were in theory as many as there are steps in the metabolic scheme, but certain areas could be excluded en bloc. Thus the breakdown of glycogen to lactic acid was unimpaired in tissues of depancreatized animals.[87,88] Pyruvate and lactate disposal rates were not lowered by the lack of insulin.[89] Effects on citrate and pyruvate oxidation either were not sufficiently uniform or were restricted to particular species[90] or strains of animals. In the whole animal or in muscle tissue large effects on the uptake of glucose and deposition of glycogen could be obtained with little or no rise in O_2 consumption or even CO_2 production. This is illustrated by the data of Gemmill's original paper (1940), on the effects of insulin on the isolated diaphragm.

Thus far we have discussed two important pathways of glucose disposal—by oxidation and by storage of glycogen. Drury[91] concluded on indirect evidence, and Stetten and co-workers demonstrated directly,[92] that the formation of fat was quantitatively a most important path of glucose utilization, that a lack of insulin retarded lipogenesis, and that insulin administration hastened the formation of fat from carbohydrate.

Taking account of the demonstration that insulin increased the rate of glucose transformations in all of the quantitatively important ways, it was reasonable to assume that directly or indirectly the hormone stimulated the formation of glucose-6-phosphate, since this ester is the branch point of the metabolic scheme.

The work from Cori's laboratory seemed to provide experimental proof for the hypothesis.[93,94] In cell-free extracts, hexokinase activity was inhibited by pituitary and adrenal factors, and this inhibition was restored by insulin. It is difficult in the framework of the concept of a single action of insulin to fit these data to the well-known positive effects of insulin in animals without hypophysis or adrenals. The expected lower (inhibited) rate of hexokinase activity in preparations made from diabetic animals could not be obtained by others.[95] The relief of inhibition by insulin proved to be not uniformly obtained.[96,97,98] The adrenal and pituitary factors shown to be inhibitory in this test did not correlate with the hormonal preparations which were diabetogenic in vivo.

And yet, logic dictated that the locus

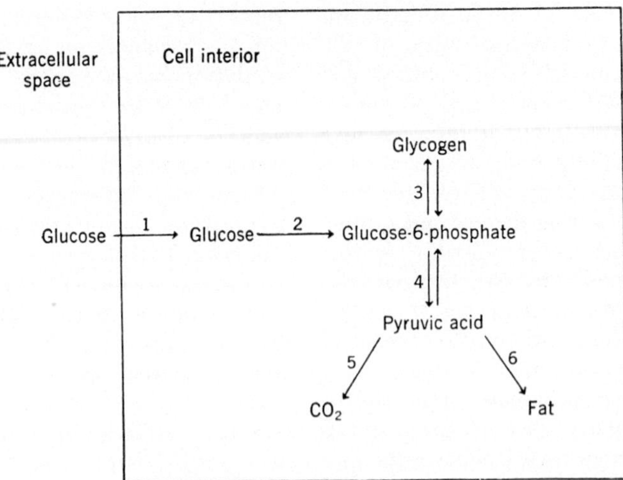

FIG. 21. The over-all reaction of glucose utilization. Any one of the numbered reactions might be rate-limiting. (From Glass, B. (ed.): Survey of Biological Progress, Vol. III. New York, Academic Press, Inc., 1957.)

of insulin action must be sought at or about the hexokinase level. In the usual presentation of the scheme of intermediary carbohydrate metabolism the first reaction is that catalyzed by hexokinase. The tacit assumption has thereby been made that the rate of glucose transfer from the extracellular compartment into the cell interior was not limiting. In the earlier years of the history of experimental diabetes the opinion had been expressed, notably by Höber and Loewi, that the metabolic disturbance of diabetes might be based upon the difficulty of glucose entry into cells. This view was insufficiently supported by the experimental evidence presented. Thus it came about that insulin was postulated to act upon an enzymatic, transforming reaction in the cell interior, and thereby to cause a "glucose vacuum," which served to "pull" more hexose in from the extracellular compartment.

It is clearly evident that the result would be the same whether the glucose was "pulled" or "pushed" into the cell, and that using glucose as the substrate one measures ordinarily the over-all rate of a chain of reactions, without determining which one of these is limiting (Fig. 21). To attack the problem it was necessary to choose a substrate which was expected to be affected by insulin, and an animal preparation in which the rate of metabolism of that substrate was as close to zero as possible. Galactose was chosen, since it is a naturally occurring isomer of glucose and also because the work of Wierzuchowski[99] had shown an influence of insulin on the galactose tolerance of dogs. The test preparation was the eviscerated nephrectomized dog, since galactose is metabolized primarily by liver, gut, and kidney. It can be demonstrated that galactose does indeed under these conditions behave like a nonutilizable substance, i.e., it equilibrates in a certain volume of distribution and is not metabolized. Its volume of distribution is about 40 to 43 per cent of the carcass weight. This volume is obtained with varying amounts of the sugar, from 0.25 to 1.00 g/kg body weight. When insulin is given to the animal, the rate of distribution is increased and the volume at equilibrium varies from 68 to 72 per cent of the body weight. This figure is close to that of total body water, and the results demonstrate that insulin has helped to transfer galactose from the extracellular compartment into the cell interior (Fig. 22). It was possible to show this action of insulin because galactose (in the preparation used) offered the opportunity of separating an entry mechanism from the intracellular chain of enzymes. Insulin could also be given at a time when a 40 per cent distribution had been reached and when it would open up an intracellular area for galactose which had previously been inaccessible. Using eviscerated nephrectomized rats, the above phenomena were reproduced, and in addition it was shown that no appreciable loss of galactose occurred during the experiment.[77]

In other experiments it was demonstrated that the described "transfer" action of insulin must be specific for a certain group of substances. It did not affect the rate or the volume of distribution of urea, alanine, creatinine, sucrose, or sodium chloride. In order to gain some insight into the system affected by the hormone the volume of distribution of a series of hexoses and pentoses was determined in the absence and presence of insulin. Of these, in addition to galactose, D-xylose and L-arabinose were insulin-responsive in the eviscerated dog; D-arabinose, D-sorbitol, and L-rhamnose were unresponsive. Of the sugars utilizable by the extrahepatic tissues of the dog, D-fructose, D-mannose, and L-sorbose were not significantly responsive to insulin action.[77] In later experiments it was shown that the volumes of distribution of glucuronic and galacturonic acids were similarly unresponsive to insulin. From these data, the general conclusion was drawn that the insulin "transfer" system was one adapted to a specific chemical configuration, namely, hexoses and pentoses which possess the "glucose" configuration about carbons 1, 2, and 3. The action of insulin seems to be independent of the utilizability of the sugar in the tissues.

The principal lines of evidence and deduction here presented have been confirmed and extended (though differing in detail) by several laboratories. Thus Ross[100] has calculated the permeability constant for glucose entry from the plasma into the aqueous humor in rabbits under varying conditions. His data show that insulin increased the rate of entry of glucose into the eye, and that the permeability constant is decreased in an established alloxan diabetes. In the first paper cited he interprets his findings to mean an influence on hexokinase, but subsequently this interpretation was modified because of results obtained in work with rabbit lens in vitro.[100] Using such a tissue, insulin increased the rate of entry of glucose from 0.2 to 0.7 mg/g/hour. In the

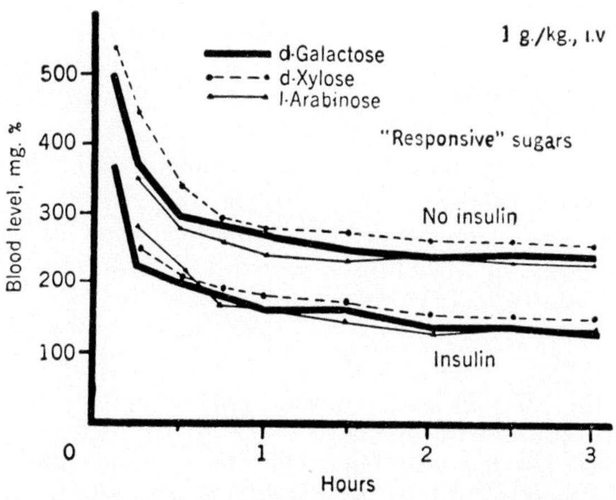

FIG. 22. The effect of insulin on the distribution of sugars in eviscerated-nephrectomized dogs. The particular sugar is given in one injection at zero time. Within a few minutes it distributes itself in the vascular system. Some time after one hour it becomes distributed, in a volume corresponding to about 40 per cent of body weight. In the presence of insulin the final volume of distribution corresponds to total body water. (From Glass, B. (ed.): Survey of Biological Progress, Vol. III. New York, Academic Press, Inc., 1957.)

absence of insulin, galactose did not enter the lens. In its presence, there was an appreciable rate of galactose uptake (0.11 mg/g/hour).

Wick and Drury[101] using galactose-C^{14} in eviscerated rabbits, showed that although in this species there is some oxidation of the galactose, the principal effect of insulin was to increase the rate of transfer of that sugar into cells. From their observation it can be concluded that glucose and galactose compete for the "transfer" system.

Haft et al., employing various sugars in the medium bathing rat diaphragm in vitro, found that insulin increased the volume of distribution of galactose, but in contrast to previous experience they noted a significant effect of insulin on the utilization of fructose. They were therefore unable to confirm the reported structural specificity of the "transfer" system. These findings, as well as the recent results with mannose reported by Wick and Drury,[102] demand a re-examination of the structural specificity hypothesis. In the light of the data of Mackler and Guest,[103] who found that an effect of insulin on fructose utilization was demonstrable only in the absence of glucose, the mutual inhibitory action of the sugars must be taken into account in studying the properties of the glucose intake system. In view of our own data showing no definitive effect of insulin on the utilization of mannose, and those of C. and G. Cori[104] on eviscerated rats showing no insulin effect on the disposal of fructose and mannose, it is possible that certain species (e.g., rabbit) possess a sugar transfer system which differs in structural specificity from that of the dog or the rat.

The hexokinase system of the extrahepatic tissues of the dog exhibits a high order of activity. Even if the blood sugar is raised to 1200 mg per cent (in the presence of insulin) there is only an insignificant amount of free glucose in the intracellular compartment of skeletal muscle. This was estimated by using the chloride space as a measure of the extracellular compartment, and glucose oxidase for the specific estimation of the free hexose.[77] Park demonstrated that under certain conditions insulin can be shown to increase the level of free glucose in skeletal muscle and heart.[14,105] This was done either by overwhelming the hexokinase system with more glucose than it could handle, or by keeping tissues at a low temperature at which hexokinase activity was strongly reduced, while the transfer action of insulin was not affected to the same degree. This was the first demonstration that the postulated action of insulin applies to glucose as well as to other sugars.

The work just summarized allows the conclusion that insulin acts (at least in the peripheral tissues of the dog, rabbit, and rat) to facilitate the transfer of extracellular free glucose into the cell. The subsequent fate of the sugar would depend upon the state of the enzymatic apparatus.

Several areas of inquiry now become pertinent:

1. What is the nature of the insulin-sensitive glucose transfer mechanism? Are any deductions possible at present, and what lines of investigation are necessary to study such mechanisms?

2. Is the effect of insulin here described actually of the primary type? Does it account for all or most of the observed effects on insulin administration or removal? How does this action of insulin relate to that of the so-called contra-insulin factors of the pituitary and of the adrenal cortex?

3. Is the action of insulin on the handling of sugar by the liver the same or similar to the one described for the extrahepatic tissues?

The work of Stadie's laboratory[76] since 1949 makes it evident that insulin and certain other hormonal factors are "fixed" by the cell (surface?) and probably exert their effects in the "fixed" state. This work has also emphasized the need for a degree of "intactness" of the cell in demonstrating certain hormonal activities. These data and views are compatible with the theory of insulin action here presented, but provide as yet no additional insight into the nature of the "transfer" system.

The nature and chemical structure of what is loosely called the cell membrane or surface is, in the case of most animal cells, still in the realm of concept and speculation. Its lipoprotein constitution is derived from studies on red cell "ghosts" and deductions based upon rates of penetration in relation to lipid solubility. Rosenberg and Wilbrandt (1952) have recently reviewed the literature on red cell permeability to the sugars. Their own work, together with that of Rothstein (1954), leads them to the conclusion that glucose is phosphorylated at the surface to a metaphosphate form, which is more lipid-soluble and thus gains entry into the cell. There is no direct evidence that phosphorylation precedes entry[106] but this work and that of Le Fevre and Davies[107] and Widdas[108] suggests that specific constituents of the cell surface are concerned with the transport of certain sugars. It is interesting to note that the structural specificity of the insulin-responsive sugars is reflected in a similar specificity of red cell permeability. Wilbrandt[109] remarks that in the case of human erythrocytes L-arabinose and D-xylose penetrate, but the cells are not permeable to D-arabinose and L-xylose. Widdas suggests that the present evidence is compatible with a "carrier" type of entry followed by phosphorylation. Inhibition by phlorhizin does not prove phosphorylation. This glucoside may be a competitive inhibitor because of its structural relation to sugars.

In muscle tissue galactose, xylose, and arabinose have not been shown to become phosphorylated. At the height of insulin action on galactose distribution, P^{32} turnover is not increased over that of the noninsulin period.

Using rat diaphragm in vitro at several temperatures between 10° C and 37.5° C it could be ascertained that the action of insulin in facilitating sugar entry had a Q_{10} of only 1.2. This suggests that the action is exerted on a system different in its behavior from an "enzyme" and that the process is attended by little or no energy exchange. It is true that muscle kept for a time in the anaerobic state shows less or no insulin activity[110] in promoting glucose uptake. But this does not necessarily argue for a process coupled with oxidation. Reaction of insulin with the specific cell constituent may be impossible in an atmosphere of N_2 because of reduction of some important group in the molecule. It should also be pointed out that glucose uptake was being measured and not rate of penetration. Glucose uptake is of course compounded of entry and metabolic transformation. Park has shown that at a low temperature at which hexokinase activity was very strongly inhibited, the action of insulin on glucose transfer could be shown readily.[14,105] Resnick and Hechter,[111] who used galactose to test the transfer reaction in rat diaphragm, found insulin activity evident in N_2 as the gas phase. They have also demonstrated by paper chromatography the presence of sufficient free glactose in the tissue to account for all of the C^{14} activity disappearing from the medium.

Even though galactose is not metabolized in the peripheral tissues of the dog, and therefore is not removed after cell entry, insulin did not lead to an accumulation against the gradient. The final concentration was at equilibrium between the cell interior and the extracellular compartment. There is therefore no evidence for a so-called "active" transfer mechanism.

The view as to the nature of the transfer system most consistent with the data is that propounded by Höber,[112] namely, that "in addition to the lipid elements one has to assume the existence of protoplasmic areas of the cell surface which form the background for a regulated or physiological permeability—a property of living tissue which it possesses over and above 'physical' permeability."

From this standpoint insulin would have the property of combining with a specific constituent of the surface of certain cells. As a consequence of such binding, a temporary distortion could

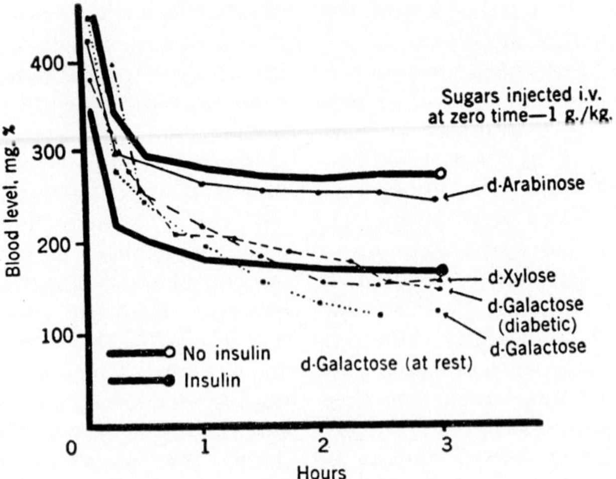

FIG. 23. Distribution of sugars in working eviscerated-nephrectomized dogs. Muscular work leads to the distribution of d-xylose and d-galactose in total body water exactly as if insulin had been given. d-Arabinose, which does not respond to insulin, is also not affected by work. (From Glass, B. (ed.): Survey of Biological Progress, Vol. III. New York, Academic Press, Inc, 1957.)

be produced in the molecular architecture of that surface, which would permit a greater rate of entry to certain materials (the sugars) which exhibit a particular kind of size, charge, etc. Brown[113] found that "reactive points" exist on the surface of plant root segments which permit entry of monosaccharides and that these "points" remain the same in number and area even though the total surface increases. Goldacre[114] discusses the possibility of changes in protein configuration in relation to osmotic work.

Insulin is not the only agent which facilitates sugar transfer. Clinical experience and the more recent experimental work of Ingle[115] have shown that glucose utilization is increased and the blood sugar is sharply reduced during muscular exercise in the complete absence of insulin. Figure 23 shows that muscular work leads to the transfer into the cell of sugars which are themselves not utilized.[77] In other words, muscular work influences the cell surface system in the same manner as does insulin (Fig. 21). It is suggested that this influence is "humoral," because stimulation of one muscle group of a hind limb leads to the distribution of galactose in the total volume of body water, and because denervation of the exercising limb has no influence on this distributive action.

The findings which indicate that in certain tissues (muscle, connective tissues) the transfer system for glucose is ordinarily fairly inactive, and that its rate of action is increased both by insulin and by muscular work, makes good biologic sense from the standpoint of the needs of the organism as a whole. During the time when no carbohydrate is being absorbed from the digestive tract, the liver maintains the blood sugar by gluconeogenesis. Over half of the hepatic glucose production is ordinarily used by the brain. If the large extent of cell surface in muscle and connective tissue were at all times open to glucose entry, the blood sugar would soon fall to levels incompatible with normal brain function. When the blood sugar is raised (after a meal), hepatic glucose production is diminished, and insulin secretion is stimulated. The insulin-sensitive tissues are "opened" to glucose, which is stored as glycogen and fat for future use. Muscular work does not raise the blood sugar. Insulin is not mobilized to open the muscle gates. Instead, some factor is released by muscle in amounts proportional to the performance of work, which has effects similar to insulin. It would be of great interest to search at what point in evolution the muscle factor emerged in relation to the point of appearance of insulin.

Those organs and tissues which work on "one gear," i.e., which do not greatly increase or decrease their energy expenditure, have an "open" glucose transfer system; while the working and storage cells, which work on several "gears," seem to have developed devices which open the gates for entry of the important blood-borne metabolite, glucose, when it is needed for work or when it is present in excess in the circulation.

At this point one can no longer avoid a statement on the controversial subject of the relation of insulin to liver cell functions. There is of course no doubt that many aspects of carbohydrate and fat metabolism in the liver are drastically affected by removal of the pancreas, and that the administration of insulin to the diabetic organism restores the metabolic changes to the normal range. The overwhelming mass of evidence in the literature indicates that these effects of insulin are not exerted directly upon processes in the liver cell. Rather it would seem that insulin, by restoring the capacity of peripheral tissues to take in glucose, sets into motion mechanisms which secondarily affect enzymic concentrations and relationships in the liver. This subject has been reviewed in detail recently and the reader is referred to that paper for examination of the evidence.[116]

De Duve[117] has recently summarized his views that there is evidence for a direct action of insulin on liver.

GLUCAGON

Not long after insulin came into general use, it was reported that the intravenous injection of insulin preparation caused an initial hyperglycemia before the characteristic lowering of the blood sugar level occurred. Two hypotheses were offered: An impurity, acting nonspecifically on the liver to cause glycogenolysis, might have been extracted with insulin; or insulin itself had an initial "irritative" effect upon the liver. A sample of crystalline insulin prepared by Abel did not show the hyperglycemic effect, although it still caused some glycogenolysis when added to blood in liver perfusions.

In 1944–45, de Duve studied the hyperglycemic action of intravenously administered insulin in rabbits and came to the conclusion that most insulin preparations contained a factor other than insulin, which he named "the hyperglycemic factor of the pancreas" (glucagon). Certain insulin preparations ("Novo insulin"), produced by a somewhat modified extraction procedure, did not show the initial blood sugar raising effect. De Duve, Sutherland, Staub, Foa, Goldner, Volk and others[118] have since worked on the chemical and physiologic aspects of the problem, the aim being to elucidate the nature of the action of glucagon and whether it plays the role of a hormone in carbohydrate regulation.

The significant work, to date, demonstrates that glucagon is protein in nature and completely separable from insulin. It causes hyperglycemia when injected intravenously into animals with adequate stores of liver glycogen. Fasting or other conditions which empty the liver of glycogen abolish the effect of glucagon. It appears, therefore, to be a factor which causes glycogenolysis but not gluconeogenesis. Because it is not effective when injected subcutaneously, it is probably destroyed rapidly by proteolytic systems in the subcutaneous tissues. Active preparations of glucagon can be extracted from the stomach and duodenum as well as from the pancreas. This distribution seemingly parallels the distribution of argentophile cells.

Glucagon causes glycogenolysis when added to liver slices in vitro. In this, it resembles epinephrine. But unlike the latter, it does not cause muscle glycogenolysis and, therefore, does not lead to a rise in lactic acid.

On the basis of presently available evidence, it is impossible completely to exclude or definitely include glucagon in the category of hormones. If it were a hormone participating in carbohydrate regulation, its hyperglycemic action might account for certain differences between alloxan and pancreatic diabetes, the greater sensitivity to insulin of totally depancreatized as compared to incompletely operated animals, the etiology of some cases of diabetes mellitus, etc. However, some considerations militate against the acceptance of glucagon as a hormone. Since it causes hepatic glycogenolysis, but not gluconeogenesis, it cannot be regarded as a diabetogenic agent in the strict sense of the word. Furthermore, whatever the nature of its action, there has, as yet, been no demonstration of a characteristic cellular site of origin in the tissues from which it can be extracted. Complete destruction of the alpha cells does not diminish the extractable glucagon of the pancreas. Finally, if the sites of origin of glucagon could be ablated from an experimental animal, one might expect a hypoglycemic syndrome (at least under certain conditions) to result. Unfortunately, however, it is not possible to remove the tissues containing glucagon without causing pancreatic diabetes.

Glucagon seems either not to affect sugar utilization in the peripheral tissues or to increase its rate to a certain extent.[118]

ADRENAL MEDULLA*

The adrenal medulla manufactures and releases two closely related, hormonally active amines, epinephrine and norepinephrine. The known effects of these materials on various organs and tissues are so numerous and varied that it would be unrewarding to attempt to get an insight into some basic action underlying all of the observed phenomena. We shall therefore select one conspicuous and functionally significant effect of epinephrine, the rise in the blood sugar level, for the more detailed survey. It has been amply demonstrated over the years that this is a regulatory action of epinephrine, since a release of the hormone from the gland is brought about by lowering the blood sugar.

The hyperglycemic effect of epinephrine depends upon the presence of an adequate amount of liver glycogen. After prolonged fasting, when the liver glycogen store is almost completely depleted, epinephrine no longer raises blood sugar levels. The known enzymatic mechanisms by which glucose is released to the blood and derived from the hepatic glycogen stores are presented in Fig. 24. The problem before us is: on which of these reactions does epinephrine directly or indirectly exert its influence? Many years ago it was demonstrated that simultaneously with the rise in blood sugar there was also a rise in blood lactic acid, following epinephrine release or administration. This response pointed to an action on muscle glycogen,[119] an action which was proved by an analysis of muscle for glycogen, hexose phosphates, and lactic acid. The reason epinephrine leads to a release of lactic acid in muscle is that this tissue does not contain the specific glucose-6-phosphatase and therefore cannot give rise to free glucose when its glycogen is being broken down (Fig. 24). Taken together, these data indicate that epinephrine must influence one or more of the reactions common to both liver and muscle, but could not exert its action on the glucose-6-phosphatase reaction, which does not exist in muscle.

The studies of Sutherland and his coworkers began with these considerations and have carried the problem ahead to its present state.[120,121] The system used consists of liver and muscle slices in vitro; most of the data were obtained with liver. The experimental observations and the conclusions drawn may be summarized as follows:

1. Neither the glucose-6-phosphatase system nor the phosphoglucomutase system, which converts glucose-6-phosphate to glucose-1-phosphate, was limit-

* From Levine, R.: On the Mechanisms of Action of Hormones on Cells. In Glass, B. (editor): Survey of Biological Progress, Volume III, New York, Academic Press, Inc., 1957, pages 202–204. By permission of the publisher.

ing in the breakdown of liver glycogen to free glucose.

2. Phosphorylase, the enzyme catalyzing the interconversion of glucose-1 phosphate and glycogen, could be the limiting system.

3. With time, a liver slice in vitro shows a progressive diminution in phosphorylase activity.

4. This loss in activity is due to a reversible "inactivation" of the phosphorylase protein. The active enzyme is itself a phosphoprotein, and loss of P from it leads to "inactivation."

5. Certain drugs and inhibitors prevent the dephosphorylation of the enzyme protein. Thus they *prevent* inactivation in vitro.

6. Epinephrine (added in vitro to the medium bathing the liver slice) stimulates the rate of reaction between phosphate and the "inactive" phosphorylase. It reactivates the system. The reactivation proceeds via an enzyme system which catalyzes formation of phosphoproteins.

The site of action of epinephrine could then, according to the above results be schematically represented as in Fig. 25.

These logically consistent and well-conceived experiments have brought us undoubtedly nearer to the "action" of epinephrine, but have not yet clearly defined it. Thus it is difficult to see why the effect of epinephrine in reactivating the phosphorylase system should invariably lead to a breakdown of glycogen. Increased glycogen synthesis would be an equally, if not more likely, result. Yet epinephrine administration is always followed by glycogen breakdown, even in the presence of added glucose.

Although epinephrine reactivates liver phosphorylase and brings its level back to the control values, there is at present no evidence that the phosphorylase is inactive under normal conditions. Since epinephrine given in vivo or added to liver slices in vitro very quickly increases the glucose output, the reactivation hypothesis does not seem to explain the phenomenon completely, unless a major portion of the system is normally in the inactive form.

It has been a controversial matter of

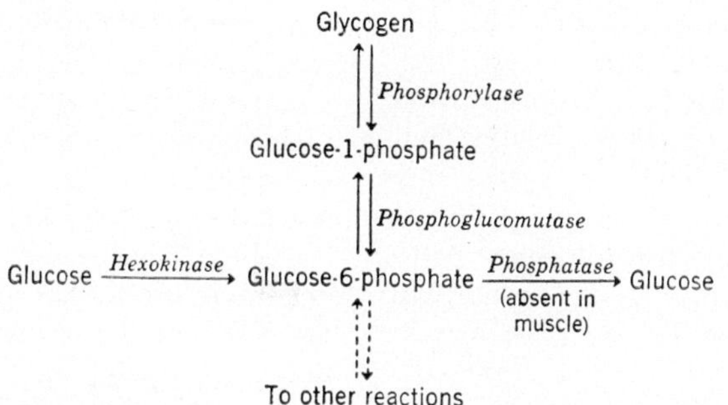

FIG. 24. Currently accepted scheme of glycogen formation and breakdown, and the enzyme systems involved therein. (From Glass, B. (ed.): Survey of Biological Progress, Vol. III. New York, Academic Press, Inc., 1957.)

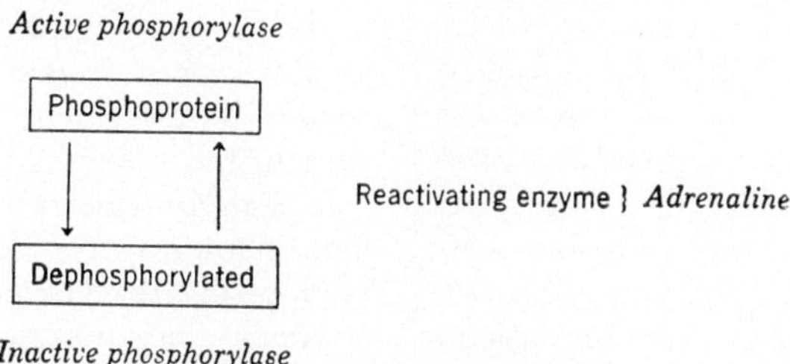

FIG. 25. Present evidence would place the action of epinephrine (adrenaline) on liver glycogenolysis, as aiding the system which reactivates the phosphorylase protein. (From Glass, B. (ed.): Survey of Biological Progress, Vol. III. New York, Academic Press, Inc., 1957.)

long standing whether epinephrine inhibits the uptake of glucose by muscle and other extrahepatic tissues. If this is so, there is a possibility that inhibition of glucose uptake would be secondary to an accumulation of glucose-6-phosphate, which may inhibit the hexokinase reaction.

ADRENAL CORTEX

The Steroids of the Adrenal Cortex

The isolation and identification of a number of steroids from the adrenal cortex and the study of their physiologic properties and those of the amorphous fractions have revealed that the various compounds or fractions have certain activities in common. However, a particular compound or fraction may exhibit one activity to the highest degree and be relatively impotent in other respects. In the absence of more precise knowledge of that vital function, the failure of which is the most urgent cause of death in untreated adrenalectomized animals, it is convenient to compare the various cortical steroids and fractions in regard to the following effects on such animals: (a) the maintenance of life, (b) the restoration of normal carbohydrate levels in all tissues, and (c) the restoration of normal sodium and potassium balance and excretion. To these effects may be added the restoration of the ability of the muscles to continue to perform work in response to prolonged stimulation. But since the activities of substances in this respect run parallel with their carbohydrate effects, these two actions may be considered together.

The relative potencies of the substances acting on carbohydrate levels maintain a similar relationship when these materials are tested on muscular work performance. Some of the earlier work with synthetic desoxycorticosterone acetate, while showing its powerful influence on the sodium and potassium balance, had revealed no action on carbohydrate metabolism. This is apparently a matter of dosage, for Harrison and Harrison have reported that 1.25 mg. daily of the substance would maintain life and a normal mineral balance in adrenalectomized rats but that it required 2.5 mg. daily to maintain a normal blood-sugar level. Similar evidence is available in the work of others, although the various authors differ from Harrison and Harrison and from each other as to the comparative potency of desoxycorticosterone on carbohydrate metabolism.[122]

Deficiencies Relieved by Salt Treatment

In spite of the qualitative difference in the prepotent activity of the various substances which may be separated from adrenal cortical extracts, it is impossible to discuss the materials concerned with the metabolism of the foodstuffs without also considering those which primarily affect the mineral balance. This is because the absence of the latter in adrenalectomized animals disturbs the normal environment of all cells and thus produces certain secondary disturbances in metabolism. The secondary effects are most readily distinguished from the primary metabolic effects of adrenalectomy by a consideration of those disturbances which are alleviated by combating the mineral imbalance with a high sodium and low potassium intake. The symptoms of adrenal cortical insufficiency which are relieved by salt treatment are as follows:

1. *Decrease in the sodium content and increase in the potassium of the blood serum.* This is accompanied by an increased excretion of sodium in the urine and a decreased excretion of potassium. The changes in excretion are known to be due to a specific effect upon the kidney tubules. The changes in the blood levels are due partly to disturbed kidney function and partly to a similar derangement of electrolyte balance in the other tissues of the body.

2. *Dehydration and hemoconcentration.* These are secondary to the loss of H_2O involved in the excessive excretion of NaCl. They are partly responsible for the rise in blood urea, although the disturbance in kidney function also contributes to this effect.

3. *Acidosis.* This is due to the retention of acid metabolites and anions, which are ordinarily neutralized and excreted by the kidneys. The failure in excretion is due in part to the circulatory failure and in part to the specific kidney disturbance. A feature of the latter is an inability to produce NH_3 for the regulation of the acid base balance.

4. *Impairment of carbohydrate absorption by the gastrointestinal tract and of the glycogen deposition from ingested carbohydrates.* These effects may be related to the movement of potassium out of all tissue cells. The passage of sugar into the cell is accompanied by a movement of potassium in the same direction.

5. *Decreased metabolic rate.* This has been demonstrated for the isolated tissues of adrenalectomized animals in vitro. In the living animal it may also depend upon the reduced blood chloride level, which interferes with the dissociation of oxygen from oxyhemoglobin, decreasing the supply of oxygen to the tissues.

6. *Anorexia and the consequent lack of gain in weight and cessation of growth.* No explanation for the loss of appetite is available.

7. *Rapid deterioration and death of the animal.* This is probably a result of the cumulative effects of dehydration and hemoconcentration, leading to a shocklike condition, plus the toxic action of high potassium levels and the hypoglycemic effects of fasting, owing to the anorexia.

The beneficial effects of salt on the above symptoms are striking and very readily demonstrated. The diminished rate of glucose absorption is completely restored to normal by the administration of NaCl in the drinking water. The same holds true for fat absorption. Similarly treated adrenalectomized rats can deposit glycogen from glucose nearly as well as normal rats and may gain weight in normal fashion. But while salt treatment enables adrenalectomized animals to survive indefinitely under favorable conditions, it does not restore them completely to normal. They are still sensitive to stresses and strains of all kinds.

Deficiencies Relieved by the C_{11} Steroids

What, then, are the primary functions of the adrenal cortex in respect to the metabolism of the foodstuffs? The answer appears in those metabolic disturbances in the adrenalectomized animal which persist despite the maintenance of a normal sodium and potassium balance. These include:

1. *Hypoglycemic effect of fasting.* Salt-treated animals which appear perfectly normal and healthy when maintained on an ample diet rapidly deteriorate when food is withdrawn, dying in hypoglycemia. The administration of sugar (in physiologic saline) rapidly restores them.

2. *Reduced levels of tissue glycogen, particularly that of liver glycogen, during fasting.* This is due to an inability to manufacture glycogen from the body stores of noncarbohydrate precursors and accounts also for the hypoglycemic effect of fasting.

3. *Diminished urinary nitrogen excretion during fasting.* In view of the fact that the protein-fed adrenalectomized animal excretes normal amounts of nitrogen, it seems likely that the difficulty in the fasted adrenalectomized animal is that of mobilization of protein from the tissues and its breakdown to the amino acid stage.

4. *Disturbance in fat mobilization.* Anterior pituitary extracts, phlorhizin administration, or phosphorus poisoning result in the accumulation of fat in the livers of normal animals but fail to do so in the absence of the adrenals.

5. *Alleviation of experimental diabetes.* The diminution of hyperglycemia, glycosuria, and ketosis in depancreatized and phlorhizinized animals which lack the adrenal cortex is readily explained by the disturbances in the mobilization of protein and fat and the consequent dearth of raw materials for gluconeogenesis.

6. *Insulin sensitivity.* This is not due

TABLE 5. EFFECTS OF ADRENALECTOMY AND OF CORTICAL STEROIDS ON THE CARBOHYDRATE LEVELS OF RATS AND MICE (LONG ET AL.[124])

SPECIES	CONDITION	HORMONAL THERAPY	BLOOD SUGAR (MG. PER CENT)	LIVER GLYCOGEN (PER CENT)	MUSCLE GLYCOGEN (MG. PER CENT)
Rats	Normal—fed	0	124	1.78	590
	Normal—48-hr. fast	0	80	0.23	507
	Normal—48-hr. fast	Cortical extract	...	1.64	536
	Adrenalectomy—fed	0	97	2.31	533
	Adrenalectomy—48-hr. fast	0	30	0.07	358
	Adrenalectomy—48-hr. fast	Cortical extract	...	1.78	411
Mice	Normal—fed	0	...	2.84	435
	Normal—fed	Cortical extract	...	9.20	1,014
	Normal—24-hr. fast	0	...	0.35	228
	Normal—24-hr. fast	Cortical extract	...	2.99	223
	Normal—24-hr. fast	Corticosterone	...	1.89	
	Normal—24-hr. fast	Dehydrocorticosterone	...	2.26	
	Adrenalectomy—fed	0	...	2.18	479
	Adrenalectomy—24-hr. fast	0	...	0.04	158
	Adrenalectomy—24-hr. fast	Cortical extract	...	2.37	182

to the lack of available liver glycogen to combat hypoglycemia, for the salt-treated adrenalectomized animal with a fairly normal hepatic glycogen level still exhibits the sensitivity.

7. *Muscular weakness and sensitivity to stress.* Because the C_{11} oxysteroids exhibit both the metabolic and anti-stress properties it has been commonly assumed that resistance to stress is in some way dependent upon the metabolic functions in question. At one time, this point of view was apparently supported by Ingle's observation that the muscular weakness of adrenalectomized animals could be relieved by the administration of carbohydrate. Subsequent work by Ingle did not confirm that finding and, as will appear later, there is now considerable doubt that the metabolic effects of the C_{11} oxysteroids are directly related to their anti-stress function.

Treatment of fasting adrenalectomized animals with corticosterone or cortin restores the normal blood-sugar level and, in large doses, may cause hyperglycemia. Such treatment also increases the liver glycogen in normal, as well as in adrenalectomized, animals.[123] The muscle glycogen is not so readily affected either by adrenalectomy or by the administration of cortical extracts (Table 5). Recent work has also confirmed the previous reports that the lack of adrenal cortical hormone diminishes the hyperglycemia and glycosuria of diabetes and that the administration of active cortical hormones restores the severity of the diabetic syndrome. Sprague et al.[125] have reported a case of a typical diabetes mellitus in a woman which disappeared completely upon the removal of an adrenal cortical tumor.

Wells[126] has reported that the injection of phlorhizin into salt-treated adrenalectomized rats causes them to excrete much smaller amounts of glucose than similarly injected normal rats. Corticosterone and 17-hydroxy-11-dehydrocorticosterone (Compound E) increase the glucose excretion of the phlorhizinized adrenalectomized animals to that of phlorhizin-treated normal rats. The amorphous fraction (cortin) and desoxycorticosterone have relatively lesser effects.

It may therefore be concluded that the primary metabolic functions of the adrenal cortex are concerned with hepatic gluconeogenesis from noncarbohydrate precursors.

Mode of Action of the C_{11} Steroids on Carbohydrate Metabolism

We have already indicated that the probable mode of action of the C_{11} oxysteroids on carbohydrate metabolism occurs partly directly and partly indirectly through the liver, and consists of the mobilization of protein and fat from the periphery, which in turn provides the raw materials for increased gluconeogenesis in the liver. However, some investigators have thought that at least some of the effect of the C_{11} oxysteroids might be due to an inhibition of glucose utilization by the peripheral tissues in a manner directly opposed to the action of insulin.

In order to maintain normal blood sugar levels, the adrenalectomized hepatectomized animal requires more glucose per unit time than does the hepatectomized normal animal. However, the better the mineral and water balance, the more do the glucose requirements of the two types of animal approximate each other, so that circulatory disturbances may obscure the issue. Working with carefully maintained eviscerated rats, Ingle[79] could not demonstrate inhibitory effects of adrenal cortical hormones on glucose utilization over a 4-hour period. There was some evidence of such an inhibition over a 24-hour period, as shown by final blood sugars. However, the differences in total sugar requirement for the whole 24-hour period are insignificant. Concordant evidence in patients suffering from Addison's disease was reported by MacBryde and de la Balze,[127] who found a very significant increase in the arteriovenous blood-sugar difference after treatment with cortical extract rich in the C_{11} steroids, despite the fact that this treatment undoubtedly increases the rate of circulation. Hence their observations indicate an increase rather than a decrease in sugar uptake by the peripheral tissues, under the influence of adrenal cortical extract.

Recently, Wick et al.[128] have used C^{14} glucose to study its oxidation in adrenalectomized rabbits and normal rabbits given C_{11} oxysteroids. In neither case was there a change in the rate of $C^{14}O_2$ production.

Intact adrenalectomized animals are extremely sensitive to insulin. It was shown by Levine et al.[129] that the eviscerated adrenalectomized rat is not abnormally sensitive to insulin. They concluded that the sensitivity depended upon the presence of the liver and not upon an adrenal-insulin antagonism in the peripheral tissues.

In view of all the above evidence which overwhelmingly indicates that the action of the C_{11} oxysteroids is central rather than peripheral, how can one explain the fact that it requires more glucose to maintain a given blood sugar level in a hepatectomized, adrenalectomized animal than in a hepatectomized normal animal? The obvious explanation is that the sugar which enters the peripheral tissues from the blood is only a portion of the carbohydrate used during the period of observation. A variable additional source of carbohydrate is the amount of glycogen present in the peripheral tissue at the beginning of the experiment. If less glycogen is broken down to supply carbohydrate intermediates, more blood sugar will be used and vice versa. This is illustrated by the work of Cohn et al.[130] who performed complete chemical balance experiments in a series of adrenalectomized, eviscerated dogs. Total carbohydrate utilization was less than normal at all blood-sugar levels tested. But muscle glycogen contributed little, if anything, to this utilization and, therefore, more glucose had to be administered to maintain desired blood levels. This behavior is similar to that found previously in hypophysectomized dogs.

The mass of evidence cited seems to indicate that the anti-insulin, hyperglycemic action of C_{11} oxysteroids is exerted directly or indirectly upon hepatic gluconeogenesis rather than on peripheral glucose utilization or "oxidation."

The impairment of muscular performance seen so characteristically in the adrenalectomized animal can be completely restored only by the C_{11} oxysteroids. Because of the action of this group of steroids on tissue carbohydrate levels and the relation of muscle work to carbohydrate turnover it was supposed that the fatigability of the adrenalectomized animal was an expression of a basic metabolic disturbance in the muscle. A reinvestigation of this problem has demonstrated, however, that the prompt muscle fatigue of adrenalectomized animals is not due to any intrinsic disturbance in the functions of the motor nerve, of the myoneural junction or of the muscle itself.[131] Preceding muscular fatigue, there is a fall in blood pressure which, of course, diminishes blood flow through the working part. Restoration of blood pressure causes an immediate return of muscle power. The C_{11} oxysteroids seem to affect the responses of the small blood vessels to reflexly produced autonomic vasomotor agents and thus affect muscle performance by a primary effect upon the blood supply. The work capacity of the muscle is thus secondarily affected, without any specific metabolic influence.

The manner in which the adrenal cortex stimulates hepatic gluconeogenesis is by no means clear, but evidence is forthcoming that it influences the mobilization and catabolism of both protein and fat. Nitrogen excretion is decreased following adrenalectomy, and the administration of cortical extracts restores the nitrogen output to normal. The increased glycosuria observed after the treatment of adrenalectomized depancreatized animals with cortical fractions or steroids is accompanied by a corresponding increase in the urinary nitrogen. Wells et al.[126] have demonstrated similar effects with the cortical substances in phlorhizinized adrenalectomized rats.

Concerning the mobilization of fat, it had been shown that various procedures which increased the fat content of the liver in normal animals usually failed to do so in the absence of the adrenals. Barnes et al. fed spectroscopically active fatty acids to fasting normal and adrenalectomized rats and were able to identify the administered fat in the livers of their normal animals, but this was not the case in the operated animals.

Recent work using isotopic glucose has shown the pronounced effect of the C_{11} corticoids on the rate of sugar production by the liver.[132] There is, as yet, little evidence that this influence is a specific one, exerted directly on the liver. The fact that salt-treated adrenalectomized animals, when fed, can maintain good carbohydrate levels suggests that the reduced carbohydrate levels of fasting may result from a disability in the mobilization of protein and fat from the peripheral stores.

THE THYROID

Metabolic Effects of Thyroid Hormone

1. The blood-sugar level in hypo- or hyperthyroid states is influenced by the effects of the lack or excess of hormone upon the gastrointestinal tract and the liver. Althausen and his co-workers have shown that the rate of absorption of hexoses from the gut is decreased during thyroid deficiency and increased when thyroid hormone is present in excess. The effect of thyroid is not limited to the intestinal mucosa but applies also to other epithelial structures, e.g., kidney tubules.[133] These effects are specific and not merely secondary to the changes in metabolic rate, for even large increases in the latter, caused by dinitrophenol administration, have no influence on the absorption of carbohydrate. The influence of the thyroid on the rate of absorption of sugar is reflected in the rise and fall of the blood-sugar level which follows the ingestion of a carbohydrate meal or the oral administration of sugar solution for testing purposes. In hyperthyroidism the oral dextrose-tolerance curve tends to be "diabetic" in nature; in hypothyroidism it tends to be "flat." The abnormalities are not seen when the factor of intestinal absorption is eliminated by administering the dextrose intravenously.

In the post-absorptive state, when the blood sugar is being supplied by the liver, the susceptibility of the latter to glycogenolytic agents or influences has a bearing on the blood-sugar level. As judged by the results of epinephrine administration, the glycogen in the liver of the hyperthyroid organism is more readily broken down than that in the normal liver. The actual outcome of this state of affairs is, of course, dependent upon the amount of hepatic glycogen present; and this may lead to apparently anomalous results. Thus, while the induction of mild hyperthyroidism leads to an exaggerated hyperglycemic response to epinephrine, severe hyperthyroidism, which depletes the hepatic glycogen stores, may lead either to no hyperglycemic response or even to hypoglycemia.

2. The glycogen content of tissues other than the liver is also affected by abnormal thyroid states. While lesser degrees of hyperthyroidism have little effect on muscle glycogen, Dambrosi has shown that the administration of large amounts of thyroid hormone definitely interferes with the rate of recovery of glycogen in exercised muscle. Hyperthyroidism also depletes the glycogen of cardiac muscle. There is some parallelism between the decreased carbohydrate stores and the increased excretion of creatine in the urine. These effects of the thyroid hormone are not simple in their mechanism, for a lack of the hormone does not produce the opposite results. Hypothyroidism is characterized only by a moderate decrease in the glycogen content of all tissues.

It has become evident recently that the amount of available vitamin B complex has a bearing upon the manifestations of hyperthyroidism—so much so, indeed, that it will require further work, in which the experimental animals or subjects are given ample supplies of vitamin B complex, to demonstrate the pure syndrome of hyperthyroidism uncomplicated by lack of the vitamin. A glimpse of the true picture has been provided in the work of Drill and his coworkers.[134] An amount of yeast concentrate approximately six times the maintenance dose for normal animals completely counteracted the glycogen-depleting effect of a dose of thyroid which caused very significant loss of glycogen in unprotected animals. It is also important to note that the extra yeast prevented loss in body weight and led to an actual increase in liver weight.

3. The increased protein catabolism and nitrogen excretion accompanying hyperthyroidism or following the administration of thyroid substances has long been recognized. The aggravation of clinical diabetes mellitus by hyperthyroidism and its amelioration in hypothyroid states have linked the thyroid activity on protein breakdown with gluconeogenesis from protein. Increased gluconeogenesis from protein has been observed by Wells et al.[126] in phlorhizinized normal, adrenalectomized and hypophysectomized rats which were treated with thyroxin or thyrotrophic hormone.

4. In view of the evidence that thyroid hormone stimulates gluconeogenesis, it is difficult to understand the relatively minor or negative results as regards carbohydrate tolerance which have been obtained either by thyroidectomy of depancreatized animals or by the administration of thyroid substance to such animals.[135]

These problems have been reinvestigated by Houssay's laboratory using both dogs and rats as experimental animals.[136] In neither of these species does thyroid treatment produce diabetes when the pancreas is intact. However, following a subtotal pancreatectomy or the administration of substances known to damage beta-cells (anterior pituitary extracts or alloxan) the animal becomes sensitive to the diabetogenic action of thyroid hormone. The severe diabetic state thus produced is reversible if the administration of thyroid hormone is not too prolonged. Otherwise, the damage to the islets becomes irreversible and a state of permanent ("metathyroid") diabetes ensues. In the rat, under certain circumstances the thyroid hormone may first aggravate a latent diabetes but then actually lead to a recovery of islet function by stimulating the production of beta-cells. This phenomenon is probably related to the well-established resistance of the rat's beta-cells to other damaging agents, and their tendency to proliferate readily.

Surgical hypothyroidism, as well as that induced by treatment with thiouracil, increases the resistance of rats to the diabetogenic action of alloxan and prevents the onset of the diabetic state which usually follows the removal of 95 per cent of the pancreas. In the dogs the effect of hypothyroidism is qualitatively similar, but not as pronounced.

The various effects of the thyroid gland on carbohydrate metabolism can perhaps be reconciled if we consider that its hormone stimulates protein and fat mobilization from the periphery, and increases the metabolic activity of the liver as well as of the peripheral tissues. Hence, the result of thyroid administration will depend upon whether ample insulin is available, or an inadequate amount is present, or whether it is entirely absent. In the presence of an amount of insulin sufficient to allow for the entry into the peripheral tissues of the increased amount of sugar manufactured by the liver in hyperthyroidism, there is no hyperglycemia, i.e., diabetes is not outwardly manifest. When insulin production becomes inadequate, hepatic gluconeogenesis begins to exceed the capacity of the peripheral tissues to take in and dispose of sugar and ketones. A frank diabetes ensues. However, following complete pancreatectomy, gluconeogenesis is already close to maximal. Its further stimulation by thyroid administration is minimal and is counterbalanced by an increase in peripheral sugar utilization and thus the hyperglycemia is not further increased.

5. There is an abnormally rapid rate of carbohydrate utilization by the peripheral tissues of hyperthyroid animals, coincident with the increased amounts of glucose entering the blood from the gastrointestinal tract and from the liver. When thyroxin-treated dogs are hepatectomized, the rate of fall of the blood-sugar level is much greater than in hepatectomized untreated animals.[137] Increased carbohydrate utilization under the influence of thyroid hormone, has been demonstrated on isolated tissues in vitro. Such tissues exhibit an increased oxygen consumption, an increased rate of glycolysis, and an increased capacity for the oxidation of lactate, pyruvate and succinate.

THE ANTERIOR PITUITARY (ADENOHYPOPHYSIS)

The effects of removal of the anterior lobe of the hypophysis in experimental animals or of the destruction of the gland by disease in human beings are as follows:[138]

1. *Trophic effects.* The removal of the pituitary is followed by an atrophy and decreased function of the thyroid gland, of the adrenal cortex and of the gonads, whether male or female. For this reason the pituitary has often been referred to as "the master-gland" of the body. However, the removal of the thyroid or the adrenal cortex or the gonads is followed by histologic changes in the pituitary. These changes have been variously interpreted, and it is still not quite certain what they mean from a functional standpoint. But there can be no doubt that the removal of these other glands does affect the structure and function of the pituitary. This is also true of the administration of the hormones or extracts of the other glands. Thus, it is clear that, while the pituitary may be more generally important than some of the other glands, it is not merely because it dominates them. It appears rather to coordinate the functions of the other glands, so that one might call it "the executive secretary" of the endocrine system rather than the master-gland.

2. *A lowering of the blood-sugar level.* The blood sugar of the hypophysectomized animal under conditions of adequate nutrition is about 20 to 30 mg. per cent lower than the blood sugar of the normal dog.

3. *The hypoglycemic effect of fasting.* A normal animal or human being may be fasted indefinitely with little or no effect on the blood-sugar level. As a matter of fact, there may be no sig-

nificant effect until a relatively short time before death from starvation, when the blood sugar may fall precipitously. However, in the absence of the hypophysis, fasting is accompanied by rapid development of hypoglycemia, so that the animal may die within a relatively short time in hypoglycemic convulsions.

4. A *decreased urine nitrogen excretion.* This is due in part to a decreased breakdown of body protein resulting from the secondary thyroid atrophy. The atrophy of the adrenal cortex may also be partly responsible.

5. A *decrease in the total metabolism of the body.* This is probably accounted for by the depression of thyroid activity, although other factors may be involved. The other factors may be the adrenal cortical atrophy and the loss of weight brought about by the marked anorexia, which is a prominent clinical feature of pituitary insufficiency.

6. *An increased sensitivity to insulin.* A small amount of insulin which would produce no noticeable effect on a normal animal will, after the removal of the hypophysis, cause prolonged and even fatal hypoglycemia.

7. A *decrease in the potassium content of the blood serum.*

8. A *decrease in the reduced glutathione content of blood, liver, and skeletal muscle.* The diminished level of reduced glutathione in the liver may be related to the insulin sensitivity.

9. A *cessation of maturation and growth.* When the pituitary is removed from immature animals, there is a cessation of maturation and growth.

The injection of crude extracts of the anterior lobe of the pituitary into hypophysectomized animals has been shown to prevent or reverse the consequences of the removal of the gland. Normal animals receiving pituitary extracts exhibit a hypertrophy and hyperfunction of the other endocrine glands. Depending upon the conditions, there may be concomitant gain in weight or increased rate of growth; or hyperglycemia, glycosuria and ketosis may develop. Under circumstances in which there is hyperglycemia and glycosuria, there is also an increased excretion of nitrogen. Where gain in weight or an increased rate of growth is a major consequence, there may be a retention of nitrogen.

The Influence of the Anterior Pituitary as a Whole on Various Aspects of Carbohydrate Metabolism

The well-fed hypophysectomized animal maintains a significantly lower blood-sugar level than the normal animal. This is due to the influence of the hypophysis on the threshold of the homeostatic mechanism for the regulation of the blood-sugar level, as will be discussed later. The profound influence of the anterior pituitary on the carbohydrate levels of blood and tissues is most clearly demonstrated by observing the effects of fasting. When food is withheld from the hypophysectomized organism, there occurs a progressive drop in the blood-sugar level, terminating in hypoglycemic convulsions and death. The glycogen content of the tissues is decreased, particularly that of the liver. This occurs even when the pancreas and the hypophysis are both removed; and the effect of fasting is exaggerated by the administration of phlorhizin.

These effects of fasting might be interpreted in one of two ways: either (1) the anterior pituitary exerts an inhibitory influence on carbohydrate utilization by the tissues, and hence hypophysectomy is followed by an excessive rate of utilization, with which the capacity of the liver for gluconeogenesis cannot keep pace; or (2) the gland exerts its primary influence on gluconeogenetic processes in the liver, and hence its removal leads to a reduced rate of sugar formation from noncarbohydrate precursors, such that the amounts of sugar necessary even for normal utilization can no longer be supplied. It is clear that these alternative explanations are similar, to the extent that they depend upon a disproportion between the rates of sugar formation and sugar utilization. But the first explanation attributes the major point of influence to the

TABLE 6. EFFECTS OF ENDOCRINE STATES AND SUBSTITUTION THERAPY ON PHLORHIZIN DIABETES IN THE RAT*

CONDITION OF ANIMALS	ENDOCRINE THERAPY	URINE SUGAR (MG. PER 100 GM. PER DAY)	URINE NPN (MG. PER 100 GM. PER DAY)	D:N	COMPARED TO THE NORMAL (= 100)	
					Sugar	NPN
Normal	....	621	182	3.4	100	100
Normal	Thyroxin	770	171	4.5	124	95
Normal	Thyrotrophic hormone	625	196	3.2	100	107
Hypophysectomized	....	148	57	2.6	24	31
Hypophysectomized	Desoxycorticosterone	323	100	3.2	52	56
Hypophysectomized	Corticosterone	449	158	2.8	72	87
Hypophysectomized	Compound E	412	170	2.4	67	94
Hypophysectomized	Compound E plus thyrotrophic hormone	625	196	3.2	100	107

* Data taken from the work of Wells and Kendall.[139]

peripheral tissues, while the second attributes it to the liver.

The work of Wells and others[139] in Kendall's laboratory confirmed the defect in gluconeogenesis in hypophysectomized animals and indicated that this influence of the hypophysis was exerted partly through the adrenal cortex and partly through the thyroid gland. These workers studied the urinary sugar and nitrogen excretion of normal, adrenalectomized, thyroidectomized, and hypophysectomized rats, respectively, treated with phlorhizin. They also included animals from which both the thyroid and the adrenal glands had been removed. By administering various hormones and combinations of hormones to the operated rats they were able to judge which hormonal factors restored the hypophysectomized animals to a normal response, so far as sugar and nitrogen excretion were concerned. Their results are summarized in Table 6. It may be seen that neither thyroid nor adrenal cortical hormone by itself was able to rectify the deficiency in hypophysectomized rats, while the combination of both hormones was successful. It may be concluded that the gluconeogenetic influence of the thyroid gland and of the adrenal cortex are each partly responsible for the total effect of the anterior pituitary.

It is generally agreed that pituitary or adrenal diabetes is at least in part due to stimulation of gluconeogenesis from protein.[140] The confusing and contradictory aspect of this field is the effect of the pituitary and of the adrenal cortex on the rate of sugar uptake by the tissues and its conversion to glycogen and/or CO_2. There seem to be unexplained species differences. Thus, the hepatectomized hypophysectomized rat or rabbit requires more sugar to maintain a normal glucose level than liverless control animals.[141] On the other hand, the hypophysectomized or Houssay dog utilizes less sugar than his normal counterpart.[142,143] Following adrenalectomy, the glucose utilization of the peripheral tissues of rats increases, but only when the animal's mineral balance and circulatory dynamics are incompletely rectified.

It might be expected that work using single tissues in vitro would be clearer and more consistent. This is not the case. The uptake of sugar and/or glycogenesis by the isolated diaphragm of hypophysectomized or adrenalectomized rats has been found by some to be increased above that of normal animals, and by others to be not at all different from normal values. Similarly inconsistent results are available for the effect of pituitary and adrenal cortical hormones when administered to normal animals or when added to the in vitro medium in which the tissues were bathed.

Samuels,[144] Wertheimer, Lundbaeck, Wilhelmi, and others showed that the type of dietary mixture (especially, the ratio of CHO:fat) seems to orient the direction of cellular metabolism along one or another pathway, thereby determining the avidity of tissues for one or another type of substrate. It is possible, therefore, that the tissues of adrenalectomized and hypophysectomized animals, in view of the known difficulties of such animals in mobilizing proteins and fats, are "oriented" toward carbohydrate. This would become especially evident when such animals did not consume a calorically adequate diet, or were placed on a high carbohydrate intake. When such animals are fed a more adequate mixed diet, they may no longer show increased uptake of sugar by their tissues. Perlmutter[145] seems to bear out this point of view directly. In the isolated diaphragms of hypophysectomized rats fed ad libitum, he observed a higher than normal uptake of glucose from the medium. When, however, he repeated his observations on rats which had been force-fed adequate amounts of a mixed diet, the sugar uptake by the diaphragms was within normal limits. Samuels' findings that the well-known insulin sensitivity of hypophysectomized animals can be abolished by dietary means is a demonstration of similar import.

The Hypophysectomized-Depancreatized (Houssay) Animal

In 1930 Houssay and his associates reported their observations in hypophysectomized-depancreatized dogs.[140] They found that such animals exhibited less severe diabetes than dogs with only the pancreas removed. The blood-sugar level varied in different animals from 320 to 113 mg. per cent. Sometimes spontaneous hypoglycemia occurred. The glycosuria was correspondingly variable and was entirely absent in some cases. Nitrogen excretion was only slightly decreased, but ketosis was either very mild or absent. The animals survived for months without insulin.

Figure 26 shows that fasting has the same hypoglycemic effect on the Houssay dog as it has on the hypophysectomized animal.[142] It also indicates the quantitative relationship between the amount of protein ingested and the consequent rise in the blood-sugar level. As might be expected, the glycosuria also depends upon the protein intake. It should be noted that, regardless of the degree of diabetic manifestations in the different animals, no ketonuria was observed.

It may be concluded that the same disturbance which causes the disability of the hypophysectomized animal as regards maintenance of his blood-sugar level, namely, the impairment of gluconeogenesis, is also responsible for the amelioration of diabetes in the Houssay animal. The extreme variability in the severity of the diabetic syndrome noted by Houssay and other authors undoubtedly resulted from the variability of the food intake of their experimental animals. The well-fed Houssay animal actually exhibits a diabetic syndrome of moderate severity, except for the lack of ketosis. The undernourished Houssay animal manifests little or no diabetes. But even under the most favorable nutritional conditions, the diabetic syndrome is not as intense as in the depancreatized animal with the hypophysis intact. This is readily understood when one considers the unavailability of its endogenous protein and fat for gluconeogenesis and the fact that, of the ingested food materials, only sugar (as such) or protein (amino acids) can contribute to the maintenance of the blood-sugar level. In other words, while the depancreatized animal with hypophysis intact can make excessive sugar at the expense of endogenous or exogenous foodstuffs, the Houssay animal can use only ingested protein for this purpose. This accounts for the hypoglycemic effects of fasting, in spite of ample fat stores; the low D:N ratios, the lack of ketosis; and the relatively long survival without insulin.

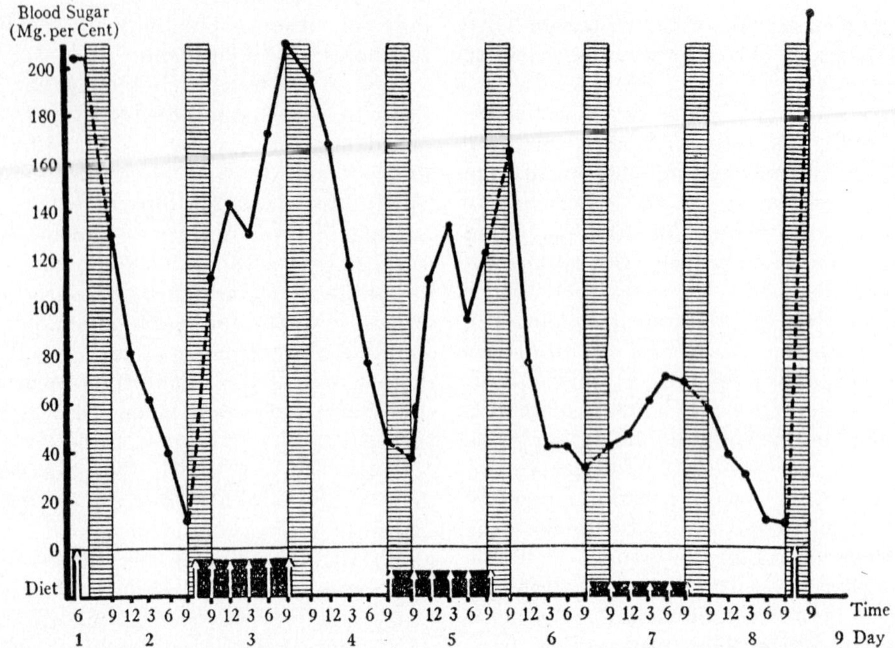

FIG. 26. Influence of the amount of protein intake on the blood-sugar level of the hypophysectomized-depancreatized dog. The black areas represent days upon which the animal was fed; the superimposed white arrows indicate the meals. The shaded strips are a foreshortened representation of the night periods, between 9:00 P.M. and 9:00 A.M. The total amount of food given on the respective days of feeding was as follows: day 1:400 gm. of lean meat, 60 gm. of cane sugar, 120 gm. of raw pancreas; day 3:378 gm. of protein as lean meat; day 5:168 gm. of protein; day 7:90 gm. of protein; evening of day 8: same as day 1. (Soskin et al.[142])

The amelioration of the diabetic syndrome in the absence of the hypophysis resembles, in many respects, that seen in depancreatized dogs maintained without insulin or undernutrition diets composed solely of protein.[146] It has been shown that carbohydrate utilization proceeds at a normal rate (because of hyperglycemia) in untreated pancreatic diabetes[60] and that hypophysectomy decreases carbohydrate utilization.[143] Hence, neither undernutrition nor hypophysectomy can be held to ameliorate the diabetic syndrome by restoring carbohydrate utilization. Undernourished depancreatized animals survive from four to six weeks and, despite the complete absence of insulin, become progressively less diabetic the longer they survive. There is a progressive lowering of the D:N ratio, a gradual increase in the R.Q., and an increasing retention of administered sugar which has both protein-sparing and antiketogenic actions. These criteria of "carbohydrate oxidation" become apparent as the fat stores of the animals are depleted. The difference between these animals and Houssay dogs consists in the means by which the diabetes is modified rather than in any difference in the final state which is reached. The undernourished depancreatized animals suffer a gradual and incomplete loss of body fat as the period of undernutrition progresses, while the Houssay animals exhibit an acute loss of ability to utilize the ample fat stores which are present. In both cases this leads to a decreased new sugar formation, so that utilization of carbohydrate is unmasked.

Interdependence of the Metabolic Factors

Table 7 summarizes the various known physiologic effects of the best-isolated components of anterior pituitary extract which together exert the so-called "diabetogenic action." It will be noted that the most important factors are the adrenotrophic, thyrotrophic and growth hormones. In general, these hormones act by mobilizing the noncarbohydrate precursors of blood sugar from the periphery and by stimulating gluconeogenesis at their expense in the liver. This seems an anomalous function to attribute to the growth hormone, since the process of growth must involve protein synthesis and nitrogen retention rather than the reverse. The fact is that the growth hormone exhibits either its anabolic or its catabolic action, depending upon the presence or absence of insulin. In the normal animal or in the depancreatized animal receiving large amounts of insulin the growth hormone causes nitrogen retention. In the untreated diabetic animal it causes increased nitrogen excretion.

Certain experiments showing the amelioration of the diabetic syndrome by adrenalectomy and its exacerbation even in the hypophysectomized animal by the administration of large amounts of adrenal cortical hormone have been interpreted as indicating that the adrenotrophic hormone is the most important factor in the diabetogenic action of the anterior pituitary. This is not necessarily so. It is true that the presence of some adrenal cortical hormone is essential for the diabetogenic action of the other anterior pituitary factors, and this may account for the amelioration of diabetes in its absence. But it has also been shown that the administration to an adrenalectomized animal of an amount of adrenal cortical hormone which by itself exerts no obvious diabetogenic effect will enable that animal to yield a significant diabetogenic response to anterior pituitary extracts.[141]

Recently de Bodo, Steele and their coworkers[157,158,159] using isotopic techniques have clarified many of the problems concerning the functions of the anterior pituitary and of the adrenal cor-

TABLE 7. ACTIONS OF VARIOUS HORMONES

HORMONE	ACTIONS	REMARKS
Growth (GH)	1. Nitrogen retention (in presence of adequate insulin)	GH and ACTH oppose each othH as far as growth is concerned; Ger and TH act synergistically
	2. Increase in glycosuria of partially depancreatized animals	
	3. Insulin resistance	
	4. Increase in ketone production	
	5. Fat mobilization	
	6. Increase in muscle glycogen	
	7. Destruction of B-cells of islets	
	8. Increase in milk production during lactation	
Adrenocorticotrophic (ACTH)	1. Increase in nitrogen excretion	
	2. Fat mobilization	
	3. Increase in glycosuria of partially depancreatized animals	
	4. Production of glycosuria in normal animals	Via adrenal cortex
	5. Insulin resistance	
	6. Increase in liver glycogen	
	7. Inhibition of growth	
Thyrotrophic (TH)	1. Increase in nitrogen excretion	
	2. Increase in B.M.R.	
	3. Increase in size of liver	Nos. 1, 2, and 3 via thyroid
	4. Decrease in tissue NPN	
	5. Accumulation of interstitial protein rich fluid (myxedema)	

tex in carbohydrate regulation. In the hypophysectomized dog they found a reduced utilization of glucose coupled with a much greater reduction in gluconeogenetic capacity. Adrenalectomy did not reduce utilization but diminished rates of gluconeogenesis. The "growth" hormone could function in the absence of the adrenals. Better regulation is achieved by the joint presence of "growth" hormone and the adrenal steroids.

REGULATION OF CARBOHYDRATE METABOLISM

We have, thus far, dealt with the storage of carbohydrate, its interconversions, and its utilization or dissimilation by the living organism. We have seen that our knowledge of the quantitative aspects of these phenomena is rather limited. It is therefore to be expected that the development of our understanding of the mechanisms which regulate carbohydrate metabolism should be correspondingly retarded. At the present time it is impossible to predict, except in the most general sort of way, what proportions of a given dose of carbohydrate will follow the various possible pathways for its disposal in the living organism under a particular set of circumstances. It is impossible to calculate how much of the carbohydrate will be stored as glycogen, how much will be converted, and how much will be dissimilated for energetic purposes.

Such partitions as might be predicted are based upon empirical data from previous experiments conducted under similar conditions. We know from experience that, when a limited amount of carbohydrate is available, it is likely to be used as a source of energy and that little of it will appear as glycogen or fat. It seems obvious that there must be fairly accurate mechanism for diverting the carbohydrate into the channel most useful for the animal, but we know little or nothing of the details of such mechanisms.

The regulation of the blood-sugar level differs somewhat from that of other carbohydrate functions. Storage, interconversions, and dissimilation vary with carbohydrate supply, whereas the blood-sugar level in the normal animal remains relatively constant under the most diverse conditions of feeding and fasting. On the other hand, the hyperglycemia and the great dependence of the blood-sugar level of the diabetic organism on the kind and amount of ingested food indicates a profound disturbance of the regulating mechanisms in diabetes.

Claude Bernard was keenly aware of the dynamic balance involved in blood-sugar regulation—the balance upon which any proper conception of regulation must be based. He clearly stated that the normal blood-sugar level represented a precise equilibrium between the rates of sugar formation in the liver and of sugar utilization in the tissues. While the role which he assigned to the liver has been confirmed by most recent workers, it has, nevertheless, been virtually ignored in the usual explanations of the various experimental or clinical states which are characterized by a persistence of abnormal blood-sugar levels. Instead, attention has been focused almost exclusively upon the utilization of sugar. This may be accounted for partly by the discovery of insulin and partly by the erstwhile predominance of the non-utilization theory of diabetes. The discovery of insulin led to overemphasis of the possible role of the pancreas in the regulation of carbohydrate metabolism; the non-utilization theory demanded that the regulating activity of the pancreas be exerted upon sugar utilization.

The Homeostatic Mechanism in the Liver

The characteristic rise and fall of the blood sugar following the administration of dextrose to normal animals represents a rapid and reproducible test of the regulating mechanisms. Wide clinical and experimental use of this test has been made. In man it has been customary to have the subject drink 300 to 500 cc. of lemonade sweetened with 50 to 100 gm. of dextrose. The test is usually performed in the morning before breakfast, for it has been found that previous food intake influences the outcome of the test. A control blood-sugar determination is made before the test, and further determinations are made at various intervals up to 3 hours after the test. The average, or "normal," blood-sugar curve obtained in the healthy subject is shown in Figure 27, where it is contrasted with the so-called "diabetic" curve from patients with diabetes mellitus and from individuals suffering from other conditions which interfere with efficient regulations.

It was customary in the past to explain the normal dextrose-tolerance curve as resulting exclusively from a stimulation of the pancreas by the administered sugar. The abnormal type of curve characteristic of the depancreatized animal and of the diabetic human was attributed to a lack of pancreatic response, with a consequent inability to dispose of the incoming sugar at the normal rate. It will be noted that this explanation did not take into account the important role of the liver in supplying sugar and the possibility that regulating might also be accomplished by controlling this supply.

Soskin and his co-workers[147] tested the fundamental basis of these explanations by substituting a constant-injection pump for the pancreas as the source of insulin in dogs. Completely depancreatized dogs received constant intravenous injections of insulin at rates just sufficient to maintain a normal, constant blood-sugar level in each particular animal. They were therefore restored to normal in a restricted experimental sense except that they could not mobilize additional insulin; they had to get along on the constant amounts of insulin supplied by their artificial substitute for a pancreas. If the previous concepts had been correct, such animals should have yielded "diabetic" dextrose-tolerance curves. But, as a matter of fact, the animals exhibited perfectly normal tolerance curves. It was evident that, provided sufficient insulin were present to maintain a constant blood-sugar level, no additional secretion was necessary for adequate regulation.

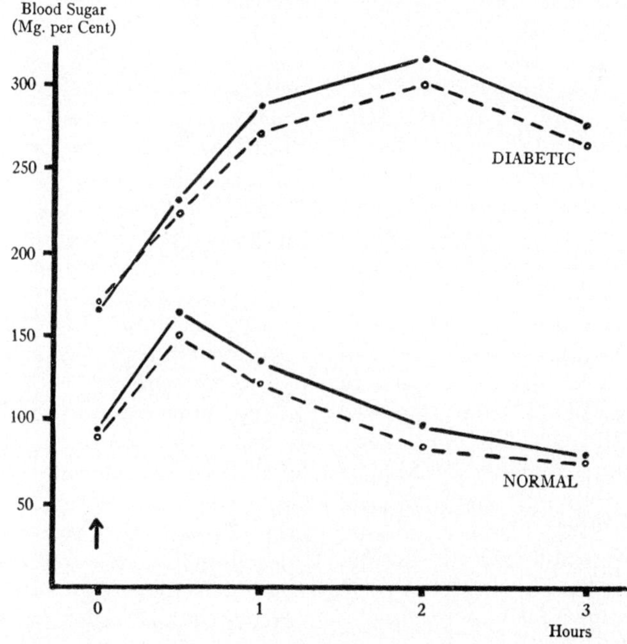

FIG. 27. Oral-dextrose-tolerance curves in normal and diabetic humans. The arrow indicates the administration of 50 gm. of glucose by mouth. The continuous lines represent arterial (capillary) blood-sugar values; the broken lines represent venous blood-sugar values.

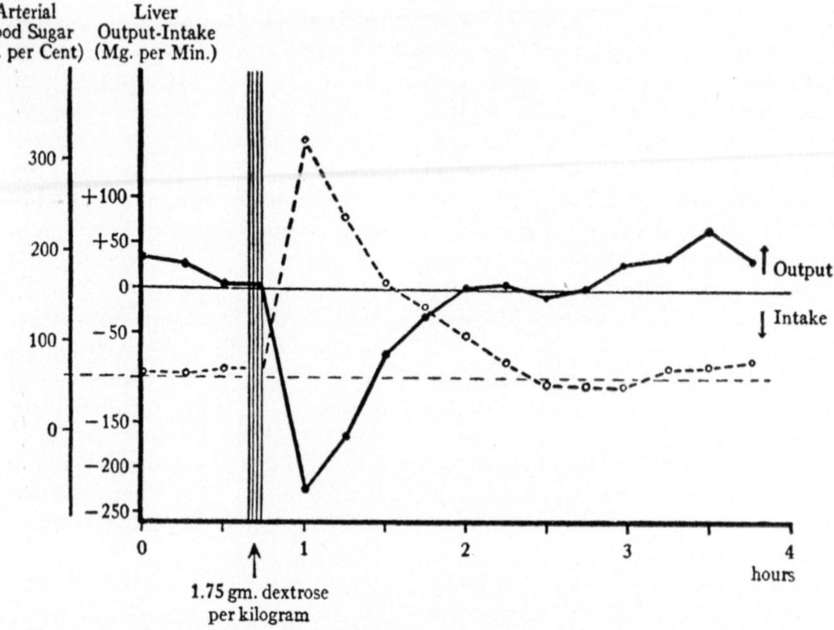

FIG. 28. Direct demonstration of the homeostatic mechanism in the liver. The effect of dextrose administration upon the output and intake of sugar by the liver of an intact dog, calculated from blood-sugar values and thermostromuhr measurements of hepatic blood flow. The broken line represents arterial blood-sugar values; the heavier, continuous line represents output or intake of sugar by the liver in milligrams per minute. Note the immediate cessation of sugar output when sugar is administered and the large intake of sugar which follows. Throughout the second hour after sugar administration the liver neither retains nor excretes sugar. During this period the level of sugar in the arterial blood falls below its original control values and does not return to normal until after the liver has resumed its output. The inhibition of the hepatic secretion of sugar is, therefore, a real and separate phenomenon from the storage of sugar. (Soskin et al.[148])

These results naturally directed attention toward the liver as possibly the factor that varied in regulation. Normal dogs were hepatectomized; and a constant injection of dextrose just sufficient to maintain a normal, constant blood-sugar level was substituted for the liver. Since the pancreas was intact, this type of animal preparation was able to mobilize insulin as required but could not alter the rate at which sugar was being delivered to the blood from the artificial liver. Such animals invariably yielded markedly "diabetic" tolerance curves. It was apparent that the pancreas was not essential to the regulating mechanisms responsible for the normal dextrose-tolerance curve, while the presence of the normal liver was essential.

This led to observations on the simultaneous blood-sugar values of the blood flowing into and out of the liver, in normal and depancreatized dogs, during the course of dextrose-tolerance tests. From these and the previous results it was postulated that (in the presence of a sufficiency of insulin, but not necessarily an extra secretion from the pancreas) the normal liver, as one of its responses to administered dextrose, decreases the output of blood sugar which it has previously been supplying from its own resources.

The homeostatic regulating mechanism for the control of the blood-sugar level was later subjected to direct proof.[148] By correlating the rate of blood flow through the liver of experimental animals with the difference in the sugar content between the blood flowing into and out of this organ, it was possible to calculate the absolute amounts of sugar entering and leaving the liver per unit of time. Figure 28 illustrates such an experiment and shows what happens when a dextrose-tolerance test is made. It may be seen that the liver, which was pouring sugar into the blood prior to the administration of the dextrose, ceased to do so almost immediately upon the administration of dextrose and started to take in large quantities of sugar. (The period following this retention of sugar is particularly worthy of note. At this time the liver neither took in nor put out sugar for a period of about an hour, showing that the inhibition of the output of sugar is a phenomenon separate from the storage of sugar.) When the period of inhibition was over, the liver again began its usual supply of sugar to the blood; and the blood-sugar level, which had fallen somewhat below the pre-test level during the inhibition, rose up to and slightly above its pre-test level. Bondy et al.[149] have since obtained essentially similar results in man, using the liver catheterization technique.

In further experiments it was also shown that completely depancreatized dogs which were receiving the appropriate constant injections of insulin exhibited at least as great a hypoglycemic reaction following the cessation of prolonged sugar administration as did normal dogs. Like the normal dextrose-tolerance curve, this phenomenon cannot be ascribed to insulin mobilization but must be accounted for by the decrease in the output of sugar by the liver in response to the influx of exogenous sugar. In other words, this period of hypoglycemia following the dextrose-tolerance curve or following the cessation of more prolonged dextrose injections corresponds to the time which elapses before the liver is able to accelerate its rate of supply of blood sugar to a point sufficient to maintain the original normal blood-sugar level.

The hepatic regulating mechanism is analogous in the system used for the regulation of temperature in many modern homes, namely, the thermostat-furnace arrangement. When the temperature of the house rises above the level at which the thermostat has been set, the furnace shuts off until the excess heat has been dissipated. When the temperature of the house falls back to the threshold of the thermostat, the furnace starts up again. This is exactly what the liver does, so far as the blood-sugar level is concerned. In this analogy the temperature is equivalent to the blood-sugar level, and the thermostat-furnace arrangement is represented by the liver. It will be noted that, just as it is the room temperature which operates the thermostat and shuts off the furnace, so it is the blood-sugar level which inhibits the output of sugar by the liver.

Accordingly the dextrose-tolerance curve and the hypoglycemic phase which often follows it resemble the fluctuations in temperature above and below the threshold of regulation when an extra quantity of heat is introduced into the temperature-regulated house. The characteristics of the curve depend upon the magnitude of the disturbing factor (the amount of sugar administered), the setting and sensitivity of the thermostat (the endocrine balance), and the capacity of the furnace (the ability of the liver to produce sugar).

The fact that the hepatectomized animal with an artificially maintained normal constant blood-sugar level (and with the pancreas and extrahepatic tissues free to exert whatever regulating powers they possess) yields "diabetic" dextrose-tolerance curves indicates the essential role of the liver in blood-sugar regulation. It is not to be supposed, however, that the hepatic mechanism is the only one involved. Glycogen deposition in both the liver and muscle and an increased utilization of sugar by the extrahepatic tissues undoubtedly play their parts. These processes, like hepatic homeostasis, are under the influence of the blood-sugar level. It seems logical to assume that smaller amounts of sugar, especially if they enter the circulation via the portal vein, may be fully compensated for by hepatic inhibition alone. Larger amounts of sugar may invoke hepatic storage as well. When the systemic blood-sugar level is raised, it will bring into play the additional factors of extrahepatic storage and increased utilization by stimulating extra insulin secretion.

The Role of the Endocrines in the Regulation of the Blood Sugar

The thermostat-furnace analogy is useful in arriving at a clear conception of the function of the endocrine glands in the regulation of the blood sugar. It is obvious that a thermostat-furnace arrangement will go through the same regulating processes at any temperature level, depending upon where the thermostat is set. In other words, it is the setting of the thermostat which determines at which temperature the furnace will shut off. Similarly, the balanced action of the endocrine secretions determines the level of blood sugar at which the liver will be inhibited. In the normal animal the endocrine balance is such that the liver is inhibited at a range between 60 and 90 mg. per cent. This, indeed, is what determines the existence of a constant normal blood-sugar level. An excess or a deficiency of any of the hormones upsets the endocrine balance and changes the threshold for the inhibition of the liver, and hence changes the blood-sugar level in a characteristic manner.

Influence of the Pancreas. It will be remembered that, while the liver turned out to be the primary organ excreting the regulating activity responsible for the dextrose-tolerance curve, it was necessary to maintain a constant supply of insulin throughout the test period. In other words, the normal endocrine balance had to be maintained in order to have regulation occur at its usual normal level. When insulin is deficient, as in experimental pancreatic diabetes, the situation is equivalent to that which would occur if the adjusting screw on a thermostat were set at an infinitely high level. If we suppose that the setting were now at 1000° F., the thermostat might just as well have been entirely removed, for all practical purposes. In the first place, the furnace is probably incapable of producing enough heat to raise the temperature of the house to 1000° F. and so to shut itself off. Secondly, even if the furnace were capable of producing that much heat, the house would burn down before the thermostat threshold was reached. What actually happens is that the furnace simply continues to produce heat in an uncontrolled manner to the limit of its capabilities. The house is overheated, and the heat is dissipated only to the extent that it can pass through the walls, doors and windows. Similarly, when insulin is deficient, the sugar output of the liver is no longer inhibited, regardless of how high the blood-sugar level rises. The result is a hyperglycemia and a glycosuria which are only aggravated by the administration of additional sugar. When the latter procedure is performed as a dextrose-tolerance test, the result is a high and prolonged curve which is not a function of the normal liver reaction but which depends upon the rate at which the sugar can be disposed of by diffusion, utilization, and excretion.

Influence of the Anterior Pituitary Gland. When the anterior pituitary gland is deficient or absent, as in the hypophysectomized animal, the situation is equivalent to that which would occur if the adjusting screw on the thermostat were turned down as far as it would go, so that the furnace would shut off even while the house was cold. This is the significance of the characteristically low blood-sugar level maintained in hypopituitarism. Conversely, the administration of anterior pituitary extracts will maintain the blood sugar at high levels. In other words, the anterior pituitary is a force tending to regulate the blood-sugar level in a direction opposite to that of insulin. To revert to our analogy, let us suppose that insulin is represented by a spring tending to pull the thermostat bar toward low-temperature regulation, while the anterior pituitary secretion is a spring pulling the bar in the opposite direction. Ordinarily, the balanced action of both springs keeps the bar floating at the desired normal-temperature setting. It will be realized, of course, that the removal of either spring will allow the other one to react violently in the opposite direction. In this connection, consider the marked sensitivity of the hypophysectomized animal to insulin. From this point of view, also, it is easy to understand the strong resemblances of hyperinsulinism to hypopituitarism and the high incidence of hyperglycemia or diabetes in hyperpituitarism.

Let us also consider what result one might expect if one were to remove the opposing springs from both sides of the thermostat. The bar would move from its normal point of balance to some other position (depending upon the force of gravity, etc.), and regulation would then occur at this fortuitous level. This situation has been duplicated in the living organism by the simultaneous removal of both the pancreas and the pituitary gland. Such an animal, when well fed, maintains a blood-sugar level in the neighborhood of 350 to 400 mg. per cent and yields perfectly normal dextrose-tolerance curves at that level.

It has been pointed out, by analogy, that the liver will go through the same regulating process at any level of blood sugar, depending upon where the threshold of the homeostatic mechanism in the liver is set by the endocrine balance. If this is so, the hypophysectomized animal or a hypopituitary human should yield a perfectly normal dextrose-tolerance curve, except that it should start from a low level and return to the same low level. This is actually the case. But a lack of understanding of all the factors involved has led to misrepresentations of the results obtained, so that the dextrose-tolerance curve in hypopituitarism has been variously reported as being abnormally low, normal, and abnormally high. Perhaps the most common error leading to the belief that "dextrose tolerance in hypopituitarism is better than normal" has been the administration of the test sugar by mouth. The low curve obtained by this procedure is a reflection of the diminished rate of absorption from the gastrointestinal tract rather than an index of the ability to handle sugar, once it has entered the blood stream.

However, even when the sugar is administered intravenously, the apparent tolerance depends upon how the data are expressed. Figure 29 shows a typical intravenous dextrose tolerance curve in a hypophysectomized dog (broken line) as compared to a similar test in a normal dog (continuous line).* If the lower initial and final levels in the hypophysectomized animal are ignored, its curve appears to be low or better than normal. If, on the other hand, the results of both curves are expressed as percentage rise above the initial level, the hypophysectomized curve appears to be high or worse than normal. When, however, the actual curves are drawn from the same base line, it can be seen that they are practically identical.

Influence of the Adrenal Cortex and the Thyroid Gland. At the present time it is difficult to separate the influences of the adrenal cortex and the thyroid gland from that of the anterior pituitary. Indeed, some of the influence of the anterior pituitary gland described above may be exerted through these other glands. At any rate, deficiency or removal of the adrenal cortex, on the one hand, or the administration of potent extracts of this gland, on the other hand, will lower or raise the blood-sugar level in a manner resembling that which occurs when the pituitary hormone is varied. To a lesser extent, this is also true of the thyroid. Presumably, then, the adrenal cortex and the thyroid influence the threshold of regulation of the sugar level in the same manner as does the anterior pituitary.

Influence of the State of the Liver on the Regulation of the Blood Sugar

Although we have compared the liver to a thermostat-furnace arrangement, we have thus far considered only those factors which operate by affecting the

* The unusual height to which the blood sugar rises and the prolonged return to initial levels (for intravenous curves) depends upon the fact that an extremely large amount of sugar was used for these tests, namely, 1.75 gm. per kilogram of body weight.

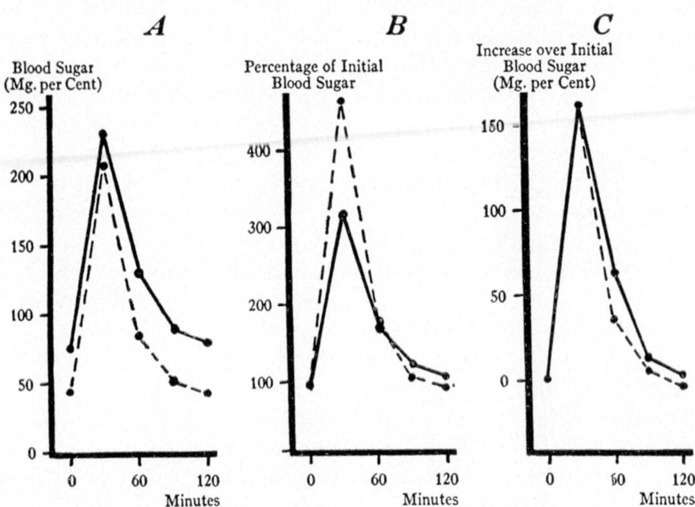

FIG. 29. Intravenous dextrose-tolerance tests in a hypophysectomized dog (*broken lines*) and in a normal dog (*continuous lines*), compared in different ways: (*A*) when absolute values are plotted, the curve of the hypophysectomized animal looks lower than normal; (*B*) when percentage increases above initial values are plotted, the curve of the hypophysectomized animal appears to be higher than normal; (*C*) when the values are superimposed by plotting absolute increases above initial values, the curves are seen to be practically identical. (Soskin.[147])

thermostat part of the mechanism. However, it is obvious that, regardless of where the thermostat is set, the state of repair and the capabilities of the furnace will have an important bearing on the degree of regulation which is achieved. For example, a thermostat setting of 80° F., would have no meaning if the furnace were incapable of producing enough heat to raise the temperature of the house to that level. Another consideration is the speed with which the rate of heat production by the furnace can be increased or diminished. Unless such adjustments are rapid, there will be a considerable overswing before the correct temperature is reached. If the thermostat on a sluggish furnace clicks over at, let us say, 80° F., the temperature may rise to 90° or 100° F., before the effect of shutting off the furnace becomes evident. Finally, even with a furnace of great capacity and high efficiency, the degree of regulation will depend upon the magnitude of the environmental temperature change for which the furnace has to compensate. In other words, the usual nightly drop of 10° to 20° F., in the outside temperature might produce practically no perceptible disturbance in the temperature of the house, while a sudden frost, dropping the outside temperature 40° to 50° F., might result in a downward dip in the house temperature before the furnace could cope with it. The analogous considerations apply to the liver as the organ which makes the blood sugar.

An example of a disturbance in sugar regulation analogous to the situation in which the furnace is incapable of raising the temperature up to the level at which the thermostat is set is the effect of fasting on the hypophysectomized animal and on the hypopituitary human. The withholding of food in the latter organisms results in a progressive hypoglycemia. This does not depend upon any change in regulation, because the resumption of food intake immediately restores the previous blood-sugar level. It does depend upon a marked reduction in the ability of the liver to make blood sugar from body stores, so that it cannot supply sufficient sugar to maintain the blood-sugar level unless additional preformed sugar or amino acids regularly enter from the gastro-intestinal tract.

The situation in the liver which is analogous to the sluggish furnace, unable to increase or decrease its rates of heat production very readily, is that where the liver is damaged by toxic agents. It is well known that the "diabetic" type of dextrose-tolerance curve is obtained in this condition.

The "diabetic" type of tolerance curve obtained in starvation or on a high-fat diet is analogous to the temporary breakdown in the temperature regulation of the house when a sudden great demand is made upon even a very efficient furnace. Both starvation and fat-feeding are alike in that no preformed carbohydrate is being received by the body, so that the liver must make all the necessary carbohydrate from its own resources. This represents a high degree of activity on the part of the liver, as compared to the normal conditions, under which it need manufacture only a small proportion of the body's requirements. The deceleration of sugar output by the liver when sugar is administered requires a longer time when the liver is working at top speed than when it is working at half- or quarter-speed.

Actual Complexity of Regulation in the Living Organism

Thus far, the analogy of the thermostat-furnace arrangement has served us well in helping to simplify the relationship between the endocrine glands and the liver in the regulation of the blood sugar. But it is necessary to realize that the mechanism which has been described is integrated with a series of other regulatory processes in the body. We have said, for example, that the threshold of regulation of the liver is determined by the endocrine balance. But what determines the characteristic rates of activity of the endocrine glands which maintain this balance? This question cannot be answered at the present time, although we do have some hints concerning certain factors. Thus there is evidence which indicates that the blood-sugar level affects not only the liver but also the activity of the anterior pituitary gland, which in turn influences the reaction of the liver to the blood-sugar level. There is also evidence that the concentration of sugar in the blood passing through the pancreas influences the rate of secretion of insulin. Furthermore, the concentration of a given hormone in the blood may have a controlling action upon the activity of the gland which secretes that hormone. Another mode of regulation may occur by the controlling effect of the hormone of one gland upon the rate of activity of another gland. An example of the latter type of effect is the excessive stimulation of the secretion of insulin by the repeated injection of massive doses of extracts of the anterior pituitary gland, eventually leading to islet exhaustion and pancreatic diabetes, as first described by Young.

It is not unusual in the study of biologic functions to find a number of overlapping mechanisms all directed toward the same end and each capable of serving the function to a considerable extent when the other mechanisms are impaired by disease or by an experimental procedure. This situation exists in regard to the regulation of the blood sugar. It has been possible to demonstrate a primitive type of regulation of sugar output by the liver, which can occur in isolated hepatic tissue in the test tube. In other words, the output of sugar is, to a certain extent, controlled by the concentration of sugar present, even in the absence of any possible endocrine adjustment. In addition to this intrinsic hepatic mechanism and its endocrine regulators, which have already been discussed, there are also certain emergency mechanisms mediated by the central nervous system and the adrenal medulla. The latter mechanisms are not evident under normal conditions, and they can be entirely eliminated experimentally without appreciably effecting the sensitivity of regulation. But when, under abnormal conditions of stress and strain, the organism is threatened by an unduly rapid or profound hypoglycemia, the emergency mechanisms rapidly come into play by breaking down liver glycogen and providing the needed blood sugar.

It may be helpful to think of the relationships between the emergency mechanisms, the endocrine glands and the intrinsic hepatic homeostasis from the phylogenetic viewpoint. The fundamental or primitive regulation may be supposed to reside in the biochemical processes of the tissue cells. The endocrine glands may represent a step up the evolutionary scale by providing a more sensitive and finely adjusted regulating mechanism, which renders the more highly developed organism less dependent upon its external environment. The emergency mechanisms may be an additional protection against hypoglycemia for the highly specialized tissues (e.g., central nervous system) of the most highly developed organisms.

The Diabetic Syndrome as a Disturbance in Regulation

During the ten years that followed the discovery of pancreatic diabetes by von Mering and Minkowski in Strassburg, the same laboratory established the classic criteria of the metabolic disturbance in experimental diabetes. These criteria comprise the quantitative excretion of administered carbohydrate in the urine of the experimental animal; the urinary dextrose-to-nitrogen ratio (D:N); the excretion in the urine of acetoacetic acid, beta-hydroxybutyric acid and acetone (ketosis); and the characteristic respiratory quotient (R.Q.).

The quantitative excretion of administered sugar by the diabetic animal suggests that the cause of the metabolic difficulty was an inability to utilize carbohydrate (the non-utilization theory). Furthermore, when Minkowski collected urine specimens from his depancreatized dogs (while fasting or when fed lean meat) and analyzed them for amounts of dextrose and nitrogen, respectively, the total amount of sugar in each 24-hour specimen seemed to bear a definite relationship to the amount of nitrogen in the same specimen. This D:N ratio averaged about 2.8:1 for his animals, from which he concluded as follows: (a) Since nitrogen is a breakdown product of protein, all the sugar which appeared in the urine was being made at the expense of protein; (b) from the apparent constancy of the D:N ratio, none of the sugar made from protein was being utilized by the diabetic animal; i.e., all of it was quantitatively excreted.

The appearance of the ketone bodies in the diabetic animal was the third basis for the non-utilization theory of diabetes. It was known that acetoacetic acid and beta-hydroxybutyric acid resulted chiefly from the breakdown of fat. Since these substances did not ordinarily appear during fasting in the normal organism (when fat was the chief metabolite), it was assumed that the ketone bodies were abnormal waste products resulting from the incomplete oxidation of fats in diabetes. From this arose the conception that a certain amount of carbohydrate had to be oxidized in order that fats could be burned completely ("fats burn in the fire of carbohydrates"). Thus the ketosis of diabetes was apparently another evidence of the lack of ability to utilize carbohydrate.

Studies of the respiratory exchange of the normal and diabetic organism apparently supported the foregoing conclusions. If the net result of complete oxidation in the body is compared to the burning of a substance in a bomb calorimeter, it is apparent that the amount of oxygen consumed and the amount of CO_2 given off in the process will depend upon the chemical nature of the substance that is being oxidized. Thus it may be calculated that, when a carbohydrate is oxidized, 1 mol. of CO_2 will result for every mol. of oxygen used, according to the reaction:

$$C_6H_{12}O_6 + 6O_2 \rightarrow 6CO_2 + 6H_2O$$

The R.Q. is the relation, expressed in volumes, between the oxygen consumed and the CO_2 given off (CO_2/O_2). Hence the R.Q. for the oxidation of carbohydrate is 1.0. In the same way, it may be calculated that the R.Q. for fat is about

0.7; for protein, about 0.8. The latter figure involves a number of assumptions, since protein is not entirely oxidized in the living organism.

It was found that the R.Q. of a normal animal under fasting conditions was in the neighborhood of 0.7. This was taken to indicate that fat was the chief fuel being used at that time. After a carbohydrate meal the R.Q. of the normal animal rose toward 1.0. This was interpreted to mean that the animal was now oxidizing the ingested carbohydrate. The diabetic organism differed from the normal in that, while its fasting R.Q. was also about 0.7, the quotient did not rise when carbohydrate was administered. This seemed to confirm the conclusion that the diabetic organism cannot utilize carbohydrate at all but derives its energy chiefly from fat.

A Crucial Experiment Opposing the Non-utilization Theory of Diabetes

On the basis of the four lines of evidence which have been outlined, the non-utilization theory of diabetes was more or less generally accepted for many years. However, as early as 1897, Kausch reported the results of removal of the liver from depancreatized geese and ducks, as compared to the results of the same procedure in normal birds. He found that, in the absence of the organ which supplies the blood sugar, the latter disappeared from the blood just as quickly in the diabetic birds as in the normal ones. There were a number of subsequent attempts to confirm this finding in mammals. Most of them showed similar results, but technical difficulties as regards complete removal of the liver and the consequent irregularity of the data rendered these findings inconclusive.

However, following the development of Mann's technique for total removal of the liver in dogs, Mann and Magath[150] reported unequivocal evidence that the completely depancreatized dog suffers just as rapid a fall in the blood sugar after hepatectomy as does the normal dog (Fig. 30). Whether orig-

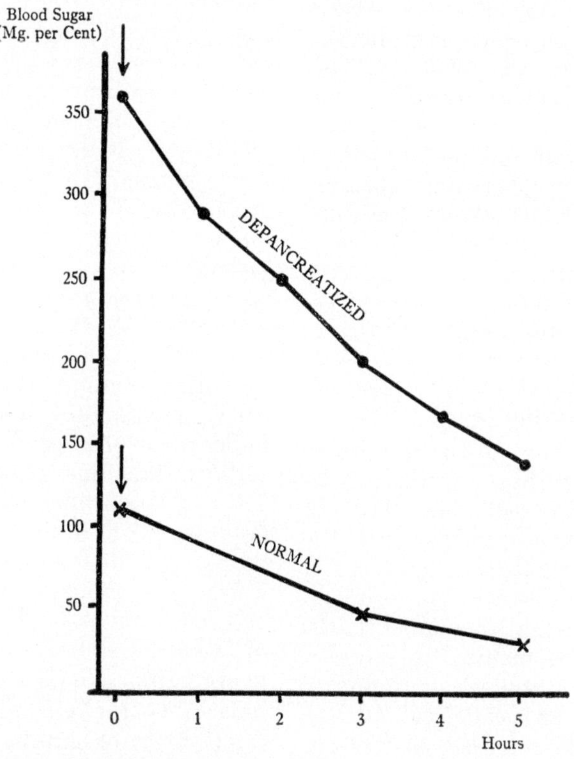

FIG. 30. Development of hypoglycemia following hepatectomy in depancreatized, as well as in normal dogs. (Mann and Magath.[150])

inally normal or diabetic, the liverless animal dies in hypoglycemic convulsions within a few hours. In either case it can be kept alive only by continuous administration of sugar or the giving of larger amounts of sugar at about 2-hour intervals. Unless one makes the rather absurd assumption that the removal of the liver suddenly restores the ability of the peripheral tissues to utilize carbohydrate, one must conclude that the diabetic animal does not entirely lack that ability. Under these circumstances it becomes important to consider all other evidence which may help to explain the diabetic syndrome without invoking the complete non-utilization of carbohydrates.

The Double Disturbance of Diabetes

In the completely depancreatized animal the disturbances in metabolism seem to be due to the lack of insulin and to the unopposed action of pituitary and adrenal hormones. The principal result of insulin lack is a diminution of the rate of sugar entry into extrahepatic tissue, i.e., a decrease in the rate of glucose use for all pathways. This is partially but not completely compensated for by the hyperglycemia. In addition, protein and fat catabolism increase leading to increased gluconeogenesis, governed largely by the pituitary and the adrenal cortex. Diabetes, then, is a disturbance in which increased hepatic sugar production is coupled with its relative underutilization.

Clinical Disturbances in the Endocrine Regulation of the Blood Sugar

The experimental diabetic syndrome is primarily a disturbance in the regulation of carbohydrate metabolism brought about by various manipulations of the endocrine glands or their hormones. But in order to avoid confusion in terminology, it is necessary to remember at the outset that diabetes mellitus, as it occurs in man, is still a clinical syndrome of obscure etiology in the individual case. The essential and minimal characteristics of this syndrome are a persistent hyperglycemia with glycosuria—all other effects, such as polyuria, dehydration, demineralization, loss of weight, ketosis and coma being secondary. In the mildest disturbances the diagnosis of diabetes mellitus often cannot be finally established until the condition has progressed in severity to the point that stable, persistent criteria develop. It often happens, also, that a mild disturbance in carbohydrate regulation is found to be accompanied by hepatic damage, hyperthyroidism, adrenal cortical tumor, etc. If the liver disease or the glandular disturbance is adequately treated by medical or surgical means and the carbohydrate disturbance is thereby eliminated, it is not customary to label the transitory hyperglycemia and glycosuria as diabetes mellitus.

It is readily understood that the foregoing terminology is merely a clinical convention. From the physiologic standpoint it is difficult to conceive of a disturbance, like diabetes mellitus, which, in some individuals, would not be found in minimal and transitory form. Nor does the presence of frank and remediable liver disease or glandular disturbance necessarily make the resulting diabetes any different from that which occurs when the etiologic disturbance cannot be detected by present clinical methods. It is this physiologic point of view which must be kept in mind in considering the possible etiologic factors involved in the recognized clinical disturbance.

We must perforce base our notions as to possible etiology upon the various experimental procedures by which a similar syndrome can be produced. These possibilities have already been indicated in the sections devoted to the various endocrine glands and the liver. Their relationships to each other are graphically illustrated in Figure 31. In the balance of forces represented there, it may readily be seen that the same end-result might be obtained in a variety of ways. A shift of regulation toward hyperglycemia might be due to a diminution in the insulin factor (an absolute lack of insulin) or to an intensification of the opposing factors (a relative lack of insulin). If the latter type of disturbance is, indeed, responsible for some cases of diabetes mellitus, it is possible that we may eventually learn to distinguish a pituitary diabetes, an adrenal cortical diabetes, and a thyroid diabetes, as well as a pancreatic diabetes. To this list must be added a possible hepatic diabetes which might occur in the absence of endocrine disturbance when the liver is no longer responding normally to its endocrine regulation. It must be emphasized that none of these considerations minimizes the importance of insulin in therapy or suggests that any other efficacious agent is known at the present time. The diagram clearly indicates that the important thing, from the therapeutic standpoint, is the maintenance of the normal balance. The administration of insulin will correct the imbalance whether it is due to an absolute or to a relative lack of this hormone.

The differentiation of the various possible types of diabetes mellitus must await the development of adequate methods for the quantitative estimation of glandular function or of the titer of the various hormones in the blood. For the present, all diabetic manifestations which are accompanied by a clinically recognizable dysfunction of some gland or of the liver are considered to be part of the syndrome associated with that clinical state.

In the overwhelming majority of cases of diabetes there is no evidence that the pituitary, adrenal or thyroid hormones are present in any but normal amounts. Nor does a primary liver dysfunction seem to play a significant role in diabetes mellitus. The diabetic state may be profoundly modified by the state of function of the above organs, but etiologically once more attention has shifted to the pancreas.

In the severe juvenile diabetic the evidence points to an inability to *produce insulin,* while the non-ketotic adult diabetic has not lost this ability but may suffer from a disturbance in the regula-

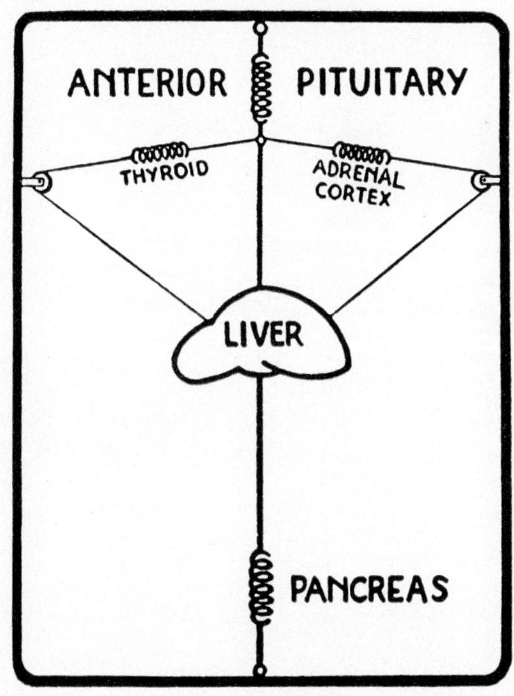

FIG. 31. Mechanical analogy to the endocrine balance. (Soskin and Levine: Carbohydrate Metabolism, Univ. of Chicago Press.)

tion of *insulin secretion* or *release*. This view has received added evidence from the variation in therapeutic efficacy of the sulfonylureas in these two groups of diabetics.[151,152,153]

When the insulin molecule is secreted into the portal blood stream it becomes subject to removal by combination with certain of the plasma proteins[154,155] and/or it may be degraded by the proteolytic system, insulinase.[156] An increase of such inactivating factors may account for the appearance of diabetes in the face of adequate insulin production and its release.

A similar situation exists as regards carbohydrate disturbances in the direction of hypoglycemia and the differentiation between hyperinsulinism and other conditions which may lead to hypoglycemia. An inspection of the following list, in conjunction with the examination of Figure 31, will relate the characteristic blood-sugar disturbances accompanying the various known endocrine syndromes with the physiologic considerations which have been outlined.

ENDOCRINE HYPERGLYCEMIAS

Anterior pituitary	Acromegaly; pituitary basophilism
Thyroid	Hyperthyroidism
Adrenal cortex	Hyperadrenocorticalism
Adrenal medulla	Pheochromocytoma
Pancreas	Diabetes mellitus

ENDOCRINE HYPOGLYCEMIAS

Anterior pituitary	Simmonds' disease; anorexia nervosa
Thyroid	Hypothyroidism
Adrenal cortex	Addison's disease; adrenal apoplexy
Pancreas	Hyperinsulinism

References

1. Cori, C. F., Cori, G. T. and Goltz, H. L.: Proc. Soc. Exper. Biol. & Med., *26:*433, 1929.
2. Crane, R. K. and Krane, S. M.: Bioch. Biophys. Acta, *20:*568, 1956.
3. Wilson, T. H.: J. Biol. Chem., *222:*751, 1956.
4. Fridhandler, L. and Quastel, J. H.: *XIX*, Intern. Physiol. Congress Abstracts, p. 365, 1953.
5. Groen, J.: J. Clin. Invest., *16:*245, 1937.
6. Russell, J. A.: Am. J. Physiol., *122:*547, 1938.
7. Althausen, T. L., Anderson, E. and Stockholm, M.: Proc. Soc. Exper. Biol. & Med., *40:*342, 1939.
8. Russell, R. S. and Nasset, E. S.: J. Nutrition, *22:*287, 1941.
9. Althausen, T. L. and Wever, G. K.: J. Clin. Invest., *16:*257, 1937.
10. Deuel, H. J.: Physiol. Rev., *16:*173, 1936.
11. Somogyi, M.: J. Biol. Chem., *75:*33, 1927.
12. Froesch, E. R. and Renold, A. E.: Diabetes, *5:*1, 1956.
13. Soskin, S., Priest, W. S. and Schutz, W. J.: Am. J. Physiol., *108:*107, 1934.
14. Park, C. R., Bornstein, J. and Post, R. L.: Am. J. Physiol., *182:*12, 1955.
15. Smith, H.: The Kidney, Oxford University Press, 1950.
16. Roe, J. H.: J. Biol. Chem., *107:*15, 1934.
17. von Crevald, S.: Klin. Wchnschr., *6:*697, 1927.
18. Good, C. A., Kramer, H. and Somogyi, M.: J. Biol. Chem., *100:*485, 1933.
19. Barker, S. B. and Summerson, W. H.: J. Biol. Chem., *138:*535, 1941.
20. Bueding, E., Stein, M. H. and Wortis, H.: J. Biol. Chem., *140:*697, 1941.
21. Friedemann, T. E. and Haugen, G. E.: J. Biol. Chem., *147:*415, 1943.
22. Gunsalus, I. C.: Fed. Proc., *13:*715, 1954.
23. Cori, G. T.: Harvey Lect., *48:*145, 1952–3.
24. Sutherland, E. W., Posternak, T. Z. and Cori, C. F.: J. Biol. Chem., *179:*501, 1949.
25. Caputto, R., Leloir, L. F., Cardini, C. E. and Paladini, A. C.: J. Biol. Chem., *184:*333, 1950.
26. Holzel, A., Komrower, G. M. and Schwarz, V.: Am. J. Med., *22:*703, 1957.
27. Park, J. T., in Phosphorus Metabolism (ed. by McElroy and Glass). Baltimore, Johns Hopkins Press, 1951, *1:*93.
28. Schoenheimer, R.: The Dynamic State of Body Constituents, Cambridge, Harvard University Press, 1942.
29. Gunsalus, I. C.: Fed. Proc., *9:*556, 1950.
30. Stern, J. R. and Ochoa, S.: J. Biol. Chem., *191:*161, 1951.
31. Stotz, E.: Cytochromes. In a symposium on respiratory enzymes, p. 149. University of Wisconsin Press, 1941.
32. Krebs, H. A.: Harvey Lect., *44:*165, 1948–49.
33. Racker, E.: Adv. Enzymol., *15:*141, 1954.
34. Hers, H. G.: Arch. internat. de physiol., *61:*426, 1953.
35. Caputto, R., Leloir, L. F., Trucco, R. E., Cardini, C. E. and Paladini, E. C.: J. Biol. Chem., *179:*497, 1949.
36. Lipmann, F.: Adv. Enzymol., *1:*99, 1941.
37. Lipmann, F.: Harvey Lect., *44:*99, 1948–49.
38. Szent-Györgyi, A.: Bioch. Biophys. Acta, *4:*38, 1950.

39. Needham, D. M.: Bioch. Biophys. Acta, *4:*42, 1950.
40. Mommaerts, W. F. H. M.: Muscular Construction. New York, Interscience Press, 1950.
41. Gemmill, C. L.: Physiol. Rev., *22:*32, 1942.
42. Goldman, D. S., Chaikoff, I. L., Reinhardt, W. O., Entenman, C. and Dauben, W. G.: J. Biol. Chem., *186:*718, 1950.
43. Drury, D. R., Wick, A. N. and MacKay, E. M.: Am. J. Physiol., *163:*655, 1950.
44. Bollman, J. L., Mann, F. C. and Magath, T. B.: Am. J. Physiol., *74:*238, 1925.
45. Soskin, S.: Am. J. Physiol., *81:*382, 1927.
46. Swanson, M. A.: J. Biol. Chem., *184:*647, 1950.
47. Geiger, E.: Fed. Proc., *10:*670, 1951.
48. Chernick, S. S., Masoro, E. J. and Chaikoff, I. L.: Proc. Soc. Exper. Biol. & Med., *73:*348, 1950.
49. Wertheimer, E. and Shapiro, B.: Physiol. Rev., *28:*451, 1948.
50. Hausberger, F. X., Milstein, S. W. and Rutman, R. J.: J. Biol. Chem., *208:*431, 1954.
51. Chaikoff, I. L.: Harvey Lect., *47:*99, 1951–52.
52. Baker, N., Chaikoff, I. L. and Schusdek, A.: J. Biol. Chem., *194:*435, 1952.
53. Rapport, D.: Physiol. Rev., *10:*349, 1930.
54. Lorber, V., Cook, M. and Meyer, J.: J. Biol. Chem., *181:*475, 1949.
55. Lifson, N., Lorber, V., Sakami, W. and Wood, H. G.: J. Biol. Chem., *176:*1263, 1948.
56. Parnes, I. and Wertheimer, E.: Biochem. J., *46:*517, 1950.
57. Parnes, I. and Wertheimer, E. Biochem. J., *46:*520, 1950.
58. Best, C. H., Dale, H. H., Hoet, J. P. and Marks, H. P.: Proc. Roy. Soc., London, s.B., *100:*55, 1926.
59. Wick, A. N. and Drury, D. R.: Am. J. Physiol., *174:*445, 1953.
60. Soskin, S. and Levine, R.: Am. J. Physiol., *120:*761, 1937.
61. Bridge, E. M.: Bull. Johns Hopkins Hosp., *62:*408, 1938.
62. Evans, G. and Bowie, M. A.: Proc. Soc. Exper. Biol. & Med., *35:*68, 1936.
63. Russell, J. A. and Bloom, W.: Endocrinology, *58:*83, 1956.
64. Adrovny, G. A. and Russell, J. A.: Fed. Proc., *13:*1, 1954.
65. Somogyi, M.: J. Biol. Chem., *141:*219, 1941.
66. Chaikoff, I. L. and Soskin, S.: Am. J. Physiol., *87:*58, 1928.
67. Gemmill, C. L. and Hamman, L.: Bull. Johns Hopkins Hosp., *68:*50, 1941.
68. Bridge, E. M.: Bull. Johns Hopkins Hosp., *61:*349, 1937.
69. Soskin, S., Levine, R. and Hechter, O.: Am. J. Physiol., *134:*40, 1941.
70. Stadie, W. C.: J. Biol. Chem., *132:*393, 1940.
71. Gaebler, O. H. and Robinson, A. R.: Endocrinology, *30:*627, 1942.
72. Mirsky, I. A.: Endocrinology, *25:*52, 1939.
73. Luck, J. M. and Morse, S. W.: Biochem. J., *27:*1648, 1933.
74. Mirsky, I. A.: Am. J. Physiol., *124:*569, 1938.
75. Soskin, S. and Levine, R.: Carbohydrate Metabolism, Chicago, University of Chicago Press, 1946, 1952.
76. Stadie, W. C.: Physiol. Rev., *34:*52, 1954.
77. Levine, R. and Goldstein, M. S.: Recent Progr. Hormone Research, *11:*343, 1955.
78. Weil-Malberbe, H.: Ergebn. Physiol. u. exptl. Pharmakol., *48:*55, 1955.
79. Sanger, F. and Thompson, E. O. P.: Biochem. J. (London), *53:*353, 1953.
80. Lundsgaard, E., Nielsen, N. A. and Orskov, S. L.: Skandinav. Arch. f. Physiol., *73:*296, 1936.
81. Lundsgaard, E., Nielsen, N. A. and Orskov, S. L.: Skandinav. Arch. f. Physiol., *81:*20, 1939.
82. Villee, C. A. and Hastings, A. B.: J. Biol. Chem., *179:*673, 1949.
83. Levine, R., Loube, S. D. and Weisberg, H. F.: Am. J. Physiol., *159:*107, 1949b.
84. Krahl, M. E.: Biol. Chem., *200:*99, 1953.
85. Levine, R., Texidor, T. A., Abrams, A. L. and Soskin, S.: Fed. Proc., *4:*45, 1945.
86. Ingle, D. J.: Am. J. Physiol., *165:*469, 1951.
87. Lukens, F. D. W.: Ann. Int. Med., *8:*727, 1934.
88. Shorr, E.: Cold Spr. Harb. Symp. Quant. Biol., *7:*323, 1939.
89. Flock, E., Bollman, J. and Mann, F. C.: J. Biol. Chem., *125:*49, 1938.
90. Shorr, E. and Barker, S. B.: Biochem. J. (London), *33:*1798, 1939.
91. Drury, D. R.: Am. J. Physiol., *131:*536, 1940.
92. Stetten, D., Jr., and Klein, B. V.: J. Biol. Chem., *162:*377, 1946.
93. Colowick, S. P., Cori, G. T. and Stein, M. W.: J. Biol. Chem., *168:*583, 1947.
94. Price, W. H., Cori, C. F. and Colowick, S. P.: J. Biol. Chem., *160:*633, 1945.
95. Stadie, W. C., Haugaard, N. and Hills, A. G.: J. Biol. Chem., *184:*617, 1950.
96. Broh-Kahn, R. H. and Mirsky, I. A.: Science, *106:*148, 1947.
97. Christensen, W. R., Plimpton, C. H. and Ball, E. G.: J. Biol. Chem., *180:*791, 1949.
98. Reid, E., Smith, R. H. and Young, F. G.: Biochem. J. (London), *42:*19, 1948.
99. Wierzuchowski, H.: Biochem. Ztschr., *237:*92, 1931.
100. Ross, E. J.: Medicine, *35:*355, 1956.
101. Wick, A. N. and Drury, D. R.: Am. J. Physiol., *173:*229, 1953.

102. Wick, A. N. and Drury, D. R.: Am. J. Physiol., *177:*535, 1954.
103. Mackler, B. and Guest, G. M.: Am. J. Physiol., *174:*487, 1953.
104. Cori, C. F. and Cori, G. T.: Proc. Soc. Exper. Biol. & Med., *26:*432, 1929.
105. Park, C. R. and Johnson, L. H.: Am. J. Physiol., *182:*17, 1955.
106. Sacks, J. and Sinex, F. M.: Am. J. Physiol., *175:*353, 1953.
107. Le Fevre, P. G. and Davies, R. I.: J. Gen. Physiol., *34:*515, 1951.
108. Widdas, W. F.: J. Physiol. (London), *125:*163, 1954.
109. Wilbrandt, W.: Arch. f. exper. Path. u. Pharmakol., *212:*9, 1950.
110. Dennis, D. J. and Rothstein, A.: Am. J. Physiol., *178:*82, 1954.
111. Resnick, O. and Hechter, O.: J. Biol. Chem., *224:*941, 1957.
112. Höber, R.: In Handbuch norm. pathol. Physiol. (Bethe, ed.). Berlin, Springer, *1:*433, 1927.
113. Brown, R.: Internat. Rev. Cytol., *1:*107, 1952.
114. Goldacre, R. J.: Internat. Rev. Cytol., *1:*135, 1952.
115. Ingle, D. J.: Am. J. Physiol., *165:*469, 1951.
116. Levine, R. and Fritz, I. B.: Diabetes, *5:*209, 1956.
117. De Duve, C.: Ciba Coll. Endocrinol. (Pancreas).
118. Foa, P. P.: Recent Progr. Hormone Res., *13:*473, 1957.
119. Walaas, O. and Walaas, E.: J. Biol. Chem., *187:*769, 1950.
120. Sutherland, E. W. and Cori, C. F.: Ann. New York Acad. Sci., *54:*639, 1951b.
121. Wosilait, W. D. and Sutherland, E. W.: J. Biol. Chem., *218:*469, 1956.
122. Sayers, G. W.: Physiol. Rev., *30:*241, 1950.
123. Long, C. N. H., Katzin, B. and Fry, E. G.: Endocrinology, *26:*309, 1940.
124. Soskin, S. and Levine, R.: Carbohydrate Metabolism, Chicago, University of Chicago Press, p. 352, 1946, 1952.
125. Sprague, R. G., Priestley, J. T. and Dockerty, M. B.: J. Clin. Endocrinol., *3:*128, 1943.
126. Wells, B. B. and Chapman, A.: Proc. Staff Meet. Mayo Clinic, *15:*503, 1940.
127. MacBryde, C. M. and de la Balze, F. A. de.: J. Clin. Endocrinol., *4:*287, 1944.
128. Wick, A. N., Drury, D. R. and MacKay, E. M.: Am. J. Physiol., *164:*224, 1951.
129. Levine, R., Simkin, B. and Cunningham, W.: Am. J. Physiol., *159:*111, 1949.
130. Cohn, C. (in preparation).
131. Levine, R., Goldstein, M. S., Ramey, E. R. and Fritz, I.: Bull. New England M. Center, *13:*114, 1951.
132. Welt, I. D., Stetten, D., Ingle, D. J. and Morley, E. H.: J. Biol. Chem., *197:*57, 1952.
133. Eiler, J. J., Althausen, T. L. and Stockholm, M.: Am. J. Physiol., *140:*600, 1944.
134. Drill, V. A., Overman, R. and Shaffer, C. B.: Endocrinology, *31:*245, 1942.
135. Lukens, F. D. W. and Dohan, F. C.: Am. J. Physiol., *129:*408, 1940.
136. Houssay, B. A.: Recent Progr. Hormone Research, *5:*141, 1949.
137. Mirsky, I. A. and Broh-Kahn, R. H.: Am. J. Physiol., *117:*6, 1936.
138. Bennett, L. L. and Evans, H. M.: in The Hormones (ed. by Pincus & Thimann) *2:*405, Academic Press, 1950.
139. Wells, B. B. and Chapman, A.: Proc. Staff Meet. Mayo Clinic, *15:*493, 1940.
140. Houssay, B. A.: New England J. Med., *214:*971, 1936.
141. Russell, J. A.: In Essays in Biology, p. 305, University of California Press, 1944.
142. Soskin, S., Mirsky, I. A., Zimmerman, L. M. and Crohn, N.: Am. J. Physiol., *114:*110, 1935.
143. Soskin, S., Levine, R. and Lehman, W.: Am. J. Physiol., *127:*463, 1939.
144. Hansen, R. G., Rutter, W. J. and Samuels, L. H.: J. Biol. Chem., *192:*243, 1951.
145. Perlmutter, M. and Greep, R. O.: J. Biol. Chem., *174:*915, 1948.
146. Soskin, S.: J. Nutrition, *3:*99, 1930.
147. Soskin, S.: J. Clin. Endocrinol., *4:*75, 1944.
148. Soskin, S., Essex, H. E., Herrick, J. F. and Mann, F. C.: Am. J. Physiol., *124:*558, 1938.
149. Bondy, P. K., Bloom, W. L., Whitner, V. S. and Farrar, B. W.: J. Clin. Invest., *28:*1126, 1949.
150. Mann, F. C. and Magath, T. B.: Arch. Int. Med., *31:*797, 1923.
151. Symposium on the Sulfonylureas. Metabolism, *5:*721, 1956.
152. Symposium on the Sulfonylureas. Diabetes, *6:*259, 1957.
153. Symposium on the Sulfonylureas. Ann. New York Acad. Sc., *71:*1, 1957.
154. Field, J. B. and Stetten, D.: Fed. Proc., *15:*815, 1956.
155. Peters, T., Burrows, B. A. and Lowell, F. C.: Fed. Proc., *15:*1982, 1956.
156. Mirsky, I. A.: Recent Progr. Hormone Res., *13:*429, 1957.
157. De Bodo, R. C., and Altszuler, N.: Vit. & Hormones, *15:*205, 1957.
158. Steele, R., Wall, J. S., de Bodo, R. C. and Altszuler, N.: Am. J. Physiol., *187:*25, 1956.
159. Altszuler, N., Steele, R., Wall, J. S. and de Bodo, R. C.: Proc. Soc. Exptl. Biol. and Med., *94:*744, 1957.

CHAPTER 3

By SAMUEL GURIN, Ph.D.

Lipid Metabolism

The field of lipid metabolism is currently going through a period of intense experimental activity. The development of new techniques such as column chromatography, countercurrent distribution and, more particularly, gas phase chromatography has provided the chemist with powerful tools capable of separating different species of lipids and of resolving complex mixtures in a quantitative and micro fashion. Together with radioisotope techniques, ultracentrifugation, electrophoresis, modern *in vitro* and perfusion techniques, these current developments have at last provided tools sufficiently powerful to stimulate the interest of investigators in the field of lipid chemistry and metabolism. As new facts become available, concepts are being altered. Major advances have been made in our knowledge of fat transport, the dynamic state of lipids in the blood, turnover of lipids in tissues, fatty acid oxidation and biosynthesis, mechanism of ketone body formation and oxidation, and cholesterol metabolism, to name but a few. The writer must be forgiven, then, if he takes the point of view that it is imperative now to re-evaluate major concepts in the light of these new developments. It is not his purpose, therefore, to review such topics as the chemistry of lipids, the fat content of foodstuffs, the lipid composition of tissues and the elementary facts of digestion. Any modern textbook of physiologic chemistry will provide this information, and there are numerous monographs for those who wish to delve further. It is proposed in this chapter to highlight new discoveries and to speculate as intelligently as possible on the impact of these findings upon our present concepts of lipid metabolism.

DIGESTION AND ABSORPTION

Triglycerides. It is now clear that the digestion and absorption of dietary fat involves (1) a stepwise hydrolysis of triglycerides to a complex mixture of tri-, di- and monoglycerides as well as free fatty acids and glycerol and (2) thorough emulsification of the products. Recent evidence suggests that pancreatic lipase predominantly accomplishes the conversions shown in [A] below. There is increasing evidence to support the view that the 2-ester linkage is less susceptible to cleavage by the lipase than are the 1 or 3 positions[1] and that the last step is essentially irreversible.[2] Borgström[3] has reviewed the evidence demonstrating that analysis of duodenal contents of human subjects indicates, on the average, some 60 to

[A]

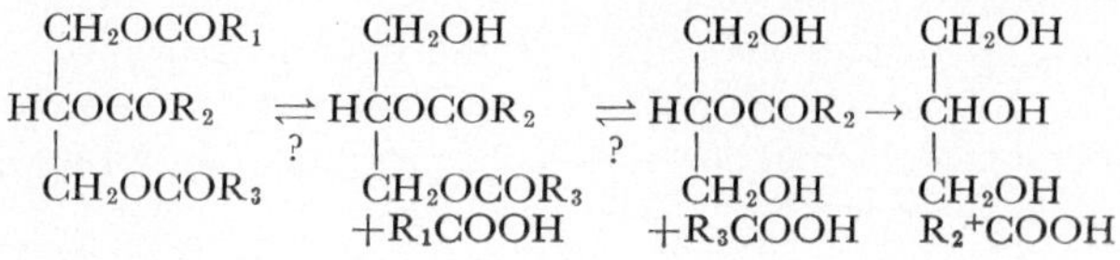

CH_2OCOR_1		CH_2OH		CH_2OH		CH_2OH
$HCOCOR_2$	$\underset{?}{\rightleftharpoons}$	$HCOCOR_2$	$\underset{?}{\rightleftharpoons}$	$HCOCOR_2$	$\rightarrow$	$CHOH$
CH_2OCOR_3		CH_2OCOR_3		CH_2OH		CH_2OH
		$+R_1COOH$		$+R_3COOH$		R_2^+COOH

70 per cent hydrolysis of administered fat. Upon analysis, 60 to 70 per cent of the triglyceride fatty acids were present in the form of free fatty acids, the remainder consisting of tri-, di- and monoglycerides. It is striking that Borgström[4] has shown that a rapid exchange can occur in the rat and *in vitro* between free fatty acids and the fatty acid portion of glycerides. Confirmatory evidence with human subjects has also been reported by Ahrens & Borgström,[5] who analyzed the chyme from the jejunum following administration of a well tolerated meal containing labeled palmitic or oleic acid. At least 50 per cent of the total recovered lipid was shown to be present as free fatty acid, the remainder being largely triglyceride with lesser amounts of di- and monoglyceride. Since all of the glycerides were found to be labeled, it is obvious that labeled free fatty acid had exchanged with unlabeled glycerides at all stages of hydrolysis. The evidence, though not conclusive, suggested that the free fatty acids were absorbed somewhat more rapidly than the glyceride fraction. When labeled mono-olein was administered, labeling was found in all three glycerides recovered from the jejunum —suggesting the possibility of reversibility of the hydrolytic process.

It has been estimated that hydrolysis of fat in the stomach is minimal (approximately 10 per cent). Gastric lipase, at the *pH* of the stomach, appears preferentially to attack triglycerides containing short chain fatty acids.[6] Although triglycerides of long chain acids are not cleaved by gastric lipase, the above mentioned phenomena explain the small amount of free fatty acids in the material leaving the stomach.

Pancreatic lipase has been partially purified by electrophoresis (paper and starch block). Borgström[7] has observed that the optimal *p*H for human pancreatic lipase is 9 (for the rat the corresponding figure was *p*H 8 and for commercial pancreatin, 8.2). The major effect observed, in addition to hydrolysis, is a rapid clearing of fine emulsions of triglyceride (tri-olein was used in this study). When only about ⅓ hydrolysis had occurred, a concomitant clearing was observed. The similarity between this effect and the clearing action of lipoprotein lipase in serum is striking. At the somewhat more acidic *p*H levels of the intestine, this clearing effect is not obtained unless bile salts are present. In the absence of lipase, bile salts were less effective as clearing agents.

The rapid exchange of labeled fatty acids with the fatty acid moieties of all types of glycerides makes it extremely difficult to determine conclusively the nature of the lipid passing through the membrane of the intestinal mucosa. The historical development of our current theories regarding the intestinal absorption of fat has been adequately described in numerous textbooks of physiologic chemistry or physiology and need not be reviewed here. Frazer[8] maintains that the intestinal mixture of tri,- di- and monoglycerides together with liberated free fatty acids and bile forms a very finely divided emulsion such that triglycerides may be absorbed along with the hydrolytic products. He was able to demonstrate that even paraffin will pass through the membrane of the intestinal mucosa provided the particle size is less than 0.5 μ, or if it is mixed with a suitable emulsifying vehicle; several other hydrocarbons were similarly absorbed after suitable emulsification. Borgström[3] is of the opinion that these hydrolytic products derived from fat are conjugated with bile salts (choleic acids) to form even more finely divided particles which are absorbed. With this reservation regarding the actual size of the absorbed particles, there is general agreement regarding the intraluminar contents prior to absorption.

The important role of the bile in fat absorption has long been recognized. Verzar[9] has provided evidence indicating that bile salts act upon water-insoluble fatty acids to bring them into solution. Frazer maintains that the role of bile is largely to produce fine emulsions without further commitments regarding how this happens or which constituents are essential. Borgström, as previously mentioned, has raised the possibility that bile salts form micelles with all of the hydrolytic products of fat digestion to form nearly clear solutions at the *p*H corresponding to that found in the small intestine. Ross *et al.*[10] have interestingly reported on a case involving a fat absorption defect in which there was no deficiency of pancreatic enzymes. The oral administration of bile produced a dramatic effect upon the steatorrhea; the level of fecal fat dropped from approximately 20 gm. per day to 8 to 9 gm. Analysis of the duodenal contents indicated that this patient had a very low level of bile salts. Glucose absorption was normal, and chylomicron studies indicated that the defect was a faulty absorption of fat. It is of interest that this patient was able to absorb some 50 per cent of administered fat in spite of the bile salt deficiency. Since in obstructive jaundice the absorptive defect may frequently be more severe, it is not certain that it is the bile salts alone that account for the total effectiveness of bile. Similarly, in patients with pancreatic lipase deficiency,[11] the rate of fat absorption is less than 50 per cent of normal. The intraduodenal administration of very finely emulsified fat (particle size 0.5 μ) to patients with such a deficiency, but having normal small-intestinal function) resulted in improved fat absorption. It is obvious that all of the above-mentioned factors are required for maximal absorption.

The amount of fat excreted in the stools is invariably increased when bile is prevented from entering the intestinal tract by a bile duct obstruction or by a bile fistula. Shapiro, Koster, Rittenberg and Schoenheimer,[12] by means of deuterium-labeled fat, demonstrated that in such states a considerable portion of administered fat is nevertheless absorbed and concluded that the increased fecal excretion of fat must in part be derived from some other source. Bergström and Blomstrand[13] have reported that in a normal subject on a diet containing about 50 gm. of triglycerides the daily output of fecal fatty acids was about 2 gm. Of this quantity, about 1 gm. was derived from the diet while the remainder probably was endogenous in origin. In a case of nontropical sprue on the same dietary, about 10.5 gm. of fatty acids were excreted, of which 7 gm. were of dietary origin. How much of the remaining fat is derived from secretion into the lumen, desquamated epithelial cells and intestinal microorganisms has not been established. Frazer[14] has reported that fecal fat can be markedly reduced by effective antibacterial therapy in certain cases of tropical sprue.

Cellular Phase. It is now clear that free fatty acids, once absorbed, can be reconverted to triglycerides and probably to a lesser extent to phospholipid. For this synthesis a metabolically active form of glycerol is required since liberated free glycerol itself is poorly utilized for this purpose.[15] In confirmation of earlier work by Verzar and Laszt[16] glycerophosphate appears to stimulate intracellular esterification of fatty acids and permits its further transit as visible particulate fat in the chyle. Sagrott (quoted by Frazer) has demonstrated a significant increase in fat absorption in the rat upon simultaneous administration of glycerophosphate.

With the rat, Gidez and Karnovsky[17] as well as Morehouse *et al.*[18] have observed that administered triglycerides labeled with C^{14} in the glycerol portion are poorly converted to phospholipids of the intestinal mucosa; this agrees with earlier concepts.[15]

There is still considerable uncertainty regarding the essential nature of phospholipid in the resynthesis and transit of fat to the lymph. Although the phospholipid content of the mucosa of the small intestine does not increase during fat absorption, there is very little doubt that the phospholipid content of the lymph does increase while fat is being absorbed.[19] Borgström[20] has reported that only 4 per cent as much C^{14}-labeled fatty acids could be recovered from lymph phospholipid as in lymph triglyceride following administration of carboxyl-labeled palmitic acid. The increase in total phospholipid of the lymph is ascribed in part to plasma phospholipids. Whether there is increased passage of plasma from capillaries of the intestinal villi during absorption of fat remains to be established. The available evidence does not point to the phospholipids as intermediates in the resynthesis of triglycerides from absorbed fatty acids. It is nevertheless still possible that some small metabolically active fraction of the intestinal phospholipids may play a significant role in the resynthesis of triglycerides.

Transit of Fat to Portal Circulation and Lymph. After administration of labeled palmitic acid (either free or as tripalmitin), approximately 70 to 90 per cent of the labeling can be recovered in the neutral fat of thoracic duct lymph.[21] Bloom, Chaikoff and Reinhardt[22] have also investigated the route of transport of saturated acids with different chain lengths. While fatty acids with 16 to 18 carbon atoms were predominantly transported via the lymph, the shorter chain acids were found present in decreasing amounts in the lymph. Later work suggested that the shorter chain acids may be transported largely by way of the portal circulation. It would appear, therefore, that the long-chain saturated and unsaturated acids[21c,23] are preferentially transported by way of the lymphatics.

Phosphatides. Because of their hydrophilic nature, it is possible that lecithins and cephalins are absorbed to a considerable extent without hydrolysis. Bloom *et al.*[24] and Blomstrand[25] have recently obtained evidence to this effect. The occurrence, however, of lecithinases in the pancreas and in intestinal mucosa suggests that significant hydrolysis may occur in the lumen as well. Recent work on ovolecithin and other phosphatides indicates that the L-α configuration must be assigned to such compounds.[26] It is also now clear that the phosphoryl choline portion is exclusively attached to the α position and not in the β position.[27] No evidence for the presence of

```
                          A
                          ¦
α'          CH2—O—COR
|             |      |
β R'OCO—C H     O
|             |      ||           +
α           CH2—O—P—OCH2CH2N(CH3)3
                     |
                     O⁻
```

naturally occurring β-lecithins has been obtained. RCO and R′CO represent long-chain fatty acyl groups attached respectively at the α' and β positions.[27b] Studies by Hanahan[28] and Long and Penny[28b] indicate that RCO (attached in the α' position) is generally an unsaturated fatty acid group while predominantly saturated acids are found in the β position. Hanahan[28] has presented evidence suggesting that there is a metabolic difference in the reactivity of the two ester positions (α' and β) of the lecithin molecule. Labeled saturated fatty acids are incorporated predominantly into the β position, while oleic acid-C^{14} is incorporated more or less equally into both positions (although the total incorporated is considerably less in the latter case). In the case of liver lecithin the α' position appeared to be associated with a greater reactivity (or turnover) as compared with the β position, while the contrary is true of lecithins of the intestinal tract. Such findings raise considerable question concerning previously reported conclusions regarding the turnover of phospholipids.

Very little phospholipid as such is found in the intestinal lumen except in the upper duodenum. Lysolecithin is, however, observed and this may be ascribed to the presence of lecithinase A in intestinal juice. This enzyme cleaves the molecule specifically at the α' position. Whether other types of phosphatides are cleaved is at the moment in doubt. There are indications of the presence in intestinal juice of other lecithinases capable of hydrolyzing lecithins at other positions. These enzymes have, however, not been well characterized or successfully separated.

Cholesterol. Although the intestine secretes enzymes capable of hydrolyzing cholesterol esters, it appears that both free and esterified cholesterol may be absorbed. Subsequent esterification of free cholesterol undoubtedly occurs in the mucosal cells since the lymph has been shown to contain significant amounts of esterified cholesterol[30] while the mucosal cells appear to contain very little in the esterified form.[31] In the absence of bile, ingested cholesterol is poorly absorbed.[32] As a consequence, attempts have been made to render the intestinal bile salts ineffective by the administration of ferric chloride, which forms insoluble iron salts of the bile acids. Apparently such therapy has been unsuccessful.

The fat content of the diet may play a role in the absorption of cholesterol, although there is no general agreement in this area. A number of investigators[33] have demonstrated in animals that appreciable absorption of cholesterol may occur with minimal fat in the diet. Pihl[34] claims that fatty acids are more effective than triglycerides. Swell *et al.*[35] have suggested that dietary fat may exert its effect upon cholesterol absorption by stimulating bile flow. The nature of the fatty acids in dietary fat appears to influence serum cholesterol levels in man; this will be discussed later.

It is striking that blood cholesterol levels are not appreciably affected by the ingestion of large amounts of cholesterol, whereas prompt effects upon the blood lipids are induced after the consumption of other types of fat. This may probably be ascribed to the relatively poor absorption of cholesterol in man. Maximal absorption has been estimated to be 10 to 20 mg. per kilogram of body weight per day.[30,36]

Although the major portion of the absorbed cholesterol is probably esterified by the time it reaches the lymph, the nature and source of the esterase have not been precisely established. Although cholesterol esterase activity has been observed in a number of tissues, the physiologic significance of these esterases has not been clearly delineated nor have the enzymes been successfully purified. Extensive work has been done on this problem by Treadwell, Swell and co-workers.[37]

Former views regarding the extreme selectivity of the intestine for cholesterol to the exclusion of plant and other steroids have been somewhat modified recently. It is clear from the work of Gould,[38] Glover *et al.*[31] and Hanahan *et al.*[39] that, in fact, small but significant quantities (up to 4 per cent) may actually be absorbed and metabolized. Hernandez *et al.*[40] have shown epi-cholesterol to be significantly absorbed while Gould *et al.*[38] have reported that tritium labeled β-sitosterol is absorbed by man in small quantities. Glover and Green[31] have suggested that absorption of cholesterol takes place at the molecular level and that cholesterol molecules entering the cell membrane can displace similar molecules which then pass into the cell via lipoprotein. According to this view, the absorption of cholesterol is actually an exchange or displacement process, and the efficiency of absorption depends upon the stereochemical requirements of the membranal and cellular lipoproteins. Thus, it is believed by these investigators that plant sterols simply do not fit the lipoproteins of the cell membrane, or, that if they do fit, they cannot be passed on to other lipoproteins of the membrane. The inhibition of cholesterol absorption in animals[41] observed with various plant sterols (β-sitosterol, stigmasterol, etc.) or cholestanol[42] could be explained if such sterols are bound in some way to the cell membrane so that they block the passage of cholesterol.

In humans, administration of plant sitosterols has been reported by several groups to lower serum cholesterol levels.[43] There is general disagreement, however, regarding the effects of such treatment in patients. While some investigators have reported moderate decreases in normal and hypercholesteremic persons,[43b,44] others have obtained doubtful effects.[45] Although cholestanol, like sitosterol, has some effect upon cholesterol absorption,[46] it is itself sufficiently well absorbed to be atherogenic.[47]

BLOOD LIPIDS

Absorbed lipids are transported via the lymphatics and enter the blood as fine droplets (chylomicra) by way of the thoracic duct. It is of interest that the removal of excessive quantities of blood fat is a much slower and apparently more difficult task than is the removal of carbohydrate and protein. In contrast to the latter two types of foodstuff, the highest level of lipid in the blood may not occur until six hours after the ingestion of a meal high in fat. Furthermore, nine to ten hours may sometimes elapse before the alimentary hyperlipemia drops to preprandial levels. It is obvious that the problem of disposing of a suspension of lipid droplets containing materials having very little solubility in water is a difficult one. In view of the high lipid content of the average American dietary, it is not amiss to stress the complex physicochemical processes that must necessarily be involved in clearing the blood of excess fat.

One of the major problems facing investigators in this field is the question of the fate and disposition of the chylomicra. This material can be obtained readily by centrifugation of chyle, serum, plasma or whole blood at 10,000 to 100,000 $\times$ g for a few minutes, as a result of which the material floats to the surface in the form of a butter-like layer. After washing the lipid fraction by repeated suspension in saline and centrifugation, a fraction is obtained which gives reasonably consistent analytic values (Table 1). Radioactive chylomicra have been prepared in this way following the administration of C^{14}-labeled triglyceride. Fredrickson *et al.*[48] have studied the fate of such chylomicra containing C^{14}-palmitic acid in the triglyceride moiety. Their results suggest that a limited hydrolysis of chylomicron triglycerides does take place in the plasma with the release of free fatty acids. This effect may probably be ascribed to the release of lipase by various tissues since appreciable hydrolysis is not observed when a specimen of plasma is allowed to stand. It is likely that chylomicra (either whole or partially degraded) are, to a considerable extent, trapped or sequestered by various organs. Friedman *et al.*[49] have obtained evidence suggesting that the reticuloendothelial cells of the liver are particularly active in this regard. Morris[50] has reported the appearance of plasma chylomicra in hepatic lymph, and French *et al.*[51] observed a decreased rate of chylomicron removal when the liver is removed. McCandless and Zilversmit[52] have presented evidence conflicting with the notion that intact chylomicra are trapped as such. Bragdon[53] has found that the labeled fatty acid of chylomicra is quickly observed in most of the tissues following its administration; this study emphasizes that some hydrolysis does occur in the blood and directs attention to those organs which are rich in lipases capable of performing this process. That such lipases can be released into the blood following heparin treatment is now well established.

After removal of the chylomicra, the bulk of the plasma lipids are present as lipoproteins. These are essentially complexes of protein with triglycerides, phospholipids and cholesterol (free and esterified). The nature of the linkages between protein and lipid is not known, and it should be emphasized that the various lipoproteins are undoubtedly complex mixtures. This point of view is emphasized because it is the writer's belief that much more research is required on the separation and characterization of individual molecular entities before meaningful clinical studies can be made. Furthermore, the manner in which they are formed is not clearly understood. Recent evidence suggests that they are probably made by the liver.[54] Whether other tissues can release lipoprotein into the blood is not known.

The various lipoproteins constitute some 12 to 15 per cent of the plasma proteins. Several methods of fractionation have yielded four distinct classes of lipoprotein ranging in density from 0.98 to 1.14. Precipitation with alcohol at low temperature and subsequent electrophoretic separations have disclosed the presence of two major groups, one migrating with the α globulins, the other with the β globulin fraction (both may be subdivided into low and high density groups).

Advantage has been taken of the differences in density of the various lipoproteins by Gofman. By means of careful fractionation in the ultracentrifuge, separations have been made depending upon their different rates of flotation in solutions of different densities. Since lipoproteins have a lower density than other serum proteins, they tend to move against the centrifugal field, and the rate of flotation or reverse sedimentation can thus be measured. Although a great deal of work of a pioneering nature has been done with this technique, it has been very difficult indeed to correlate the onset of various cardiovascular disturbances with changes in plasma lipoprotein pattern. This is not too surprising if one remembers that the empirical fractions thus obtained probably represent very complex mixtures.[55]

There is good evidence that the various lipoproteins do not represent a continuous spectrum of molecular species. Immunologic evidence suggests, for example, that the two β-lipoproteins of densities 0.98 and 1.03 are similar so far as the protein components are concerned; furthermore, they are different, in this sense, from the α-lipoproteins.[56] The proteins of the two β-lipoproteins have identical amino acid patterns, and similarly the α-lipoproteins of density 1.09 and 1.14 are identical.[57] A number of molecular weight estimations,[55,57,58] particularly upon the low density β-lipoproteins, suggest that this fraction is quite heterogenous with respect to molecular size even though the protein may be the same.

Of particular interest is the high triglyceride content of the chylomicra as well as the low density (0.98) β-lipoprotein fraction. If this low density fraction is labeled with radioiodine (I^{131}) and injected into human subjects, the radioisotope is quickly found in the β-lipoprotein of density 1.03, but not in the α-lipoproteins or chylomicra.[59] Conversely, labeled α-lipoproteins are not converted in the plasma to labeled β-lipoproteins (or chylomicra). These experiments suggest that β-lipoprotein of density 0.98 is predominantly converted into the β-species of density 1.03; this change is primarily due to a loss of triglyceride.

Recent work on "clearing factor" and, more particularly, lipoprotein lipase has helped to explain how low-density lipoproteins can be converted in blood to lipoproteins of higher density as a result of the action of this enzyme.[60] According to Korn,[61] lipoprotein lipase which can be liberated into the blood by heparin accounts for the so-called

TABLE 1. COMPOSITION OF CHYLOMICRA AND LIPOPROTEINS*

	CHYLOMICRA	β_1	β_2	α_1	α_2
Density (25°C.)	0.94	0.98	1.03	1.09	1.14
Molec. wt.	—	$5–25 \times 10^7$	$1.3–3.2 \times 10^6$	$3.6–4.3 \times 10^5$	$1.6–2 \times 10^5$
S_f (density 1.063)	—	10–400	2–10	−1	−2
Plasma conc. (mg. %)	—	150	320	80	380
Composition %	—	—	—	—	—
Peptide	2	9	21	33	57
Triglyceride	83–87	50	10	8	5
Phospholipid	6–7	18	22	29	21
Cholesterol	1–2	7	8	7	3
Cholesterol ester	3.5–6	15	38	23	14

* Data taken from Oncley.[55]

clearing action ascribed to this substance. Apparently the enzyme is confined mainly to the tissues, particularly in heart and adipose tissue, somewhat less in lung and muscle; the appearance in the blood or release from the tissues is stimulated by heparin. What is of interest is that the enzyme apparently requires lipoprotein as its substrate. Furthermore, it is primarily the triglyceride portion which is attacked by this lipase; the reaction is quite similar to the action of pancreatic lipase. The one and three linkages of the triglycerides are preferentially cleaved just as in the intestine. The products are free fatty acids, mono- and diglycerides and high-density lipoprotein. When some 50 per cent of the triglyceride has been hydrolyzed, the typical clearing effect is seen.[61]

It might be added that *in vivo* studies by Havel and Fredrickson[62] as well as by Zilversmit[52] indicate that the triglycerides of the lipoproteins are quickly converted into circulating free fatty acids (in contrast to the phospholipid portion); such results are compatible with the function ascribed to lipoprotein lipase. It should also be emphasized that the amount of circulating lipase is normally too small to account for the clearing of chylomicra; if lipoprotein lipase activity is involved in this process, it must function extravascularly.

The stimulating effect of heparin on the release of lipoprotein lipase into the blood has clarified the clearing effect associated with heparin. There is, incidentally, some evidence that the enzyme itself may contain heparin or a heparin-like polysaccharide as a prosthetic group.[61] The fact that lipoprotein-lipase concentration is appreciable in tissues raises many interesting questions concerning its intracellular action, as well as its possible role in the release of lipid from tissues into the blood.

Since the clearing phenomenon is associated with the enzymatic hydrolysis of the triglyceride of lipoproteins, it is not surprising that the onset of clearing parallels the release of free fatty acids into the plasma.[61] It has been known for a number of years that there is a small amount of free fatty acid in the blood. For example, Kendall in 1941[63] prepared crystalline serum albumin from human serum which contained 2 per cent of free fatty acid. This fatty acid could be freed from the protein only by denaturation. Since then, a number of investigators have confirmed the fact that albumin has a strong binding capacity for anions and, therefore, for fatty acids. The actual amount of free fatty acid in plasma amounts to approximately 0.5 milliequivalents per liter. If all of the acid is assumed to be stearic acid, one may calculate this value to be equivalent to approximately 10 mg. of stearic acid per 100 ml. This fatty acid fraction of the plasma has been called NEFA (nonesterified fatty acid) or UFA (unesterified acid).[64,65] The fatty acid is tightly bound to the albumin, moves with it during electrophoresis and precipitates with the protein upon treatment with the usual precipitating agents. The free fatty acid may be extracted by organic solvents. It has been calculated that approximately three moles of fatty acid can combine with one mole of albumin.[66] Although the total amount is relatively small, the metabolic significance of this fraction is probably very great, particularly since the half-life of this fraction has now been found to be approximately 2 to 3 minutes in both man and the dog.[62,67] It is obvious that if half of this material is replaced every 2 to 3 minutes, this fraction represents an extremely active and dynamic metabolic material. In fact, one can calculate that this rate of turnover is rapid enough to take care of most of the energy needs of the tissues for lipid.[48] Although it has long been known that excessive free fatty acid is toxic to tissues, numerous investigators have found that small amounts of free fatty acid may be emulsified with albumin and subsequently injected with impunity. Furthermore, experiments with radioactive palmitic acid indicate that, following suitable preparation with albumin, this material may be injected into experimental animals intravenously without damage; such injected material is very rapidly removed from the blood by the tissues.[62] All of these facts fit very nicely with what has been discovered concerning the albumin-bound fatty acid fraction of the blood. Evidence obtained by Dole[68] suggests that the fatty acids are rapidly absorbed by the tissues and that the tissues in turn can release albumin-bound fatty acids (NEFA) to the blood. The release of fatty acids to the blood by the tissues appears to be diminished when lipogenesis is active in tissues (when glucose is being well utilized), or following treatment with insulin. Contrarily, the amount of albumin-bound fatty acid released to the blood may be increased in the diabetic state and during ketosis. For example, injection of insulin can produce a marked drop in the free fatty acid fraction after some 20 minutes, whereas in diabetics exhibiting a diabetic tolerance curve the effect is delayed but nevertheless significant.[68] Dole believes that insulin actually influences the output of fatty acid into the blood rather than accelerates the utilization of free fatty acid in the tissues. Finally, the discovery that this free fatty acid fraction is metabolically very reactive and the realization that free fatty acids are very efficiently taken up by the tissues fit very nicely with our knowledge of the subsequent oxidation of fatty acids within the tissues. Recent reports[69] that some free fatty acid is also found to be associated with the lipoproteins suggest that there may be several methods for transporting fatty acids in the blood.

From what has been said, it is obvious that the variation in the concentration of certain blood lipids (particularly triglycerides) may be very great in normal persons. Obviously in the postabsorptive state the plasma-lipid concentration will depend upon a number of factors such as fat intake, rate of absorption, rate of removal of chylomicra from the blood, rate of formation of the lipoproteins and probably a host of other physiochemical phenomena. To make matters worse, the lipoproteins are undoubtedly complex mixtures. Finally, we do not have definitive evidence concerning the exact amount and nature of the various lipid substances present in the blood. For example, there have been almost no quantitative studies of the nature of the fatty acids present in the various blood lipid components of man. Recent improvements in column chromatography and in the technique of gas-liquid-phase chromatography have made more likely the possibility that we may soon achieve such analytic determinations of the nature and amount of the fatty acids present in the triglycerides, the free fatty acids, cholesterol esters, phosphatides and other lipid components of blood. James[70] has recently reported preliminary data concerning the nature of the fatty acids found in human plasma. Analysis of the fatty acids derived from the plasma triglycerides indicated the presence of a very complex pattern of fatty acids. In addition to the usual long-chain fatty acids there were found small amounts of short-chain fatty acids, fatty acids with an odd number of carbon atoms, as well as monounsaturated and polyunsaturated acids. It is clear that the pattern is very complex and that considerable study and attention must be given to this problem. Analysis of the polyunsaturated essential fatty acids of human plasma by the techniques of gas-liquid-phase chromatography has revealed in preliminary studies, for example, that there appears to be very little correlation between the essential fatty acids of plasma and coronary disease.[70]

There is no doubt that the lipoprotein pattern can change significantly in certain disorders, such as obesity, diabetes mellitus, nephrosis, thyroid disease, liver disease, atherosclerosis and a host of other abnormalities of lipid metabolism. There are also important effects of sex, age and hormones upon this pattern of lipoproteins.[71] What these changes in pattern mean in terms of diagnosis as well as the treatment of disease must probably await further knowledge concerning the identity, chemical nature and metabolism of these complex substances. There is also need for further insight into the nature of the physiologic events leading to changes in the pattern of the blood lipoproteins.

There is by now very little doubt that the liver plays a predominant role in the release of lipoprotein to the blood. It is also clear that the liver is the main tissue which supplies cholesterol rapidly and in appreciable quantities to the blood. Friedman *et al.*[72] have demonstrated that absorbed cholesterol is promptly and predominantly deposited in the liver. Hepatectomy in the dog virtually abolishes the appearance in the plasma of biosynthetic cholesterol derived from radioactive precursors.[73,74,75] There seems to be general agreement also that the liver is required for the conversion of chylomicron cholesterol into plasma lipoproteins. It has previously been mentioned that Friedman and Byers have reported evidence for the trapping of chylomicra by hepatic reticuloendothelial cells. It is likely, therefore, that the liver plays a very important role in the release of both exogenous and endogenous cholesterol to the blood in the form of lipoprotein. Since this organ is the major source of the plasma phospholipids[76,77] as well as the plasma proteins,[78] it is apparent that it probably plays a predominant role in the biosynthesis of the lipoproteins.

INTERMEDIARY METABOLISM

Fatty Acids

Oxidation of Fatty Acids. Although it has long been known that fragments containing two carbon atoms are produced upon oxidation of fatty acids, the details have not been clear until the last few years.[79,80] It is now agreed that fatty acids must first be activated by an enzymatic process requiring adenosine triphosphate (ATP) and coenzyme A (CoA) as cofactors. The primary reaction may be represented by [A] below. The expenditure of energy (ATP) is required in order to activate the carboxyl group of the fatty acid prior to oxidation. Adenylic acid (AMP) and pyrophosphate (PP) are produced in the reaction. All of the subsequent oxidative steps occur with the carboxyl group attached to coenzyme A in the form of the thioester represented by [B] below.

A number of dehydrogenases capable of removing two hydrogen atoms from fatty acid thioesters have been separated. These are mainly flavoenzymes which utilize flavine adenine dinucleotide (FAD) as the cofactor or hydrogen acceptor represented by [C] below.

Following hydration of the double bond which results in the formation of a β-hydroxyacylcoenzyme A derivative, a subsequent dehydrogenation yields a β-keto derivative. This series of events is quite similar to the classic beta-oxidation mechanism with the one important

[A]

$$1.\ RCH_2CH_2COOH + HSCoA + ATP \xrightleftharpoons{\text{thiokinase}} RCH_2CH_2CO{-}SCoA + AMP + PP$$

[B]

$$2.\ RCH_2CH_2CO{-}SCoA \xrightleftharpoons{\text{dehydrogenase}} RCH = CHCO{-}SCoA$$

[C]

$$3.\ RCH = CHCO{-}SCoA + H_2O \xrightleftharpoons{\text{crotonase}} RCH(OH)CH_2CO{-}SCoA$$

$$4.\ RCH(OH)CH_2CO{-}SCoA \xrightleftharpoons{\text{dehydrogenase}} \underset{\beta\ \ \alpha}{RCOCH_2CO{-}SCoA}$$

difference that coenzyme A remains attached to the carboxyl group throughout the process represented by [A] below.

Finally the β-keto derivative is cleaved by an enzyme known variously as thiolase or β-ketothiolase. A novel feature of this cleavage involves the addition of a second coenzyme A molecule (RSH is added rather than H_2O). This results in a thiolytic cleavage rather than hydrolytic. The result is the production of a fatty acid CoA derivative which is now shorter by two carbon atoms and which can go through the same cyclic process again. The other product of the reaction is acetyl coenzyme A. The latter substance is the metabolically active 2-carbon fragment whose identity has been the subject of extensive investigation for a half a century. As a result of the pioneering investigations of Lippman and of Lynen[79,80] it is now clear that acetyl coenzyme A is the major product derived from fatty acid oxidation *via* this series of reactions. Starting with stearic acid (18 carbon atoms), this series of reactions would have to be repeated a total of eight times in order to produce 9 molecules of acetyl coenzyme A. The last turn of the cycle would begin with butyryl coenzyme A represented by [B] below.

This cycle of events explains how fatty acids may be converted quantitatively to acetyl coenzyme A. There are also a number of other metabolic implications. It is the acetyl CoA which is subsequently oxidized to CO_2 and H_2O by means of the citric acid cycle (see below). If the reactions of the fatty acid oxidation cycle are reversible, then the main outlines of fatty acid synthesis are clear. Two molecules of acetyl CoA can condense to form acetoacetyl CoA which may subsequently be converted to butyryl CoA (4 carbon acid). In analogous fashion butyryl CoA may condense with another molecule of acetyl CoA to give rise to a 6-carbon derivative and so on until the long-chain fatty acids are eventually produced.

Since acetyl CoA is derived not only from fatty acids, but from pyruvate (major glycolytic product of carbohydrate), represented by [C] below, it becomes clear that acetyl CoA is a key intermediate in oxidative metabolism. It should also be pointed out that the glycogenic amino acids and some

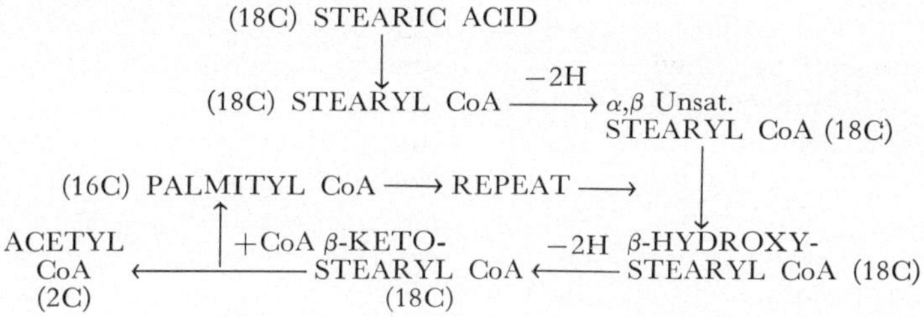

(18C) STEARIC ACID
↓
(18C) STEARYL CoA —(−2H)→ α,β Unsat. STEARYL CoA (18C)
↓
β-HYDROXY-STEARYL CoA (18C) —(−2H)→ β-KETO-STEARYL CoA (18C) —(+CoA)→ ACETYL CoA (2C) + (16C) PALMITYL CoA → REPEAT →

FIG. 1. Fatty acid oxidation cycle.

[A]

$$5.\ RCOCH_2CO{-}SCoA + HSCoA \xrightleftharpoons{\text{thiolase}} RCO{-}SCoA + CH_3CO{-}SCoA$$

[B]

$CH_3CH_2CH_2CO{-}SCoA$ (butyryl CoA) ⇄ $CH_3CH{=}CHCO{-}SCoA$ (crotonyl CoA)

⇅

$CH_3COCH_2CO{-}SCoA$ (acetoacetyl CoA) ⇄ $CH_3CH(OH)CH_2CO{-}SCoA$ (β-hydroxy butyryl CoA)

⇅

$2\ CH_3CO{-}SCoA$ (Acetyl CoA)

[C]

$$\text{(Glucose) } C_6H_{12}O_6 \rightleftharpoons 2\ CH_3COCOOH \text{ (pyruvate)} \xrightarrow{-CO_2} 2\ CH_3CO{-}SCoA \text{ (acetyl CoA)}$$

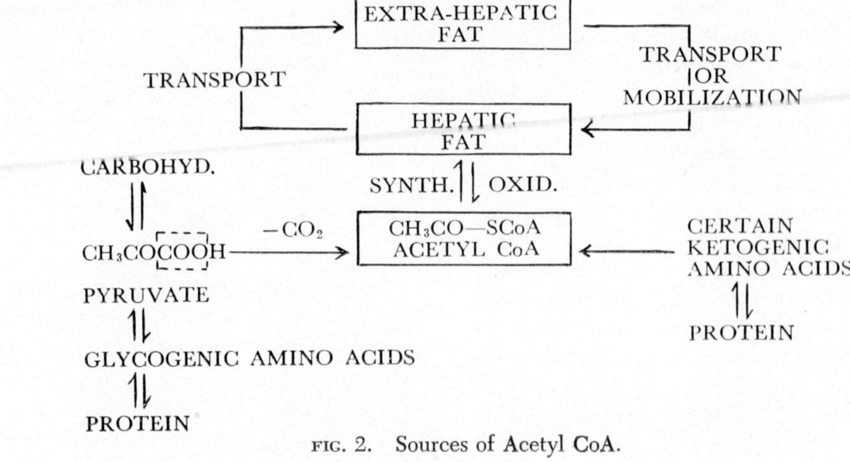

FIG. 2. Sources of Acetyl CoA.

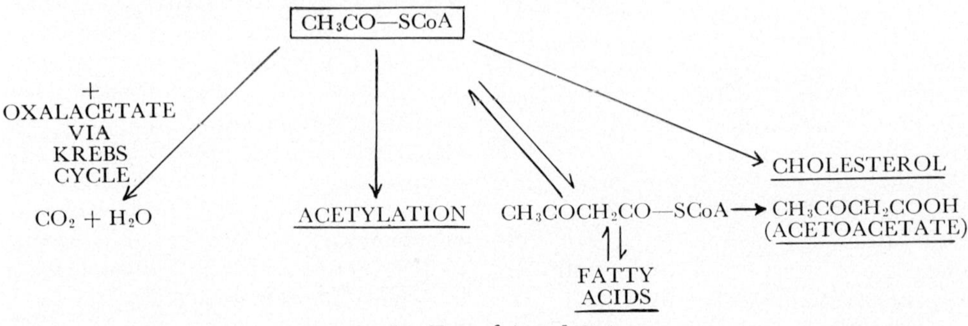

FIG. 3. Fate of Acetyl CoA.

of the ketogenic amino acids as well can also yield acetyl CoA. For a clear understanding of intermediary metabolism, it is therefore vital to know all we can concerning the sources of and rate of formation of acetyl CoA, as well as its fate.

Although acetyl CoA can be produced in all tissues, it is the liver which can, upon demand, form acetyl CoA at a tremendously increased rate. The important role of the liver in fat metabolism has long been known. The lipid content of the liver can promptly rise as a result of mobilization of fat from the fat depots produced by a number of causes. Mobilization of fat during starvation or untreated diabetes, to name but two causes, results in increased fat content of the liver. It is known that high fat diets frequently produce an accumulation of liver fat. The liver actively oxidizes and synthesizes fatty acids; in addition, the rate of oxidation can be rapidly increased when glucose utilization is depressed as, for example, in diabetes. The liver is the major organ capable of synthesizing plasma phospholipids; it is able to synthesize cholesterol and cholesterol esters at a rapid rate.

Metabolic Fate of Acetyl CoA. Acetyl CoA is the primary fuel of the Krebs citric acid or tricarboxylic acid cycle.[81] The mechanism by which this process is initiated involves the condensation represented by [A] below. Acetyl CoA (from any source) can condense with

---

[A]

$$\begin{array}{l} CO—COOH \\ | \\ CH_2—COOH \\ \text{(oxalacetic acid)} \end{array} + CH_3CO—SCoA \rightarrow HO—\begin{array}{c} CH_2—COOH \\ | \\ C—COOH \\ | \\ CH_2—COOH \\ \text{(citric acid)} \end{array} + CoA$$

oxalacetate under the influence of a condensing enzyme (present in all tissues) to produce citrate.[82] The resulting citrate is converted by the enzymes of the aerobic citric acid cycle to oxalacetate with a concomitant formation of 2 moles of CO_2 and H_2O. The net result is the complete oxidation of two carbon atoms: $CH_3COOH + 2O_2 \rightarrow 2CO_2 + 2H_2O$ + energy. It should be emphasized that the process is cyclic and that the oxalacetate is regenerated (used catalytically). So long as there is an adequate supply of oxalacetate, relatively large quantities of acetyl CoA can be oxidized to CO_2 and H_2O. It must be kept in mind, however, that oxalacetic acid is quite unstable since it tends to decarboxylate very readily as shown in [A] below. Normally, oxalacetate may be replenished in several ways: (1) Pyruvate plus CO_2 yields malate, which is readily converted to oxalacetate as in [B] below. (2) Phosphopyruvate can react reversibly with CO_2 + IDP (inosine diphosphate) to yield oxalacetate + ITP. (3) Aspartic and glutamic acids can be metabolized to oxalacetate and α-ketoglutarate respectively. The latter substance can yield oxalacetate by way of the Krebs cycle. If one looks at the citric acid cycle, it is clear that there is no net gain or loss of oxalacetate. In order to produce *more* oxalacetate, (1) it is necessary to provide a source of pyruvate (carbohydrate or glycogenic amino acids) which can fix CO_2 to form malate or oxalacetate as described above and (2) it is necessary to provide an *increased amount* of any member of the citric acid cycle. This point is emphasized because there are occasions when the oxidation of fatty acids to acetyl CoA may be tremendously accelerated in the face of a limited supply of oxalacetate (starvation, diabetes; see Fig. 3).

From the previous discussion of fatty acid oxidation, it is apparent that acetyl CoA, under the influence of thiolase, can yield acetoacetyl CoA as the first step in the biosynthesis of fatty acids as shown in [C] below. In addition, there appears to be present in liver a deacy-

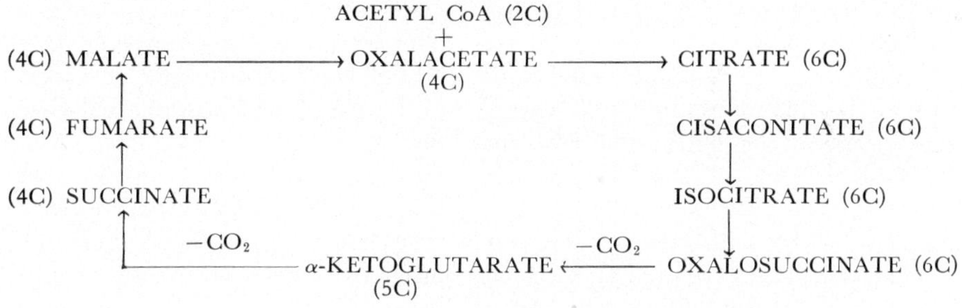

```
                         ACETYL CoA (2C)
                               +
(4C) MALATE ──────────→ OXALACETATE ──────────→ CITRATE (6C)
        ↑                   (4C)                      ↓
(4C) FUMARATE                                   CISACONITATE (6C)
        ↑                                             ↓
(4C) SUCCINATE                                  ISOCITRATE (6C)
        ↑                                             ↓
        └──── −CO2 ──── α-KETOGLUTARATE ←── −CO2 ── OXALOSUCCINATE (6C)
                              (5C)
```

FIG. 4. Citric acid cycle.

[A]

$$\begin{matrix} CO{-}COOH \\ | \\ CH_2{-}COOH \end{matrix} \xrightarrow{-CO_2} CH_3{-}CO{-}COOH \text{ (pyruvate)}$$

[B]

$$CH_3COCOOH + CO_2 \underset{TPN}{\overset{TPNH_2}{\rightleftharpoons}} \underset{\text{(malic)}}{\begin{matrix} HOCH{-}COOH \\ | \\ CH_2{-}COOH \end{matrix}} \rightleftharpoons \underset{\text{(oxalacetic)}}{\begin{matrix} OC{-}COOH \\ | \\ CH_2{-}COOH \end{matrix}}$$

[C]

$$2\ CH_3CO{-}SCoA \xrightarrow{\text{thiolase}} CH_3COCH_2CO{-}SCoA + Co\ ASH$$

lase system which is capable of hydrolyzing acetoacetyl CoA to free acetoacetate (see [A] below). An important point here is that in liver this reaction is essentially irreversible. In other words, the liver has no efficient mechanism for reconverting acetoacetate to acetoacetyl CoA and therefore to acetyl CoA. Since the liver is unable to convert acetoacetate to acetyl CoA in more than trace quantities, it is not surprising that acetoacetate is relatively inert in liver (except for its reduction to D(—) β-hydroxybutyrate). Although this explains why the liver is able to form "ketone bodies," one may well ask why extrahepatic tissues cannot similarly form ketone bodies since the same enzymes are present. In such tissues there is an efficient mechanism for reactivating free acetoacetate[83] (see [B] below). Therefore acetoacetate can be readily oxidized to CO_2 in peripheral tissues since there are enzymes present for the conversion of acetoacetate to acetoacetyl CoA, and therefore to acetyl CoA. Viewed in this light one can consider that excessive acetoacetate production by the liver represents, in a sense, a storage form of acetyl CoA particularly in situations where excessive acetyl Co A accumulates. The amount of free acetoacetate produced by the liver would therefore be dependent upon (1) the rate of breakdown of fatty acids to acetyl CoA, (2) the availability of oxalacetate, (3) possible inhibition of cleavage of acetoacetyl CoA to acetyl CoA as a result of an accumulation of excessive acetyl CoA and (4) deacylase activity. Other possible explanations of ketogenesis can, of course, be invoked. At any rate, it is now clear why most mammalian tissues which can convert fatty acids to acetyl CoA are capable of oxidizing fatty acids completely to CO_2 and H_2O, whereas the liver can, in addition, produce ketone bodies from fatty acids.

Since acetate can furnish all of the carbon atoms for the biosynthesis of cholesterol, this provides another metabolic outlet for acetyl CoA. Although it is believed by a number of investigators that acetoacetate is involved in this biosynthesis, this has not been definitely established. Again, it is not surprising that cholesterol biosynthesis may be accelerated by the liver in conditions where there may be an accumulation of acetyl CoA and, more particularly, "ketone bodies."

Finally, it has been well established that acetyl CoA is an important acetylating agent in biologic systems. Nachmansohn has clearly demonstrated its role in the formation of acetyl choline, and there is little doubt that a similar role is played in the biosynthesis of acetylated hexosamines and mucopolysaccharides.

Site of Fatty Acid Oxidation. The ability to oxidize fatty acids to CO_2 and H_2O is widespread. This has been demonstrated for liver, kidney, heart, lung, spleen, brain and skeletal muscle. In contrast to other tissues, however, the liver is capable of increasing enormously the rate of oxidation of fatty acids, particularly in conditions in which carbohydrate utilization is diminished (fasting, diabetes, high fat-low carbohydrate diets). It has long been known that liver preparations obtained from previously fasted or experimentally diabetic animals produce increased amounts of "ketone bodies" from fatty acids.[84] It has also been established that in the diabetic state, extrahepatic tissues are not able to accelerate significantly their oxidation of fatty acids.

The details of fatty acid oxidation and ketone body production have been clarified and delineated by the develop-

---

[A]

$$CH_3COCH_2CO\text{—}SCoA + H_2O \xrightarrow{\text{deacylase}} CH_3COCH_2COOH + CoASH$$

[B]

$$\text{Acetoacetate} + \text{Succinyl CoA} \rightleftharpoons \text{Acetoacetyl CoA} + \text{Succinate}$$

ment of improved *in vitro* techniques (tissue slices, minces, homogenates, etc.). Using modern techniques, it is possible with some tissues to shear cell membranes and thus obtain cell-free suspensions capable of performing many of the metabolic reactions characteristic of intact tissues. Such homogenates may be subsequently fractionated by centrifugation at different speeds to yield distinct particulate fractions representing cell debris, nuclei, mitochondria, microsomes and finally a water-clear supernatant fluid.

Kennedy and Lehninger[85] and, independently, Schneider[86] demonstrated clearly that mitochondria represent the only subcellular fraction of liver capable of oxidizing fatty acids to CO_2 and H_2O. If washed mitochondria are employed, complete oxidation is achieved provided adenosine triphosphate (ATP) is supplied for activation of the fatty acids (to obtain the fatty acid CoA derivatives) and provided a source of oxalacetate is furnished to maintain the citric acid cycle. In the absence of such a source of oxalacetate, the citric acid cycle cannot function, and very little CO_2 can be produced. In such circumstances, only ketone bodies are formed. It is obvious, therefore, that such washed mitochondria can convert fatty acid CoA derivatives to acetyl CoA even though the citric acid cycle is not functioning because of lack of substrate (oxalacetate). It is quite clear that mitochondria contain not only the enzymes required for fatty acid oxidation, but also a full complement of citric acid cycle enzymes as well as the cytochrome system which permits the ultimate transfer of electrons to oxygen. The mitochondrion is therefore a highly organized particle which respires since it can generate CO_2 (citric acid cycle) and utilize O_2 (cytochrome system). It should be emphasized that although certain enzymes of the fatty acid cycle as well as the citric acid cycle may also be found in the supernatant water-soluble fraction, the cytochrome system is confined to the mitochondria. Mitochondria obtained from several tissues have similarly been found capable of oxidizing fatty acids.

Langdon[87] has obtained evidence that most of the fatty acid oxidizing enzymes (fatty acid to acetyl CoA) are also present in the water-soluble supernatant fraction. He believes that, while fatty acid oxidation occurs predominantly in the mitochondria, the reverse process of lipogenesis is accomplished to a significant degree outside the mitochondria where a reducing environment required for the biosynthesis of long-chain fatty acids is provided.

Lipogenesis. FATTY ACIDS. That mammals can synthesize fat or fatty acids from nonlipid sources has long been known. The limitations of space, however, prevent a lengthy discussion of the historical development of this field. With the advent of isotopes it was possible for Schoenheimer[88] and Rittenberg[89] to demonstrate that fatty acids are synthesized biologically by multiple condensation of small molecules. Bloch[90] and Brady *et al.*[91] observed the biosynthesis of labeled fatty acids by liver slices and liver homogenates upon incubation with C^{13}- or C^{14}-labeled acetate and other precursors. Other workers[92,93] investigated aqueous extracts or slices and homogenates of liver which were capable of incorporating labeled acetate, acetyl CoA, pyruvate and glucose into long-chain fatty acids. It became quite clear that fatty acids can be synthesized from any precursor which is capable of forming acetate or acetyl CoA. Pyruvate, for example, can be incorporated into fatty acids when either its alpha or beta carbons are labeled with C^{13} or C^{14}, but not when it is labeled in the carboxyl position (the carboxyl group is lost as CO_2 prior to formation of acetyl CoA). Experiments with labeled glucose are also in accord with the concept that carbohydrate must first undergo glycolysis to pyruvate and subsequent decarboxylation to acetyl CoA prior to fatty acid synthesis (see diagram). It should be mentioned in passing that many tissues are capable of synthesizing fatty acids in similar fashion. Those possessing considerable activity are liver, skin, intestine, kidney and adipose tissue. In general, most tissues appear to have some fat-synthesiz-

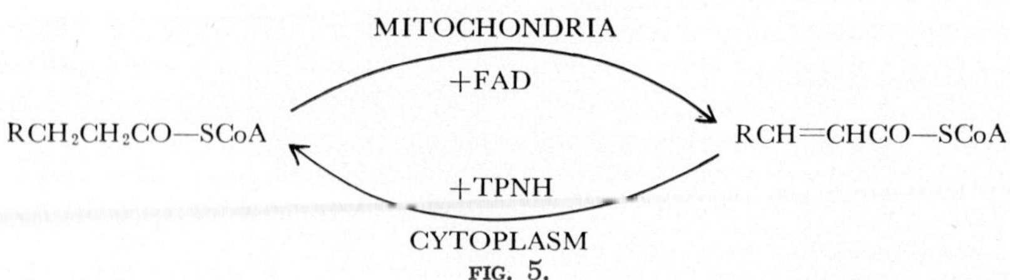

FIG. 5.

ing ability, although liver, intestine and adipose tissue are particularly active.

In each turn of the fatty acid cycle (see Fig. 1), four hydrogen atoms are removed by dehydrogenase systems and converted to H_2O. It is apparent that if the process is to be reversed in the direction of fatty acid synthesis, a source of hydrogen atoms must be supplied. This is now known to be furnished by reduced di- and triphosphopyridine nucleotides (DPNH and TPNH). Working with aqueous extracts of liver, it has been shown[92c,94] that lipogenesis from labeled acetyl CoA or 2-C^{14} pyruvate will proceed only when DPN, TPN, citrate or isocitrate, fructose diphosphate and CoA are provided. The citrate or isocitrate provides a source of reduced TPN, and fructose diphosphate generates reduced DPN.

Evidence has accumulated suggesting that the biosynthesis of fat, and therefore of fatty acids, is somehow dependent upon efficient utilization of carbohydrate. Drury[95] and, more definitively, Stetten and co-workers[96] demonstrated that, although large amounts of carbohydrate can be converted into fat by the normal animal, the process is nearly abolished in the "diabetic" state. The administration of insulin *in vivo* once again restores lipogenesis. Liver slices, homogenates or extracts obtained from diabetic animals show a similar inability to synthesize fat from glucose pyruvate or acetate;[93,97,98] other tissues have been shown to behave similarly. Even fasting for 24 hours is sufficient to reduce lipogenesis (in liver slices) to 5 to 10 per cent of that observed on a standard dietary.[99] Furthermore, a change from a high carbohydrate diet to one high in protein and fat produces some inhibition of lipogenesis from glucose.

Why is there, then, an inability to synthesize fat in such states? It cannot be ascribed to a lack of acetyl CoA since the fatty acid oxidative cycle and ketogenesis proceed at an accelerated rate in both the "diabetic" and fasting states. Chaikoff and his co-workers[100,101] have suggested that rapid lipogenesis by the liver requires the simultaneous participation of efficient glycolysis (efficient utilization of glucose). Shaw *et al.*[98,102] prepared particle-free extracts of livers from alloxan-diabetic rats which recovered considerable lipogenic activity upon addition of glycolytic intermediates such as fructose diphosphate. This dependency upon glycolysis becomes clear once it is recognized that the glycolytic conversion of glucose to pyruvate yields reduced DPN which is required for lipogenesis (discussed above). In addition to fructose diphosphate, supplementation with citrate[94] or isocitrate[103] is essential. The necessity for the latter two substances was not clarified until Langdon[87] reported the additional requirement for reduced TPN. Citric and isocitric acids can act as excellent reductants for TPN in such systems.

There is some indication that the dehydrogenation of saturated fatty acid CoA compounds to their corresponding α, β unsaturated derivatives in mitochondria may be dependent upon flavoenzymes (FAD), while the reverse process which occurs predominantly outside the mitochondria requires TPNH for at least one of the steps. Langdon suggests, therefore, that lipogenesis occurs most efficiently in the cytoplasm, where one finds metabolic processes capable of forming reduced DPN and reduced TPN.

Figure 6 illustrates the two processes: (1) glycolysis to pyruvate, yielding

DPNH, and (2) the hexose monophosphate oxidative pathway to 6-phosphogluconate and ribulose-5-phosphate, which yields TPNH. If this interpretation is correct, it becomes clear why efficient utilization of glucose is important for lipogenesis. It has recently been reported[104] that the enzyme systems involved in the conversion of glucose-6-P to 6-P-gluconate and ribulose-5-P are less active in livers of alloxan-diabetic animals. This would depress the amount of available TPNH. The report that glucose-6-phosphatase activity is enhanced in livers of diabetic animals[105,106] suggests also that less glucose-6-P is available in such states. This would provide less glucose-6-P for glycolysis or for oxidation to 6-P-gluconate. Recent reports

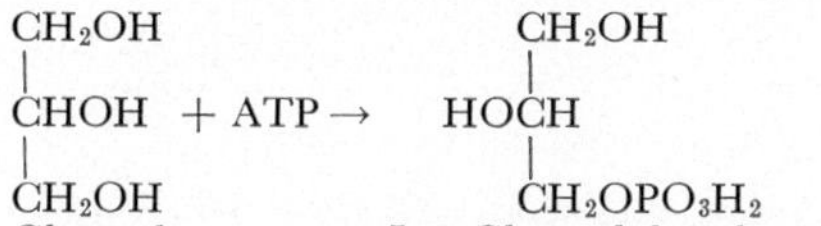

$$\begin{array}{l} CH_2OH \\ | \\ CHOH \\ | \\ CH_2OH \\ \text{Glycerol} \end{array} + ATP \rightarrow \begin{array}{l} CH_2OH \\ | \\ HOCH \\ | \\ CH_2OPO_3H_2 \\ \text{L-}\alpha\text{ Glycerolphosphate} \end{array}$$

by Siperstein, who employed homogenates of normal and "diabetic" livers, confirm the fact that stimulation of glucose utilization and, in addition, enhancement of the 6-P-gluconate pathway will restore lipogenesis in "diabetic" preparations.[107]

Triglycerides

Most of the *in vitro* work so far reported indicates clearly that the reversal of the fatty acid oxidative cycle yields fatty acid coenzyme A derivatives which are rapidly hydrolyzed to free fatty acids.[91] The manner in which these free fatty acids (or their coenzyme A derivatives) can be incorporated into triglycerides has until recently remained obscure. Although lipases can hydrolyze triglycerides, and although there is isotopic evidence (previously described) that there may be some reversal of this process during digestion, there is great doubt that this pathway can account for the rapid intracellular synthesis of triglycerides. The evidence suggesting that L-α glycerophosphate is more readily utilized than glycerol for triglyceride synthesis is more in accord with recent experiments dealing with the metabolism of phosphatidic acids and phospholipids.

It has been demonstrated that the following metabolic reactions do occur; furthermore, they have been shown to proceed with net synthesis of the product and therefore cannot simply be exchange reactions (see [A] below).

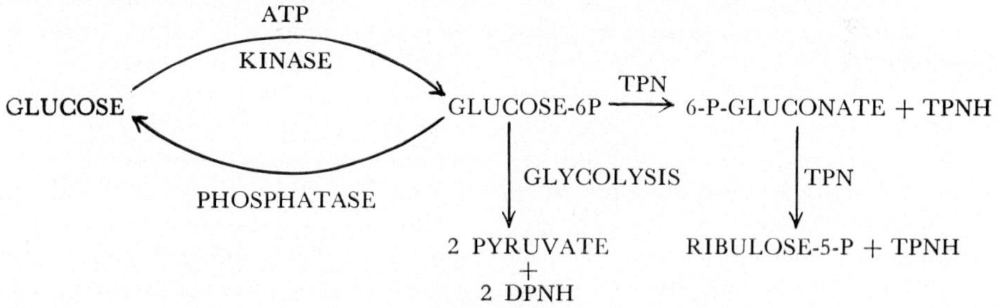

$$\text{GLUCOSE} \underset{\text{PHOSPHATASE}}{\overset{\text{ATP, KINASE}}{\rightleftarrows}} \text{GLUCOSE-6P} \xrightarrow{\text{TPN}} \text{6-P-GLUCONATE} + \text{TPNH}$$

$$\text{GLUCOSE-6P} \xrightarrow{\text{GLYCOLYSIS}} 2\ \text{PYRUVATE} + 2\ \text{DPNH}$$

$$\text{6-P-GLUCONATE} \xrightarrow{\text{TPN}} \text{RIBULOSE-5-P} + \text{TPNH}$$

FIG. 6.

[A]

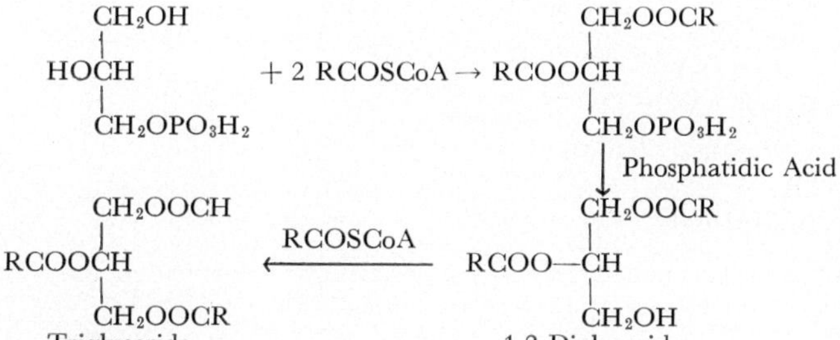

$$\begin{array}{l} CH_2OH \\ | \\ HOCH \\ | \\ CH_2OPO_3H_2 \end{array} + 2\ RCOSCoA \rightarrow \begin{array}{l} CH_2OOCR \\ | \\ RCOOCH \\ | \\ CH_2OPO_3H_2 \\ \text{Phosphatidic Acid} \end{array}$$

$$\downarrow$$

$$\begin{array}{l} CH_2OOCH \\ | \\ RCOOCH \\ | \\ CH_2OOCR \\ \text{Triglyceride} \end{array} \xleftarrow{RCOSCoA} \begin{array}{l} CH_2OOCR \\ | \\ RCOO{-}CH \\ | \\ CH_2OH \\ \text{1,2-Diglyceride} \end{array}$$

The synthesis of phosphatidic acids has been demonstrated by Kornberg and Pricer[108] as well as by Kennedy.[109] Although phosphatidic acids have not been detected in significant quantities in mammalian tissue because they are difficult to isolate and are unstable, the fact that they can be shown to be formed at a rapid rate by extracts or homogenates of liver is most significant. If it can be shown that phosphatidic acids are metabolically very reactive, this would explain the low abundance in tissues. Recently, Kennedy[110] has found an enzyme present in chicken liver and in various tissues of the rat which is capable of cleaving phosphatidic acids to inorganic phosphate and diglyceride. Weiss and Kennedy[111] subsequently reported the presence in liver of an enzyme capable of coupling 1,2 diglycerides with palmityl CoA to yield triglyceride. In these particular experiments, a net synthesis of triglyceride was obtained. All attempts to demonstrate a reaction between glycerol and fatty acid CoA derivatives have been unsuccessful. The evidence is in accord with the notion that (1) glycerol is not as efficiently used as L-α glycerophosphate (see previous discussion) and (2) a requirement for ATP is mandatory since glycerol must be phosphorylated and the fatty acids activated. Tietz and Shapiro[112] demonstrated that the incorporation of labeled fatty acid into neutral fat by liver homogenates requires ATP. In later experiments Stein and Shapiro[113] reported that glycerophosphate and not glycerol is the precursor of the glycerol moiety of the neutral fat produced by their enzyme system. Whether the same enzymes and metabolic sequences are to be found in all the tissues which are known to synthesize triglycerides has not been established. There is no reason to presume that there would be any major differences.

Phospholipids

Although the ability to synthesize phospholipid is widespread, the liver is undoubtedly one of the chief organs involved in the production of this group of compounds. Chaikoff and co-workers[76,77] have demonstrated, for example, that the plasma phospholipids are derived almost exclusively from the liver. It is of interest that the liver appears to contain a variety of such compounds including phosphatidyl choline (lecithins), phosphatidyl ethanolamine (cephalins), phosphatidyl serine and similar derivatives of inositol and sphingosine. Intestine, kidney, muscle, brain and nerve tissue, to name but a few, have been demonstrated to have the capacity to synthesize phospholipids. It is probably safe to say that all cells have, in varying degree, the ability to manufacture some or all of these substances. That there are significant qualitative differences in the enzymes present in various tissues is undoubtedly true if one considers the distribution and nature of the phospholipids found in brain, nerve, spleen, muscle, adipose tissue, etc.

The biosynthesis of phospholipid has been studied predominantly with liver preparations, although other tissues are undoubtedly active. Wittenberg and Kornberg[114] have demonstrated that choline can be phosphorylated by liver (and a number of other tissues) to form phosphoryl choline (see [A] below).

A coenzyme necessary for the next biosynthetic step has been found by Kennedy[115] to be cytidine triphosphate*

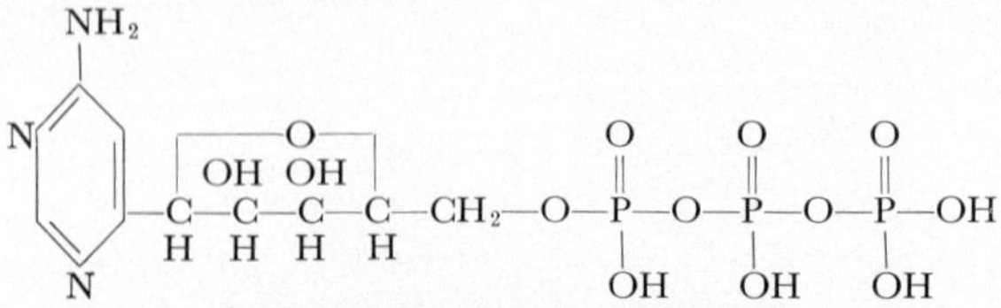

* [Structure: pyrimidine ring with NH_2 and N atoms, attached to ribose —C—C—C—C— (H H H H; OH OH; ring —O—) —CH_2—O—P(=O)(OH)—O—P(=O)(OH)—O—P(=O)(OH)—OH]

(CYTIDINE TRIPHOSPHATE)
CyPPP

[A]

$$ATP + HOCH_2CH_2\overset{+}{N}(CH_3)_3 \longrightarrow H_2O_3POCH_2\overset{+}{N}(CH_3)_3$$

(Choline) (Phosphoryl Choline)

(cytosine-ribose-triphosphate, CyPPP). Liver and brain as well as other tissues contain enzyme systems capable of performing the conversions shown in [A] below.

The products of this series of reactions are lecithin and cytidine monophosphate. The latter substance can presumably react with ATP to regenerate CyPPP. The significant features of this important metabolic pathway, which have been so clearly developed by Kennedy, need to be emphasized: (1) The reactive forms of choline are phosphoryl choline and cytidine diphosphate choline. (2) Diglycerides appear to be the important acceptor substances which are capable of reacting with cytidine diphosphate choline to accept the phosphoryl choline moiety.

This information, together with what has previously been said about triglyceride formation, places diglycerides in a key metabolic position as the major precursors of both neutral fat and phospholipids (see [B] below).

Kennedy suggests that a deficiency of CyPPcholine would result in an increased formation of triglyceride from diglyceride. This appears to be precisely what happens when hepatic synthesis of phospholipid is inhibited for one reason or another. It has long been recognized that a choline deficiency (or methionine deficiency, since this amino acid provides the methyl groups for choline) will, in some species, produce fatty livers. It is apparent that such a deficiency will result in a decrease in available CyPPcholine and, therefore, increased hepatic synthesis of triglyceride.

As is commonly known, a deficiency of the highly unsaturated fatty acids frequently results in the development of fatty livers. It is therefore of interest that diglycerides containing saturated fatty acids in the 1,2 positions will not react with CyPPcholine to form phospholipid.[110] It is only when the 1 position of the diglyceride is occupied by an unsaturated acid that appreciable synthesis of lecithin takes place. These metabolic phenomena help to explain (or at least to clarify) many of the physiologic events associated with the development of fatty livers. Just why the inability of the liver to synthesize (and perhaps to break down) phospholipid results in an accumulation of fat is not clear. It is possible that the release of fat from the liver to the plasma requires the preliminary formation of lipoprotein, and there is certainly good circumstantial evidence that phospholipid is required for the biosynthesis of lipoprotein.

Since every modern textbook of biochemistry as well as numerous monographs and review articles contain abundant information on fatty liver, the writer proposes not to expand further on this important problem.

The metabolic reactions leading to the biosynthesis of the lecithins have been described in some detail because

---

[A]

$$1.\ \mathrm{CyP{-}P{-}P} + \underset{\text{Phosphoryl Choline}}{\mathrm{P{-}OCH_2CH_2\overset{+}{N}(CH_3)_3}} \longrightarrow \underset{\text{Cytidine Diphosphate Choline}}{\mathrm{CyP{-}P{-}OCH_2CH_2\overset{+}{N}(CH_3)_3}} + \mathrm{PP}$$

$$2.\ \mathrm{CyP{-}P{-}OCH_2CH_2\overset{+}{N}(CH_3)_3} + \underset{\text{Diglyceride}}{\begin{array}{l}\mathrm{CH_2OOCR}\\ \mathrm{RCOOCH}\\ \mathrm{CH_2OH}\end{array}} \rightleftharpoons \underset{\text{Phosphatidyl Choline (Lecithin)}}{\begin{array}{l}\mathrm{CH_2OOCH}\\ \mathrm{RCOOCH}\quad \mathrm{O}\\ \mathrm{CH_2O\overset{\|}{P}{-}OCH_2CH_2\overset{+}{N}(CH_3)_3}\\ \qquad\ \ \mathrm{O^-}\end{array}} + \mathrm{CyP}$$

[B]

$$\underset{\text{Choline}}{\text{Phosphatidyl}} \xleftarrow{\text{CyPPcholine}} \overset{\text{Phosphatidic Acids}\ \downarrow}{\text{Diglycerides}} \xrightarrow{\text{RCO—SCoA}} \text{Triglycerides}$$

similar considerations apply to the biosynthesis of the cephalins and sphingomyelins. For example, Kennedy and Weiss[115] have described a similar series of reactions for ethanolamine ($HOCH_2$-CH_2NH_2) involving intermediate formation of CyPPethanolamine. Further propriate diglycerides leads to the subsequent formation of phosphatidylethanolamine (cephalins).

Since sphingomyelins contain a phosphoryl choline group, it might be predicted that CyPPcholine is also involved in this synthetic pathway. It is of interest, therefore, that Sribney and Kennedy[116] have provided evidence for the reaction represented in [A] below. These investigators have obtained evidence of the presence in chicken liver of an enzyme which catalyzes this reaction with the formation of a phospholipid having the properties of sphingomyelin.

Emerging from these studies is the first clear light concerning the manner in which a wide variety of phosphatides may be synthesized in mammalian tissues. It is obvious, of course, that this information will lead to significant studies of those clinical diseases involving abnormal phospholipid metabolism. One should not forget, however, that the simple metabolic outlines presented here represent only a beginning, and that much more needs to be explained from a metabolic point of view. Saturated lecithins, for example, have been found in brain and lung;[117] in addition, the phosphatidic acids need to be put on a sounder basis. Finally, it would be surprising to find identical metabolic pathways or enzyme systems in such widely diverse tissues as brain, nerve, spleen, liver and intestine.

Little is known about the metabolic pathways by which the phospholipids are catabolized in mammalian tissues. It is clear that the liver is a site of intense activity so far as turnover (synthesis and breakdown) of phospholipid is concerned. Fasting, for example, produces a profound drop in liver phospholipids of several species.[118] Experiments with radioactive inorganic phosphate or organic compounds labeled with radioactive carbon have provided information regarding the turnover (or rate of replacement) in various tissues. The evidence suggests a wide variation in rates, ranging from very rapid turnover in liver to an extremely slow rate in brain, with small intestine, kidney and muscle exhibiting intermediate values.[119] Accurate estimations of phospholipid turnover (particularly in the liver) have been difficult to obtain because of the limitations inherent in the isotopic techniques employed; e.g., the use of C^{14}-labeled unsaturated fatty acids is complicated by the metabolic activity or exchangeability of the fatty acid residue in the α' position of phospholipids. Furthermore, most of the fractions isolated in experiments of this nature must inevitably be heterogeneous. There is some evidence, however, that phospholipids are to some degree degraded to glycerylphosphorylcholine and to the ethanolamine analogue.[120] This, of course, suggests the presence of enzymes corresponding to lecithinases A and B (or more properly phospholipase A and B) which would cleave the fatty acid residues from lecithins and cephalins to yield glycerylphosphorylcholine, etc. It has, furthermore, been found by Dawson[121] that the resulting products can be further degraded by liver homogenates to L-α glycerophosphate.

Kennedy's work (previously described) suggests that another major pathway for the catabolism of phospholipids must be considered. The reversible nature of the reaction as in [B] below

---

[A]

N-acylsphingosine + CyPPcholine → Sphingomyelin + Cy P

[B]

CyPPcholine + diglyceride ↔ Phosphatidyl choline + Cy P

suggests that important intermediates in the catabolism of the phospholipids may be 1,2 diglycerides.

Unsaturated Acids

The ability of the mammalian organism to introduce double bonds into fatty acid molecules is limited. Normal oxidation of fatty acyl CoA derivatives yields α,β unsaturated intermediates, which are readily metabolized further (as previously described). Stetten and Schoenheimer[122] demonstrated with isotopic techniques that stearic acid can be converted metabolically to oleic acid ($\Delta^{9,10}$-octadecenoic acid), and palmitic acid to palmitoleic ($\Delta^{9,10}$-hexadecenoic) acid. Since these two acids represent the predominant monounsaturated acids found in mammalian tissues, it is clear that the requirements for these unsaturated acids can be met endogenously. The dehydrogenase necessary for this conversion appears to be widely distributed.

The discovery by Burr and Burr in 1929[123] that linoleic acid ($\Delta^{9,12}$ octadecadienoic) is essential for the nutrition of the rat led to subsequent experiments by Bernhard and Schoenheimer[124] which demonstrated that this acid cannot be synthesized endogenously. Although linoleic, linolenic ($\Delta^{9,12,15}$ octadecatrienoic) and arachidonic ($\Delta^{5,8,11,14}$ eicosatetraenoic) acids have been heretofore considered to be the main "essential fatty acids," it is now known that linoleic acid is a precursor of the C_{20} acid, arachidonic acid.[125] Furthermore, it has been demonstrated by Mead *et al.*[126] that 1-C^{14} acetate is incorporated into arachidonic acid when linoleate is administered to a deficient animal. Similarly, C^{14}-linoleate has been found by Steinberg *et al.*[127] to be incorporated into arachidonate. It is also of interest that linolenic acid can be converted into acids containing four (tetraenoic) and six double bonds (hexaenoic acids); the tetraenoic acid is, however, not identical with arachidonic acid.

Although the effects of a deficiency of the essential fatty acids have not been clearly delineated for man, nevertheless the multiplicity of effects in animals (maintenance of skin, growth, reproduction, cholesterol transport) suggest that further studies in man will reveal requirements for the essential fatty acids. This area has been fully reviewed by Holman.[128]

Perhaps greatest interest in this field is aroused by the relationship of the polyunsaturated acids to cholesterol transport and blood levels. It is known that cholesterol esters contain a high proportion of polyunsaturated acids, and that, in rats on a fat-free diet, plasma cholesterol decreases while the content of cholesterol in the liver increases.[129] Since under such circumstances the cholesterol which accumulates in the liver is mainly in the esterified form, Alfin-Slater and co-workers[129] suggest that it is largely the nonessential fatty acids which have in this case esterified the cholesterol producing a faulty cholesterol metabolism.

Since the original report of Kinsell in 1952,[130] which demonstrated that dietary vegetable and animal fats exert different effects on human serum cholesterol levels, considerable effort has been expended in an attempt to determine the nature of this phenomenon. Hardinge and Stare[131] reported that complete vegetarians had lower serum cholesterol levels than those consuming dairy products. Groen *et al.*,[132] studying 60 volunteers, each of whom served as his own control, provided evidence that the highest cholesterol levels were obtained on high animal-fat diets while the lowest were observed on a completely vegetarian diet containing nearly isocaloric quantities of fat. Ahrens *et al.*[133] have reviewed the numerous studies made with widely different population groups which have strengthened the belief that certain fats can elevate while other fats can lower serum levels of cholesterol and phospholipid. It is still uncertain, however, whether these results can be ascribed to the preponderance of unsaturated fatty acids in certain types of fat or to the presence of plant sterols which might be expected to interfere with absorption. Ahrens[133] has analyzed the fatty acids of the serum triglycerides in a patient during two successive feeding periods when butter and corn oil respectively composed the sole dietary fat. During the latter feeding period, the linoleic acid content was found to have increased some tenfold while the serum cholesterol levels dropped significantly. Whether these two findings bear any significant relationship to each other remains to be established. It is of interest in this connection that James[70] utilizing the techniques of liquid-gas-phase chromatography estimated the per cent composition of linoleic and arachidonic acid in the acids derived from (1) phospholipids of the red blood cells, (2) plasma phospholipids and (3) plasma neutral fat in a series of patients with coronary artery disease. These levels were compared with a group of "normal controls" matched for age and sex. No significant difference was found between the two groups. Although there has been a vast amount of literature on the subject, it can be stated only that there are good grounds for believing that numerous factors are undoubtedly involved in the etiology of atherosclerosis and coronary disease. Although total caloric intake, type and quality of the diet, and the qualitative and quantitative aspects of fat intake are undoubtedly significant, basic research in this difficult area will have to provide much more meaningful information before significant relationships can be discerned. This whole subject has been reviewed in various articles and texts.

CHOLESTEROL METABOLISM

Numerous studies suggest that many factors may play a role in atherosclerosis and coronary artery disease (endocrine, dietary, disturbances of lipid transport, tissue damage, thrombosis, etc.). There is very little doubt, however, that coronary artery disease is frequently associated with high levels of blood cholesterol. Although analysis of serum cholesterol may have very little significance so far as diagnosis or prognosis of individual cases is concerned, nevertheless statistical data with large groups suggest some kind of correlation.

Regardless of whether there is a direct connection or not, great interest has centered about those nutritional factors which appear to influence serum cholesterol levels. Keys[134] and others[135] have reported that in men, the levels of serum cholesterol are relatively independent of intake of dietary cholesterol. Since in such persons, elimination of cholesterol-rich foods from the dietary produced no lowering of the serum levels, it is quite apparent that endogenous production of cholesterol must account for such findings. Reports by numerous investigators[133] suggest that serum cholesterol levels are influenced by the amount and character of the fat consumed rather than the cholesterol intake. Severe restriction of fat intake frequently results in a lowering of serum cholesterol levels. There is some suggestion, as previously described, that replacement of animal fat by certain vegetable fats effectively reduces cholesterol levels.[130,133] Whether this is so or not, judicious lowering of the American high fat intake would appear to be a wise maneuver in persons with elevated serum cholesterol levels. It seems clear that wherever very low-fat diets prevail, serum cholesterol levels do not rise appreciably after the age of thirty.

Endogenous Synthesis

All mammalian cells, with the possible exception of mature nerve cells, appear to be capable of synthesizing cholesterol from acetyl coenzyme A and consequently from any substance capable of being converted into this important metabolite. It has previously been pointed out that fat, carbohydrate and many amino acids can be metabolically converted to acetyl coenzyme A. It is no surprise, therefore, that cholesterol-free diets are relatively ineffective in lowering serum cholesterol.

Considerable evidence concerning the mechanism of biosynthesis of cholesterol has come from experiments involving incubation of tissue slices or homogenates with cholesterol precursors that have been labeled with isotopic carbon (heavy carbon C^{13} or radioactive C^{14}). It is now well established that the two carbon atoms of acetate can provide all the carbon atoms of cholesterol.

By incubating liver slices with methyl-labeled acetate or carboxyl-labeled acetate, Bloch and his co-workers[136] demonstrated that both carbon atoms could be incorporated into cholesterol and were furthermore able to conclude that, of the 27 carbon atoms of cholesterol, 15 were derived from the methyl carbon (M) and 12 from the carboxyl carbon (C) of acetate. As a result of the brilliant investigations of Cornforth and co-workers[137] as well as of Bloch *et al.*,[136] the origin of every carbon atom of cholesterol has been determined.

If one considers the structure of the cholesterol molecule, it becomes obvious that branched-chain intermediates must somehow be synthesized from acetate prior to formation of cholesterol. The finding that radioactive acetoacetate can be incorporated by liver slices into cholesterol[138] suggested the possibility that the liver is capable of condensing acetoacetate with acetate to form a branched-chain acid containing 6 carbon atoms. It was soon established that such an acid (β-hydroxy-β-methyl glutaric) could be readily synthesized by rat liver homogenates from acetate.[139] Rudney[140] has provided more detailed evidence for this synthesis by demonstrating that acetyl coenzyme A can condense with acetoacetyl coenzyme A to form the same 6-carbon branched-chain acid (HMG) as represented in [A] below.

Recently Ferguson *et al.*[141] have demonstrated that this acid can be reduced by yeast enzymes to mevalonic acid.

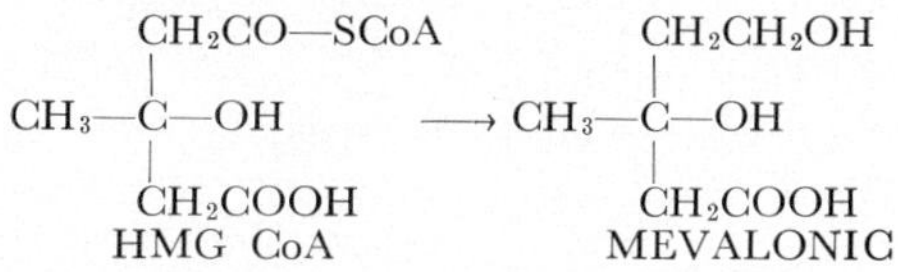

$$CH_3-\underset{\underset{CH_2COOH}{|}}{\overset{\overset{CH_2CO-SCoA}{|}}{C}}-OH \longrightarrow CH_3-\underset{\underset{CH_2COOH}{|}}{\overset{\overset{CH_2CH_2OH}{|}}{C}}-OH$$

HMG CoA　　　　MEVALONIC

2-C^{14} mevalonate (labeled in the carbon α to the carboxyl) has been found by Tavormina *et al.*[142] to be an extremely potent precursor of cholesterol when incubated with rat liver homogenates. Numerous laboratories have confirmed this finding as well as the fact that the carboxyl group of mevalonate is not incorporated into cholesterol but is converted to CO_2. Although mevalonate has not as yet been isolated from mammalian tissue, the fact that it

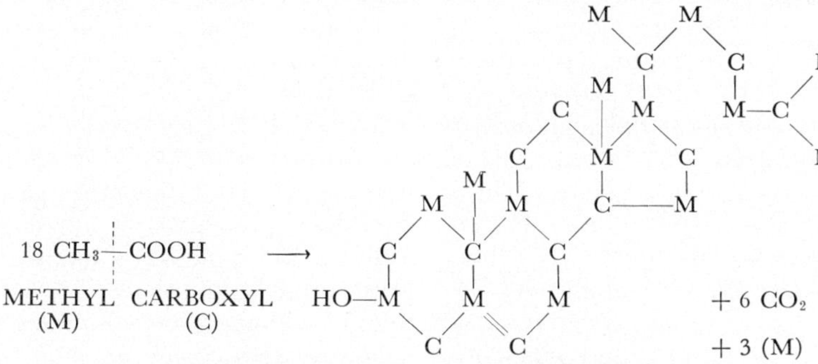

18 CH_3 ⁞ COOH ⟶ [cholesterol skeleton with each carbon labeled M or C; HO—M at position 3] + 6 CO_2 + 3 (M)

METHYL (M)　CARBOXYL (C)

18 MOLES ACETATE → 1 CHOLESTEROL

FIG. 7.

[A]

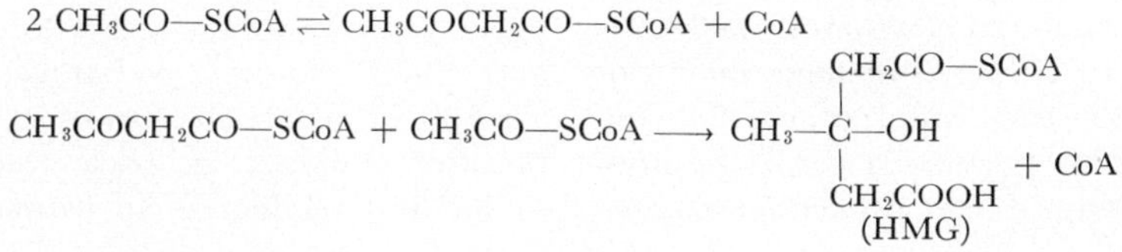

$$2\ CH_3CO-SCoA \rightleftharpoons CH_3COCH_2CO-SCoA + CoA$$

$$CH_3COCH_2CO-SCoA + CH_3CO-SCoA \longrightarrow CH_3-\underset{\underset{CH_2COOH}{|}}{\overset{\overset{CH_2CO-SCoA}{|}}{C}}-OH + CoA$$

(HMG)

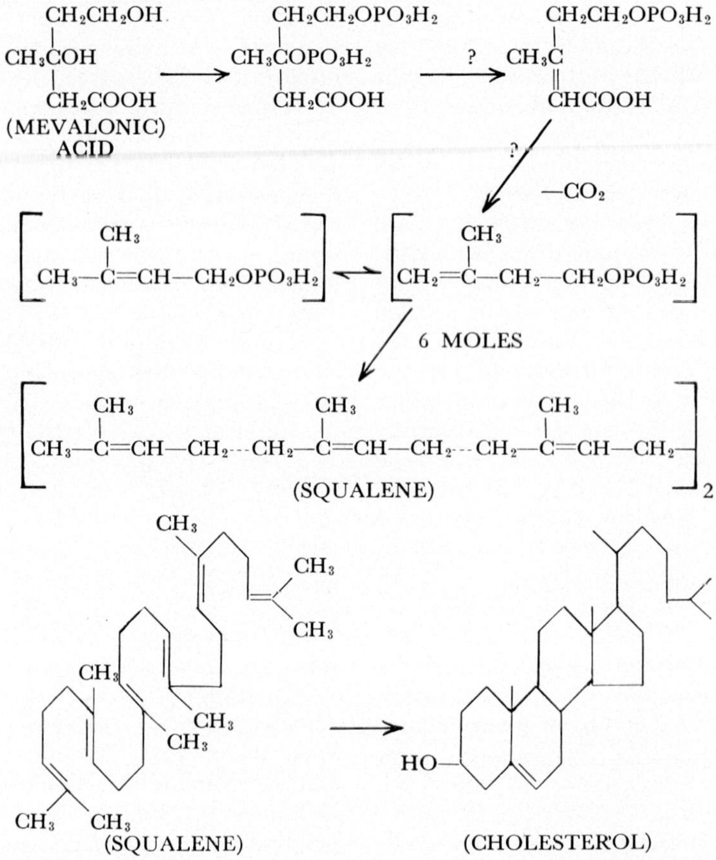

CH_2CH_2OH / CH_3COH / CH_2COOH (MEVALONIC ACID) → $CH_2CH_2OPO_3H_2$ / $CH_3COPO_3H_2$ / CH_2COOH ? → $CH_2CH_2OPO_3H_2$ / CH_3C ‖ $CHCOOH$

? $-CO_2$

$[CH_3-C(CH_3)=CH-CH_2OPO_3H_2]$ ⇌ $[CH_2=C(CH_3)-CH_2-CH_2OPO_3H_2]$

6 MOLES

$[CH_3-C(CH_3)=CH-CH_2 \cdots CH_2-C(CH_3)=CH-CH_2 \cdots CH_2-C(CH_3)=CH-CH_2-]_2$

(SQUALENE)

CH₃ CH₃ CH₃ CH₃ CH₃ CH₃ CH₃ CH₃

(SQUALENE) → HO— (CHOLESTEROL)

FIG. 8. Postulated scheme for conversion of mevalonate to cholesterol.

is present in certain microorganisms and is formed by yeast from HMG CoA suggests that further experiments will demonstrate its formation by mammalian tissue. The fact remains that mevalonate is the most efficient precursor of cholesterol yet found when tested with mammalian tissues.

The conversion of mevalonate to cholesterol proceeds via squalene, a noncyclic hydrocarbon containing 30 carbon atoms.[143]

Mevalonate is rapidly and efficiently converted to squalene by rat liver slices, homogenates[142] and even by the supernatant fluid obtained after centrifugation of all of the particulate matter present in such homogenates. Yields as high as 15 to 20 per cent have been obtained with the supernatant enzyme system.[144] This portion of the biosynthesis of cholesterol can proceed anaerobically and requires ATP, Mg^{++} ions, DPN and TPN. Phillips *et al.*[145] have presented evidence suggesting that mevalonate is phosphorylated (probably to the diphospho-ester). Since it is known that the carboxyl group is readily converted to CO_2, it becomes possible to speculate about the nature of the 5-carbon precursor or "biological isoprene unit." One such likely possibility is isoprenyl phosphate. (A large number of known 5-carbon branched-chain acids, aldehydes and alcohols have been tested without success.) The biologic importance and nature of this 5-carbon precursor can hardly be overemphasized since it undoubtedly serves as a precursor of rubber, terpenes, carotenes and plant steroids. Whatever the nature of the 5-carbon "isoprene unit" may be, the evidence is clear that 6 such molecules polymerize to form squalene.

As early as 1926 Channon and Marrian[146] had isolated squalene from fish liver; this was confirmed by Thannhauser.[147] Both Channon[148] and Heilbron[149] conceived the notion that there might be a biogenetic relationship between squalene and steroids, and Robinson[150] in 1934 proposed that the squalene structure could be folded in such a way as to resemble the steroid nucleus. Woodward and Bloch[151] suggested a different kind of folding (see diagram) which fitted the experimental facts better, and then demonstrated that their ideas were correct. If one compares the structure of cholesterol with squalene (suitably folded), it is apparent that cyclization, reduction, loss of 3 methyl groups and introduction of an alcohol group must occur.

That squalene is an important intermediate in cholesterol synthesis now rests on secure grounds. Channon[148] originally observed an accumulation in liver after feeding squalene. Although the amount of squalene normally present in mammalian liver is too small for direct isolation, Bloch and his colleagues[143] noted that after administration of squalene to rats, substantial amounts of the substance could subsequently be recovered from the liver. If, along with the squalene which served as a carrier, either carboxyl- or methyl-labeled C^{14} acetate was fed, the squalene recovered from the liver was found to be radioactive. When this biosynthetic radioactive squalene was in turn fed to mice, at least 20 per cent of the absorbed squalene was converted to cholesterol. It has also been possible to demonstrate the conversion of squalene to cholesterol in cell-free preparations.[152] More recently, small amounts of squalene have been found in pork liver, skin, hair fat and in ovarian or dermoid cysts.

Apparently intact microsomes plus supernatant fluid (obtained from homogenates of rat liver) are required for the efficient conversion of squalene to cholesterol. This phase of the biosynthesis requires oxygen. Bloch and co-workers[152] have obtained evidence implicating lanosterol as an intermediate in this process. Comparison of the structure of lanosterol with the folded structure of squalene (see diagram) will show the close relationship of the two.

It is obvious that a number of intermediate steroids are involved in cholesterol synthesis and that the manner in which the three extra methyl groups are eliminated will be the subject of considerable study.

The ability to synthesize cholesterol from acetyl CoA or from substances capable of conversion to this substance appears to be widespread among mammalian tissues. For example, *in vitro* studies with animal tissues such as skin, small intestine, adrenal cortex, testes, ovaries, mammary gland, kidney, aorta and brain (new-born) have confirmed this belief.

In the tissues, cholesterol is found in both the free and esterified forms. The ratio of the free to the esterified form varies considerably among the different organs, but remans fairly constant for each tissue under normal conditions. Sperry,[153] for example, has reported on

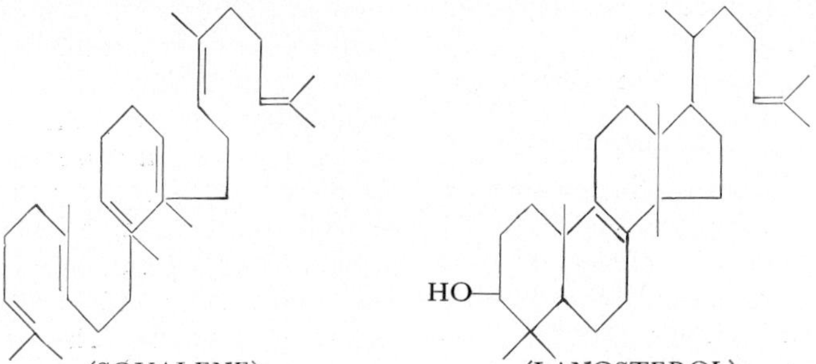

(SQUALENE) HO (LANOSTEROL)

FIG. 9.

the constancy of this ratio in normal blood plasma. There is no longer any doubt that in the tissues some of this material must be bound to intracellular lipoproteins, which are currently being extensively investigated. Recent work on the nature and distribution of tissue lipoproteins has been reviewed by Cohen,[154] Chargaff[155] and Lovern.[156]

Although enzyme fractions with cholesterol esterase activity have been obtained from several tissues, it is still uncertain that only one enzyme or a variety of esterases are involved. Furthermore, the physiologic significance of the cholesterol esters is not obvious; in general a high ratio of esterified to non-esterified cholesterol is characteristic of tissues exhibiting a rapid turnover of cholesterol. In brain, for example, where cholesterol is relatively inert metabolically, almost no cholesterol esters are present.

Precise analytic data are also lacking on the nature of the fatty acids which are normally esterified with cholesterol. In general, highly unsaturated fatty acids predominate in this lipid component. In some species very high iodine numbers have been obtained, with good evidence that linoleic, linolenic, oleic, palmitoleic and arachidonic acids are present in appreciable quantities; lesser amounts of the saturated fatty acids are found.[157] Iodine numbers of approximately 130 have been obtained for the acids present in human plasma cholesterol ester preparations.[158] Although there is very little doubt that the "essential fatty acids" are normally associated with this fraction, it should be noted that Kinsell *et al.*[159] have demonstrated that the iodine number (or degree of unsaturation) can vary over a wide range depending upon the nature of the dietary fat.

Both liver and pancreas have been implicated as sources of the cholesterol esterase present in serum. Active preparations of pancreatic cholesterol esterase have been obtained by a number of investigators.[160] Liver esterases appear to be particularly important since labeled cholesterol esters are found promptly in the liver following administration of labeled acetate.[74,75] It has been mentioned elsewhere that hepatectomy, shortly after the administration of C^{14}-acetate, virtually abolishes the appearance of labeled cholesterol in the sterol ester fraction of blood and several other tissues; the appearance of free C^{14}-cholesterol is not so affected.

Catabolism of Cholesterol

Although the side-chain of cholesterol is readily oxidized in the living organism, the nucleus or ring system is not. When cholesterol labeled with C^{14} in carbon 26 is administered to animals, considerable isotope is promptly observed in the respiratory CO_2.[161] On the other hand, no labeled CO_2 is obtained when one of the ring carbons is made radioactive. As a matter of fact, following intravenous administration of cholesterol labeled in carbon 4 to rats, Siperstein and Chaikoff[162] recovered 95 per cent of the radioactivity from the feces in the subsequent 15 days. Of this recovered activity, 10 per cent was found to be in the fecal sterols and 85 per cent in the form of steroid acids.

It is believed that these steroid acids are products resulting from bacterial action upon the bile acids. The evidence by now has become overwhelming that cholesterol is converted to bile acids by the liver. Intravenous or intraperitoneal injection of labeled cholesterol into animals with a bile fistula has usually resulted in the recovery of very high yields of isotope in the accumulated bile acids. Thus, Bergstrom[163] after intraperitoneal injection of C^{14} cholesterol into rats recovered 22 per cent as pure cholic acid from the bile. Following intravenous injection, Siperstein *et al.*[162] found that approximately 38 per cent of the administered isotope (in cholesterol) could be recovered in the collected bile within 48 hours; similar results were obtained after feeding the radioactive cholesterol. Since very little radioactivity could be recovered from the urine, intestinal contents and acholic feces, these investigators were able to conclude that of the cholesterol-C^{14} normally excreted from the body, over 90 per cent passes through the bile. Of this 90 per cent which is excreted by way of the bile, more than 95 per cent was identified as bile acids.

Since similar results have been observed following administration of labeled cholesterol to a patient with a bile fistula,[164] it is apparent that this is a widespread phenomenon, and that fecal steroids (coprosterol and dihydrocholesterol) are not the only quantitatively important end products of cholesterol metabolism in man. In this particular case 40 per cent of an administered dose of 4-C^{14}-cholesterol was excreted in 50 hours; of this amount 98.5 per cent was found in the bile, whereas only 1.3 and 0.2 per cent were found in the acholic feces and urine respectively. Only a small fraction of the cholesterol which is lost from the body does so as intact sterol by way of the bile or by secretion through the intestinal wall.

Since the conversion of cholesterol to bile acids appears to be a major catabolic pathway for cholesterol, it is of interest to follow the fate of the bile salts following their entrance into the intestinal lumen. Apparently reabsorption occurs very rapidly and efficiently. In rats, 80 to 90 per cent of the C^{14} excreted through the bile was promptly reabsorbed when the material was reinfused into the duodenum. This fraction is then carried by way of the portal blood to the liver where it is quickly re-excreted into the bile.[165] Although the enterohepatic circulation in the whole animal thus allows only a small portion of the bile salts to escape into the feces with each cycle, it is apparent that the sum of these small losses can account for the bulk of the C^{14} of administered cholesterol which is excreted in the feces. It should be understood that bile salt excretion studies carried out with bile fistula animals represent a state of maximal conversion by the liver of cholesterol to bile acids.[166]

Linstedt[167] has studied bile acid formation in humans by administering cholic acid labeled with C^{14} followed by isolation of bile samples at various time intervals. From the dilution of the isotope by endogenous bile acids, he was able to estimate the total body pool of cholic acid to be from 0.58 to 1.3 gm. It has been calculated that the normal person converts about 1 gm. of cholesterol to bile acids per day.

The main factor influencing the rate of bile acid excretion from the body appears to involve the action of intestinal bacteria upon bile salts which results in the formation of metabolic products that can no longer be reabsorbed. In the absence of intestinal bacteria, bile acids are retained longer; it is of interest also that when the intestine is sterile, bile salts can be detected in the feces, whereas normally a complex mixture of hydroxy and keto acids (steroid acids?) is produced by the action of the intestinal bacteria upon the bile acids.[168]

The mechanism by which cholesterol is converted to bile salts has not been completely elucidated. If one compares the chemical structures of cholesterol and cholic acid, it is clear that the liver is able to cleave only three terminal carbons from the side-chain. Evidence for this has been obtained by Zabin and

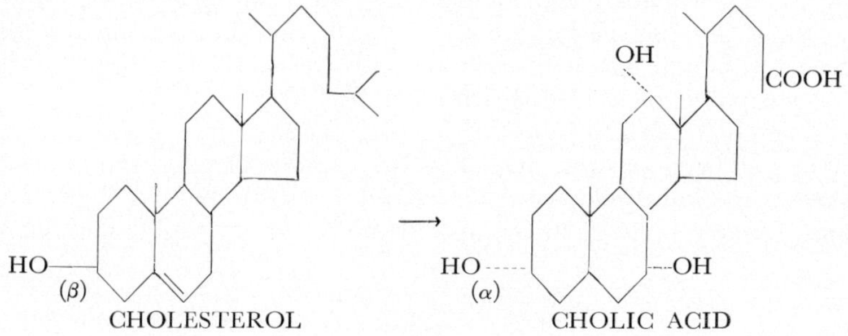

HO— (β) CHOLESTEROL → HO---- (α) ---OH OH COOH CHOLIC ACID

FIG. 10.

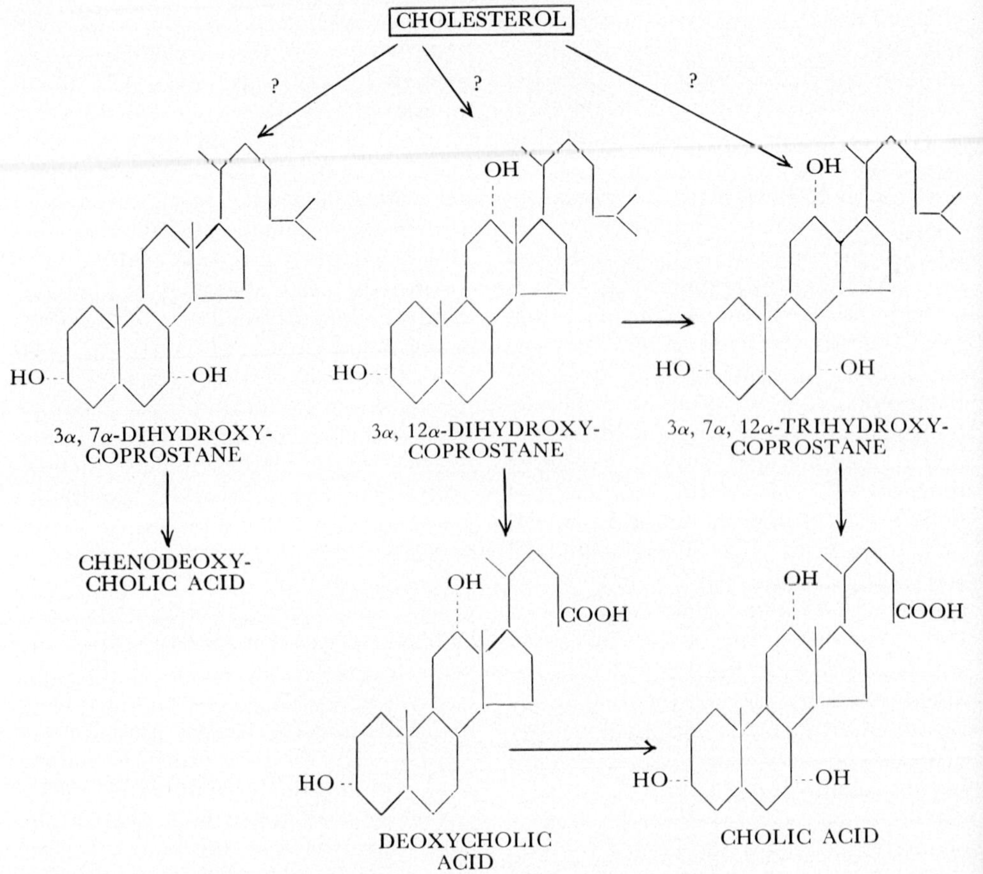

CHOLESTEROL

3α, 7α-DIHYDROXY-COPROSTANE → CHENODEOXYCHOLIC ACID

3α, 12α-DIHYDROXY-COPROSTANE → DEOXYCHOLIC ACID

3α, 7α, 12α-TRIHYDROXY-COPROSTANE → CHOLIC ACID

FIG. 11.

Barker[169] and Staple *et al.*[170] In addition, the alcohol group at carbon 3 must be inverted to the α configuration, two other alcohol groups (α configuration) are introduced at positions 7 and 12, and the double bond of cholesterol is reduced to yield cholic acid. Bergström and his coworkers[166,171] have obtained evidence that the three hydroxyl groups are introduced (in the proper configuration) and the double bond is reduced to yield 3α, 7α, 12α trihydroxycoprostane before the three terminal carbon atoms are removed. Although rat liver mitochondria are capable of oxidizing carbon 26 or 27 of cholesterol to CO_2,[170b,172] it has not as yet been possible to convert cholesterol to cholic acid with such preparations. Deoxycholic acid is apparently not produced in the liver of man[173] but is probably formed from cholic acid in the intestine as a result of bacterial action. It may then be reabsorbed and excreted in the bile in the conjugated form. Deoxycholic acid can also be hydroxylated on carbon 7 by rat liver homogenates to yield cholic acid.[174] The product actually isolated in this case is the conjugated form of the acid, taurocholic acid. Before cholic acid can combine with taurine or glycine to yield taurocholic and glycocholic acids respectively, the carboxyl group must first be activated. Cell-free liver preparations have been obtained which are capable of performing this activation and condensation.[162,175] As might be expected Mg^{++}, ATP and CoA are re-

A

Cholic Acid + ATP + CoA → Cholyl CoA + AMP + PP

quired. It is probable that cholyl CoA may also be actually formed as a result of a thiolytic cleavage of the three terminal side-chain carbons of 3α, 7α, 12α trihydroxycoprostane[170b] during the biosynthesis of bile acids by the liver.

It seems clear that the conversion of cholesterol to bile acids is an irreversible process. Byers and Biggs[176] demonstrated that labeled cholic acid cannot be converted to cholesterol in the rat. Although there have been reports suggesting that cholesterol may not be the only precursor of the bile acids, there is at present no definitive evidence ruling out cholesterol as the major source of the bile acids.

Intestinal Excretion. Cook *et al.*[168b] have reported that adult man on a mixed diet excretes approximately 0.5 gm. of fecal sterols daily. Since plant sterols are poorly absorbed, obviously these substances will be found in varying quantity with changes in the diet. Although coprostanol (coprosterol) is the major saturated sterol present, a number of unsaturated C_{27} compounds are also excreted, among them 7-dehydrocholesterol and Δ^7-cholestanol. In addition cholestanol (dihydrocholesterol), coprostanone[177] and smaller amounts of other ketones[178] as well as several di- and tri-hydroxysterols have also been identified.[168b]

Although the origin of all these sterols is not completely clear, there is very little doubt that the intestinal mucosa is capable of secreting sterol. The cholesterol of the bile is largely reabsorbed. The formation of coprostanol probably occurs as a result of bacterial action in the large intestine[179] since it has recently been demonstrated that bacterial cultures isolated from feces can convert cholesterol to coprostanol.[177,180]

As a result of the experiments of Schoenheimer *et al.*[181] it was formerly believed that Δ^4-cholestenone was an obligatory intermediate in this conversion via coprostanone. Recently it has been demonstrated, however, that this may not be the case.[177] A direct microbial reduction has been reported for the conversion of cholesterol to coprostanol without the intermediate formation of cholestenone. Probably both pathways may be involved since liver can transform Δ^4-cholestenone to cholestanone and cholestanol.

Mention has already been made of

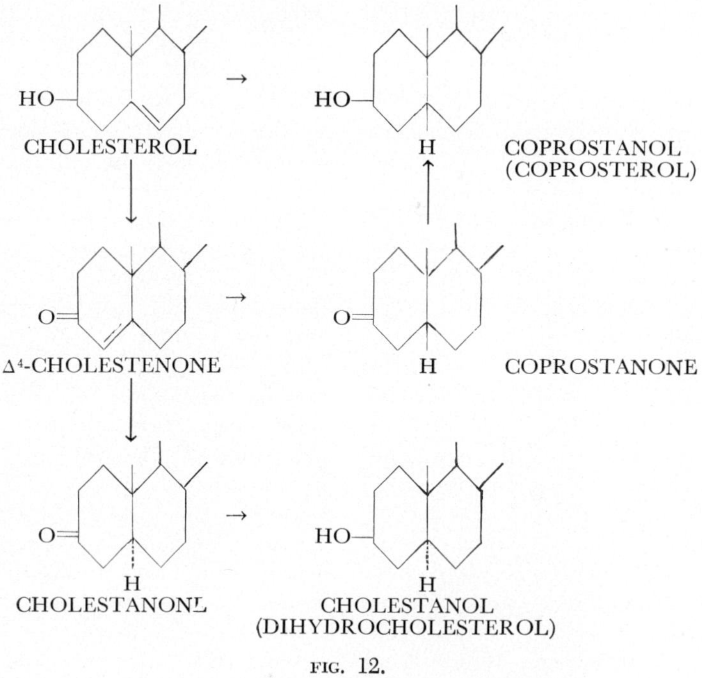

HO— CHOLESTEROL → HO— H COPROSTANOL (COPROSTEROL)

O= Δ^4-CHOLESTENONE → O= H COPROSTANONE

O= H CHOLESTANONE → HO— H CHOLESTANOL (DIHYDROCHOLESTEROL)

FIG. 12.

the presence in fecal lipids of steroid acids produced by the action of intestinal microorganisms upon the bile acids. These steroid acids may be formed in amounts up to 250 mg. per day.[168b] It should be remembered that deoxycholic acid is probably formed in the intestine and that a portion of this acid and its bacterial products are excreted along with the steroid acids.

Adrenocortical Steroids and Sex Hormones

It has long been suspected that cholesterol is a precursor of the adrenocortical steroids and sex hormones. The administration of deuterium-labeled cholesterol to a pregnant woman resulted in the urinary excretion of labeled pregnanediol.[182] It is also established that stimulation of the adrenals to produce increased amounts of steroid is accompanied by a concomitant decrease in the cholesterol content of the gland. Not only can adrenal tissue incorporate labeled acetate into cholesterol,[184] but, as Haines[185] has shown, the tissue can incorporate acetate into adrenocortical steroids. Subsequent work has shown that labeled cholesterol is converted by adrenal tissue into pregnenolone, a precursor of progesterone,[186] and to corticosterone and cortisol.[187] Additional evidence with adrenal perfusion techniques and adrenal homogenates has provided further proof that labeled cholesterol can serve as a good source of the adrenocortical steroids.[188] The first major reaction of cholesterol which has been identified in adrenal tissue involves cleavage of a 6-carbon fragment from the side-chain. Staple, Lynn *et al.*[189] have found that this reaction occurs in the water-soluble cytoplasmic fraction obtained from adrenal glands, testes and ovaries, but not in liver.

Δ^5-Pregnenolone is readily converted to progesterone by enzymes found in the microsomal fraction of adrenal tissue; the same reaction is known to occur in placenta and ovaries as well as in the testis.[190] Since progesterone serves as a precursor of 17-hydroxyprogesterone, cortisol and corticosterone[191] as well as testosterone,[192] the major pathways in the biosynthesis of the steroid hormones are now clear.

Once the 17α-hydroxy group has been introduced, the remaining 2-carbon side-chain can be cleaved to yield androstenedione.[192a] This product can be converted in the adrenals or the gonads to testosterone and to androsterone as well as its isomers. Undoubtedly the amount of androgens formed in those tissues is a reflection of competitive metabolic reactions. If, for example, 17-hydroxyprogesterone is converted rapidly to cortisol, or if progesterone is largely diverted to corticosterone (and perhaps aldosterone), less will be converted to androstenedione and the androgens. Conversely, the pathway may be shifted in the gonads in the direction of increased synthesis of the sex hormones. It is by now well established that human ovarian tissue slices can convert labeled testosterone to estradiol-17β.[193] Although there has been some evidence suggesting that acetate may be incorporated into steroid hormones without obligatory formation of cholesterol, the evidence is somewhat indirect and is complicated by the fact that good metabolic mixing of cholesterol may not have occurred. If one part of a cell (or tissue) contains cholesterol which is metabolically inert (or turns over slowly) because of its low solubility, it would be easy to conclude, on the basis of radioactivity studies, that cholesterol was not involved as an intermediate. At the moment, the known metabolic pathways which have been established for cholesterol are sufficient to support the belief that the adrenocortical steroids and sex hormones are largely derived from cholesterol. Many details regarding the biosynthesis of these physiologically important steroids have been painstakingly discovered. It is not proposed here to discuss such details extensively, but rather to refer those who are interested to the numerous review articles and monographs that are available. Although the clinician is also interested in the urinary excretory products derived from the adrenocortical and sex hormones, the variations in the excretion of the neutral 17-keto steroids as well as the α ketolic steroids and pregnanediol (from progesterone) have been adequately described elsewhere. It is sufficient here to recall that, in the normal person relatively small amounts of urinary steroids are excreted. If cholesterol is thought to be the major source of this important group of substances, it is clear that on a quantitative basis they represent very little drain on the body supplies of cholesterol. Only in abnormal states (for example adrenal and testicular tumors or hyperadrenocortical activity) would the effect upon

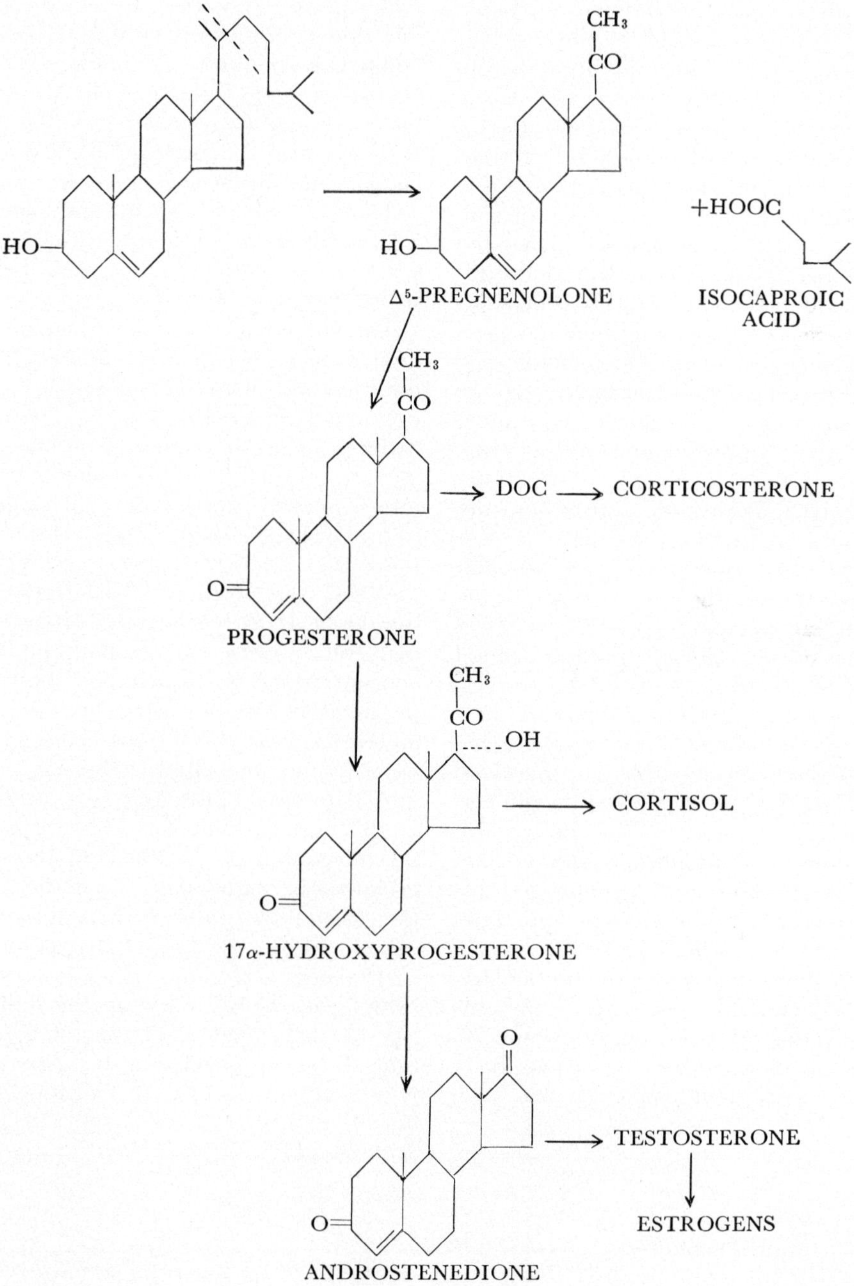

CH_3 CO HO— HO— +HOOC

Δ^5-PREGNENOLONE

ISOCAPROIC ACID

CH_3 CO

→ DOC → CORTICOSTERONE

O=

PROGESTERONE

CH_3 CO OH

→ CORTISOL

O=

17α-HYDROXYPROGESTERONE

O

→ TESTOSTERONE

↓

ESTROGENS

O=

ANDROSTENEDIONE

FIG. 13. Biosynthesis of steroid hormones.

the catabolism of cholesterol be expected to be quantitatively significant.

DYNAMIC ASPECTS OF LIPID METABOLISM

Experimental Techniques

Until the advent of isotopic techniques, knowledge concerning the rates of synthesis and breakdown of tissue components was difficult to obtain. This was particularly true in situations in which the quantity of certain tissue components remained constant. If, for example, the serum cholesterol concentration is maintained at a reasonably constant level, or if the cholesterol content of the liver remains unchanged over a period of time, it would be difficult to decide whether this represents an unreactive static condition or a dynamic steady state in which inflow just balances outflow. Obviously there is no problem when the organism is gaining weight, depositing fat or suffering from a wasting disease. In these situations, simple balance studies and a few observations are sufficient to make it clear that the total quantity of a particular component is either increasing or decreasing at an appreciable rate. At this juncture, a few relevant questions might be asked. Is an increased deposition ascribable to accelerated inflow or to a diminished outflow? Does a severe hypercholesteremia result from increased inflow of cholesterol (excessive dietary intake, accelerated endogenous synthesis) or from diminished outflow (inhibition of catabolism, diminished excretion)? These questions are sometimes difficult to answer.

With the aid of isotopes, particularly of hydrogen and carbon, it is possible to study the rates of deposition and replacement of molecules in various body compartments *while the organism is in a steady state* (caloric balance). If, for example, one wishes to study depot fat in a series of experimental animals that are not growing and not obviously depositing fat, it is possible to label the fat by administering a small dose of some isotopic precursor. For example, acetate labeled with C^{14} in one or both carbons might be employed. Since acetate can be converted into fatty acids, the depot lipids will in time become labeled; it should be remembered, however, that nonisotopic as well as isotopic fat is simultaneously being synthesized. If it is *assumed* that rapid mixing of labeled and unlabeled molecules occurs, discontinuance of the isotopic acetate will result in a continuous drop in the isotopic content of the depot fat as shown below in [A] below.

The following data may then be obtained in experimental animals: (1) total amount of fat by analysis, (2) isotope content of the fat, e.g., specific activity or isotope concentration. This may be observed at a number of time intervals (zero time, at time of maximal isotope concentration and at varying times thereafter).

When the isotope concentration of the depot lipids has dropped from maximal concentration to one half maximal concentration, it is assumed that approximately 50 per cent of the lipid molecules have been replaced by new nonisotopic molecules. The time required to accomplish this is referred to as the *biologic half-life*. The half-life of the fatty acids of the depot lipids is approximately eight days (for the rat); that of the liver fatty acids is about two days, and of the brain fatty acids 10 to 15 days.

Since in the steady state the half-life can be determined and the total quantity of fat involved can be estimated, it is relatively simple to calculate how

[A]

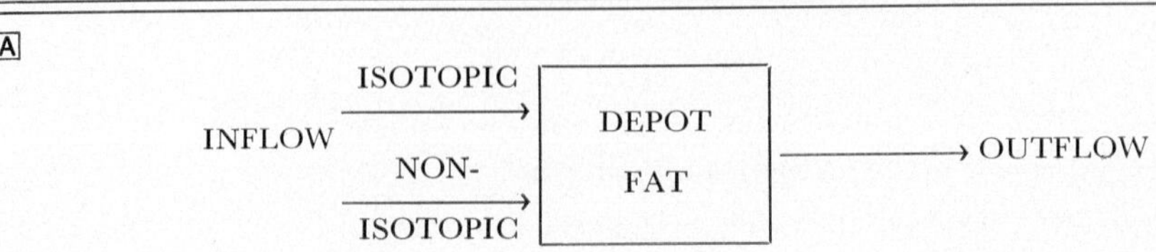

many grams have been replaced per day (turnover rate = grams synthesized and broken down per day). The percentage of the total replaced per day is the turnover rate constant.

Another technique involves giving a constant and uniform dose of isotopic material daily, followed by measurements of the rate at which the incorporation of isotope into the product or tissue component increases with time. In such cases, a curve such as that in Figure 14 is usually obtained.

The half-life may be thus determined, or the isotope may then be discontinued and the rate of fall in isotope concentration measured as in the previous illustration.

As a result of numerous experiments of this type, it has become quite clear that most tissue components are continuously being broken down and replaced by new molecules (turnover). The turnover varies considerably; cholesterol in brain is replaced very slowly (half-life > 100 days) while the turnover in intestine or liver may be very much more rapid. Such techniques have proved to be very helpful in developing our concepts concerning the dynamic state of many tissue components. It should be kept in mind, however, that such measurements are only approximations since (1) the subject may not be in the steady state, (2) there may not be rapid and complete mixing in the tissue being studied, and (3) the particular tissues under study may be equilibrating rapidly with some other compartment (liver cholesterol and blood cholesterol, or liver phospholipid and blood phospholipid). In spite of these difficulties, techniques of this sort have proved remarkably useful.

The term "turnover" is generally restricted to animals in the steady state (when the rate of entry of a substance equals the rate of exit). When these two rates are not equal and the total quantity under study increases or decreases, the term loses much of its meaning. Compare, for example, two animals in which the amount of depot lipid of one is twice as great as the other. Assuming that they are both in the steady state and that both are synthesizing and breaking down fat at the same rate, it is apparent that the fraction turned over per day will be twice as great in one as in the other. Such problems have been discussed by Zilversmit,[194] Solomon,[195] Comar,[196a] and Russell.[196b]

In the case of cholesterol, interesting results have been obtained with techniques of this sort. For example, if one follows the appearance of labeled cholesterol in the blood of humans who have received C^{14}-acetate,[197] the free cholesterol of plasma appears to be labeled before the cholesterol esters (2 to 4 hours for maximal radioactivity). This cholesterol equilibrates rapidly with erythrocyte cholesterol, the process having a half-time of 1 to 2 hours. It is only after several days that the plasma cholesterol esters reach the same level of radioactivity as the free cholesterol.[197b] The disappearance of labeled cholesterol from human plasma has been studied by Kurland *et al.*,[198] who found that the half-time for this process is 8 to 12 days. London and Rittenberg,[199]

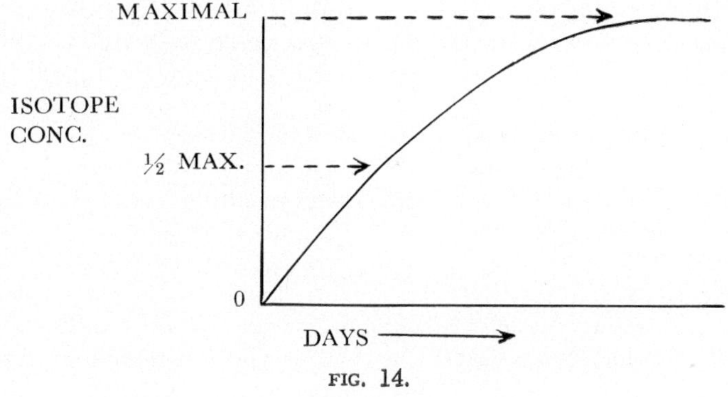

FIG. 14.

using deuterium-labeled water, previously reported a half-time of 8 days. Orally administered cholesterol-C^{14} appears more slowly in the plasma, the peak activity appearing 24 to 48 hours after administration (probably because of slow absorption). There seems to be very little doubt that the cholesterol which is absorbed from the intestine becomes indistinguishable from that which is synthesized by the liver. Free cholesterol from the liver equilibrates promptly with that of the plasma, which in turn equilibrates with the erythrocyte cholesterol; the transformation of free to esterified cholesterol appears to be a slower process.

The liver seems to be the main organ concerned with the regulation of both the total body content of cholesterol and the plasma cholesterol level. The total body content appears to depend upon a balance between the quantity formed endogenously plus that acquired from the diet on the one hand and the amount excreted and catabolized on the other. As the dietary intake of cholesterol increases (at least in some species), cholesterol biosynthesis in the liver decreases; this has been determined experimentally by Gould and Taylor,[200] Alfin-Slater *et al.*,[201] Tomkins *et al.*,[202] Langdon and Bloch[203] and Frantz *et al.*[204] Other tissues do not respond in the same way to high cholesterol diets. A diet high in fat does not have a similar homeostatic effect on liver cholesterogenesis.

As has previously been mentioned, the major catabolic products of cholesterol (75 per cent or more) appear to be the bile acids produced in the liver. The rate of formation of the bile acids appears to be regulated by the body content of bile salts and can be increased markedly by loss of such substances resulting, for example, from a bile fistula. The more efficient the reabsorption of bile salts, the slower their turnover and the slower the conversion of cholesterol to bile acids.

The manner in which the liver regulates serum cholesterol levels is not clear. Whenever it has been studied, it has always been found true that there is a very rapid interchange of free cholesterol molecules between liver and plasma. Surprisingly enough, the serum cholesterol levels do not always reflect the concentration of cholesterol in the liver; on the other hand, as cited above there is an inverse relationship between the rate of hepatic synthesis and liver cholesterol levels. A high cholesterol diet in experimental animals usually increases the liver cholesterol level first (particularly the esterified fraction), and eventually the plasma level. On the other hand, hypothyroidism frequently is associated with hypercholesteremia with very little change in liver content. In the rat, fat-free diets are reported by Alfin-Slater[129] to produce a decrease in plasma level but an increase in liver content. It may be guessed that the release of cholesterol into the blood by the liver is intimately concerned with the mechanism of hepatic synthesis and release of lipoprotein. If this is correct, then the turnover of phospholipids and the triglycerides in the liver must bear a significant relationship to the homeostatic regulation of blood cholesterol. In this connection, it is of some interest that a change in the plasma levels of any one of the three types of blood lipid (triglycerides, phospholipids and cholesterol) is usually associated with changes in the others. Deuel[205] has extensively reviewed those physiologic factors (age, sex, race, pregnancy, lactation) which have a bearing on blood lipid levels.

The manner in which adipose tissue is capable of releasing lipid into the blood is unknown; triglyceride appears to be the major component involved, although there is evidence[206] that it contains lipoprotein lipase and can release fatty acids into the blood. It is generally believed that in man fatty liver arises frequently from excessive mobilization of depot lipid. A transport lipemia usually resulting from such depot mobilization is frequently observed in some types of liver poisoning, starvation, high-fat low-carbohydrate diets, diabetes mellitus, hypothyroidism and certain other chronic infectious diseases. There is some support for the notion that regulation of this process of mobilization is under endocrine control, particularly by the anterior pituitary.

The production of fatty liver resulting from choline or methionine deficiency has been previously discussed in the section on phospholipids. This topic is adequately reviewed in numerous texts and monographs.

Effects of Abnormal States

Starvation. It has previously been pointed out that the biosynthesis of fatty acids is profoundly depressed in the fasting state and that lipogenesis is dependent upon effective utilization of glucose *via* glycolysis and the hexose monophosphate oxidative pathway. Decreased hepatic synthesis of cholesterol is also observed in fasted rats.[207] Since cholesterogenesis also requires reduced DPN and TPN, it is possible that similar considerations apply in the case of cholesterol synthesis. This point is not clear, as the following discussion indicates.

Diabetes Mellitus. In alloxan-diabetic rats or pancreatectomized cats, cholesterol synthesis (liver slices) occurs at a normal or accelerated rate.[208,209] This is in decided contrast to the diminished synthesis of fatty acids in the diabetic state. The reasons for this discrepancy are not clear. In both the fasting and diabetic state a transport lipemia delivers increased quantities of fat to the liver, which responds by accelerating the oxidation of fatty acids to acetyl CoA. In both cases one would therefore expect an accelerated rate of production of acetyl CoA and acetoacetyl CoA. Although the hypothesis explains the increased production of ketone bodies (deacylation of acetoacetyl CoA) in each instance, there is no obvious way to account for the differences in cholesterogenesis. One clue suggests itself as a result of some recent experiments by Lynen,[210] who has reported that the deacylation of acetoacetyl CoA to acetoacetate is not a direct hydrolysis but involves the intermediate formation of HMG CoA as represented in [A] below. The net result of this series of reactions is the removal of coenzyme A from acetoacetyl CoA. It will be remembered that the biosynthesis of fatty acids cannot proceed unless butyryl CoA is formed from acetoacetyl CoA, this reaction requires reduced TPN, which will be in short supply in both states. If, on the other hand, HMG CoA (or a closely related compound) is required for cholesterol synthesis, the accelerated production or turnover of HMG CoA should result in an increased or at least normal rate of synthesis of cholesterol provided that subsequent requirements for reduced TPN are satisfied. Why this is so in the diabetic but not in the fasting state is a problem for future investigation.

Thyroid. Although elevated serum cholesterol levels are frequently observed in the hypothyroid state, a number of investigators[211] have concluded that hepatic synthesis of cholesterol in thiouracil-treated or thyroidectomized animals is actually depressed. Conversely, hyperthyroidism results in accelerated hepatic cholesterogenesis.

Since many metabolic reactions are frequently retarded in the hypothyroid state, it is not surprising that this is also true of hepatic cholesterogenesis. The rise in serum cholesterol levels must therefore be ascribed to a defect in

---

[A]

$$CH_3COCH_2CO{-}SCoA + CH_3CO{-}SCoA \rightarrow CH_3{-}\underset{\displaystyle CH_2{-}COOH}{\overset{\displaystyle CH_2{-}CO{-}SCoA}{\underset{|}{\overset{|}{C}}}}{-}OH$$

(HMG CoA)

$$CH_3{-}\underset{\displaystyle CH_2{-}COOH}{\overset{\displaystyle CH_3{-}CO{-}SCoA}{\underset{|}{\overset{|}{C}}}}{-}OH \rightarrow CH_3COCH_2COOH + CH_3CO{-}SCoA$$

either the rate or manner of removal of this substance from the blood. Total carcass cholesterol appears, however, not to be significantly altered in experimentally induced hypothyroidism. The major change seems to be restricted primarily to the blood. Weiss and Marx[212] have reported that the rate of disappearance of labeled cholesterol from the blood is decreased in hypothyroid animals and increased in the hyperthyroid states. Friedman, Byers and co-workers,[213] as well as Thompson and Vars,[214] have studied extensively the biliary excretion of cholesterol and bile acids in the hypothyroid state. The results suggest that there is a diminished excretion of cholesterol and bile acids in hypothyroidism and that the rate of elimination by this route increases upon administration of thyroid hormones.

Gould[197b] has reported that, whereas normal humans can convert administered C^{14}-labeled acetate to blood cholesterol at a significant rate, severely myxedematous patients show a marked inability to perform the same process. Lipsky *et al.*[215] have obtained similar results. Therapy with thyroid hormone produced a rapid return to normal synthetic rates. Kurland and Lucas[216] have also observed a depressed rate of disappearance of injected C^{14}-cholesterol from the blood of patients with myxedema.

Adrenal. Serum cholesterol levels are significantly depressed in experimental stress or upon administration of ACTH to animals[183,217] or man.[218] The change is primarily in the cholesterol ester fraction. Whether this decrease in blood levels results from a rapid uptake by the adrenal glands which cannot be adequately compensated or whether the entire effect may be ascribed to the independent action of the adrenocortical steroids is not clear.

There is not complete agreement on the role of the adrenals upon fatty acid synthesis. In Houssay animals the administration of cortisone reduced lipogenesis;[208b] furthermore, Welt and Wilhelmi[219] have reported that administration of ACTH produces a similar inhibition of lipogenesis. Altman *et al.*,[220] however, claim that cortisone acts synergistically upon insulin when lipogenesis is studied in perfused livers. Perry and Bowen[221] have reported that hepatic synthesis of fatty acids is depressed in adrenalectomized animals; furthermore, these investigators report that hepatic synthesis of cholesterol is also reduced following adrenalectomy.

Pancreas and Pituitary. It has previously been indicated that efficient lipogenesis requires an adequate supply of reduced DPN and TPN. Wenner and Weinhouse[222] have demonstrated that the *in vitro* utilization of glucose by liver preparations is stimulated by DPN (increased glycolysis), whereas addition of TPN stimulates utilization of glucose by way of the hexose monophosphate pathway. Siperstein[107] has studied fatty acid and cholesterol synthesis in such preparations obtained from normal and "diabetic" animals. The addition of both cofactors was observed to stimulate fatty acid and cholesterol synthesis to a remarkable degree, particularly in the "diabetic" preparations. So far as fatty acid synthesis is concerned, there is no doubt that the increased utilization of glucose produced by insulin can accelerate lipogenesis. Stadie[223] has reviewed this field. Brady *et al.*[208b] have reported that pancreatectomy reduces lipogenesis (fatty acids) by the liver, whereas in the hypophysectomized animal the process appears to continue at an accelerated rate. Although the latter finding has been questioned by Baruch *et al.*,[224] the difference reported may possibly be due to a nutritional defect since such animals do not maintain weight well. The inhibiting effect of pancreatectomy upon lipogenesis can be abolished by subsequent hypophysectomy. This has been interpreted by Brady *et al.*[208] to mean that the pituitary possibly secretes a principle which blocks lipogenesis directly or indirectly through some other endocrine organ. Insulin appears to antagonize this inhibiting principle.

Although hypophysectomy appears to depress cholesterol synthesis,[224,225] it is claimed again that this may be ascribed to a nutritional effect, since increasing the glucose content of the diet from 25 to 60 per cent restored hepatic cholesterogenesis.[226]

Nephrosis. Hyperlipemia and hypercholesteremia are seen in human nephrosis as well as in experimental nephrosis. That these phenomena are intimately associated with the profound hypoalbuminemia seems abundantly clear from the reports of Heymann and Hackel[227] and of Rosenman *et al.*[228] London and co-workers[229] have concluded that the nephrotic patient does not exhibit an increased hepatic synthesis of cholesterol; furthermore, the increased blood cholesterol could not have been derived from dietary sources.[230] Rosenman and his co-workers[231] have stated that they believe the hypercholesteremia may be ascribed to a trapping of cholesterol in the plasma. Undoubtedly this involves a mobilization lipemia. Whether the hyperlipemic effect produced by a deficiency of serum albumin may be related to the binding capacity of albumin for free fatty acids is an open question at the present time.

Concluding Remarks

It is abundantly clear that much more investigation will be required before the complex processes involved in lipid physiology can be adequately described and explained. Not only is the regulation of blood lipids dependent upon a number of unknown forces which are involved in the release and uptake of blood lipids by the liver and other organs, but it is also important to recognize the very complex metabolic processes occurring within the organs and tissues themselves. This interplay represents a most complex pattern which will have to be laboriously untangled.

Turnover studies and radioisotope techniques, with all their limitations, are at least providing some information even though the measurements may not be very precise. Slowly, such techniques along with refinements in the methods of isolation and quantitative estimation are yielding information which should help the clinician. A better understanding of the clinical problems involving abnormalities of triglyceride, phospholipid, cholesterol and cerebroside metabolism will depend upon this painstaking research of the clinician, the biologist and the chemist.

References

GENERAL READING

Deuel, H. J., Jr.: The Lipids. 3 vols. New York, Interscience Publishers, 1957.

Hilditch, T. P.: The Chemical Constitution of Natural Fats. New York, John Wiley & Sons, 1956.

Lovern, J. A.: The Chemistry of Lipids of Biochemical Significance. London, Methuen & Co., 1955.

MONOGRAPHS AND SYMPOSIA

Page, I. H. (ed.): Chemistry of Lipides as Related to Atherosclerosis. Springfield, Illinois, Charles C Thomas, 1958.

Biochemical Problems of Lipids. London, Butterworths Publications Ltd., 1956.

Progress in the Chemistry of Fats and Other Lipids. London and New York, Pergamon Press, 1952–1955.

Najjar, V. A. (ed.): Fat Metabolism. Baltimore, The Johns Hopkins Press, 1954.

Cook, R. P.: Cholesterol. New York, Academic Press, 1958.

TEXT REFERENCES

1. Mattson, F. H. and Beck, L. W.: J. Biol. Chem., *214:*115, 1955.
2. Borgström, B.: Biochim. et biophys. acta, *13:*491, 1954.
3. Borgström, B.: Chemistry of Lipides as Related to Atherosclerosis, Symposium. Springfield, Illinois, Charles C Thomas, 1958, p. 137.
4. Borgström, B.: Acta physiol. scandinav., *25:*101, 111, 328, 1952.
5. Ahrens, E. H. and Borgström, B.: Biochemical Problems of Lipids. London, Butterworths Publications Ltd., 1956, p. 315.
6. Schönheyder, F. and Volqvartz, K.: Acta physiol. scandinav., *11:*349, 1946.
7. Borgström, B.: Biochemical Problems of Lipids. London, Butterworths Publications Ltd., 1956, p. 179.

8a. Frazer, A. C., Pover, W. F. R. and Sammons, H. G.: Biochemical Problems of Lipids. London, Butterworths Publications Ltd., 1953, p. 137.

b. Frazer, A. C., Pover, W. F. R., Sammons, H. G. and Schneider, R.: Biochemical Problems of Lipids. London, Butterworths Publications Ltd., 1956, p. 331.

9. Verzar, F. and McDougall, E. J.: Absorption from the Intestine. New York, Longmans, Green & Co., 1936.

10. Ross, C. A. C., Frazer, A. C., French, J. M., Gerrard, J. W., Sammons, H. G. and Smellie, J. M.: Lancet, *1:*1087, 1955.
11. Frazer, A. C.: Proc. III Europ. Congress Nat. Soc. Gastroent. 1953, p. 60.
12. Shapiro, A., Koster, H., Rittenberg, D. and Schoenheimer, R.: Am. J. Physiol., *117:*525, 1936.
13. Bergström, S. and Blomstrand, R.: Biochemical Problems of Lipids. London, Butterworths Publications Ltd., 1956, p. 323.
14. Frazer, A. C.: Biochemical Problems of Lipids. London, Butterworths Publications Ltd., 1956, p. 329.
15a.Reiser, R., Bryson, M. J., Carr, M. J. and Kuiken, K. A.: J. Biol. Chem., *194:*131, 1952.
b.Favarger, P., Collet, R. A. and Cherbuliez, E.: Helvet. chim. acta, *34:*1651, 1951.
c.Karnovsky, M. and Gidez, L. I.: Fed. Proc., *10:*205, 1951.
16. Verzar, F. and Laszt, L.: Biochem. Ztschr., *270:*24, 1934.
17. Gidez, L. I. and Karnovsky, M. L.: Biochemical Problems of Lipids. London, Butterworths Publications Ltd., 1956, p. 301.
18. Morehouse, M. G., Skipski, W. P., Searcy, R. L. and Spolter, L.: Biochemical Problems of Lipids. London, Butterworths Publications Ltd., 1956, p. 341.
19a.Zilversmit, D. B., Chaikoff, I. L. and Entenman, C.: J. Biol. Chem., *172:* 637, 1948.
b.Bollman, J. L., Flock, E. V., Cain, J. C. and Grindley, J. H.: Am. J. Physiol., *163:*41, 1950.
20. Borgström, B.: Acta physiol. scandinav., *25:*291, 1952.
21a.Bloom, B., Chaikoff, I. L., Reinhardt, W. O., Entenman, C. and Dauben, W. G.: J. Biol. Chem., *184;*1, 1950.
b.Bergström, S. *et al.:* Acta chem. scandinav., *4:*1142, 1950.
c.Reiser, R. and Bryson, M. J.: J. Biol. Chem., *189:*87, 1951.
d.Borgström, B.: Acta chem. scandinav., *5:*643, 1951.
22. Bloom, B., Chaikoff, I. L. and Reinhardt, W. O.: Am. J. Physiol., *166:*451, 1951.
23. Bergström, S., Blomstrand, R. and Borgström, B.: Biochem. J., *58:*600, 1954.
24. Bloom, B., Kiyasu, J. Y., Reinhardt, W. O. and Chaikoff, I. L.: Am. J. Physiol., *177:*84, 1954.
25. Blomstrand, R.: Acta physiol. scandinav., *34:*147, 1953; also Artom, C., and Swanson, M. A.: J. Biol. Chem., *175:* 871, 1948.
26. Baer, E., Bucknea, D. and Newcombe, A. G.: J. Am. Chem. Soc., *78:*232, 1956.
27a.Baer, E. and Kates, M.: J. Biol. Chem., *185:*615, 1950.
b.Long, C. and Maguire, M. F.: Biochem. J., *54:*612, 1953; *57:*223, 1954.
28a.Hanahan, D. J.: J. Biol. Chem., *207:*879, 1954.
b.Hanahan, D. J.: Biochemical Problems of Lipids. London, Butterworths Publications Ltd., 1956, p. 274.
29. Long, C. and Penny, I. F.: Biochem. J., *58:*15, 1954.
30. Favarger, P. and Metzger, E. F.: Helvet. chim. acta, *35:*1811, 1952.
31. Glover, J. and Green, C.: Biochemical Problems of Lipids. London, Butterworths Publications Ltd., 1956, p. 359.
32. Siperstein, M. D., Chaikoff, I. L. and Reinhardt, W. O.: J. Biol. Chem., *198:* 111, 1952.
33a.Popjak, G.: Biochem. J., *40:*608, 1946.
b.Bollman, J. L. and Flock, E. V.: Am. J. Physiol., *164:*480, 1951.
c.Pihl, A.: Acta physiol. scandinav., *34:* 183, 1955.
34. Pihl, A.: Acta physiol. scandinav. *34:* 197, 1955.
35. Swell, L., Flick, D. F., Field, H., Jr. and Treadwell, C. R.: Am. J. Physiol., *180:* 124, 1955.
36. Biggs, M. W. *et al.*: Circulation, *6:*359, 1952.
37a.Swell, L., Byron, J. E. and Treadwell, C. R.: J. Biol. Chem., *186:*543, 1950.
b.Swell, L., Boiter, T. A., Field, H., Jr. and Treadwell, C. R.: Am. J. Physiol., *181:* 193, 1955.
38. Gould, R. G., Lotz, L. V. and Lilly, E. M.: Biochemical Problems of Lipids. London, Butterworths Publications Ltd., 1956, p. 353.
39. Hanahan, D. J. and Al-Wakil, S. J.: Arch. Biochem., *44:*150, 1953.
40. Hernandez, H. H., Chaikoff, I. L., Dauben, W. G. and Abraham, S.: J. Biol. Chem., *206:*757, 1954.
41. Peterson, D. W.: Proc. Soc. Exper. Biol. & Med., *78:*143, 1954.
42. Siperstein, M. D., Nichols, C. W. and Chaikoff, I. L.: Circulation, *7:*37, 1953.
43a.Pollak, O. J.: Circulation, *7:*702, 1953.
b.Joyner, C., Jr. and Kuo, P. T.: Am. J. M. Sc., *230:*636, 1955.
c.Farquhar, J. W., Smith, R. E. and Dempsey, M. E.: Circulation, *14:*77, 1956.
d.Best, M. M. and Duncan, C. H.: Circulation, *14:*334, 1956.
44a.Barber, J. M. and Grant, A. P.: Brit. Heart J., *17:*296, 1955.
b.Best, M. M., Duncan, C. H., Wathen, J. D., Van Loon, E. J. and Shipley, R. E.: Circulation, *10:*590, 1954.
45a.Friedman, M., Homer, R. and Byers, S. O.: Circulation, *12:*709, 1955.
b.Steiner, A. and Riley, F. P.: Circulation, *12:*483, 1955.

c. Wilkinson, C. F., Jr., Boyle, E., Jackson, R. S. and Benjamin, M. R.: Circulation, *4:*302, 1955.
46. Rosenman, R. H., Byers, S. O. and Friedman, M.: Circulation Res., *2:*45, 1954.
47. Nichols, C. W., Lindsay, S. and Chaikoff, I. L.: Proc. Soc. Exper. Biol. & Med., *89:*609, 1955.
48. Fredrickson, D. S., McCollester, D. L., Havel, R. J. and Ono, K.: In Page, I. H. (ed.): Chemistry of Lipides Related to Atherosclerosis, Springfield, Illinois, Charles C Thomas, 1958, p. 205.
49a. Friedman, M., Byers, S. O. and St. George, S.: Am. J. Physiol., *184:*141, 1956.
b. Friedman, M., Byers, S. O. and Roseman, R. H.: Am. J. Physiol., *177:*77, 1954.
50. Morris, B.: Quoted by Fredrickson, ref. 48.
51. French, J. E., Morris, B. and Robinson, D. S.: Quoted by Fredrickson, ref. 48.
52. McCandless, E. L. and Zilversmit, D. B.: Fed. Proc., *16:*85, 1957.
53. Bragdon, J. H.: Quoted by Fredrickson, ref. 48.
54. Marsh, J. B.: Fed. Proc., *17:*270, 1958.
55. Oncley, J. L.: In Page, I. H. (ed.): Chemistry of Lipides as Related to Atherosclerosis. Springfield, Illinois, Charles C Thomas, 1958, p. 114.
56. Gitlin, D.: Quoted by Oncley, ref. 55.
57a. Shore, B. and Shore, V. G.: Plasma, *2:* 621, 1954.
b. Shore, B.: Biochem. et biophys. acta, in press.
58. Avigan, J., Redfield, R. and Steinberg, D.: Biochim. et biophys. acta, *20:*557, 1956.
59. Gitlin, D., Cornwell, D. G., Nakasato, D., Oncley, J. L., Hughes, W. L. and Janeway, C. A.: J. Clin. Invest., *37:*172, 1958.
60. Shore, B., Nichols, A. V. and Freeman, N. K.: Proc. Soc. Exper. Biol. & Med., *83:*216, 1953.
61. Korn, E. D.: In Page, I. H. (ed.): Chemistry of Lipides Related to Atherosclerosis. Springfield, Illinois, Charles C Thomas, 1958, p. 169.
62. Havel, R. and Fredrickson, D. S.: J. Clin. Invest., *35:*1025, 1956.
63. Kendall, F. E.: J. Biol. Chem., *138:*97, 1941.
64. Dole, V. P.: J. Clin. Invest., *35:*150, 1956.
65. Gordon, R. S., Jr. and Cherkes, A.: J. Clin. Invest., *35:*206, 1956.
66. Goodman, D. S.: In Page, I. H. (ed.): Chemistry of Lipides as Related to Atherosclerosis. Springfield, Illinois, Charles C Thomas, 1958, p. 199; also Gordon, R. S.: quoted by Dole in same reference.
67. Fredrickson, D. S. and Gordon, R. J.: Quoted by Fredrickson, ref. 48.
68. Dole, V. P.: In Page, I. H. (ed.): Chemistry of Lipides as Related to Atherosclerosis. Springfield, Illinois, Charles C Thomas, 1958, p. 189.
69. Lindgren, F. T.: In Page, I. H. (ed.): Chemistry of Lipides as Related to Atherosclerosis. Springfield, Illinois, Charles C Thomas, 1958, p. 203.
70. James, A. T.: In Page, I. H. (ed.): Chemistry of Lipides as Related to Atherosclerosis. Springfield, Illinois, Charles C Thomas, 1958, p. 19.
71a. Barr, D. P., Russ, E. M. and Eder, H. A.: Tr. A. Am. Physicians, *65:*102, 1952.
b. Barr, D. P., Russ, E. M. and Eder, H. A.: Blood Cells and Plasma Proteins. New York, Academic Press, Inc., 1953, p. 332.
72. Byers, S. O., Friedman, M. and Gunning, B.: Am. J. Physiol., *175:*375, 1953.
73. Gould, R. G.: Am. J. Med., *11:*209, 1951.
74. Harper, P. V., Neal, W. B. and Hlavacek, G. R.: Metabolism, *2:*69, 1953.
75. Eckles, N. E., Taylor, C. B., Campbell, D. J. and Gould, R. G.: J. Lab. & Clin. Med., *46:*359, 1955.
76. Fishler, M. C., Entenman, C., Montgomery, M. L. and Chaikoff, I. L.: J. Biol. Chem., *150:*47, 1943.
77. Goldman, D. S., Chaikoff, I. L., Reinhardt, W. O., Entenman, C. and Dauben, W. G.: J. Biol. Chem., *184:*727, 1950.
78. Miller, L. L., Bly, C. G., Watson, M. L. and Bale, W. F.: J. Exper. Med., *94:* 431, 1951.
79. Lynen, F.: Ann. Rev. Biochem., *24:*653, 1955.
80. Lehninger, A. L.: In Page, I. H. (ed.): Chemistry of Lipides as Related to Atherosclerosis. Springfield, Illinois, Charles C Thomas, 1958, p. 265.
81. Krebs, H. A. and Johnson, W. A.: Enzymologia, *4:*148, 1937.
82a. Kaplan, N. O. and Lipmann, F.: J. Biol. Chem., *174:*37, 1948.
b. Stern, J. R., Shapiro, B. and Ochoa, S.: Nature, *166:*403, 1950.
83. Stern, J. R., Coon, M. J. and Del Campillo, A.: Nature, *171:*28, 1953.
84. Stadie, W. C.: Physiol. Rev., *25:*395, 1945.
85. Kennedy, E. P. and Lehninger, A. L.: J. Biol. Chem., *172:*487, 1948; *179:*957, 1949.
86. Schneider, W. C.: J. Biol. Chem., *176:* 259, 1948.
87. Langdon, R. G.: In Page, I. H. (ed.): Chemistry of Lipides as Related to Atherosclerosis. Springfield, Illinois, Charles C Thomas, 1958, p. 291.
88. Schoenheimer, R.: The Dynamic State of Body Constituents. Cambridge, Harvard University Press, 1942.

89. Rittenberg, D. and Bloch, K.: J. Biol. Chem., *160:*417, 1945.
90. Bloch, K.: Cold Spring Harbor Symp. Quant. Biol., *13:*29, 1948.
91. Brady, R. O. and Gurin, S.: J. Biol. Chem., *186:*461, 1950.
92a. Gurin, S.: In Najjar, V. A. (ed.): Fat Metabolism. Baltimore, Johns Hopkins Press, 1954, p. 138.
b. Brady, R. O. and Gurin, S.: J. Biol. Chem., *199:*421, 1952.
c. Dituri, F. and Gurin, S.: Arch. Biochem., *43:*231, 1953.
93. Chernick, S. S., Chaikoff, I. L., Masoro, E. J. and Iseaf, E.: J. Biol. Chem., *186:*527, 1950.
94a. Deuel, H. J., Jr.: The Lipids. New York, Interscience Publishers, 1957, vol. 3, p. 9.
b. Brady, R. O., Mamoon, A. and Stadtman, E. R.: J. Biol. Chem., *222:*795, 1956.
95. Drury, D. R.: Am. J. Physiol., *131:*536, 1940–41.
96a. Stetten, D., Jr. and Boxer, G. E.: J. Biol. Chem., *156:*271, 1944.
b. Stetten, D., Jr. and Klein, B. V.: J. Biol. Chem., *159:*593, 1946; *162:*377, 1946.
97. Brady, R. O. and Gurin, S.: J. Biol. Chem., *187:*589, 1950.
98. Shaw, W. and Gurin, S.: Arch. Biochem., *47:*220, 1953.
99. Masoro, E. J., Chaikoff, I. L., Chernick, S. S. and Felts, J. M.: J. Biol. Chem., *185:*845, 1950.
100. Baker, N., Chaikoff, I. L. and Schusdek, A.: J. Biol. Chem., *194:*435, 1952.
101a. Chernick, S. S. and Chaikoff, I. L.: J. Biol. Chem., *188:*389, 1951.
b. Chernick, S. S., Chaikoff, I. L. and Abraham, S.: J. Biol. Chem., *193:*793, 1951.
102. Shaw, W. N., Dituri, F. and Gurin, S.: J. Biol. Chem., *226:*417, 1957.
103a. Dituri, F., Shaw, W. N., Warms, J. V. B. and Gurin, S.: J. Biol. Chem., *226:* 407, 1957.
b. Tietz, A.: Biochim. et biophys. acta, *25:*303, 1957.
c. Langdon, R. G.: J. Biol. Chem., *226:* 615, 1957.
104. Glock, G. E. and McLean, P.: Biochem. J., *61:*390, 1955.
105. Ashmore, J., Hastings, A. B. and Nesbett, F. B.: Proc. Nat. Acad. Sc., *40:*673, 1954.
106. Langdon, R. G. and Weakley, D. R.: J. Biol. Chem., *214:*167, 1955.
107. Siperstein, M. D. and Fagan, V. M.: Science, *126:*1012, 1957.
108. Kornberg, A. and Pricer, W. E.: J. Biol. Chem., *204:*345, 1953.
109. Kennedy, E. P.: J. Biol. Chem., *201:*399, 1953.
110. Weiss, S. B., Smith, S. W. and Kennedy, E. P.: Nature, *178:*594, 1956.
111. Weiss, S. B. and Kennedy, E. P.: J. Am. Chem. Soc., *78:*3550, 1956.
112. Tietz, A. and Shapiro, E. P.: Biochim. et biophys. acta, *19:*374, 1956.
113. Stein, Y. and Shapiro, B.: Biochim. et biophys. acta, *24:*197, 1957.
114. Wittenberg, J. and Kornberg, A.: J. Biol. Chem., *202:*431, 1953.
115. Kennedy, E. P. and Weiss, S. B.: J. Biol. Chem., *222:*193, 1956.
116. Sribney, M. and Kennedy, E. P.: Fed. Proc., *16:*253, 1957.
117. Kennedy, E. P.: In Page, I. H. (ed.): Chemistry of Lipides as Related to Atherosclerosis. Springfield, Illinois, Charles C Thomas, 1958, p. 325.
118. Hodge, H. C., McLachlan, P. L., Bloor, W. R., Welsh, E., Kornberg, S. L. and Falkenheim, M.: Proc. Soc. Exper. Biol. & Med., *68:*332, 1948.
119. Fishler, M. C.: Physiol. Rev., *22:*302, 1942.
120. Dawson, R. M.: Biochem. J., *59:*5, 1955.
121. Dawson, R. M.: In Biochemical Problems of Lipids. London, Butterworths Publications Ltd., 1956, p. 280.
122. Stetten, D., Jr. and Schoenheimer, R.: J. Biol. Chem., *133:*329, 1940.
123. Burr, G. O. and Burr, M. M.: J. Biol. Chem., *82:*345, 1929.
124. Bernhard, K. and Schoenheimer, R.: J. Biol. Chem., *133:*707, 1940.
125a. Rieckehoff, I. G., Holman, R. T. and Burr, G. O.: Arch. Biochem., *20:*331, 1949.
b. Witten, P. W. and Holman, R. T.: Arch. Biochem., *37:*90, 1952.
126. Mead, J. F., Steinberg, G. and Howton, D. R.: J. Biol. Chem., *205:*683, 1953.
127. Steinberg, G., Slayton, W. H., Howton, D. R. and Mead, J. F.: Fed. Proc., *14:*286, 1955.
128. Holman, R. T.: In Biochemical Problems of Lipids. London, Butterworths Publications Ltd., 1956, p. 463.
129. Alfin-Slater, R. B., Aftergood, L., Wells, G. F. and Deuel, H. J.: Arch. Biochem., *52:*180, 1954.
130. Kinsell, L. W., Partridge, J., Boling, L., Margen, S. and Michaels, G. D.: J. Clin. Endocrinol., *12:*909, 1952.
131. Hardinge, M. G. and Stare, F. J.: J. Clin. Nutrition, *2:*83, 1954.
132. Groen, J., Tjiong, B. K., Kamminga, C. E. and Willebrands, A. F.: Voeding, *13:*556, 1952.
133. Ahrens, E. H., Hirsch, J., Insull, W., Jr. and Peterson, M. L.: In Page, I. H. (ed.): Chemistry of Lipides as Related to Atherosclerosis. Springfield, Illinois, Charles C Thomas, 1958, p. 222.
134. Keys, A.: Science, *112:*79, 1950.
135. Gardner, J. A. and Gainsborough, H.: Biochem. J., *22:*1048, 1928.
136. Bloch, K.: Harvey Lect., *48:*68, 1954.

137. Cornforth, J. W. and Gore, I. Y.: Biochem. J., *65*:94, 1957.
138a.Brady, R. O. and Gurin, S.: J. Biol. Chem. *189*:371, 1951.
b.Curran, G. L.: J. Biol. Chem., *191*:775, 1951.
139a.Rabinowitz, J. L. and Gurin, S.: J. Biol. Chem., *208*:307, 1954.
b.Rudney, H.: J. Am. Chem. Soc., *76*: 2595, 1954.
140a.Rudney, H.: Fed. Proc., *15*:342, 1956.
b.Ferguson, J. J. and Rudney, H.: Fed. Proc., *16*:179, 1957.
141. Ferguson, J. J., Durr, I. F. and Rudney, H.: Fed. Proc., *17*:219, 1958.
142. Tavormina, P. A., Gibbs, M. H. and Huff, J. W.: J. Am. Chem. Soc., *98*: 4498, 1956.
143a.Langdon, R. G. and Bloch, K.: J. Am. Chem. Soc., *74*:1869, 1952.
b.Langdon, R. G. and Bloch, K.: J. Biol. Chem., *200*:129, 135, 179, 1953.
144. Dituri, F., Rabinowitz, J. L., Hullin, R. P. and Gurin, S.: J. Biol. Chem., *229*:825, 1957.
145. Phillips, A. H., Tchen, T. T. and Bloch, K.: Fed. Proc., *17*:289, 1958.
146. Channon, H. J. and Marrian, G. F.: Biochem. J., *20*:409, 1926.
147. Thannhauser, S. J. and Fromm, F.: Ztschr. f. physiol. Chem., *187*:173, 1930.
148. Channon, H. J.: Biochem. J., *20*:400, 1926.
149. Heilbron, I. M., Kamm, E. D. and Owens, W. M.: J. Chem. Soc., p. 1630, 1926.
150. Robinson, R.: J. Soc. Chem. Ind., *53*: 1062, 1934.
151. Woodward, R. B. and Bloch, K.: J. Am. Chem. Soc., *75*:2023, 1953.
152. Tchen, T. T. and Bloch, K.: J. Am. Chem. Soc., *77*:6085, 1955.
153. Sperry, W. M.: J. Biol. Chem., *114*:125, 1936.
154. Cohen, P. P.: In Page, I. H. (ed.): Chemistry of Lipides as Related to Atherosclerosis. Springfield, Illinois, Charles C Thomas, 1958, p. 95.
155. Chargaff, E.: Advances in Protein Chemistry. Vol. I. New York, Academic Press, Inc., 1944.
156. Lovern, J. A.: The Chemistry of Lipids of Biochemical Significance. London, Methuen and Co., 1955.
157. Lough, A. K., Garton, G. A. and Duncan, W. R. H.: Biochem. J., *65*:31, 1957.
158. Clement, G., Clement, J. and Louedec, A.: Arch. Sc. physiol., *8*:233, 1954.
159. Kinsell, L. W., Michaels, G. D., Dailey, J. P., Splitter, S. and Talpers, S. J.: Proc. Soc. Exper. Biol. & Med., in press.
160a.Klein, W.: Ztschr. f. physiol. Chem., *259*: 268, 1939.
b.Le Breton, E. and Pantaleon, J.: Arch. sc. physiol., *1*:63, 1947.
c.Yamamato, R. S., Goldstein, N. P. and Treadwell, C. R.: J. Biol. Chem., *180*: 615, 1949.
d.Swell, L., Byron, J. E. and Treadwell, C. R.: J. Biol. Chem., *186*:543, 1950; Swell, L. and Treadwell, C. R.: J. Biol. Chem., *212*:141, 1955.
e.Korzenovsky, M., Vesely, B. M. and Diller, E. R.: Fed. Proc., *15*:292, 1956.
161. Chaikoff, I. L. *et al.*: J. Biol. Chem., *194*: 413, 1952.
162. Siperstein, M. D. and Chaikoff, I. L.: Fed. Proc., *14*:767, 1955.
163. Bergström, S.: Kgl. fisiograph. sallskap. Lund, *22*: No. 16, p. 1, 1952.
164. Siperstein, M. D. and Murray, A. W.: J. Clin. Invest., *34*:1449, 1955.
165. Deuel, H.: The Lipids. New York, Interscience Publishers, 1955, vol. 2, p. 111.
166. Bergström, S. and Borgström, B.: Ann. Rev. Biochem., *25*:177, 1956.
167. Linstedt, S.: Acta chem. scandinav., *10*: 1051, 1956.
168a.Gustafsson, B. C., Bergström, S., Linstedt, S. and Norman, A.: Proc. Soc. Exper. Biol. & Med., *94*:467, 1957.
b.Cook, R. P., Edwards, D. C. and Riddell, C.: Biochem. J., *62*:225, 1956.
c.Edwards, D. C. and Cook, R. P.: Biochem. J., *61*:671, 1955.
169. Zabin, I. and Barker, W. F.: J. Biol. Chem., *205*:633, 1953.
170a.Staple, E. and Gurin, S.: Biochim. et biophys. acta, *15*:372, 1954.
b.Lynn, W. S., Jr., Staple, E. and Gurin, S.: Fed. Proc., *14*:783, 1955.
171a.Bergström, S., Paabo, K. and Rumpf, J. A.: Acta chem. scandinav., *8*:1109, 1954.
b.Bergström, S. and Linstedt, S.: Biochem. et biophys. acta, *19*:556, 1956.
172a.Anfinsen, C. B. and Horning, M. C.: J. Am. Chem. Soc., *75*:1511, 1953.
b.Fredrickson, D. S. and Ono, K.: Biochem. et biophys. acta, *22*:183, 1956.
173. Linstedt, S.: Ark. kemi., *11*:145, 1957.
174. Bergström, S. and Gloor, U.: Acta chem. scandinav., *8*:1373, 1954; *9*:1545, 1955.
175a.Bremer, J.: Acta chem. scandinav., *10*: 56, 1956; Biochem. J., *63*:507, 1956.
b.Elliott, W. H.: Biochem. J., *62*:427, 433, 1956.
c.Siperstein, M. D. and Murray, A. W.: Science, *123*:377, 1956.
176. Byers, S. O. and Biggs, M. W.: Arch. Biochem., *39*:301, 1952.
177. Rosenfeld, R. S., Fukushima, D. K., Hellman, L. and Gallagher, T. F.: J. Biol. Chem., *211*:301, 1954.
178. Robertson, D. M.: Biochem. J., *61*:681, 1955.
179. Gardner, J. A., Gainsborough, H. and Murray, R. M.: Biochem. J., *29*:1139, 1935.

180. Rosenheim, O. and Webster, T. A.: Biochem. J., *37*:580, 1943.
181a.Schoenheimer, R., Rittenberg, D. and Graff, M.: J. Biol. Chem., *111*:183, 1935.
b.Anchel, M. and Schoenheimer, R.: J. Biol. Chem., *125*:28, 1938.
182. Bloch, K.: J. Biol. Chem., *157*:661, 1945.
183. Sayers, G.: Physiol. Rev., *30*:241, 1950.
184. Srere, P. A., Chaikoff, I. L., Treitman, S. S. and Burstein, L. S.: J. Biol. Chem., *182*:629, 1950.
185. Haines, W. I.: In Recent Progress in Hormone Research. New York, Academic Press, Inc., 1952, vol. 7, p. 255.
186. Saba, N., Hechter, O. and Stone, D.: J. Am. Chem. Soc., *76*:3682, 1954; Arch. Biochem., *58*:249, 1955.
187. Zafferoni, A., Hechter, O. and Pincus, G.: Fed. Proc., *10*:150, 1951; J. Am. Chem. Soc., *73*:1300, 1951.
188. Hechter, O. and Pincus, G.: Physiol. Rev., *34*:459, 1954.
189. Staple, E., Lynn, W. S., Jr. and Gurin, S.: J. Biol. Chem., *219*:845, 1956.
190. Dorfman, R. L.: Ann. Rev. Biochem., *26*:523, 1957.
191. Levy, H., Jeanloz, R. W., Jacobsen, R. P., Hechter, O., Schenker, V. and Pincus, G.: J. Biol. Chem., *211*:867, 1954.
192a.Lynn, W. S., Jr. and Brown, R.: Biochem. et biophys. acta, *21*:403, 1956.
b.Slaunwhite, W. R., Jr. and Samuels, L. T.: J. Biol. Chem., *220*:341, 1956.
c.Brady, R. O.: J. Biol. Chem., *193*:145, 1951.
d.Wotiz, H. H.: J. Biol. Chem., *216*:677, 1955.
193. Baggett, B., Engel, L. L., Savard, K. and Dorfman, R. I.: J. Biol. Chem., *221*: 931, 1956.
194. Zilversmit, D. B.: Nature, *175*:863, 1955.
195. Solomon, A. K.: J. Clin. Invest., *28*:1297, 1949.
196a.Comar, C. L.: Radioisotopes in Biology and Agriculture. New York, McGraw-Hill Book Co., 1955.
b.Russell, J.: Persp. in Biol. & Med., *1*:138, 1958.
197a.Hellman, L., Rosenfeld, R. S. and Gallagher, T. F.: J. Clin. Invest., *33*:142, 1954.
b.Gould, R. G., Le Roy, G. V., Okita, G. T., Kabara, J. J., Keegan, P. and Bergenstal, D. M.: J. Lab. & Clin. Med., *46*:374, 1955.
198. Kurland, G. S., Lucas, J. L. and Freedburg, A. S.: J. Clin. Invest., *33*:950, 1954.
199. London, I. M. and Rittenberg, D.: J. Biol. Chem., *184*:687, 1950.
200a.Gould, R. G. and Taylor, C. B.: Fed. Proc., *9*:179, 1950.
b.Taylor, C. B. and Gould, R. G.: Circulation, *2*:467, 1950.
201. Alfin-Slater, R. B., Schotz, M. C., Shimoda, F. and Deuel, H. J.: J. Biol. Chem., *195*:311, 1952.
202. Tomkins, G. M., Sheppard, H. and Chaikoff, I. L.: J. Biol. Chem., *201*: 137, 1953; *203*:781, 1953.
203. Langdon, R. G. and Bloch, K.: J. Biol. Chem., *202*:77, 1953.
204. Frantz, I. D., Schneider, H. S. and Hinkelman, B. T.: J. Biol. Chem., *206*:465, 1954.
205. Deuel, H. J.: The Lipids. New York, Interscience Publishers, 1955, Vol. 2.
206. Korn, E. D. and Quigley, T. W.: Biochim. et biophys. acta, *18*:143, 1955; J. Biol. Chem., *226*:833, 1957.
207. Tomkins, G. M. and Chaikoff, I. L.: J. Biol. Chem., *196*:569, 1952.
208a.Brady, R. O. and Gurin, S.: J. Biol. Chem., *187*:589, 1950.
b.Brady, R. O., Lukens, F. D. W. and Gurin, S.: J. Biol. Chem., *193*:683, 1951.
209. Hotta, S. and Chaikoff, I. L.: J. Biol. Chem., *198*:895, 1952.
210. Lynen, F.: Unpublished.
211a.Karp, A. and Stetten, D., Jr.: J. Biol. Chem., *179*:819, 1949.
b.Byers, S. O., Rosenman, R. H., Friedman, M. and Biggs, M. W.: J. Exper. Med., *96*:513, 1952.
c.Marx, W., Gustin, S. T. and Levi, C.: Proc. Soc. Exper. Biol. & Med., *83*:143, 1953.
212. Weiss, S. B. and Marx, W.: J. Biol. Chem., *213*:349, 1955.
213a.Byers, S. O. and Friedman, M.: Am. J. Physiol., *168*:297, 1952.
b.Rosenman, R. H., Friedman, M. and Byers, S. O.: Circulation, *5*:589, 1952; J. Clin. Endocrin., *12*:1287, 1952.
214. Thompson, J. C. and Vars, H. M.: Proc. Soc. Exper. Biol. & Med., *83*:246, 1953.
215. Lipsky, S. R., Bondy, P. K., Man, E. B. and McGuire, J. S.: J. Clin. Invest., *34*:950, 1955.
216. Kurland, G. S. and Lucas, J. L.: J. Clin. Invest., *34*:947, 1955.
217. Mann, G. V. and White, H. S.: Metabolism, *2*:47, 1953.
218. Conn, J. W., Vogel, W. C., Louis, L. H. and Fajans, S. S.: J. Lab. & Clin. Med., *35*:504, 1950.
219. Welt, I. D. and Wilhelmi, A. E.: Yale J. Biol. & Med., *23*:99, 1950.
220. Altman, K. I., Miller, L. L. and Bly, C. C.: Arch. Biochem., *31*:329, 1951.
221. Perry, W. F. and Bowen, H. F.: Am. J. Physiol., *184*:59, 1956.
222. Wenner, C. E., Dunn, D. F. and Weinhouse, S.: J. Biol. Chem., *205*:409, 1953.
223. Stadie, W. C.: Diabetes, *5*:263, 1956.
224. Baruch, H. and Chaikoff, I. L.: Endocrinology, *56*:609, 1955.

225. Tomkins, G. M., Chaikoff, I. L. and Bennett, L. L.: J. Biol. Chem., *199*:543, 1952.
226. Hill, R., Bauman, J. W. and Chaikoff, I. L.: Endocrinology, *57*:316, 1955.
227. Heymann, W. and Hackel, D. B.: Proc. Soc. Exper. Biol. & Med., *89*:329, 1955.
228. Rosenman, R. H., Friedman, M. and Byers, S. O.: J. Clin. Invest., *35*:522, 1956.
229. London, I. M., Sabella, G. F. and Yamasaki, M. M.: J. Clin. Invest., *30*:657, 1951.
230. Friedman, M., Rosenman, R. H. and Byers, S. O.: J. Clin. Invest., *33*:1103, 1954.
231. Rosenman, R. H., Friedman, M. and Byers, S. O.: J. Clin. Invest., *34*:700, 1955.

CHAPTER 4

By ABRAHAM CANTAROW, M.D.

Mineral Metabolism

CALCIUM AND PHOSPHORUS METABOLISM

Functions

CALCIUM

Although over 99 per cent of the body Ca and 80 to 85 per cent of its P are in the bones (p. 200), important functions of these elements are exerted in directions other than preservation of skeletal structure. Ca ions (1) decrease capillary and cell membrane permeability, (2) decrease neuromuscular excitability, and are necessary for (3) muscle contraction, (4) normal transmission of nerve impulses, and (5) blood coagulation. Ca ions also activate certain enzymes, including lipase, succinic dehydrogenase, adenosine triphosphatase, and some proteases.

Coagulation of Blood. Calcium is necessary for normal coagulation of blood (and milk), although it may be replaced in this capacity, but less efficiently, by strontium, barium and magnesium. It appears likely that ionized calcium is essential for the formation of thrombin from its inactive precursors in the blood and tissues and that this process depends upon the formation of an intermediary colloidal complex containing prothrombin, cephalin and calcium.

Neuromuscular Irritability. Ionic concentrations exert an important if not a controlling influence upon neuromuscular irritability, which is enhanced by an increase in Na or K ions and diminished by an increase in Ca, Mg and H ions. This relationship may be expressed as follows:

$$\text{Irritability} \propto \frac{[Na^+] + [K^+]}{[Ca^{++}] + [Mg^{++}] + [H^+]}.$$

The exact site of action of these factors in this connection is not known (nerve cell, muscle cell, or myoneural junction) but it is probably within the nervous mechanism or at the myoneural junction.

The inhibitory influence of calcium is not limited to skeletal muscle and the voluntary nervous system but extends also to unstriated muscle and autonomic nerves. Its importance in the production of normal cardiac contractions and rhythmicity has long been recognized. The *effect of calcium on the heart* resembles that of sympathetic stimulation, although studies suggest that it acts upon (a) the contractile elements, (b) the idioventricular centers, (c) the conduction system, (d) the cardiac nerves and (e) the coronary arteries. The chief effects of an excess of calcium are the development of more forceful contractions, the degree of diastolic relaxation diminishing progressively until the heart stops beating in a state of tonic contraction or systolic standstill (*calcium rigor*). Withdrawal of calcium results in diastolic standstill. Studies of the relationship between the various cations and the autonomic nervous system suggest that, in general, as in the case of the heart, the effect of calcium resembles that of sympathetic stimulation, in contrast to that of K, which resembles parasympathetic stimulation.

Membrane Permeability. There is reason to regard increase in cell membrane permeability as an intimate part of the excitatory process, inhibition, as the opposite process, being associated with decreased permeability. Since the cell membrane is impervious to cations under ordinary conditions, the action of the calcium ion is probably exerted at the surface of the cell and is probably attributable to its effect in diminishing membrane permeability and in consolidating or stabilizing colloidal systems. Sodium and potassium have an opposite effect in this connection, increasing permeability and colloidal dispersion and normal cell function is dependent upon the presence of these and other ions in balanced proportions.

PHOSPHORUS

Phosphorus is widely distributed throughout the organism, being present in all cells and body fluids in a variety of organic and inorganic combinations.

The vital functions of P in various phases of organic metabolism are referred to repeatedly elsewhere. It is necessary merely to recall here the fundamental role of high-energy phosphate bonds in the storage, liberation and transfer of energy (e.g., ATP, phosphocreatine), the importance of hexose and triose-phosphates in the intermediary metabolism of carbohydrate, and the metabolic significance of such P-containing substances as phospholipids, nucleic acids, and nucleotides (DPN, TPN, etc.). We are concerned here only with the metabolism of *inorganic phosphate,* which may be ingested as such or may be liberated from ester combination by the activity of phosphatase enzymes during the period of digestion or intermediary metabolism.

The **phosphate buffer system,** consisting of a mixture of monosodium and disodium phosphates, is important in the regulation of the acid-base equilibrium in the tissue fluids, the addition of strong acids or alkalies to such a system causing relatively little change in the *p*H of the fluid.

Requirements[1,2]

The requirement of the organism for *calcium* varies considerably under different physiologic conditions. The normal adult requires a minimum daily intake of 0.45 to 0.55 gm. (7 to 8.5 mg. per kg.) for maintenance of equilibrium; for purposes of safety it is advisable to provide an excess of about 50 per cent above this figure (0.7 to 0.85 gm. Ca, 1.0 to 1.2 gm. CaO). The daily *phosphorus* requirement for normal adults is about 0.88 to 0.91 gm. (12 to 14 mg. per kg.). Allowing an excess of 50 per cent, the recommended intake for maintenance of equilibrium is about 1.32 to 1.36 gm. daily, constituting approximately 1/40 to 1/50 of the protein requirement.

Age. The breast-fed infant is maintained by about 45 mg. Ca per kg. daily and the artificially-fed infant by about 150 mg. per kg. This discrepancy is due largely to the fact that 50 to 70 per cent of the calcium of human milk is retained, as compared to about 30 to 35 per cent of that of cow's milk. The requirement during childhood and adolescence is less definitely established. According to some, there is gradual decrease from values of 70 mg. per kg. at three years to 12 mg. at sixteen years. Others place the minimum gross requirements as follows: six months to two years, 0.8 gm. daily; two to nine years, 0.9 gm.; nine years, 1 gm., increasing to 2 gm. at fifteen to sixteen years and subsequently decreasing steadily to the adult level (0.55 gm.).

Breast-fed infants require about 25 mg. P per kg. daily (average retention 55 per cent), and artificially-fed infants 95 mg. per kg. (retention 25 per cent). These figures are based upon the assumption of an adequate vitamin D intake. As in the case with calcium, the requirement for phosphorus decreases from about 79 mg. per kg. at three years to 35 mg. at sixteen years.

The Ca:P intake ratio is about 0.7 to 0.8 during infancy, approximately 0.77 during childhood and adolescence and about 0.53 during adult life. The high requirement of children as compared with that of adults is due largely to the necessity for providing for skeletal growth. This disproportion is actually greater than is indicated by the figures quoted above, since the percentage retention of calcium decreases with advancing years.

Food Factors. The most important and only good natural source of calcium is milk and milk products. About 0.7 gm. Ca is provided by one quart of milk or one-quarter pound of cheese. Meat is a poor source and fruits and vegetables only slightly better from a practical standpoint. Moreover, much of the calcium of vegetables is lost in the discarded water during the process of cooking. The calcium of milk is better absorbed and retained than is that of vegetables, and some variation in this regard exists among vegetables: e.g., the high oxalate content of spinach and other leafy vegetables renders their calcium relatively unavailable.

Although normal nutrition depends more upon an adequate intake of both Ca and P than upon the Ca:P ratio, the latter acquires more significance as the absolute values for either element approach the minimum requirement levels. Under such circumstances, abnormally high or low intake ratios result in impaired utilization of both Ca and P. Proper assimilation is also favored by a simultaneous adequate intake of vitamins D and C. Diets unusually high in fat may tend to inhibit absorption of Ca from the intestine due to the formation of insoluble calcium soaps. Lactose appears to favor absorption of Ca, probably through the development of increased acidity by lactic acid fermentation.

Phosphorus is present in all natural foodstuffs, in largest quantity in milk and milk products, meat, liver, egg yolk, cereals, nuts and leguminous vegetables. Diets high in milk and protein, especially nucleoprotein, will readily provide an adequate P intake. Although there is evidence that the P of vegetables, milk and meats is capable of meeting normal requirements, probably not all forms of combination are equally well utilized. The availability depends in part upon the type of the P compound and upon other constituents of the diet. Infants retain 55 per cent of the P of human milk and 25 per cent of that of cow's milk.

Pregnancy and Lactation. The requirement and retention of calcium are considerably increased during *pregnancy,* particularly during the late months. The quantity retained is more than can be accounted for by fetal utilization, and perhaps represents the establishment of a reserve supply which may be called upon during subsequent emergencies. The calcium content of the fetus increases from about 5 gm. at the twenty-eighth week to 30 gm. at the fortieth week. It has been estimated that the Ca requirement during pregnancy is 1.5 to 3.0 gm. daily and that the total retention under conditions of adequate intake is about 50 gm. The excess, above that utilized by the fetus, is stored in the maternal skeleton. This storage amounts to about 200 mg. daily from the fourth to the ninth month, and 300 mg. during the last week of pregnancy. If the supply is not adequate for the needs of the fetus, its mineral requirements will be met by Ca and P mobilized from the maternal skeleton, with consequent demineralization of the latter.

The onset of *lactation* is marked by a sudden change from a positive to a negative calcium balance. The loss of Ca is due not only to the large quantities present in the milk but also to excessive excretion, particularly in the feces. Negative balances may occur with daily intakes of as much as 3 gm. and may continue for several months after cessation of lactation. This loss of Ca may be diminished by administration of increased amounts of vitamin D.

The P requirement is also increased during pregnancy, a daily intake of 2.5 to 3 gm. being generally adequate. Under these conditions, if the supply of Ca and vitamin D is adequate, about 35 to 40 gm. of P are retained during the period of pregnancy. A portion of this is stored (with Ca) in the bones, the remainder participating in the intermediary metabolism of carbohydrate, fat and protein. Although a negative balance may occur with the onset of lactation, this is not so pronounced nor so persistent as in the case of Ca.

Absorption

Calcium and phosphate are absorbed in the small intestine, more readily in the upper than in the lower portions. In the course of digestion of nucleoproteins and phosphoproteins, phosphate may be split off and absorbed as such. If ester forms are present, they may undergo hydrolysis (enzymes of pancreatic and intestinal juice) prior to absorption. It has been suggested that because of this fact a considerable fraction of the dietary phosphate is absorbed later than the major portion of the Ca. This may permit better absorption of both elements, especially in regions of relatively low acidity.

Factors Influencing Degree of Absorption. Several factors influence the degree of absorption of Ca:

(a) CONCENTRATION IN INTESTINE. Other factors being equal, absorption of Ca is roughly proportional to its concentration in the intestine. The same appears to be true of phosphate.

(b) REQUIREMENT OF ORGANISM. As in the case of iron, but not to the same extent, the amount of Ca absorbed varies somewhat with the requirement of the organism for this element.

(c) INTESTINAL *p*H. Calcium salts, particularly phosphates and carbonates, are quite soluble in acid solutions and are relatively insoluble in alkaline solutions. Consequently, factors which increase intestinal acidity favor absorption of Ca, and vice versa. Under conditions of normal gastric acidity, Ca salts of weak organic acids are converted to the soluble chloride and, if retained in the stomach for a sufficient period, even the less soluble basic phosphate may go into solution. The acidity in the duodenum, normally *p*H 2.3 to 7.0, is of considerable importance, determining whether more of the Ca is in the form of the more soluble acid phosphate or less soluble basic phosphate. Calcium chloride and acid phosphate are probably absorbed from the duodenum before the gastric juice acidity is neutralized. Subsequently, absorption of Ca may be favored by the presence of organic acids (e.g., lactic, citric, amino acids, fatty acids).

(d) OTHER SUBSTANCES IN THE FOOD MIXTURE. An excess of Mg apparently diminishes absorption of Ca, especially if the latter is not present in adequate amounts. Considerable interest has centered in the Ca:P ratio, the optimum ratio for absorption of both elements being about 1:1 (1:2 to 2:1). An excessively high ratio is accompanied by decreased absorption of phosphate. It is stated that a low ratio does not result in decreased Ca absorption. This effect is apparently related to the influence on solubility of the products (calcium phosphates) formed under these conditions. Such substances as iron, beryllium, aluminum and strontium, which form insoluble phosphates, likewise interfere with absorption of phosphate, and can induce rickets.

Calcium salts (chloride, gluconate, lactate) are absorbed most efficiently in interdigestive periods, i.e., when the stomach and duodenum contain no food. When given for therapeutic purposes, therefore, these salts should be administered about one-half to three-quarters of an hour before meals and eating between meals should be avoided. Disturbance of fatty acid absorption limits absorption of Ca, in part through formation of insoluble soaps in the intestine and also perhaps by interference with absorption of vitamin D. Inadequate absorption may also result from protracted diarrhea, and from gastrocolic fistula, following the rapid passage of intestinal contents through the bowel.

Phytic acid (inositol hexaphosphate), which occurs in cereal grains, forms insoluble salts (phytin) with Ca and Mg (insoluble above *p*H 3 to 4), with consequent impairment of absorption of these elements. This phemonenon is regarded as the basis of the rachitogenic effect of such cereals as oatmeal. Hydroxyacids such as lactic, citric and tar-

taric shift the precipitation point of Ca phytate toward a higher *p*H (see also action of vitamin D).

(e) VITAMIN D. Vitamin D promotes absorption of Ca from the distal ileum, where absorption is otherwise relatively poor, but not from the upper ileum, where Ca is absorbed more readily. Intestinal absorption of phosphate is apparently increased somewhat. This may be a result of increased Ca absorption, maintaining an optimum local Ca:P ratio.

Vitamin D apparently counteracts the effect of phytic acid in binding the Ca ions and thus diminishing Ca absorption. In adequate amounts and with a high Ca intake, it suppresses the rachitogenic and anticalcifying effect of phytic acid. The mechanism of its action in this connection is not known.

Vitamin D lowers the *p*H in the distal ileum, cecum and colon. This may facilitate Ca absorption or, on the other hand, may be a result, in part at least, of the increased absorption, due to associated decrease in basic anions in the intestinal contents.

Simple phosphates (Ca, Na, K) are absorbed as such, largely in the small intestine and more readily in its upper than its lower portion. Factors which influence the absorption of calcium phosphate have been referred to previously. In the course of gastric and intestinal digestion of nucleoproteins and phosphoproteins, phosphate is split off and is absorbed as such. If ester forms are present, they must undergo hydrolysis by phosphatases prior to absorption. For example, liberation of phosphate from such substances as lecithin and the carbohydrate esters of phosphoric acid does not occur until they have been subjected to the action of pancreatic and intestinal secretions. It has been suggested that because of this fact, a considerable fraction of the ingested phosphate is absorbed later than the major part of the calcium. This permits absorption of portions of both of these elements which would not otherwise be absorbed, especially in regions of low acidity. It is also probable that a part of the phosphorus excreted into upper levels of the intestine is absorbed at lower levels.

Excretion

Calcium is excreted by the kidneys, the liver, and the epithelium of the large bowel. The fact that the fecal Ca includes that portion of the ingested Ca that has escaped absorption and has passed through the gastrointestinal tract has rendered difficult the exact quantitative determination of intestinal excretion of Ca. With low and moderate levels of intake (0.1 to 0.5 gm. daily) about 30 to 50 per cent is eliminated in the urine, while with high levels (1 gm.) about 10 to 25 per cent is so excreted. However, considerable deviations from these values occur, dependent probably upon variable dietary, metabolic and gastrointestinal factors. The renal threshold for excretion of Ca probably lies between 6.5 and 8.0 mg. per 100 cc. of serum, little being eliminated in the urine at serum levels below these values.[3] This threshold is raised in the presence of renal functional impairment, the urinary Ca constituting a steadily diminishing fraction of the total excretion in progressive kidney damage.

The proportion *excreted* in the feces is increased by factors which diminish absorption (p. 195); among the most important of these are steatorrhea, diarrhea and vitamin D deficiency. An increase in both urinary and fecal Ca occurs in hyperthyroidism and after administration of thyroxin. Increased urinary excretion of Ca results chiefly from the operation of factors that increase the rate of its mobilization from the bones. These include (a) acidosis or administration of an excess of acid-forming substances, (b) thyroxin, (c) parathyroid hormone, (d) excessively large doses of vitamin D (20,000 units or more). In the presence of thyroid, parathyroid and vitamin D deficiencies the urinary excretion of Ca is decreased. In *idiopathic hypercalciuria*, a condition responsible for a large proportion of cases of urinary lithiasis, there is apparently a genetic defect in the renal tubular mechanism for reabsorption of calcium from the glomerular filtrate.

Inorganic P is excreted by the kidneys and bowel, usually somewhat more in the urine than in the feces, the relative proportions varying considerably under different conditions. The source of inorganic P in the urine is the inorganic P of the plasma, although there is evidence that it may be contributed to by hydrolysis of phosphoric acid esters through phosphatase activity. The renal threshold is about 2 to 3 mg. of P per 100 cc. of plasma, excretion falling to a minimum at concentrations below this level.

On a balanced diet the urinary P constitutes about 60 per cent of the total excretion. As the Ca intake is decreased the proportion of P eliminated in the urine increases, being about 75 per cent of the total with a moderately low intake and about 85 per cent with a low Ca-moderately high P intake. The proportion excreted in the feces is increased by dietary factors which inhibit absorption, including a high intake of Ca (p. 195). In the presence of renal functional impairment, as in chronic glomerulonephritis, the urine phosphate is decreased and the fecal phosphate correspondingly increased. Urine P is increased after administration of parathyroid hormone, thyroxin, acids or acid-forming substances, dihydrotachysterol and extremely large amounts of vitamin D. Therapeutic doses of vitamin D cause a decrease in fecal P, which is increased under conditions of vitamin D deficiency. Vitamin D increases and parathyroid hormone decreases reabsorption of phosphorus by the renal tubular epithelium, the former thus diminishing and the latter increasing urinary excretion of phosphorus. The urinary acidity is regulated to a large extent by the relative proportions of acid (BH_2PO_4) and alkaline (B_2HPO_4) phosphates excreted; this constitutes an important part of the mechanism whereby the kidneys conserve base and regulate the acid-base balance of the body fluids.

Blood Calcium[4,5,6,7]

There is no Ca in erythrocytes. The Ca content of plasma (usually determined in serum) is 8.5 to 11.5 mg/100 ml. (usually 9 to 11 mg., or 4.5 to 5.5 mEq./liter). During infancy and early childhood (to 12 years) the average values approach the upper limit of this range, falling with advancing years.

Calcium exists in the plasma in two physiologically distinct fractions, designated (1) diffusible or ionized and (2) nondiffusible or nonionized. The diffusible fraction (50 to 60 per cent of total) is capable of passing through an artificial semipermeable membrane (cellophane, collodion) and through the living capillary wall; the nondiffusible fraction (40 to 50 per cent of total) cannot pass through, owing to its combination with plasma proteins. Although the two fractions may vary independently of each other under certain abnormal circumstances (e.g., hypoproteinemia, in which the nondiffusible Ca alone may be decreased; hypoparathyroidism, in which the diffusible fraction alone may be decreased), they seem to be in a state of rather unstable equilibrium. The parathyroid hormone exerts its influence primarily and almost entirely on the diffusible (ionized) fraction, which probably is the only physiologically active portion of the serum calcium.

Maintenance of the plasma Ca concentration within a narrow range is of vital concern to the well-being of the organism inasmuch as this ion has a profound influence on certain fundamental processes affecting cell function (e.g., membrane permeability, neuromuscular excitability). A few of the factors concerned in the preservation of the normal level of Ca in the plasma deserve special mention.

(a) **Parathyroid Hormone.** In the fasting state (i.e., no absorption from intestine), the plasma Ca concentration is maintained primarily by the mobilization of Ca from the bones through the action of the parathyroid hormone, which is one of the most important factors in the regulation of the concentration of Ca ions in the body fluids.

The metabolic actions of the parathyroid hormone, which are exerted primarily in the metabolism of calcium and phosphorus, are reflected in the consequences of (1) removal of the parathyroid glands and (2) injection of extracts of these glands.

EFFECTS OF PARATHYROIDECTOMY. The following phenomena occur after removal of all parathyroid tissue: (1) decreased urinary excretion of inorganic phosphorus; (2) increase in serum inorganic phosphorus concentration; (3) decreased urinary excretion of calcium; (4) decrease in serum calcium concentration, largely if not entirely in the diffusible (ionized) fraction.

As the concentration of calcium in the extracellular fluids falls, manifestations of neuromuscular hyperexcitability develop, eventuating in death with the clinical picture of tetany. Fibrillary muscle twitchings pass successively into generalized tremors, increased muscle tonus, painful clonic, and finally, tonic spasms and violent generalized convulsions, with laryngeal spasm and asphyxia. The autonomic nerves and smooth muscles are also affected, with involvement of the heart and gastrointestinal and urinary tracts.

EFFECTS OF PARATHYROID HORMONE INJECTION. The chief consequences of administration of this hormone are: (1) increased urinary excretion of inorganic phosphate; (2) decrease in serum inorganic phosphorus concentration; (3) increased urinary excretion of calcium; (4) increase in serum calcium concentration; (5) increased serum alkaline phosphatase activity. There is also an increase in the concentration of citrate and glucosamine in the blood, and in urinary excretion of citrate.

The skeleton is the source of the increased urinary calcium and phosphate. Continued, repeated injection of parathyroid hormone results in the characteristic skeletal picture of diffuse osteitis fibrosa cystica, with resorption of trabecular and cortical bone, fractures and deformities, appearance of numerous giant cells and osteoclasts, and necrosis, hemorrhage, and replacement fibrosis of the marrow. Healing processes, which progress simultaneously, are accompanied by the appearance of numerous osteoblasts. The action of parathyroid hormone is exerted not only on the mineral but also on the organic components of bone; it apparently regulates the rate of degradation of this tissue.

There is direct evidence of a primary direct action on bone. Pieces of bone, transplanted in contact with parathyroid tissue, undergo reabsorption in the area of contact, and deposition of new bone on the opposite side. Less direct, but nevertheless highly suggestive evidence is furnished by the observation that parathyroid hormone produces rapid depolymerization of bone mucopolysaccharide, with increase in glycoprotein in the blood and urine. There seems to be little doubt that this hormone influences, and perhaps regulates the rate of dissolution of both the organic (i.e., osteoid) and mineral components of bone, in the course of which calcium is released from both stable and labile fractions of the bone mineral. It is not known whether the hormone acts directly or by stimulating osteoclasts.

The general consensus is that parathyroid extract increases urinary phosphate excretion in man as well as in laboratory animals. By the use of clearance techniques, this phosphaturia has been shown to be due mainly to depression of renal tubular reabsorption of phosphate, glomerular filtration being only slightly increased. This increased urinary loss is probably the direct cause of the hypophosphatemia which is a consistent consequence of parathyroid hormone administration.

The increased concentration of calcium in the body fluids is often followed by deposition of calcium phosphate in various tissues, including the myocardium, kidneys, stomach, arteries, bronchi and pulmonary alveoli. Calculi may develop in the kidneys or lower urinary tract as a result of the high concentration of calcium and phosphate in the urine.

MECHANISM OF ACTION. Present evidence suggests that parathyroid extract exerts a dual effect. (1) It decreases renal tubular reabsorption of inorganic phosphate from the glomerular filtrate, with consequent excessive loss of phosphate in the urine and a fall in its concentration in the plasma. (2) It accelerates mobilization of calcium and phosphate and other compounds from the skeleton, with consequent increase in the concentration of calcium in the plasma and increased urinary excretion of calcium and phosphate. Although it has generally been assumed that the parathyroid glands secrete a single hormone with this dual action (i.e., on bones and kidneys), there have been suggestions that two hormones may be secreted, one perhaps acting on the bones ("calcium-mobilizing"), the other on the kidneys ("phosphaturic"). The increase in serum alkaline phosphatase activity in hyperparathyroidism is a reflection of increased osteoblastic activity in areas of healing in the bones.

CONTROL OF PARATHYROID SECRETORY ACTIVITY. There is no conclusive evidence to indicate nervous or hormonal control of parathyroid function, although certain observations suggest that the anterior pituitary may influence parathyroid activity in some way. Secretory activity is apparently regulated mainly by the plasma calcium concentration, a decrease in which stimulates parathyroid hormone secretion. This phenomenon plays an important role in the mechanism of maintenance of a relatively normal serum calcium concentration in a variety of clinical disorders characterized by a tendency toward hypocalcemia. This compensatory state of "secondary hyperparathyroidism" (p. 215) occurs consistently in such conditions as renal failure, rickets, chronic steatorrhea, the Fanconi syndrome, etc., and also perhaps in normal pregnancy. Conversely, increase in serum calcium concentration depresses parathyroid activity.

The parathyroid hormone increases the rate of mobilization of calcium from the skeleton into the extracellular fluids. Consequently, regulation of its secretion by the level of calcium in the blood plasma constitutes a very efficient autoregulatory mechanism; i.e., in effect, the serum calcium concentration regulates itself through the medium of parathyroid stimulation or depression. There is also controversial evidence that parathyroid activity is stimulated by an increase in plasma phosphate concentration, independently of any associated change in calcium concentration. Some believe that this "phosphate-controlled mechanism" may affect secretion of a hormone that acts only on the kidney, depressing tubular reabsorption of phosphate.

(b) **Vitamin D.** Vitamin D appears to act principally by increasing the absorption of Ca from the intestine and by facilitating the deposition of Ca and P in the bones (zones of provisional calcification). This factor exerts a greater and more immediate influence upon P than Ca in the blood serum. The mechanism of its action is not clearly understood. The view that it acts through stimulation of the parathyroid glands is contradicted by several facts. The parathyroid hormone has no antirachitic effect, causes a primary decrease in serum P and corpuscular ester P, and an increase in serum phosphatase activity and negative Ca and P balance, whereas vitamin D, in physiologic dosage, produces directly opposite effects. Moreover, the characteristic histologic picture of osteitis fibrosa cystica, which has been observed in experimental hyperparathyroidism, has not been seen in experimental hypervitaminosis D. Phosphate clearance studies have also revealed an important difference in the effects of vitamin D and parathyroid hormone. Administration of vitamin D to dogs was found to result in a marked increase in the maximum rate of absorption of phosphate by the renal tubular epithelium, increasing the concentration of inorganic phosphate in the plasma.[8] Administration of parathyroid hormone was followed by a considerable decrease in the rate of reabsorption of phosphate by the renal tubules and a consequent reduction in the plasma phosphate concentration.[8]

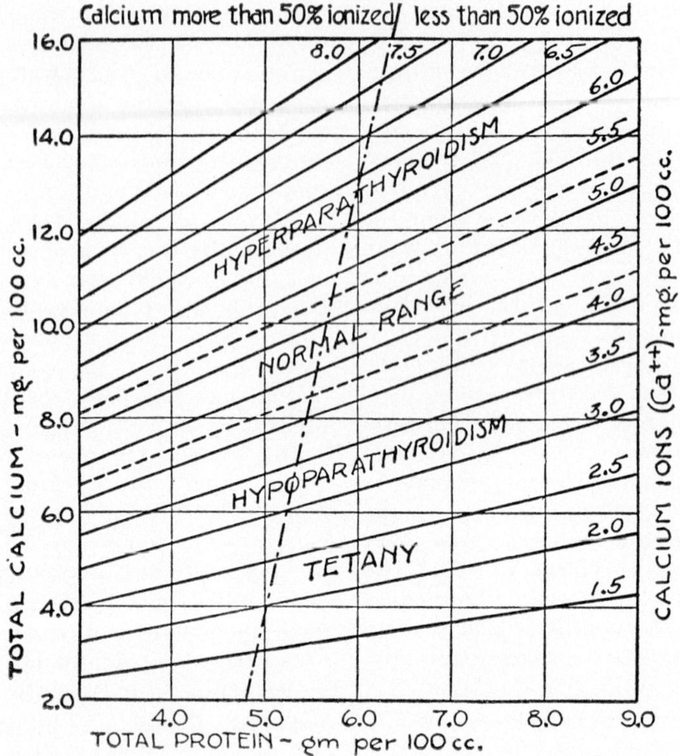

FIG. 1. Chart for calculation of [Ca^{++}] from total protein and total calcium of serum or plasma. (McLean, F. C. and Hastings, A. B.: Am. J. Med. Sc., *189:*601, 1935.)

(c) **Plasma Proteins.** Calcium exists in the plasma in higher concentration than would be possible in the absence of protein. As indicated above, about half of the plasma Ca (nondiffusible fraction) is bound to plasma protein, principally albumin, decrease in which may be accompanied by a decrease in the serum Ca concentration (Fig. 1). The calcium-binding potentialities of the plasma proteins may not be "saturated" under normal conditions, so that frequently no significant fall in serum Ca occurs at slight or moderate levels of hypoproteinemia. Such variations, since they are confined to the nondiffusible Ca fraction, are not accompanied by manifestations of altered Ca metabolism or neuromuscular excitability (e.g., tetany), and hypocalcemia of this type (i.e., due to hypoproteinemia) does not cause stimulation of parathyroid function.

(d) **Plasma Phosphate.** There is a roughly reciprocal relationship between the concentrations of Ca^{++} and $PO_4^{\equiv}$ ions in solutions in vitro. In the body fluids this relationship is exhibited to a limited extent and usually only in one direction; i.e., rather marked increase in serum $PO_4^{\equiv}$ may cause a fall in serum Ca^{++} concentration. This is encountered clinically in advanced renal failure with high serum PO_4 concentrations. Tetany may occur under these circumstances.

Deposition and Mobilization of Bone Minerals.[7] There is no complete unanimity of opinion regarding either the essential chemical nature or the mechanism of deposition of the mineral components of bone. The most important of the ionic constituents are Ca (about 26 per cent of the dry weight). PO_4 (about 12 per cent), CO_3 (about 3.5 per cent), and smaller amounts of Mg, Na, F, and citrate. On the basis of chemical analysis and X-ray diffraction studies, it would appear that the basic bone mineral has a crystal structure similar to that of the apatite group of phosphate minerals, probably a hydroxyapatite. As the crystal grows it is exposed to other elements and molecular groupings which cannot be incorporated in the lattice, the most important of which are carbonate, citrate, Mg, Na, F, Sr. These, with additional Ca and PO_4, are deposited on the surface of the hydroxyapatite crystal, stopping its growth. In bone, a new surface is started by the development of an independent crystal. In the case of dental enamel, a new surface is started by covering over the previous one.

The surface deposits are not part of the chemical structure of the fundamental bone mineral and are therefore more readily removed than the latter without actual dissolution of bone substance. Studies with radioactive elements indicate that these materials may be divided into two categories: (1) elements or molecular groupings which can displace or replace normal constituents of bone both on the surface and in the interior of the crystals; metabolic turnover of these components is relatively slow; (2) elements or molecular groupings which can enter a surface reaction with bone crystals, but which cannot be incorporated in the crystal lattice; metabolic turnover of these components is relatively rapid. It is believed that not more than 12 per cent of the skeletal Ca can be mobilized without actual dissolution of bone substance, including the matrix. This readily exchangeable Ca is in the form of salts (carbonate, citrate, phosphate) on the surface of the bone crystals, not in the actual lattice.

Mineralization of Bone. Bone formation involves two distinct fundamental processes: (1) construction of an organic matrix and (2) deposition of bone salts in this matrix. In areas of developing bone, reticular cells of the invading marrow turn into osteoblasts, which appear to be responsible for laying down the intercellular organic matrix (osteoid), which is largely protein in nature. Ascorbic acid is essential for the normal formation of this organic matrix. Its role (p. 470) and that of vitamin A (p. 381) in this connection are considered elsewhere. The osteoblasts subsequently turn into osteocytes, the mature bone cells. When bone undergoes destruction, the osteocytes and osteoblasts form osteoclasts, which are actively involved in the breakdown of bone; these can in turn be transformed to osteoblasts or reticular cells.

Proper mineralization requires provision of Ca^{++} and $Po_4^{\equiv}$ ions, at the site, in their proportions in the mineral matter of bone. Mineralization will not occur if there is a deficit in one of these ions even though the other is present in adequate amounts. These ions are provided in the concentrations present in the interstitial fluid in which they, of course, exist in solution. Understanding of the process of mineralization of bone must involve an explanation of the mechanism underlying the precipitation of calcium phosphate at this site. This is not entirely clear.

Alkaline phosphatase is present invariably in areas of active mineralization, suggesting that it is involved in this process. It is present in particularly high concentration in osteoblasts and, in skeletal disorders, its concentration in the blood plasma reflects the degree of osteoblastic activity (p. 205). It was originally believed that this enzyme hydrolyzes organic esters of phosphoric acid in the developing bone, producing a local increase in $PO_4^{\equiv}$ ion concentration with consequent precipitation of calcium phosphate (local supersaturation). However, there is no evidence that such esters are present in these situations in amounts adequate to produce this effect. It has been suggested that phosphatase favors mineralization: (1) by increasing the concentration of $PO_4^{\equiv}$ ion; (2) by increasing the concentration of Ca^{++} ion by removing a complexing agent (phosphoric esters); (3) by preventing absorption of ester phosphate, thereby eliminating a process which inhibits growth of the mineral crystals. Evidence is growing that this enzyme is primarily concerned with production of the organic matrix rather than directly with the deposition of bone salt.

Recently, attention has been directed toward the possibility that glycolysis may be involved in bone mineralization. Pre-osseous cartilage contains glycogen, phosphorylase, ATP and lactic acid, important components of the glycolytic cycle. Cartilage cells preparatory to mineralization accumulate large amounts of glycogen, which disappears abruptly just before or during the course of deposition of bone salts. Whether glycolysis provides a source of phosphoric ester substrate for phosphatase, or whether its main purpose is the provision of energy for some phase of the mechanism of bone formation is not clear. Although, in vitro, cartilage matrix may become calcified after all enzymes have been inactivated, there are important quantitative differences which suggest that glycolysis assists in some as yet unknown way in calcification of the matrix in the living organism.

Vitamin D is necessary for normal skeletal mineralization. The mode of its action in this connection is not known; it may perhaps provide optimum conditions of Ca^{++} and $PO_4^{\equiv}$ concentration in the bone. It is also essential for the normal growth of bones, exerting a specific effect at the zone of provisional calcification in long bones and at corresponding sites in membranous bones. Defects in this mechanism result in rickets.

It is convenient to divide the conditions necessary for normal calcification into two categories, viz., (1) local and (2) humoral. The local mechanism includes those factors, enzymatic and nonenzymatic, present in the bone matrix, that determine its calcifiability; these are largely unknown. The humoral mechanism includes the factors involved in the supply and transport, in proper form and concentration, of the mineral elements necessary for calcification. This classification is useful in approaching the differential diagnosis of generalized skeletal disorders, which may be classified conveniently, on the basis of pathogenesis, as (1) osteoporosis (primary defect in local mechanism, i.e., osteoid matrix) and (2) osteomalacia (primary defect in humoral mechanism, e.g., serum calcium or phosphate concentrations [p. 207]).

Interrelations of Citrate and Calcium Metabolism. Skeletal citrate comprises a large portion of the total body citrate (about 70 per cent in the mouse). Its ultimate relation to the metabolism of calcium may be indicated as follows:

(1) Citrate forms a soluble, poorly ionized complex with calcium, and therefore can effectively remove calcium ions from solution (basis of anticoagulant and tetanic effects).

(2) Local increases in citrate concentration resulting from cellular activity might conceivably be a factor in promoting dissolution of bone salt, even at comparatively high *p*H levels.

(3) In general, changes in plasma citrate are paralleled by changes in calcium, e.g., after nephrectomy, parathyroid hormone or vitamin D administration, and after injection of calcium chloride or neutral citrate.

Mobilization of Calcium. In common with other tissues, bone undergoes continual metabolic turnover, its various components undergoing degradation, mobilization and replacement. This is true also of its mineral constituents. Studies with radioactive Ca have shown, as mentioned above, that this element occurs in two types of deposit (i.e., bone salt and surface deposit) which differ in their lability. Less than 12 per cent of the skeletal Ca is readily mobilizable and replaceable, probably without dissolution of the osteoid matrix; the remainder is much more stable and probably cannot be mobilized without simultaneous breakdown of osteoid tissue. Moreover, the mineral constituents of the trabecular portions of bone are more labile than those of the cortex.

Regulation of Serum Calcium Concentration. There is good evidence of a very rapid exchange of calcium between the extracellular fluids, including blood plasma, and the bones. The concentration of calcium in these fluids is maintained within quite narrow limits, even in the face of extensive loss of this element, so long as the regulatory mechanisms and the skeletal stores remain adequate.

According to current concepts, calcium deposits in the bones may be regarded as in two different categories, morphologically and functionally. One, the "stable" calcium, comprising 88 to 96 per cent of the total, is a component of the true "bone salt," a hydroxyapatite, the crystals of which are intimately incorporated in the osteoid matrix. It is probable that release of this calcium, as well as of other constituents of the "bone salt," requires dissolution of the organic matrix. This is accomplished by the parathyroid hormone. The other type of deposit, the "labile" calcium (4 to 12 per cent of total bone calcium) is loosely held on the surfaces of the apatite crystals, and readily undergoes resolution or exchange with other ions, the crystal structure itself remaining undisturbed. This deposit is potentially in equilibrium with the calcium ions in the extracellular fluid, and can be mobilized very rapidly.

In the absence of parathyroid hormone, the concentration of calcium in the extracellular fluid is maintained at a rather constant but subnormal level by simple chemical equilibrium with the labile fraction of the bone mineral. This rapidly acting mechanism suffices to maintain a serum calcium concentration of 4 to 7 mg. per 100 cc. The other mechanism, mediated by the parathyroid hormone, regulates the rate of degradation of the organic and stable mineral components of bone, perhaps by stimulating osteoclastic activity, liberating "stable" calcium (and other ions) from the hydroxyapatite crystals and also "labile" calcium from the surface deposits. This is necessary for maintenance of the normal plasma calcium concentration (i.e., 8.5 to 11.5 mg. per 100 ml.).

The influence on Ca metabolism of other factors, such as the anterior hypophysis, thyroid, adrenal cortex, gonads and renal function, is evidenced chiefly under abnormal conditions, and will be considered subsequently. Ingestion of adequate amounts of soluble Ca salts in the postabsorptive state results in distinct elevation of serum Ca, which reaches a maximum in about two to three hours and returns to the previous level in about four hours. After intravenous injection, the peak is reached in a few minutes, with a subsequent fall to normal, usually within one to two hours, depending upon the quantity administered. Following intramuscular injection (Ca gluconate) the serum Ca rises to a maximum level in about one hour and falls gradually over a period of three to four hours. Intravenous or intramuscular injection of Mg. salts may cause a fall in serum Ca, at times to tetanic levels.[9]

Miscellaneous Factors. Estrogens exert an influence in Ca metabolism which varies widely in different species. Marked hypercalcemia occurs in birds during and just before ovulation, and may also be induced by administration of estrogen. This increase is largely in the non-diffusible fraction. Although this phenomenon does not occur in mammals, in rats estrogens produce hyperossification of the proximal epiphyseal zone of the tibia and thickening of the trabeculae, filling the upper fifth of the diaphyseal marrow cavities. This may be prevented by administration of androgens. It is questionable whether these observations are applicable to man. However, after the menopause, a type of osteoporosis often develops, with negative Ca balance, which may be benefited by administration of estrogen and/or androgen.

Androgens, too, influence skeletal mineralization. Being protein anabolic hormones, enhancing protein synthesis, they stimulate formation of the osteoid matrix (largely protein), with consequent retention of calcium and phosphate for its subsequent mineralization.

Osteoporosis and negative Ca balance may occur in subjects with hyperthyroidism or hyperfunction of the adrenal cortex. This may be due to the protein catabolic action of excessive amounts of thyroid hormone and the adrenal 11-oxysteroids, affecting primarily the osteoid matrix and secondarily, therefore, skeletal mineralization.

Decreased alkalinity of the body fluids (acidosis), due to any cause, may result in increased urinary excretion of Ca. The excess is presumably removed from the bones because of the increased solubility of the labile Ca deposits in a more acid medium.

Defective skeletal growth (in children) and undermineralization of the skeleton occur in the presence of disturbances of fat absorption (steatorrhea) from the intestine (sprue, celiac disease). There may be hypocalcemia and hypophosphatemia. These abnormalities are probably due in large measure to inadequate absorption of vitamin D under these conditions. The increased amounts of fatty acid in the intestine in these disorders, by binding Ca^{++} in the form of insoluble soaps, together with the incident diarrhea, may also contribute to the decreased absorption of Ca (increased excretion in feces).

Similar skeletal disorders also occur in the presence of hypophosphatemia tribute to the decreased absorption of phosphate by the renal tubular epithelium, with consequent increased urinary excretion (Fanconi syndrome).

Tetany (increased neuromuscular excitability) occurs whenever the concentration of Ca^{++} ions in the plasma and tissue fluids falls to sufficiently low levels, regardless of the cause of the hypocalcemia. It also occurs as a characteristic manifestation of alkalosis, without hypocalcemia, owing perhaps to decreased ionization of the plasma Ca at decreased H^+ ion concentrations.

Phosphatase Activity[5,6,7,10,11]

Definition and Distribution. Phosphatase is an enzyme which hydrolyzes monophosphoric esters, with the liberation of inorganic phosphate. It is present in practically all tissues, body fluids and cells, including red blood cells and leukocytes. In the fetus and during the period of growth it is present in greatest concentration in the bones and teeth. It occurs in largest amount in ossifying cartilage but is absent from resting epiphyseal cartilage, from nonossifying cartilage in other situations and from bones before the appearance of ossification centers. In adults, the intestinal mucosa contains the largest amount (per unit of wet weight), followed in approximate order by the renal cortex, bone, thyroid, spleen, lungs, suprarenal glands, blood vessels and pancreas, with some variation in different species. Four types of phosphomonoesterases of biologic significance may be differentiated on the basis of their activity in different *p*H ranges:[12] (1) a type (alkaline phosphatase) with optimal activity at about *p*H 9.3, present in blood plasma or serum, bone, kidney, intestine, mammary gland, spleen, lung, leukocytes, adrenal cortex and seminiferous tubules; (2) a type (acid phosphatase) with optimal activity at *p*H 6, occurring in mammalian erythrocytes and yeast; (3) a type (acid phosphatase) with optimal activity at *p*H 5, occurring in prostatic epithelium, spleen, kidney, blood plasma, liver, pancreas and rice bran; (4) a type (acid phosphatase) with optimal activity at about *p*H 3 to 4, obtained from taka-diastase. Alkaline phosphatases are variously activated by a number of substances, including Mg, Fe, Mn, Co, Ni, ascorbic acid and glycine, and are inhibited by Cu, Zn and cholic acid.

The bones are apparently the chief if not the only source of the "alkaline" phosphatase of plasma, which is not appreciably reduced after removal of practically all abdominal viscera. However, some believe that other organs, especially the liver, may be additional sources of plasma phosphatase. Normal plasma or serum contains small amounts of acid phosphatase (*p*H 4.9) (less than 4 Gutman-King-Armstrong units per 100 cc.). This may have its origin in the liver, spleen, bones, kidneys and prostate, but is not entirely or even largely of prostatic origin (p. 206), since it is present in women and children in essentially the same amounts as in adult men.[13] This is of interest because of the increase in this factor in prostatic carcinoma. Because of the presence of large amounts of an acid phosphatase in the red blood cells, care must be taken to avoid hemolysis in plasma or serum in which this determination is to be made. The acid phosphatase of prostatic origin is inhibited by L-tartrate. This permits separation of serum acid phosphatase activity into "prostatic" and "nonprostatic" components. The normal concentration of "prostatic acid phosphatase," determined in this manner, is less than 0.6 King-Armstrong units.

Functions of Phosphatase. By virtue of their power to liberate inorganic phosphorus from ester combinations, phosphatases play an important part in the absorption and excretion of P and in its intermediary metabolism. It seems significant in this connection that they are usually present in large quantity in the intestinal mucosa (absorption), kidney (excretion) and bones (ossification). Phosphatases also play an essential part in fermentation reactions and in the chemical reactions in various phases of muscular activity. Their relation to the phenomenon of calcification is of particular interest, and is considered elsewhere (p. 201).

Serum Alkaline Phosphatase Activity. According to the method of Bodansky,[14] a unit of alkaline phosphatase activity is defined as "equivalent to the actual or calculated liberation of 1 mg. of phosphorus as the phosphate ion during the first hour of incubation at 37° C. and *p*H 8.6, with the substrate containing sodium beta-glycerophosphate, hydrolysis not exceeding 10 per cent of the substrate." The range of normal values for plasma or serum alkaline phosphatase activity in adults by this method is 1.5 to 4 units per 100 cc. and for children 5 to 14 units. With the King-Armstrong procedure, the normal values for adults range from 3.7 to 13.1 units and for children from 15 to 20 units. Corresponding values with the Kay procedure are 0.1 to 0.2 and 0.17 to 0.34 units, respectively. Phosphatase activity is low at birth, rises to a maximum during the first month of life and remains fairly high during the second year, the values in later childhood falling gradually to adult levels. High protein diets cause a decrease and high carbohydrate diets an increase in phosphatase activity of the serum. Some observers have reported a slight increase in the last few months of pregnancy, but the statistical significance of such findings is questionable.

Increased Serum Alkaline Phosphatase Activity.[5] Serum alkaline phosphatase activity is increased chiefly in certain diseases of bone and in certain hepatic and biliary tract disorders. In the former, it appears to be related in most instances to the extent of osteoblastic activity or to the intensity of attempts at bone formation. The mechanism of increase in diseases of the liver and bile passages has not been established, although some attribute it to retention in the blood as a result of impaired excretion.

Serum phosphatase activity is consistently increased in active *rickets* (20 to 190 units). The degree of increase may be regarded as a reliable criterion of the severity of the condition, a decrease occurring within a few days after institution of antirachitic therapy and normal values being gradually restored during the period of active repair. High values (15 to 125 units) are obtained rather consistently in polyostotic forms of *osteitis deformans* (Paget's disease). Normal or slightly increased activity (to 25 units) may occur in cases with localized involvement of one or two bones. The values tend to be lower in older subjects. A moderate increase (20 to 40 units) is observed in clinical and experimental *hyperparathyroidism.* Slightly elevated values (5 to 15 units) have been reported occasionally in patients with generalized osteoporosis, marked hyperthyroidism, osteomalacia, metastatic carcinoma involving bone, osteogenic sarcoma, cases of Hodgkin's disease, lymphosarcoma and leukemia with bone involvement, polyostotic fibrous dysplasia, during the period of healing of fractures, Gaucher's disease with bone resorption and osteosclerosis fragilis generalisata (marble-bone disease), and, rarely, in renal rickets and multiple myeloma. The statement appears justified that an increase in serum alkaline phosphatase activity in skeletal disorders is a reflection chiefly of osteoblastic activity. In the light of this fact one may readily understand the lack of consistent relationship between serum phosphatase activity and the extent of skeletal demineralization in various bone diseases.

Serum phosphatase activity is increased in a large proportion of patients with obstructive and hepatocellular types of *jaundice* (to 60 units). Values above 20 units are obtained much more often in the former than the latter form, but this factor is of limited value in differential diagnosis because of a wide overlapping of values in the two groups of cases. High figures are also observed in certain patients with portal cirrhosis, metastatic carcinoma involving the liver, sarcoidosis, histoplasmosis, liver abscess, echinococcus cyst, single bile duct obstruction, and biliary fistula. On the other hand, normal values have been reported in infants with congenital atresia of the bile ducts. No increase occurs in hemolytic types of jaundice. In patients with intra-abdominal malignancy of various types, significant increase in alkaline phosphatase activity of the serum, in the absence of evidence of skeletal metastases, suggests metastasis to the liver.

Increased serum phosphatase activity has been reported in the following conditions: during periods of calcification of hemorrhages in scurvy, in active tuberculosis and Boeck's sarcoid, and in chronic myeloid leukemia. Increased phosphatase activity has also been demonstrated in tumor cells, in heterotopic bone, in muscle and fibrous tissue in preossification stages of myositis ossificans and in the liver, spleen, and kidneys in myelogenous leukemia.

Determination of serum alkaline phosphatase activity is useful in distinguishing between conditions characterized by osteoporosis and those characterized by osteomalacia. In osteoporosis, the fundamental defect is in bone formation, with inadequate construction of bone matrix and, therefore, subnormal osteoblastic activity; under such circumstances, there is no increase in serum alkaline phosphatase activity. In osteomalacia, the defect lies in inadequate mineralization of the bone matrix (osteoid tissue), with consequent increased susceptibility of the bone to injury and active attempts at repair, with increased osteoblastic activity and increased serum alkaline phosphatase activity.

Increased Serum Acid Phosphatase. Determinations of serum acid phosphatase activity have been shown to be of clinical value in carcinoma of the prostate, especially with metastases.[13,15–19] The source of this enzyme under these circumstances is the acinar epithelium of the prostate gland, which contains 500 to 2500 units per gram of fresh tissue (human and monkey) after puberty. A high concentration may be induced in the prostates of immature rhesus monkeys by administration of androgens.[20] Carcinomatous prostate tissue also may contain large amounts of acid phosphatase, and when metastases occur, with invasion of lymph or blood channels, large amounts of the enzyme may enter the circulation. Normal values are obtained in about 95 per cent of cases of nonprostatic disease, including skeletal disorders accompanied by high values for serum alkaline phosphatase. A slight increase (rarely over 6 and not over 10 units) may occur in advanced Paget's disease (osteitis deformans), osteopetrosis, hyperparathyroidism and carcinoma of the breast with extensive skeletal metastases. Care must be exercised to avoid hemolysis in the serum, which increases its acid phosphatase activity.

As stated by Gutman,[21] normal values may be obtained in metastasizing prostatic carcinoma for the following reasons: (a) the prostatic cells may elaborate very little enzyme because of anaplasia or very low androgen levels; (b) there may not be sufficient invasion of the blood or lymph channels to permit entrance into the circulation of significant amounts of the enzyme; (c) depression of acid phosphatase activity may follow castration, administration of estrogens, intensive irradiation or radical prostatectomy.

Increasing experience indicates that significantly elevated total serum acid phosphatase values (above 4.0 Gutman-King-Armstrong units per 100 cc.) are obtained in only 50 to 60 per cent of cases of metastatic prostatic cancer, and seldom in the absence of metastases. However, when tartrate-sensitive serum acid phosphatase is measured (i.e., "prostatic acid phosphatase"), much closer positive correlations are observed. Values above 0.6 units have been obtained in 85 to 90 per cent of cases of metastatic prostatic cancer, and in 50 to 70 per cent without demonstrable metastases. This procedure has increased the clinical usefulness of acid phosphatase determinations.[18,19]

Disturbances of Bone Formation and Mineralization. Abnormalities may occur in both phases of bone construction, i.e., (a) in the formation of the osteoid matrix and (b) in the subsequent process of mineralization. Accurate diagnosis and proper therapy require that these two classes of skeletal disorders be clearly differentiated.

TABLE 1. OSTEOPOROSIS

1. *Congenital*
   - Osteogenesis imperfecta
2. *Inadequate stimulation* (stress and strain)
   - Disuse atrophy
3. *Degenerative*
   - Senile osteoporosis
4. *Nutritional*
   - Malnutrition (especially protein)
   - Vitamin C deficiency
   - Vitamin A deficiency
5. *Endocrine*
   - Estrogen deficiency (postmenopausal)
   - Androgen deficiency (eunuchoidism)
   - Adrenal hyperfunction (Cushing's syndrome)
   - Hyperthyroidism
   - Hypothyroidism
   - Acromegaly
   - Panhypopituitarism (Simmonds' disease)
6. *Idiopathic*

Defective osteoid formation, designated *osteoporosis* (Table 1), is not due to disturbance in calcium or phosphorus metabolism, and there is no consistent alteration in serum calcium or phosphate in conditions in this category. The fundamental defects usually consist in inadequate protein synthesis (generalized), excessive protein catabolism (generalized), or nutritional inadequacies more specifically affecting osteoid formation (e.g., disuse atrophy, vitamin A deficiency), and defective osteoblastic function (e.g., scurvy, osteogenesis imperfecta). Inasmuch as these disorders are characterized by inadequate regenerative capacity of the bones, i.e., inadequate osteoblastic proliferation and/or function, there is no increase in serum alkaline phosphatase, which is a reflection of osteoblastic activity.

TABLE 2. OSTEOMALACIA

1. *Nutritional*
   - Vitamin deficiency (Disturbance in absorption of Ca or P) (rickets)
   - Calcium and/or phosphorus deficiency
   - Steatorrhea
   - Chronic diarrhea (ulcerative colitis)
   - Gastrocolic fistula, intestinal resections, etc.
   - Insoluble phosphate complexes, e.g., with Al, Fe, Pb, Be, etc.
2. *Renal Functional Impairment*
   - Glomerular damage ("renal rickets")
   - Tubular malfunction
     - Fanconi syndrome
     - Renal tubular acidosis
     - Idiopathic hypercalciuria
3. *Endocrine*
   - Hyperparathyroidism
4. *Hypervitaminosis D* (mechanism obscure)

On the other hand, in the conditions included under the designation osteomalacia, the fundamental defect is in the metabolism of calcium and/or phosphorus (Table 2). There is no necessary abnormality in osteoid formation. Indeed, this is usually excessive, because of the increased stimulation resulting from weakening and injury of the bones. The nature of the metabolic aberration varies, but the effect in each instance is inadequate mineralization of the osteoid matrix. In these conditions, in addition to alterations in serum calcium and phosphorus, which are often quite characteristic, there is often an increase in serum alkaline phosphatase activity, a reflection of increased osteoblastic activity. This may be absent in conditions such as glomerulonephritis, because of the coexistence of serious impairment of protein nutrition. In general, however, increase in serum alkaline phosphatase is of great value in distinguishing osteomalacia from osteoporosis.

Hypercalcemia[4,5,6]

Hyperparathyroidism. Increase in the serum calcium concentration is one of the most striking and constant features of hyperparathyroidism, either spontaneous or induced by administration of parathyroid hormone. Values as high as 29.5 mg. per 100 cc. have been observed. The mechanism underlying the production of this phenomenon as well as the associated metabolic and clinical manifestations are described elsewhere (pp. 217, 220).

Hypervitaminosis D. Hypercalcemia may result from administration of excessive amounts of vitamin D. This condition is now rarely encountered clinically. However, there is a wide range of individual susceptibility to the action of this factor, and the coincident administration of large quantities of calcium increases the tendency toward the development of hypercalcemia. Vitamin D is usually well tolerated in doses many times the normal requirement. However, seriously deleterious effects may be produced by extremely large amounts (500 to 1000 times the normal requirement). The early symptoms are due chiefly to the induced hypercalcemia (increased intestinal absorption of calcium, and possibly increased skeletal mobilization). These include anorexia, thirst, lassitude, constipation and polyuria, followed later by nausea, vomiting and diarrhea. Hyperphosphatemia may occur.

Increased urinary excretion of calcium and phosphorus may lead to urinary lithiasis, and the hypercalcemia and hyperphosphatemia to metastatic calcification. The kidneys, arteries, bronchi, pulmonary alveoli, muscles and gastric mucosa are principally involved. Renal failure may develop, leading to death. In growing children there may be excessive mineralization of the zone of provisional calcification at the expense of the diaphysis, which undergoes demineralization (with extremely large doses).

Dihydrotachysterol (A.T. 10). The administration of therapeutic doses of this substance, a photochemical derivative of ergosterol, results in an increase in serum calcium (p. 234). Its physiologic effect appears to be more closely analogous to that of parathyroid hormone than is that of vitamin D, since it causes greater urinary excretion of phosphate and rise in serum calcium than does the latter. It has no significant antirachitic properties.

Multiple Myeloma. Serum calcium values ranging from normal to over 20 mg. per 100 cc. have been observed in patients with multiple myeloma. Hypercalcemia has been reported in about 50 per cent of cases in which mention was made of the serum calcium concentration, above 12 mg. in 20 to 45 per cent. Some have attributed this to a state of hyperparathyroidism, but the serum phosphate is usually normal or increased (renal functional impairment) and the serum alkaline phosphatase activity is usually normal. There is no consistent correlation with hyperproteinemia. It seems probable that the hypercalcemia is due primarily to active bone destruction by the progressing skeletal lesion, being contributed to, perhaps, by renal functional impairment (decreased calcium excretion), a common feature of this disease.

Skeletal Neoplasm. The serum Ca concentration is usually normal in the great majority of cases of primary and metastatic neoplasms of bone, although urinary calcium excretion may be increased. However, values as high as 22 mg. per 100 cc. have been observed, with increasing hypercalciuria, particularly in cases of extensive metastatic involvement of the skeleton. In such cases, values for serum P and phosphatase activity are usually within normal limits, except in osteogenic sarcoma, in which the serum phosphatase activity may be increased.

Androgens and estrogens are being employed extensively in the treatment of inoperable breast cancer with skeletal metastases, often with striking temporary improvement, remineralization of the skeletal lesions, and diminishing urine calcium excretion. However, severe hypercalcemia and increasing hypercalciuria occasionally develop, usually with rapid progression of the osteolytic lesions, presumably the source of the added calcium. The serum calcium may rise rapidly (few days) to extremely high levels, i.e., over 20 mg./100 cc. The hypercalcemia is accompanied by nausea, vomiting, and dehydration, and, in severe cases, progressive and fatal renal functional impairment and kidney damage.

Acute Bone Atrophy. Hypercalcemia, with increased urinary excretion of calcium and phosphorus, may occur as a result of rapid demineralization of bones, especially in the presence of simultaneously impaired renal function. This has been observed particularly in children, during periods of immobilization of the extremities due to fractures or paralysis (poliomyelitis). In contrast to hyperparathyroidism, the serum phosphate is either normal or increased. Similarly, hypercalcemia has been observed occasionally in patients with osteitis deformans with rapid and extensive demineralization.

Milk and Alkali Intoxication.[22,23,24] A rather characteristic syndrome may occur in subjects, usually with peptic ulcer, who ingest excessive amounts of milk and absorbable alkalies. This is marked by hypercalcemia, alkalosis, renal functional impairment and abnormal calcium deposits, without hypophosphatemia or increase in urine calcium. Practically all patients have band keratitis and calcium deposits in the conjunctivae.

It is believed that the hypercalcemia is the result of the excessively high intake of calcium in the presence of renal functional impairment induced or aggravated by alkalosis due to the high alkali intake. This condition superficially resembles hyperparathyroidism complicated by renal failure, but the differential diagnosis is usually easy. In addition to the characteristic history, in this syndrome there is no increase in urine calcium. The clinical and laboratory manifestations improve dramatically when milk and alkalies are withdrawn and the alkalosis and the hypochloremia and hypopotassemia (due to vomiting) are treated by parenteral administration of proper solutions of electrolytes, unless irreversible kidney damage has occurred.

It must be remembered, however, that duodenal ulcer occurs rather frequently in subjects with hyperparathyroidism (p. 219). Administration of milk and absorbable alkalies to such patients may precipitate acute hyperparathyroidism, with nausea, vomiting, lethargy, prostration and azotemia, which may terminate fatally if not recognized promptly.

Sarcoidosis.[25] Hypercalcemia and hypercalciuria occur occasionally in patients with sarcoidosis, the cause being obscure. There may be associated renal calculi, nephrocalcinosis (with renal insufficiency), generalized calcinosis, band keratitis and other manifestations of hypercalcemia. These findings may so dominate the clinical picture as to suggest hyperparathyroidism. Balance studies in such cases have revealed increased intestinal absorption of calcium, which, however, was inadequate to account for the increase in urine calcium. It has been suggested that the fundamental defect may be increased sensitivity to vitamin D in sarcoidosis. Good results have been reported with cortisone therapy. Administration of sodium phytate has also been recommended (decreasing Ca absorption).

Idiopathic Infantile Hypercalcemia.[26] This condition has been detected usually between the ages of four months and 2 years. Two forms have been described: (a) a mild (benign) form, with recovery, apparently complete, in a few months or years; (b) a severe form, either progressing to death from renal failure or eventuating in permanent mental retardation.

The chief symptoms include anorexia and vomiting, with consequent malnutrition and underdevelopment, constipation, hypotonia, lethargy and mental retardation. There is a rather characteristic "elfin" facial appearance, with low-set ears, prominent epicanthic folds, wide mouth, overhanging upper and large lower lip, underdevelopment of the bridge of the nose, and, at times, strabismus.

In severe cases the hypercalcemia almost invariably produces renal impairment, at times with nephrocalcinosis and complicating kidney infection and also calcific deposits in the lungs and muscles. There is reduction in size of the brain and skull and increased radiologic density of the base of the skull and the epiphyses, at times of sufficient degree to be mistaken for osteopetrosis.

The cause is unknown. The possibility of increased sensitivity to vitamin D has been suggested. It may be desirable to reduce the calcium intake. Cortisone has been reported to produce improvement.

Miscellaneous. Ingestion of adequate amounts of soluble calcium salts in the post-absorptive state results in an elevation of serum calcium, which reaches a maximum in two to three hours and returns to the previous level in about four hours. After intravenous injection, the peak is reached in a few minutes, with a subsequent fall to normal, usually within two to three hours, depending upon the quantity given. After intramuscular injection (calcium glucogalactogluconate), a maximum level is reached in about one hour, with a subsequent fall over a period of three to four hours. Intravenous or intramuscular injection of magnesium salts may cause a fall in serum calcium, at times to tetanic levels (p. 212).

The serum Ca may be increased in rare instances of advanced nephritis with uremia, although any deviation from the normal in this condition is usually in the opposite direction (p. 211). The hypercalcemia is difficult to explain; some believe that chronic nephritis is accompanied by a state of hyperparathyroidism, because of the rather common observation of enlargement of the parathyroid glands (p. 215).

Hypercalcemia has been observed occasionally in leukemia and polycythemia vera, the mechanism of its production being unknown. Slight elevations may occur in conditions in which the CO_2 content of the blood is increased, thereby enhancing its capacity for maintaining Ca in solution (asphyxia, chronic emphysema, pneumonia, silicosis, congestive heart failure).

Administration of anterior hypophyseal extracts to experimental animals has resulted in hypercalcemia. This has been attributed to the action of a "parathyrotrophic" principle. However, except for the possible hypophyseal origin of hyperparathyroidism due to diffuse hyperplasia or hypertrophy of the parathyroid glands, elevation of the serum Ca concentration has not been observed in uncomplicated clinical pituitary disorders. Borderline high values occur occasionally in patients with pituitary basophilism. A similar effect has followed administration of gonadotropic hormone and certain estrogens to experimental animals. Marked hypercalcemia (20 to 28 mg. per 100 cc.) occurs in birds just before and during ovulation. This phenomenon has been produced by artificial distention of the oviduct.

Hypocalcemia[4,5,6]

Hypoparathyroidism. Hypocalcemia is one of the most constant and characteristic features of diminished parathyroid function. Both diffusible and nondiffusible fractions are decreased. The clinical and metabolic features of this condition are described elsewhere (p. 228).

Pseudohypoparathyroidism.[6] Cases have been observed which present the metabolic and clinical picture of hypoparathyroidism, but in which the fundamental disturbance appears to be diminished end organ (bones, kidneys) responsiveness rather than merely lack of hormone. In contrast to true hypoparathyroidism, large doses of parathyroid hormone exert little or no effect on the serum calcium and phosphorus concentrations or calcium and phosphorus excretion in the urine in such cases. They are also somewhat resistant to dihydrotachysterol and vitamin D, but not completely so.

Children with this condition present a rather characteristic appearance, with short stature, shortness of the extremities in relation to the trunk, round face with thick neck, fat, stubby hands, short fingers, and short metacarpal and metatarsal bones.

Vitamin D Deficiency (Rickets, Osteomalacia). Deficiency in vitamin D results characteristically in rickets in young children and in osteomalacia in older children and adults. In the majority of early cases the serum calcium is within normal limits, the serum phosphate being characteristically decreased and the serum alkaline phosphatase activity increased. In some instances, however, especially later, and if the calcium intake is low, hypocalcemia occurs (4 to 7.5 mg./100 cc.), with manifestations of tetany (infantile tetany, spasmophilia, osteomalacic tetany).

Although the primary effect of vitamin D deficiency is diminished absorption of calcium from the intestine, hypocalcemia is usually not an early manifestation. This is due presumably to the fact that the tendency toward lowering of the serum calcium concentration stimulates the parathyroids (enlargement and hypersecretion), with consequent increased mobilization of skeletal calcium and lowering of the serum phosphate concentration. Hypocalcemia appears when this compensatory mechanism becomes inadequate, i.e., when the readily mobilizable calcium of the bones has been exhausted. There is also probably diminished intestinal absorption of phosphate (secondary to diminished calcium absorption).

Maternal Tetany. The serum calcium concentration tends to fall, but not to subnormal levels, during the late months of normal pregnancy and during lactation. It may occasionally become subnormal, with mild tetanic manifestations. This condition, maternal tetany, is discussed elsewhere (p. 235).

Neonatal Tetany. "Tetany of the newborn" appears to be related to the existence of tetany in the mother. It is discussed elsewhere (p. 236).

Acute Pancreatitis. Hypocalcemia has been reported to occur in the majority of cases of acute hemorrhagic pancreatitis (up to 70 per cent), the values usually ranging between 7 and 8 mg./100 cc., but occasionally falling below 7 mg. This has been attributed to sudden removal of large amounts of calcium from the extracellular fluids, including the blood plasma, as a result of its fixation as insoluble calcium soaps by fatty acids in areas of fat necrosis. The validity of this explanation has not been established.

Steatorrhea. This condition is encountered in celiac disease, in sprue and occasionally in prolonged obstructive jaundice (p. 236). The outstanding feature is defective absorption of fat from the intestine, as a result of which large quantities of insoluble calcium soaps are formed with consequent inadequate absorption of Ca and also of vitamin D, aggravated by the associated diarrhea. The serum Ca may be low and tetany, delayed ossification (in infants) and osteoporosis occur frequently.

Inadequate Intake. This condition is due to a diet deficient in total caloric value and in Ca, P and vitamin D, and resembles a slowly progressive osteomalacia.

Hypoproteinemia. Serum Ca values as low as 5.7 mg. per 100 cc. have been observed in association with hypoproteinemia accompanying the nephrotic syndrome, obstructive jaundice, kala-azar, malignancy and other cachectic states. The diminution in serum Ca occurs entirely in the nondiffusible fraction and is apparently due to the decrease in serum albumin concentration and not to any disturbance of calcium metabolism. There is no significant alteration in diffusible Ca and no increase in neuromuscular excitability.

Chronic Glomerulonephritis. Hypocalcemia is occasionally observed in non-nephrotic forms of chronic glomerulonephritis in the stage of renal functional failure. It occurs usually in the late stages of this condition and is associated with and perhaps dependent upon the increase in serum P which is present in such cases (see p. 213). The concentration of Ca varies roughly inversely with that of P, values as low as 4 to 6 mg. being observed occasionally, at times with manifestations of tetany. In many cases the decrease in serum Ca is contributed to by the presence of hypoproteinemia. It is believed by some that hypocalcemia may be responsible for certain of the manifestations of uremia.

Skeletal changes may occur in chronic nephritis or in congenital urinary tract defects, their character varying from generalized osteoporosis to cyst formation and deformities, with extensive metastatic calcification. When occurring during the period of skeletal growth the condition has been termed renal rickets or renal dwarfism. A similar condition may occur in adults, with fibrocystic changes in all bones and metastatic calcification, particularly in the media of the arteries (Mönckeberg type) and in the neighborhood of joints. This has been termed *renal osteitis fibrosa cystica*, and is regarded as the adult counterpart of renal rickets. In both forms there are evidences of long existing renal failure, usually marked acidosis, hyperphosphatemia, usually normal or slightly reduced serum Ca concentration and generally normal serum phosphatase activity. *Parathyroid hyperplasia*, involving principally the chief cells, has been found in a large proportion of such cases, being probably compensatory in nature and induced by the prolonged decrease in serum Ca. All the parathyroid glands are increased in size when hyperplasia is present. The nature and extent of the skeletal changes are not directly proportional to the degree of hyperplasia, suggesting that the bone lesions are not due entirely to hyperparathyroidism in such cases. It appears probable that the bone changes are contributed to also by (a) acidosis and (b) inadequate absorption of Ca resulting from the excretion into the intestine of large amounts of P which would have been eliminated in the urine under conditions of normal renal function. Differentiation of this condition from hyperparathyroidism is considered elsewhere (p. 215).

Magnesium, Phosphate, Oxalate and Citrate Tetany. Intravenous injection of magnesium salts may cause a fall in serum calcium, at times to tetanic levels (p. 236).

A fall in serum calcium, with signs of tetany, may follow intravenous injection of neutral or alkaline sodium phosphate. The hypocalcemia of chronic renal failure probably results chiefly from phosphate retention.

Parenteral administration of soluble oxalates and of citrates produces tetany, the former through the formation of insoluble calcium oxalate, with hypocalcemia, the latter by formation of poorly ionized calcium citrate, without hypocalcemia. Citrate intoxication has been observed during replacement of large volumes of blood in exchange transfusions, hemorrhage and cardiovascular surgery.

Inorganic Phosphorus in Blood[2,4,5,6]

The inorganic phosphorus of the blood probably exists almost entirely in the plasma. The chief difficulty in determining its concentration in the red blood cells arises from the fact that a portion of the phosphoric esters in these cells undergoes hydrolysis in the process of analysis, with the consequent liberation of phosphate.

The *serum inorganic P* ranges from 5 to 6.5 mg. per 100 cc. in infancy and gradually diminishes until it reaches 3 to 4.5 mg. in normal adults. The concentration is usually highest in summer and lowest in winter, varying with the concentration of ultraviolet rays. A slight increase follows the ingestion of calcium and a considerable drop follows parenteral administration of Mg salts. Under normal conditions, ingestion of carbohydrate results in a progressive fall in serum P which persists during the period of increased glucose utilization, returning to normal in four to five hours. This is due to the fact that combinations of carbohydrate and phosphoric acid (hexose-phosphate) play an important part in the intermediary metabolism of carbohydrate. A similar drop follows administration of insulin and epinephrine.

Hyperphosphatemia. The serum P concentration may be increased by therapeutic and excessive doses of vitamin D. Slightly increased values are also observed in hypoparathyroidism, the degree of increase being approximately proportional to the degree of hypocalcemia. A rise also occurs at times during the period of healing of fractures. Highest values (8 to 40 mg. per 100 cc.) are observed in renal failure (chronic glomerulonephritis, pyelonephritis, nephrosclerosis, urinary obstruction, polycystic disease and destructive kidney lesions). An increase has also been reported in acute intestinal obstruction and following injection of histamine. Phosphate retention in renal failure may contribute to the development of acidosis, but the latter may exist in the absence of the former.

Hypophosphatemia. Vitamin D deficiency is one of the most important causes of hypophosphatemia, values of 1 to 3 mg. per 100 cc. being obtained frequently in children with rickets. The exact mode of action of vitamin D is not clearly understood, but deficiency in this factor probably results in inability to utilize Ca and P properly in the process of ossification, with increased excretion of P in the feces. The fall in serum P is most marked when the P intake is inadequate. The serum Ca concentration may be normal or subnormal (p. 211). It has been pointed out that if the concentration of Ca be multiplied by that of P, each being expressed in mg. per 100 cc., a product is obtained which, in the normal child, ranges from 50 to 60. When the product is below 30, *rickets* is usually present and when it is above 40, either healing is occurring or rickets has probably not been present. These observations cannot be relied upon absolutely.

Diminished serum P concentration occurs in osteomalacia, being here, as in rickets, a manifestation of vitamin D deficiency. It occurs also in steatorrhea (sprue, celiac disease), probably as a result of defective intestinal absorption of Ca, P and vitamin D, due to the excessive amount of fat in the intestine. The characteristic fatty diarrhea in these conditions is frequently accompanied by skeletal demineralization, dwarfism, low serum Ca and P and manifestations of rickets and tetany.

Hypophosphatemia may occur as a feature of a partial or complete Fanconi syndrome.[27] This designation is applied to a group of conditions, exhibiting a familial tendency, characterized by inadequate renal tubular reabsorption of certain constituents of the glomerular filtrate, due presumably to inherent defects in certain enzymatic transport mechanisms in the tubular epithelial cells. This does not include functional derangements associated with morphologic tubular damage, e.g., nephrosis. The following substances, singly or in various combinations, are excreted in the urine in abnormally large amounts: glucose (p. 757), various amino acids, lactic acid, β-hydroxybutyric acid, ammonia and phosphate. There are frequently acidosis, hypophosphatemia and rickets or osteomalacia. The serum calcium concentration is usually within normal limits and the serum alkaline phosphatase activity increased. We are concerned here only with the abnormality in phosphate.

The increased urinary excretion of phosphate, due to its inadequate tubular reabsorption from the glomerular filtrate, is believed to be the direct cause of the lowered serum phosphate concentration. If this falls to a sufficiently low level, the Ca:PO_4 ratio becomes unfavorable for deposition of bone mineral, with consequent development of rickets (growing children) or osteomalacia (adults).

Hyperphosphaturia, hypercalciuria, hypophosphatemia, increased alkaline phosphatase and rickets or osteomalacia may occur without any of the other characteristic features of the Fanconi syndrome in the typical form, e.g., aminoaciduria. The designation "tubular insufficiency without glomerular insufficiency" has been applied to this condition (a form of "renal tubular acidosis"). It has been suggested that the underlying defect may be an inadequate amount of phosphatase in the renal tubular cells. It has been reported that phosphatase activity in these cells is increased by vitamin D, and there are reports of improvement in several of the manifestations of the Fanconi syndrome following administration of this agent.

The term "hypophosphatasia" has been applied to what appears to be a developmental anomaly characterized by multiple abnormalities and defective mineralization of the skeleton, hypercalcemia and low levels of phosphatase in the plasma, liver, kidneys, intestine, and especially in the bones, which are largely uncalcified. The condition differs from rickets, therefore, in certain essential respects.[28]

Injection of *parathyroid hormone* is followed by a decrease in serum P which probably results from its increased elimination in the urine. A similar change occurs characteristically in uncomplicated clinical hyperparathyroidism (p. 220). This decrease is roughly proportional to the degree of hypercalcemia. With the supervention of renal failure in this condition, the urinary excretion of P diminishes and the serum P rises to normal or supernormal levels (p. 220).

Hypophosphatemia can be produced experimentally by oral administration of cations that combine with PO_4 to form insoluble phosphates; among these are beryllium and aluminum.

Calcium and Phosphorus in Other Body Fluids[5]

The electrolyte composition of the interstitial fluid of the body is the result of a Donnan distribution between the fluid and the blood plasma. The Ca and P in this fluid are therefore in a state of equilibrium with their diffusible fractions in the plasma, plus an additional variable amount roughly proportional to the protein content of the fluid. Thus the Ca content ranges from 4.5 to 5.5 mg. per 100 cc. in the case of protein-free fluids and transudates and from 5 to 11 mg. in transudates and exudates with high protein contents and in synovial fluid, which has a protein content of 4.2 to 7.3 gm. per 100 cc. The Ca content of ocular fluid is about 6 to 7 mg. per 100 cc. and that of cerebrospinal fluid 4.5 to 6 mg. Although the latter is quantitatively identical with the diffusible fraction of serum Ca under normal conditions, this is not the case in abnormal states. For example, very little change occurs in cerebrospinal fluid Ca following parathyroidectomy, although the serum Ca concentration may be markedly diminished. In some instances the values for Ca in the serum and cerebrospinal fluid may be practically identical. This is not true of other body fluids.

The inorganic P of the blood plasma is practically entirely diffusible and, consequently, its concentration in the water of the interstitial fluids of the body is practically the same as in the water of the plasma. The actual concentration is slightly higher than in equivalent volumes of plasma because of the relatively high protein content of the latter. The P content of aqueous humor and of cerebrospinal fluid averages about 50 per cent of that of the plasma, suggesting that these fluids are not in diffusion equilibrium with the blood.

Clinical Manifestations of Abnormal Calcium and Phosphorus Metabolism

The most important clinical conditions characterized by disturbance of Ca and P metabolism are those dependent upon or associated with abnormalities of *parathyroid function* and of *vitamin D supply* or utilization. In these conditions, characteristic changes in the metabolism of these elements can usually be demonstrated. There are many other clinical disorders, not primarily dependent upon disturbance in Ca or P metabolism, in which significant changes may occur in the Ca content of and distribution in various tissues. In certain of these, as in renal disease and hyperthyroidism, the pathogenesis of these changes is fairly well understood. In others, however, as in certain skeletal disorders (osteitis deformans, polyostotic fibrous dysplasia, marble-bone disease, fragilitas ossium, etc.) and in calcinosis universalis, little or no disturbance of Ca and P metabolism can be demonstrated. The former will be discussed in detail and the latter mentioned only briefly in their relation to problems of differential diagnosis.

HYPERPARATHYROIDISM[4,5,6,29]

Excessive secretion of parathyroid hormone has been demonstrated in association with (a) adenoma of one or more parathyroid glands and (b) diffuse hyperplasia or hypertrophy of all parathyroid glands. These may be regarded as primary forms of hyperparathyroidism, although it has been suggested that diffuse hyperplasia may be the result of hypophyseal hyperfunction, with excessive stimulation of the parathyroids, presumably by an undemonstrated parathyrotropic principle of the pituitary gland.

The existence of a state of hyperparathyroidism has been implied or affirmed in a number of other conditions in which parathyroid hyperplasia is present occasionally or consistently. These include:

1. Chronic glomerulonephritis and other forms of renal disease associated with "renal rickets."
2. True rickets and osteomalacia (vitamin D deficiency).
3. Chronic steatorrhea (sprue, celiac disease).
4. Pregnancy and lactation.
5. Certain cases of senile osteoporosis, multiple myeloma, pituitary basophilism, metastatic malignancy involving the skeleton, osteogenesis imperfecta, chronic hypertrophic arthritis, acromegaly and "marble-bone disease."

Except perhaps in the latter group, the parathyroid enlargement and hypersecretion occur in response to decrease in the plasma calcium concentration, the normal stimulus to parathyroid activity. In some cases, this results from decreased absorption from the intestine (vitamin D deficiency, steatorrhea), in others from hyperphosphatemia (renal failure). In pregnancy, it is a consequence of the increased requirement for calcium during the period of growth of the fetal skeleton. During lactation, the serum calcium tends to decrease as a result of excretion of calcium in the milk.

There should be no confusion between primary hyperparathyroidism and these conditions of "secondary hyperparathyroidism." With the exception of the last-named group of miscellaneous skeletal diseases, which probably do not belong in this category, hypercalcemia does not occur in these disorders. The enlargement and hyperactivity of the parathyroid glands constitute a mechanism designed to maintain a normal plasma calcium level in the face of a tendency toward hypocalcemia. If the blood calcium concentration should rise above normal, parathyroid activity would be depressed automatically, with prompt decrease in the serum calcium. This fact, together with differences in serum phosphate and phosphatase activity, usually aids materially in distinguishing between true, i.e., primary hyperparathyroidism and "secondary hyperparathyroidism."

Hyperparathyroidism has also been implicated as an etiologic factor in *scleroderma.* This association has been predicated on the basis of the occasional occurrence of calcinosis in scleroderma and the experimental production of scleroderma-like lesions by administration of parathyroid hormone. However, there is no substantial evidence that this condition is accompanied by a state of hyperparathyroidism.

A state of hyperparathyroidism (*primary hyperparathyroidism*) is the functional basis for the development of the condition variously designated as generalized osteitis fibrosa cystica, von Recklinghausen's disease of bone, parathyroid osteosis, osteodystrophia cystica and osteodystrophia fibrosa. The term "hyperparathyroidism" is to be preferred inasmuch as it indicates the essential nature of the disorder and not only do the other designations emphasize only a single aspect of the pathologic changes, but they may give an erroneous impression of the character of the skeletal lesions. Moreover, all of these lesions may occur in other conditions in which the factor of hyperparathyroidism is not implicated.

Etiology. The condition has been produced in experimental animals by administration of parathyroid hormone. Excessive secretion of this hormone is the cause of the subjective and objective manifestations of clinical forms of the disease. It is due to either (1) focal hyperplasia (adenoma) of one or more parathyroid glands or (2) hyperplasia or hypertrophy of all parathyroid glands.

Pathology.[30] One or more parathyroid glands are practically invariably involved in a neoplastic, hyperplastic or hypertrophic process. Adenomas have been found in about 86 per cent of cases and diffuse hyperplasia in about 14 per cent. In the neoplastic group, a single gland is involved in over 90 per cent of instances, the lower parathyroids being affected about five times as frequently as the upper. Tumors of aberrant parathyroid tissue have been found within the thyroid and the thymus glands and in the mediastinum (retrosternal). A few cases have been reported of *carcinoma* of the parathyroid glands accompanied by metabolic features of hyperparathyroidism. Occasionally the syndrome may occur in the absence of demonstrable morphologic abnormality of the parathyroids, but in such cases the possibility of aberrant parathyroid tissue must be considered. It should also be emphasized that enlargement of these glands (hyperplasia) frequently occurs as a secondary phenomenon, without clinical or metabolic manifestations of hyperparathyroidism, in such conditions as rickets, osteomalacia, renal disease, skeletal carcinomatosis, multiple myeloma and pregnancy.

In cases of diffuse hypertrophy or hyperplasia the total *weight* of the parathyroid glands may be as great as 19 gm., more than 100 times normal. Adenomatous glands weighing as much as 300 gm. have been reported, but characteristic manifestations have been observed with tumors only twice the size of a normal gland. In contrast to the neoplastic cases, in those with diffuse hyperplasia or hypertrophy there appears to be a distinct correlation between weight of parathyroid tissue and degree of hyperparathyroidism. Histologically, these glands are characterized by the uniformity of their structure, the enormous size of the cells, the extreme clearness of the cytoplasm (wasserhelle Zelle) and the tendency to glandular formation. Rarely the dominant cell type is the so-called "chief cell." In the localized tumors, involving a portion of one gland, a whole gland or, occasionally, portions of two glands, the histologic picture is much less uniform. The tumors may be composed almost entirely of chief cells, wasserhelle cells or oxyphil cells or any combination of these elements, with gland formation in one area, broad anastomosing cords in another and solid cell masses elsewhere. Acute necrosis and hemorrhage may occur within these tumors. This has been suggested as an explanation for the spontaneous remissions that occur occasionally.

Parathyroid adenomas, usually multiple, have been reported, in association with multiple pancreatic islet tumors, in subjects with pituitary tumors, mainly eosinophilic (acromegaly), but also chromophobic. The basis for these relationships is not known.

The *skeletal lesions*[6] vary considerably and include generalized demineralization, multiple foci of osteitis fibrosa with or without benign giant cell tumors and single or multilocular cysts, hemorrhages, cortical thinning, and localized expansion of the bones leading to fracture and deformity, which may be of extreme grade. Every conceivable variation may occur, from mild osteoporosis, with slight fibrosis, to extensive cystic change with giant cell tumor. The periosteum may be thinned and the medullary cavity filled with grayish white fibrous tissue interspersed with fine reticulated bone. Decalcification may be of so extreme a grade that the affected bones can be readily cut with a knife. The long tubular bones are usually the seat of earliest and most extensive involvement. Next in order of involvement are the vertebrae, sacrum, pelvis, skull, jaw bones, flat bones of the thorax and the short tubular bones of the hands and feet.

On histologic examination there is an increase in the number of osteoclasts, connective tissue proliferation, and fibrosis of the marrow. These areas of fibrosis may contain giant cells, fresh or old extravasated blood, single or multiple cystic spaces, giant cell tumors and finely reticulated bone. In the long bones, the greatest amount of regeneration and repair usually occurs in the diaphyses, the epiphyses showing no change or only osteoporosis.

Changes may occur in other tissues. The majority result from the direct action of excessive amounts of parathyroid hormone or from precipitation of calcium phosphate, or are the consequences of these phenomena. In acute forms of hyperparathyroidism, which are rare clinically, degenerative changes may be found in the renal tubular epithelium, heart muscle and gastric mucosa. Calcific deposits, probably erroneously termed "metastatic" calcification, may occur in these situations and also in the lungs and walls of the arteries. Serious pathologic changes in the kidneys are perhaps the most common of the extra-skeletal lesions, occurring in about 50 per cent of cases. These consist of nephrolithiasis (calcium phosphate calculi), pyelonephritis, and calcific deposits in the lumen of the tubules and in the peritubular and interstitial tissue, with interstitial fibrosis and contraction.[29]

Compression of the spinal cord has been observed as a result of collapse or fracture of thoracic or lumbar vertebrae. Decubitus ulcers, pneumonia and urinary tract infection may develop in the terminal stages.

Duodenal ulcer has been present in 20 to 25 per cent of a few reported series of cases of hyperparathyroidism, and symptoms strongly suggestive of peptic ulcer in an additional 15 to 20 per cent.[31] The basis of this relationship is not clear, but it seems to be more than coincidental. The parathyroid hormone has been reported to stimulate gastric secretion of pepsin.

Clinical Features. SEX AND AGE. About 70 per cent of the reported cases have been in women, the predominance of females over males being slightly greater in the adenoma than in the hyperplastic group. The condition occurs most commonly between the ages of twenty and sixty years, but has been observed at two years of age, probably beginning in the first year. Such cases are rare.

The frequency of most important early and late symptoms and signs is outlined in Table 5. The most striking and important clinical features are usually referable to involvement of the skeleton and kidneys and to the level of calcium in the body fluids. It is important to appreciate the fact that certain patients with hyperparathyroidism may present few or no skeletal manifestations, and others few if any urinary tract symptoms. Some have no demonstrable involvement of either of these systems when first seen, despite the presence of characteristic metabolic features.

SKELETAL CHANGES. There may be no symptoms referable to the skeleton. In the majority of instances, however, one or more of the following are present: bone pain and tenderness, bone tumor, kyphosis or other deformity, spontaneous fractures, clubbing of the fingers (due to loss of supporting substance), waddling gait and limp. At times, the earliest clinical indication of the presence of this condition is the discovery of a giant cell tumor of the jaw (*epulis*). Pain may be severe and, being frequently referred to the joints of the lower extremities and to the spine, is often erroneously regarded as arthritic. Demonstrable changes may be minimal or absent in early stages or in the rarely encountered instances of rapidly pro-

TABLE 3. SEX INCIDENCE OF HYPERPARATHYROIDISM*

	PER CENT Females	Males
Total cases	70	30
Adenoma (88 per cent)	70.6	29.4
Hyperplasia (12 per cent)	66.7	33.3

* After Castleman and Mallory.[30]

the findings are not pathognomonic, except perhaps in advanced and classic forms of the disease.[4] The important *radiographic manifestations* include generalized osteoporosis, cysts, fractures, tumors, deformities and a granular, mottled appearance of the calvarium. There may be no demonstrable skeletal abnormality, or only a slight degree of demineralization. In advanced cases the most marked changes are usually ob-

TABLE 4. AGE INCIDENCE OF HYPERPARATHYROIDISM

	AGE IN YEARS 0–9	10–19	20–29	30–39	40–49	50–59	60–69	70–79	80–89
Total cases	0	12	29	29	46	45	12	8	1
Adenoma	2	11	26	27	39	40	11	5	1
Hyperplasia	0	1	3	2	7	5	1	3	0

TABLE 5. SYMPTOMS OF HYPERPARATHYROIDISM

	PER CENT Early	Late
Skeletal		
Pain in back or extremities	47	40
Deformities	27	35
Fractures	18	24
Difficult gait	15	14
Muscle weakness	14	15
Bedfast	2	18
Enlarged skull	0	1
Renal		
Polyuria, polydipsia	6	8
Colic	6	2
Gastrointestinal		
Nausea, vomiting, anorexia	8	14
Epigastric pain	2	4
Miscellaneous		
Marked weight loss	8	12
Deafness	0	1
Paresthesias	0	2

gressive acute hyperparathyroidism. There is reason to believe that the extent of bone involvement is an index of the duration rather than of the severity of the disease.

The x-ray is of great value in diagnosis, but it must be emphasized that

served in the long bones. The order of involvement of the remainder of the skeleton is as follows: vertebrae, pelvis, calvarium, jaw bones, thorax and bones of the hands and feet. Obviously, the effect of the hyperparathyroid state in promoting mobilization of Ca and P must be exerted upon the entire skeleton and, therefore, more or less generalized decalcification is an absolutely essential feature of the x-ray picture, regardless of the presence or extent of other changes.

The *long bones* show cortical thinning, the trabeculae becoming indistinct and the shadow light and homogeneous, or the medullary cavity may appear to be expanded. If new trabeculae are formed, the bone may present a finely mottled, granular appearance. There may be single or multilocular cysts, often accompanied by marked localized expansion and surrounded by only a thin shell of bone. Fractures are common and tend to unite readily. Giant-cell tumors are not uncommon in both long and short tubular bones. Cysts, too, are seen in the small bones of the hands and feet. These changes may be associated with a variable degree of deformity. Similar manifestations may be observed in the spine; biconcavity of the vertebrae may result from extreme softening.

The calvarium may be thinned and porotic, it may present a finely mottled granular appearance, or it may be irregularly or generally thickened, resembling the changes in Paget's disease. The remainder of the skull usually shows evidence of osteoporosis, occasionally with cysts and giant cell tumors in the mandible and maxillae. The pelvis and scapulae often show decalcification and cyst formation, with deformities and fractures in the former, due probably to the excessive strain to which it is subjected.

Calcific deposits may be observed in soft tissues, especially in the kidneys and lower urinary passages (calculi) or, occasionally, in the arteries.

GASTROINTESTINAL SYMPTOMS. Anorexia and constipation are often troublesome features, due probably to the existing hypercalcemia, with consequent gastrointestinal atony. There may be periodic, recurring bouts of nausea and vomiting, at times with severe abdominal pain, these attacks usually lasting from a few days to two weeks. These manifestations are generally attributed to acute parathyroid intoxication.

Typical duodenal ulcer symptoms may be present. This condition (peptic ulcer) apparently occurs with unusual frequency in patients with hyperparathyroidism (20 to 25 per cent).[31] The basis for this association is not clear, although parathyroid hormone has been reported to increase gastric pepsin. Cases of this type must not be confused with peptic ulcer patients presenting the syndrome of hypercalcemia and alkalosis due to excessive ingestion of milk and absorbable alkalies (p. 209).

URINARY TRACT SYMPTOMS. These include polyuria, polydipsia, frequency of urination, enuresis, nocturia, dysuria, renal colic, hematuria, pyuria, ureteral obstruction and other manifestations of stone in the urinary passages or renal failure. These symptoms are due primarily to the increased excretion of Ca and P by the kidneys and, perhaps, to deposition of calcium salts in the kidneys as a result of hypercalcemia and degenerative changes in the tubular epithelium. Renal complications have been reported in 30 to 70 per cent of cases of hyperparathyroidism. These may be classified under three headings:

1. Precipitation of calcium phosphate in the renal pelvis with calculus formation and resulting pyelonephritis.

2. Precipitation in the uriniferous tubules (nephrocalcinosis), with resulting nephrosclerosis, contraction and renal functional impairment, with or without hypertension. In some cases the calcium deposits in the kidneys are demonstrable by x-rays.

3. Precipitation in the kidneys as a part of the process of precipitation in various soft tissues, with acute renal failure and death in a few hours or days. This seldom occurs clinically, and only in very acute forms of hyperparathyroidism. Death in such cases is associated with circulatory collapse; this feature and the rapidly progressive renal failure have been attributed to dehydration and marked plasma sodium and chloride deficit resulting from the excessive loss of these elements in the urine.

It is important to note that these renal lesions can occur in the absence of demonstrable skeletal changes, the former being an index of the severity and the latter of the duration of the disease. It has been estimated that hyperparathyroidism is the etiologic factor in about 0.3 per cent of cases of urinary lithiasis. The latter may be the first clinical evidence of this condition.

MISCELLANEOUS SYMPTOMS. Lassitude and muscular weakness are common early symptoms, and there may be difficulty in muscular coordination. These are probably dependent upon muscular hypotonia due to hypercalcemia. This is evidenced objectively by diminished electrical excitability of muscles and nerves (p. 192). Another interesting manifestation is shortening of the R-T interval in the electrocardiogram, which may be reduced to about 0.22 second (normally 0.26 to 0.28 second; in hypocalcemic tetany, 0.30 to 0.34 second).

There may be a variety of rather bizarre neurotic, psychotic and neurologic manifestations, including disorientation, blindness, convulsions and coma. These are most pronounced usually in cases with extreme grades of hypercalcemia and have been attributed to deposition of calcium salts in the brain.

Loss of appetite and loss of weight are nearly always present and may lead to profound emaciation. There may be extreme dehydration and base deficit as a result of prolonged polyuria and loss of sodium and other electrolytes in the urine. Respiratory difficulty and reduction in height may result from deformities in the thorax (kyphosis and scoliosis) and extremities (bowing, knock-knee, etc.), due to softening and fractures. Stunting of growth has been observed in cases in which the skeletal changes had progressed before full physiologic growth had been attained. Occasionally, a parathyroid tumor may be palpable in the neck, but owing to their position behind the thyroid or in the mediastinum, even extremely large parathyroid glands may not be visible or palpable from the surface. The trachea or esophagus may be displaced by enlarged glands. Metastatic calcification and visceral hemorrhages may occur in very acute phases of the disease.

Metabolic Manifestations. The characteristic, indeed, almost pathognomic metabolic manifestations are: (a) hypercalcemia, (b) hypophosphatemia, (c) increased urinary excretion of Ca and (d) increased serum phosphatase activity. It is the combination of all these rather than the presence of any one that is of diagnostic significance.

In typical cases the serum Ca has ranged from 12.5 to 29.4 mg. per 100 cc. Values above 20 mg. are rare. Occasionally, the serum Ca may be within normal limits, but repeated determinations usually reveal hypercalcemia at some time during the course of the disease. Hypercalcemia is probably invariably present during periods of progression of the skeletal lesions and in the presence of active symptoms. It is possible that there may be periods of temporary latency of the condition, as in the case of hyperthyroidism; under such circumstances the characteristic metabolic features will be lacking and accurate diagnosis may be impossible. Spontaneous remission may possibly occur as a result of necrosis or hemorrhage in adenomatous glands.[32] Such remissions may be preceded by a brief period of severe acute exacerbation of the disease. There is also experimental basis for the possibility that the serum Ca concentration may return to normal or even subnormal levels following a period of hypercalcemia with exhaustion of the mobilizable Ca reserves in the bones, particularly if the Ca intake is inadequate. Occasionally, relatively low or normal values may be obtained in cases complicated by renal failure, with high serum P levels. Similar difficulty in producing hypercalcemia by parathyroid hormone has been reported in nephrectomized animals. Accurate diagnosis is difficult under such circumstances (p. 222).

The *serum inorganic P concentration* is subnormal in typical uncomplicated cases, ranging from 1 to 2.5 mg. per 100 cc. in adults and to 3.5 mg. in young children. This finding is not as constant as is hypercalcemia, chiefly perhaps because of the frequent coexistence of a variable degree of renal functional impairment, which tends to produce an increase in serum P. In advanced renal failure increased concentrations may be observed, accompanied by nitrogen retention and a tendency toward lowering of the previously elevated serum Ca values, at times to subnormal levels. Under such circumstances the condition may be confused with "renal rickets" (p. 223).

The *serum phosphatase activity* is usually, but not invariably increased, usually ranging from 6.5 to 25 Bodansky units, and occasionally as high as 60 units. The relatively slight increase in the majority of instances (as compared, for example, to the findings in Paget's disease) contrasts strikingly with the extent of the skeletal changes. This is due to the fact that the phosphatase activity is probably a reflection of the degree of osteoblastic activity, which is usually rather low in hyperparathyroidism.

Abnormally large amounts of Ca are eliminated in the urine, especially under conditions of low Ca and comparatively low P intake. Under such circumstances the urinary Ca may exceed the quantity ingested and may constitute 70 to 90 per cent of the total output. The organism is in a state of negative Ca and usually also negative P balance, this being most readily demonstrated when the intake of these elements is maintained at a low level for test periods of at least three days (calcium 0.11 gm., phosphorus 0.4 gm. daily). In contrast to other conditions accompanied by negative Ca and P balance (rickets, osteomalacia), the loss occurs chiefly by way of the kidneys rather than the bowel.

Other Laboratory Findings. Extensive fibrosis and cystic changes in the bone marrow may result in an aplastic type of anemia, with leukopenia and, occasionally, thrombopenia. During periods of severe acute hyperparathyroidism there may be manifestations of hemoconcentration (increased plasma protein concentration and increasing hematocrit values), hypochloremia, and evidences of renal failure (hyperphosphatemia, nitrogen retention, acidosis). Prolonged vomiting may be accompanied by oliguria. Bence Jones proteinuria has been reported. In the presence of urinary tract complications the urine may contain albumin, casts, leukocytes, red blood cells and bacteria. Small calcium phosphate calculi may be passed.

Prognosis. Hyperparathyroidism is an insidious disease, usually of long duration. Except in rare instances of the very acute form, death results usually from complications such as renal failure, respiratory and urinary tract and other infections, cardiac failure, inanition, etc. Temporary spontaneous remissions may occur, but the condition tends to become progressively worse unless proper treatment is instituted. In many reported instances of apparently spontaneous remission there is considerable question as to the accuracy of the diagnosis. Permanent and complete cure, with healing of the bone lesions, has followed surgical removal of affected glands.

Diagnosis.[34,35] Cases of hyperparathyroidism may be roughly classified under four headings on the basis of the predominant clinical manifestations:[29]

1. CLASSIC HYPERPARATHYROIDISM (VON RECKLINGHAUSEN). In this form there are pain, spontaneous fractures, skeletal deformities, bone cysts and tumors and generalized decalcification.

2. OSTEOPOROTIC FORM. The bone changes in this type are practically identical with those of hyperthyroidism, osteomalacia, inactivity or senile osteoporosis. Significant symptoms may be absent.

3. RENAL FORM. The presenting symptoms may be those of urinary lithiasis, pyelonephritis or renal functional insufficiency. Skeletal changes may be absent, minimal, or extreme. Diffuse nephrocalcinosis may be demonstrable by the x-ray.

4. ACUTE HYPERPARATHYROIDISM. This form is rarely encountered clinically. The manifestations are those of acute experimental parathyroid intoxication, and include nausea, vomiting, prostration, hematemesis, melena, diarrhea, visceral hemorrhages, the shock syndrome and renal failure. Manifestations suggestive of this condition have been observed to occur for a brief period immediately following acute necrosis of adenomatous glands. This has been followed by remission of all symptoms and return of the serum calcium to a normal level.[32]

Because of the variability of the clinical manifestations and skeletal changes, the diagnosis of hyperparathyroidism must rest finally upon demonstration of the characteristic group of metabolic features, namely, (a) hypercalcemia, (b) hypophosphatemia, (c) excessive calcinuria on a low Ca, relatively low P intake, (d) increased serum phosphatase activity and, although unsatisfactory in our experience, an excessive quantity of parathyroid hormone in the blood (Hamilton and Schwartz).[33] In the absence of one or more of these findings, particularly the first three, accurate diagnosis is difficult. This difficulty arises most commonly in those cases accompanied by advanced renal insufficiency, in which the serum Ca may be normal or subnormal, the serum P increased and urinary Ca excretion relatively low.

The following procedures may be useful in selected cases.

CALCIUM TOLERANCE.[36] 1. The subject is given an identical diet for three successive days, with breakfast at 8 A.M. Urine is collected in 24-hour periods from (a) 8 A.M. of the second day to 8 A.M. of the third day and (b) from 8 A.M. of the third day to 8 A.M. (before breakfast) of the fourth day.

2. On the third day, one hour after breakfast, infuse intravenously, over a four-hour period, 1 liter of 0.85 per cent NaCl solution containing calcium gluconate-glucoheptonate in an amount that will provide 15 mg. Ca per kilogram body weight. Meals are given as on the preceding days.

3. Five samples of blood are obtained (for determinations of calcium, inorganic phosphorus and total protein concentrations) as follows: (a) before starting the infusion; (b) in the middle (two hours); (c) at the end; (d) four hours after the end; (e) twenty-four hours after the start of the infusion.

4. The inorganic phosphorus excretion is determined for each of the two 24-hour urine collections.

Interpretation. This test procedure is based on the principle that, in normal subjects, elevation of the serum Ca concentration depresses secretion of parathyroid hormone, with consequent rise in serum inorganic phosphorus concentration and sharp decrease in phosphorus excretion in the urine (p. 198).

In subjects with hyperparathyroidism, the average rise in serum Ca and P is smaller, and the urine excretion of phosphate extremely variable, being smaller, unchanged, or actually larger, as compared with the pre-injection level.

PARATHYROID ACTIVITY INDEX.[37] The extent of renal tubular reabsorption of inorganic phosphate is calculated on the basis of the following determinations: (1) glomerular filtration rate (inulin or creatinine clearance); (2) plasma inorganic phosphorus concentration; (3) urinary phosphorus excretion.

Interpretation. This test procedure is based upon the principle that the extent of tubular reabsorption of phosphorus is an index of the level of circulating parathyroid hormone. In subjects with normal parathyroid function, 50 to 75 per cent of the phosphorus of the glomerular filtrate is reabsorbed in the tubules. In those with hypoparathyroidism, a larger proportion is reabsorbed, and in hyperparathyroidism a smaller proportion. The value of this procedure in the diagnosis of hyperparathyroidism is limited by the frequent co-existence of kidney damage.

Hyperparathyroidism must be differentiated from a number of skeletal disorders with which it may be confused if careful metabolic studies are not made, and also from other conditions accompanied by hypercalcemia.

Differential Diagnosis. POLYOSTOTIC FIBROUS DYSPLASIA.[38,39] This condition has been described in the literature under a variety of designations, including osteodystrophia fibrosa unilateralis, osteitis fibrosa localisata, osteodystrophia fibrosa cystica generalisata, fibrous osteodystrophy and osteitis fibrosa disseminata. It is probably much more common than hyperparathyroidism and the majority of cases have undoubtedly in the past been erroneously regarded as the latter, to which it is entirely unrelated etiologically. The following features differentiate it from hyperparathyroidism:

1. It occurs most often in children and young adults, more frequently in females.

2. Symptoms commonly date back to early childhood, the condition evolving very slowly over a period of years or decades.

3. The characteristic pathologic feature is apparently a disturbed development or function of the bone-forming mesenchyme, resulting in filling of the medullary cavity of the affected bones by fibrous tissue, with areas of collagenous differentiation, hyaline cartilage

or spicules of primitive fiber bone. These bones may present an x-ray picture indistinguishable from that of true osteitis fibrosa cystica (hyperparathyroidism). Epiphyses as well as diaphyses may be affected.

4. The progress of the condition tends to become less active with advancing years and a condition of equilibrium may be established with restoration of function, although the normal bone structure is not restored.

5. The involvement is predominantly unilateral, but lesions may occur on the opposite side.

6. Unaffected portions of the skeleton show no evidence of demineralization, except that resulting from disuse.

7. In girls, there may be precocious puberty and some cases have shown areas of cutaneous pigmentation having a distribution related to the osseous changes.

8. Except for the very occasional occurrence of slight hypercalcemia and slightly increased serum phosphatase activity, there is no evidence of abnormality of Ca or P metabolism.

MULTIPLE MYELOMA. Multiple myeloma may simulate hyperparathyroidism clinically, roentgenographically, and chemically. However, the distribution of the skeletal lesions is usually somewhat different and demineralization is rarely, if ever, generalized. Hypercalcemia may be present, often to a marked degree, but it is frequently accompanied by increase in serum globulins. The serum P concentration is rarely subnormal and is frequently increased (renal failure). The serum phosphatase activity is rarely increased. Excessive calcinuria may occur in the presence of hypercalcemia. Bence Jones proteinuria is present in the majority of cases, while it is observed rarely in hyperparathyroidism. Secondary enlargement of the parathyroid glands has been described. In doubtful cases, marrow puncture or bone biopsy is the only certain way to establish the correct diagnosis.

GENERALIZED SKELETAL XANTHOMATOSIS. Typical forms of the Hand-Schüller-Christian syndrome present no difficulty in diagnosis. Cases of xanthomatosis involving only the long bones, pelvis or calvarium may, however, be confused with hyperparathyroidism on the basis of the x-ray appearance of the bones and the occurrence of spontaneous fractures. However, diffuse demineralization is absent, as are the usual metabolic manifestations of hyperparathyroidism, there is often an increase in plasma cholesterol esters, cutaneous lesions are common, and histologic examination of the affected bones (biopsy) reveals the characteristic vacuolated "foam" cells containing cholesterol.

The bone changes in *Gaucher's* and in *Niemann-Pick's* disease may present an x-ray picture resembling that of hyperparathyroidism. These conditions, however, usually present other characteristic features, including splenomegaly, hepatomegaly and pulmonary involvement; there is rarely evidence of abnormality of Ca and P metabolism, the serum phosphatase activity is normal, and examination of material obtained by marrow or splenic puncture or bone biopsy usually reveals the lipid-containing cells typical of those conditions.

RENAL RICKETS. Renal rickets may present all of the cardinal clinical and laboratory features of the osteoporotic type of hyperparathyroidism complicated by renal functional impairment. It usually differs from the latter, however, in the following respects:

1. The renal impairment antedates the bone changes and, frequently, there is a long history of renal disease, often with hypertension and its attendant cardiovascular manifestations. If the onset occurs in early childhood, growth may be stunted (dwarfism).

2. The underlying cause is usually chronic glomerulonephritis, chronic pyelonephritis or renal hypogenesis. Consequently, urinary lithiasis or nephrocalcinosis are rare in this condition, whereas they constitute a common basis for the development of advanced renal functional impairment in hyperparathyroidism.

Parathyroid hyperplasia, at times of marked degree, may occur in advanced renal insufficiency. It has been regarded as a response to hyperphosphatemia and the skeletal demineralization has been attributed to chronic acidosis, the excretion of abnormally large amounts of Ca and P by the bowel and, perhaps, to the development of a state of secondary hyperparathyroidism, especially in cases of congenital urinary tract defect, when the exact time of onset of renal functional impairment cannot be established. Metastatic calcification, especially in the arteries, has been observed in renal rickets and, occasionally, there may be changes in the bones resembling the cysts and giant cell tumors of osteitis fibrosa cystica. The serum Ca concentration is usually normal or subnormal, and the serum P concentration is increased. However, the significance of these findings in differential diagnosis is diminished by the fact that the supervention of renal failure in true primary hyperparathyroidism tends to produce an increase in the previously low serum P and a fall in the previously elevated serum Ca concentration. Frequently the only possible means of differentiating the two conditions is to decipher the course of events leading to the combination of skeletal lesions and renal impairment.

VITAMIN D DEFICIENCY (OSTEOMALACIA.) The term osteomalacia, which was formerly applied to a variety of dissimilar bone disorders, should now be applied only to that condition dependent upon and associated with deficiency in Ca, P and vitamin D. It is the adult counterpart of childhood rickets (p. 238). The parathyroid glands may be somewhat enlarged. It differs from hyperparathyroidism in the following respects:

1. The serum Ca is normal or subnormal, the urinary Ca excretion is not increased, and excessive amounts of Ca and P are lost in the feces.

2. Although the appearance of the bones may resemble superficially that in the osteoporotic form of hyperparathyroidism, fibrosis is minimal, the trabeculae have wide osteoid borders and there are few osteoclasts.

3. Osteomalacia responds promptly to administration of adequate amounts of Ca, P and vitamin D, which have no beneficial effect on the course of hyperparathyroidism.

The skeletal lesions of late rickets in adolescent children may resemble osteitis fibrosa cystica, particularly in bowing of the lower extremities and widening of the metaphyses. The criteria useful in differential diagnosis are identical with those outlined for osteomalacia.

PAGET'S DISEASE (OSTEITIS DEFORMANS). Formerly, osteitis deformans and osteitis fibrosa cystica were regarded by many as variants of the same fundamental process. This opinion was based largely upon occasional superficial similarities in the x-ray appearance of the bones; among these are thickening and mottling of the calvarium, and diffuse sclerosis, cortical thickening, and coarsely striated trabeculation at times observed in the bones of the extremities in hyperparathyroidism. In some instances confusion has undoubtedly resulted from the coexistence of the two conditions. However, there is no valid evidence that the parathyroids are implicated in the pathogenesis or etiology of Paget's disease. Hypercalcemia and hypophosphatemia rarely occur, Ca and P balances are normal, serum phosphatase activity is usually greatly increased (in the polyostotic form), the skeletal lesions are localized, the periosteum is almost always involved, giant cell tumors are usually absent, and the cortex of the long tubular bones is usually lamellated. Enlargement of the parathyroid glands is rare and fractures seldom occur. Hypercalcemia has been reported in occasional cases in which there is extensive and rapid demineralization, but the serum phosphorus concentration is normal or elevated in such cases. The condition has also been reported in association with true hyperparathyroidism.

METASTATIC MALIGNANCY. Metastatic malignancy of the bones may be mistaken for hyperparathyroidism. This, as in other skeletal lesions, is due chiefly to the x-ray appearance of the bones, but also in some cases to the occurrence of hypercalcemia. However, the differentiation should be made readily on the bases of (a) age, (b) demonstration of a primary site of the malignant process, (c) distribution of the skeletal lesions, which are seldom below the knees or elbows in metastatic carcinoma, and (d) the normal appearance of the rest of the skeleton and the absence of hypophosphatemia. In rare instances the parathyroid glands may be the seat of metastases. The development of hypercalcemia during the course of sex steroid therapy of breast cancer is referred to elsewhere (p. 208).

OSTEOPOROSIS OF OTHER ORIGIN. The osteoporotic lesions of hyperparathyroidism may be simulated roentgenographically by similar changes resulting from a variety of causes. These include senile osteoporosis, and that associated with disuse or inactivity, hyperthyroidism, pituitary basophilism and hypercorticoadrenalism. In the great majority of instances these conditions present few if any diagnostic difficulties.

In *senile osteoporosis* the serum and urinary Ca and P and serum phosphatase activity are normal. The skeletal lesion is characterized by chronic atrophy of the marrow, absence of osteoid borders, and occasionally brown areas of hemosiderin and oil cysts in the long bones resulting from liquefaction of the fatty marrow. The parathyroid glands may be slightly enlarged. A type of osteoporosis occurring in women after the menopause (natural or artificial) and, occasionally in men also, has been termed postmenopausal osteoporosis.[40] The spine and pelvis are most commonly and most extensively involved, the long bones less frequently, and the skull almost never, in contrast to hyperparathyroidism. There is often fracture or crushing of the vertebrae and herniation of the nucleus pulposus through the vertebral end plates. The serum calcium concentration is normal in uncomplicated cases and the serum phosphorus is usually normal, occasionally slightly low.

Acute bone atrophy, occurring, especially in children, during periods of rapid demineralization, as in immobilization of the extremities due to fracture or paralysis (poliomyelitis) (p. 209), may occasionally present some difficulty in differential diagnosis because of the occasional elevation of serum calcium concentration, particularly in the presence of simultaneous renal functional impairment. However, the attendant circumstances and the absence of hypophosphatemia should enable the differentiation from hyperparathyroidism to be made readily. In *pituitary basophilism*, adrenal cortical tumor and hyperthyroidism, the diagnosis is usually made readily on the basis of the characteristic features of those conditions. The urinary Ca excretion may be increased but the other metabolic manifestations of hyperparathyroidism are lacking. Hyperplasia of the parathyroid glands has been reported in pituitary basophilism; in this condition and in cortical tumor, demineralization is usually confined chiefly to the vertebrae.

MISCELLANEOUS CONDITIONS. Localized skeletal lesions may simulate hyperparathyroidism roentgenographically. These include solitary giant cell tumors, focal osteitis fibrosa cystica, solitary cysts and multiple enchondromata. In these disorders there is no evidence of abnormality of Ca or P metabolism, and serum phosphatase activity is normal, as are the bones except for the areas involved in the local processes.

A syndrome has been described, characterized by (a) multiple bone cysts with a distribution suggesting a relation to nerve roots or to an embryologic defect in the myotomes; (b) areas of pigmentation with a distribution suggesting some connection with the bone cysts; (c) precocious puberty in females but apparently not in males.[41] The bone lesions appear to be of the nature of fibrous osseous dysplasia (p. 222), and the condition is not accompanied by demonstrable evidence of abnormality in calcium of phosphorus metabolism.

Neurofibromatosis (von Recklinghausen) may be accompanied by a variety of osseous changes, cystic, atrophic, and demineralization and deformity. These changes may occur in the skull, vertebrae and long bones, and have been observed in the absence of cutaneous and subcutaneous lesions. There is no abnormality in serum calcium or phosphorus.[42]

The occurrence of hypercalcemia in sarcoidosis is referred to elsewhere (p. 209). The combination of hypercalcemia, increased serum alkaline phosphatase activity, hypercalciuria, urinary calculi, nephrocalcinosis, renal failure and skeletal lesions may superficially be suggestive of hyperparathyroidism. This possibility can usually be eliminated readily by the following features of sarcoidosis: (a) absence of hypophosphatemia; (b) presence, usually, of hyperglobulinemia; (c) absence of generalized demineralization; (4) rather characteristic localization of chief bone lesions in hands and feet.

Osteoporosis and other lesions of hyperparathyroidism may be simulated roentgenographically by bone changes in certain cases of leukemia, Hodgkin's disease, polycythemia vera, erythroblastic and hemolytic anemias, osteomyelitis, radium poisoning and osteogenesis imperfecta. In certain experimental animals the administration of large doses of parathyroid hormone over long periods may result in skeletal changes resembling those of "marble bone" disease (Albers-Schönberg), in which condition parathyroid hyperplasia has been reported.[43] This has prompted the suggestion that this rare disorder may represent a special form of hyperparathyroidism, but there is no metabolic evidence that such is the case. Hypercalcemia may occur occasionally in leukemia and in polycythemia vera. However, with occasional exceptions, none of these conditions is accompanied by abnormality of Ca or P metabolism, and their differentiation from hyperparathyroidism can usually be made readily on the basis of the rather typical clinical and laboratory manifestations in each instance.

Hypervitaminosis D, due to administration of excessive amounts of vitamin D, may superficially mimic hyperparathyroidism in certain respects. The important features of this condition are discussed elsewhere (p. 240).

Treatment. *Roentgen therapy* has been practically entirely unsatisfactory in cases due to adenoma, resulting in neither symptomatic nor metabolic improvement. There is some indication, however, that better results may be obtained in those due to generalized hyperplasia or hypertrophy. Unfortunately, the distinction between the two forms can be made only by surgical exploration. It has been suggested that irradiation therapy may be useful under the following conditions: (a) when operative procedures are contraindicated; (b) when a tumor has not been found at operation; (c) when part of an adenoma has been left behind at operation.

Medical treatment consists essentially in administration of a diet high in Ca and P, usually supplemented by Ca and P salts. This has resulted in some cases in definite improvement in the skeletal lesions, which is usually only temporary. Moreover, it is not without danger, since it aggravates the existing tendency toward deposition of lime salts in soft tissues, the development of renal complications, dangerous hypercalcemia and circulatory failure.

The treatment of acute fulminating hyperparathyroidism (p. 221) consists essentially in intravenous administration of solutions of sodium chloride and dextrose for the purpose of replenishing Na and Cl and maintaining renal function. In this condition, in which an extremely high serum calcium concentration may be of immediate concern, a procedure may be resorted to, as a temporary measure, which has been suggested for the management of hypercalcemia occurring in the course of treatment of patients with breast cancer (p. 208).[44] This consists in intravenous infusion of 250 cc. of 2.5 per cent sodium citrate solution, repeated if necessary. This may serve to minimize precipitation of calcium salts in the kidneys and urinary tract, through the formation of a poorly dissociable calcium citrate complex, thus reducing the concentration of calcium ions.

There have been attempts to use the active chelating agent, ethylenediaminetetraacetic acid (EDTA) in the management of the hypercalcemia. This compound forms a complex with calcium ions that is almost entirely non-ionized at *p*H 7.4, the calcium atom of the complex being therefore inactive physiologically. Intravenous injection of large amounts of the sodium salt of EDTA can readily induce hypocalcemia in laboratory animals. However, although reduction in serum calcium has been produced by this means in patients with hypercalcemia, the effect is quite transient (up to a few hours).[45] No significant clinical benefits have been observed. It is conceivable, however, that this form of therapy may be useful in acute hyperparathyroidism. The dosage employed has been about 200 mg./kg. of sodium-EDTA in 3 per cent solution injected intravenously over a period of 30 to 60 minutes.

Surgical treatment offers the only hope of permanent benefit. Because of the great difficulty of locating and identifying a parathyroid tumor at operation, it is advisable to attempt to locate it preoperatively by means of roentgenograms designed to demonstrate (a) calcification of the capsule, (b) displacement of the trachea or (c) displacement or filling defect of the esophagus (after swallowing barium). Moreover, it must be realized that parathyroid glands may be present anywhere from the pharynx to the mediastinum, and may be buried in the thyroid gland. At operation, a frozen section from a biopsy specimen should be examined to determine (a) whether it is parathyroid tissue and (b) whether it is normal, adenomatous or hyperplastic. If adenomatous, the affected gland should be removed, provided no normal glands had been removed previously. If this had been done, a piece of the gland somewhat larger than a normal gland should be left and its location marked by a silver suture to facilitate subsequent removal, if necessary. If histologic examination reveals hyperplasia, an attempt must be made to locate all parathyroid glands since all are involved in such cases. It appears advisable to remove about three-fourths of the parathyroid tissue identified.

Postoperative Course. Improvement occurs promptly following removal of diseased parathyroid tissue. Within a few hours the urinary excretion of Ca and P diminishes sharply, as does the urine volume. There may be transitory anuria with manifestations of renal failure. The serum Ca falls rapidly, reaching normal or subnormal levels in twelve to twenty-four hours. The normal serum P and phosphatase activity are restored more gradually, usually after a period of several weeks or months. In some cases the serum P remains low indefinitely. Subjective improvement is likewise prompt. The skeletal lesions gradually disappear over a period of months, bone cysts being the only permanent abnormality, apart from preexisting deformities. Nephrocalcinosis and other renal and urinary tract changes also persist, as do other calcific deposits in soft tissues.

Tetany is the most common complication of parathyroidectomy. It may occur even in cases in which adequate amounts of parathyroid tissue were left and at serum Ca levels as high as 8 mg. per 100 cc. The development of tetany may be dependent upon (a) the extremely rapid fall in serum Ca, (b) atrophy and functional insufficiency of the remaining parathyroids after sudden removal of a hyperfunctioning gland, (c) inadequate amounts of Ca or an excess of P in the diet, and (d) removal of too much parathyroid tissue. Except when due to the latter, the condition is transitory. Treatment is essentially the same as in all forms of parathyroid tetany (p. 232) except that larger amounts of Ca should be administered because of the excessive demand incident to the necessity for skeletal recalcification. Even in the absence of tetany, calcium should be administered orally and parenterally if a large portion of the parathyroid tissue has been removed. Parathyroid hormone or dihydrotachysterol may be required (p. 233). During the period of skeletal recalcification, an optimal or high Ca intake (1 to 1.5 gm.) and an optimal P intake (0.75 to 1 gm.) should be provided, supplemented by 3 to 5 gm. of secondary calcium phosphate ($CaHPO_4$) or other Ca salts (gluconate or lactate) if the bone changes have been extensive. Phosphorus should be administered cautiously in the presence of tetany or hypocalcemia (p. 233). In the absence of the latter, vitamin D may be administered in conjunction with Ca salts in an attempt to facilitate recalcification of the skeleton.

HYPOPARATHYROIDISM AND TETANY[4,5,6]

Tetany is the outstanding clinical manifestation of hypoparathyroidism. Since this symptom complex may be produced by a variety of causes, it seems advisable to consider it here as a clinical entity and to discuss its varied etiology from the standpoint of differential diagnosis.

Tetany is a syndrome characterized by an abnormally increased reaction of the somatic and autonomic motor and sensory nerves to stimuli and by painful, tonic spasms of groups of muscles or even of the entire musculature of the body. This hyperirritability is dependent upon or associated with one or more of the following phenomena: (a) hypocalcemia, with a decrease in the ionized fraction of the serum Ca and also in the nondiffusible fraction; (b) hyperphosphatemia, the increase in serum P perhaps operating to bind and thus inactivate a portion of the serum Ca; (c) alkalosis, which acts probably by depressing Ca ionization; (d) depression of Ca ionization by other factors, such as administration of citrate; (e) hypomagnesemia, which may produce hyperirritability in itself or may act through the medium of causing a portion of the Ca to be bound by phosphate ordinarily bound to Mg.

Clinically, all forms of tetany may be divided into two stages—latent and manifest. The former presents no frank symptoms, but these may be elicited by stimulation of peripheral nerves; the latter is manifested by spontaneous muscular spasms and other manifestations of nervous hyperirritability.

Latent Tetany. The presence of this condition is demonstrated by mechanical or electrical excitation of the hyperexcitable nerves.

ERB PHENOMENON. This important sign depends upon the fact that the neuro-muscular response to galvanic stimulation can be obtained with weaker currents in tetany than under normal conditions. Measurements are usually made on the peroneal or median nerves, the indifferent electrode (50 sq. cm.) being placed on the abdomen and the stimulating electrode (3 sq. cm.) over the nerve. The galvanic battery should be graduated in fifths up to 5 milliamperes. Contractions occur by making or breaking the current (closing or opening contractions) and vary according to the different poles employed (anode or cathode). There are, therefore, four different types of response, *viz.*, cathodal closing (C.C.C.), anodal closing (A.C.C.), cathodal opening (C.O.C.) and anodal opening (A.O.C.) contractions. Typical electrical thresholds in normal subjects are presented in Table 6.

TABLE 6. ELECTRICAL THRESHOLDS IN MILLIAMPERES

AGE	C.C.C.	A.C.C.	C.O.C.	A.O.C.
Under 6 months	3.5	7.0	10.0	9.0
1–2 years	2.5	5.0	8.0	6.0
Over 5 years	1.8	4.0	6.5	3.5

Clinically, the C.O.C. is the most useful reaction, a contraction elicited by less than 5 ma. being highly suggestive of tetany. The A.O.C. is more delicate but more difficult to interpret. Attainment of an A.O.C. with currents less than that required to produce an A.C.C. (anodal reversibility) is also of significance up to the fifth year. These reactions are not infallible. They may vary considerably from time to time and even in normal subjects, and bear no consistent relation to the serum Ca concentration. Nevertheless, the Erb phenomenon is of great value in the diagnosis of latent tetany.

CHRONAXIE. Chronaxie is the length of time necessary to elicit a reaction when a current is employed, the strength of which is twice the rheobase. The rheobase is the minimal galvanic current which, continued indefinitely, suffices to produce a reaction. Normally, it takes about 0.024 second (24 sigma) to elicit a reaction from the flexor pollicis. In tetany it may take only 12 to 14 sigma; in hyperparathyroidism it may take as long as 50 sigma.

CHVOSTEK SIGN (FACIAL PHENOMENON). Hyperexcitability of the facial nerve to mechanical stimulation is elicited by tapping the trunk of the facial nerve (a) immediately anterior to the external auditory meatus or (b) just below the zygomatic process. A positive reaction consists in momentary contraction of the lip, the lip and nose, or the entire side of the face. This sign is most dependable before the second year, after which time it may occur in normal subjects. It may occur also in meningitis. Dorsal flexion and abduction of the foot may be produced by tapping the peroneal nerve on the lateral surface of the fibula just below the head (peroneal sign).

TROUSSEAU PHENOMENON. This sign is elicited by making pressure upon the blood vessels and nerves of the upper arm (tourniquet or sphygmomanometer) with sufficient force to stop the circulation. A positive reaction consists in the production of the typical "tetanic" contraction of the fingers and hand in the obstetric position. A bilateral response may follow application of the pressure to one arm. This sign is not pathognomonic of tetany and is less reliable than the Chvostek sign.

OTHER SIGNS. A number of other signs have been described, depending on stimulation of various nerves or muscles. Dimpling of the tongue may be produced by tapping it lightly (also in myotonia). Plantar flexion of the foot and spasm of the extensor muscles of the knee may be produced by grasping the ankle and forcibly flexing the thigh at the hip joint (tension of sciatic nerve). Carpal spasm may follow forcible abduction of the arm (tension of brachial plexus).

Hyperexcitability of sensory nerves is also present, but is not easily demonstrated. The "Hoffman phenomenon" consists in the manifestation of hyperirritability of peripheral sensory nerves to galvanic and faradic currents. Hypersensitivity of the optic, acoustic, vagus, glossopharyngeal and other nerves has been demonstrated.

Chemical changes in the blood are among the most significant features of all forms of tetany. Inasmuch as the changes in latent tetany differ from those in manifest tetany only in degree, they will be described subsequently in the discussion of that condition.

Manifest Tetany. ACUTE TETANY. After a variable period of latency, neuromuscular irritability increases to the point where spontaneous manifestations appear. Among the most important of these are carpopedal spasm, laryngospasm, and convulsions. These may be preceded and accompanied by paresthesias and intense pain.

In *carpal spasm* the thumb is inserted into the palm, the fingers extended at the distal joints, are flexed at the metacarpophalangeal joints ("obstetric hand"), and the wrist is flexed and the hand drawn to the ulnar side. In pedal spasm the feet are bent downward, often in the position of equinovarus. There may be stiffness or spasm and pain in other muscle groups of the extremities. Facial spasm may produce stiffness and rigidity, with a fixed expression ("tetany facies"), the corners of the mouth being drawn downward ("carp mouth"). There may be rigidity of the entire body, especially of the neck and back, strabismus, nystagmus, inequality of the pupils and difficulty in speech and swallowing.

Laryngospasm occurs most frequently in children and is precipitated by very slight reflex irritation (cold, emotional disturbance, sudden awakening, etc.). It is characterized by a loud inspiratory crow due to spasm of the glottis. The attacks vary in severity and frequency and, if repeated, may be accompanied by dyspnea, cyanosis, coma, and respiratory failure, which may terminate fatally. Usually the glottic spasm relaxes in a few minutes. Diaphragmatic spasm may cause inspiratory or, rarely, expiratory apnea, which may cause death. Broncho-tetany may produce attacks simulating asthma; in severe cases there is dyspnea, with areas of pulmonary atelectasis and emphysema. This condition responds well to calcium but is not relieved by epinephrine.

Autonomic nerves and smooth muscles may be extensively involved. Spasm has been observed in the iris, ciliary muscle, esophagus, throughout the gastrointestinal tract (often with pain, vomiting, constipation or diarrhea), the bladder (with urinary retention or enuresis), the bronchi and the heart. *Cardiac spasm* (probably vagus stimulation) may cause sudden death, with precipitate pallor and apnea. Palpitation, tachycardia, and cardiac irregularity occur frequently. The R-T interval may be prolonged to 0.30 to 0.34 second (normal, 0.25 to 0.28 second). *Angiospasm* results in pallor, especially of the fingers and toes, dermographia and muscle pain. There may be localized areas of puffiness of the skin or frank edema, usually limited to the face or the dorsum of the hands and feet, but at times generalized. This occurs more frequently in young infants than in adults.

Convulsions, usually generalized, but sometimes limited to one side of the body (hemitetany) or to single muscle groups, occur most frequently in infants. They may appear suddenly and spontaneously or may be precipitated by slight stimulation. Premonitory manifestations may occur, including paresthesias, joint pains, muscular twitching, carpopedal spasm, laryngospasm, etc. Death may occur if the convulsions are prolonged and repeated frequently (status eclampticus).

There may be *mental symptoms,* such as irritability, apprehension, disorientation, hallucinations and confusion, moodiness, loss of memory and dulness. These phenomena are usually of brief duration and, since they occur most frequently in tetany following thyroidectomy, they may be dependent in part upon a state of hypothyroidism. Loss of consciousness during convulsions occurs rarely, if ever.

CHRONIC TETANY. Chronic tetany develops most commonly in conditions which do not respond particularly to specific forms of therapy. Hypoparathyroidism is the most important of these, although recently introduced therapeutic measures have greatly diminished the chronicity of tetany in this condition, as in infantile tetany, spruc, celiac disease and osteomalacia. However, in cases of very mild or latent tetany, particularly in hypoparathyroidism, the progress of the metabolic abnormalities characteristic of chronic tetany may escape recognition because of the absence of acute manifestations. These consist largely in trophic changes in structures of ectodermal origin, notably the hair, skin, nails, teeth, and the crystalline lens of the eye.

The hair becomes coarse in texture and is lost in patches or almost completely. The skin is thickened and roughened and the nails become brittle, ridged and may be shed. These changes are believed to be due to spasm of the vessels of the nail beds. Defects appear in the dentin and enamel of the teeth, which may exhibit small pits and horizontal grooves. These changes are particularly striking in infantile tetany, in which the disturbance in Ca and P metabolism occurs during the period of dental development. They are observed much less commonly at present than formerly, because of the introduction of improved methods of treatment and diagnosis. Lenticular opacities, both nuclear and cortical, have been observed in a large proportion of cases, their true incidence being appreciated more widely with the increased use of the slit lamp for their early demonstration.

Etiologic Classification of Tetany.[4] The several forms of tetany may be classified as follows (Shelling):

I. Tetany due to reduction in concentration or inactivation of a portion of the serum Ca.

(a) Parathyroprivic tetany, idiopathic and postoperative.
(b) Infantile tetany, usually associated with rickets.
(c) Osteomalacic tetany.
(d) Maternal tetany.
(e) Neonatal tetany.
(f) Tetany due to loss or lack of absorption of calcium, as in sprue, celiac disease and other forms of steatorrhea.
(g) Pseudohypoparathyroidism.

II. Tetany due to inactivation or precipitation of calcium, as in citrate, oxalate and phosphate tetany.

III. Tetany due to alkalosis. Hyperventilation, bicarbonate and gastric tetany.

IV. Tetany due to magnesium deprivation.

(a) Experimental Mg deprivation.
(b) "Grass tetany" of cattle.

Parathyroprivic Tetany (Hypoparathyroidism). Clinically, this occurs in two forms, (a) postoperative, following thyroidectomy or parathyroidectomy, and (b) idiopathic, a condition analogous to spontaneous hypothyroidism. A third variety may follow hemorrhage or inflammation in the deep cervical tissues or in the glands themselves; this form is rare.

Postoperative tetany may result from accidental removal of one or more parathyroid glands during thyroidectomy, or from excision of too much parathyroid tissue in parathyroidectomy for hyperparathyroidism. In most cases, however, following thyroidectomy, it is probably due to temporary suppression of parathyroid function, as a result of trauma, edema or hemorrhage or interference with the blood supply. In such cases the condition is usually mild and of brief duration.

Manifestations of latent or manifest tetany appear usually within a few hours or days after operation. In some instances in which an interval of several days to a few weeks elapse, disturbance of blood supply to the parathyroid glands is often due to fibrous organization of inflammatory exudate or hemorrhagic extravasations, and the tetany is frequently prolonged or even permanent.

Manifestations of hypoparathyroidism have been reported in cases in which the parathyroid glands have been involved in tuberculosis and amyloid disease. Extensive hemorrhage into the glands has been observed in infants dying of tetany. However, there is no consistent relationship between the presence of inflammation, fibrosis, degeneration, hemorrhage or cystic changes in the glands and the occurrence of manifestations of hypoparathyroidism.

Idiopathic hypoparathyroidism (juvenile or adult) is a comparatively rare condition. Its cause is unknown, although it has been attributed to inflammation of or hemorrhage into the glands. It is practically always chronic in nature and presents essentially the same clinical and metabolic features as are seen in postoperative tetany. Autopsy in a few cases has revealed either apparent absence of parathyroid tissue or complete aplasia of parathyroid epithelial cells, with replacement by fat cells. Reports of several instances of the simultaneous occurrence of idiopathic hypoparathyroidism and chronic moniliasis raised the question of a possible relation between the two conditions. Although there is no clear evidence of a hereditary factor, cases have been observed in as many as three siblings. There have been several instances of coexisting Addison's disease.

Tetany following parathyroidectomy for hyperparathyroidism is due in many instances to the fact that the remaining glands are in a state of atrophy or functional suppression as a result of the presence of a hyperfunctioning adenomatous gland. This condition is usually transitory.

The characteristic *metabolic features*

TABLE 7. METABOLIC FEATURES IN CLINICAL FORMS OF TETANY

TYPE	CALCIUM	BLOOD PHOSPHORUS	*p*H	URINE CALCIUM	FECES CALCIUM
Parathyroid	Low	High	Normal	Low	Normal
Infantile	Low	Usually low; may be high or normal	Normal	Low	High
Osteomalacic	Low	Usually low; may be normal	Normal	Low	High
Steatorrhea	Low	Usually low; may be normal	Normal	Low	High
Maternal	Low	Variable	Normal	Low	Variable
Alkalotic	Normal	Normal	High	Normal	Normal
Nephritis	Low	High	Low	Low	High

of parathyroprivic tetany are: (a) hypocalcemia, (b) normal or increased serum P concentration, (c) decreased urinary excretion of Ca and P, with positive Ca and P balances, (d) normal serum phosphatase activity, (e) normal acid-base equilibrium, and (f) no significant skeletal abnormality.

One of the most important manifestations is the diminished serum Ca concentration. This is usually between 7 and 8 mg. per 100 cc. in latent and between 4 and 6 mg. per 100 cc. in manifest tetany. However, this close parallelism between the severity of symptoms and the degree of hypocalcemia is not constant. Latent tetany may be present at normal or at low (6 to 7 mg. per cent) serum Ca levels and manifest tetany may occur at concentrations as high as 8 mg. per 100 cc. Such discrepancies indicate that other factors must participate in the pathogenesis of neuromuscular hyperirritability in this condition. Perhaps the most important of these is the serum P concentration. This is at times normal, but is usually increased (5 to 10 mg. per cent). Even when it is not elevated, the serum Ca–P ratio is decreased. It appears likely that this absolute or relative increase in serum P plays a significant role in determining the precipitation of clinical symptoms of tetany. From the standpoint of differential diagnosis, particularly from tetany due to vitamin D deficiency, the elevated or normal serum P concentration, positive Ca and P balances, normal serum phosphatase activity and absence of skeletal abnormality are of paramount importance.

Treatment. Rational therapy consists in correction of the existing metabolic errors: (a) hypocalcemia, (b) phosphate retention and hyperphosphatemia and (c) parathyroid deficiency. This may be accomplished by (1) administration of Ca salts, (2) restriction of intake of P, (3) specific substitution therapy (parathyroid transplants or parathyroid hormone administration), and (4) administration of dihydrotachysterol (A.T. 10) or large doses of vitamin D.

CALCIUM THERAPY. Calcium salts may be administered orally (chloride, lactate, gluconate), intramuscularly (gluconate) or intravenously (chloride, gluconate). The chloride contains 36 per cent, the lactate 18 per cent and the gluconate about 9 per cent calcium. The phosphate may be administered orally, but is much less effective because of the effect of the phosphate ion. Oral Ca administration constitutes the mainstay of the therapeutic regimen in parathyroid tetany. The usual dosage for adults is: gluconate, 4 gm., chloride and lactate, 2 gm., four times daily. To ensure maximum absorption, calcium salts should be given in interdigestive periods, that is, about one-half to three-quarters of an hour before meals and at bedtime. The chloride is perhaps the most effective but is also the most irritating, and the gluconate can usually be taken over long periods with a minimum of gastrointestinal disturbance.

In the presence of acute spastic or

convulsive phenomena, Ca should be given intravenously, the chloride in doses of 5 to 10 cc. of a 10 per cent solution, the gluconate in doses of 10 to 30 cc. of a 10 per cent solution and the glucogalactogluconate, 10 to 20 cc. of a 20 per cent solution. These, given at a rate of 2 to 3 cc. per minute, produce prompt relief (within a few minutes), but the hypercalcemic effect usually lasts only about one to two hours. The injection may be repeated three or four times daily, if necessary, and should be supplemented by oral or intramuscular therapy. Calcium gluconate (10 per cent) may be given intramuscularly (10 to 20 cc.), the hypercalcemic response being obtained in fifteen to thirty minutes and lasting four to eight hours. This route may be employed twice daily, if necessary to prevent acute manifestations, or if oral therapy is not feasible. Caution must be exercised in parenteral administration of calcium salts to patients receiving digitalis, because of the danger of cardiac arrest.

LOW PHOSPHORUS THERAPY. Increase in P intake causes an increase in the requirement for both Ca and parathyroid hormone in hypoparathyroidism. Consequently, it is advisable to restrict the daily intake of P to 0.3 to 0.6 gm., according to the total caloric protein intake. For this reason, milk, despite its high Ca content, often causes an exacerbation of tetanic manifestations and increased refractoriness to parathyroid hormone, since each quart contains about 0.93 gm. P. It is therefore not advisable to use milk or milk products as a source of extra Ca in such cases. Absorption of phosphate from the intestine may be decreased by administration of aluminum hydroxide gel, 30 to 40 cc. with each meal.

PARATHYROID THERAPY. Transplantation of parathyroid tissue has not met with great success, although some cases have been reported in which good results have been obtained following growth of parathyroid tissue in the plasma of the recipient.[46] Apparent cure (postoperative tetany) has followed transplantation of the thyroid and parathyroid glands of a 25 day old infant by vascular anastomosis in the lower abdominal wall.[47] In the great majority of instances, substitution therapy consists in the subcutaneous or intramuscular administration of parathyroid hormone. One unit of the hormone is defined as "one one-hundredth of the amount which produces, on an average, 1 mg. rise in the blood serum Ca in 20-kilogram dogs, over fifteen hours." One cubic centimeter contains 100 such units. The dosage depends upon the degree of hypocalcemia and the severity of the manifestations of tetany. This agent is most effective when the intake of Ca is increased and that of P is maintained at a relatively low level (0.3 to 0.6 gm.). In very acute cases, 500 units (5 cc.) of the hormone may be given daily in divided doses of 100 units. The quantity needed for maintenance must be determined in each case by repeated determinations of the serum Ca concentrations, which may increase rapidly and to dangerous levels, especially if the hormone is injected at relatively short intervals. The usual maintenance dose, except in cases of virtual aparathyroidism, is from 50 to 200 units daily. If more than 100 units are required, it is advisable to administer equal doses at twelve-hour intervals.

The increase in serum Ca occurs gradually, reaching a maximum in eight to fifteen hours, and then subsides, reaching preinjection levels in about twenty-four hours. A step-ladder effect may be obtained, if the hormone is injected repeatedly at intervals of four to eight hours, and dangerous hypercalcemia may result. It has been observed that symptomatic relief may occur at times within one hour after injection, although there is little or no change in serum Ca concentration at that time. This may be due to the possibility that the primary effect is to increase the diffusible, ionized fraction in the blood and tissue fluids at the expense of the non-diffusible fraction. A state of "refractoriness" or "immunity" to the effects of the hormone develops in subjects to whom it has been given continuously over long periods. The serious objections to the prolonged use of the parathyroid hormone are (a) that it must be given parenterally, (b) that spontaneous activity of remaining parathyroid tissue may be suppressed or inhibited, and (c) that a refractory state develops. For these reasons it is seldom employed except for brief periods.

DIHYDROTACHYSTEROL (A.T. 10).[29,48–50] Dihydrotachysterol is a photochemical derivative of ergosterol which has a pronounced hypercalcemic effect but practically no antirachitic properties. It is effective when given orally in an oil solvent (1.25 mg. per cc.) and therefore represents a distinct advance in the therapy of tetany of parathyroid origin. It appears to increase absorption of Ca from the bowel and to increase urinary excretion of phosphorus, resembling vitamin D in the former respect and parathyroid hormone in the latter.[29] As is the case with the hormone, its hypercalcemic effect is so marked that, until the dosage necessary for maintenance has been established, the level of serum Ca must be determined frequently if dangerous hypercalcemia is to be avoided. The necessity for this procedure may be diminished, if it is not feasible, by the daily application of a qualitative test for Ca in the urine (Sulkowitch).[29] If no precipitate (calcium oxalate) appears, there is no Ca and the serum Ca is probably below 7.5 mg. per cent. If there is a fine white cloud, the serum Ca concentration is probably within normal limits, while if a dense milky precipitate appears hypercalcemia is present. The serum Ca determination is much superior to this procedure for accurate regulation. The metabolic effects of dihydrotachysterol persist for seven to ten days after discontinuing its administration.

The *dosage* varies considerably, depending upon the degree of hypocalcemia. Ca salts should be given simultaneously. Initially, 3 to 10 cc. may be required daily for two or three days, then 1 to 2 cc. daily for one or two weeks, depending upon the degree of elevation of serum Ca. In many cases, after the latter has returned to normal, it may be maintained within satisfactory limits by as little as 1 to 2 cc. two or three times weekly, or even by smaller amounts. The maintenance requirement for dihydrostachysterol seems to be independent of the original severity of the clinical manifestations. Patients occasionally are refractory to this agent, requiring relatively large doses for control of tetany and maintenance of normal serum Ca and P concentrations. The cause of this hyposensitivity is not clear. In certain cases it is due to poor absorption from the intestine, e.g., in chronic pancreatitis.

Many recommend the use of vitamin D in rather large doses (50,000 to 300,000 I.U. daily), in conjunction with a high Ca, low P intake. The most effective means of securing this high dosage is by use of crystalline preparations, which contain 20,000 to 40,000 I.U. per milligram. In many cases this has resulted in restoration of normal Ca and P concentrations in the serum. Calcium salts must be given in adequate dosage if a satisfactory increase in serum Ca is to be maintained. Precautions must be observed as in the case of dihydrotachysterol.

Administration of thyroid extract is of value in raising the serum Ca in hypoparathyroidism, probably by accelerating its mobilization from the bones. The addition of lactose to the diet is also of benefit in many cases. It acts perhaps by furthering Ca absorption by increasing intestinal acidity and by lowering the plasma phosphate (increased carbohydrate utilization).

Although seldom necessary, sedatives such as chloral hydrate, phenobarbital or sodium amytal may be beneficial in relieving severe convulsions or dangerous laryngospasm.

Because of its depressant action, magnesium has been used as an emergency measure in the treatment of severe parathyroid tetany (0.5 to 1 gm. $MgSO_4$ intravenously, in 2 to 5 per cent solution; 0.2 cc. of 8 per cent $MgSO_4$ solution per kg. intramuscularly). A syringe containing 10 cc. of 10 per cent calcium chloride or gluconate must be available for administration promptly if circulatory or respiratory embarrassment develops. However, the use of magnesium is not advisable since it may actually further lower the serum Ca concentration.

Pseudohypoparathyroidism. This designation has been applied to a condition with metabolic manifestations indistinguishable from those of hypoparathyroidism, in which parathyroid function is normal but in which the responsiveness of the target organs (bones, kidneys) to the parathyroid hormone is diminished. The important features of this condition are discussed elsewhere (p. 210).

Infantile Tetany. This is due characteristically to vitamin D deficiency and inadequate intake of calcium. It is usually associated with rickets, but may occur in the absence of clinical manifestations of that condition. The serum Ca is decreased. The serum P is usually subnormal in the presence of rickets, but may be normal or elevated in its absence. The Ca and P balances are negative or subnormal, due to excessive loss of these elements in the feces. The serum phosphatase activity is usually increased in proportion to the severity of the skeletal lesions, which vary from simple demineralization to typical rachitic manifestations.

As for *treatment,* this condition usually responds well to the addition of extra amounts of Ca to the antirachitic regimen. It is given in the same manner as in hypoparathyroidism (p. 234). Vitamin D may be given in the form of cod liver oil or other fish liver oils, irradiated ergosterol or ultraviolet irradiation of the skin. The action of cod liver oil is rather slow and it is usually necessary to employ more concentrated forms of the vitamin (p. 234). The quantity required naturally varies with the severity of the deficiency; 10,000 to 100,000 international units may be required daily. In the majority of cases a high P intake is advisable. It is essential that Ca be given, particularly in the first several days of vitamin D administration, since otherwise there is a primary fall in serum Ca, with aggravation of tetanic manifestations, due probably to rather sharp elevation of the serum P concentration.

Osteomalacic Tetany. This form of tetany is due to Ca and vitamin D deprivation and, occurring in adults with osteomalacia, may be regarded as the counterpart of infantile tetany. In the past, occurring most commonly during the winter months and in the early spring, and in subjects living and working under conditions which deprived them of adequate nutrition and exposure to sunlight, this condition was variously termed idiopathic tetany, workmen's tetany, shoemaker's, tailor's, seamstress's, carpenter's, housemaid's tetany, etc. The metabolic manifestations are the same as those of infantile tetany, although the serum P concentration is more consistently subnormal and x-ray examination reveals generalized skeletal demineralization. Treatment is essentially the same as in infantile tetany.

Maternal Tetany. The requirement for Ca, P, and vitamin D is increased in pregnancy, and the occurrence of parathyroid hyperplasia indicates increased demand upon those structures. Under normal conditions the serum Ca does not fall to subnormal levels, but it may do so occasionally, particularly in the late months and during lactation, accompanied by manifestations of tetany, mild or latent. These consist usually of muscle cramps, insomnia, irritability, tingling or burning sensations and other paresthesias in the extremities, and the signs of latent tetany (p. 228). The etiology of this condition is not clear, but it appears to be dependent, in some instances, upon deficiency in Ca and vitamin D intake and in others upon parathyroid deficiency operating alone or in conjunction with the other factors.

Maternal tetany is best *prevented* or *treated* by administration of Ca salts (orally or parenterally) and vitamin D in adequate dosage. In cases in which the serum P concentration is increased, parathyroid hormone or dihydrotachysterol may be employed, as in parathyroid tetany. Tetany of the newborn usually responds well to administration of Ca salts parenterally and, if necessary, parathyroid hormone.

Neonatal Tetany. Tetany in the newborn, neonatal tetany, a rare condition, appears to be related usually to the existence of tetany in the mother, although this relationship is not definitely established. It has been explained on the assumption that the fetal parathyroids are not fully functioning in such cases, and that the overburdened maternal parathyroids are not able to compensate adequately for this deficiency. This condition has occurred also in newborn children of women with hyperparathyroidism. This has been attributed to depression of parathyroid activity in utero by the elevated calcium level in the maternal, and therefore in the fetal, blood plasma. It is claimed that the parathyroid hormone cannot cross the placental barrier.

Neonatal tetany appears to differ fundamentally from the more common form of infantile tetany, which rarely occurs before the third or fourth month. It occurs usually in formula-fed babies, rarely in breast-fed infants, owing presumably to the higher proportion of phosphorus to calcium in cow's milk, in conjunction with hypofunction or immaturity of the parathyroids.

Tetany in Steatorrhea. Tetany, latent or manifest, is a rather common manifestation of celiac disease, sprue and so-called "idiopathic" steatorrhea. It is due to impaired intestinal absorption of fats, resulting in the formation of relatively insoluble calcium soaps and, therefore, inadequate assimilation of calcium. There is probably also inadequate absorption of vitamin D. Impaired absorption is also contributed to by the increased intestinal motility. These abnormalities eventuate in osteoporosis, rickets, dwarfism, osteomalacia, hypocalcemia and tetany. The serum P concentration is also frequently diminished and excessive amounts of Ca and P are lost in the feces. These conditions are usually easily differentiated from other forms of tetany by the characteristically high fat content of the feces, the presence of anemia of various types, and gastrointestinal abnormalities.

Treatment of tetany of this variety consists primarily in treatment of the underlying steatorrhea, plus administration of vitamin D and calcium salts, parenterally if oral administration is not feasible. Dihydrotachysterol may be useful in refractory cases.

Phosphate, Citrate and Oxalate Tetany (p. 212). Parenteral administration of soluble oxalates and of citrates produces tetany, the former by the production of hypocalcemia through the formation of insoluble calcium oxalate, the latter by formation of a poorly ionizable calcium citrate compound, without hypocalcemia. Tetanic manifestations may also follow the intravenous injection of neutral, alkaline or slightly acid sodium phosphate, with a concomitant fall in serum Ca concentration. That tetany does not occur after injection of acid sodium phosphate even though the serum Ca falls is probably due to an increase in ionization of Ca incident to the accompanying acidosis. There is evidence that increase in serum P in various forms of tetany is accompanied by increase in neuromuscular irritability and, in parathyroid tetany, by increased resistance to parathyroid hormone. This suggests a relationship between hypocalcemia and hyperphosphatemia and the severity of tetany, which is due to the possibility that phosphate, like bicarbonate and citrate, depresses Ca ionization. Tetany occurs occasionally in advanced forms of renal failure. It is associated with hypocalcemia and hyperphosphatemia, the latter probably being the cause of the former. This condition thus probably represents a true primary "phosphate" tetany. In this condition, manifestations of tetany are often absent, despite the low serum Ca concentration, because of the almost invariably accompanying acidosis.

Alkalotic Tetany. As is indicated in the formula,

$$\text{Irritability} \propto \frac{[Na^+] + [K^+]}{[Ca^{++}] + [Mg^{++}] + [H^+]},$$

decrease in the hydrogen ion concentration results in increased neuromuscular irritability with no accompanying change in serum Ca concentration. Thus, tetany may be present in alkalosis. This may occur clinically in the following conditions: (a) following ingestion of excessive quantities of alkali, especially bicarbonate; (b) after prolonged periods of pulmonary hyperventilation, with lowering of alveolar and plasma CO_2 tension (voluntary, hysteria, certain cases of encephalitis); and (c) after excessive gastric lavage or protracted vomiting (gastric tetany), as in pyloric or upper intestinal obstruction. The excessive loss of HCl results in lowering of the plasma Cl and increase in bicarbonate, with consequent tendency toward a more alkaline reaction in the blood and tissue fluids.

In bicarbonate and gastric tetany, in addition to the history and clinical findings, significant observations include: increase in plasma CO_2 combining power, decrease in plasma Cl concentration (gastric tetany), increase in *p*H of the blood, and normal serum Ca concentration.

In hyperventilation tetany, the significant chemical changes are: fall in alveolar and plasma CO_2 combining power, increase in plasma *p*H, increase in alkalinity and decrease in ammonia in the urine, and normal serum Ca concentration.

Treatment of these types of tetany is, of course, removal or correction of the underlying cause. Administration of sodium chloride, by restoring the normal plasma Cl, promptly relieves tetany due to excessive vomiting or gastric lavage. It is seldom necessary to resort to the use of acidifying agents such as dilute HCl or ammonium chloride. If desirable, ammonium chloride may be given in doses of 1 to 2 gm., three or four times daily, and HCl, in N/10 solution, mixed with milk or fruit juices, in divided doses up to 250 cc. daily.

Low Magnesium Tetany. As has been indicated (irritability formula, p. 192), the magnesium ion has essentially the same effect as the calcium ion upon neuromuscular irritability. Hyperexcitability, convulsions, and low serum Mg concentration have been produced in experimental animals (rat and dog) by feeding diets practically free of magnesium.[51] A similar condition, accompanied by defective ossification, occurs spontaneously in cattle grazing on pastures poor in Mg ("grass tetany"). No comparable disorder has been reported in man. Hypocalcemia occurs occasionally but not consistently. The tetany may be due directly to the hypomagnesemia or, indirectly, to relative inactivation of Ca by an excess of P which would normally have been bound by Mg. The condition is cured by administration of adequate amounts of magnesium.

Conditions Simulating Tetany. Manifestations of nervous hyperirritability, including convulsions, may occur, particularly in infants and young children, at the onset of acute infectious diseases. In the absence of vitamin D deficiency or of alkalosis, which may follow prolonged vomiting, these have no relation to true tetany, from which they may be differentiated by the absence of the characteristic chemical findings. The same is true of such conditions as meningitis, tetanus, uremia, and poisoning with chemical agents, including atropine, strychnine, lead and guanidine.

VITAMIN D (ANTIRACHITIC VITAMIN)[52]

The role of vitamin D in nutrition and the clinical manifestations of deficient and excessive supply of this factor are described elsewhere (pp. 394–400). It is necessary here only to summarize its influence upon Ca and P metabolism.

The multiple nature of vitamin D is now well established, at least ten different sterol derivatives having been shown to possess antirachitic properties in varying degree. The two of greatest practical significance are vitamin D_2 (calciferol, irradiated ergosterol of yeast, viosterol) and vitamin D_3 (activated 7-dehydrocholesterol, present in cod liver oil and produced by irradiation of milk or of the skin). The various forms of vitamin D have qualitatively the same effect physiologically, and can be detected only by their action in the prevention or cure of rickets. Consequently, the mode of action of this factor can be best illustrated by reviewing the consequences of its withdrawal from the diet and of its subsequent readministration.

Vitamin D Deficiency. Under ordinary conditions, vitamin D is necessary for normal calcification of bone, although this is not the case in vitro. The absence of adequate amounts from the diet results in the development of rickets in infants and osteomalacia in adults, other factors, particularly the Ca and P intake and the rate of body growth being also of great importance.

RICKETS. In normal, growing long bones, the epiphyseal cartilage is a narrow plate, supported by transverse trabeculae or a thin fenestrated plate of bone on the epiphyseal side and uniformly penetrated by capillaries on the diaphyseal side. Growth takes place by continuous proliferation of orderly columns of cartilage cells on the epiphyseal side and by simultaneous degeneration of mature cartilage cells on the diaphyseal side. The latter are replaced by capillaries and osteoblasts, which are responsible for the deposition of the bony matrix (zone of preparatory calcification). One of the characteristic features of normal growth is the presence, on the diaphyseal side of the plate of cartilage, of a continuous layer of clear cartilage cells in an almost straight line.

The *first visible changes* in rickets are in the cessation of degeneration in the diaphyseal cartilage cells, the absence of a straight layer of clear cells, and the absence of capillaries and osteoblasts in this zone. The proliferating epiphyseal cartilage becomes wider and its diaphyseal border irregular, the cells losing their columnar arrangement. Cartilage cells and osteoid tissue (poorly calcified) extend toward the shaft of the bone. These changes, i.e., defective calcification at the points of growth and enlargement of the epiphyseal cartilages, result in softening of the bones and the development of the characteristic rachitic deformities (p. 394). In experimental animals these changes may be demonstrated histologically and by means of the *"line test."* The latter consists essentially in staining the split bone with silver nitrate to demonstrate the line of new calcification. Chemical analysis of rachitic bone reveals a decrease in calcium, phosphate and carbonate, and an increase in magnesium and organic matter (normal ratio of ash to organic matter, 3:2; rachitic, 1:2 or 1:3).

Clinically, the diagnosis is made on the basis of clinical findings (p. 394), x-ray examination and chemical studies. The bone shadows are less dense than normally and the ends of the bones present a moth-eaten appearance, the outline being indistinct and the ends frequently concave rather than straight or convex. The *serum Ca and P concentrations* vary considerably in different stages of the disease and under different conditions of Ca and P intake. In the majority of cases in infants on modified milk diets, the serum Ca is essentially normal and the serum P is low, frequently 1 to 3 mg. per 100 cc. The ester P of the red blood cells is low also. During the initial stage of recovery, particularly if vitamin D is given inadequately and the Ca intake is relatively low and the P intake high, the serum Ca may be low and the serum P elevated and tetany may develop (p. 233). Occasionally, especially in premature infants, the serum Ca and P are both low. In experimental animals, by varying the Ca/P ratio in the diet, rickets may be produced with high Ca, low P or low Ca, high P values in the serum.

The serum phosphatase activity is increased in rickets, being perhaps the earliest metabolic manifestation of the condition. The degree of increase is roughly indicative of the severity of the defect. Repair is accompanied by a decrease in this factor, normal values being restored usually only after all other manifestations have disappeared. Ca and P balances are subnormal and may even be negative in severe cases. The excretion of P and Ca in the feces is considerably increased and the urinary Ca and P decreased. It is of interest that the parathyroid glands frequently enlarge and the cells hypertrophy. The significance of this observation is questionable.

When vitamin D is given to rachitic subjects the metabolic abnormalities are corrected and the zones of provisional calcification reassume a more normal appearance. Histologic evidence of beginning repair may be noted within twenty-four to forty-eight hours. The manner in which vitamin D produces this effect is not clearly understood. The hypothesis that it operates through stimulation of parathyroid activity has no basis in fact. Metabolic studies indicate that it increases absorption of Ca from the intestine, increases retention of P in the organism and facilitates utilization of both Ca and P in the process of calcification of bone. Recent studies suggest that it aids also in the liberation of inorganic P from organic compounds, thus rendering more available for bone formation. Vitamin D appears to be necessary for the occurrence of the proper type of cartilage degeneration preliminary to normal calcification and, in clinical rickets, for the maintenance of a Ca and P content of the blood plasma and tissue fluids favorable for the deposition of the normal calcium-phosphate complex in the osteoid matrix (p. 201).

LATE RICKETS AND OSTEOMALACIA. Rickets usually occurs before the second year, during the period of most active bone growth and development. Occasionally it may occur in older children (four to sixteen years); then it is termed late or *juvenile rickets*. The etiology, pathogenesis, metabolic features and morphologic changes are essentially the same as in infantile rickets except that the histologic changes in the bones are modified by the difference in the stage of their development.

Deficiency in vitamin D, Ca and P intakes in adults results in osteomalacia, which may be regarded as *adult rickets*. It differs from ordinary rickets in that, skeletal growth having been completed, the characteristic rachitic abnormalities occurring in the zones of provisional calcification are, of course, lacking. The entire bone is softer than in rickets, the mineral content being greatly diminished, although the Mg is usually increased, constituting a state of generalized skeletal demineralization. This is evident by x-ray examination. The serum Ca and P concentrations are lowered and fecal excretion of Ca and P is increased. Changes in Ca metabolism are usually more pronounced than those in P metabolism and tetany may develop (p. 235). Marked deformities may develop as a result of the extreme pliability of the bones. This condition has become rare in civilized countries, but still occurs in times of famine and under other conditions of inadequate vitamin D and Ca intake, especially when exposure to sunlight is simultaneously restricted. Osteomalacia, like rickets, is cured by an adequate supply of vitamin D, Ca and P.

MISCELLANEOUS. Rachitic and osteomalacic changes may occur in infants with celiac disease and in adults with sprue or "idiopathic" steatorrhea. The skeletal abnormalities in these conditions are dependent upon inadequate absorption of Ca and probably of vitamin D, which results from impaired absorption of fat and increased intestinal motility (fatty diarrhea). The essential features with regard to Ca and P metabolism and skeletal changes are the same as those of rickets, in children, and osteomalacia, in adults. Tetany may develop (p. 235). Successful treatment depends upon correction of the underlying condition, but administration of Ca and vitamin D is frequently beneficial.

Absorption and utilization of vitamin D are impaired in the presence of hepatocellular damage and in the absence of bile salts from the intestine (obstructive jaundice and bile fistula). In the latter case, absorption of Ca is also interfered with because of the disturbance of fat digestion and absorption, with consequent formation of insoluble calcium soaps. When these hepatic or biliary tract disturbances occur in children (congenital or juvenile cirrhosis), growth is stunted (hepatic rickets).

The condition known as renal rickets is described elsewhere (p. 223). It is dependent primarily upon retention of phosphorus, with high serum P concentration, increased P excretion into the intestine and consequent interference with Ca absorption. Acidosis also contributes to the development of skeletal demineralization. When renal functional insufficiency occurs during the period of skeletal growth, growth is stunted (renal dwarfism). Deficiency of vitamin D is not involved in the pathogenesis of this condition.

Hypervitaminosis D. Manifestations of vitamin D excess have been rarely encountered clinically in the past because of the wide margin between ordinary therapeutic and toxic doses. However, with the increasing employment of very large amounts of this agent in various conditions, evidences of hypervitaminosis are observed occasionally. Toxic manifestations should be watched for in infants receiving more than 30,000 international units, in children receiving more than 50,000 international units, and in adults receiving more than 200,000 international units daily over protracted periods. As much as 1,000,000 international units daily has been given for several weeks with little or no evidence of toxicity.

The concentrations of Ca and P in the blood and their excretion in the urine are increased, the Ca and P balances becoming negative unless large amounts of these elements are administered. In children, there is increased deposition of lime salts in the zones of provisional calcification. If the intake is inadequate, demineralization occurs in the shafts of the bones, with continued deposition at the epiphyses. Thus, in infants, osteoporosis may progress simultaneously with the healing of rachitic lesions. In experimental animals, bone changes have been produced which superficially resemble those of hyperparathyroidism but are not histologically identical with the latter. Degenerative changes occur in renal tubular epithelium, blood vessels, heart, stomach, intestines, liver and bronchi, with metastatic or dystrophic calcification in many of these tissues (pp. 217, 243). Degeneration and abnormal calcification are most readily produced when the diet is high in P and adequate in Ca. The *symptoms* of vitamin D excess include nausea, vomiting, anorexia, loss of weight, diarrhea, headache, polyuria, increased urinary frequency, weakness, urinary abnormalities (albumin, casts, hematuria) and evidences of renal functional impairment.

Miscellaneous. By virtue of its relationship to the state of "intercellular material," vitamin C (ascorbic acid) plays an important part in growth and repair of bones and teeth (p. 471). It appears to be necessary for the proper functioning and development of osteoblasts (also ameloblasts and odontoblasts), which in its absence are unable to form osteoid tissue and revert to their prototype (fibroblasts). The resulting bone lesions are quite characteristic and the diagnosis of scorbutic skeletal lesions may usually be made readily by x-ray or histologic examination (p. 471). There is no evidence of disturbance of Ca or P metabolism in vitamin C deficiency and serum phosphatase activity is normal, except during periods of calcification of hemorrhagic extravasations. Mention is made here of this condition because it may at times complicate the picture of rickets.

Lead resembles calcium in its deposition in and mobilization from the bones and, in both of these respects, it is influenced in the same manner by factors which influence the latter. In other words, the deposition of lead in the bones is favored by factors which favor the deposition of Ca (high Ca and P intake, adequate vitamin D intake) and its liberation is facilitated by factors which accelerate mobilization of Ca (parathyroid hormone, excessive doses of vitamin D, inadequate Ca and P intake, acidosis, thyroxin). The *administration of lead* has no significant effect on Ca or P metabolism that can be demonstrated by alteration in Ca and P balance or excretion, or in serum Ca and P concentrations. During the process of deposition of lead in the skeleton, Ca is liberated from the calcium phosphate of the bones and is replaced by lead, which is retained as the relatively inert and insoluble (at resting *p*H) tri-lead phosphate. Flat bones (skull, pelvis, scapula) contain more lead than tubular bones, the ends of long bones containing more than the shafts and the teeth (principally in the dentin) proportionately more than the bones. During the period of active growth, lead is deposited chiefly in the zones of provisional calcification and in the subperiosteal zones. In *children* with lead poisoning this is evidenced by the x-ray as a series of transverse lines in the diaphyses and linear rings of density in ossification centers of the epiphyseal cartilages and carpal bones. These may resemble changes that occur in healing rickets. In *adults,* the distribution resembles that in children, but the characteristic changes in the zones of provisional calcification are, of course, lacking, and retention in the bones does not occur as avidly as in embryonal or growing bone. It is stored in relatively high concentration in the trabeculae, especially at the epiphyses. These facts are taken advantage of in the treatment of lead poisoning. During acute episodes, the flow of lead toward the bones, where it is stored in inert form, is stimulated by high Ca and P intake. After subsidence of acute manifestations, if gradual mobilization and excretion of lead is desired, this may be accomplished by administration of a diet low in Ca and P, acids or acid-forming substances (dilute HCl or ammonium chloride) or parathyroid hormone, among other agents.

Radium resembles lead in its storage in and mobilization from the skeleton. It is deposited most readily in newly formed trabeculae and undergoes gradual mobilization and redeposition until it is redistributed throughout the bones. It differs from lead, however, in that, because of its destructive action, prompt removal from the body is desirable. This may be facilitated by the use of agents which favor mobilization and excretion of Ca and lead, but their effect is not so striking as in the case of these elements.

MINERAL METABOLISM AND TEETH

In considering the effects of disturbances of mineral metabolism on dental structure, one must draw a distinction between the period of dental development and that of adult tooth structure. Calcification of growing teeth may be influenced by a number of factors. Hypoparathyroidism (parathyroid tetany) may be accompanied by defective calcification of the dentin and enamel hypoplasia (p. 230). In experimental animals, hypophysectomy or adrenalectomy result in rather characteristic changes in calcification of the dentin, which is denser than normal. Similar changes have not been described in man. *Vitamin A deficiency* in rats and guinea pigs results in atrophy and metaplasia of the enamel-forming organ, atrophy and depression of function of odontoblasts, cessation of enamel formation and defective formation of dentin. Similar changes have been described in the tooth germ during infancy, and it seems probable that vitamin A is of the greatest importance in contributing to normal dental development during the formative period. Vitamin C deficiency in animals is characterized by *defects in enamel, cementum and dentin.*[53] This factor appears to be necessary for proper development and functioning of odontoblasts and ameloblasts (enamel). In C deficiency, the pulp becomes atrophied and hyperemic, odontoblasts show evidence of degeneration, with small cysts and foci of abnormal calcification and, in complete deficiency, the matrix is undifferentiated. Although evidence of similar changes in humans is meager, the consensus is that an adequate intake of vitamin C is probably essential for normal dental growth and structure. There seems to be no doubt that vitamin D deficiency *in infancy* may result in defective calcification, hypoplastic defects and caries in deciduous teeth. It probably has little or no influence upon the development of caries in permanent teeth although, since the latter develop during the entire period of growth, there may be enamel hypoplasia and abnormal calcification of dentin.

It is generally believed that the adult tooth is a fixed structure, unaffected by metabolic factors which influence the Ca and P deposits in the bones. This question has aroused considerable discussion, especially in its relation to the important problem of dental caries. The statement seems justified that there is no substantial evidence that adult teeth are subject to active withdrawal of calcium, even in such extreme conditions as experimental and clinical hyperparathyroidism, in which enormous quantities of Ca and P may be withdrawn from the skeleton. On the other hand, it has been found that radium, which is deposited in situations and in a manner similar to that of calcium, is deposited in adult teeth. Furthermore, when radioactive P is administered, a very small amount enters the nongrowing tooth, and it has been calculated that 1 per cent of the P content of a human tooth is replaced by P from the food in about 250 days. Therefore, it cannot be maintained that the teeth are metabolically inert. However, the available evidence suggests that the fully erupted adult tooth, unlike bone, is not significantly subject to modification in structure or calcification by changes in Ca or P metabolism.

The teeth may be affected by other minerals. *Lead* is known to be deposited in the teeth in relatively high concentration in lead poisoning. Its relation to the occurrence of dental defects has not been established. Ingestion of excessive amounts of *fluorine* (fluorosis) results in a condition known as "mottled enamel." The occurrence of this disorder is related to the amount of fluorine in drinking water and is endemic in certain districts.[54] The fluorine is retained also in the bones, and the Ca balance has been found to be diminished and the serum phosphatase activity lowered. In acute fluorine poisoning the serum Ca concentration may be diminished (formation of calcium fluoride). Although *chronic fluorosis* exerts a marked effect on skeletal development, enzyme action, body growth, respiration and reproduction, the growing tooth shows the most striking effects. These teeth, as well as adult teeth, become an opaque, chalky white and then brown, and the enamel becomes pitted. The enamel-forming cells (ameloblasts) are first affected and enamel formation is disturbed, probably by the deposition of calcium fluoride instead of the normal phosphate and carbonate, and perhaps by disturbance in the phosphatase mechanism. Deciduous teeth are affected only by much larger doses of fluorine than are required to produce characteristic changes in permanent teeth.

Of special importance is the observation that ingestion of amounts of fluoride (1.0 to 1.5 parts per million in drinking water) too small to produce mottling renders the teeth more resistant to caries. This has led to widespread fluoridation of water supplies, with encouraging results. Topical application is apparently also somewhat effective. It is believed that fluorine may undergo surface adsorption by the hydroxyapatite crystals of the enamel, forming a protective layer of acid-resistant fluoroapatite. The F^- ion may also act by inhibiting the metabolism of oral bacterial enzymes, diminishing local production of acids (from carbohydrate) that are believed by many to be important in the production of dental caries. It is known to inhibit enzymes requiring Ca, Mg, Zn, and Cu, e.g., enolase, certain esterases and bone alkaline phosphatase.

PATHOLOGIC CALCIFICATION[55]

Calcification may occur in abnormal situations under a variety of circumstances. These may be classified as (1) metastatic calcification, (2) dystrophic calcification, (3) calcinosis, (4) arterial calcification, (5) lithiasis (renal, biliary, salivary, etc.) and (6) heteropic bone formation. Abnormalities of Ca and P metabolism are implicated in the etiology of certain forms of metastatic and dystrophic calcification and perhaps also in calcinosis.

Metastatic Calcification. This term is applied to the deposition of lime salts in tissues which have not been the site of preceding regressive changes. The lesions occur chiefly in the kidneys (especially tubular epithelium), gastric mucosa (chiefly about acid-secreting glands), and lungs (alveolar walls and vessels); less frequently there is calcification of the pulmonary veins and wall of the left auricle and, rarely, of the peripheral arteries, trachea and liver. Occasionally, virtually all tissues are affected. In some instances, especially in cases of renal "osteitis fibrosa" (p. 224), there is an extreme degree of calcification of practically the entire arterial system, readily demonstrable by the x-ray. Occasionally the media is primarily or exclusively involved (Mönckeberg's sclerosis). These deposits have approximately the same mineral composition as bone, except perhaps for a slightly higher Ca/P ratio. In some instances actual bone formation may occur.

It is significant that the tissues most commonly affected (kidneys, stomach, lungs) are those in which acid secretion takes place, the cells themselves being relatively alkaline in reaction. This relatively high local alkalinity favors precipitation of Ca and P from the blood plasma in the form of calcium phosphate. Obviously, if the previous condition of the tissues is assumed to be normal, precipitation of Ca and P from the plasma presupposes that the capacity of the latter for maintaining them in solution has been exceeded. Phenomena that might produce this effect are (a) increase in the concentration of Ca or P or of both, (b) increased alkalinity, and, perhaps, (c) decrease in total electrolyte concentration and (d) decrease in protein content of the plasma. Impairment of renal function may also be a contributory factor, the accompanying acidosis increasing mobilization of Ca from the bones and the elevation of serum P probably increasing the quantity of colloidal calcium phosphate in the blood.

Metastatic calcification has been observed clinically in the following conditions: hyperparathyroidism, hypervitaminosis D and renal rickets and renal "osteitis fibrosa," and, less frequently, in multiple myeloma, myelogenous leukemia, extensive skeletal metastases of sarcoma and carcinoma, "marble-bone disease" and widespread osteomyelitis. Although no cases have as yet been reported, it may also follow administration of excessive amounts of dihydrotachysterol (A.T. 10). These are generally regarded as examples of true metastatic calcification. However, although conditions favorable for the occurrence of this phenomenon are often present in such conditions, i.e., hypercalcemia, hyperphosphatemia, destructive bone lesions and renal functional impairment, it is probable that frequently local tissue changes precede and facilitate the precipitation of lime salts. Under such circumstances, the condition should be regarded more properly, in part at least, as one of dystrophic calcification. Thus, regressive changes in the renal tubular epithelium, heart muscle and other tissues have been found to precede the occurrence of demonstrable calcification in these situations in experimental hyperparathyroidism and hypervitaminosis D.[56]

Dystrophic Calcification. This term is applied to deposits of lime salts in dead, degenerated, or devitalized tissue, as in infarcts, areas of necrosis and fatty degeneration, inspissated collections of pus, hyalinized scar tissue, caseating tubercles, and atheromatous patches in the intima of vessels. This constitutes the most common type of pathologic calcification, may occur in any organ or tissue and, in the vast majority of cases, is not dependent upon or associated with abnormality of Ca or P metabolism. However, as stated above, precipitation of lime salts in the soft tissues in hyperparathyroidism and hypervitaminosis D may represent a process of dystrophic calcification superimposed upon one of true metastatic calcification. It is believed that deposition of calcium phosphate is facilitated in dead or devitalized tissues by virtue of the lowered CO_2 tension and increased alkalinity in such areas. Naturally, this phenomenon becomes more marked and more extensive in the presence of such aggravating factors as hypercalcemia, hyperphosphatemia, destructive bone lesions and renal functional impairment, such as occur in hyperparathyroidism, hypervitaminosis D, renal osteitis fibrosa, and after administration of dihydrotachysterol.

Calcinosis.[57,58] In this rather rare condition, lime salts are deposited in and beneath the skin. Two forms have been described: (1) *Calcinosis circumscripta,* the more common, in which calcification is superficial, localized to the skin, occurs at any age, almost invariably in the upper extremities, particularly in the fingers and, because of the resemblance of the deposits to tophi, has been called "calcium gout." (2) *Calcinosis universalis,* occurring most frequently in the first two decades, in which, in addition to the skin, widespread deposits occur subcutaneously and in the connective tissue of muscles, tendons, fascia and nerves, with serious impairment of health. Calcification has also been observed in the capsules of lymph nodes, but not in the usual visceral situations in which metastatic calcification is usually observed. The nodules often coalesce and may break down and ulcerate, extruding a chalk-like material. True bone formation may occur. When the muscles are extensively involved the condition is termed "myositis ossificans." The etiology is unknown. Scleroderma, or manifestations of the Raynaud syndrome, occur in a large proportion of cases. Although evidence of previous tissue damage has not been demonstrated, it seems significant that this process involves portions of the body liable to trauma and most subject to muscular activity. Serum Ca and P concentrations and serum phosphatase activity are normal, but balance studies have revealed a striking tendency to retain Ca and P. This has been ascribed to an increased affinity of the affected tissues for these elements. It may be significant that increased phosphatase activity has been demonstrated in muscle and fibrous tissue in preossification stages of myositis ossificans. Spontaneous disappearance of the calcific deposits has been reported, rarely, however, in the generalized form. The course is chronic, with spontaneous remissions and exacerbations. Calcinosis circumscripta causes little or no interference with function, but in calcinosis universalis contraction of tendons and muscles interferes with joint and muscle function and ulcerations of the skin may lead to local infections, septicemia, or bacteremia.

Treatment is unsatisfactory. Attempts have been made to mobilize the abnormal deposits of calcium by the production of acidosis (ketogenic diet, ammonium chloride), parathyroid hormone, low Ca intake and administration of di-sodium hydrogen phosphate. Physical therapy, heliotherapy, radiotherapy, insulin, acetylcholine and pilocarpine have been used, without consistently significant effect.

References

1. Stearns, G.: *J.A.M.A., 142:*478, 1950.
2. Shohl, A. T.: Mineral Metabolism. New York, Reinhold Publishing Corp., 1939.
3. Albright, F.: J.A.M.A., *112:*2592, 1939.
4. Shelling, D. H.: The Parathyroids in Health and Disease. St. Louis, C. V. Mosby Co., 1935.
5. Cantarow, A. and Trumper, M.: Clinical Biochemistry. 5th Ed. Philadelphia, W. B. Saunders Co., 1955.
6. Albright, F. and Reifenstein, E. C.: The Parathyroid Glands and Metabolic Bone Diseases. Baltimore, Williams and Wilkins Co., 1948.
7. Bourne, G. H. (ed.): The Biochemistry and Physiology of Bone. New York, Academic Press, Inc., 1956.
8. Harrison, H. E. and Harrison, H. C.: J. Clin. Invest., *22:*603, 1943.
9. Haury, V. G. and Cantarow, A.: Proc. Soc. Exper. Biol. & Med., *43:*335, 1940.
10. Kay, H. D.: Physiol. Rev., *12:*384, 1932.
11. Robison, R.: Herter Lectures. New York, New York University Press, 1932.
12. Sunderman, F. W.: Am. J. Clin. Path., *12:*404, 1942.
13. Gutman, A. B.: J.A.M.A.: *120:*1112, 1942.
14. Bodansky, A.: J. Biol. Chem., *101:*93, 1933; *104:*473, 1934.

15. Sullivan, T. J., Gutman, E. B. and Gutman, A. B.: J. Urol., *48:*426, 1942.
16. Huggins, C. and Hodges, C. V.: Cancer Research, *1:*293, 1941.
17. Emmett, J. L. and Greene, L. F.: J.A.M.A., *127:*63, 1945.
18. Fishman, W. H. et al.: N. England J. Med., *255:*925, 1956.
19. Bonner, C. D. et al.: J.A.M.A., *164:*1070, 1957.
20. Gutman, A. B. and Gutman, E. B.: Proc. Soc. Exper. Biol. & Med., *41:*277, 1939.
21. Gutman, A. B. and Gutman, E. B.: J. Clin. Invest., *17:*473, 1938.
22. Burnett, C. H. et al.: New England J. Med., *240:*787, 1949.
23. Scholz, D. E.: J. Clin. Endocrinol., *14:* 1076, 1954.
24. Albright, F. and Kerr, R. C.: J.A.M.A., *148:*1218, 1952.
25. Henneman, P. H. et al.: J. Clin. Invest., *35:*1229, 1956.
26. Schlesinger, B. E. et al.: Brit. M. J., *1:*127, 1956.
27. Fanconi, G.: Jahrb. f. Kinderh., *147:*299, 1936.
28. McCance, R. A. et al.: Quart. J. Med., *25:*523, 1956.
29. (a) Albright, F., Aub, J. C. and Bauer, W.: J.A.M.A., *102:*1276, 1934.
    (b) Albright, F. et al.: Arch. Int. Med., *54:*315, 1934.
    (c) Albright, F. et al.: Am. J. M. Sc., *187:*49, 1934.
    (d) Albright, F., Sulkowitch, H. W. and Bloomberg, E.: Arch. Int. Med., *62:*199, 1938; Am. J. M. Sc., *193:* 800, 1937.
    (e) Albright, F., Drake, T. G. and Sulkowitch, H. W.: Bull. Johns Hopkins Hosp., *60:*377, 1937.
30. Castleman, B. and Mallory, T. B.: Am. J. Path. *11:*1, 1935.
31. Tsumori, H. et al.: J. Clin. Endocrinol., *15:*1141, 1955.
32. Howard, J. E. et al.: J. Clin. Endocrinol., *13:*997, 1953.
33. (a) Hamilton, B. and Schwartz, C.: J. Pharmacol. & Exper. Therap., *46:* 285, 1932.
    (b) Hamilton, B. and Highman, W. J., Jr.: J. Clin. Invest., *15:*99, 1936.
34. Chambers, E. L., Jr., et al.: J. Clin. Endocrinol., *16:*1507, 1956.
35. Bogdonoff, M. D. et al.: Am. J. Med., *21:* 583, 1956.
36. Howard, J. E. et al.: J. Clin. Endocrinol., *13:*1, 1953.
37. Crawford, J. D. et al.: J. Clin. Invest. *29:*1488, 1950.
38. Lichtenstein, L.: Arch. Surg., *36:*874, 1938.
39. Horwitz, T. and Cantarow, A.: Arch. Int. Med., *64:*280, 1939.
40. Albright, F., Smith, P. H. and Richardson, A. M.: J.A.M.A., *116:*2465, 1941.
41. Albright, F. et al.: New England J. Med., *216:*727, 1937; Endocrinology, *22:*411, 1938.
42. Uhlmann, E. and Grossman, A.: Ann. Int. Med., *14:*255, 1940.
43. Selye, H.: Endocrinology, *16:*547, 1932.
44. Shorr, E.: Proc. First Conference on Steroid Hormones and Mammary Cancer, A.M.A., p. 100, 1949.
45. Holland, J. F. et al.: Proc. Soc. Exper. Biol. & Med., *84:*359, 1953.
46. Stone, H. B., Owings, J. C. and Gey, G. O.: Am. J. Surg., *24:*387, 1934.
47. Sterling, J. A. and Goldsmith, R.: Surgery, *35:*624, 1954.
48. (a) Albright, F., Bloomberg, E., Drake, T. and Sulkowitch, H. W.: J. Clin. Invest., *17:*317, 1938.
    (b) Albright, F.: J.A.M.A., *112:*2592, 1939.
49. Snapper, I.: Lancet, *1:*728, 1934.
50. MacBryde, C. M.: J.A.M.A., *111:*304, 1938.
51. Greenberg, D. M. and Tufts, E. V.: Am. J. Physiol., *121:*311, 1938.
52. Jeans, P. C.: J.A.M.A., *143:*177, 1950.
53. King, C. G.: J.A.M.A., *142:*363, 1950.
54. Greenwood, D. A.: Physiol. Rev., *20:*582, 1940.
55. Barr, D. P.: Physiol. Rev. *12:*593, 1932.
56. Cantarow, A., Stewart, H. L. and Housel, E. L.: Endocrinology, *22:*13, 1938.
57. Rothstein, J. L. and Welt, S.: Am. J. Dis. Child., *52:*368, 1936.
58. Bauer, W., Marble, A. and Bennett, G. A.: Am. J. M. Sc., *182:*237, 1931.

MAGNESIUM METABOLISM[1,2,3]

Experimental observations in recent years have thrown considerable light upon the role of magnesium in animal nutrition. However, little is known as yet of its functions in the human organism and of the relation of disturbance of Mg metabolism to clinical observable abnormalities in man. The few such disturbances that have been demonstrated and the possibility of future developments in this field justify a brief resumé of present knowledge of this subject.

Functions

These cannot be stated definitely but must be merely inferred from the physiologic properties of Mg as demonstrated experimentally. Mg is present in all cells and body fluids, its chief deposits being in the bones and muscles. It is a probably important constituent of bone, constituting 0.5 to 0.7 per cent of the ash. An excess has been shown to inhibit calcification, in vivo and in vitro. In other respects, too, it acts as an antagonist to calcium (pharmacologically). It activates the alkaline phosphatase of plasma, bone, etc., and may thus play a part in the functioning of many enzyme systems concerned with the intermediary metabolism of phosphorus and carbohydrate and in muscular contraction. Muscle contains much more Mg than Ca, but the significance of this fact is not apparent. It plays a role similar to that of Ca in the control of neuromuscular irritability but, peculiarly, its action in this respect is counteracted by Ca. For example, the narcosis produced by parenteral injection of Mg salts may be prevented or relieved by administration of Ca. Moreover, the effects of Mg deficiency in experimental animals are enhanced by Ca administration and ameliorated by a simultaneous low Ca intake.

Absorption, Excretion, Requirement

The *absorption* of Mg from the bowel resembles that of Ca in many respects (p. 195). It is diminished by a high intake of fat, phosphate, Ca and alkalis, due probably to their influence on the solubility of Mg salts. Vitamin D apparently exerts no influence upon absorption of Mg.

Under normal conditions, 50 to 80 per cent is *excreted* in the feces (bile and intestinal secretions) and the remainder in the urine. The quantity in the urine is increased somewhat following administration of acidifying substances (HCl, NH_4Cl), and slightly and very temporarily after parathyroid hormone. No significant alteration occurs in hyperthyroidism or hyperparathyroidism, indicating an essential difference between Ca and Mg metabolism. After parenteral administration of Mg salts, 70 to 90 per cent is eliminated in the urine.

The *requirement* for Mg is not known exactly, since equilibrium may be established, in adults at least, on relatively low or high intakes, whereas infants and children show extremely variable balances regardless of the intake. It has been estimated, however, that 0.2 to 0.6 gm. daily is adequate for adults. Because of the high Mg content of chlorophyll, green vegetables constitute an important dietary source of this element.

Blood Magnesium[1,4]

Mg is present in both red cells and plasma, about 5.4 to 7.8 mg. per 100 grams in the former and 1.8 to 3.6 mg. per 100 cc. (1.5 to 3.0 mEq./liter) in the latter. A decrease has been reported during menstruation and in the late months of pregnancy. About 75 to 90 per cent (average 85 per cent) of the serum Mg is in diffusible form, the remainder being probably bound to protein (see Calcium, p. 197). The Mg content of cerebrospinal fluid is higher than that of blood serum, averaging about 3.3 mg. per 100 cc. (2.7 mEq./liter).

Little is known regarding the factors involved in the regulation of Mg metabolism or the Mg content of the blood. The latter is relatively unaffected by phosphate, protein, vitamin D or parathyroid hormone, although the last apparently causes a slight and brief elevation of serum Mg. There is in some respects a reciprocal relationship between Mg and Ca in the serum; e.g., in oxalate poisoning, the decrease in serum Ca is accompanied by an increase in Mg, while the hypermagnesemia induced by parenteral administration of Mg salts is accompanied by a fall in serum Ca concentration, even to tetanic levels.

Slight *increases* have been reported in chronic infections, atherosclerosis, hypertrophic arthritis, essential hypertension and oxalate poisoning. A slight decrease has been reported in uremia, epilepsy, rickets and hypervitaminosis B. However, many of the values regarded as abnormal by some fall within the range regarded as normal by others, and the general opinion is that significant deviations from the normal do not occur consistently enough to be of clinical importance. Increase in serum Mg occurs rather frequently in renal failure, but rarely to values more than twice normal. The danger has been emphasized of administration of Mg salts as purgatives or for other reasons in such cases because of the possibility of consequent elevation of the serum Mg to dangerous levels.[5] It seems questionable whether this occurs frequently enough to constitute a real hazard. *Hypermagnesemia* is accompanied first by sedation and mild hypnosis (at 5 mg. per 100 cc.) and later by profound coma (18 to 20 mg. per 100 cc.) This effect may be counteracted by parenteral administration of soluble Ca salts. The rise in Mg is usually accompanied by a fall in Ca and an increase in blood sugar, with glycosuria.

Marked *decrease* in serum Mg concentration (to 10 per cent of normal) has been produced in experimental animals by virtual withdrawal of Mg from the diet; it occurs also in the so-called "grass tetany" of cattle.[6] These conditions are accompanied by manifestations of increased neuromuscular excitability (electrical reactions, restlessness, convulsions) and later coma. In the experimental animals the chief manifestations include vasodilatation, hyperemia and hyperexcitability and, later, cachexia, kidney damage (nephrosis, periglomerular fibrosis, calcification) and myocardial degeneration and fibrosis. The Ca content of the soft tissues is increased (50 to 100 per cent in heart and muscle; fifteen times normal in kidney). Although no such condition has yet been observed in man, these observations indicate the indispensability of Mg for the animal organism. There is a relative increase in the Mg content of the ash of bones in rickets and osteomalacia.

An increase in the nondiffusible fraction of serum magnesium (25 to 60 per cent of the total) has been reported in hyperthyroidism, normal values (15 to 30 per cent of the total) being restored by adequate treatment with iodine or subtotal thyroidectomy. Very low values for nondiffusible magnesium, below 5 per cent of the total, have been obtained at times in patients with myxedema, an increase occurring after administration of thyroid extract.[7,8] The significance of these changes is not known.

References

1. Schmidt, C. L. A. and Greenberg, D. M.: Physiol. Rev. *15:*297, 1935.
2. Shohl, A. T.: Mineral Metabolism. New York, Reinhold Publishing Corp., 1939.
3. McClure, F. J.: J.A.M.A., *139:*711, 1949.
4. Haury, V. G. and Cantarow, A.: J. Lab. & Clin. Med., *27:*616, 1942.
5. Hirschfelder, A. D. and Haury, V. G.: J.A.M.A., *102:*1138, 1934; J. Biol. Chem., *104:*647, 1934.
6. Greenberg, D. M. and Tufts, E. V.: Am. J. Physiol., *121:*311, 1938.
7. Soffer, L. J., Cohn, C., Grossman, E. B., Jacobs, M. and Sobotka, H.: J. Clin. Invest., *20:*429, 1941.
8. Dine, R. F. and Lavietes, P. H.: J. Clin. Invest., *21:*781, 1942.

IRON METABOLISM[1,2,3]

Function

Although present in the body in relatively small amounts, iron is of great importance to the life and function of all cells and of the organism as a whole. It is an essential component of hemoglobin and its chief functions lie in the transport of oxygen to the tissues (hemoglobin) and in cellular respiration or oxidation processes (cytochrome system, catalase, peroxidase).

Requirement, Absorption

Normal adults may be maintained in approximate iron equilibrium with intakes of as little as 5 mg. daily, but it is believed that 10 to 15 mg. constitute a more satisfactory allowance. This amount appears to be adequate to meet the demands of menstruation, pregnancy and lactation in the absence of digestive disturbances that might interfere with absorption of iron. Young children (four to eight years) require daily about 0.6 mg. per kg. of weight and infants (up to one year) 1 to 2 mg. per kg. Under normal conditions the requirement may be met by the iron of foodstuffs, particularly liver, meats, egg-yolk, green leafy vegetables and legumes.

Iron differs from practically all other electrolytes in that the quantity in the

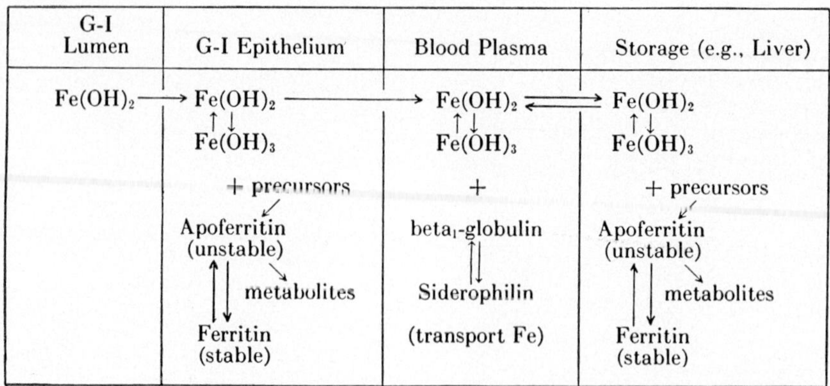

FIG. 2. Mechanism of absorption, transport, storage and mobilization of iron. (Cantarow & Schepartz: Biochemistry, 2nd Ed.)

body is controlled by regulation not of its excretion, but rather of its absorption into the organism. The body stores of Fe are conserved very efficiently, only minute amounts being excreted in the urine and feces, usually less than 1 mg. daily. Relatively large amounts are, of course, lost in the menstrual flow. That present in the body in various substances, e.g., hemoglobin, is almost completely reutilized following its liberation in the course of metabolic degradation of these substances. The bulk of the Fe of the feces is unabsorbed food Fe; a very small amount enters the intestine in the bile and escapes in the feces.

Several factors make absorption of Fe difficult, regardless of the form in which it is ingested: (1) the relatively high *p*H in the jejunum favors the formation of insoluble basic Fe compounds; (2) Fe salts of bile acids are relatively insoluble; (3) the presence of relatively large amounts of phosphate favors the formation of insoluble Fe phosphates; (4) absorption of Fe is interfered with, therefore, in the absence of free HCl in the stomach (achlorhydria) and by administration of alkalies.

Absorption occurs chiefly in the upper duodenum and stomach, but, to a lesser extent, throughout the small intestine. Absorption of inorganic salts of Fe compares favorably with that of the Fe of foodstuffs, which is chiefly a colloidal ferric hydroxide. In general, ferrous Fe is better absorbed than ferric.

Normal gastric acidity facilitates the ionization and solution of ingested Fe and delays the formation of insoluble, undissociable compounds which may form above *p*H 5. At the slightly acid reaction usually encountered in the duodenum, ionizable Fe compounds are converted chiefly to ferrous or ferric hydroxides, the former being favored at higher acidities and by the presence of reducing agents in the digestive mixture (glutathione, ascorbic acid, SH-groups of proteins and digestion products).

The normal organism absorbs Fe only in proportion to its needs, the quantity absorbed being determined by the magnitude of the body reserves of this element. However, under unusual conditions, excessive amounts can be absorbed. Apparently the gastrointestinal mucosa is the tissue immediately responsible for its acceptance or rejection, which is regulated by the amount of ferritin in the mucosal epithelial cells. This is an Fe-protein complex (25 per cent Fe) containing aggregates of ferric hydroxide and a protein, apoferritin (m.w. 450,000). Apoferritin has vasodepressor and antidiuretic properties, the latter being mediated by the neurohypophysis. Ferritin occurs also in other parenchymal cells, e.g., the liver and spleen, and in the bone marrow and reticuloendothelial cells generally. It is believed to be the chief storage form of iron.

Ferrous iron, on entering the mucosal

epithelial cell, is oxidized, forming ferric hydroxide, which combines with the protein, apoferritin, synthesized in the cell, forming ferritin (Fig. 2). Apoferritin is present in very small amounts and is apparently unstable, breaking down quickly unless Fe is present to convert it to ferritin, which is more stable. The equilibrium between these intracellular forms of Fe is potentially reversible. Entrance of Fe into the cell ceases when its capacity for storing ferritin is exhausted. The amount of ferritin in the mucosal cells therefore regulates Fe absorption from the gastrointestinal tract.

Transport

In accordance with body needs, the reactions in the mucosal cell, outlined above, are reversed, the mechanism being unknown. It has been suggested that slight decrease in circulating Hb, with a fall in O_2 content, may favor reduction of ferric to ferrous iron, causing breakdown of ferritin to apoferritin and permitting absorption of additional Fe. The ferrous iron thus mobilized passes into the blood plasma, undergoes reoxidation to the ferric state, and combines with one of the plasma β-globulins. This compound, termed "siderophilin" ("transferrin"), is present in a concentration of about 0.25 g./100 ml. plasma. Each molecule can combine with two atoms of iron. The Fe content of plasma is 50 to 180 μg./100 ml.; this is the transport Fe (ferric).

The Fe content of whole blood is normally 40 to 60 mg./100 ml., averaging 45 in women and 52 in men. Practically all of this is in organic form, as hemoglobin, which contains about 0.335 per cent Fe (ferrous), all of which is in the red blood cells.

Utilization, Storage

In the tissues, as needed, the plasma Fe is apparently released from siderophilin, passes out of the capillary and into the cells, where it may be utilized or stored (as ferritin). Although the plasma contains only a small amount of iron, the turnover rate is rapid, averaging about 0.56 mg./kg. body weight per day, or, in a 70-kg. man, about 40 mg./day. The storage mechanism is identical with that described for the formation of ferritin in the gastrointestinal mucosal cells. The liver, spleen, and intestinal mucosa are the chief storage sites, but other organs (e.g., pancreas, adrenals) and all reticuloendothelial cells contain ferritin. When Fe is deposited in abnormally large amounts, hemosiderin may be formed, a compound similar to ferritin, but containing more Fe (up to 35 per cent).

Iron is utilized chiefly in the synthesis of hemoglobin, myoglobin (muscle Hb), and certain respiratory enzymes (cytochromes, peroxidase, catalase). The latter are probably formed in all cells, myoglobin in muscle cells, and hemoglobin in the developing red blood cells (normoblasts, reticulocytes) in the erythropoietic tissues, principally the bone marrow in man. The approximate distribution of Fe in the body is as follows (Fig. 3): (1) circulating Hb, 70 per cent; (2) myoglobin, 5 per cent; (3) storage Fe, 20 per cent; (4) functional tissue Fe (respiratory enzymes), 5 per cent. Thus, about 75 per cent of the body Fe is in the form of hemoglobin, 20 per cent is in storage form, available for utilization, and 5 per cent is functional tissue Fe, not readily available for other purposes. The Fe of erythrocyte hemoglobin is readily available, but not that of myoglobin.

The quantity of Fe mobilized in the organism daily far exceeds the exogenous supply. About 0.8 per cent of the circulating erythrocytes undergo disintegration daily (life one hundred twenty-five days), liberating about 7 to 8 grams of Hb (0.34 per cent Fe). In the course of its degradation, this gives rise to about 25 mg. of Fe, the bulk of which is immediately utilized in the resynthesis of Hb, but some may enter the blood plasma for transport to other tissues. Synthesis of Hb, and consequently utilization of Fe for this purpose, require among other things adequate amounts of pteroylglutamic acid and vitamin B_{12}.

Mobilization of Fe from ferritin in

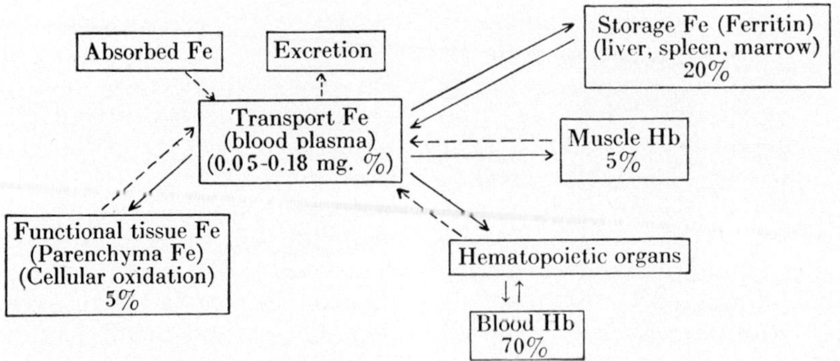

FIG. 3. Approximate distribution of iron in the body. (Cantarow & Schepartz. Biochemistry, 2nd Ed.).

storage sites, e.g., liver, is accomplished by reversal of the reactions involved in its storage. As in the case of the gastrointestinal epithelium, this may involve initial reduction of ferric to ferrous Fe, the latter passing out of the cell into the blood stream; this disturbs the intracellular Fe equilibrium, ferritin breaking down to Fe and apoferritin. The latter, being unstable, continues to break down until equilibrium is restored and loss of Fe from the cell ceases. The reaction can then be reversed in the direction of ferritin formation.

Excretion

The efficiency of utilization of endogenous iron is such that only small quantities are lost under normal conditions, averaging about 0.5 to 1.5 mg./day in men and approximately double this amount in women (menstrual loss). Small amounts are lost in the sweat (<0.5 or 1.0 mg.), minute quantities in the hair, and the remainder largely in the feces (0.3 to 0.75 mg.). The latter (fecal) is contributed to by (1) true excretion, (2) desquamated mucosal cells, and (3) incompletely reabsorbed biliary iron.

Abnormal Iron Metabolism

Disturbances in the metabolism of iron are evidenced by (a) decreased hemoglobin formation, (b) decrease in circulating hemoglobin, or (c) abnormal deposition of iron-containing pigment in the tissues (hemosiderin). A consideration of the pathogenesis and treatment of the various types of anemia is beyond the scope of the present discussion. It must be pointed out, however, that certain forms of hypochromic and microcytic *anemia* are dependent upon inadequate supply or absorption of iron, the latter occurring particularly in the presence of gastric anacidity (plus other factors). Iron deficiency may also occur as a result of *hemorrhage,* with consequent exhaustion of the available tissue reserves of this element. Low values for plasma or serum iron have been reported in hemorrhagic and hypochromic types of anemia. High values are present in forms of anemia characterized by diminished hemoglobin formation not due to iron deficiency (pernicious anemia).

Because they are absorbed more readily from the intestine, ferrous salts are more effective than ferric salts (with the exception of iron and ammonium citrate) in the *treatment* of iron-deficiency anemias. The usual daily dosage of the preparations employed most commonly are: iron and ammonium citrate, 6 gm. (1000 mg. iron); reduced iron, 3 gm. (2800 mg. iron); ferrous carbonate, 4 gm. (360 mg. iron); ferrous sulfate, 1 gm. (200 mg. iron).

Deposition of excessive amounts of iron-containing pigment (hemosiderin) in the tissues occurs (a) as a result of excessive breakdown of red blood cells in hemolytic types of anemia, (b) in conditions in which hemoglobin synthesis is inadequate because of factors other than iron deficiency (pernicious anemia), (c) in transfusion hemosiderosis, and (d) in hemochromatosis. In the latter condition, relatively enormous amounts of iron may be deposited in the tissues, particularly in the liver, pancreas and retroperitoneal lymph nodes, over 50 gm. having been found in the body (exclusive of the blood) in some cases.[4] This iron overload is frequently associated with bronze pigmentation of the skin, hepatic cirrhosis, diabetes and evidence of myocardial damage, attributed, in part at least, to the cytotoxic effects of the high concentration of iron. The pathogenesis of idiopathic hemochromatosis is not clear. It appears likely that, for some unknown reason, excessive absorption of iron occurs over periods of many years.[5] In the late stages, saturation of the tissues with iron may so retard its assimilation that excessive absorption is no longer demonstrable. On the basis of the presence of an exaggerated positive iron balance, repeated phlebotomy has been suggested as a rational therapeutic procedure, at times with reinfusion of the withdrawn plasma.

Similar iron overload and cutaneous pigmentation, usually, however, without cirrhosis or diabetes, may occur in patients receiving frequent transfusions of whole blood over long periods, e.g., for refractory or hypoplastic anemias. It may also result from prolonged excessive parenteral iron therapy.

References

1. Moore, C. V. and Dubach, R.: J.A.M.A., *162:*197, 1956.
2. Gubler, C. J.: Science, *123:*87, 1956.
3. Granick, S.: Physiol. Rev., *31:*489, 1951.
4. Sheldon, J. H.: Hemochromatosis, London, Oxford University Press, 1935.
5. Finch, S. C. and Finch, C. A.: Medicine, *34:*381, 1955.

COPPER METABOLISM[1,2]

Absorption, Excretion

Only small amounts of copper are absorbed, apparently only from the upper small intestine. Under normal conditions, 85 to 99 per cent of the quantity ingested is excreted in the feces, partly via the bile; 0 to 15 per cent escapes in the urine (0 to 0.7 mg./day). The concentration in milk, except in colostrum, is lower than in blood plasma. The amount retained in the body apparently depends mainly on the copper status of the tissues, being influenced relatively slightly by the intake.

In the blood, copper is distributed approximately equally between erythrocytes and plasma, except in late pregnancy, when the concentration rises in the plasma (but not the cells). It is present in the erythrocytes in the form of erythrocuprein. About 96 per cent of the plasma Cu is firmly bound to α_2-globulin (8 atoms Cu per molecule) as ceruloplasmin, the main transport form; a variable but smaller amount is less firmly bound to albumin; a very small quantity is dialyzable. The normal concentration in the plasma is 65 to 165 (av. 115) μg./100 ml. in adults, and 45 to 100 (av. 75) μg./100 ml. in the newborn. It increases during pregnancy, from the third month on, being approximately doubled at term.

Copper is distributed widely throughout the tissues; the highest concentrations are in the liver (hepatocuprein), kidneys, heart, bone marrow, brain and hair. The amount in the tissues decreases with inadequate intake; the liver is apparently the main storage site, its Cu content reflecting the state of Cu nutrition under most circumstances.

Function, Deficiency Manifestations

Copper is an essential component of the respiratory pigments (hemocyanins) of certain marine "blue-blooded" species, i.e., gastropods and arthropods, and of phenol oxidases in plants; the only representative of this category of importance in mammals is tyrosinase. It is present also in butyryl CoA dehydrogenase.

All available evidence points to a role in hemopoiesis as the main function of copper, the exact nature of which is unknown. Copper deficiency results in a microcytic anemia, similar to that resulting from iron deficiency, which, however, cannot be corrected by administration of iron. There are impairment of erythropoiesis and decrease in erythrocyte survival time. Associated reductions in tissue catalase and cytochrome-c and in cytochrome oxidase activity suggest that copper is involved in the metabolism of iron, acting perhaps as a catalyst for its incorporation into these substances, and also into hemoglobin.

In certain species, in addition to anemia, copper deficiency is accompanied by impaired growth, coarsening and depigmentation of hair, decreased reproductive capacity and milk production, and, e.g., in sheep, symmetrical demyelination in the cerebral hemispheres and motor tracts of the cord, producing a characteristic incoordination of gait.

In man, a condition of hepatolenticular degeneration (Wilson's disease) is characterized by abnormally large accumulations of copper in the brain and liver, increase in urine copper, decrease in ceruloplasmin and increase in the loosely bound copper fraction in the plasma, and positive copper balance. There is also increased urinary excretion of amino acids and dicarboxylic amino acid peptides. It is not known whether the abnormality in copper metabolism is primary or secondary to changes in amino acid metabolism. However, synthesis of ceruloplasmin is impaired and it has been suggested that this may be the primary defect, the consequent low level in the plasma resulting in some way in increased absorption of copper from the intestine and, eventually, in excessive storage in the tissues. The frequently increased urinary excretion of copper has been related by some to the excretion of excessive amounts of amino acids and peptides with which it may be chelated.

Certain therapeutic procedures have been suggested, based on these biochemical observations. Absorption of copper can be reduced by oral administration of ion exchange resins or potassium sulfide, whereas its mobilization from the tissues may be accomplished by parenteral administration of chelating agents, e.g., the calcium disodium salt of ethylenediaminetetraacetic acid, or of dimercaprol. The clinical value of such procedures is still uncertain.

Requirement

The average daily diet, adequate in other respects, contains about 1.5 to 4 mg. Cu. The minimum daily requirement for man is not known, but has been estimated to be 0.6 to 2 mg. It has been found that, in infants, administration of 1 to 2 mg./day is distinctly superior to administration of iron alone in maintaining normal hemoglobin levels.

COBALT METABOLISM[1]

Cobalt is readily absorbed from the intestine (70 to 80 per cent), about 65 per cent of the amount ingested being excreted in the urine, the remainder in the feces. Only minute amounts are present in tissues, the largest in the liver (storage site). Its nutritional importance in man apparently arises mainly from the fact that it is an essential component of vitamin B_{12} (4.5 per cent Co).

In ruminants, but not other species, Co deficiency results in anorexia, wasting, a profound macrocytic anemia, fatty liver and hemosiderosis of the spleen. In certain species, a moderately excessive intake of Co results in polycythemia. This may be a pharmacologic effect due to the action of Co in inhibiting certain respiratory enzymes, e.g., cytochrome oxidase, succinic dehydrogenase.

As indicated above, the only established function of cobalt is in hemopoiesis, by virtue of its presence in the vitamin B_{12} molecule, which, an essential substance for animals, originates apparently only in microorganisms. Co is firmly bound in the B_{12} molecule and in this form undergoes no significant interchange with inorganic cobalt.

If Co is required in man only for vitamin B_{12} formation (by intestinal bacteria), its requirement is much lower than for any other trace mineral. As little as 1 to 2 μg. of B_{12} daily, containing 0.045 to 0.09 μg. Co, suffices to maintain normal bone marrow function in pernicious anemia. An average American diet supplies many times this amount. In contrast, the requirement for ruminants is relatively high (0.1 mg./day for sheep); these are the only species in which Co deficiency has been demonstrated.

References

COPPER

1. Gubler, C. J.: J.A.M.A., *161*:530, 1956.
2. Marston, H. R.: Physiol. Rev., *32*:66, 1952.

COBALT

1. Marston, H. R.: Physiol. Rev., *32*:66, 1952.

CHAPTER 5 *By* LOUIS G. WELT, M. D.

Water Balance in Health and Disease

PHYSIOLOGIC CONSIDERATIONS

Volumes of the Body Fluids

The total volume of the fluids of the body varies between the approximate limits of 50 and 70 per cent of the body weight. Since adipose tissue is relatively free of water the percentage of the body weight that is water is less in obese than in lean persons. This total volume of body water is divided into two major compartments: the intracellular, which accounts for approximately two thirds of the total, and the extracellular, which constitutes the remaining third. The latter is further subdivided into several smaller components: the interstitial fluid and plasma, and several very specialized volumes which include the lymph, the cerebrospinal fluid, the utricular endolymph and the aqueous humor of the eyes.

The volume of any particular compartment may be estimated[1] if a substance is available which will assume a uniform distribution within that component of the body fluids. The test substance must be nontoxic, it must not enter metabolic pathways within the time interval necessary for its distribution, its excretory pathway is ideally limited to urine during the time interval necessary for complete mixing, and it must be subject to quantitative chemical analysis in serum as well as in urine. If a substance has these characteristics, a known amount, A, may be administered; the amount lost from the body, E, during the time necessary for complete mixing can be determined; the concentration per liter, C, at the time of equilibration can be estimated by analysis; and the volume of distribution of the substance, V, can be calculated from the equation:

$$V = \frac{A - E}{C} \qquad (1)$$

The total volume of body water[2,3] can be estimated by using water labelled with deuterium or tritium,[4,5,6] or by the use of antipyrine and derivatives thereof.[7,8,9] The volume of the intracellular compartment cannot be estimated directly, but it may be inferred as the difference between the volumes of total body water and that of the extracellular phase. The volume of this latter compartment has been estimated with a variety of substances and by different techniques. The materials that have been used include inulin, sucrose, sulfate, thiosulfate, mannitol, bromide, thiocyanate and isotopic chloride.[10–21] These substances may provide different values, and the "space" which is accepted as most truly representative of the extracellular fluid as a physiologic entity depends on the definition of this unit of volume.[22–25] The definition which appears most reasonable to many is: that volume of fluid which is external to the cells and within which there is (except for large molecular species) diffusion equilibrium. This definition would exclude fluid in the major urinary collecting system, the gastrointestinal tract and the ducts of the exocrine glands. These fluids are frequently referred to as transcellular. This definition would also exclude the special fluids such as the aqueous humor, the utricular endolymph[26] and the cerebrospinal fluid.

Most of the substances listed above, except chloride, bromide and thiocyanate* occupy a volume of distribution of approximately 16 per cent of the body weight. The volumes of distribution calculated from the use of chloride and bromide are close to 20 per cent of the body weight. Most of this difference can be accounted for by the fact that substances such as inulin, sucrose, etc., do not penetrate the connective tissue fluid freely. In vitro studies of muscle tissue suspended in fluid containing isotopic chloride and inulin suggest that inulin ultimately occupies almost the same volume of distribution as chloride but takes a much longer time to achieve complete equilibration.[12] Many investigators feel that the "chloride space" is the closest approximation to the extracellular phase within the context of the definition presented above.

Chloride Space. This concept forms the basis for the estimation of the extracellular space of excised tissue and for the calculation of *changes* in the volume of extracellular fluids in the intact patient or experimental animal.[25,27–34] The calculation, which assumes that virtually all of the chloride in a tissue is in an extracellular site, is probably most valid with respect to muscle as an isolated tissue. Since muscle represents the largest single mass of tissue, and since exchanges of chloride between cells and their environment are not large over short intervals of time, the estimation of *acute changes* of the extracellular volume (calculated in terms of the "chloride space") is considered a reasonable approximation.

The total tissue water (T) of excised tissue and the fractions which may be assigned to the extra- and intracellular phases can be estimated. The total tissue water is the difference in weight between the fresh wet tissue and the weight after it has been dried for 72 hours at a temperature between 95° C. and 105° C. This volume (actually weight) of water is most conveniently expressed in terms of dry tissue. This latter frame of reference will be more useful if the fat content of the tissue is estimated so that the reference can be to "fat-free dry solids" (FFDS). This is, of course, virtually all cellular solids. The tissue and serum are then analyzed for chloride and this is expressed as mEq. per 100 grams of FFDS for tissue, and per one liter of serum *water*. If one assumes that all of the chloride in the tissue is extracellular and in diffusion equilibrium with the chloride in the water of serum, the following formula defines the quantity of water in the extracellular phase:

$$E = \frac{Cl_{FFDS}}{Cl_E} \times 1000^* \qquad (2)$$

where E is the volume of the extracellular phase per 100 gm. FFDS. Cl_E represents the concentration of the chloride in the extracellular water and is derived from the formula:

$$Cl_E = \frac{Cl_s}{W_s \times 0.95}^{\dagger} \qquad (3)$$

where Cl_s is the concentration of the chloride in serum, W_s is the water of serum, and 0.95 is the Gibbs-Donnan factor. Obviously the intracellular water

* Thiocyanate is known to enter cells and, in fact, has the largest volume of distribution of those materials used to estimate the magnitude of the extracellular space.

* Several studies have suggested that about one milliequivalent of the chloride in 100 grams FFDS is not in diffusion equilibrium with the chloride in serum water. For this reason, Yannet and Darrow have suggested that the formula be corrected by subtracting one milliequivalent from Cl_{FFDS} in the calculation of E.

† The value for W_s, the water of serum, can be estimated directly from the difference between the wet and dry weight of serum obtained under the same circumstances as those described for the water of tissue. The solids of serum are represented almost entirely by proteins and lipids. The latter is usually a fairly constant fraction and, hence, in instances where hyperlipemia is unlikely the value for serum water may be estimated from a regression equation:[35]

$$W_s = 98.4 - 0.718P_s \qquad (4)$$

where W_s is serum water expressed as ml. per 100 ml. serum, and P_s is the concentration of total proteins in grams per cent.

(I) per 100 grams FFDS is the difference between T and E.

Acute changes in the volume of the extracellular fluid can be estimated in the intact preparation if information is available concerning the concentrations of chloride in the extracellular water (Cl_E) at the two times representing the limits of the interval during which the change occurred, and if the net gain or loss of chloride by the subject (the external balance or $\pm b_{Cl}$) is known. A reasonable value for the initial volume of E is *assumed.* Since the calculation represents the *change* in volume, the value *assumed* for the initial volume is not crucial. The equation for the calculation is:

$$E_2 = \frac{(E_1 \times [Cl_{E_1}]) \pm b_{Cl}}{[Cl_{E_2}]} \tag{5}$$

where E_1 and E_2 and Cl_{E_1} and Cl_{E_2} represent the initial and final volumes and the initial and final concentrations of chloride in the extracellular water, respectively. The difference between E_1 and E_2 is the change (ΔE) in volume of the extracellular fluid. Acute changes in body weight, ΔW, can be approximately equated with acute changes in total body water. Since

$$\Delta W = \Delta E + \Delta I, \tag{6}$$

ΔI (the change in volume of the intracellular space) can be inferred as the difference between ΔW and ΔE.

Blood Volume. The plasma volume which approximates 5 per cent of the body weight has been calculated from the volume of distribution of protein-bound dyes such as T-1824, and albumin tagged with I^{131}.[36-38] Since the proteins, particularly albumin, are not wholly confined to the vascular compartment but gain access to the interstitial fluid, the lymph and other extravascular components of the body protein pool, the volume of distribution of albumin tagged with dye or I^{131} is likely to be in excess of the true plasma volume. This extravascular distribution is likely to be exaggerated in disease states, and its use under these circumstances may be particularly suspect.

The estimation of the red cell mass is considered to be more reliable and has been measured with red cells labeled with carbon monoxide,[36] two different isotopes of iron[39] and the isotopes of phosphorus and chromium.[40-43] Red cells tagged with iron require a donor, whereas the erythrocytes can be labeled with the isotopes of phosphorus and chromium in vitro. The chromium tag is more stable since this element does not enter metabolic pathways so far as is known and, hence, is probably the best label available for this estimate. The total blood volume may be calculated from the red cell mass and the packed cell volume. Some criticisms have been raised of the validity of using the value for packed cell volume of blood obtained from a large vessel to represent this function for the average of the entire vascular system. Despite these criticisms, this technique probably gives the closest approximations of total blood and plasma volumes.

Each of these measurements of spaces has been of value in the investigation of the normal and pathologic physiology of water and electrolytes in health and disease and in experimental animals. Moreover, there is no doubt that such measurements would provide help in the management of patients whose illness is accompanied by a disorder of hydration and of electrolyte imbalance, but unfortunately most of these techniques are not applicable as routine clinical tools. However, the information that has been obtained from their use in the meticulous study of small groups of patients provides important insights into the pathogenesis and management of these disorders. When this background information is accompanied by the more crude data which the clinician may derive from the history, physical examination and the intelligent use of laboratory techniques that are available, a fairly shrewd appraisal of deficits and excesses of fluid volume may be made.[24]

Composition of the Body Fluids

There are major differences in the compositions of the intra- and extracellular fluids; and, of course, there are significant differences among the several types of cellular fluid and minor differences among the several components of the extracellular fluid. The composition of the latter is much better understood and more completely described both because it is basically the simpler of the two major fluids and because it is available for direct analysis in the form of serum and transudates into serous cavities. The only cells that are available in bulk in relatively pure form are the erythrocytes. Since these are unique, non-nucleated and highly specialized cells, it would, of course, be most hazardous to generalize from their characteristics to all cells.

Extracellular Fluid. SERUM. The commonly accepted normal range of concentrations of the electrolytes in serum is as follows:

CATIONS	
Sodium	132 to 142 mEq./L.
Potassium	3.5 to 5.0 mEq./L.
Calcium	4.5 to 6.0 mEq./L.
Magnesium	1.5 to 3.0 mEq./L.

ANIONS	
Chloride	98 to 106 mEq./L.
Total CO_2	26 to 30 mM./L.
Phosphate and Sulfate	2 to 5 mEq./L.
Nonprotein Organic Anions	3 to 6 mEq./L.
Proteins	15 to 19 mEq./L.

The average sum of the concentrations of all the cations is 150 mEq./L. and this is considered to be identical with the total anion concentration. These concentrations are conventionally expressed in relation to a unit volume of serum, but since these ions are distributed in the *aqueous* phase of the serum it must be appreciated that it would be more precise to express these concentrations per liter (or, even more accurately, per kilogram) of the water of serum. The average water content of serum is about 93 per cent and, hence, the average concentration in the water of serum can be calculated by dividing the serum concentration by 0.93.

INTERSTITIAL FLUID. The interstitial fluid of the extracellular compartment is an ultrafiltrate of serum and differs from the latter in that the concentrations of large molecular species such as the proteins and lipids are much lower. Furthermore, the concentrations of diffusible ions are not identical with their concentrations in the water of serum. This is due, in part, to the fact that a fraction of some ions such as calcium and magnesium are bound to the proteins. In addition, the concentrations in the interstitial fluid of the freely diffusible ions must be corrected by the Gibbs-Donnan factor to account for the asymmetric distribution of these ions across the capillary membrane.

The Gibbs-Donnan equilibrium will be described a little later. The calculation for the conversion of the concentration of chloride in serum to that in the water of extracellular fluid was presented as equation 3. The employment of the Gibbs-Donnan factor for a similar calculation to convert the concentration of sodium in the serum to that in E is

$$Na_E = \frac{Na_s \times 0.95}{W_s} \qquad (7)$$

Intracellular Fluid. The composition of the intracellular fluids cannot be investigated directly[23] and, therefore, the characteristics of these fluids are inferred from analyses of whole tissue. For example, if one proceeds with the analysis of muscle tissue as described earlier, and adds data with respect to the concentrations of sodium and potassium in serum and tissue, one can partition the total sodium and potassium between E and I, and with the derived data for the volumes of these two phases one can calculate the concentrations of these cations in cell water. The values for Na_{FFDS} and K_{FFDS} are obtained by direct analysis, the values for Na_E and K_E from direct analyses of these cations in serum and a value obtained directly or inferred for serum water. The total quantity of sodium in 100 gm. of fat-free dry solids is composed of a fraction in the extra- and the intracellular water, and the quantity in each compartment, in turn, may be represented by the product of the concentration in a particular phase and the volume of that same phase, thus:

$$Na_{FFDS} = ([Na_E] \times E) + ([Na_I] \times I) \quad (8)$$

and,

$$Na_{FFDS} - ([Na_E] \times E) = ([Na_I] \times I) \quad (9)$$

The volume for I is calculated from the total tissue water (obtained from the difference between wet and dry weights) and the volume for E calculated from equation 2. From these data the concentration of sodium in cell water may be calculated. A similar calculation can be made with respect to potassium. However, the difference between the total quantity of potassium in fat-free dry solids and that which may be ascribed to the cellular phase is so small that the correction for that which is contained in the extracellular phase may be neglected. Similar calculations can be made for magnesium, proteins, phosphate, sulfate and bicarbonate. In this last instance, however, certain assumptions have to be made with respect to the CO_2 within the cells that may be present as carbamino-CO_2 rather than as bicarbonate. However, if one makes assumptions for the values of intracellular pK and pCO_2 (see later under Acid-Base Equilibrium), the intracellular pH can be estimated.[29] Within the limits of the validity of the framework underlying these calculations and of the techniques involved, the following average composition of muscle cell fluid is inferred:

CATIONS	
Sodium	10 mEq./L.
Potassium	150 mEq./L.
Magnesium	40 mEq./L
ANIONS	
Bicarbonate	10 mM./L.
Phosphate and Sulfate	150 mEq./L
Proteins	40 mEq./L

Even if one grants the reasonableness of these calculations, this gross description of composition tells one nothing concerning the physicochemical characteristics of these materials. The size, complexity and number of molecular species in which phosphate, sulfate and proteins participate are unknown, yet these features are critical with respect to information concerning electrochemical equivalence and equilibria. It is implicit that the cations may not be as completely dissociated and ionized in cell fluid as they are in the extracellular water. As noted before, it is even unrealistic to speak of intracellular fluid as an entity, since the cells of different tissues obviously have differences in composition which are associated with their different structures and functions. Furthermore, the intracellular fluid of a single species of cell is not an indivisible entity since it, in turn, is compartmented at least into extra- and intranuclear and mitochondrial fluids.

The complex characteristics of cell composition and the striking differences between it and the extracellular environment serve to emphasize the highly specialized physiologic functions of cells, the intricate mechanisms that must be available to maintain these compositional differences with large concentration gradients, the opportunities for alterations in metabolic reactions that may result from even subtle modifications in composition, and the changes in this very composition that may be induced by alterations of reaction rates. This will be referred to again in the discussions related to internal exchanges of electrolytes and active transport.

Internal Exchanges of Water and the Concept of Osmotic Uniformity

In contrast to the marked differences in the composition of the several major and minor compartments of the body's fluids, it is believed that the total solute concentration in each of these fluids is approximately equal. This is presumed to be a consequence of the characteristic of the membranes separating the fluids, namely, free permeability to water.

Chemical Potential of Water. When two compartments containing aqueous solutions are separated by such a membrane, molecules of water will move from one compartment to the other. Equilibrium with respect to the movement of water will obtain when the same number of water molecules pass in each direction per unit time and there is no net alteration in volume of either compartment. This tendency for the molecules of water to pass from one compartment to the other—spoken of as "escaping tendency" by Clark[44]—is related to the average energy of the molecules of water per mol and is referred to as the *chemical potential* of the water. Whenever the chemical potentials of the water[45,46] of two contiguous solutions differ, there will be a net movement of water from the phase with the higher chemical potential to that of the lower until equilibrium is again reached.

The chemical potential or "escaping tendency" of water molecules may be influenced by the addition of solutes to water and by changes in pressure and temperature. The chemical potential of water is reduced when solute is added, and the reduction is proportional to the concentration of solutes in the aqueous solution. In contrast, the "escaping tendency" of water molecules is enhanced by an increase in hydrostatic pressure and temperature.

Figure 1 may help to illustrate these principles. This depicts the familiar U tube, separated into compartments I and II by a membrane in its midsection. The membrane is completely permeable to water. In A there is noted the effect of the addition of a volume of pure water. Since there is no solute in this water, and since it is assumed that the temperature is uniform throughout the system, the only factor that could produce a difference in the chemical potential of the water between I and II is pressure and, therefore, at equilibrium it is noted that the pressures (which are equated with the heights of the columns) are identical. In this state of equilibrium the molecules of water are moving from I to II and from II to I at an identical rate and there is no net alteration in the volume of either compartment.

It is next assumed (with reference to Figure 1B) that the membrane is freely permeable to molecules of urea, and that some of this substance had been

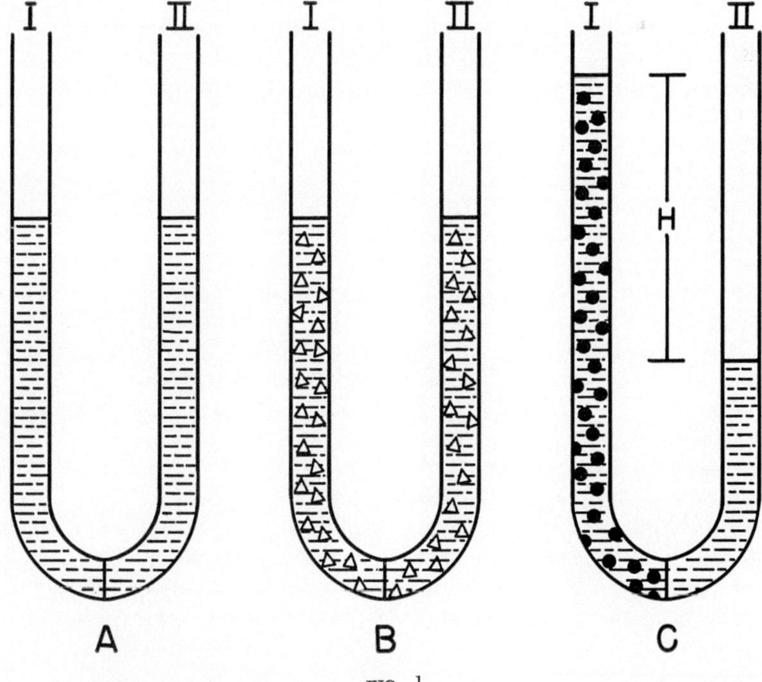

FIG. 1.

added to one or the other of these two compartments. Since urea can penetrate the membrane, it soon is distributed in a uniform fashion throughout the entire volumes of I and II. The addition of the urea has decreased the chemical potential of the water, but since the concentration of urea is identical in both compartments, the chemical potentials of the water of each compartment have been reduced equally. Since there is no *difference* in the chemical potentials of the water in I and II there is a state of equilibrium and the same number of molecules of water pass in each direction across the membrane in unit time. The only difference between the states of equilibrium in A and B is that the *rate* of exchange of water molecules is less in B because the "escaping tendency" of these molecules of water has been reduced by the addition of the solute, urea.

Osmotic Pressure. It may next be assumed (with reference to Figure 1C) that the membrane has an additional characteristic: it is *im*permeable to glucose molecules. Therefore, if glucose were added to side I it would be confined to that compartment. The addition of this solute, in contrast to urea, diminishes the chemical potential of the water on side I only. Under this circumstance the "escaping tendency" of the water molecules on side I is less than on side II and as a consequence more molecules of water pass from II to I than from I to II in unit time. This promotes a redisposition of volume between the two compartments. A result of this net change in volume is to establish a difference in hydrostatic pressures between these two fluids such that the pressure on side I exceeds that on side II. It will be recalled that an increase in hydrostatic pressure on an aqueous solution will increase the chemical potential of the water. Eventually the difference in the hydrostatic pressures on sides I and II will be sufficient to make the chemical potentials of the water of each compartment identical once again. At this point a state of equilibrium is re-established; the same number of water molecules pass in each direction across the membrane per unit time, and there will be no further alteration in the volume of the two fluids. This difference in hydrostatic pressure, H, between the two fluids at equilibrium is a *measure* of the influence of the solute, glucose, on the activity of the molecules of water; it is referred to as the *osmotic pressure,* and it is approximately proportional to the molal concentration of solutes. It is, therefore, inaccurate to speak of a solution as *exerting a pressure;* rather, the osmotic *pressure* is that force that must be applied to a solution to restore the chemical potential of the water molecules to that of pure water at the same temperature. The *difference* in osmotic pressure between two fluids composed of water and solutes is that pressure that would have to be imposed on the solution with the higher concentration of solutes (lower chemical potential of water) to increase its chemical potential to equal that of the other fluid. The equation for the calculation of osmotic pressure of dilute solutions is *similar* to that for the calculation of a gas pressure and is

$$P = CRT$$

where P is osmotic pressure, C is the activity of the solute, R is the gas constant, and T is the absolute temperature. In a manner similar to the behavior of a mixture of gases, the *total osmotic pressure* of a solution with several solutes is the sum of the individual *partial pressures.*

Within the context of the examples given with Figure 1, urea contributed to the total osmotic pressure (i.e., diminished the chemical potential of the water) but it did not contribute an "*effective osmotic pressure.*" This latter was contributed by the glucose and is referred to in this fashion because it was, in fact, effective in promoting a redistribution of water between the two compartments. With respect to biologic fluids and membranes (most of which are freely permeable to water), it may be said that an increase or decrease in the concentration of those solutes that permeate membranes freely increases or decreases the total osmotic pressure (i.e., decreases or increases the chemical potential of the water) in an identical fashion on both sides of the membrane. However, an increase or decrease in the concentration of a solute that cannot penetrate a membrane freely will increase or decrease the *effective osmotic pressure* as well as the total (i.e., will decrease or increase the chemical potential of the water) in the fluid in which its concentration has been altered. In subsequent discussions the more familiar term *effective osmolality* will be used; it should constantly be recalled that an increase or decrease in this function is equated with a reciprocal change in the chemical potential of the water of that fluid and that unless a hydrostatic force is applied to the solution with the decreased chemical potential (i.e., with the increased effective osmolality) the differential rate of movement of water across the separating membrane will favor an accession of water to the fluid with the increased effective osmotic pressure (i.e., diminished chemical potential of water) until a state of equilibrium is re-established and the effective osmolalities (chemical potentials of water) of the two solutions are again identical.

The concept of a uniform osmotic pressure throughout the fluids of the body has been challenged in recent years.[47-49] Much of the data presented with respect to this problem has to do with the osmolality of the solutions in which slices of tissue, which have been immersed therein, neither gain nor lose weight. It has been inferred that a gain in weight by a tissue implies an accession of fluid to the cellular space and, since this occurs when the tissues are bathed in solutions with higher osmolalities than extracellular fluid, it is concluded that the intracellular fluid has a higher total solute concentration than the extracellular fluid. Leaf[50] described similar studies but presented an alternative interpretation involving the movements of both solutes and water into cells whose membranes behaved less selectively in vitro than in vivo. Conway and his colleagues[51] reported data on depression of the freezing point of tissues which suggest that the intra- and extracellular fluids had the same osmolality. Critics claim that the technique of grinding the frozen tissue does not effectively destroy the cell membranes and that the fluid whose freezing point is being determined is, in essence, extracellular fluid.[49] In a subsequent publication, Appelboom and Brodsky[52] reported studies of the osmotic activities of tissue water and concluded that these are isosmotic with plasma. Although a categorical statement concerning this problem is not appropriate, the preponderance of the evidence continues to support the concept that the cellular fluids are, in fact, isotonic with respect to their environmental fluid.[53,54] This, of course, could hardly be the case for those cells that secrete a hypotonic fluid such as the sweat and salivary glands, for the renal tubular cells that tolerate a hypotonic tubular fluid, and for those cells of the nephron which are able to abstract water from luminal fluid up to a four- to five-fold concentration gradient.

Exchanges of Water between the Intra- and Extracellular Compartments. The concept that most cell membranes are freely permeable to water and that there is, therefore, an isotonic relationship between the cellular and extracellular fluids carries the very important implication alluded to above that a change in the effective osmolality of the fluid of either compartment will promote a redistribution of water between these two phases. Primary changes in the osmolality of the extracellular fluid occur commonly. There are data to suggest that such changes may originate in the cellular fluid as well, but it is not clear how often this may occur in a clinical context.[32,55,56]

Sodium and its salts represent almost all of the solutes that usually contribute to the effective osmolality of the extracellular fluid. Therefore, in most instances an increase or a decrease in the concentration of sodium in the serum

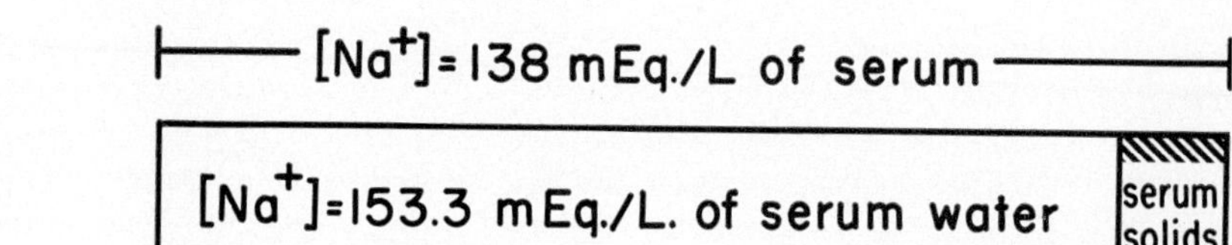

[Na+] = 115 mEq./L of serum

B. Hyperlipemia [Na+] = 153.3 mEq./L. of serum water serum solids

FIG. 2.

represents an increase or decrease in the effective osmolality of the extracellular fluid which, in turn, will promote a redistribution of water from or into the cellular compartment. Hypernatremia may be accompanied by a decrease or an increase in the volume of the extracellular fluid. This space will be diminished if the hypernatremia has developed as a consequence of the loss of water in excess of sodium salts, and it will be expanded if the increased concentration of sodium may be ascribed to the administration of sodium in excess of water. In either instance the volume of the *intra*cellular compartment is presumed to be decreased when there is hypernatremia. Likewise, hyponatremia may be associated with a contraction or an expansion of the volume of extracellular fluid. It will be contracted if sodium salts have been lost in excess of water and expanded if there has been a positive balance of water in excess of salt. In either event the volume of the *intra*cellular compartment is assumed to be expanded when there is hyponatremia.[24,25,57]

There are, however, two circumstances when a depressed concentration of sodium in the serum may not necessarily represent a diminution of the effective osmolality of the extracellular fluid. It will be remembered that it would be more precise to speak of the concentration of an ion such as sodium in terms of its concentration in the water of serum. The determination is, of course, performed on a diluted aliquot of serum, and since the percentage of serum that is water is so large and fairly constant, the convention is to refer the concentration to a unit of volume of serum. In circumstances characterized by hyperlipemia,[58] the lipids may occupy a more significant volume of the serum and the percentage of serum that is water may be drastically reduced to as low as 70 to 80 per cent. An average concentration of sodium of 138 mEq./L. in a serum whose content of water was 90 per cent would represent a concentration of 153.3 mEq. per *liter* of serum *water* (138/0.90). If this same concentration obtained in the *water* of a *lipemic* serum whose water content was only 75 per cent, the concentration per liter of *serum* would be 115 mEq. (153.3 $\times$ 0.75) (see Figure 2). Thus, in this instance a striking hyponatremia does not mean that there is an increased chemical potential of the *water* of serum.

Although glucose contributes to the effective osmolality of the extracellular fluid, the magnitude is usually small. At a concentration of 80 mg. per cent (800 mg./L.) this would amount to 4.4 mOsm./L. However, if hyperglycemia supervenes, the corresponding increase in the effective osmotic pressure will promote a movement of water from the cells.[59] This will dilute the concentration of sodium and the other electrolytes and may depress the level to the point of frank hyponatremia. In this instance the interpretation that the hyponatremia signifies a diminished effective osmotic pressure would be in error. For these reasons any concentration of sodium in a patient with diabetes mellitus should be interpreted with knowledge of the simultaneous concentration of glucose in the serum.

Exchanges of Water between Plasma and Interstitial Fluid Compartments. The distribution of the fluid between these two components of the extracellular space is determined by the several factors that affect the chemical potentials of the water of these two phases. Most of the solutes of the extracellular fluid do not contribute to a *difference* in the effective osmolality between the plasma and interstitial fluid because the bulk of these can traverse the capillary endothelial membrane with freedom. However, the large molecules such as the proteins are confined, for the most part, to the intravascular space and, therefore, depress the chemical potential of the plasma water alone. In turn, the hydrostatic pressure of the blood vessels tends to increase the chemical potential of the plasma water. Likewise, the small concentration of proteins of the interstitial fluid and the tissue tension influence the chemical potential of the water of the interstitial fluid.[60] The influence of the proteins is referred to as the *colloid osmotic pressure.* In addition to the effect of the concentration of the colloidal molecules themselves, there is an additional factor due to an asymmetric distribution of ions as a result of the ionized state of the nondiffusible proteins.

GIBBS-DONNAN EQUILIBRIUM. This is an example of the manner in which there may be an unequal distribution of ions across a membrane despite the fact that the membrane is permeable to them. The phenomenon is dependent on the presence of another ion to which the membrane is not permeable. Assume a system in which there are two phases, I and II, separated by a membrane M. It will be stated that there is a solution of NaCl in each phase. The rate at which either sodium or chloride can move from I to II is dependent on the frequency with which the particular ion makes contact with the membrane, and this, of course, is proportional to its concentration. However, the demand of electroneutrality restricts the diffusion of one ion across the membrane without the other. Therefore, the rate of diffusion of the ions is proportional to the frequency with which the two ions have simultaneous contact with the membrane. From statistical theory it may be stated that this is proportional to the product of the concentrations of the two ions. When there is equilibrium and there is no net movement of the salt, the rate of diffusion of NaCl from I to II will equal the rate from II to I and the products of the concentrations of ions in each phase at that time must be equal:

$$[Na_I][Cl_I] = [Na_{II}][Cl_{II}] \quad (10)$$

or

$$\frac{[Na_I]}{[Na_{II}]} = \frac{[Cl_{II}]}{[Cl_I]} \quad (11)$$

A different system is now assumed, as in Figure 3*A*, in which there is initially a solution of NaP on side I and NaCl on side II, the concentrations indicated by the lower case letters alongside each ion. The membrane will be assumed to be freely permeable to Na^+ and Cl^- but not to P^-. Since the concentration of chloride is higher in II than in I it will tend to diffuse into I (in association with sodium) and if the amount of NaCl that moves from II to I is indicated by x, the situation at equilibrium will be as depicted in Figure 3*B*. It will further be stated that any change in volume will be opposed by the imposition of the necessary hydrostatic pressure. Since there is said to be a state of equilibrium with respect to sodium and chloride, the products of their concentrations in each phase must be equal, and

$$[a + x][x] = [b - x][b - x] \quad (12)$$

A

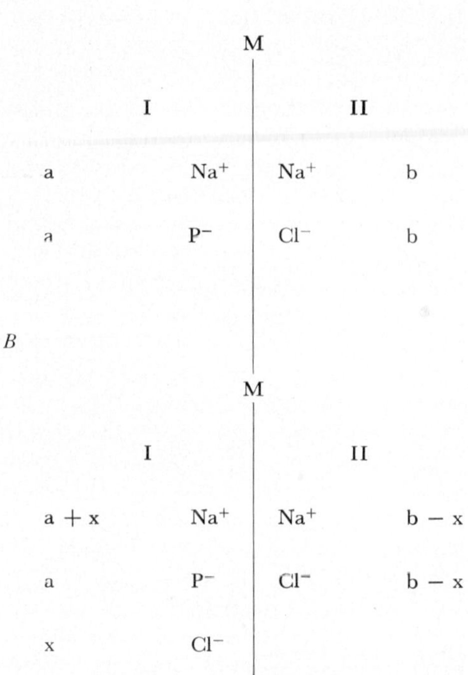

FIG. 3. Illustration of Gibbs-Donnan equilibrium.

Since the two factors on the left hand side of this equation are unequal, [a + x] must be greater than [b — x], and the latter must be larger than [x]. This implies that the concentration of sodium is higher on side I and the concentration of chloride is higher on side II. A concentration gradient for two ions has been established across a membrane that is freely permeable to each of the ions.

The sums of the concentration of sodium and chloride on the two sides of the membrane are also unequal. The sum of the factors in a square is less than the sum of unequal factors which provide the same product as the square; therefore,

$$[a + x] + [x] > [b - x] + [b - x] \quad (13)$$

Thus, the sum of sodium and chloride on side I exceeds the sum of the concentrations of these two ions on side II. This difference in total solute concentration is in addition to that contributed by the concentration of the colloid itself, and the sum of the two is frequently referred to as the *colloid oncotic pressure.*

STARLING FORCES. The net movement of fluid across the capillary endothelium is, then, conditioned by these several factors.[60] Those favoring transudation from the plasma to the interstitial fluid include the factors that increase the chemical potential of the plasma water (the hydrostatic pressure) and decrease the chemical potential of the water of the interstitial fluid (the concentration of proteins in this fluid). In contrast, those factors which favor reabsorption into the blood stream include the concentration of proteins in plasma, the excess in concentration of the diffusible ions (which diminish the chemical potential of the water of plasma) and the tissue tension (which increases the chemical potential of the water of interstitial fluid). These were described by Starling and are frequently referred to as the Starling forces. In general, about one-fourth of the extracellular fluid is confined to the plasma and the remainder to the interstitial fluid. Furthermore, the adjustment of the forces noted above is such as to favor a net movement of fluid from the vascular system at the arteriolar end of the capillaries into the vascular system at the venous end of these minute vessels. Although the *net* exchange of volume across the vascular endothelium is usually minimal, if any, from day to day, the total exchange is tremendous. Hence, a small change in one or more of the Starling forces can result in a large change in net movement of fluid. An increase in the hydrostatic pressure of the capillaries or a diminished concentration of proteins in plasma can easily promote a redistribution of fluid from plasma to the interstitial fluid.

At the same time it should be emphasized that a net change in the Starling forces need not necessarily promote a redisposition of volume since there is an alternative route, the lymphatic vessels, by which fluid may be returned from the interstitial fluid to the plasma.

LYMPHATICS. The lymphatic system originates as capillaries with blind ends.

These vessels are unique in that they represent virtually the only efficient mechanism for returning the large molecular species, such as proteins and lipids, to the blood stream from the interstitial fluid and the gastrointestinal tract. The proteins gain access to but appear to be restrained from leaving the lymph vessels and, hence, are transported from the periphery centrally to empty into the veins. The tissue tension external to the lymphatics and the colloid osmotic pressure of the lymph favor the net movement of water (and electrolytes) from the interstitial spaces to the lymph vessels. The volume of lymph draining an area appears to be influenced in part by the volume of the interstitial fluid in that area. The flow of lymph is conditioned by gravity, the contraction of the skeletal muscles, and by valves that reside in the larger lymphatic vessels.

The volume of fluid that traverses this route is significant, and since it is increased when the interstitial volume is expanded, it may play a most important role in modifying the effects of alterations in the Starling forces that would otherwise lead to a more gross collection of edema. When the lymphatic vessels to a part are occluded, the small quantities of protein that do leave the vascular capillaries accumulate in the interstitial fluid. This diminishes the difference in the colloid osmotic pressure between plasma and interstitial fluid and promotes a net accumulation of fluid in that localized portion of the interstitial compartment.

Internal Exchanges of Electrolytes

The exchange of electrolytes across the membranes separating the intracellular from the extracellular fluid is a complex and poorly understood area of electrolyte physiology. This matter is a subject of intense study in many laboratories, and the reader is referred to several excellent reviews and symposia for original discussions of these problems.[61,73]

The striking differences between the composition of cells and their environment (and, in turn, between cells and subcellular structures such as nuclei and mitochondria) are related to specialization of tissue functions. The large concentration gradients that exist across cell membranes, as for example with respect to potassium, sodium and chloride, were at one time considered to be a consequence of impermeability of the cell membrane to these ions. It was necessary to view this theory with suspicion from the start since it neglected to provide some mechanism for the initial access to the cell interior of those solutes that accumulate therein. This concept was more thoroughly invalidated when it was shown, using radioactive isotopes, that cations such as potassium move across the cell membranes in a constant state of exchange with potassium on the other side of the membrane.

Active Transport. Since the ions can permeate the membrane and the direction of net exchange may be against a concentration gradient, it is implicit that the maintenance of the concentration gradients and the net movement contrary to the gradient are energy-requiring phenomena to which the term *active transport* is applied. Although the demonstration of the transport of a solute from a lower to a higher concentration is clear evidence of the participation of forces other than that of simple diffusion and, hence, is an *active transport,* Rosenberg considers this definition too narrow and states: "A broader definition could be . . . formulated in the following manner: active transport is the movement of a substance which is influenced by other forces in addition to the chemical (or analogous) potential gradient of this substance. An advantage of this definition would be that it would roughly cover the usual concept and permit a theoretical treatment, whereas a disadvantage would be the difficulty of the experimental determination of whether a given transport is active if it is not an uphill transport."[69]

The active transport of solutes appears to be linked with special anatomic and spatial characteristics of membranes, specific enzyme systems and the optimal concentrations of ions for their activation, utilization of oxygen, intermediary metabolic pathways which presumably involve coupled reactions such as oxidation and phosphorylation, hormones, and other factors. Some visualize the movement of ions against a concentration gradient in a system of transport that has the following characteristics: (a) a compound called a "carrier" which forms a reasonably stable compound or complex with the ion, and (b) a chemical system which reacts with the carrier compound resulting in the release of the ion from the carrier. The release of the ion could be achieved by altering the chemical nature of the carrier, or by implementing an exchange for some other ion of similar charge. The carrier might act, for example, in a fashion akin to exchange resins. In fact, one special example of the movement of ions from one compartment to the other is spoken of as the *ion exchange* mechanism. In such a system there may be an exchange of sodium for potassium or hydrogen ion, etc. These exchanges will be commented on later in relation to potassium depletion, responses to distortions in acid-base relationships and the renal regulation of electrolyte balance.

Bone. Although the chemical and physical characteristics of bone have been studied for some time, it is only in recent years that there has been considerable interest in the participation of bone sodium and potassium in the dynamic alterations that occur in response to depletions or excesses of these ions as well as their contribution (along with bone carbonate) to the maintenance of a normal acid-base equilibrium.[74–78] The composition of bone differs strikingly from that of other tissues in that only about one fifth is water, and that only about one third of the bone solids is protein. Two thirds of the solid component of bone is composed of inorganic salts which are organized in a crystal lattice structure. Approximately a third to a little less than a half of the total body sodium is in bone; of this only about 15 per cent can be ascribed to the extracellular fluid, and less than 1 per cent to the intracellular phase of bone. The major fraction is believed to be part of the crystal structure of the bone salts, and approximately 30 to 40 per cent of this is exchangeable with a circulating isotope of sodium within twenty-four hours of its administration. There is considerably less potassium than sodium in the mineral phase of bone.

It has been demonstrated that sodium and, perhaps, potassium deficits are shared by the bones, and that these cations appear to exchange for hydrogen ions (and vice versa) in opposing distortions in acid-base relationships. It has been claimed that sodium may leave bone in response to hyponatremia, but each time this has been reported the experimental design has included the complication of a metabolic acidosis. Other studies in which extreme dilutional hyponatremia has been induced in rats for twenty-four hours with water loads as large as 15 per cent of the body weight have revealed no significant change in bone sodium.

It has also been demonstrated that the chronic administration of large loads of sodium salts may promote an increase in bone sodium. In view of the observations that significant quantities of sodium may leave or enter bone minerals, it is clear that calculations of exchanges of cations between the extracellular fluid and some other compartment cannot necessarily be interpreted as an exchange with the intracellular phase. In many instances these shifts may represent exchanges between the extracellular fluid and bone solids.

Extrarenal External Exchanges of Electrolytes and Water

Thirst. One of the essential elements in the regulation of the balance of water is its ingestion. Under most circumstances the quantity of water which is imbibed is regulated with almost as much precision as the mechanisms responsible for its excretion. The subjective sensory impression which motivates the desire for and the acquisition of water is thirst. Although thirst is admittedly a subjective phenomena and, hence, impossible to quantitate in a precise manner, considerable insight may be gained from observations of the quantity of water which is voluntarily ingested by man and other animals under specific circumstances.

It had been observed on innumerable occasions that the loss of fluid from the body was usually accompanied by thirst. Gilman,[82] however, established the fact that a deficit of fluid was not essential to the development of thirst when he reported that the intravenous administration of a hypertonic solution of NaCl to dogs in a normal state of hydration was followed by the ingestion of large quantities of water. In fact, the volume of water ingested was adequate to restore the effective osmolality of the body fluids close to the initial level. In the same investigation it was also reported that the injection of a concentrated solution of urea, isosmolar with the solution of salt, promoted much less voluntary drinking. Since both solutes should have affected the total solute concentration of the body fluids in an identical fashion, an increase in the osmolality of the fluids per se appears not to be the stimulus to thirst. The discriminatory response to the administration of salt as opposed to urea implies that an increase in the effective osmolality of the extracellular fluids, or the consequence thereof, namely a contraction of the intracellular volume, is the primary alteration inducing a sensation of thirst. This appears to hold whether the hypertonicity of the extracellular fluid is promoted by a loss of water without or in excess of salt or by the administration of salt in excess of water.

Although *cellular* dehydration, therefore, appears to be the primary stimulus to thirst,[83–85] other stimuli must also operate since humans and experimental animals exhibit thirst when they are salt depleted and the body fluids are hypotonic (implying that the cells are increased in volume).[79,86] The thirst in these circumstances appears to be abated when the concentration of sodium is restored toward normal. Thirst is also noted when dehydration is associated with a normal concentration of sodium, and is a common complaint following acute blood loss. The common denominator among these last several circumstances appears to be a contraction of the volume of the extracellular fluid. It may be stated, therefore, that the primary and secondary stimuli to thirst are contraction of the intracellular and extracellular volume respectively.

There are data which implicate certain areas in the hypothalamus as the site of cells which respond to these alterations in the internal environment. Hypodipsia has been noted in rats with electrolytic lesions in the ventromedian nuclei of the hypothalamus.[87] Andersson has made very significant contributions in this field and has demonstrated that the injection of tiny amounts of a hypertonic solution of salt directly into a particular area of the hypothalamus promotes an intense drinking response in goats.[88] The injection of *isotonic* saline in the same area fails to evoke this thirst response. Stimulation of this area also causes the ingestion of water. Greer[89] noted a polydipsic response to electrical stimulation of the hypothalamus of a rat. It is not clear thus far that the same centers respond to both the osmometric and volumetric stimuli.

Many other factors are involved in thirst. For example, the responses to cellular or extracellular dehydration may be modified by the distention of the stomach[90] and by the ingestion of water that escapes immediately by way of an esophagostomy. Conditioned reflexes, emotional stimuli, and in man, at least, sociological factors also influence the regulatory mechanisms involved in thirst.[24,91]

Although probably obvious, it should be emphasized that the central nervous system conditions the reception of and response to stimuli provoking thirst in a less specific sense.[91] These comments refer to the level of the state of consciousness. The frequency with which patients with coma or a clouded state of consciousness develop significant deficits of water while under medical observation is sufficient justification for emphasizing the obvious fact that such patients can neither appreciate nor respond to their own thirst mechanisms.

Insensible Perspiration. Water is continuously lost in the expired air from the lungs and from the surface of the skin. This evaporative loss of water is referred to as *insensible perspiration.* The inspired air is exposed to a large surface in the pulmonary alveoli where its temperature is raised to that of blood and it becomes almost saturated with water vapor. The rate of loss of water from the skin is conditioned by the surface area of the skin, the difference in temperature between the evaporating surface of the skin and the environmental air, and the vapor pressure of the latter. In addition, the rate of loss of water as insensible perspiration appears to be conditioned by the effective osmotic pressure of the body fluids. Gilman and Barbour[92] have reported data which imply that the rate of insensible loss is inversely correlated with the concentration of sodium in the extracellular fluids. Since water is lost from the skin in this fashion as vapor, the loss is regulated in part by the chemical potential of the water of the body's fluids.

The total insensible loss per day is approximately 600 to 1000 ml. in an average adult, and it is responsible at rest for the loss of about 25 per cent of the heat produced in the body each day. The interrelationships between the insensible loss of water and heat are further emphasized by pointing out that the rate of loss of water is accelerated by increase in the metabolic rate (fever, exercise).

This insensible loss consists of water without solute.

Sensible Perspiration (Sweat). Sweat differs from insensible perspiration in that it contains solutes. The sweat is always a hypotonic solution except in some instances of adrenal cortical insufficiency and in patients with mucoviscidosis. An average composition of sweat is as follows:[93–95]

Sodium.	48.0 mM./L.
Potassium.	5.9 "
Chloride.	40.0 "
Ammonia.	3.5 "
Urea.	8.6 "

The production of sweat appears to be primarily responsive to heat. It does not appear to be equated with skin temperature but rather with the internal temperature, which presumably evokes afferent impulses to centers located in the anterolateral portions of the hypothalamus which, in turn, regulate the motor activities necessary to eliminate body heat.

The rate of production of sweat is related, in part, to the effective osmolality of the body fluids. As is the rate of loss of insensible perspiration, the rate of loss of sweat is diminished by increasing the concentration of sodium in the extracellular fluids.[93]

It has already been inferred that the secretions of the adrenal cortex may play a role in regulating the salt content of sweat. It would appear that salt depletion induces a diminished concentration of sodium and chloride in sweat; this regulatory influence is presumably mediated through the adrenal cortical hormones.[96] Inadequate secretion of these hormones is responsible for increased concentrations of sodium and chloride in the sweat of patients with adrenal cortical insufficiency, whereas the excessive losses of salt in the sweat of subjects with mucoviscidosis is due to an abnormality of the sweat glands and they are poorly responsive to these hormones.

Gastrointestinal Tract. The factors that condition the characteristics of the fluid in the various segments of the gastrointestinal tract include the composition of the fluid that is secreted in each of these areas and the responses that are elicited with respect to the influx and outflux of solutes and water when various exogenous solutions gain access to the gastrointestinal lumen. Complex problems are involved in analyzing the specific rates of absorption and secretion of water and each of the various solutes which, when summated, represent the net changes that may be observed in the luminal fluid.[80]

All of the gastrointestinal secretions are approximately isosmotic with plasma except for saliva, which is hypotonic.[98] Aside from the hydrogen ion secretion of the stomach,[99] the major cation of the gastrointestinal secretions is sodium, but its concentration diminishes and reciprocates with potassium as the caudal end of the bowel is approached. Chloride is the major anion of the fluids in most of the upper tract secretions (pancreatic fluid is an exception) and diminishes as the concentration of bicarbonate increases toward the distal large colon.[100] The average concentrations for the various ions along the tract are listed in Table 1. The total volume of fluid secreted into the gastrointestinal tract is estimated by Gamble[22] to average 8 liters per day. Since there is a more or less continuous process of secretion and reabsorption, there is very little net exchange. Data have been reported by Edelman and his co-workers[101–104] concerning the volume of water and the quantities of several ions in the human gastrointestinal tract. The data were derived from an examination of the intestinal tract at postmortem, and the authors emphasize that agonal changes may have been responsible for the observations and, hence, may not be representative of the situation in health. Their data suggest that the gastrointestinal tract contains 1.5 per cent of the total body water, 1.6 per cent of the total exchangeable sodium, 1 per cent of the total exchangeable potassium, and almost 2 per cent of the total exchangeable chloride. These data are presented in Table 2. Thus, although there are only small fractions of the total body water and ions in the gastrointestinal tract under the circumstances of these studies, it is clear how quickly one may sustain significant deficits of water and electrolytes if these secretions are lost by vomiting, diarrhea, tube drainage or ileostomy. Moreover, in diseased states the rate of secretion may be increased.

The net exchange of water between the intestinal tract and the extracellular fluid is conditioned by the difference in the chemical potentials of the water in these two fluids, but it is clear that this is not the sole regulatory mechanism. It has been demonstrated, for example, that the rate of secretion of water into the lumen of an ileal loop is essentially constant despite marked variation in the concentrations of solutions of NaCl instilled into the lumen. On the other hand, the rate of absorption of water from the gut varies inversely with the concentration of salt in the luminal fluid. Thus, despite some dependence on the differences in osmotic pressure, the net exchange cannot be predicted on the basis of osmotic or hydrostatic forces alone.

Since the intestinal secretions deviate significantly in specific ionic concentrations from that of extracellular fluid, and solutes can be reabsorbed and secreted against concentration gradients, it is obvious that active transport and, perhaps, ion-exchange mechanisms are involved in these processes. The secretion of HCl by the stomach is dependent on neural and humoral stimuli, an enzyme (carbonic anhydrase), oxygen and metabolic substrates. Transport of ions in other parts of the intestinal tract appears to

Table 1. Composition of Gastrointestinal Fluids

Fluid	Na^+	K^+	HCO_3^-	Cl^-
		mM./L.		
Stomach	20–100	5–25	......	90–155
Pancreas	110–150	3–10	70–110	40–80
Bile	120–150	3–12	30–50	80–120
Small Intestine	80–150	2–10	20–40	90–130

TABLE 2. PER CENT OF TOTAL EXCHANGEABLE WATER, Na^+, K^+, AND Cl^- IN VARIOUS SEGMENTS OF GASTROINTESTINAL TRACT

SEGMENT	WATER	Na^+	K^+	Cl^-
	Per Cent			
Stomach	0.40	0.45	0.14	0.91
Small intestine	0.70	0.74	0.42	0.67
Proximal large bowel	0.30	0.36	0.43	0.32

be modified by hormonal influences, specifically the secretions of the adrenal cortex.

Acid-base Relationship

An understanding of the factors regulating acid-base equilibrium is frequently made needlessly difficult by the multiple uses and misuses of the terms *acid* and *base* themselves. In much of the clinical literature these terms have been used interchangeably with *anion* and *cation* respectively, and through long usage have acquired a certain degree of respectability. This is not a minor consideration, since the misuse of these terms tends to obfuscate the very nature of the problems that are involved. In the discussion presented here the term *acid* will be used to refer to any substance that is able to provide a hydrogen ion (H^+), and *base* will refer to any substance that is able to accept a hydrogen ion.[44,105] Thus an acid tends to increase the concentration of hydrogen ions in a solution, and a base tends to diminish their numbers. This may be represented as follows:

$$\text{Acid} \rightleftarrows \text{Base} + H^+ \qquad (14)$$

Certain substances can serve as either an acid or a base; for example, $H_2PO_4^-$ can dissociate to H^+ and $HPO_4^=$, or it can accept a hydrogen ion and become H_3PO_4. In the first instance it served as an acid by providing a hydrogen ion, and in the second instance it served as a base and accepted a hydrogen ion from the solution. These statements should serve to focus attention on the central role of the hydrogen ion in acid-base relationships. For these reasons it becomes important to understand the manner in which the concentration of hydrogen ions may be expressed and the inferences that may be drawn from this manner of expression.

The dissociation of an acid, such as HA, is usually stated in the following manner:

$$HA \rightleftarrows H^+ + A^- \qquad (15)$$

The rate at which this reaction proceeds towards the right is proportional to the concentration of the acid, HA, and may be described as equivalent to $k_1[HA]$. In a similar fashion, the rate at which the reaction proceeds in the opposite direction is proportional to the product of the molar concentrations of the two reaction products, H^+ and A^-, and this may be expressed as $k_2[H^+][A^-]$. At equilibrium the two rates are equal. Thus, the following expression obtains:

$$k_1[HA] = k_2[H^+][A^-] \qquad (16)$$

This equation can be restated as:

$$\frac{k_1}{k_2} = \frac{[H^+][A^-]}{[HA]} \qquad (17)$$

The ratio of the two constants can be represented by a new constant, K, and then the entire statement can be rearranged in a manner designed to express the concentration of hydrogen ions, as follows:

$$[H^+] = K\frac{[HA]}{[A^-]} \qquad (18)$$

An alternative method of expressing the concentration of hydrogen ions was introduced by Sørenson, wherein this concentration is represented as the negative logarithm. This latter is referred to as *p*H and the negative logarithm of the constant, K, is referred to as *p*K. When these conventions are applied to equation (18), a new equation emerges:

$$pH = pK + \log\frac{[A^-]}{[HA]} \qquad (19)$$

This, in turn, may be stated in a more general form as:

$$pH = pK + \log\frac{[\text{Base}]}{[\text{Acid}]} \qquad (20)$$

This is the *Henderson-Hasselbalch equation*. Since the logarithm of 1.0 is zero, the pH equals pK when the ratio of the molar concentrations of base and acid is one.

Physiologic solutions are characterized in part by the presence of several poorly dissociated acids and their more dissociable salts. In such a situation the function A^- of equation (19) derives virtually entirely from the particular salt involved. The salt may be referred to as BA, and if the salt were, in fact, completely dissociated, the term BA could be incorporated directly into equation (19) as a substitute for $[A^-]$. However, although the quantity of A^- that may derive from BA is proportional to its molal concentration, the salt is not completely dissociated, and the factor describing its degree of dissociation may be incorporated into the constant, pK, in which case this is changed to pK′. In turn, the salt to which the pK′ refers is noted by adding a subscript, as for example pK'_{HCO_3}. The new equation is now:

$$pH = pK'_A + \log \frac{[BA]}{[HA]} \qquad (21)$$

Buffers. A buffered solution is one that has the capacity to minimize a deviation in pH when a strong acid or base is added to it. The buffer consists of a pair of compounds represented either by a weak acid and a highly dissociated salt of that acid, or a weak base and a highly dissociated salt of that base. The buffering effect is due to the formation of a quantity of weak acid or base approximately equivalent to the quantity of strong acid or base added to the solution. In this fashion the strong acid or base is substituted for with weak acid or base, and, hence, a change in hydrogen ion concentration is not prevented but it is certainly minimized. This buffering effect may be illustrated by the reactions that might be anticipated if a strong acid such as HCl were added to a solution containing the weak acid, HA, and its highly dissociated salt, BA:

$$2HA + 2BA + HCl \rightarrow 3HA + BA + BCl \qquad (22)$$

It is noted that the hydrochloric acid reacted in such a way as to increase the concentration of HA and decrease the concentration of BA. The increase in the concentration of HA implies a small but definite increase in the concentration of hydrogen ions, but certainly much less than would have obtained had the HCl been added to a solution with no buffer activity. It will also be noted that equation (22), as written, reveals that there were equal molar concentrations of HA and BA initially, and, hence, the pH prior to the addition of the HCl was equal to the pK'_A. The reaction described in equation (22) also reveals that there was a decrease in the concentration of BA as well as an increase in the concentration of HA. This dictates a change in the buffer ratio from 1.0 to 0.33, and the pH must now be less than the pK'_A.

This illustrates the principle that a deviation of pH depends on the change of the ratio of the buffer pair. This fact has several important implications. The first of these is that the nearer the ratio of the buffer pair is to 1.0, the less change in pH will take place when a given quantity of acid is added to the buffered solution. Thus the buffer system may be said to be most efficient when the pH of the soluton is identical with the pK′ of the particular buffer in question. Secondly, it must be clear that at any ratio of the buffer pair, there will be a smaller change in that ratio following the addition of a given increment of acid if the *concentrations* of the components of the buffer system are high rather than low. Lastly, it is apparent that the capacity to buffer added acid is no longer possible when there is no base (hydrogen ion acceptor) left.

Biologic fluids contain several buffer systems (proteins, phosphates, bicarbonate-carbonic acid, etc.). The ratio of the components of each of the buffer pairs will be determined by the pH and, in turn, these several ratios determine the pH. If the ratio of any one of several buffer pairs alters, all of the ratios of the other buffer pairs must change. This is frequently referred to as the isohydric principle.

As noted earlier in the chapter, the

body fluid most accessible for analysis is the plasma, and the pH of the extracellular fluid may be estimated from a direct determination on this fluid, or from knowledge of the relationship between the molar concentrations of bicarbonate and the sum of the dissolved CO_2 and carbonic acid. This relationship is expressed by the equation:

$$pH = pK'_{HCO_3^-} + \log \frac{[HCO_3^-]}{[H_2CO_3] + [\text{dissolved } CO_2]} \quad (23)$$

The denominator of this buffer ratio is actually almost entirely dissolved CO_2 (the ratio between dissolved CO_2 and H_2CO_3 is approximately 800 to 1), and the quantity of dissolved CO_2 is, in turn, proportional to the tension or partial pressure pCO_2,* of the gas.

The pK' for bicarbonate is 6.1 in plasma at body temperature.[107,108] Under usual circumstances the ratio of bicarbonate to the sum of carbonic acid and dissolved carbon dioxide is 20:1. The log of 20 is 1.301. Thus, under these circumstances the pH is the sum of 6.1 and 1.301, or 7.40.

At first glance it might be assumed that the bicarbonate-carbonic acid buffer pair is highly inefficient (in the usual chemical sense) at the pH of the extracellular fluids, since it was emphasized that a buffer pair is most efficient when the ratio of its components is close to one. However, this is more than counterbalanced by the unique characteristic that the concentration of one of the components, carbonic acid, is determined by the tension of the gas CO_2. The hydration and dehydration of carbon dioxide allows this gas to obtain hydrogen ions from and return them to water. Furthermore, the gas is unique in that it is ubiquitous since it is constantly being formed as a product of metabolism. Lastly, since it is a gas, its rate of elimination from the body can be drastically altered by changes in the depth and the rate of the respirations.

Although the buffer activity within the body is reflected in the bicarbonate-carbonic acid system, and although it is the one which has received considerable attention not only because of its importance but as noted above because of the ease of access of plasma for study, it is by no means the only important buffer system in the body. The hemoglobin of the erythrocytes, the proteins of the plasma, and the phosphates, bicarbonates and proteins of the intracellular fluids each make significant contributions to the over-all buffering activity. It is clear that the first line of defense in minimizing a deviation in pH is the activity of the buffers. The magnitude of this activity could be estimated if one were able to sum the anions of the buffer salts (the total of *base*) which are capable of accepting hydrogen ions. It is not possible to estimate this total with any ease; it includes contributions from bone as well as from the extra- and the intracellular fluid. However, it is possible to gain some insight concerning their magnitude by considering the buffers which are present in whole blood.[109] Whole blood buffers include bicarbonate, proteins and phosphate of plasma, and the hemoglobin, phosphate and bicarbonate of the red blood cells. The quantity of each of these in a liter of whole blood is dependent on its concentration in plasma and red cells and on the fraction of the total volume represented by each medium in whole blood. The anionic properties of hemoglobin vary in the oxygenated and the reduced forms and, therefore, the degree of oxygen saturation of hemoglobin is a necessary datum. The sum of these buffers has been referred to by Singer and Hastings as *buffer bases*,[109] and its range of normal

* The expression pCO_2 refers to the tension or partial pressure of the gas, carbon dioxide. In usual circumstances it is close to 40 mm. Hg. The quantity of a gas such as carbon dioxide that is dissolved in a liquid is proportional to its tension, pCO_2, and this quantity can be expressed in mM./L. as being equal to $\alpha \times pCO_2$. The term α is equal to 0.0301 (mM./L. per mm. Hg.) for plasma at a temperature of 38° C. Dissolved CO_2 is, in turn, in equilibrium with carbonic acid and, hence, the sum of dissolved CO_2 and carbonic acid can be said to be proportional to the pCO_2. A pCO_2 of 40 mm. Hg. would be equal to $0.0301 \times 40 = 1.2$ mM./L. of dissolved carbon dioxide and carbonic acid.

values is 46 to 52 mM./L. Singer and Hastings[109] have prepared a nomogram from which the value for buffer base may be read along with the value for pCO_2 if the pH of the blood, the packed cell volume, and the total CO_2 content of whole blood or plasma are known. The particular clinical value of having information with respect to the quantity of whole blood buffer base is concerned with those circumstances in which it may be difficult to distinguish between various forms of acid-base disturbances. For example, the anionic properties of the plasma proteins vary indirectly with pH; therefore, the retention of carbon dioxide will raise the concentration of bicarbonate, but the anionic equivalence of the proteins will be reciprocally reduced. As a result, a depressed pH due to the retention of CO_2 should be unaccompanied by a change in the value for buffer base. There should likewise be no change in the value for buffer base when an alkalosis has been induced by hyperventilation. Furthermore, this use of buffer base values may help to elucidate instances of more complicated mixtures of acid-base disturbances. In uncomplicated instances of metabolic acidosis and alkalosis the values for buffer bases are diminished and elevated respectively.

Actually the same information may usually be obtained in a less elegant fashion by examining the interrelationships between the concentration of sodium and the sums of the concentrations of total carbon dioxide content and chloride. Under ordinary circumstances the difference between the concentration of sodium and the sum of the concentrations of the two major anions is between 5 and 10 mM./L. Since the retention or excessive elimination of carbon dioxide will be accompanied by a reciprocal change in the concentration of chloride, the difference continues to be approximately 5 to 10 mM./L. in respiratory disturbances of acid-base equilibrium. In contrast, when there is a metabolic acidosis and bicarbonate has been displaced by some undetermined anion, the difference will be increased. These matters will be discussed at greater length in relation to more detailed analysis of distortions of acid-base balance.

Acidosis and Alkalosis. Acidosis and alkalosis have frequently been defined in terms of the concentration of CO_2 in the serum. It should be clear from the above discussion that this is not proper since the state of acid-base relationships, if it is to be defined in relation to CO_2, must be able to discriminate between that fraction of the total CO_2 which is carbon dioxide gas plus carbonic acid and that fraction which is bicarbonate. The estimation of total CO_2 content does not provide this information. Moreover, the total CO_2 content of the serum may be depressed or elevated in the face of an acidosis or an alkalosis. It is frequently possible to infer the state of acid-base relationship from knowledge of the total CO_2 content of the serum and the clinical picture, but ultimately information concerning the pH of the blood is essential for proper documentation whenever there is any doubt. It is best to have pH determined on arterial blood (or blood obtained from a limb vein without stasis after the part has been warmed for about ten minutes at 45° C.). The pH may be more or less disturbed than the concentration of carbon dioxide or other electrolytes in the serum. This depends on the rate and character of the pathogenesis of the particular distortion in acid-base relationships, and on the degree of success which may have attended the physiologic mechanisms that operate to minimize the deviation in pH. These mechanisms include the activity of the buffer systems which have already been referred to, the role of ion exchange processes, respiratory regulation and the contribution of the kidneys.

Anion Exchange. The regulation of acid-base equilibrium revolves around the central problem of maintaining the pH of the extracellular fluids around 7.40, and usually within the limits of 7.35 and 7.45. The exchange of *anions* across cell membranes appears to be restricted to the erythrocyte and, perhaps, the renal tubular cells. Bicarbonate and chloride ions can and do diffuse across the red cell membrane, and the ratio of the concentrations of these ions in red cell and plasma water is responsive to changes in *p*H. Thus, an increase in the tension of carbon dioxide as this occurs as the blood passes from artery to vein through tissue is followed by the diffusion of CO_2 into the red blood cell where it is, in part, hydrated to carbonic acid. The dissociation of this acid augments the concentration of bicarbonate and this, in turn, promotes a diffusion of bicarbonate ions from the red cell to plasma water. This is coupled with a movement of chloride from the plasma to red cell water.[22,44,105] It will be noted that the net effect of this sequence has been to increase the concentration of bicarbonate in the plasma in consequence of the increased concentration of CO_2 in the plasma. This tends to maintain the ratio of bicarbonate to carbon dioxide and carbonic acid closer to twenty than would be the case without this shift. Furthermore, the diffusion of CO_2 into the red cell, its subsequent hydration to carbonic acid, and the dissociation of this latter provides a mechanism for the accession of hydrogen ions to the intracellular fluid where they may be buffered. In the circumstance of the unique red cell and its hemoglobin, it should be noted that as CO_2 accumulates in the plasma as the blood courses through the tissues, the hemoglobin loses oxygen and in the reduced state is better able to buffer the hydrogen ions made available by the accession of the CO_2. This is a very oversimplified illustration of an amazingly complex series of events, each of which appears to reciprocate and interdigitate in such a fashion as to subserve the interests of minimizing a deviation in *p*H with only minor consequences in terms of disturbing the other characteristics of the internal environment.

Cation Exchange. The exchange of *cations* such as potassium, sodium, and perhaps calcium for hydrogen ions across cell membranes and between bone and the extracellular fluid for hydrogen ions appears to play an important role among those factors which operate to maintain *p*H within narrow limits.[110-122] Most of the data with respect to this particular aspect of the problem have been derived in experimental designs in which the individual tissues have not actually been analyzed. The exchanges among the several compartments have been calculated from estimates of change in concentrations of ions in the extracellular fluid, changes in the volume of the extracellular compartment, observations of the external balance of ions, and, lastly, with the assumption that exchanges of hydrogen ion can be accounted for from changes in the concentration of bicarbonate in the extracellular fluid and red cell water which may occur because of the loss of carbon dioxide (or the retention of this gas) by way of the lungs. Reference to a previous section dealing with the measurements of the extracellular space and the problems that are involved makes it clear that such calculations are subject to certain intrinsic errors and limitations. In addition, the assumption that changes in hydrogen ions may be equated with changes in the concentrations of bicarbonate due to loss or gain of CO_2 via the respiratory tract depends on the premise that no change in the production of CO_2 occurs when acid-base equilibrium is altered. If, in fact, the metabolic production of carbon dioxide increases or decreases with alkalosis and acidosis, these calculations may be subject to great error. Nevertheless, to the extent that these techniques of study have some validity it has been estimated that about 50 per cent of an acid load administered to dogs was neutralized by an exchange of hydrogen ions for sodium and potassium ions. In another investigation it was reported that 25 per cent of the "neutralization" of administered sodium bicarbonate had been accomplished by the exchange of intracellular (including bone) hydrogen ions for extracellular sodium ions. Exchanges of a similar nature are reported in studies in which the gain or loss of acid is conditioned by breathing high concentrations of carbon dioxide or by hyperventilation. These latter states are equivalent, of course, to clinical conditions of respiratory acidosis and alkalosis respectively.

Repiratory Regulation of Acid-base Equilibrium. As implied above, the lungs play an important role in the regulation of acid-base balance by altering the excretion of acid as carbon dioxide.[123,124] Furthermore, the centers which regulate the depth and frequency of ventilation are quite sensitive to minor alterations in the chemical composition of the blood and the extravascular fluids. The receptors which are located in the medullary respiratory centers appear to be responsive to the pCO_2 and the pH of their environment in such a fashion that an increase in the tension of carbon dioxide or in the hydrogen ion concentration promotes an increase in pulmonary ventilation, and a decrease in these two functions inhibits ventilation. In each instance it would appear that the alteration in respiratory activity is in a direction which would tend to correct the initial deviation in the pCO_2 or pH. When these two factors are considered as stimuli, the pCO_2 appears to be a more potent agent than the pH of the extracellular fluids. However, it must be emphasized that alterations in pCO_2 may actually influence the rate and depth of respirations by changes in the intracellular pH inasmuch as the cell membranes appear to be completely permeable to carbon dioxide. In addition to these central chemoreceptors, there are peripheral sites in the carotid and aortic bodies which are quite sensitive to pO_2, and much less so to pCO_2 and pH.

One very interesting aspect of chemoregulation of respiratory activity that will be referred to later in more detail concerns the phenomenon of altered sensitivity of the central chemoreceptors to a particular pCO_2.[125–129] A period characterized by hypercapnia appears to diminish the sensitivity of the respiratory centers to a specific level of pCO_2, and, in contrast, a period of hypocapnia seems to enhance the sensitivity of the respiratory center to a given level of CO_2 tension. The mechanism of this altered response is not clear. However, as will be noted later, one of the adjustments to a chronically elevated pCO_2 is an increase in the concentration of bicarbonate in the extracellular fluids. It will be recalled that in the discussion of buffer activity it was noted from a consideration of the Henderson-Hasselbalch equation that at any ratio of the buffer pair the change in the ratio will be less for a given increment of acid if the concentrations of the components of the buffer pair are high rather than low. Thus, if both pCO_2 and bicarbonate concentration are high, a specific increment in pCO_2 will affect the ratio (and, hence, the pH) less than if these concentrations were low. If a similar situation exists within the cells, the explanation of the altered sensitivity may lie in the fact that the intracellular environment is more or less capable of buffering a change in pH. This buffering capacity will be augmented if the concentrations of the two components of the ratio are high as they are in respiratory acidosis and metabolic alkalosis and will be diminished if the concentrations of the two components are low as they would be in respiratory alkalosis and metabolic acidosis.

Renal Physiology[22,24,25,130–136]

The secretion of urine represents the summation of a complex series of mechanisms beginning with the formation of a volume of ultrafiltrate of plasma which is many times larger than the bladder urine formed during the same interval of time. The reabsorption of the bulk of the filtered solutes and water, and, in turn, the secretion of certain solutes, are regulated in such a discriminatory fashion that the internal environment is maintained remarkably constant with respect to the volume, disposition, composition and acid-base relationships of the body fluids. The study of the precise mechanisms underlying these processes continues to be a fascinating and challenging problem. The mechanisms involved appear to interrelate anatomic and chemical structure, physicochemical attributes of composition, with organization of subcellular structure; enzymes, hormones and intermediary metabolic pathways with bio-energetics and active transport of solutes; hemodynamic forces initiated by the contraction of the myocardium with the hydrostatic pressure which promotes filtration at the glomerulus and the rate of perfusion of the renal parenchyma. The variety of scientific disciplines and techniques which is represented by those investigators interested in the function of this organ is in itself an articulate expression of its complexity.

Whereas most of the functions subserved by those organs and tissues discussed in the section on extrarenal external exchanges of electrolytes and water are concerned with rather specialized interests, the kidneys are responsible for many and, at the same time, frequently subtle considerations. The speed and the precision with which the kidneys react to deviations in the internal environment is responsible, in great part at least, for the ability of the organism to survive the ordinary events of day-to-day living and the more complicated problems imposed by the stress of disease. The most eloquent eulogy of the kidney was presented by Dr. Homer Smith when he wrote: "Recognizing that we have the kind of blood we have because we have the kind of kidneys that we have, we must acknowledge that our kidneys constitute the major foundation of our physiological freedom. Only because they work the way they do has it become possible for us to have bones, muscles, glands, and brains. Superficially, it might be said that the function of the kidneys is to make urine; but in a more considered view one can say that the kidneys make the stuff of philosophy itself."[137]

The functional unit of the kidney is the nephron, which consists of a glomerulus, a proximal tubule, the loop of Henle and a distal tubule beyond which the nephron connects with others to join a collecting tubule. The major details of the gross and microscopic anatomy of the renal tissue have been described for many years, although there is undoubtedly more to be learned about them. The more subtle details of structure which have been revealed with the aid of the electron microscope are most exciting, and the reader is urged to consult the descriptions which are available.[133]

Glomerular Filtration. The first step in the elaboration of urine is the formation of an almost protein-free filtrate of the plasma at the glomerulus. The capillary endothelium is freely permeable to water and the solutes of small molecular size. The quantity of water filtered per unit time is conditioned by the difference in the chemical potential of the water of the plasma and that of the ultrafiltrate, and the volume of plasma exposed to the filtering surface per unit time. The colloidal solutes diminish the chemical potential of the plasma water, but this is more than overcome by the hydrostatic pressure in the glomerular vessels; consequently, there is a net movement of water out of the glomerular capillaries into the proximal tubule. The pressure also enhances the chemical potential of the solutes, and those which can permeate the endothelial membrane move at such a rate that a net exchange transpires.

In this regard, it is important to mention a new concept introduced by Pappenheimer and Kinter[138–140] which provides alternative explanations for certain observations in the study of renal physiology. They suggest that as the interlobular arteries divide in the renal circulation the first off-shoots receive a preponderance of the peripherally located plasma and little of the central stream of erythrocytes, a process called plasma-skimming. Thus, certain vessels will carry plasma-rich blood and other vessels will carry plasma-poor (or cell-rich blood). They postulate that the latter blood passes through the more cortical glomeruli and is short-circuited around the peritubular capillaries. This has certain implications with respect to the rate of filtration at the glomerulus. If the total volume of blood within a glomerulus is reasonably constant, the filtration of a given volume of fluid will cause a lesser increase in the concentration of the nondiffusible solutes (proteins) if the fraction of the glomerular vascular volume which is plasma is initially large rather than small. Since the efficiency of plasma-skimming is greater with an increase in hydrostatic pressure, an increase in renal arterial pressure will promote perfusion of the glomeruli with a fluid that is richer in plasma. Even if the hydrostatic pressure in the glomerular vessels themselves had not changed, the filtration of more fluid would be favored. However, this would tend to be counterbalanced in the glomeruli receiving cell-rich blood and, hence, GFR may be somewhat independent of changes in arterial pressure.

Glomerular Filtration Rate. An estimate of the rate of filtration at the glomerulus is of great importance in the investigation of many aspects of renal physiology and is of considerable value in the evaluation of selected patients with problems which include renal disease. Measurement of the rate of glomerular filtration (GFR) is based on the concept of renal *clearance*. This latter term is defined as the volume of plasma which contains the quantity of a particular substance that is excreted in the urine in a unit of time (which is usually one minute). In other words, it is the virtual volume of plasma which is "cleared" of that substance by the kidney in one minute. If one knows the rate of excretion of urine and the simultaneous concentrations of a particular substance in the plasma and urine, the *clearance* may be calculated from the formula:

$$\text{Clearance} = \frac{UV}{P} \qquad (24)$$

where U and P represent the concentration of the substance in urine and plasma respectively, and V is the rate of excretion of urine per minute. The clearance is usually referred to as C, and a subscript may be employed to denote the particular substance whose clearance is under consideration. The clearance of a particular substance would be an estimate of the rate of filtration at the glomeruli if it had the following characteristics: (1) freely filtered at the glomerulus, (2) neither reabsorbed nor secreted by the renal tubular cells, (3) neither synthesized nor altered by the kidney, (4) subject to accurate analysis in both plasma and urine. A variety of substances have been employed for this purpose, including creatinine, thiosulfate, mannitol and others. The most widely accepted substance for use in man is inulin. Exogenous creatinine is valid in most other animals. Endogenous creatinine clearance usually varies with inulin clearance in healthy man, although the calculated values may differ considerably. In disease the endogenous creatinine clearance is less reliable.

The clearance of substances which are filtered but also reabsorbed and, in some instances, secreted is an abstraction and really has little meaning except when estimated simultaneously with the GFR in an effort to understand some of the net quantitative aspects of the several operations which are involved in the renal excretion of the particular substance. For example, if the rate of excretion of a compound or ion were in excess of that which could have been filtered, the implication is clear that some fraction of this material that appeared in the urine must have been secreted by the tubular cells. It is in this fashion that it was demonstrated that potassium can be secreted by the renal tubular cells.[141–143] When the clearance of a substance that is filtered is less than the GFR, it is clear that some of the material must have been reabsorbed by the renal tubular cells. However, it is also possible that a substance which is filtered, reabsorbed *and* secreted may have a clearance less than the GFR under many circumstances.

The clearance of urea was once used frequently as a measure of renal function. It is believed that urea is filtered and reabsorbed, although there is some suggestion that it might even be secreted as well.[144] At rates of excretion of urine which are 2 ml./min. or a little more, the clearance of urea is approximately one half that of the GFR. This is, however, only an approximation since the rate of excretion of urea is conditioned by the rate of excretion of water as well as the filtration rate. For these reasons, the use of the urea clearance is not recommended as a valuable tool in investigating the status of renal function; if it is deemed important to estimate GFR, it would be much more desirable to estimate the clearance of inulin, C_{In}. The normal value for inulin clearance in the human is approximately 125 ml./min. per 1.73 sq. m. surface area in males and about 110 ml./min. in females.

Renal Plasma Flow.[131–133] If one had access to a substance which could be maintained at a reasonably steady concentration in the plasma by continuous infusion, and if the material had the following characteristics: (1) it were not altered, destroyed, nor synthesized by the kidneys, (2) it were entirely removed from the plasma as the blood traversed the kidney in single passage from the renal artery to the renal vein, (3) it were completely excreted into the urine as it was removed from the plasma, (4) its concentration in urine and plasma could be estimated accurately, then its *clearance* would be a measure of the volume of plasma that coursed through the kidney in a unit of time (usually referred to as one minute). The volume of whole blood that perfused the kidney per unit of time could then be calculated from information concerning the packed cell volume of the whole blood.

There are substances that almost conform to the qualities listed above, and of these Diodrast and para-aminohippurate (PAH) have been the most widely used to measure these parameters of renal function in man and the lower animals. Direct catheterization of the renal vein has made it clear that extraction of these substances is not actually 100 per cent during a single course through the kidney, but that in normal subjects it approximates 92 per cent. This would suggest that an average of 8 per cent of the plasma traversing the renal mass did not have contact with tissue, such as the glomerular filter or the renal tubular cells, which could dispose of the material.* When Diodrast or PAH is used to measure renal plasma flow, it is usually not accompanied by a direct estimate of the extraction ratio, and, therefore, the value calculated as the clearance represents the volume of plasma flowing through functional renal tissue; this is frequently referred to as the *effective* renal plasma flow. The average value for the clearance of PAH in humans is 654 and 592 ml. per minute per 1.73 sq. m. of surface area in males and females respectively.

Concept of Tubular Maxima. Many of the processes with which the renal tubular cells are concerned represent reactions which require the expenditure of energy since they involve the active transport of ions and molecules against concentration gradients.[62] It is not surprising, therefore, to find that there are maximal rates at which some of these processes may transpire. Certain specific reabsorptive and secretory functions may be examined with respect to the maximum rates that may be achieved, and these may be utilized to study some of the characteristics of the transport mechanisms, to provide information about disorders that have their origin remote from the kidney but in which the kidneys participate through an alteration in a tubular transport mechanism, and to evaluate the quantitative aspects of renal tubular function as this may be correlated with the extent and type of renal disease. The maximal rate of reabsorption or secretion of a substance is referred to as a Tm, and a subscript is added to denote the substance under consideration. For exam-

* This could be ascribed to renal parenchyma other than the glomeruli and tubules, such as the capsule and the collecting system of the kidney. In addition, it could be due in part to "shunting" of blood such as has been proposed by Trueta et al.[145] and more recently by Pappenheimer and Kinter.[138–140] In these latter terms, alterations in the degree to which a substance such as PAH is extracted might be associated with variations in the degree of "plasma-skimming" referred to in the earlier phase of the discussion of renal physiology.

ple, the maximal rate of reabsorption of glucose[146] or phosphate is referred to as Tm_G or Tm_P respectively, and the maximal rate of *secretion* of PAH is referred to as Tm_{AH}. The nature of the tubular maximum as a measurement may be illustrated by the maximal rate of reabsorption of glucose, or Tm_G. Under ordinary circumstances the quantity of glucose that is filtered per minute, which is equivalent to the product of its concentration in plasma and the volume of the GFR, is small enough so that the tubules are able to reabsorb all of it and none escapes into the urine. If the concentration of glucose in plasma is progressively increased, a point is reached where some glucose gains access to the urine; if the concentration in the plasma is increased enough, a point is reached where every increment in the quantity of glucose filtered finds its way into the urine. The difference between the amount that is filtered and the amount that is excreted is the amount reabsorbed. Under the circumstances just cited, the amount reabsorbed is the maximum or Tm_G. Similar calculations may be made for other substances that are filtered and reabsorbed, such as phosphate, or for substances that are secreted.

Although reference is frequently made to tubular maxima for other substances such as water, and ions such as chloride and sodium, their definition is not as easily established, and there is some question as to how one may be certain that a mechanism for the reabsorption of any of these materials has, in fact, been saturated. Moreover, since many of these materials are reabsorbed by several different processes, and their rates of excretion are highly conditioned phenomena, the precise description of rate factors is still quite incomplete. Some of the reasons for this will become apparent in the discussion of the problems related to the excretion of water and salts and to the acidification of the urine.

Excretion of Water. It is presumed that the rate of excretion of water is the net difference between the volume that is filtered and the quantity that is reabsorbed per unit time. This implies that water is not secreted by the renal tubules, an hypothesis which has been suggested but which is untestable at this time. The conceptual framework concerning the operations that are involved in the reabsorption of water is at best only an approximation, but there are adequate data to support the general characteristics of the description that follows. Some of these data are highly inferential, whereas fewer but very important data have been contributed by careful investigations involving micropunctures of renal tubules, initially by the group working with Richards at Philadelphia,[147-149] and more recently independently by Wirz[150-153] and by Gottschalk.[154]

The reabsorption of the water that is filtered at the glomerulus is thought to be accomplished at several anatomic levels in the nephron by mechanisms which differ from each other in certain essential features.[155-160] The first and the largest in terms of volume occurs in the proximal portion of the renal tubule, where the reabsorption of water is thought to be a passive consequence of the active reabsorption of solutes. The abstraction of solutes in the proximal nephron creates a dilute or hypotonic tubular fluid (increasing the chemical potential of the water), and water is then thought to diffuse across the tubular epithelium along the established osmotic gradient. The volume of fluid that reaches the end of the proximal tubule is therefore primarily conditioned by the volume that is filtered and the rate at which solutes are extracted. It is believed that under most circumstances approximately 85 to 90 per cent of the filtered solutes and water are removed as the fluid proceeds along the proximal tubule. Since the abstraction of solutes is the active process and the reabsorption of water is a passive consequence, the fluid at the end of this first portion of the nephron is presumed to be isosmotic with filtrate, *although its specific composition has been drastically altered.* Independent micropuncture studies by Walker, Bott, Oliver and McDowell, by Wirz, and by Gottschalk all confirm the fact that fluid obtained from the proximal tubule is isosmotic with filtrate. However, none of these punctures have been in the last third of the proximal tubule, and the character of the fluid in this last third has not been defined by actual observation.

The second phase in the reabsorption of water has been ascribed to the distal tubule. It has been suggested by Smith[131,133] on theoretical grounds, and subsequently proved by cryoscopic examination of fluid obtained by micropuncture of mammalian distal tubules by Wirz[151–153] and by Gottschalk,[154] that the active reabsorption of solutes from the loop of Henle and the distal tubule is followed by an isosmotic reabsorption of water in the distal tubule only when there is maximal activity of the antidiuretic hormone (ADH). It is further implied, and now partially supported by direct observations, that the distal tubular fluid is made maximally dilute by the abstraction of solutes without water in the complete absence of ADH. With intermediate quantities of antidiuretic hormone between none and a maximum, more and more water may be reabsorbed up to the point where the urine is isosmotic with the filtrate. Thus, the volume of water that may be reabsorbed is limited in the first phase by the rate of reabsorption of solutes, and in the second phase by the action of the antidiuretic hormone as well.

In this fashion a varyingly hypotonic or isosmotic fluid reaches the next phase, which is beyond the distal tubule and is believed to be in the early segment of the collecting system. At this site water is reabsorbed without (or, at least, in excess of) solutes, and probably independently of ADH. The quantity of water reabsorbed at this site is thought to be limited by at least two parameters: namely, a rate and an osmotic gradient. In man the limiting rate is 5 to 7 ml. per minute, and the maximal concentration of human urine approaches a limit at 1400 milliosmolal. This third phase of reabsorption of water is frequently referred to as $T^{c}_{H_2O}$, and similarly the first and second phases may be referred to as $T^{p}_{H_2O}$ and $T^{d}_{H_2O}$ respectively.

There are data from a variety of sources which support the major aspects of this description. The earlier micropuncture studies established the approximate volume of the reabsorbate in the proximal tubules, and the identity of the osmolality (by vapor pressure studies) of the proximal tubular fluid and the filtrate. Wirz has reported observations concerning the osmolality (utilizing a cryoscopic technique) of proximal and distal tubular fluid under circumstances of a water diuresis and the antidiuresis induced by water deprivation. He confirmed the observation that the fluid in the proximal tubule was isosmotic with filtrate during water diuresis. He also noted that the fluid obtained from the first portion of the distal tubule was hypotonic in either circumstance and that it remained dilute when the animal was experiencing a water diuresis, whereas the distal tubular fluid became isosmotic with filtrate along the course of the distal tubule when the activity of the antidiuretic hormone was maximal. However, the osmolality of the distal tubular fluid did not exceed that of the filtrate despite the fact that the bladder urine was simultaneously concentrated. These observations have been confirmed by Gottschalk and Mylle and lend strong support to the description presented above.

Although the site of urine concentration is unknown, it is apparent that it is beyond the distal tubule, and there are reasons to believe that it may be in the collecting tubules. One of these reasons is the observation that the desert rodent manufactures the most highly concentrated urine and has an unusually large system of collecting tubules. A second reason is the fact that animals with potassium depletion are unable to concentrate the urine properly and have a structural lesion in the collecting tubule.[161,162] Although these observations do not constitute proof concerning the locus of the concentrating mechanism, they are certainly highly suggestive.

The probability that the third phase of the reabsorption of water is partly independent of ADH is suggested by data from two major sources. Shannon[163] observed the excretion of concentrated urines in dogs with experimental diabetes insipidus when they had been subjected to dehydration. It cannot be concluded with confidence that this represented an ADH-independent concentrating mechanism, since it is never safe to assume that experimental or clinical diabetes insipidus is complete and that there is a total inability to secrete any antidiuretic hormone. More recently Berliner and Davidson[164] have reported a beautifully designed experiment with data that seem to leave little question concerning the fact that a hypertonic urine can be formed in the absence of the antidiuretic hormone. They induced a water diuresis in dogs and examined the characteristics of the urine collected from each kidney separately. When a steady rate of excretion of a hypotonic urine was established, they constricted one renal artery so as to reduce the rate of filtration at the glomerulus on that side. This was accompanied by a drastic reduction in the rate of urine flow on that side, and the urine itself was found to be slightly hypertonic to the plasma, whereas the urine issuing from the other kidney continued to be as dilute as it had been before. This latter observation supports the contention that the procedures employed did not induce a secretion of ADH; despite this there was hypertonic urine on the ipsilateral side. The production of a hypertonic urine in the absence of ADH is ascribed to the accession of a markedly reduced volume of dilute tubular fluid to the $T^c_{H_2O}$ site, so that even though this fluid was dilute, the abstraction of some water without solutes was great enough to convert the osmolality of the fluid to a value in excess of that of the filtrate.

The mechanism for the abstraction of water without (or in excess of) solutes at the $T^c_{H_2O}$ site is unknown. It is not clear whether or not it operates in the absence of ADH, although the study of Berliner and Davidson cited above is compatible with the theory that this phase of the reabsorption of water is independent of the antidiuretic hormone. Some suggestions, along with supporting data, have been presented by Berliner,[165] Wirz,[150–153] Uhlrich,[166,167] and Gottschalk[154] concerning this problem, and they merit very serious consideration. It was noted above that the fluid in the earliest part of the distal tubule was hypotonic whether or not ADH was active. If the secretion of water is discounted, the implication is clear that solutes without, or in excess of, water were transported out of the luminal fluid somewhere between the last third of the proximal tubule and the beginning of the distal tubule.[168–170] If it is assumed that the fluid remains isosmotic with filtrate all along the proximal tubule, the active transport of solutes that dilutes the fluid between the proximal and distal tubules must be in the loops of Henle, of which a certain number dip down deep into the medulla and lie adjacent to the collecting tubules. The rapid active transport of solutes (presumably preponderantly sodium and chloride) from this portion of the nephron tends to increase the osmolality of the interstitial fluid at these sites.[165] If the rate of active transport into the interstitium is greater than the rate at which these solutes diffuse away, a mechanism is available to maintain the fluid in those areas at a high osmolality. If the collecting tubular cells are freely permeable to water, the difference in the osmolality of the fluids within and outside of the collecting tubules would promote a redistribution of water from the tubule to the interstitium and thence into the blood vascular system.

Ullrich[166,167] and his co-workers and Berliner et al.[165] have demonstrated a gradient in the osmolality and the concentration of sodium in the tissue fluid of kidney slices as one proceeds from cortex to medulla. This gradient is present whether the urine is being concentrated or not, although it is considerably more striking when a concentrated urine is being formed. Moreover, Berliner has observed that the concentration of sodium in the tissue fluid of the medulla is highest when the urine is concentrated and that the concentration of sodium in the total tissue water of the medulla is higher than in the simultaneous urine, thus proving that the high concentration of this cation in the medullary water cannot be ascribed solely to its concentration in the fluid within the tubules and ducts. Berliner[165] also suggests that the anatomic characteristics of the blood vessels which accompany the thin limb and loop of Henle, which makes a hairpin turn, help to diminish the effect of diffusion of solutes away from this area and, hence, tend to sustain the osmotic gradient that is established by the active transport of solutes into the interstitial fluid.[171] Lastly, Gottschalk[154] raises the question of the importance of the rate of flow of blood in these areas in relation to the maintenance and magnitude of the osmotic gradient.

In addition to the fact that this general hypothesis provides an explanation for the formation of a hypertonic urine in the absence of ADH, it also permits an explanation for the formation of minimally concentrated urine despite maximal antidiuretic hormone activity when the rate of excretion of solutes is large in what is usually referred to as a solute or osmotic diuresis.[24,25,58,81,131–133,172–175] An osmotic diuresis supervenes in any circumstance in which there is a decrease in the fraction of the filtered solutes that is reabsorbed. This, in turn, may obtain whenever the composition of the filtrate is altered in such a way that there is an increase in the concentration of some solute(s) the reabsorption of which is limited. This may occur as a consequence of a greater production of urea during the course of an increased rate of catabolism of protein, an increase in the intake of salt or hyperglycemia. It may be readily induced by the infusion of concentrated solutions of glucose, urea and sodium chloride, or by the intravenous administration of solutes the reabsorption of which is markedly limited, such as sulfate, or those solutes which are virtually nonreabsorbable by the renal tubules, such as mannitol, sucrose and other sugars.* In each of these circumstances an unusually large volume of fluid gains access to the distal tubule, and even if this event promotes an augmented reabsorption of solutes at this site, the quantity of solutes that escape reabsorption is enhanced. Since the reabsorption of water in the distal tubule under the influence of maximum ADH activity does not proceed beyond the point where the fluid is made isosmotic with filtrate, it is clear that an unusually large volume of presumably isosmotic fluid will gain access to the $T^c_{H_2O}$ site. Under this circumstance the quantity of water reabsorbed at this third site is limited by rate rather than by osmotic gradient, since the abstraction of 5 to 7 ml. per minute will not raise the total solute concentration of this fluid to the limiting osmolality of 1400 mOsm./Kg. of water. Moreover, as the rate of excretion of solutes increases and more and more fluid is brought to this last site, the abstraction of a constant volume of water affects the final concentration of the intratubular fluid less and less. If the osmolality of the urine is plotted against the rate of excretion of solutes it will be noted that urine osmolality approaches that of plasma in an asymptotic fashion as the rate of excretion of solutes increases.

In many discussions concerned with its excretion, water is treated as two fractions or clearances, spoken of as free and osmolar water,[131,133,155,156] and

$$V = C_{osm} + C_{H_2O} \qquad (25)$$

where V is the rate of excretion of water, C_{osm} is the clearance of osmolar water, and C_{H_2O} is the clearance of free water. The osmolar water is that vol-

* Other factors which will enhance the rate of excretion of solutes and thereby induce an osmotic diuresis include an augmented filtration rate[176,177] and the administration of pharmacologic agents such as organic mercurial compounds and carbonic anhydrase inhibitors which interfere specifically with the rate of reabsorption of ions by the renal tubular cells.

ume which could contain the solutes, excreted per minute, at a concentration identical with that of the filtrate. Thus, C_{H_2O} has a positive value only when the bladder urine is hypotonic to plasma, and it has a negative value when the bladder urine is hypertonic to plasma. A negative free water clearance may be equated with the third operation, and its magnitude can be estimated when it can be certified that there is maximal ADH activity. Under this latter circumstance the urine that gains access to the third site is already isosmotic so that a negative value for free water clearance may be interpreted as the volume of water abstracted at the final site. In contrast, if ADH activity is present but less than maximal, the free water clearance may still be positive; if it is negative, it is compounded of factors that are concerned with the volume and the tonicity of the fluid brought to the final site. The maximal rate at which $T^c_{H_2O}$ may operate can be estimated only when there is maximal ADH activity and the rate of excretion of solutes is sufficiently large to insure that the limiting parameter will be *rate* and not the osmotic ceiling. In order to assign a positive value to $T^c_{H_2O}$ when the urine is hypertonic the equation reads:

$$T^c_{H_2O} = C_{osm} - V \qquad (26)$$

Although there is obviously much to recommend this general formulation, the hypothesis as stated must at least be incomplete. Among the features which are difficult to resolve are the factors regulating $T^c_{H_2O}$. If this were truly limited only by a rate and an osmotic ceiling, then the maximal osmotic gradient should be achieved whenever the urine flow is less than the maximal $T^c_{H_2O}$ (referred to as $T^c_{mH_2O}$). This seems not to be the case, however, and maximal concentrations of the urine are noted only when the rate of excretion of solutes is small. The gradual rather than abrupt change from a maximally concentrated urine as the rate of solute excretion increases under circumstances of maximal ADH activity remains unexplained. A factor of time which might interfere with the attainment of osmotic equilibrium when the rate of flow of fluid was increased has been suggested but discarded by Robinson.[132] Another difficulty with the hypothesis is that urea appears to obligate less urine water than other solutes. There are several explanations for this, including the possibility that urea may be actively secreted at a site beyond the third phase of reabsorption of water.[144] If urea is secreted distal to the third phase of water reabsorption, the entire calculation of free and osmolar water becomes meaningless. The calculation is equally meaningless if the fluid that reaches the $T^c_{H_2O}$ site is not isosmotic with filtrate.

Antidiuretic Hormone. Although this discussion has emphasized the relationships between the rates of excretion of solutes and water, it should be borne in mind that under usual conditions, when modest rates of solute excretion obtain, the conservation or rejection of water by the kidneys is largely conditioned by the presence or absence of the *antidiuretic hormone*. The secretion of this hormone is influenced by circumstances concerned with the internal environment.[24,81,84,157,159,160] Verney demonstrated some time ago that secretion of the antidiuretic hormone was induced by the intracarotid arterial injection of hypertonic solutions of salt, glucose and sucrose, but not by urea.[178] The discriminatory response between salt, glucose and sucrose on the one hand and a solution of urea on the other implies that the receptor organ is responsive to alterations in the *effective* rather than the total osmolality of its environmental fluid. This, in turn, implies that the stimulus to the secretion of ADH is, in fact, the decrease in intracellular volume induced by a *relative* deficit of water of the fluids bathing the osmoreceptors in the anterior hypothalamus.[179–181] These observations have been confirmed and amplified and it now appears clear that the primary factor that serves to stimulate or suppress the secretion of ADH is a relative deficit or excess of water respectively. More recently von Euler[182] measured potential differences with an electrode placed in the Ringer-agar filled frontal sinus and an exploring electrode in the supraoptic nucleus in cats. A slow potential change was recorded in response to an injection of a 2 per cent solution of NaCl into the carotid artery, and a potential difference of opposite direction was noted when the same volume of solute-free water was injected in lieu of the strong salt solution. There are many sources of data to support the contention that the supraoptic and paraventricular nuclei are involved in the mechanisms leading to the release of ADH. In fact, it is now believed that these two nuclei are the sites at which the hormone is secreted and from which it is carried by way of the axones of the cells that make up these nuclei to the median eminence of the hypophyseal stalk and then to the posterior lobe of the pituitary gland, where the hormone is stored before it is released into the general circulation.[183]

In addition to the stimulus to secretion of ADH by a relative deficit of water, there are data which suggest that a diminished volume, or some function thereof, in a key portion of the body fluids may also promote the secretion of this hormone.[184–189] The locus or loci of such presumed "volume receptors" are unknown but would most likely be in some component of the extracellular space. Since a relative deficit of water is of necessity accompanied by an increase in the effective osmolality of the body fluids and, hence, a diminution in the volume of the cells, it may be stated that the primary and secondary stimuli for the secretion of ADH are diminutions in the volume of the intra- and extracellular compartments respectively.

Other stimuli which provoke the secretion of this hormone include unpleasant and painful experiences[190–192] and a variety of drugs including histamine, nicotine, acetylcholine, ferritin, morphine, anesthetic drugs and other agents.[24,193–196] Ethyl alcohol appears to be unique in its ability to suppress the secretion of this hormone.[197–199]

The chemical characteristics of the hormone have been defined in a brilliant series of investigations reported by du Vigneaud and his collaborators.[200–202] They report that the hormone is an octopeptide amide containing the eight amino acids, aspartic acid, cystine, glutamic acid, glycine, proline, tyrosine, phenylalanine and arginine.

The manner in which the antidiuretic hormone promotes the reabsorption of water is unknown. The effect of neurohypophyseal hormones on the transport of water across the skin of the toad and frog has been known for some time, and Koefoed-Johnsen and Ussing[203] have recently suggested that these agents may influence this process by changing the number or size of pores in the membrane. It is conceivable that the hormone might act in this way with respect to pores in the renal epithelium of the distal tubule.[204]

The quantitative relationship between the dose of hormone administered as a constant rate of infusion of an aqueous solution of vasopressin and the antidiuretic response calculated as the change in the clearance of free water has been investigated in normal humans.[204] These data fit several regression equations, one of which relates the magnitude of the response to an approximately square root function of the dose of hormone. Another equally good regression equation was defined which related the reciprocal of the response to the reciprocal of the dose. This relationship would conform to any one of several theories which include: (1) an hypothesis suggested by Ussing that the hormone molecule influences the size or number of pores, (2) an hypothesis which supposes that the hormone causes a specific increment in the osmotic pressure of certain renal tubular cells that is so oriented as to promote the osmotic reabsorption of water.

Among the factors which could condition the dose-response relationship of this hormone is the manner in which it gains access to its locus of action. If it is filtered and acts on the distal tubular cells, the concentration at which it gains access to the distal tubular fluid will be determined not only by the level of the hormone in the plasma but by the degree to which it is concentrated en route to the distal nephron by the abstraction of a large volume of the filtered water. If, on the other hand, it is not filtered but gains access to the site of action from the contraluminal side of the tubule, the amount that reaches a particular site in a unit of time might be related, in part, to the rate at which plasma perfuses the kidney and hence might be influenced by the renal plasma flow as well as the concentration of the hormone in the plasma. Although the composition and structure of the antidiuretic hormone have been described, it is not clear whether it circulates as the free polypeptide or is combined in some fashion to a larger molecular species.[205] It has been reported that the antidiuretic activity in rat plasma is not found in an ultrafiltrate, and that it is associated with the beta globulin fraction when the plasma proteins are separated by electrophoresis.[206]

There have been suggestions in times past that hormones other than the antidiuretic hormone influence the rate of excretion of water. A diuretic hormone secreted by the anterior pituitary gland has been postulated, and there have been discussions of the role of the thyroid hormone and the adrenal cortical hormones in the regulation of the rate of excretion of water.[207] It is unlikely that these hormones have any effect on the reabsorption of water per se; rather they probably exert an influence on its rate of excretion by altering the rate of filtration at the glomerulus, the rate of excretion of solutes, and, in part, by redistribution of the quantities of solutes reabsorbed in the proximal and the distal portions of the tubules.[208-209] Interestingly enough, the oxytocic hormone which differs from ADH only in the character of two of its eight amino acids and which is thought to play a role primarily in relation to the initiation and course of parturition, seems also to have an influence on renal hemodynamics. It has been reported by one group that animals with diabetes insipidus have a diminution in the GFR, in the renal plasma flow and in the maximal ability to secrete PAH, and that these functions are restored toward normal not by vasopressin (which does correct the defect in concentrating ability) but by oxytocin.[210]

Excretion of Salt.[24,25,79,81,131-133,135,211] The factors that are responsible for the regulation of the rate of excretion of salt are poorly understood. The mechanisms responsible for the reabsorption of sodium and chloride are in part intimately interrelated and in part completely independent of one another. They are probably reabsorbed at several sites within the nephron and are responsive to situations that operate locally within the nephron as well as to stimuli that arise at a distance from the kidneys. The reabsorption of sodium is conditioned by many factors, including the status of the volume and composition of the body fluids, acid-base equilibrium, the rate of excretion of potassium, the rate of excretion of all other solutes, and hormones.

In general it may be stated that, all other conditions being equal and controlled, the rate of excretion of sodium is influenced by the rate of filtration of this cation at the glomerulus, whether this is altered by a gross change in the rate of formation of filtrate at the glomeruli, or by a change in the concentration of sodium in the filtrate itself.[176,212,213] However, it would appear that this is not a prominent influence in man, and factors other than the rate at which sodium is filtered take precedence in the regulation of the rate of excretion.

Among the factors which seem especially important in this regard is the status of the volume of some component of the extracellular fluids or of some function thereof.[24,81,83,214,215] The importance of some physiologic function which may be equated in some fashion with volume becomes immediately apparent when one considers the many observations in the literature concerning the conditions under which marked alterations in the rate of excretion of salt may be made manifest. Patients with cirrhosis of the liver and ascites may excrete a urine that is virtually free of salt despite normal concentrations of sodium in the serum and normal rates of GFR. A change from the supine to the quiet erect posture is accompanied by a diminution in the rate of excretion of salt.[216,217] It is true that this is also accompanied by a decrease in the GFR but, in fact, the diminished rate of excretion of salt persists when the rate of filtration at the glomerulus is maintained by the infusion of a strong solution of salt. The assumption of the sitting posture after reclining is also associated with a diminished salt excretion. The infusion of *hypo*tonic solution of salt will augment the rate of excretion of salt.[218] The sudden manual closure of an arteriovenous fistula will be followed by a saluresis despite the lack of significant alterations in GFR, and an antisaluresis is noted when the fistula is allowed to open, again without alterations in renal hemodynamics.[219] It has also been noted that an increase or decrease in the renal artery perfusion pressure may be accompanied by changes in the rate of excretion of salt without alterations in the rate of filtration at the glomerulus. The rate of excretion of salt is diminished in the face of an absolute deficit of water despite the fact that this is simultaneously associated with a striking increase in the concentration of sodium in the serum.[30] Each of the items noted above suggests most strongly that one of the primary influences on salt excretion is, in fact, somehow related to the volume of fluid in some key segment of the body. The search for this so-called "volume receptor" has engaged the interest of several laboratories over the past years. It is unlikely that "volume" actually expresses itself as such, but, perhaps, its influence is made known by alterations in pressure, rate of flow of blood, viscosity of blood, concentration of the colloid components of the blood, etc. There are some reasons for suggesting that a "volume receptor" may reside in the pulmonary circulation,[220] in the left atrium of the heart,[221] in the intracranial area, in the arterial side of the circulation, and, perhaps, in the circulation of the kidney itself. There is one study which might be interpreted to suggest that the interstitial compartment is the segment of the body fluids of which the volume is significant in this context. This concerns the observation that there is a reduction in salt excretion when infusions of concentrated albumin are administered.[222,223] In contrast with most of the other data which suggest that antisaluresis is associated with a contraction of blood volume or a sequestration of part of the blood volume, this procedure is accompanied by an expanded intravascular volume at the expense of the volume of the interstitial fluid. An alternative interpretation has been offered suggesting the possibility that some mechanism responsible for the renal tubular reabsorption of salt might be influenced by alterations in the oncotic pressure of the plasma.[186]

However, even if it were freely granted that renal tubular activity were responsive somehow to "volume," the question remains as to how an alteration in volume initiates abrupt changes in the rate of reabsorption of sodium and its salts by the renal tubule. These stimuli could operate through neurogenic and hormonal mechanisms, among others.

There are many reasons to suspect that neurogenic influences may modify the rate of excretion of sodium by the kidneys. Bernard and later Jungmann and Meyer[224] induced an increase in the rate of excretion of salt by puncturing the floor of the medulla. Subsequently, Jungmann and Meyer demonstrated that renal denervation resulted in an augmented rate of excretion of salt, and this finding has been confirmed many times by many experimental groups. There is less agreement as to whether the "denervation diuresis" is due to altered renal hemodynamics and vasoregulation or to a direct effect on the specific tubular mechanisms responsible for the reabsorption of ions.[225-235] The possibility that direct neural influences may be significant is emphasized by the observation that some patients with lesions of the central nervous system appear to develop a "salt-wasting syndrome" which may be severe; it may require as much as 50 to 60 grams of NaCl per day to prevent the development of a negative balance.[91,236,237] If left unattended these patients may develop all of the consequences of salt depletion dehydration but do not develop the striking hyperkalemia of adrenal cortical insufficiency. The renal tubules of such patients are able to respond to DOCA, and the adrenal cortices appear to be able to respond to stimulation with ACTH. The precise location of the lesion in the central nervous system with which this is associated is difficult to establish since most of the patients have had rather widespread disease, although a few with reasonably well localized brain tumors have been noted. There are recent data which link the central nervous system with the regulation of the secretion of aldosterone, the salt-retaining hormone of the adrenal cortex.[238,239] These observations point to the diencephalon as the site of secretion of a neurohumor that serves to stimulate the secretion of aldosterone. Although this is an attractive alternative hypothesis to the concept of a more direct neurologic control of renal tubular activity, it seems somewhat unconvincing in view of the fact that the cerebral salt-wasting syndrome differs rather strikingly from aldosterone insufficiency in terms of the quantities of salt that are required to maintain balance and the absence of a tendency to retain potassium. The question of whether there is or is not direct neurogenic control of renal tubular reabsorption of salt therefore remains in doubt. Positive evidence for neuroregulation will demand an experimental design wherein renal denervation is accompanied by an unequivocal increase in the rate of excretion of salt in association with a diminished GFR.

The influence of the adrenal cortical hormone(s) has already been alluded to. It is now reasonably well established that the important adrenal cortical hormone with respect to the reabsorption of sodium is aldosterone.[240–243] The secretion of this hormone appears to be relatively independent of ACTH. The physiologic stimuli that appear to be responsible for the secretion of this hormone include a contraction of the extracellular volume and hyperkalemia.[244–248] Hyponatremia appears to have little influence. The rate of secretion of aldosterone from the adrenal cortex of the dog appears to be increased when the blood volume is specifically diminished. It is exciting to speculate that "volume," or some function thereof, may make itself known through those mechanisms that control the rate of secretion of this hormone, and that it is, perhaps, in this way that volume plays a critical role in the regulation of the rate of excretion of sodium insofar as this is an alteration of renal tubular activity in contradistinction to an influence of volume on renal hemodynamics.

Virtually nothing is known concerning the site of action in the nephron of this salt-retaining hormone. Data on the effects of cortisone and hydrocortisone suggest that they act primarily on the distal portion of the tubule.[24] The influence of this hormone on renal hemodynamics and its site of action are, of course, crucial questions, and data with respect to these problems would allow a more definitive analysis of some of the secondary consequences of adrenal cortical insufficiency. These will be discussed in more detail later in this chapter when Addison's disease is considered.

Much has been written of the influence of the antidiuretic hormone on the rate of excretion of Na, Cl and other ions. It seems reasonably clear from perusal of the data that there is no evidence that ADH in physiologic doses plays any role in the regulation of the rate of excretion of salt. In large doses it may influence salt excretion in lower animals and man through pressor effects and alterations in renal hemodynamics. With chronic administration of vasopressin (as Pitressin in Oil) Leaf et al.[249] demonstrated that the rate of excretion of salt was increased only when the volume of the body fluids had become expanded by the development of a positive balance of water. When the subjects received the same amount of vasopressin but limited the intake of fluids so that a positive balance of water was avoided and, hence, there was no increase in the volume of fluid, there was also no increase in the rate of excretion of salt.

The rate of excretion of salt may be enhanced during a *solute* or *osmotic diuresis*.[59,155,156,172–175,250] The intensity of the saluresis is conditioned primarily by the increased rate of excretion of the loading solute. Several explanations have been advanced for the enhanced excretion of salt, and the most reasonable of these may be illustrated by comparing the consequences of the reabsorption of solutes in the proximal tubule in ordinary circumstances with the events that transpire when an infusion of mannitol is administered. Under ordinary circumstances sodium and its salts represent more than 90 per cent of the filtered solutes. Therefore, when sodium salts are actively reabsorbed from the proximal tubule and water diffuses as a passive consequence, the concentration of the sodium remaining in the tubular fluid does not fall very low. This is implicit in the statement that the fluid at the end of the proximal tubule is isosmotic with filtrate and contains no glucose. The major solutes are obviously sodium salts and urea. In contrast, when mannitol is present in the tubular fluid the volume of water reabsorbed is limited because mannitol cannot be reabsorbed and pre-empts a volume to maintain this tubular fluid isosmotic with filtrate. Sodium is reabsorbed, and as this occurs there is an isosmotic reabsorption of water. However, as more and more sodium is removed the fluid that remains has a higher and higher concentration of mannitol and a lower and lower concentration of sodium. It is suggested that, perhaps, there is a gradient in the concentrations of sodium between the luminal and interstitial fluids above which the active transport of sodium cannot be achieved. This would result in the delivery of a large volume of fluid containing a supernormal quantity of sodium (but at an unusually low concentration) to the distal tubule. Although the distal tubular mechanisms for the reabsorption of sodium may accelerate, they are usually inadequate to cope with the large quantities of this cation that gain access to this portion of the nephron and, hence, a varying amount escapes reabsorption completely.

Arguments have been raised against this interpretation of the effects of a solute diuresis on the rate of excretion of salt. In particular, it has been stated that this hypothesis fails as a generalization since sodium sulfate and urea do not promote a saluresis in a consistent fashion. However, it is probably fair to state that when urea and sulfate are administered in such a way as to augment the rate of excretion of solutes in much the same quantitative fashion as glucose, mannitol, etc., there is an augmented rate of excretion of salt as well. It has also been claimed that the effects of solute loading in respect to the augmented rate of excretion of salt are initiated in a stimulus that originates remote from the kidney. It has been suggested that the infusion of hypertonic solutions of glucose or mannitol promotes an increased rate of excretion of salt because their administration increases the effective osmotic pressure of the extracellular fluids (or diminishes the volume of the intracellular fluids), and that the reason urea is ineffective is that it does not influence the *effective* osmotic pressure or the distribution of the body fluids. This argument appears invalid for the reasons given above plus the fact that the administration of a hypotonic solution of mannitol also promotes an augmented rate of excretion of salt.[251] This could hardly operate by altering the effective osmotic pressure of the extracellular fluids since the concentration at which the solution was administered was such as to prevent this change.

Although it seems clear that solute diureses exert their influence on salt excretion by an effect on intratubular conditions, it does not follow that a saluresis is an inevitable consequence of the administration of mannitol or the accession of a significant hyperglycemia. A solute load does not promote a significant saluresis in patients who are suffering with disorders characterized by avid reabsorption of salt such as those with congestive heart failure with edema and cirrhosis with ascites.[252] This in no way implies that intratubular factors are not important in the regulation of the rate of excretion of salt, but it does imply that intratubular forces are only some of the conditioning factors involved. Other stimuli originating from dislocations of the internal environment may have sufficiently profound effects on the activity of the renal tubular cells so that the usual response to a particular set of intratubular circumstances is almost completely negated.

Excretion of Potassium. The rate of excretion of potassium is the net result of the quantities that are filtered, reabsorbed and secreted. The conclusion that a solute which is filtered is also secreted depends on the demonstration of a rate of excretion of that solute in excess of the amount that is simultaneously filtered. This has been reported by several groups of investigators in the case of potassium.[141–143,253] Although the fact that potassium is secreted can be proved only under the circumstances cited above, it is believed by most that this mechanism is in continuous operation. There are data which must be interpreted to imply that potassium is at least partially reabsorbed in the proximal tubule. Some suggest that perhaps all of the filtered potassium is reabsorbed and that all that gains access to the bladder urine is, in fact, secreted.

The secretion of potassium appears to operate through a mechanism referred to as "ion exchange" in which an ion of similar and equal charge is reabsorbed in a reaction that is somehow coupled with the secretion of potassium into the tubular fluid.[143,254] It is believed that this particular ion exchange mechanism operates in relation to the reabsorption of sodium, that it probably transpires in the distal tubule, that it may be in part activated through the influence of the hormone aldosterone, and that, in a sense, potassium is in a competitive position with hydrogen ions in this exchange for sodium. This will be discussed in more detail in the section dealing with acidification of the urine. However, it may be stated in a general way that under ordinary circumstances the reabsorption of sodium at a particular site in the nephron is associated with the exchange for a specific quantity of potassium and hydrogen ions, and that when the availability of one ion diminishes, the other competes more favorably in the exchange process.

It was once thought that the hormones of the adrenal cortex that had an influence on the electrolytes promoted both an increased reabsorption of sodium and an augmented excretion of potassium as specific and independent events. This has been demonstrated not to be true for DOCA and cortisone;[255] no data are available for aldosterone with respect to this particular point. However, it has been clearly demonstrated that DOCA and cortisone do not have a primary action of promoting the excretion of potassium, but that alterations in the rate of excretion of the latter are primarily dependent on changes in the rate of reabsorption of sodium.[255] For example, animals and human subjects on completely sodium-free regimens who are already reabsorbing all the filtered sodium do not demonstrate an increased rate of excretion of potassium when DOCA or cortisone is administered. Since under these circumstances the reabsorption of sodium is already 100 per cent, it cannot be augmented by the administration of these agents.

There are several implications with respect to the rate of excretion of potassium if this function is, in fact, in large part a consequence of an ion exchange mechanism with sodium. The first of these has already been alluded to in relation to the availability of potassium and its "competitive" position with respect to hydrogen ions. The availability of one or the other is, in turn, a reflection of the concentrations of potassium and hydrogen ions within the renal tubular cells. Another implication is that the amount of potassium that can be exchanged for sodium at a specific site is conditioned in the first instance by the amount of filtered sodium that reaches the exchange site. If, for example, this site is in the distal tubule, it must follow that the exchange will be compromised to the extent that the delivery of sodium from the proximal tubule is diminished,[256] or that distal tubular reabsorption of sodium is inadequate owing to insufficiency of the adrenal cortical hormone(s). Therefore, it may be anticipated that in circumstances of dehydration in which there has been a diminished GFR or other influences that would tend to promote a more avid reabsorption of sodium in the proximal tubule, the accession of less sodium to the site where it has the opportunity to exchange for potassium may well be accompanied by a diminished rate of secretion of this cation. The hyperkalemia of adrenal cortical insufficiency attests to the probability that secretion(s) of this gland may well be involved in effecting this exchange mechanism.

There are some data that have been interpreted to mean that intracellular dehydration may have an influence promoting the excretion of potassium.[142] However, close inspection of these reports suggests that this is true only when the loss of fluid from the cells has been accomplished through an increase in the effective osmotic pressure of the extracellular fluids due to an increase in the concentration of sodium and its salts, but not when the loading solute is mannitol or glucose. Hence, this fails as a generalization, and it may well be that the initial observation may be explained as the consequence of a large load of filtered sodium leading to the availability of an unusual quantity of this cation for reabsorption in the distal tubule in an exchange for potassium. The induction of hyponatremia with a water load is associated with a diminished rate of excretion of potassium.[213]

Solute and water diureses do not have a specific influence on the rate of excretion of potassium. However, the concentration of potassium in the urine does not usually fall below that of the serum except in circumstances of such diureses, or in circumstances wherein potassium depletion has developed as a result of disorders other than renal disease. The conservation of potassium by the kidneys is more efficient than it was once thought to be, but the urine is never as free of potassium as it may be of sodium.

Acidification of the Urine.[24,25,113,114,131,257–259] The kidneys make a significant contribution to the regulation of acid-base equilibrium by promoting alterations in the net rate of excretion of hydrogen ions, and by processes of selective reabsorption and rejection of cations and anions by the renal tubular cells. These two processes, as alluded to in the prior discussions, are interdependent to the extent that sodium reabsorption is coupled with the secretion of hydrogen or potassium ions. The total rate of secretion of hydrogen ions by the renal tubular cells can be calculated from the sum of the titratable acid, ammonium ions and a fraction which is equivalent to the difference between the bicarbonate that is filtered and excreted. The titratable acid may be equated with the quantity of sodium hydroxide that must be added to the urine to restore its *p*H to that of the parent filtrate.

Some acids may be excreted as such but this excretion is limited in a quantitative sense since the lowest *p*H of the urine appears to be 4.5, and at that level only minor concentrations of even poorly dissociated acids can exist as such. Caution must be exercised to avoid the error of necessarily equating a low urinary *p*H with a high rate of excretion of acid. A small quantity of a dissociated acid in a poorly buffered urine will cause considerable lowering of the *p*H of the urine. The same quantity of titratable acid in a buffered solution might be associated with very little depression of the *p*H.

The urinary buffers play an important

role in the processes that are involved in the acidification of the urine. The most important of these are the bicarbonate-carbonic acid pair and the monosodium and disodium phosphate systems. It was initially believed that the acid that was excreted was present originally in the filtrate. This theory implied that acidification of the urine was accomplished by the preferential reabsorption of the bicarbonate and the disodium phosphate components of the buffer systems noted above.[260] However, Pitts and his collaborators[113,114,261,262] reported in a group of highly significant papers that experiments could be designed in which the quantity of acid excreted per minute was in excess of the amount that could have been filtered in the same time interval. They developed the hypothesis that hydrogen ions were *secreted* into the tubular fluid in exchange for sodium. The source of the hydrogen ions for this secretory process is not known for certain, although it is usually represented as having been derived from carbonic acid. The latter, in turn, is represented as having been formed from the hydration of carbon dioxide which is either produced by the metabolic activity of the tubular cell or gains access to it from the blood brought to the kidney. Since the rate of production of hydrogen ions would be slow if it were dependent on the uncatalyzed hydration of carbon dioxide, it was reassuring to note that Davenport and Wilhelmi observed that the cortex of the kidney was rich in carbonic anhydrase, and it is now assumed that this enzyme is responsible for the rapid hydration of carbon dioxide to carbonic acid.[263,264] The dissociation of the latter, then, provides the ultimate source for the hydrogen ions utilized in the exchange process. These reactions may be represented in the following manner:

$$H_2O + CO_2 \downarrow H_2CO_3 \downarrow H^+ + HCO_3^-$$

(This reaction is accelerated by the enzyme carbonic anhydrase)

The reactions that are involved in the exchange of hydrogen ions for sodium and the net effect of this operation on the acidification of the urine may be illustrated in the following series. The first of these describes the exchange of hydrogen ions for the sodium ions associated with bicarbonate as filtered and shown in A below. In this series of events it is noted that the bicarbonate which returns to the interstitial fluid is not the bicarbonate that was filtered but rather has its origin from the bicarbonate within the cell, which in turn is represented to have been derived from the dissociation of carbonic acid. It is further noted that the carbonic acid formed from the reaction between the secreted hydrogen ion and the filtered bicarbonate ion is dehydrated, and the carbon dioxide is pictured as returning to the interstitial fluid by diffusion through the renal tubular cell. Although there is good evidence that this diffusion occurs, the fact remains that the carbon dioxide tension of the urine may exceed that in the plasma; this would not be true if the renal epithelium were completely permeable to carbon dioxide. There have been two opposing views concerning this seeming paradox. Kennedy, Orloff and Berliner[265] believed

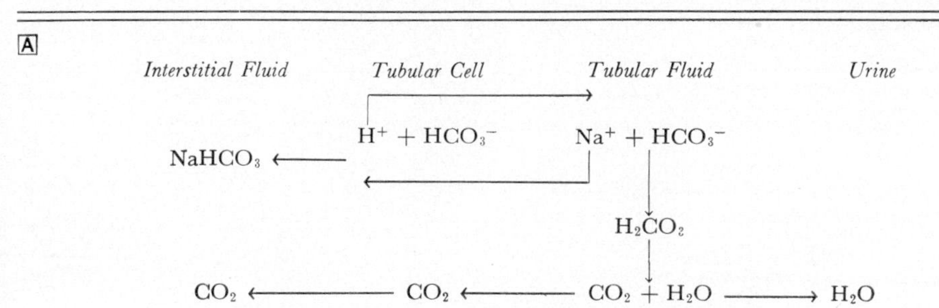

that the high pCO_2 of bladder urine could be explained by the mixing of urines with different pH issuing from different tubules at a point in the collecting system where the physical factors were unfavorable for the easy diffusion of CO_2 back into the plasma. Pitts suggested that in the absence of carbonic anhydrase in the tubular fluid, the dehydration of carbonic acid might be delayed so that some of the carbon dioxide was not made available until a point had been reached in the nephron where the renal epithelium was no longer permeable to carbon dioxide. Ochwadt and Pitts[266] made this thesis more acceptable by demonstrating that an increased tension of carbon dioxide in the urine could be reduced by the intravenous administration of the enzyme carbonic anhydrase. Presumably the enzyme gained access to the tubular fluid and hastened the dehydration of the carbonic acid so that the carbon dioxide was available for back diffusion at a point in the nephron where the epithelium was permeable to CO_2.

Another phase of the acidification of the urine concerns the exchange of hydrogen ions for the sodium associated with the phosphate salts, and this may be depicted as in the sequence represented in [A] below. It will be noted that the net effects of these reactions include the reabsorption of sodium, the extrusion of a hydrogen ion which reacts with the phosphate buffer to convert disodium to monosodium phosphate, the reabsorption of *bicarbonate*, and, to the extent that the ratios of the di- and monosodium phosphate and bicarbonate-carbonic acid buffers have been changed in the urine, the pH of this fluid must have been altered.

It should be clear from the discussion thus far that the quantity of hydrogen ions secreted into the tubular fluid may be in excess of the quantity that gains access to the bladder urine. If the reabsorption of bicarbonate is accomplished by the reactions described above, it is clear that for each filtered bicarbonate ion that is reabsorbed, one hydrogen ion must be secreted. However, if a fair amount of the carbonic acid formed in the tubular lumen is dehydrated and the carbon dioxide is re-cycled, the quantity of hydrogen ions that have been secreted in the interest of reabsorption of bicarbonate must be calculated from knowledge of the quantity of bicarbonate ion that has been filtered and excreted per unit time. The difference between these two values represents one part of the quantity of hydrogen ions secreted in that time.

The rate of secretion of hydrogen ions by the renal tubular cells is conditioned by many factors, including the pH of the renal tubular cell fluid, the pCO_2 of the extracellular fluid,[267,268] the availability of buffers in the tubular lumen, the intensity of the stimuli that are responsible for the reabsorption of sodium[269] (by the exchange process), and the status of the stores of potassium in certain key renal tubular cells. A decreased pH of the tubular cell fluid and hypercapnia, both of which could readily make more hydrogen ions available for secretion, appear to be factors which do, in fact, accelerate the rate of secretion of hydrogen ions. The manner in which a diminished content of potassium in renal tubular cells might favor the exchange of hydrogen ions in lieu of potassium for sodium has already been discussed.[143,270–273] In addition, there appears to be a limiting gradient

[A]

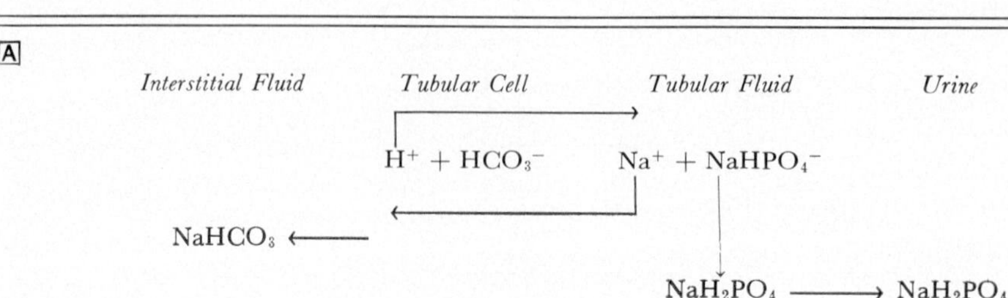

against which hydrogen ions can be secreted into the tubular fluid, which is approximately 800:1. If there is a large quantity of buffer in the urine to minimize the concentration of free hydrogen ions, this gradient is not approached and, therefore, does not of itself impose a restriction on the quantity of hydrogen ions that can be secreted. In contrast, limited quantities of buffer will impose a restriction on the rate of secretion of hydrogen ions by failing to resist the decrease in *p*H consequent to their accumulation in the tubular fluid.

The rate of excretion of ammonia does not usually change as abruptly as does that of titratable acid, but in proper circumstances the excretion of ammonia may make a greater contribution in quantitative terms. Ammonia is formed in the kidney, and it is believed that the greatest fraction is derived from glutamine.[274] The de-amidation of glutamine is accelerated by the enzyme glutaminase, which has been demonstrated in the kidneys. However, ammonia may be formed from other precursor amino acids, and it has not been proved that glutamine is, in fact, the major source of urinary ammonia in the human. Factors other than the rate of *production* of ammonia are relevant to its rate of *excretion;* among these are the *p*H of the urine, the rate of flow of urine and the permeability characteristics of the membrane of the renal tubular cell.[275-278] It is not clear whether ammonia diffuses into the tubular fluid and reacts with hydrogen ions to become ammonium ion, or whether ammonium ion as such is formed within the renal tubular cell and then secreted. An inverse relationship between the *p*H of the urine and the rate of excretion of ammonia has been described by many observers. These data strongly suggest that ammonia diffuses into the tubular fluid as such and forms ammonium ion. The quantity of ammonium ion formed in this way would be limited by the *p*H of the tubular fluid if it is assumed that the rate of production of ammonia is not a limiting factor. Moreover, so long as the tubular fluid was acid, as much ammonia as could diffuse from the cells would react with hydrogen ions to form ammonium and a state of equilibrium would not be reached. Thus, when the urinary *p*H is low, the rate of flow of urine has little effect on the rate of excretion of ammonia. In contrast, when the urinary *p*H is not low, and the diffusion of ammonia and its reaction with hydrogen ions approach a state of equilibrium, the flow of urine past the point of addition of ammonia may become crucial in the regulation of the rate of excretion of ammonia. Within the context of the view that ammonia diffuses from the renal tubular cells and is "trapped" within the lumen by virtue of its reaction with hydrogen ion, the accession of ammonia to the luminal fluid and its reaction with hydrogen ion may be looked upon as a buffering action.[278] In this instance ammonia is the base, or proton acceptor. Since this buffering activity will minimize the fall in *p*H, thereby diminishing the gradient for hydrogen ions between cell and luminal fluid, the further secretion of hydrogen ions (in exchange for sodium) will be favored. In this sense, the secondary factors that may be considered to condition the increased rate of excretion of ammonia would be a decrease in the quantity of buffer in the tubular fluid, an intense stimulus for the reabsorption of sodium (in a cation exchange process) and a diminished availability of potassium ions for secretion. If one examines the events that precede the acceleration of the excretion of ammonia when ammonium chloride is ingested, the following are noted: (a) a negative balance of sodium obtains; (b) the reabsorption of the diminished quantities of filtered bicarbonate becomes virtually complete; (c) a negative balance of potassium develops. These three events set the stage for: (a) an avid reabsorption of sodium, (b) a diminished quantity of buffer in the tubular luminal fluid, and (c) a decreased availability of potassium to exchange for the reabsorbed sodium. The addition of ammonia to the urine and its consequences can be illustrated in a manner similar to that used above in detailing the events involved in the reabsorption of bicarbonate and the addition of hydrogen ions to the phosphate buffer system as in [A] below. In this instance it is seen that sodium is again reabsorbed as the bicarbonate, the anion is contributed by the carbonic acid formed within the tubular cell, ammonia derived from glutamine diffuses into the luminal fluid where it is trapped as ammonium, and ammonium chloride is excreted into the urine, whereas sodium chloride had been filtered.

If each of the mechanisms that have been described with respect to the acidification of the urine is examined closely, a very important implication emerges: namely, that more bicarbonate may be reabsorbed than is filtered at the glomerulus. This circumstance is a corollary of the observation of Pitts and his colleagues that more hydrogen ions may gain access to the urine than are filtered at the glomerulus.

The administration of a carbonic anhydrase inhibitor suppresses all of those reactions which are dependent on a readily available source of hydrogen ions. A carbonic anhydrase inhibitor promotes an augmented rate of excretion of sodium, bicarbonate and potassium, and diminishes the rate of excretion of titratable acid and ammonia.[168,258,279]

The sites within the nephron where the secretion of hydrogen ions occurs are not known. The few observations that are available with respect to the *p*H of tubular fluid suggests that the site of acidification of the urine is in the distal tubule.[280] However, no observations of the *p*H of tubular fluid have been made under circumstances of an acidosis. Moreover, there are reasons to suspect that at least one site of secretion of hydrogen ions is actually in the proximal portion of the tubule. If a carbonic anhydrase inhibitor such as acetazolamide is administered to normal human subjects while they are undergoing a maximal excretion of water in a design characterized as physiologic diabetes insipidus, the rate of excretion of water is increased as well as the rates of excretion of sodium, bicarbonate, etc. The augmented rate of excretion of $NaHCO_3$ is interpreted to mean a diminution of bicarbonate reabsorption due to inhibition of carbonic anhydrase and, hence, lesser availability of hydrogen ions to exchange with sodium. Since in a state of physiologic diabetes insipidus virtually all the urine that gains access to the distal tubule is excreted save for that fraction which is reabsorbed at the $T^{c}_{H_2O}$ site, an increased flow of urine implies that a larger volume of fluid had gained access to the distal tubule. This could readily occur because the obligatory reabsorption of water in the proximal tubule was diminished owing to the decreased reabsorption of solutes (sodium bicarbonate). Moreover, if this is due to inhibition of carbonic anhydrase, it implies that the latter is, in fact, operative in the proximal tubule and that hydrogen ions are secreted at that site.[168]

It might be anticipated that any factor that would diminish the rate of re-

---

[A]

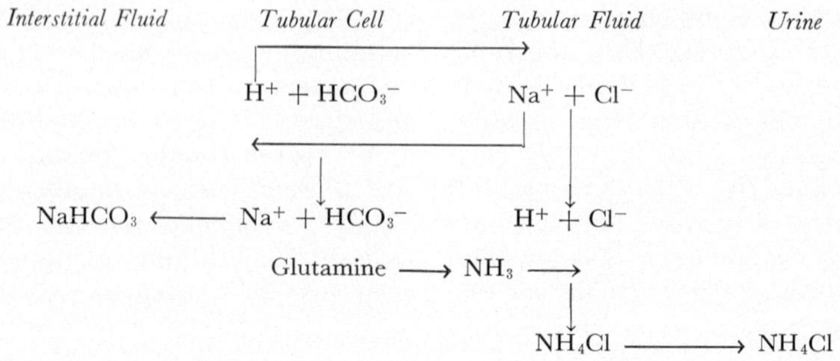

Interstitial Fluid	*Tubular Cell*	*Tubular Fluid*	*Urine*
	$H^+ + HCO_3^-$ →	$Na^+ + Cl^-$	
	← (Na⁺ exchanged) ↓	↓	
$NaHCO_3$ ⟵	$Na^+ + HCO_3^-$	$H^+ + Cl^-$	
	Glutamine ⟶ NH_3 ⟶	↓	
		NH_4Cl ⟶	NH_4Cl

absorption of sodium might interfere with the acidification of the urine. A defect in the manner in which an acid load is handled might therefore be anticipated in adrenal cortical insufficiency, and this has been observed both in the naturally occurring disease and in experimental circumstances.[24,281,282] The defect in the excretion of an acid load in chronic renal insufficiency may be in part due to an inability to reabsorb sodium properly. It is also probable that there are specific tubular defects characterized by an inability to secrete hydrogen ions properly; this may be the mechanism for the development of a metabolic acidosis both in acquired and in some infrequent instances of congenital renal tubular disease.

Many of the problems which have been referred to in this brief discussion of renal physiology will be discussed in other sections of this chapter, and in more specific terms as these are relevant to an understanding of clinical problems. There are obviously many unanswered questions concerning the manner in which the kidneys are able to subserve the many demands to maintain a nearly normal internal environment with respect to volume, composition and acid-base equilibrium. The mechanisms responsible for these activities are triggered by stimuli that arise in remote sites, as well as by specific intrarenal deviations that function as conditioning factors regulating gross operations as well as their rates.

CLINICAL DISORDERS

The discussion of the clinical disorders of the metabolism of water, electrolytes and acid-base equilibrium will be presented for the most part in general terms that befit phenomena that may *accompany* many and varied disorders, rather than in terms of individual diseases. The latter will be analyzed in detail only when a disorder of water or electrolyte balance is the dominant feature of the disease, or when it appears profitable to do so in the interests of illustrating a general principle.

An appreciation of the factors involved in the pathogenesis and management of disorders of fluid and electrolyte balance is dependent on an understanding of the qualitative and quantitative character of the net exchange of the several ions and water that may have developed during the course of the patient's illness. Most of the problems of interpretation and management of disorders of hydration are resolved by the simple method of establishing a balance sheet on which the total estimated losses of water and ions are tabulated, the total intake of each of these is recorded and summated, and the *net* exchange of each is calculated. Although these estimates are not precise, this procedure usually allows one to define the qualitative character of the alterations and the approximate quantities involved. Most of this information is available from the history or from a hospital chart in which these data have been carefully recorded. The physical examination and the laboratory tests, which include a careful urinalysis as well as the more elegant chemical analyses of the serum and urine, will provide additional data which permit a more precise analysis of the patient's status. The therapeutic problem is, then, largely one of providing those materials in appropriate quantities which will restore the normal state of hydration. It is truly not an oversimplification to state that an understanding of most of the clinical disorders of hydration and electrolyte balance is achieved with the use of simple arithmetic. However, this arithmetic must be applied in an informed manner and the clinician must be aware of certain mandatory and basal requirements for water and electrolytes and, furthermore, must have some insight as to how these may be modified by a variety of conditioning influences.

Basal Requirements[24,25]

In this discussion it will be assumed that for one reason or another the patient must receive the necessary water, electrolytes, etc., by a parenteral route, that he has accumulated no antecedent deficits, that he will sustain no unusual losses, and that kidney function is normal. In addition, the problem will be of short duration and, hence, the need for the provision of calories, proteins, and other essential food substances can be disregarded. The problem is then refined to the prescription of a regimen which will maintain a normal state of hydration, avoid the depletion or excess accumulation of the major minerals and minimize the most immediate consequences of starvation.

Water. The recommendation for the daily volume of water to be administered is based on the mandatory and desirable losses that may be anticipated. The approximate daily volume of insensible perspiration is about 600 to 1000 ml. for the average adult. However, about 200 to 400 ml. may be subtracted from this figure since this latter volume is approximately that which is supplied by the endogenous production of the water of metabolism. Although a small solute load such as that to be anticipated from the regimen that is being described could be excreted at high concentration in a small volume of urine, there seems little advantage (and some disadvantage) in promoting the excretion of a continuously highly concentrated urine. A reasonable daily volume of urine for the anticipated solute load would be approximately 1000 ml. Lastly, it might be desirable to include an additional volume of 200 to 300 ml. to anticipate other losses such as sweat, etc., which if not lost by an extrarenal route could be readily excreted as additional urine. These several components of daily water loss add up to about 1800 ml.

NaCl. If the patient who serves as the model for this discussion had been ingesting a usual diet prior to the start of this regimen, he would have been receiving 8 to 10 grams (135 to 170 mM.) of NaCl each day. If this intake of salt were suddenly discontinued he would excrete a urine virtually free of salt in four to nine days. However, in the interval a negative balance of NaCl would develop. This, in turn, would almost certainly be accompanied by an equivalent loss of water and the net effect would be an approximately isotonic contraction of the volume of the extracellular fluid with the preservation of a normal concentration of sodium in the serum. This deficit of volume in itself is almost certainly not harmful, but it does prejudice the patient's ability to withstand further losses which might readily occur during the course of his illness. Thus, unless there is some specific reason why salt should not be administered to this patient, it is recommended that he receive 3 to 5 grams (52 to 85 mM.) of sodium chloride each day. This quantity should be sufficient to avoid a negative balance by way of the urine and sweat, and if for any reason salt retention supervenes and an equivalent volume of water is retained, it is unlikely that the volume of the extracellular fluid will expand by more than a third to one half a liter each day. Moreover, this accession of volume would be recognized quickly and at this time the administration of salt could be eliminated before an untoward expansion of the extracellular volume could obtain.

Potassium. It was pointed out earlier that the conservation of potassium is not quite as efficient as that for sodium, and a deficit will develop unless the potassium excreted is replaced. Approximately 40 to 60 mM. of potassium a day is safe to administer and will usually be sufficient to avoid a significant depletion of this ion.

Carbohydrate. Approximately 100 grams of carbohydrate per day are necessary for the Krebs cycle. If this quantity is not made available from an exogenous or an endogenous source of pre-formed carbohydrate, the catabolism of protein and fat will be accelerated and will provide an accession of organic acid end-products to the extracellular fluid. The acids will be buffered but will contribute to a metabolic acidosis, and the excretion of the anions of these acids involves another drain on the body's store of sodium. These consequences of carbohydrate starvation can be minimized by the administration of at least 100 grams of glucose per day so long as its administration is distributed over some significant fraction of the twenty-four hours.

In summary, it may be stated that the total *basal* requirements for an average adult per twenty-four hours are as follows:

Water	1500 to 1800 ml.
NaCl	52 to 85 mM. (3 to 5 grams)
KCl	40 to 60 mM. (3 to 4.5 grams)
Glucose	minimum of 100 grams

These requirements can be readily supplied in the following fluid prescription:

1000 to 1300 ml. 10% glucose in water
300 to 500 ml. 5% glucose in isotonic saline
4 grams KCl (added to the total volume of fluid to be administered).

It must be emphasized that this is not a universally applicable prescription; it applies specifically to an adult patient with the limiting characteristics listed in the initial paragraph of this section.

Since the requirements for water and minerals are related more closely to the rate of metabolism than to size or age, the following values, which are referred to a base of 100 calories expended, may be of value in both pediatric and adult practice:[283]

Water	100 ml.
Na	2 to 3 mM.
K	2 to 3 mM.
Cl	1 to 2 mM.

In turn, the probable average caloric expenditure per 24 hours may be estimated from body weight in the following fashion:

0 to 10 Kg.—100 cal./Kg.
10 to 20 Kg.—1000 cal. plus 50 cal./Kg. for each Kg. in excess of 10.
20 Kg. and over—1500 cal. plus 20 cal./Kg. for each Kg. in excess of 20.

In addition, carbohydrate must be supplied as previously indicated.

Modifications of Basal Requirements. Many circumstances may demand revision of the prescription presented above, which is designed simply to compensate for ordinary losses. The management of patients with antecedent deficits will be discussed later in relation to the general problems of dehydration. However, in addition to dehydration itself there are a variety of circumstances that may well condition the need for the administration of larger volumes of water and solutions of electrolytes, and a few circumstances wherein these might be restricted to some advantage.

INSENSIBLE PERSPIRATION. The volume of water that is lost as insensible perspiration is increased by anything that augments the metabolic rate such as fever, increased muscular activity or specific disease entities, and by factors that increase the volume of air exchanged by the lungs. Since insensible perspiration is solute-free water, all losses by this route should be replaced as water without salt. Fever or an increase in the environmental temperature will promote sweating.

SWEAT. The volume of sweat that a patient may lose is quite difficult to estimate; it is even more difficult to estimate in a dry climate where evaporation is so rapid that one may easily underestimate the volume or even conclude that the patient is not sweating at all. The general order of the magnitude of loss that may be achieved as sweat may be appreciated from data reported in several studies. Gamble[284] observed the loss of 2400 ml. of sweat in a six hour period in a normal subject lying quietly in the nude unprotected from the sun on a "moderately hot summer day." Workmen have been known to lose eight to ten liters a day. It will be recalled that sweat is a hypotonic fluid; therefore, these losses should be replaced with a solution that contains approximately 50 mM. of NaCl per liter. This can be prepared for intravenous administration as a solution composed of one part isotonic saline and two parts of glucose in water.

GASTROINTESTINAL SECRETIONS. Water and electrolytes may be lost from the gastrointestinal tract in copious quantities by vomiting, diarrhea, ileostomy, fistulous drainage, or by constant tube suction. These losses should be considered to be isotonic with the extracellular fluid in terms of the total electrolyte content, although, as noted earlier, their composition differs from serum in several respects. Despite this the loss of gastrointestinal fluid can usually be successfully replaced as isotonic saline along with appropriate quantities of potassium. This is especially true if renal function is not compromised, since the normal kidney will selectively retain and reject ions in such a fashion as to restore the composition of the body fluids to normal. Furthermore, it must be emphasized that the replacement fluid must be chosen with regard to the total impact of a particular loss on the state of hydration and acid-base equilibrium. For example, the fluid lost from the stomach by vomiting due to pyloric obstruction associated with a peptic ulcer may contain considerable hydrochloric acid, and only small quantities of sodium and potassium. However, the initial effect of the loss of HCl is the development of a metabolic alkalosis, and the initial responses to this include an augmented rate of excretion of sodium bicarbonate and potassium into the urine. Hence, the net loss of sodium and potassium from the body is in excess of that lost in the vomitus per se.

LARGE VOLUMES OF URINE. There are several factors which condition the excretion of unusually large volumes of urine, and among these is an increased quantity of solutes destined for excretion. The influence of large solute loads on the rates of excretion of water and salt has already been described in the section on Renal Physiology. The most frequent cause of a *solute diuresis* in patients is uncontrolled glycosuria of diabetes mellitus. Other circumstances include the excretion of large amounts of urea consequent to the administration of diets with high protein content[91,285] to patients who are unable to achieve a positive nitrogen balance owing to the catabolic state which accompanies many forms of "injury."[286-289] The solute diuresis due to glycosuria may require additional volumes of water and added quantities of salt in the daily fluid prescription if dehydration is to be avoided. The osmotic diuresis due to urea is not likely to promote significant salt depletion, but may lead to large deficits of water if adequate volumes are not added to the daily allotment. In this regard, it may be suggested that if protein is to be administered to patients in a period when they are probably unable to store nitrogen, a minimum of a liter of water should be added to the basal requirements for every 100 grams of protein administered.

Patients with *chronic renal insufficiency* are usually unable to concentrate the urine appropriately and the conservation of sodium may be less efficient than in patients with normal kidneys. Hence, the requirements for water and salt may exceed those suggested under basal requirements. The quantity of salt lost in the urine in patients with chronic renal insufficiency is obviously best determined by chemical analysis of a urine sample. In many instances of severe renal insufficiency it is found that the *concentration* of sodium in the urine is somewhere between 50 and 90 millimols per liter. In addition, patients with chronic renal insufficiency frequently vomit and have diarrhea. The loss of gastrointestinal secretions must be considered in terms of the maintenance of fluid balance in these patients.

EDEMA. It is assumed that salt will not be administered to patients with complications such as congestive heart failure, cirrhosis with ascites, the nephrotic syndrome, and other states characterized by the formation of edema unless some special circumstance supervenes. In rare instances the volume of water required may be less than that noted in the discussion of basal requirements if it is observed that a positive balance of water develops.

POSTOPERATIVE PERIOD. The other circumstance wherein the quantities of salt and water *may* be profitably reduced below those suggested is in the immediate postoperative period, provided that the patient has a normal state of hydration initially and provided that the threat of a volume deficit from bleeding or other source of loss is not great.[290] It seems clear that the retention of salt and water are among the responses to the stress, medication and anesthesia which accompany surgery. This does not necessarily mean that the administration of salt and water should be sharply curtailed, since there are often co-existing deficits of volume or threats thereof that make it desirable for the physician to administer and the patient to retain adequate quantities of salt and water. There is, perhaps, no other single clinical circumstance in which the issues of management have been more clouded and confused by a lack of logic and an excess of dogma and routinization. The requirements of the patient in the postoperative period demand as much individualization in terms of the development of a proper fluid prescription for the particular problem at hand as in any other circumstance. The plea is made that "rules" of procedure be abandoned and that the individual patient be treated in terms of the special problems he presents with due consideration of the probability that there is a tendency to retain salt and water in the immediate postoperative period. Categorical statements concerning the management of the problems of fluid balance in the postoperative period are as ill-advised as they are in any other clinical context.

Fluids Available for Parenteral Administration

In the same vein, some comments are appropriate with respect to "special" solutions for parenteral administration, the composition of which is designed to meet the requirements of particular losses such as "gastric replacement fluids," "intestinal replacement fluids," etc. Their use is discouraged because therapy must be individualized. The intelligent management of disorders of hydration and acid-base equilibrium demands an analysis of the particular nature of the distortions that are observed in the clinical problem of the specific patient. The routinization of therapy that follows the use of mass-produced special solutions tends to minimize the diligence with which this analysis is made. This is not in any sense whatsoever to be interpreted as an implication that solutions other than glucose in water or isotonic saline are not frequently indicated. It should be interpreted as an implication that when the need arises an appropriate fluid be designed for the particular patient and his special problem. Virtually every problem can be adequately handled with a fluid fabricated from the following list of raw materials:

5%, 10%, 50%	glucose in water
0.9% NaCl	(154 mM./L.)
5% NaCl	(855 mM./L.)
7.5% $NaHCO_3$	(900 mM./L.)
14.9% KCl	(2000 mM./L., i.e., 2 mM./ml.)

This solution of KCl is highly concentrated and should be administered only after it has been appropriately diluted.

Techniques of Administration of Fluids

Fluids may be administered by mouth, by intermittent or continuous gavage, by vein or by the subcutaneous route (hypodermoclysis). The oral route has all of the obvious advantages. Administration by gavage allows the provision of adequate calories, proteins and other essential nutrients in addition to water and electrolytes. The intravenous route is convenient, and the technique of threading a large vein with a plastic tube has eliminated some of the technical problems. The rate of the administration of fluids is of some significance when the intravenous route is employed. This is of especial importance with patients who may have cardiovascular disease in whom the rapid infusion of fluid may precipitate pulmonary edema and other manifestations of congestive heart failure. Such patients should be observed most carefully so that the earliest evidence of an untoward response may be recognized. The hazards which attend the administration of fluids to patients with cardiovascular disease will frequently modify the characteristics of the fluid prescription and the speed with which the fluid is administered, but they should not be allowed to interfere unduly with the proper management of dehydration. Patients with heart disease are certainly not immune to the evil consequences of dehydration and disturbances of acid-base equilibrium. Furthermore, in addition to the precautions concerning the quantity of fluids and the rate of their administration, it is well to take the time to explain to these (as well as other) patients what is planned so that anxiety may be allayed and the patient reassured with respect to the often frightening experience of the infusion procedure.

The alternative subcutaneous route may occasionally have some advantages over intravenous infusions, especially in patients with heart disease. The accession of fluid from the subcutaneous tissue to the vascular system is, of course, slower than when the fluid is introduced directly into the vein, and if the central and peripheral venous pressures should rise as a result of myocardial incompetence, the absorption of fluid from the subcutaneous depot will be delayed even more. This may well provide an added factor of safety. The hypodermoclysis may also be useful on occasion when there is some delay in the administration of fluids by vein because of technical difficulties. Two precautions should be observed if one considers administering fluids by the subcutaneous route: (1) The fluid should be isotonic with plasma. If it is hypertonic, it will promote a redistribution of water from the vascular compartment to the interstitial fluid, thus transiently reducing the plasma volume.[291] If the patient is already dehydrated this may be a most undesirable complication. Furthermore, a hypertonic solution may be irritating to the subcutaneous tissues. (2) Solutions of 5 per cent glucose and water (although approximately isotonic with plasma) should not be administered by this route if the patient is dehydrated.[292] When 5 per cent glucose in water is introduced into the subcutaneous tissue, two gradients are established between the plasma and the interstitial fluid. One is a gradient for the diffusion of glucose from the interstitial fluid to plasma; the second is a gradient for the diffusion of sodium salts from the plasma to the interstitial fluid. Sodium and its salts diffuse more quickly than glucose and, hence, the clysis pool will become hypertonic to plasma water prior to its reabsorption. This will promote the accession of a volume of fluid from the plasma to the interstitial compartment. If plasma volume is already reduced, as is usually the case in dehydration, this further reduction may be sufficient to induce a state of peripheral vascular collapse. The use of hyaluronidase does not minimize this exchange but, in contrast, has been reported to aggravate the situation, presumably by promoting a larger area for the exchange.

Dehydration

The literal interpretation of the word *dehydration* is a loss of water; hence, as applied to clinical circumstances, it is hardly ever a complete description of the situation. In fact, the term is misleading in this regard since most instances of what is referred to as "clinical dehydration" represent deficits of sodium salts as well as water and may also be complicated by other deficits and abnormalities such as potassium depletion and alterations in acid-base balance. Dehydration does imply a contraction of the extracellular volume which is usually shared by both components of this compartment: the plasma and interstitial volumes. The cellular space may be contracted, expanded or normal in volume depending on the relationship between the volume of water and quantity of sodium that has been lost from the body. Hemoconcentration and dehydration are not synonymous. The former refers specifically to a contraction of the plasma volume and is characterized by an increase in the concentration of the cellular and nondiffusible components such as red cells and proteins. Hemoconcentration frequently accompanies dehydration, but may be present in the absence of dehydration whenever there is an imbalance of the Starling forces which favor a redistribution of fluid between the plasma and the interstitial fluid compartment such as to contract the former and expand the latter.

Although, as noted above, clinical dehydration is almost invariably associated with deficits of both water and sodium salts, one may profitably classify dehydration in terms of the relationship between the quantities of each that is lost in the following terms: (1) loss of water in excess of sodium, (2) loss of sodium in excess of water, (3) isotonic loss of sodium and water. These three general types of dehydration may also be referred to as hypertonic, hypotonic and isotonic contractions of the body fluid. Each of these may or may not be accompanied by other deficits and disorders, and it should be emphasized that the classification of a particular state of dehydration is a reflection of the *net* losses. This, in turn, implies the importance of eliciting from the history not only what the patient may have lost in the way of water and electrolytes but what may have been ingested or administered prior to the time of observation.

General Considerations. Before proceeding further with the discussion of some of the details of the various pathogeneses and mechanisms underlying the development of states of dehydration, it may be profitable to consider some of the more general features that help one to evaluate the state of hydration and the character of the deficits which may be present. An analysis of that phase of a patient's problem that deals with disorders of hydration is dependent on the same tools used throughout clinical medicine: namely, the history, the physical examination and the intelligent selection and interpretation of laboratory data. In a later discussion the various pathogeneses of dehydration will be discussed in somewhat isolated terms in the interests of clarity, but it must be emphasized that in most instances patients will have experienced a variety of insults of different magnitude, for longer and shorter periods of time, in a variety of clinical contexts. The very essence of the analysis of the character of dehydration requires an evaluation of all the available data both in qualitative and quantitative terms.

HISTORY. The history which includes a careful review of the entire sequence of events during the course of the illness, will provide very important data with respect to the quality and magnitude of the deficit of electrolytes and water. It is exceedingly worth while to tabulate these data in the form of a simple balance sheet whenever there is the possibility that a disorder of hydration is a significant feature of the patient's illness. A balance sheet with simple headings as indicated below will be adequate and is often of great value as an aid in following the course of the patient in hospital as one proceeds with management.

Intake				Output					
Date / Time	Weight	Character of Fluid	Volume	Urine	Insensible Loss	Sweat	Vomitus	Diarrhea	Blood

This systematic treatment of the data should allow the physician to make a fair estimate of the deficits in terms of volume, salt, potassium and the probable nature of the alterations, if any, in acid-base equilibrium. Acute changes in body weight can usually be ascribed primarily to a loss or gain in fluid. Facts concerning fever and sweating are relevant, as is information concerning the possibility of renal insufficiency or diabetes mellitus. Knowledge of the usual level of blood pressure is helpful since a blood pressure in the normal range might actually be hypotensive for a patient who had pre-existing hypertension. Thirst is a very significant symptom and may be most helpful in calling the attention of the physician to a disorder of hydration which might otherwise be neglected. Thirst is most commonly due to a primary deficit of water, although, as alluded to earlier, it may also arise from the contracted volume of the extracellular compartment even when this is accompanied by hyponatremia and expansion of the volume of the intracellular fluids.

Dehydration may develop during the course of hospitalization, and the data referred to above should certainly be available in the hospital record. The administration of parenteral fluids should be recorded in the hospital chart with as much attention to detail as drugs and other forms of therapy. Furthermore, it is likely that the very process of recording the data concerning the intake and output of fluids would serve to focus the attention of the responsible physician on the quality and the quantity of fluids that would be most appropriate as replacement for the daily losses of the particular patient in question.

PHYSICAL EXAMINATION. The physical examination may well provide signs that contribute information concerning the analysis of the deficit of electrolytes and water. The appearance, elasticity, texture, temperature and color of the skin, the moisture of the mucous membranes, the intraocular pressure, the level of blood pressure and the pulse rate all contribute information which may be of some use in an estimation of the quantitative aspects of the deficit of volume. In addition, the state of consciousness may have some relation to the magnitude of this deficit. Muscular weakness and the character of the deep tendon reflexes may suggest potassium depletion. The nature of the respiratory activity may suggest an alteration in acid-base equilibrium. In metabolic acidosis, which is very commonly associated with dehydration, the respirations are deep and are frequently accelerated as well. A positive Chvostek reflex may suggest a systemic alkalosis, but it may also be present if the patient has hypocalcemia even if this is coincident with an acidosis. An odor of acetone on the breath implies an elevated level of serum ketones. Some have stated that an imprint of the finger left on the skin signifies hyponatremia with intracellular edema. This is a grossly unreliable sign since it can be frequently observed in patients with normal concentrations of sodium in the serum and has been noted even with hypernatremia. In addition to the information noted above, the physical examination supplies invaluable information with respect to underlying disorders of which the dehydration and disturbance of acid-base equilibrium may be only one important concomitant.

LABORATORY DATA. The laboratory data, when intelligently selected and properly interpreted, can be of enormous help in a proper appreciation of a problem in hydration and will frequently dictate certain aspects of the program of management.

The packed cell volume, the level of hemoglobin in blood and the total protein concentration in serum can be quite helpful in evaluating the degree of contraction or expansion of the plasma volume. However, the inferences to be derived from these data are dependent on *changes* in the concentration and, hence, they are of most help when the disorder of hydration has developed while the patient has been under observation. They are usually of only limited usefulness upon admission to the hospital because it is not always safe to assume that these values were at normal levels prior to the onset of illness, but they can be of inestimable aid in interpreting a situation which has developed during the course of that phase of the illness which may have transpired in the hospital. The *concentration of sodium* in the serum is a significant datum in the analysis of the state of dehydration but it should be made clear that it, too, has limitations in terms of interpretation. In this regard, it is worth while to emphasize the fact that the concentration of sodium in the serum per se cannot possibly be automatically equated with the presence or absence of a state of dehydration. The *concentration* of sodium in the serum is simply a statement of the quantity of sodium in some unit of volume of the extracellular fluid; it is usually expressed as milliequivalents per liter. Patients with normal concentrations of sodium in the serum may have no disorder of hydration, or, in contrast, they may have gained or lost many liters of fluid. The true significance of a normal concentration of sodium lies in the fact that if the patient has gained or lost fluid the gain or loss of water was associated with a gain or loss of sodium approximately equal to 140 millimols per liter of the water that was gained or lost. In the same manner, a variety of states of hydration may be accompanied by hypo- or hypernatremia. Hyponatremia is a frequent accompaniment of certain types of dehydration and implies that there has been a loss of salt in excess of water; however, patients with edema may also have hyponatremia. This will be discussed in some detail later, but the fact should be emphasized here that hyponatremia per se does not necessarily imply dehydration *or* edema but simply states that in either instance there has been a disproportionate loss or gain of water and salt. Hypernatremia implies a gain of salt in excess of water or a loss of water in excess of salt, and once again may be compatible with either dehydration or an expansion of the extracellular fluid volume.

The level of potassium in the serum and the total content of CO_2 may be altered, and these abnormalities are usually accompanied by disturbances in acid-base equilibrium. A more complete discussion of these particular abnormalities will be deferred for presentation in the section on acid-base equilibrium.

The renal excretion of urea is the net result of the amount that is filtered less the amount that is passively reabsorbed by diffusion through the renal tubules. This process of reabsorption is favored by high concentration gradients between the tubular luminal and interstitial fluids; therefore, a diminished rate of filtration at the glomerulus or a highly concentrated urine, or both, will favor a reduced rate of excretion and an increase in the concentration of urea in the body fluids. One of the consequences of dehydration is an impaired perfusion of the kidney, and this, in turn, frequently results in a diminished filtration rate; hence, the concentration of urea in the blood may serve as one index of the severity of the dehydration. In addition, it may be a token of antecedent renal disease which will modify the character of the dehydration and may imply alterations in the approach to management.

Considerable information may be obtained from a careful *urinalysis*. It may readily provide useful information with respect to the probability of kidney disease. In the absence of glycosuria or proteinuria a high specific gravity is evidence for good renal function and an antidiuretic response.* This has certain inferences with respect to the state of hydration and may be helpful in guiding therapy. The excretion of salt in the urine despite hyponatremia is the definition of a "salt-wasting syndrome" and carries very important implications. An inability to concentrate the urine is seen commonly with many types of chronic renal disease but may be an accompaniment of the renal defect in acute potassium depletion and may be a clue to its existence.

The levels of concentration of other substances in the blood may frequently be of significant aid in a more complete understanding of the pathogenesis of a state of dehydration and in management, but the laboratory examinations listed above provide the most useful in-

* Regression equations have been calculated from a large number of determinations of the specific gravity and freezing point depression of the same urines. In these equations, Y refers to milli-osmolality and X refers to the specific gravity of the urines. The equation which applies to urines that contain neither glucose nor protein is:

$$Y = -37{,}233.72 + 37{,}270.09X;$$

the equation which applies to urines containing protein is:

$$Y = -27{,}169.88 + 27{,}219.97X;$$

and the equation which applies to urines containing glucose is:

$$Y = -32{,}285.91 + 32{,}337.98X.$$

formation and are certainly the most critical from the standpoint of an estimate of the nature of the problem and immediate management.

With these general comments in mind, it is now appropriate to return to a somewhat more detailed discussion of dehydration. In the interests of clarity this discussion will be presented in terms of the classification listed earlier. This will tend to oversimplify some of the problems. The reader should be reminded that not only are there many different avenues by which dehydration may develop but, in addition, several may be simultaneously operative. Ultimately, the most significant problem is to understand the character of the *net* deficits, since this is one of the major considerations in therapy.

Loss of Water in Excess of Sodium. This type of dehydration is characterized by a contraction of the body water in such a way that the deficit of volume is shared by all compartments. The loss of water without or in excess of salt must be accompanied by an increase in the concentration of sodium in the serum (and extracellular fluid). Since this represents an increase in the effective osmolality of the extracellular fluid, there will be a redistribution of water between the cells and the extracellular compartment so that there is a net movement of water from the cells to the extracellular fluid. In this fashion the total solute concentration of all compartments of body water is again equalized. Not only does the increased concentration of sodium promote the redistribution of water so that the deficit of volume is shared by all compartments, but it also serves as a stimulus to thirst, to the secretion of the antidiuretic hormone and to diminishing the loss of water by way of insensible and sensible perspiration. Thus, there is an automatic feed-back mechanism whereby the deficit of water promotes the ingestion and retention of water. Furthermore, the contraction of volume (or some function thereof) promotes the retention of sodium (despite its high concentration in the serum), and this response tends to conserve urinary water and sustains the desirable consequences of the hypernatremia noted above.

The less specific characteristics of this type of dehydration correlate with the severity of the contraction of the extracellular compartment. Since the loss of volume is shared by all compartments of the body fluid, it is clear that in this type of dehydration the largest deficit of total body water may obtain with the smallest diminution of the interstitial fluid and plasma volumes. There are many routes by which this type of dehydration may supervene.

LACK OF INGESTION OF WATER. The lack of ingestion of water is probably the most common cause of a deficit and is observed most frequently in infants and in patients who are unable to appreciate or respond to the sensation of thirst because of weakness and debility, clouding of consciousness or frank coma.[91] This may happen when the patient is unattended at home and, on occasion, may develop in the hospital as well. The patient who is unable to appreciate, respond to or even communicate the fact of thirst is completely dependent on his physician(s) for the proper measures to insure the maintenance of a normal state of hydration. It should be emphasized that significant deficits of water may develop in such situations despite the fact that no *unusual* losses of water obtain.

UNUSUAL LOSSES OF WATER. Among the conditions that may be responsible for unusual losses of water are excessive sweating, solute diureses, diabetes insipidus and water-losing renal disease, both congenital and acquired.

Sweat. The loss of sweat represents a deficit of water in excess of sodium (except in patients with adrenal cortical insufficiency or mucoviscidosis, in which the concentration of sodium in sweat may approach that in the serum). However, the *net* deficits that are noted as a result of sweating are related not only to the qualitative character of sweat itself and the volume that is lost but also to what the sweating subject may have ingested during the course of the time interval prior to observation. If he has refrained from the ingestion of fluid and food the net deficits will clearly represent a loss of water in excess of salt. On the other hand, if the sweating subject drinks water the net deficits may represent proportionate losses of water and salt or even a loss of salt in excess of water.

Solute Diuresis. Patients with the solute diuresis of uncontrolled glycosuria will excrete unusual quantities of water and salt. However, so long as they remain conscious and are able to ingest and retain fluid and food they usually manage to replace these losses, and significant dehydration does not develop. The clinical reflection of the loss and replacement of large volumes of water is noted in the classic complaints of polyuria and polydipsia. The degree of the dehydration that supervenes when diabetic acidosis develops is contributed to not only by the urinary losses but also by increased losses of insensible perspiration owing to increased respiratory activity and by losses from vomiting.[294] Almost invariably the net deficits in diabetic acidosis represent a loss of water in excess of sodium. However, because of the hyperglycemia and hyperlipemia the concentration of sodium in the serum is rarely elevated and is usually normal or depressed to frankly hyponatremic levels. (See Exchanges of Water Between the Intra- and Extracellular Compartments.)

Solute diuresis due to the excretion of large amounts of urea arising from the use of gavage feedings with large quantities of proteins in patients who are unable to store nitrogen was commented on earlier.[91,285] If these patients are fully conscious they are probably able to communicate the fact that they are thirsty. However, the administration of food and fluid by gavage is frequently a part of the regimen of a patient who is unable to ingest food and fluid because of debility or because of varying degrees of clouded sensorium or frank coma. Under these circumstances the brisk flow of unconcentrated urine due to the large rate of excretion of urea is interpreted as evidence of a normal state of hydration and renal function when, in fact, the large urine flow is promoting a state of water deficit dehydration. There are many reasons to conclude that the administration of large amounts of protein under certain circumstances is fruitless and undesirable. However, there are those who contend that it is proper to make what is usually a futile effort to promote a positive balance of nitrogen. The pros and cons of this argument will not be discussed here, but it should be emphasized that if protein is to be administered under these circumstances, then adequate volumes of water should be made available to allow the inevitable excretion of large quantities of urea without compromising the state of hydration. The administration of a minimum of one liter of water per 100 grams of protein in addition to the other requirements for water should be adequate for this purpose.

Many reports have appeared in the literature describing instances of hypernatremia in patients with lesions of the central nervous system.[91,295,296] Some have suggested that there were special relationships between some function of the central nervous system (other than diabetes insipidus) and the hypernatremia. Although this may be true, the evidence to support this contention is not convincing. Whenever the data have been presented in sufficient detail to allow a satisfactory evaluation, the hypernatremia has appeared to be due to a negative balance of water (in excess of sodium) as a result of inadequate ingestion or administration, or excess losses such as obtain in solute diureses and diabetes insipidus.[91]

DIABETES INSIPIDUS.[84,160,297–299] Diabetes insipidus is the clinical expression of partial or total insufficiency of the antidiuretic hormone. It is characterized by an inability to concentrate the urine and may certainly be responsible for very large deficits of water. Since acute diabetes insipidus may be associated with trauma (accidental or surgical) or infection of the central nervous system, it may be accompanied by a clouded sensorium or a comatose state. Under these circumstances, major deficits of water may occur in a matter of hours and remain unrecognized. More commonly, diabetes insipidus is of a more chronic nature and is associated with a normal sensorium; in these instances the polydipsia almost always manages to replace the deficits of water. There has been discussion over the years concerning whether polydipsia or polyuria is primary in diabetes insipidus. It seems clear now, however, that when a lesion in the central nervous system is such as to interfere solely with the neurohypophyseal system the defect is primarily a failure to conserve water and that the polydipsia is the response to thirst which in turn has been stimulated by the loss of water in excess of solutes and a consequent increase in the effective osmolality of the extracellular fluids. Since the mechanisms within the central nervous system which determine the appreciation and response to thirst are anatomically close to the neurohypophyseal system, it is easy to understand how experimental and clinical lesions responsible for diabetes insipidus may on occasion be complicated by lesions which alter the thirst mechanism in a primary way as well.

NEPHROGENIC DIABETES INSIPIDUS. In addition to diabetes insipidus[300] there is a disease frequently referred to as nephrogenic diabetes insipidus, which may mimic the syndrome due to insufficiency of the antidiuretic hormone. However, in this instance the secretion of ADH is presumably quite normal, but the renal tubules are unable to respond appropriately and these patients excrete copious quantities of water. This appears to be a congenital abnormality which has been observed in both sexes. In addition there are several acquired renal diseases which are characterized by an inability to conserve water appropriately. One of these is quite rare and has been referred to as "water-losing nephritis."[301-303] The patients who have been reported thus far have had obstructive uropathy or multiple myeloma, have developed severe thirst and polyuria and have been unresponsive to Pitressin. Lastly, the renal lesion which accompanies potassium depletion[161,162,304-307] has as one of its manifestations an inability to conserve water appropriately. Any of these circumstances may be responsible for an unusual loss of water and if uncorrected may give rise to a dehydration characterized by a deficit of water in excess of salt.

CORRECTION OF HYPERNATREMIA.[24] As pointed out earlier in this discussion, the hallmark of a loss of water in excess of salt is hypernatremia (except in some instances of hyperlipemia or hyperglycemia). The responses which are elicited as a consequence of the hypernatremia have also been listed. In addition, the intensity of the hypernatremia may be used to estimate the magnitude of the deficit of pure water. To the extent that hypernatremia has been provoked by the loss of water without solutes, the ratio of the average normal concentration of serum sodium and the elevated value represents the fraction of the normal total body water (TBW) that remains. Thus, if one considers the average normal concentration of sodium in the serum to be 138 mM./L. and a value of 175 mM./L. is found in a patient with a probable normal total body water of 42 liters (e.g., 60 per cent of the weight of a 70 Kg. male of average build), one may calculate the deficit of water in the following fashion:

$$\frac{\text{Normal Conc. Na}_s\ (138\ \text{mM./L.})}{\text{Elevated Conc. Na}_s} = \frac{\text{X (current TBW)}}{\text{Normal Vol. TBW}},$$

or:

$$\frac{138}{175} = \frac{X}{42}$$
$$X = {}^{138}\!/_{175} \times 42$$
$$X = 33.1\ \text{L.}$$

Thus, the *deficit* of water is 42 − 33.1 = 8.9 liters. In this hypothetical instance one would have to achieve a *positive balance* of 8.9 liters of water before the concentration of sodium in the serum had been restored to normal. If the dehydration had been purely a deficit of water this procedure would correct the situation.* If some salt had been lost in addition to the water, the administration of water to restore the concentration of sodium to normal would merely have corrected the *relative* deficit of water, and the second phase of management would involve the administration of a sufficient quantity of an isotonic solution of sodium salts to restore the volume of the extracellular compartment to normal.

Loss of Sodium in Excess of Water. This type of dehydration is characterized by a contraction of the extracellular compartment and *expansion* of the *intracellular compartment*. The loss of sodium in excess of water results in a diminution in the concentration of sodium in the serum and extracellular fluid; this is equated with a diminished effective osmolality of the extracellular fluid and a redistribution of water between the cells and the extracellular compartment such that the former gains from the latter. Thus, not only does the extracellular compartment suffer a deficit in volume to the exterior but, in addition, this loss is compounded by an additional loss of volume to the cells as well. It is clear, therefore, why for a given quantity of water lost to the exterior this type of dehydration is the most severe in terms of a contraction of the interstitial and plasma volumes. In addition, the dilution of the cellular fluids per se may add complicating clinical features of which an altered state of consciousness is outstanding. Further insights into the significance of hyponatremia as this reflects the severity of a dehydration may be provided by considering some of the general principles that may be involved in the pathogenesis of this type of fluid disorder.

Although a primary loss of salt in excess of water would always be expected to be associated with hyponatremia, a *significant* depression of the concentration of sodium in the serum is not always found in the early phase of the development of the dehydration. The reasons for this will be clear if the pathologic physiology is considered. An initial loss of sodium in excess of water will almost certainly have induced some degree of hyponatremia even if this is not readily detected by the ordinary chemical analyses of serum. This slight but definite depression in the concentration of sodium which is equated with a slight but definite decrease in the effective osmolality of the extracellular fluid may be expected to suppress the secretion of the antidiuretic hormone. This, in turn, will diminish the rate of reabsorption of water by the renal tubular cells and a sufficient quantity of water will be excreted to restore the concentration of sodium in the serum to normal. The net effect at this point is an isotonic contraction of the extracellular compartment. As sodium continues to be lost in the urine this same sequence repeats itself until the contraction in volume of the extracellular compartment is such as to be a stimulus in itself for the secretion of ADH, and the hormone will be available to enhance the renal tubular reabsorption of water despite the presence of hyponatremia. Since a contraction in volume of the extracellular compartment must be of some significance before it serves to stimulate the secretion of ADH, it is apparent that when dehydration is noted with hyponatremia, the intensity of the volume contraction must already be significant. The initial response is frequently referred to as a "sacrifice in volume in the interests of maintaining tonicity of the body fluids."

As in water deficit dehydration, there are many avenues by which a dehydration characterized by the loss of salt in excess of water may come about. These include adrenal cortical insufficiency, cerebral salt wasting, renal disease with salt wasting, and all losses of salt and water in which water is *replaced* without salt.

ADRENAL CORTICAL INSUFFICIENCY.[308–311] Adrenal cortical insufficiency is not a common disease but serves perhaps as the classic example of a disorder in

*It should be cautioned that the too rapid correction of a water deficit in infants may be associated with convulsive seizures and, perhaps, neurologic sequelae.

which salt is lost in excess of water. This loss results presumably from an inability on the part of the renal tubules to conserve salt properly owing to inadequate secretion of aldosterone and, perhaps, hydrocortisone as well. The loss of salt in excess of water from the extracellular compartment is due primarily to a loss via the urine. However, there are data which make it appear unlikely that this is the sole route of removal of sodium from the extracellular compartment, and it is suspected that there is an associated movement of sodium to some bony and perhaps cellular depot as well.[312–314]

In addition to the usual consequences of severe dehydration such as impaired peripheral flow with diminution in the renal plasma flow and filtration rate, secondary increases in the concentration of urea nitrogen and some degree of metabolic acidosis, an outstanding feature of the salt depletion dehydration of adrenal cortical insufficiency is the co-existing striking hyperkalemia. The precise cause of this is not clear, but there are many reasons to suspect that at least one phase of sodium reabsorption which is influenced by the adrenal cortical hormone is the reabsorption of sodium in exchange for potassium. If, in fact, most of the potassium which is excreted in the urine is secreted in such an exchange process, one can readily see how the failure to reabsorb sodium would be interrelated with the failure to secrete potassium appropriately. Hypoglycemia may accompany the dehydration of adrenal cortical insufficiency.

CHRONIC RENAL INSUFFICIENCY. Patients with chronic renal insufficiency may have considerable difficulty in reabsorbing sodium adequately despite a diminished filtered load of this cation. On occasion this may be of sufficient magnitude to mimic and be misinterpreted as adrenal cortical insufficiency.[315–317] The disease process is quite different, however, and represents a failure in function of the renal tubular cells. This particular tubular defect has been found in association with several types of advanced renal disease. Although a defect in salt reabsorption sufficiently severe to be mistaken for adrenal cortical insufficiency is rare, a much less intense disability is common. The precise nature of the defect is not clear; the several possibilities that must be considered include an interference with a specific transport mechanism that is primarily involved in the reabsorption of sodium or some secondary mechanism, such as an inability to secrete hydrogen or potassium ions. It is possible that some instances of salt wasting may be due to the effect of an "osmotic diuresis." It has been suggested that in many instances chronic renal insufficiency is characterized by virtually total destruction of a certain proportion of nephrons, a smaller proportion remaining intact. It is further suggested that although the over-all filtration rate of the two kidneys is diminished, the GFR per functioning nephron is actually increased and that as a consequence of the augmented filtered load of sodium per nephron some of this cation escapes into the urine. In addition, when the concentration of urea increases (as the result of over-all diminution in GFR) this is additive to the influence of an increased filtration rate per nephron in the promotion of a solute diuresis with the escape of sodium into the urine.[160,318–321]

The defect may be present but not clinically significant because the patient ingests sufficient salt each day to prevent the development of a negative balance. The defect may be unmasked only when the patient is advised to restrict the dietary intake of salt to very low levels. Such a regimen is frequently recommended because of the mistaken view that patients with chronic renal insufficiency tend to retain salt. This is not true unless they have some complication such as severe hypoalbuminemia or congestive heart failure. The error of this concept needs emphasis. The loss of salt each day may not be great when the patients are on a regimen of salt restriction, but in the course of days or weeks the deficit may become of great significance with the development of dehydration with hyponatremia. When patients with chronic renal disease develop dehydration with the consequences of further impairment of renal perfusion, and renal decompensation supervenes upon renal insufficiency, their status may be very seriously compromised. Such patients may have drastic reduction in renal function, and, unless corrected, the dehydration may be directly or indirectly responsible for a fatal outcome. This hazard of salt restriction in patients with chronic renal disease should be recognized by all. If, despite this, it is considered advisable for one reason or another to prescribe such a regimen, it is the responsibility of the physician to make certain that the patient can tolerate this limitation of dietary salt. Observations of change in body weight, urine flow, blood urea nitrogen, concentration of sodium in the serum and the concentration of sodium in the urine will make it clear whether the program is safe.

CEREBRAL SALT-WASTING SYNDROME.[91,236] A cerebral salt-wasting syndrome with all the consequences of dehydration may be observed in certain patients with disease of the central nervous system. It has been observed most commonly in patients with cerebral vascular accidents including subarachnoid hemorrhage, in encephalitis, bulbar poliomyelitis, and in a very few instances in which the lesion has been more localized, as with a brain tumor. The defect is characterized by an extraordinary rate of excretion of salt which may require the administration of more than 50 grams a day to prevent the development of a negative balance. Despite the dehydration with hyponatremia and evidences of renal decompensation such as azotemia, hyperkalemia is not common and, in fact, the disorder may be associated with a concomitant deficit of potassium.

The mechanisms underlying the inability to conserve salt properly are not clear. The evidence concerning the possibility of a direct neurogenic influence on the renal tubules was briefly summarized in the section dealing with renal physiology. One alternative hypothesis is that there is an interference with the orderly sequence of events leading to the secretion of a hormone that implements the reabsorption of sodium. There is some evidence that there is a measure of control of the secretion of aldosterone by a humoral agent secreted in the central nervous system, perhaps in the diencephalon. One major objection to this interpretation is that hyperkalemia is not commonly observed in this type of salt wasting, and the quantity of salt that is necessary to prevent a negative balance is much more than is usually needed in adrenal cortical insufficiency. Another alternative is that there may be an excessive secretion of a hormone that is responsible for inhibiting the reabsorption of sodium. Genest and his group[322] have reported some evidence for the secretion of such a compound. There is little information which would allow a preference for any of these hypotheses at this time. The facts accumulated thus far are compatible with the thesis that something interferes with the reabsorption of sodium in the proximal tubule which in turn promotes the accession of an unusually large quantity of salt to the distal tubule and that, although sodium reabsorption is enhanced at this latter site, some spills over into the urine. The augmented reabsorption of sodium at the distal site would allow a normal or even increased rate of secretion (and excretion) of potassium and would explain both the salt wasting and the lack of hyperkalemia.

A net deficit of salt in excess of water may arise despite the fact that the characteristic of the *primary source of loss* is water in excess of salt or losses of salt and water in an isotonic relationship. The latter may result whenever the water deficit is more adequately replaced than is the deficiency of salt. This may arise if the patient drinks water or if a physician administers water without salt. If the loss of volume is not large the extra water may be excreted owing to the fact that the diminution in the effective osmolality of the extracellular fluid suppresses the secretion of ADH. However, if the deficit of volume is larger this suppressive influence of the hypotonicity is more than counterbalanced by a stimulus to the secretion of ADH that arises from the volume deficit or some one of its functions.

The management of dehydration accompanied by hyponatremia is directed as in all other instances of dehydration toward the restoration of a normal volume and tonicity of the body fluids. In many circumstances, especially when renal function is basically normal, both goals of therapy may be realized by providing adequate quantities of an isotonic solution of sodium salts. In some instances when the dehydration is extreme it may be desirable to restore the concentration of sodium to normal more quickly by the administration of sodium salts in a hypertonic rather than an isotonic solution. Certainly hypotonic fluids should be avoided until normal tonicity is achieved.

CORRECTION OF HYPONATREMIA.[24,323] If it is considered desirable to correct the hyponatremia promptly, the amount of sodium that must be administered is equivalent to the deficit in the concentration per liter multiplied by the estimated number of liters of *total body water*. This follows from the facts that the cell membranes are freely permeable to water and that the effective osmolality of one compartment cannot be altered without inducing an identical change in the other. Although the administered sodium will be largely confined to the extracellular compartment, the total solute concentration of the cells will rise as a result of the net movement of water from the cellular to the extracellular space. The amount of sodium that must be administered to restore the concentration to normal is equal to:

Normal concentration Na_s (138 mM./L.)
— current concentration of Na_s
× Total volume of body water

For example: In a patient with an assumed volume of total body water of 40 liters and a concentration of sodium in the serum of 128 mM./L.:

$$138 - 128 \times 40 = 400 \text{ mM. Na}$$

If all of the sodium were to be administered as sodium chloride one would need: $400 \times 58.5 = 23.4$ grams NaCl (since one millimol of NaCl equals 58.5 mg.). This could be administered as 468 ml. of a 5 per cent solution of NaCl. In contrast, if one elected to administer half the Na as NaCl and the other half as $NaHCO_3$, the following calculation would be appropriate:

$$200 \times 58.5 = 11.7 \text{ gm. NaCl}$$
$$200 \times 84 = 16.8 \text{ gm. } NaHCO_3$$

This could be satisfied by 234 ml. of 5 per cent NaCl and 224 ml. of 7.5 per cent $NaHCO_3$.

Loss of Sodium and Water in Isotonic Proportions. A dehydration with net deficits of sodium and water in the same proportion as they exist in the extracellular fluid will obviously be characterized by a normal concentration of sodium in the serum, contraction of the extracellular compartment and no significant change in the volume of the intracellular fluid. Since the extracellular compartment bears the total loss of volume, this type of dehydration is midway between primary water deficit and primary sodium deficit in severity for equal losses of volume to the exterior.

Since the character of the *net* deficit is a consequence of loss and gain, such a dehydration may develop in many ways, but perhaps the most common is the loss of gastrointestinal fluids with little or no replacement by the patient or physician. However, a net isotonic loss of salt and water may be an early phase of adrenal cortical insufficiency or renal salt wasting, or may result from excessive sweating with *partial* replacement with water and no salt, etc.

The correction of the dehydration per se is easily achieved by the administration of isotonic solutions of sodium salts until the volume of the extracellular compartment is expanded to normal followed by the institution of measures designed to maintain a normal state of hydration.

The Principles of Management of Dehydration.[24,25] The primary goals of therapy of dehydration are simple. They include the restoration of the body fluids to normal with respect to volume, effective osmolality, composition and acid-base relationships. The character and volume of fluid necessary to satisfy these goals are dependent on the analysis of the characteristics of the dehydration in question. A course of action should follow the interpretation of the character of the dehydration, and, although the analysis cannot be expected to be precise, it can serve as a framework with the precaution that the plan of therapy will be interrupted at appropriate intervals to allow a re-evaluation of the status of the patient. This reappraisal should employ all of the available clinical and laboratory data that are relevant to the problem at hand. At this time the initial plan of management may be altered in accord with the results of the first phase of therapy and the second analysis. As is true in the management of most other clinical problems, the management of dehydration calls for a combination of logic, information and considerable empiricism. In many instances the restoration of a normal volume and effective osmolality of the body fluids and the repair of a deficit of potassium, if present, will allow the correction of other complicating disturbances. This is especially true if renal function is basically normal and if any effect of renal decompensation is removed by improvement of the state of hydration.

When the initial goals of therapy as outlined above have been realized, plans must immediately be made to maintain the normal state of hydration. A fluid prescription must be developed within the framework of the principles outlined in the initial phase of this discussion of dehydration. In particular, one must pay attention not only to the usual basal requirements but to any characteristic in the patient's clinical status that may justifiably dictate an alteration in these basal requirements.

The restoration of the effective osmolality of the extracellular fluids can be achieved by utilizing the equations listed in the discussion of deficits of water in excess of salt and deficits of salt in excess of water. The volume of fluid to be administered when the contraction is isotonic or after alterations in tonicity per se have been corrected must be based on a gross appreciation of the quantitative character of the volume deficit. This will be assessed in a limited fashion by the history, by the physical examination and by the information from laboratory data.

No attempt will be made to discuss the problems of management of dehydration in further detail. The very essence of the message which this discussion should impart is the fact that the *details* of management must be defined in relation to the particular patient and cannot be discussed beyond general principles and generalizations. The treatment must be designed to meet the specific problems of the individual patient not only in terms of quality and quantity of fluids to be administered but also in terms of the route and the speed of administration. These details can be appreciated only when the specific requirements for repair of the dehydration in a particular patient are considered. The special elements associated with the etiology, diagnosis and management of disorders such as diabetes insipidus and adrenal cortical insufficiency will be found in other chapters of this volume.

Disorders of Acid-Base Equilibrium[105,106,109,120,259]

Certain of the basic principles underlying acid-base relationships and the mechanisms available for the preservation of acid-base equilibrium were presented in the first half of this chapter. Those sections summarized the nature of the activity and composition of buffer systems, the exchanges of ions that tend to mitigate alterations in acid-base equilibrium, the role of respiratory regulation, and finally the impact of renal tubular functions on the maintenance of a reasonably stable internal environment in these terms. The discussion to follow will attempt to present the general characteristics of the clinical abnormalities in acid-base disturbances with respect to pathogenesis, compensatory responses, nature of the compositional changes and management. Much of the discussion must center around the impact of these disturbances on the Henderson-Hasselbalch equation, and, hence, this expression is re-presented here specifically in terms of the bicarbonate-carbonic acid system. Reference to this equation, which defines *p*H, will be helpful in visualizing the sequences and consequences of the primary and secondary factors involved in the development of acidosis and alkalosis:

$$pH = 6.1 + \log \frac{[NaHCO_3]}{[H_2CO_3 + \text{dissolved } CO_2]}$$

It will be recalled that at a *p*H of 7.40 the ratio of this buffer pair is equal to 20.

There are four major categories of acid-base disturbance: respiratory and metabolic acidosis and respiratory and metabolic alkalosis. These will be discussed for the most part as separate entities, but it should be mentioned here and will be emphasized later that mixed disturbances are not uncommon. The clinician must be alert to this possibility since their recognition may well modify his approach to management.

Respiratory Acidosis. Respiratory acidoses develop as a consequence of the improper elimination of carbon dioxide by way of the lungs due either to hypoventilation or to ventilation which is uneven with respect to blood flow.[123,124,324] Impaired diffusion across the alveolar-capillary membrane may contribute to its development, but it is unlikely to be the sole cause since the diffusion of carbon dioxide is so rapid. Respiratory acidosis is commonly observed in patients with pulmonary emphysema and fibrosis, cardiopulmonary diseases, and may be noted more acutely when respiratory exchange is suddenly limited by disorders such as severe central nervous system depression, acute injuries to the chest wall, spontaneous pneumothorax, atelectasis and widespread pneumonitis.

If the rate of production of carbon dioxide is unaltered, the failure to eliminate this gas adequately must result in an increased tension of carbon dioxide and an increased concentration of carbonic acid; the value of the denominator of the buffer pair is increased and the value of the ratio itself is diminished to something less than 20, and this, in turn, defines a decrease in the *p*H.

Carbon dioxide appears to permeate most cell membranes with ease and it is therefore distributed throughout all the fluids of the body.[117,118] This permits a large share of the retained CO_2 to be buffered by the cell fluids. In addition, some may be incorporated in bone as carbonate.

The disturbance in acid-base equilibrium can be minimized by those measures which tend to buffer and dispose of the increment of hydrogen ions and those which result in an increase in the concentration of bicarbonate, thereby restoring the value for the buffer ratio back toward 20. The exchange of hydrogen ions for sodium and potassium of cells and bone permits some increase in the bicarbonate concentration in the extracellular fluid. In addition, there may be some exchange of chloride for bicarbonate in an anion exchange across cell membranes, although this is known to occur with certainty only across the membrane of the red blood cell. A more important mechanism by which chloride is replaced with bicarbonate relates to alterations in renal tubular activity characterized by an increased rate of excretion of titratable acid, ammonium and chloride, and a diminished rate of excretion of bicarbonate.[267,325-327] These responses imply a net increase in the rate of secretion and excretion of hydrogen ions, and in this manner the kidneys not only eliminate more acid but alter composition in such a way as to restore the buffer activity and the ratio of the buffer pair. In effect, more bicarbonate is reabsorbed by the tubules than is filtered at the glomeruli due to a larger exchange of hydrogen ions for sodium as proposed in the schema presented in the section dealing with acidification of the urine. The increased tension of CO_2 is responsible, in part at least, for the increased availability and rate of secretion of hydrogen ions.

The increase in the pCO_2 and the diminution in pH each stimulate respiratory activity and this, in turn, serves to prevent or retard further accumulation of carbon dioxide. The net effects of all of these mechanisms may be such as to allow only a minor deviation in pH; however, the alterations in composition may be quite striking. A typical pattern of electrolyte composition in a patient with respiratory acidosis is as follows:

Na	139 mM./L.
K	4.3 mM./L.
Total CO_2	38 mM./L.
Cl	93 mM./L.
pH	7.34
pCO_2	70 mm. Hg

The major features of these alterations are an increase in the concentration of total CO_2, a depressed concentration of chloride, a modestly diminished pH and an elevation of the pCO_2. The sum of the concentrations of carbon dioxide and chloride is 131 mM./L., and this differs from the concentration of sodium in the serum by 8 mM./L. The usual difference between the sum of the concentrations of total CO_2 and chloride on the one hand and sodium on the other varies between 5 and 10 mM./L. and is a rough guide to the concentration of other anions in the extracellular fluid. It is significant that this value is normal in *respiratory* acidosis where the accumulation of acid is due virtually entirely to the retention of CO_2 itself.

Another significant feature of these compositional changes is the fact that the pH is only slightly depressed despite the marked elevation of pCO_2. The ability to tolerate a pCO_2 of this magnitude has certain advantages in that a greater quantity of carbon dioxide can be excreted per unit volume of ventilatory exchange when the pCO_2 is high rather than low, and in these circumstances there will be no further increase in CO_2 tension unless the primary disease worsens.

It has been noted in several instances in this discussion that the increase in the tension of CO_2 served to stimulate respiratory activity; however, as the elevation in pCO_2 is maintained, the respiratory centers seem to develop some diminution in sensitivity to this stimulus of hypercapnia.[126,127] As the sensitivity to the hypercapnia diminishes, the ventilatory drive may be lessened, and this, in turn, promotes the retention of more carbon dioxide. The next increment in pCO_2 subsequent to this event will tend to drive ventilation a little more, but each increment becomes less and less effective; ultimately, the hypercapnia becomes extreme and the increased pCO_2 no longer serves as an *effective* stimulus to augment ventilatory exchange.

MANAGEMENT. The management of patients with this disorder includes all of those measures that tend to improve the underlying pulmonary or cardiopulmonary disease such as the elimination of infections, relief of bronchospasm, treatment of cardiac failure with digitalis preparations, venesections to diminish the packed cell volume and to decrease the viscosity of the circulating blood, rest, and improvement of the hypoxia by the administration of oxygen. The use of oxygen therapy carries certain risks in these patients. It has already been mentioned that sustained hypercapnia is accompanied by a diminished response to specific levels of CO_2 tension, and in these circumstances hypoxia may be the only important stimulus for respiratory activity. If the patient is then exposed to a breathing mixture with a high oxygen content, the hypoxia may be relieved, this last stimulus to ventilation is minimized, and a decreased ventilatory exchange permits further accumulation of carbon dioxide with the development of more extreme hypercapnia and a more acute reduction in pH. The patient may quickly become confused, lapse into coma and die.[328-330] This discussion should certainly not be interpreted to imply that such patients should never be treated with oxygen. However, it should serve to emphasize the need for some caution and close observation when oxygen is administered so that the earliest phase of such a complication may be recognized. In addition, it should be mentioned that drugs such as morphine sulfate and barbiturates, which tend to depress the respiratory center, are generally contraindicated.

In many instances the general measures of management noted above will be found quite adequate to deal with this problem. However, these may fail or the basic disease process may progress to the point where hypercapnia and hypoxia are extreme and more drastic measures may be indicated. In these situations the use of mechanical respirators offers a valuable therapeutic approach.[331] If ventilatory exchange can be increased by these devices, the hypoxia and hypercapnia are both improved and, hence, a material benefit is promptly achieved. In addition, if the pCO_2 is maintained at a reduced level for some time, the respiratory center may regain a normal degree of sensitivity to specific levels of pCO_2 and an increased tension of carbon dioxide may once again serve as an appropriate stimulus to ventilation.

In recent years several drugs have been used in the management of this disorder. Although *carbonic anhydrase inhibitors* such as Diamox have not been uniformly successful, some patients seem definitely to have been helped by their use. However, even in those instances when it appears to have benefited the patients, the data are too inadequate and inconsistent to provide an explanation of its mode of action with any security.[332] One hypothesis suggests that the decrease in pH of the blood (owing to the diminished rate of secretion of hydrogen ions by the renal tubules which is accompanied by an increased elimination of bicarbonate in the urine and the consequent reduction of the concentration of bicarbonate in the extracellular fluid) serves to stimulate an increase in ventilatory exchange and an accelerated elimination of carbon dioxide. Another hypothesis suggests some direct action on the respiratory center which renders it more sensitive to specific levels of carbon dioxide. In any event the increased elimination of CO_2 that is sometimes noted promotes a diminution in the hypercapnia and this, in turn, may be expected to restore the sensitivity of the respiratory center in a manner similar to that suggested with respect to the use of mechanical respirators.

A second agent that has been recently investigated is *salicylate,*[333–335] which may be administered orally as aspirin or intravenously as the sodium salt. It has been clearly established both in normal subjects and in patients with chronic pulmonary disease that salicylates somehow increase the sensitivity of the respiratory center to carbon dioxide. Thus, when patients with chronic hypercapnia whose respiratory center is somewhat insensitive to CO_2 are given salicylates, ventilation may be increased sufficiently to accelerate the rate of elimination of carbon dioxide and promote more nearly complete saturation of hemoglobin with oxygen. This agent has not had wide enough application for us to be certain as to how often it may be used successfully without inducing side reactions, which may include psychoses. Furthermore, salicylates increase CO_2 production as well, and if the bellows action of the chest cannot respond to the stimulating effect of the drug, the level of pCO_2 may increase and the respiratory acidosis may worsen.

Metabolic Acidosis. A metabolic acidosis results from an accumulation of endogenously produced acids, from the excessive administration of exogenous acids or from a primary loss of bicarbonate. An accumulation of acids is observed classically in diabetic acidosis, in which 4-carbon ketone acids are formed more rapidly than they can be siphoned off into the Kreb's cycle, and in chronic renal insufficiency, in which acids accumulate because of incompetent renal function. In some instances of chronic renal insufficiency there is an excessive loss of bicarbonate into the urine because of a defect in the secretion and exchange of hydrogen for sodium ions, thus leading to a diminished rate of reabsorption of bicarbonate.

DIABETIC ACIDOSIS. Many features of a metabolic acidosis can be illustrated by examining in some detail the sequence of events that may be noted in the development of and recovery from diabetic acidosis. It has already been stated that the accumulated acid is almost entirely represented by the 4-carbon ketones which may be symbolized as HK. The first consequence of their accession to the extracellular fluid may be visualized as follows:

$$HK + NaHCO_3 \rightleftharpoons NaK + H_2CO_3$$

If this reaction is now considered in relation to the Henderson-Hasselbalch equation, it is immediately noted that the concentration of bicarbonate must have diminished and the concentration of carbonic acid and the pCO_2 must have increased. These changes, which are due primarily to an increase in hydrogen ions, result in a decrease in the concentration of the numerator and an increase in the concentration of the denominator of the buffer ratio of the Henderson-Hasselbalch equation and define a decrease in the pH. An increase in the pCO_2 is not actually observed during the course of the development of the metabolic acidosis if the respiratory system is intact, since as soon as the pCO_2 and pH are minimally elevated and depressed respectively, ventilation is increased, the elimination of carbon dioxide is accelerated, and the pCO_2 falls. The diminution in pCO_2 tends to restore the buffer ratio back toward 20, and to the extent that this occurs the deviation in pH is minimized. The respiratory response to these changes in pCO_2 and pH is characterized first by an increase in depth and later in the frequency of respirations and is spoken of as Kussmaul breathing.

It will be noted that at the time of a full blown metabolic acidosis both the pCO_2 and the pH are depressed, and some question may be raised as to whether the diminution in pH is now the major drive to respiratory activity. This seems unlikely since Winters et al.[128] have noted that during the recovery from diabetic acidosis (and other metabolic acidoses as well) the pH returns to normal before the total CO_2 content of the serum is restored to its original value. This situation is clearly associated with a reduction in pCO_2, and it has been inferred that when there has been a period of hypocapnia, the respiratory center may become sensitized to lower levels of pCO_2. This is recognized as the antithesis of the desensitization of the respiratory center to pCO_2 during exposure to hypercapnia. The precise mechanisms responsible for these alterations in what is referred to as "sensitivity" are certainly not clear. However, it will be recalled from the discussion of buffers that the degree to which the pH may be altered by the addition of a specific increment of acid is related not only to the value of the ratio of the buffer pair but to the concentration of the two components as well. Thus, when the concentration of bicarbonate and the tension of CO_2 are high, a given increment of acid will influence the pH less than if the same quantity of acid gained access to the body fluids when the concentrations of the components of the buffer pair were initially low. It is reasonable to suggest that there may be a reflection of these alterations in composition, concentration and response in the fluids that compose the specific chemoreceptor organ.

The response of the kidneys to such a metabolic acidosis is characterized by virtual total reabsorption of all the filtered bicarbonate and an increase in the net rate of excretion of acid in the form of titratable acid and ammonium ions. The increase in the net rate of excretion of acid does not necessarily imply that there has been an increase in the net rate of *secretion* of hydrogen ions.[259] For example, if the rate of filtration of bicarbonate is 1 mM./min. and this is totally reabsorbed by exchange of hydrogen ions for sodium, less hydrogen ion must be secreted than if the rate of filtration of bicarbonate is 2.5 mM./min. and only one half of the filtered load of bicarbonate is reabsorbed. This distinction between the net rates of *secretion* and *excretion* of acid is made to emphasize the fact that the diminution in pCO_2 characteristic of a metabolic acidosis does not jeopardize the ability of the kidney to increase the net *excretion* of acid. A fairly typical pattern for the concentrations of electrolytes and the pH and pCO_2 of the serum of a patient with diabetic acidosis may be illustrated by the following data:

Na	120 mM./L.
K	4.8 mM./L.
Total CO_2	7 mM./L.
Cl	85 mM./L.
Glucose	900 mg. %
pH	7.12
pCO_2	20 mm. Hg

The sum of the concentrations of chloride and CO_2 in the serum is 92 mM./L. and the difference between this value and the concentration of sodium is 28 mM./L. This is significantly in excess of the usual difference of 5 to 10 mM./L., and in diabetic acidosis this excess is almost all represented by the 4-carbon ketone anions. The pCO_2 and pH are both significantly depressed. The concentration of potassium does not reflect the fact of a potassium deficit. The depressed concentration of sodium cannot be equated with a decrease in the effective osmolality of the extracellular fluid since the concentration of glucose is 50 milliosmolal (see discussion of Exchanges of water between the intra- and extracellular compartments).

The management of the acid-base disturbance in diabetic acidosis is usually not a major concern since the administration of insulin and the correction of the defect in carbohydrate utilization is accompanied by a diminished rate of production of ketone acids. Those that have accumulated are dissipated by utilization and excretion, and as they disappear, bicarbonate concentration is automatically restored toward normal. It was noted previously that in the recovery phase the pH frequently returns to normal prior to the restoration of the concentration of total CO_2. If significant quantities of bicarbonate were to be administered early in the management of diabetic acidosis, it may be readily appreciated that a mixed metabolic and respiratory alkalosis might very easily complicate the recovery phase of this disorder.

RENAL INSUFFICIENCY. A metabolic acidosis associated with renal insufficiency may obtain in several ways. In many instances a metabolic acidosis supervenes during the course of chronic renal insufficiency in consequence of a diminished rate of glomerular filtration and an impaired rate of excretion of the fixed anions of acid end-products of metabolism.[336] Among these are phosphate, sulfate and other unknown and undetermined products. These acids of phosphate and sulfate are more highly dissociated than carbonic acid; hence, as was noted in the case of the ketone acids, they displace bicarbonate to form sodium salts of the fixed anions. In addition to these accumulations, the renal tubules may develop specific defects characterized by an inability to reabsorb bicarbonate appropriately. For example, there might be a specific inability to secrete hydrogen ions, or the reactions involved in the formation of ammonia from its precursors might be jeopardized, or that phase of the active transport of sodium which is coupled with the exchange for hydrogen ions might be at fault. On occasion an inability to effect the exchange of hydrogen ions for sodium may be almost solely responsible for the development of a metabolic acidosis. In these circumstances the depression of filtration rate may be slight and insufficient to account for the accession of undetermined fixed anions to the extracellular fluid. In this situation the metabolic acidosis is due virtually entirely to the failure to reabsorb bicarbonate, and if the concentration of sodium in the serum is maintained at a normal level the deficit of bicarbonate in the anion column is replaced by chloride. This type of disorder is frequently referred to as *renal tubular acidosis*[337–340] and in rare instances is unassociated with *glomerular insufficiency*. More commonly it is a phase during the course of a variety of chronic renal disorders and is, perhaps, most frequently noted in chronic pyelonephritis. In this particular type of acidosis the primary defect is the reduction in the concentration of bicarbonate, which diminishes buffer activity and is accompanied by an increase in hydrogen ions. This is reflected in a decreased *p*H which is defined by the reduced value of the ratio of the buffer pair. This is, in turn, associated with an increase in ventilatory exchange with increased elimination of carbon dioxide and a tendency to restore the *p*H of the blood toward normal. A characteristic set of chemical data in such a circumstance is as follows:

Na	137 mM./L.
K	3.3 mM./L.
Total CO_2	15 mM./L.
Cl	116 mM./L.
*p*H	7.29
pCO_2	30 mm. Hg

The striking features of these compositional changes include the depressed concentration of bicarbonate, the elevated concentration of chloride and a diminution in the *p*H and pCO_2. In addition it should be emphasized that the sum of the concentrations of CO_2 and chloride is 131 mM./L., which differs only by 6 mM./L. from the concentration of sodium. Thus, one can tell at a glance that this acidosis is not due to the accumulation of acids of phosphate or sulfate, etc. It could be the response, however, to the administration of an acid such as HCl or its equivalent NH_4Cl, in which case the bicarbonate would have been displaced by this highly dissociated acid. In the absence of a history of the administration of either of these drugs, the acidosis must be due to a defect in the reabsorption of bicarbonate due to some intrinsic renal tubular defect or to the administration of a drug such as a carbonic anhydrase inhibitor which impairs the ability to secrete hydrogen ions in exchange for sodium. If one did not know the *p*H, another alternative would have to be considered, namely, respiratory alkalosis.

In instances of chronic renal insufficiency in which a metabolic acidosis is due to the accumulation of acidic end-products of metabolism (owing to impaired filtration rate as well as to specific defects in the rate of secretion of hydrogen ions), the pattern of concentrations of electrolytes would be similar to the following:

Na	137 mM./L.
K	5 mM./L.
Total CO_2	15 mM./L.
Cl	90 mM./L.
*p*H	7.29
pCO_2	30 mm. Hg

There are several differences between these figures and those presented in the previous discussion. The most significant difference lies in the fact that the sum of the concentrations of CO_2 and chloride in this last instance is 105 mM./L., which is 32 mM./L. less than the concentration of sodium. This is considerably larger than the usual difference of 5 to 10 mM./L. The excess is represented by phosphate, sulfate and other anions. In this instance the blood urea nitrogen would certainly be elevated because of the impaired rate of filtration at the glomeruli, whereas in the former instance it might or might not have been elevated, depending on the degree to which GFR had been diminished.

One other difference between these two sets of chemical data is the concentration of potassium which was depressed in the former instance. Since hydrogen and potassium ions compete with one another in exchange for sodium, it may be readily appreciated that when the ability to secrete hydrogen ions is impaired there might well be an increased urinary excretion of potassium with consequent hypokalemia. This, in fact, is not infrequently noted and in some instances may be a prominent feature of the renal dysfunction. It is referred to as potassium-losing renal disease.[341] (Some cases of "potassium-losing renal disease" have subsequently been found to be instances of primary hyperaldosteronism.)[342–344]

MANAGEMENT. The metabolic acidosis associated with renal insufficiency can be modified by the administration of sodium bicarbonate. When the problem is one of long range chronic management the patient can be instructed to ingest a few grams of sodium bicarbonate a day (and if necessary, diminish the intake of sodium chloride). In this fashion the concentration of bicarbonate can be increased at the expense of chloride, buffer activity is increased, the value for the buffer ratio can be raised, and the *p*H can be restored toward a more normal value. The appropriate amount of sodium bicarbonate to be ingested daily is difficult to predict and must be evaluated empirically. One should observe the caution that it is possible to alter acid-base relationships with bicarbonate administration so rapidly that latent tetany associated with hypocalcemia may progress to frank carpopedal spasm. It is recommended that 2 to 4 grams of sodium bicarbonate be ingested daily at first and that the dose be varied depending on the response. The complication of manifest hypocalcemic tetany may be prevented by the daily ingestion of several grams of calcium lactate. Lastly, it is suggested that the daily ingestion of aluminum hydroxide may promote the excretion of phosphorus in the stool, thus modifying the degree of the acidosis and the intensity of the hypocalcemia. In addition to whatever advantages may accrue from the restoration of the *p*H toward a more nearly normal level, the increase in the concentration of bicarbonate allows the restoration of the internal environment toward a normal composition which is better able to cope with further increments of acid because of increased buffer capacity, may relieve the troublesome symptom of hyperpnea, and may diminish the excessive rate of excretion of potassium and calcium in the urine.

Thus far the management of the metabolic acidosis which accompanies renal insufficiency has been discussed in relation to a fairly stable chronic status. In addition, patients with chronic renal insufficiency may develop acute episodes of deteriorating function accompanied by more drastic disturbances in acid-base equilibrium, and metabolic acidosis is a prominent feature of all types of acute renal insufficiency. It is in these circumstances that the correction of metabolic acidosis may be more significant in terms of ultimate recovery from the acute disorder. The restoration of a more nearly normal acid-base equilibrium in such patients is dependent on efforts aimed toward increasing the concentration of bicarbonate in the extracellular fluids. This can be accomplished most efficiently when the disorder is accompanied by hyponatremia, for in this circumstance one can restore the concentration of sodium to more nearly normal levels with sodium bicarbonate in lieu of sodium chloride. The use of hypertonic or isotonic solutions of sodium bicarbonate must be decided on the basis of the associated problem. If the patient's state of hydration is such that there is no deficit of total volume, the solution employed should be hypertonic in concentration. If, on the other hand, there is a deficit in volume as well as in the concentration of sodium, one may achieve an appropriate correction with the use of isotonic solutions of sodium bicarbonate. It should be emphasized, however, that the patient with renal insufficiency usually lacks the fine discriminatory control which characterizes normal renal tubular function. It is frequently more desirable and successful to attempt correction of a disordered internal environment by the use of fluids whose specific composition is designed toward this end, rather than simply to provide the raw materials in appropriate bulk and rely on the function of the renal tubules selectively to reabsorb and reject ions and water in appropriate quantities. If there are hyponatremia and acidosis and one wishes to restore the concentration of both sodium and bicarbonate, the quantity of sodium as bicarbonate to be used may be calculated in a manner similar to that discussed in the section dealing with hyponatremia and dehydration. This should represent an excessive quantity of bicarbonate because, as administered, the ratio of bicarbonate to sodium is much higher than that in the extracellular fluids. However, for reasons which are not altogether clear, such an excess can rarely be demonstrated.[119] If the patient has acidosis with dehydration accompanied by a normal concentration of sodium, a measure of correction can be achieved simply by expanding the volume of the extracellular fluids with an isotonic solution of sodium bicarbonate. The most unsatisfactory circumstance is characterized by a reduction in the concentration of bicarbonate with a normal concentration of sodium and a normal or expanded volume of the extracellular fluids. On rare occasions the hyperpnea may be so uncomfortable as to warrant an attempt to increase the concentration of bicarbonate by the administration of a hypertonic solution of sodium bicarbonate. However, hypernatremia will accompany any significant increase in bicarbonate concentration, and the thirst engendered thereby may be as uncomfortable as the hyperpnea for which the solution of bicarbonate was administered.

The complication of frank hypocalcemic tetany must always be considered as a hazard when the metabolic acidosis of renal insufficiency is to be treated with the intravenous administration of solutions of bicarbonate. This can usually be avoided by the injection of at least 10 cc. of a 10 per cent solution of calcium gluconate prior to the administration of bicarbonate. The solution of calcium should not be admixed with the bicarbonate since the precipitation of calcium carbonate will result.

The principles underlying the management of a severe acidosis resulting from the administration of drugs such as ammonium chloride or Diamox are essentially those presented above. Most commonly, such acidoses clear quite promptly once the administration of the drug has been discontinued if renal function is intact.

Respiratory Alkalosis. A respiratory alkalosis is the consequence of the excretion of carbon dioxide by way of the lungs at a rate which exceeds its production. This reduces the pCO_2, which, in turn decreases the concentration of hydrogen ions and increases the value for the ratio of the buffer pair of bicarbonate-carbonic acid to a value in excess of 20 and defines an increase in the pH. This disorder may be noted in the *early* stage of pulmonary and cardiopulmonary disease when an increase in ventilatory exchange is conditioned by the development of hypoxia. It will be recalled that the diffusion of carbon dioxide is much faster than that of oxygen; hence, when there is a barrier to diffusion and hypoxia is compensated for by hyperventilation, the excretion of CO_2 is likely to be augmented. It is also noted in more extreme degree on rare occasions when there is a lesion of the central nervous system which is irritative to the respiratory center and disorganizes the control of respiratory exchange in such a fashion as to provoke hyperventilation. It is also characteristic of the early stage of salicylate intoxication when the drug has stimulated the respiratory mechanism directly, prior to the time when the salicylates induce a ketonemia. The latter event promotes a dissipation of bicarbonate and the net result may be what is referred to as a mixed acid-base disturbance composed of respiratory alkalosis and metabolic acidosis. It has also been reported in patients with severe hepatic disease[345] and is partially correlated with but not necessarily caused by increased levels of blood ammonia.

Respiratory alkalosis, however, is most commonly observed in an anxious and tense person (more commonly a female) who develops the habit of hyperventilation as a response to minor emotional stresses and strains.[125,346,347] These patients usually have some constant degree of hyperventilation and then, in response to an emotional situation, will increase ventilation to the point where there is an acute decrease in pCO_2 and elevation of pH. These episodes are accompanied by a variety of symptoms which include giddiness and light-headedness (frequently referred to by the patient as dizziness), circumoral and peripheral paresthesias, tremulousness of muscles, and, on occasion, frank carpopedal spasm. Despite the fact that these symptoms develop because of ineffectiveness of compensatory mechanisms due to inadequate time for the renal responses, the chemical changes in the blood may be quite subtle; if one depended solely on the concentrations of the electrolytes, one might discern no significant abnormalities. However, a determination of the *p*H and calculation of the pCO_2 from this datum plus the concentration of total CO_2 in the serum will reveal the nature of the disturbance.

When there is a more sustained hyperventilation, as may be the case with an appropriately placed lesion of the central nervous system, compensatory responses and the consequent compositional changes become more prominent features. The major compensation is achieved through renal mechanisms characterized by a diminished rate of secretion and excretion of acid, which is accompanied by increased urinary elimination of sodium and potassium bicarbonate and retention of chloride. In this fashion the concentration of bicarbonate is decreased (and is replaced by chloride) so that the value for the buffer ratio is reduced toward 20 and the *p*H restored to a level more closely approximating 7.40. A pattern of chemical data typifying the changes seen in respiratory alkalosis which has been sustained is as follows:

Na	141 mM./L.
K	3.5 mM./L.
Total CO_2	18 mM./L.
Cl	114 mM./L.
*p*H	7.46
pCO_2	25 mm. Hg

It will be noted that the major alterations in the concentrations of electrolytes are a depression of the total CO_2 content and an increase in the level of chloride, which will be recognized as characteristic of the first pattern described under metabolic acidosis. In addition, the sum of the concentrations of CO_2 and chloride is 132 mM./L. and the difference between this and the concentration of sodium is only 9 mM./L. which is within the usual limits. In fact, the similarity between these two patterns extends to the fact that the pCO_2 is depressed in each instance, and the only distinguishing characteristic is the *p*H. If the value for buffer base were calculated or read from the nomogram of Singer and Hastings[109] it would be noted to be normal in this instance but depressed in the circumstance of the previously described metabolic acidosis. It is important to recognize and discriminate between respiratory alkalosis and metabolic acidosis when chemical data may mimic one another, since the administration of bicarbonate to a patient with respiratory alkalosis will worsen the clinical condition.

MANAGEMENT. The management of a patient with the hyperventilation syndrome resulting from a reaction pattern to emotional stimuli must be directed primarily toward education of the patient concerning the mechanism of the production of her symptoms. In this regard it is most helpful to have the patient voluntarily hyperventilate to reproduce the symptoms which formed the complaints and then to demonstrate how these can be abated by re-breathing into a paper bag or by breath-holding. Such a demonstration is frequently quite convincing and is most helpful in providing the motivation for the patient to train herself to discard this reaction pattern. When hyperventilation has provoked frank tetany with carpopedal spasm, the immediate need is to increase the tension of CO_2. This can be accomplished by having the patient rebreathe into a paper bag. The administration of a solution of calcium is unlikely to be of benefit.

Metabolic Alkalosis. A metabolic alkalosis is characterized by an increase in the concentration of bicarbonate in the extracellular fluid unattended by a proportionate increase in the pCO_2, so that there is increased buffer activity, the value of the buffer ratio is in excess of 20, and the *p*H is increased. The pathways along which a metabolic alkalosis may develop are multiple and include the administration of sodium bicarbonate (or sodium salts of readily metabolized organic acids such as lactate, citrate, acetate, etc., which are equivalent to equimolar quantities of sodium bicarbonate); the loss of hydrochloric acid from the stomach; the loss of chloride with sodium in a relationship in excess of that which obtains normally in the extracellular fluid; an excessive excretion of acid in the urine; and the movement of hydrogen ions from the extracellular fluid to cellular depots in response to a deficiency of potassium. Not only are there a variety of pathways which lead to metabolic alkalosis, but in addition each episode may serve as the primary event and may elicit interdependent responses characteristic of the other pathways so that it is quite rare to encounter a metabolic alkalosis which is due to a single sequence; almost all instances are multicausal. This interplay among the primary events and secondary responses can best be illustrated by tracing the sequences which may follow each of the possible primary events.[24,25]

The compensatory mechanisms which would tend to minimize the deviation of pH, as these may be anticipated from the characteristics of the Henderson-Hasselbalch equation, should be borne in mind throughout this discussion. In brief, the basic alterations which would tend to reduce the buffer ratio toward 20 and the pH toward 7.40 are a reduction in the concentration of bicarbonate and an increase in the tension of CO_2. Both might be accomplished by the addition of acids stronger than carbonic acid (such as lactic, ketone and others) from the cellular fluids to the extracellular space. The exchange of sodium from the extracellular fluid for hydrogen ions from the cells would have similar consequences. The tension of CO_2 would theoretically be decreased initially, but by the time such patients are seen, the pCO_2 is usually slightly elevated presumably because of some slight hypoventilation. This response is limited, however, perhaps by hypoxia, and by the hypercapnia itself, since both of these are stimuli to increased ventilatory exchange. An increased excretion of bicarbonate and increased reabsorption of chloride would tend to diminish the concentration of bicarbonate in the extracellular fluid, but this may be limited by the hypercapnia, which makes hydrogen ions more available for secretion and promotes more efficient reabsorption of bicarbonate. There are other serious limitations that may be imposed on each of the compensatory mechanisms, and, in addition, there may be anatomic as well as functional deterioration of the kidneys as a result of certain features of metabolic alkalosis. Among these are the specific alterations imposed by the potassium depletion which almost invariably accompanies metabolic alkalosis. It is also possible that anatomic disturbances within the nephron are caused by alkalosis per se, but this has not yet been clearly defined.

ALKALOSIS DUE TO THE ADMINISTRATION OF SODIUM BICARBONATE.[348-350] The administration of sodium bicarbonate by mouth or by vein will in itself induce a mild metabolic alkalosis. A severe degree of metabolic alkalosis is unlikely to result because the ability to excrete excessive loads of bicarbonate by the kidney is so great that it is difficult to sustain an increased concentration of bicarbonate in the extracellular fluid unless the administration of bicarbonate is accompanied by some other complicating feature which tends to contribute to the alkalosis or minimize the efficiency of the mechanisms responsible for compensation. The administration of sodium bicarbonate does nevertheless induce some degree of metabolic alkalosis, and one of the consequences is an augmented rate of excretion of potassium. This is, presumably, a consequence of the nature of the competition between potassium and hydrogen ions for the reabsorption of sodium by the exchange process discussed in the section dealing with the problems of acidification of the urine. If the increased rate of excretion of potassium exceeds intake of this cation, a deficit of potassium will be induced. The development of potassium depletion may be expected to have several consequences which will tend to increase rather than minimize the intensity of the metabolic alkalosis induced initially by the administration of sodium bicarbonate.

A deficit of potassium owing to an increased excretion of this ion in the urine will induce some reduction in the concentration of potassium in the extracellular fluid. This, in turn, seems somehow to be followed by the movement of potassium from the cells to the extracellular space. The loss of potassium from the cell is associated with a movement of other cations from the extracellular space into the cells. In most experimental studies the character of the cation exchange is such that for every three potassium ions lost from the cells, two sodium ions and one hydrogen ion gain access to the cellular fluid. It can be readily appreciated that the loss of hydrogen ions from the extracellular compartment will intensify the alkalosis in that fluid.[111,351-354]

Furthermore, it is believed that as the loss of potassium proceeds the deficit is shared by the renal tubular cells. Anderson and Mudge[272] have reported on the direct relationship between potassium and bicarbonate in kidney slices, and their data support the assumption that the deficit of potassium in the renal tubular cells is accompanied by an intracellular acidosis. This provides a more secure background for an explanation of the favorable competitive position of hydrogen ions for exchange with sodium in the reabsorptive process despite the extracellular alkalosis. It would account for a further loss of hydrogen ions into the urine, for an increased renal tubular reabsorption of bicarbonate and a consequent intensification of the extracellular alkalosis. Thus, although the administration of sodium bicarbonate will not in itself induce a severe metabolic alkalosis, the latter will supervene in those instances when a deficit of potassium develops.

ALKALOSIS DUE TO THE LOSS OF GASTRIC SECRETIONS.[355-357] The initial event predominantly responsible for the development of a metabolic alkalosis when gastric secretions are lost by vomiting or suction is the loss of hydrochloric acid. In addition to the loss of hydrogen ions with chloride, there is a loss of chloride in excess of sodium so that the concentration of bicarbonate in the extracellular fluid is increased. This provides more buffer activity, tends further to diminish the concentration of hydrogen ions, increases the value for the buffer ratio, and defines an increase in the *p*H. Potassium is lost in the vomitus and in the urine; since the very nature of the gastrointestinal disorder makes it unlikely that the patient can ingest and retain potassium-containing food and fluid, a deficit of potassium develops quickly. In addition to the deficit of potassium, which tends to sustain and intensify the metabolic alkalosis, there are other factors which impose limitations on the mechanisms of compensation. Sodium deficiency due to the loss of NaCl in the vomitus and $NaHCO_3$ in the urine imposes specific limitations on the mechanisms that might operate to modify the intensity of the alkalosis.

The deficit of sodium is accompanied by a loss of water. If no water is administered the net deficit is likely to be characterized by a loss of water in excess of sodium because of insensible loss which will not have been replaced; if water is administered the net characteristic of the deficit will be a loss of salt in excess of water. In either event the volume of the extracellular fluid will be contracted and the rate of excretion of sodium in the urine will diminish. A reduction in the rate of excretion of sodium clearly limits the rate of excretion of bicarbonate and to this extent limits the ability of the kidneys to rid the body fluid of the excessive quantity of bicarbonate.[358] Furthermore, if potassium depletion is coincidental with virtually total reabsorption of filtered sodium, that fraction of the sodium which is reabsorbed by an exchange mechanism will be inter-related with the secretion of hydrogen ions rather than potassium and the net rate of excretion of acid into the urine will be increased despite the systemic alkalosis. The urine will no longer be alkaline, and since this condition develops despite the extracellular alkalosis, it is referred to as "paradoxical aciduria." It is probable that this aciduria is conditioned not only by the deficit of potassium but by the fact that the reabsorption of sodium is complete in the context of potassium deficiency, necessitating the secretion and excretion of hydrogen and ammonium ions.

Each of these factors involved in the pathogenesis of the alkalosis and dehydration have significant implications with regard to management. It should be clear that the administration of ammonium chloride, which might well correct the alkalosis, would do little to improve the other important features of the situation, namely, the severe dehydration, potassium depletion and sodium deficit. In fact, the administration of ammonium chloride might well aggravate each of these factors and worsen the clinical status of the patient. The therapeutic measures that are indicated in the management of a situation such as this are as follows:

(1) The dehydration should be corrected by the administration of salt and water in quantities and concentrations dictated by the intensity of the volume deficit and the relative proportion in which the two have been lost. These judgments must be made according to the principles outlined in the discussion of dehydration.

(2) The potassium depletion should be corrected. The manner in which this may be accomplished with safety will be presented in a later section dealing primarily with potassium depletion.

(3) Adequate quantities of carbohydrate must be administered to diminish protein catabolism and allay ketonemia.

(4) Once the dehydration and potassium deficiency have been corrected current losses must be replaced as indicated.

ALKALOSIS DUE TO ALTERATION IN RENAL TUBULAR FUNCTION. Organic mercurial compounds which are so useful in the management of many types of edema influence the edema by augmenting the rate of excretion of sodium and chloride in the urine. It is not clear in what manner these compounds influence urinary composition, where in the tubule they exert their influence, or whether the primary effect is on chloride or sodium. However, the net effect of their administration is usually to promote the excretion of sodium and chloride in a ratio of 1:1 or even less. If water is lost from the extracellular space in relation to the quantity of sodium excreted it will be apparent that in addition to a contraction in the volume of the extracellular fluid there will be a diminished concentration of chloride and a reciprocal increase in the concentration of bicarbonate.[359] Furthermore, to the extent that chloride is excreted in excess of sodium there will be a loss of potassium and ammonium into the urine. These events result in a metabolic alkalosis produced primarily by the excessive loss of chloride and the increased concentration of bicarbonate and sustained, in part, by additional losses of hydrogen ions (as ammonium) and the secondary effects of a deficit of potassium. Since conditions characterized by edema are associated with avid renal tubular reabsorption of sodium, it is impossible to compensate for the alkalosis by the excretion of sodium bicarbonate and this, too, tends to sustain the state of acid base disequilibrium. In addition to the undesirable consequences of metabolic alkalosis in general, it specifically inhibits further responses to organic mercurial diuretics and is one of the common causes of a refractory state to these agents.[360–362] There are special reasons, therefore, to recognize this state of affairs and to correct it so that the patient may again have the benefits of the action of these diuretics. The administration of ammonium chloride will usually correct the acid-base disturbance and if the alkalosis was the sole reason for the refractory state, the latter is also simultaneously repaired. Furthermore, to the extent that metabolic alkalosis is associated with potassium depletion, there are serious implications with respect to the response to preparations of digitalis, since a deficit of potassium makes a patient more sensitive to a given dose of these drugs. The appearance of evidences of digitalis intoxication following the exhibition of mercurial diuretics may be interpreted to imply some degree of potassium depletion, and the evidences of digitalis intoxication may be reversed by the careful administration of potassium salts.

ALKALOSIS DUE TO DEFICIT OF POTASSIUM. The manner in which potassium depletion may initiate, sustain and interrelate with metabolic alkaloses has been discussed above. A deficit of potassium can develop in a variety of ways including diarrhea (due to primary disease of the bowel or excessive use of laxatives),[363] losses of fluid from other parts of the gastrointestinal tract with inadequate dietary replacement, chronic renal insufficiency,[364] treatment with organic mercurial diuretics, adrenal cortical steroid therapy,[365] or as part of the syndrome due to excessive adrenal cortical secretions such as in Cushing's syndrome[366] and primary hyperaldosteronism.[342-344]

The development of potassium deficit from the action of excessive amounts of adrenal cortical hormones is due presumably to the fact that these agents promote the reabsorption of sodium in part by a mechanism which involves exchange with potassium or hydrogen ions. The excessive secretion of both potassium and hydrogen ions promotes the development of a metabolic alkalosis, which, in turn, may induce further excretion of potassium, and a vicious cycle is induced and perpetuated. In addition to a deficit of potassium and a metabolic alkalosis, patients with primary hyperaldosteronism usually have elevated concentrations of sodium in the serum, hypomagnesemia, latent tetany and hypertension.

Since potassium is the major intracellular cation, it is not surprising that depletion of this element is associated with many examples of functional and structural abnormalities. Among the commonly noted abnormalities which accompany potassium depletion are: impaired neuromuscular function, including skeletal, smooth and cardiac musculature; abnormalities in the ECG and cardiac arrhythmias; impaired carbohydrate tolerance; alterations in the kidneys, which appear to involve primarily the collecting tubules with an associated inability to concentrate the urine appropriately; a decrease in the GFR and a defect in the transport of PAH; polydipsia; alterations in the characteristics of gastric secretion and intestinal motility; and others.[162,367-380]

Although it is quite apparent from this brief recounting of the effects of potassium depletion that this state may have serious consequences, it is wise to proceed cautiously with *restitution of potassium* so as to avoid the complications of therapy. The most hazardous of these is the possibility of achieving cardiotoxic levels by the administration of potassium salts too rapidly or in too large a quantity. This may be especially true when a deficit of potassium coexists with a state of dehydration characterized by a significant contraction of the extracellular fluid volume. In such circumstances the excretion of excesses of administered potassium cannot be relied upon because the dehydration may have induced renal decompensation. It is wise, therefore, not to attempt the correction of a deficit of potassium until the coincident dehydration has been repaired, urine flow is well established, and the concentration of potassium in the serum is known to be depressed. The route of administration of potassium salts should be considered with respect to the safety with which a deficit may be repaired. Whenever possible it is desirable to use the oral route since this imposes a restraint on the rapidity with which potassium gains access to the circulation, and represents a safeguard against hyperkalemia if ingestion is at a rate not in excess of 20 mM. per hour. This discussion should not be interpreted to mean that it is necessarily unsafe to administer potassium by vein; rather, judgment and caution should be exercised when this is done.

Unfortunately there is no way to estimate the intensity of a deficit of potassium with any precision. Some inferences may be drawn from the level of potassium in the serum, although even in the absence of the complicating feature of dehydration the serum concentration is only poorly correlated with the cellular stores of this cation. The degree of alkalosis, as this may be equated with the increase in the concentration of bicarbonate in the serum, provides some guide, but it must be emphasized that potassium depletion can and does occur in the absence of alkalosis and, hence, this also fails as a safe guide to the intensity of a potassium deficit. The alterations in the ECG, characterized by a prolongation of the QT interval, a broad flat T wave, inversion of the T wave, depression of the ST segment and defects in conduction, may be of some aid if other causes of such changes can be ignored.

Since the quantity of potassium necessary to repair the deficit is unknown, the response to the administration of potassium must be noted and the plan of therapy in this regard must be reevaluated at intervals. When there is potassium depletion in adults, the level of potassium in the serum is depressed, and renal function is normal, it is safe to administer potassium at a rate of 20 millimols per hour, but it is, perhaps, desirable to limit the first replacement to 60 to 100 mM. At that time a new set of chemical data, an ECG and an evaluation of the clinical status will provide reasonably good information concerning a safe dose to be administered in the next phase of treatment. Unfortunately, the rate of infusion may vary owing to changes in the position of a needle in the vein, the position of the limb, etc. In order to make certain that the rate of administration of potassium does not exceed approximately 20 mM./hour it is wise to adjust the concentration in the infusate to a level that will make this unlikely; a reasonably safe figure would be 50 mM./L.

It must be restated that this discussion of acid-base equilibrium has been presented in terms of four distinct and separate entities. This was considered desirable in the interests of clarity. It would be a disservice, however, to leave the impression that clinical disturbances of acid-base equilibrium are usually as neatly classified as this. Quite commonly the disturbance is mixed and in a given disorder may pass progressively from one kind to another. This is, perhaps, best illustrated by the sequence which may be observed in salicylate intoxication in children, which probably starts as a respiratory alkalosis, may quickly become complicated by a metabolic acidosis due to the development of ketonemia resulting from the influence of salicylates on intermediary metabolic pathways, may then be modified by an element of alkalosis contributed by potassium depletion, and finally may terminate with a contribution of respiratory acidosis due to disorganization and failure of the respiratory centers. The particular classification at a specific point in time during the course of such an illness must be defined by the *p*H, the pCO_2, the interrelationships between the sum of the concentrations of CO_2 and chloride and the concentration of sodium, and the value for buffer base. Most instances of acid-base equilibrium are, however, less complicated than this and should not defy ready analysis if the principles which have been presented are recalled.

Lastly it should be emphasized that a disturbance of acid-base equilibrium is usually only one of many coincidental disorders and not necessarily the most significant of these. Furthermore, in many instances the disequilibrium of acid-base balance will be automatically corrected if the underlying disease is corrected, if hydration is restored, if potassium deficits are replaced, or if other appropriate aspects of the primary disturbance are improved.

Familial Periodic Paralysis.[381-385] This rare condition is an example of a disorder of potassium metabolism which is frequently associated with hypokalemia but without evidence of a metabolic alkalosis. The condition is characterized by intermittent episodes of weakness and paralysis of the skeletal muscles of the limbs and trunk. In very severe forms the muscles of the face, pharynx and respiration may be involved as well. The paralysis is attended by absent deep tendon reflexes. The majority of the cases are of the familial type and many, but certainly not all, are accompanied by hypopotassemia* during the paralytic episode. Despite this association with a depressed concentration of potassium in the serum and the fact that attacks may be prevented and treated with potassium salts, there is no evidence that these patients have a deficit of this cation. Balance studies performed during the development of paralysis reveal a decreased rate of excretion of potassium in the urine and the hypokalemia must be explained as a transfer of potassium from the extracellular fluid to some cellular depot.

Attacks may be precipitated by the administration of glucose and insulin and by the injection of epinephrine. Hyperthyroidism[386] seems to sensitize patients with this disease to more frequent episodes. The author has seen a patient whose only attack thus far was during the last trimester of pregnancy. Some attacks are unassociated with hypokalemia, and when a depressed level of potassium in the serum is a feature of the disorder there is little correlation between the concentration of serum potassium and the intensity of the muscular weakness.

Conn and his colleagues[387] have recently reported a very interesting and important group of observations on several patients with familial periodic paralysis. They noted that attacks of paralysis could be readily induced with glucose and insulin or by the administration of 2-methyl-9-α-fluorohydrocortisone when the patients were on a diet which contained more than 200 mM. of sodium per day. The glucose and insulin somehow promoted an increased secretion of aldosterone which caused a retention of sodium, followed by hypokalemia, a reduced urinary excretion of potassium and paralysis. The same procedure did not induce an episode of paralysis when the patients were eating a diet containing only 27 mM. of sodium per day. Since the daily excretion of aldosterone was higher when the patients were on the lower sodium intake, it is clear that the aldosterone was not responsible per se for the sequestration of potassium into some cellular repository. They conclude that the primary event in the sequence leading to the episode of paralysis was the retention of sodium.

There are obviously still many unanswered questions about this disorder, but it would appear that salt restriction combined with an adequate dietary intake of potassium may be very important in the prevention of attacks of paralysis in some of these patients.

Edema

Edema is an increase in the volume of the interstitial fluid component of the extracellular compartment. It may be associated with an increase or a decrease in the plasma volume. The increase in the interstitial fluid volume may be generalized as in severe hypoalbuminemia of the nephrotic syndrome, it may be a more segregated collection as in obstruction to the venous or lymphatic drainage from a limb, or it may be seen solely as a collection of ascitic fluid as in cirrhosis of the liver. The presence of edema, generalized or localized, implies that there is a significant disturbance in the interplay of the Starling forces in such a fashion that the rate of transudation of fluid from the vascular compartment to the interstitial spaces exceeds its return to the blood stream either directly or via the lymphatics.

The forces that tend to promote a rate of transudation from the vascular system in excess of reabsorption are: (1) an increase in the hydrostatic pressure in the capillary bed, (2) a decrease in the colloid oncotic pressure of the plasma, (3) an increase in the colloid oncotic pressure of the interstitial fluid, and (4) a diminution in tissue tension. A heightened pressure in the minute vessels through which fluid is exchanged between the vascular system and the

* There are very likely several different disease entities characterized by episodes of muscle weakness and paralysis, and it is possible that only one of these is commonly associated with hypokalemia.

interstitial space results from an increase in venous pressure which, in turn, may be due to a variety of causes, varying from simple mechanical obstructions as in a venous thrombosis to congestive heart failure with venous congestion or to the accession of a larger volume of fluid to the circulation resulting from the ingestion or administration of large quantities of fluid. Examples of diminished colloid osmotic pressure in the plasma are as varied as are the causes for hypoalbuminemia, which include malnutrition, liver failure, an increased rate of catabolism of albumin, and an unusual loss of protein into the urine as in the nephrotic syndrome. An increase in the colloid osmotic pressure of the interstitial fluid is usually associated with some element of obstruction to the lymphatic drainage from a part.

In attemping to understand the pathogenesis of edema it is important to discriminate between the primary events involving those mechanisms responsible for the maldistribution of fluid between the two major components of the extracellular space and the renal response in terms of the retention of salt and water. In some instances the abnormal retention of salt and water may, in fact, be the primary disturbance; the edema is then simply a secondary manifestation of the generalized increase in the volume of the extracellular fluid, of which the interstitial space is one component. These probably represent (a) rather special circumstances characterized primarily by acute reduction in renal function so that the excretion of salt and water is drastically curtailed and, perhaps, (b) certain instances in which abnormal secretions of salt-retaining hormones promote the accumulation of edema.[388] Aside from these instances, which will be discussed separately, an attempt will be made to interrelate the normal physiology of the metabolism of salt and water with the responses which characterize a state of edema. The general *hypothesis* which will be offered is that in *most instances* the initial defect is one which promotes a redistribution of fluid volume between the vascular and extravascular components of the extracellular space, and that the renal responses are secondary and predictable physiologic consequences.

Obstruction of Venous or Lymphatic Drainage. Perhaps the most simple example is the situation wherein a large collection of fluid is retained in the interstitial phase of a limb because of obstruction of the venous and lymphatic drainage. The obstruction of the venous return will increase the hydrostatic pressure in the distal capillary bed; as a result, the rate of transudation of fluid from the arteriolar end of the minute vessels will exceed the rate of reabsorption at their venous end. In addition, the small quantities of protein that permeate these vessels cannot leave the interstitial space because their usual avenue of escape, the lymphatics, is also blocked. This will tend to increase the concentration of protein in the interstitial fluid, and, to the extent that it does, a restraining force is imposed on the return of fluid to the vascular system. The net result of these several defects is that the volume of interstitial fluid in the limb is increased at the expense of the vascular compartment. It will be recalled that, for reasons which are certainly not clear, a decrease in plasma volume, or some function thereof, operates to promote a diminished rate of excretion of sodium.[214–219] This may be implemented in part by a decrease in glomerular filtration rate, but it seems also to be due to an altered rate of tubular reabsorption of sodium. In turn, it is possible that the increased renal tubular reabsorption of sodium due to the contracted volume is implemented through an increased secretion of the self-retaining hormone of the adrenal cortex, aldosterone.[241–247,389] The increased rate of reabsorption of sodium may be simultaneously accompanied by an isosmotic reabsorption of water; if not, the increased reabsorption of sodium will tend to increase the concentration of this cation in the extracellular fluid, which, in turn, will provoke thirst and an increased secretion of ADH. The water ingested in response to thirst will be retained as a consequence of the antidiuretic hormone and the net result will be an isotonic expansion of the extracellular space. If sufficient salt and water are retained to allow the plasma volume to re-expand to normal despite the increased accession of fluid to the interstitial phase of the limb, the stimulus to the retention of sodium no longer obtains and the patient then may be expected to excrete into the urine the quantity of salt ingested each day. In other words, a new steady state will have been established characterized by an expanded interstitial fluid space in the limb whose venous and lymphatic drainage has been obstructed and by a plasma volume which is again normal because of the retention of some extra salt and water.

Nephrotic Syndrome. This thesis may be presented in essentially the same terms in relation to the generalized edema which characterizes the nephrotic syndrome. In this instance it may be said that the initial defect (so far as the production of edema is concerned) is the excretion of protein into the urine owing to disease of the glomeruli.[390] The loss of protein in this fashion results in a severe hypoproteinemia with hypoalbuminemia which reduces the colloid osmotic pressure of the plasma and, hence, promotes a redistribution of volume between the vascular and extravascular components of the extracellular space and the appearance of generalized edema. This, in turn, should result in a reduced plasma volume, which is frequently reflected in increased values for packed cell volume. The diminished plasma volume promotes a retention of salt and water, which is presumably aided and abetted by increased secretion of aldosterone and the antidiuretic hormone. Despite the retention of large quantities of salt and a large volume of water, it is probable that in many instances the plasma volume is never quite restored to normal since the retained fluid cannot be confined within the vessels but escapes immediately into the interstitial spaces (including the peritoneal and the pleural spaces). The probability of this thesis is supported not only by the fact that the administration of a hyperoncotic solution of albumin will promote a diuresis, but by the fact that the sequence of events in which this diuresis unfolds is almost precisely the reverse of the pathway described for the pathogenesis of the edema.[391]

If the degree of hypoalbuminemia is less striking it is probable that sufficient salt and water may be retained so that, although a large fraction of the increment gains access to the interstitial space, a sufficient quantity may remain within the vascular volume and, hence, dissipate the stimuli for further retention of salt and water by the kidneys.

It has been assumed thus far that the retention of sodium is primary to the retention of water. This is attested to by the success with which edema may be modified when the ingestion of sodium is minimized, since under most circumstances of edema formation (as in most instances of dehydration as well) the factors that influence the regulation of the concentration of sodium in the extracellular fluid are such that water will be retained only in proportion to sodium.[83,392] However, it will be recalled from the discussion of the sequence of events in dehydration characterized primarily by a loss of salt, that, although water is lost to maintain a normal concentration of sodium in the serum in the early phases of development of the dehydration, there comes a point when the diminution in plasma volume is such as to serve as a stimulus to the secretion of the antidiuretic hormone, and at this point water is retained and "tonicity is sacrificed in favor of volume." If the development of edema has as its initial event the loss of plasma volume to the interstitial fluid because of a disequilibrium of the Starling forces, it is possible that the diminution in plasma volume (or the significant function thereof) may serve as a stimulus to the secretion of ADH so that even if no salt is available in the diet, water will be retained and the syndrome of edema with *dilutional hyponatremia* is observed.[160,188,323,393] It will be recalled that among the significant inferences to be drawn with respect to hyponatremia associated with dehydration was the fact that this implied a severe state of dehydration. Likewise, the presence of hyponatremia associated with edema indicates a severely disordered internal environment and carries the implication of a very grave prognosis. (See later discussion of Hyponatremia.)

This proposal, which is a preliminary attempt to provide a unifying concept concerning the origin of edema, meets more serious challenges when one makes these interrelations with the edema of congestive heart failure or severe cirrhosis with ascites when these two clinical disorders are associated with an *expanded* rather than a *contracted* plasma volume. However, it is possible to resolve this dilemma if one further assumption is made to the effect that the receptor organs which respond to some function of a diminished plasma volume are on the arterial side of the circulation. It is possible to conceive of the situation wherein *total* blood volume is expanded but the disposition of volume between the arterial and venous circulation is such as to represent a diminished arterial volume despite a significant expansion of the venous volume.

Cirrhosis with Ascites. Measurements of blood volume are reported to be increased in cirrhosis with ascites when there is a fairly large system of dilated venous radicles, usually accompanied by varices. If the initial event in the formation of ascites involves obstruction to the portal venous system (and the lymphatic drainage from the liver as well), the initial consequence should be an enlarged portal venous bed plus an increased hydrostatic pressure therein which favors transudation into the ascitic sac. If the enlarged portal bed is, in fact, an early stage in the pathogenesis, it is not difficult to assume that this has involved a redisposition of some volume of blood from the arterial to the portal venous portion of the circulation. In this sense, then, the arterial volume may have become contracted. The latter then promotes the retention of salt, which is followed by the ingestion and retention of water. If the basic disease is far advanced, the retained fluid is distributed predominantly into the expanding venous system and the ascitic fluid, and the arterial volume may never re-expand to the point where it no longer serves as a stimulus to the retention of salt. Of course, there are less intense situations in which a new balance is reached characterized by some ascites, some increase in plasma volume and no further stimuli for the retention of the raw materials of edema fluid. There has been considerable comment in the past concerning the role of the liver in the conjugation or other means of inactivation of hormones, and it has been suggested that the retention of fluid in patients with hepatic insufficiency is due to inadequate inactivation of those hormones which implement fluid retention.[394,395] This seems unlikely on several grounds. In the first place, if these hormones were inadequately destroyed, their high circulating level would be expected to shut off further secretion by the gland either by some direct feedback mechanism or as a consequence of the effects they would have produced. Thus, if there are high levels of ADH in the presence of hyponatremia one must assume not only that the liver has failed to inactivate the hormone but that the neurohypophyseal mechanism continues to secrete ADH in the absence of an appropriate stimulus. This is a more complicated and less tenable theory than that there is some feature of the disease process which leads to an unusually *intense* but *normal* stimulus for the secretion of ADH.[189] The diureses observed following the infusion of hyperoncotic solutions of albumin in the nephrotic and after establishment of a communication between the peritoneal cavity and the subcutaneous tissue in the cirrhotic certainly suggest that the hormones and the kidneys are playing purely secondary roles and are not primarily responsible for the edema in these patients;[396,397] furthermore, Laragh and his co-workers[398] were able to produce massive ascites in control and diabetes insipidus dogs with equal ease by constriction of the inferior vena cava in the thorax.

Congestive Heart Failure. Lastly, one may consider the manner in which congestive heart failure may fit into this general thesis. There is little doubt that the plasma volume is expanded in patients with significant degrees of congestive heart failure.[399–401] However, as in cirrhosis and ascites, it is quite possible to visualize the probability that there is a redistribution of volume between the arterial and venous circulation so that the former is contracted, the latter is expanded, and the total is in excess of normal. The diminution in cardiac output may be responsible for this maldistribution, and as a result of the diminished arterial volume there are two effects on renal function. The first of these is direct, in that the diminished rate of perfusion of the kidneys leading to a decreased filtration rate and renal plasma flow promotes a smaller filtered load of sodium, and this may be associated with a lessened rate of excretion of this cation.[402,403] In addition, the diminished volume somehow influences renal tubular activity in such a fashion that there is a more avid reabsorption of salt.[404,405] The retention of water may be considered to be secondary to the retention of salt except in extreme instances when the "diminished volume" is significant enough in itself to serve as a stimulus to the secretion of ADH through some nonosmotic mechanism. Under these circumstances, the patient with congestive heart failure would have edema and dilutional hyponatremia which, as noted earlier, is most significant in terms of the severity of the disorder and the prognosis. The retained fluid would be distributed within the circulation and the extravascular portion of the extracellular space according to the new steady state of the Starling forces engendered by the consequences of the heart failure as these are reflected in the levels of hydrostatic pressure in the pulmonary capillaries and the peripheral minute vessels. It is possible that with less severe degrees of failure a new state would be reached wherein no *further* accumulation of salt and water would obtain because arterial volume had been restored to normal. This thesis, in relation to cardiac failure, is supported by the observations of Eichna et al.,[406] who studied the responses to rapid digitalization of patients with severe congestive heart failure. They noted prompt changes characterized by increase in cardiac output, decrease in the right auricular and peripheral venous pressures, increase in systolic blood pressure and widening of the pulse pressure, and increase in the rates of excretion of salt and water. The diureses of salt and water were not dependent on renal hemodynamic changes and, hence, it is strongly suggested that among the immediate effects of the improved cardiac function was a diminution in the renal tubular reabsorption of salt and water. Since an increase in cardiac output and decrease in venous pressure were the first events, it is not altogether unreasonable to suggest that among the earliest effects was a redisposition of blood volume in such a way as to expand the arterial volume of the circulation.

This general hypothesis regarding the pathogenesis of edema may be summarized as follows: The primary defect is a disturbance which leads to a diminution in the blood (arterial) volume. This may come about as a consequence of: (1) local obstruction to venous and/or lymphatic drainage from a limb or the portal system; (2) hypoalbuminemia with diminished colloid osmotic pressure of the plasma and an increased rate of transudation of fluid from and diminished rate of reabsorption of fluid into the circulation; (3) diminished competence of the myocardium, which leads to a decrease in cardiac output (in terms of need if not in absolute value) and a redisposition of the blood volume from the arterial to the venous circulation. The increased venous filling will increase capillary pressure and promote an increased rate of transudation of fluid from the vascular system.

The consequences of a diminished (arterial) blood volume are:

(1) Increased renal tubular reabsorption of salt implemented by: (a) hormones (e.g., aldosterone) and (b) a decreased filtered load of sodium owing to a diminution of glomerular filtration rate.

(2) The retention of sodium must be coincidentally associated with an equivalent reabsorption of water (an isosmotic reabsorption) or it must induce a subtle increase in the concentration of sodium in the extracellular fluids. This, in turn, promotes: (a) thirst and the ingestion of water and (b) secretion of ADH and increased renal tubular reabsorption of water.

(3) The retained isotonic fluid is then distributed within the extracellular compartment in a manner dictated by the new level of the Starling forces. There are several alternatives: (a) All of the retained fluid may gain access to the interstitial space and the stimuli for further retention of salt and water persist. (b) The fluid may gain access to the venous circulation where some of it may be retained in the expanding venous system, and some may be dissipated into the interstitial space because of the increased hydrostatic pressure transmitted to the peripheral minute vessels by the enhanced venous volume. (c) Enough of the retained fluid may remain in the arterial circulation to re-expand that volume to the point where it no longer serves as a stimulus to the renal retention of salt and water.

(4) The further retention of sodium may be prevented by lack of ingestion. In this circumstance there will be no stimulus for the further accumulation of water. The net result is an isotonic expansion of the extracellular compartment with redisposition of fluid as dictated by the net vector of the Starling forces. Alternatively, the "diminished volume" may be of significant enough magnitude to promote the continued secretion of ADH and the retention of water in excess of salt with resultant *chronic dilutional hyponatremia*.

(5) Any factor which will tend to correct the initial defect leading to the diminished blood (arterial) volume will tend to block this series of responses and will result in a re-expansion of volume and consequent diuresis of salt and water. For example: (a) Elevation of the limb whose venous drainage is blocked will allow the interstitial fluid to gravitate to an area where the mean capillary pressure is lower and where the excess fluid can be reabsorbed into the circulation. (b) A communication between the peritoneal cavity and the subcutaneous tissue in patients with cirrhosis and ascites allows the fluid to gain access to areas where the vascular pressure is lower and where it can be reabsorbed into the blood stream.* (c) The administration of a solution of 25 per cent albumin to patients with severe hypoalbuminemia, as in the nephrotic syndrome, will increase the concentration of circulating albumin, raise the colloid osmotic pressure of the plasma, promote the reabsorption of fluid from the interstitial space to the circulation, expand plasma volume and promote a diuresis of water and salt. (d) The improvement in cardiac competence by digitalization increases cardiac output and redisposes blood from the venous to the arterial circulation. This, in turn, allows the interstitial fluid to be reabsorbed into the circulation and the expanded arterial volume promotes an increased rate of excretion of salt and water into the urine.

There are certainly groups of patients in whom edema appears to result from a primary disturbance in renal function due either to renal disease or to the response of the kidneys to a primary disturbance in the secretion of hormones which implement the retention of salt (and water). The most obvious of the first group are patients with acute renal insufficiency characterized by severe oliguria (acute glomerulonephritis, acute tubular necrosis, some instances of severe toxemia of pregnancy, etc.)

* Unfortunately, these devices are soon surrounded by tissue and the communication is closed within a few days or weeks.

who continue to ingest or are given usual quantities of salt and water. Since the major pathway for excretion is not available, the excess fluid will be distributed between the extra- and intracellular space on the basis of the quantitative relationship between the retained salt and water. To the extent that the fluid is retained within the extracellular space, the disposition between the plasma and interstitial fluid will be determined by the net effect of the Starling forces. In other situations the retention of sodium (and water) is the primary event in the formation of edema. This is noted, for example, when adrenal steroids are administered as therapeutic agents and the diet is not restricted with respect to sodium. Interestingly enough, the edema that develops is not massive and appears to be somewhat self-limiting. Perhaps the accumulation of salt and water, with the consequent expansion of the interstitial fluid and plasma volumes, tends to promote an increased rate of excretion of sodium which counteracts the influence of the steroid on sodium retention.

It would be grossly misleading not to emphasize that this discussion of the pathogenesis of edema is admittedly tentative and, at least, incomplete. Furthermore, it is an oversimplification. It is offered as a framework for considering the problems of patients with edema in the hope of increasing our understanding of the manner in which edema develops and the implications which this must have for therapy.

Management of Patients with Edema. The management of a patient with edema must be concerned with all aspects of the patient's disorder. It is possible to become so preoccupied with the treatment of the abnormal collection of fluid that more significant features of the illness are left unattended. Overly aggressive attention to the delivery of the edema itself may, in turn, promote significant harm and worsen the patient's clinical status. The treatment of these patients may be discussed under two general categories: (1) rather general measures the aim of which is to promote a negative balance of salt and water by one means or another, and (2) more specific therapy which may promote improvement in some basic primary disorder of which the edema is merely a secondary consequence.

1. GENERAL MEASURES. (a) *Dietary Restriction of Salt.* Since edema is extracellular fluid and, as noted before, is ordinarily an isotonic expansion in which one liter of water is retained along with approximately 140 mM. of sodium, it is possible to limit the further accession of fluid volume by the simple expedient of eliminating sodium from the dietary intake. With modern food processing and appropriate advice it is quite possible for patients to restrict the intake of sodium to as little as 8 to 10 mM./day even at home. This is certainly one of the most efficacious methods of limiting the accumulation of edema, although it does impose some hardships on the patient and the personnel responsible for the preparation of meals. In addition to its value in the prevention of further accumulation of fluid, dietary restriction of this magnitude may lead to the delivery of edema. The more severe disturbances associated with edema formation may be accompanied by the excretion of a urine that is virtually free of salt. However, there are many examples of a less severe disorder in which the renal tubular reabsorption of sodium is less avid and the daily excretion of sodium may readily exceed 8 to 10 mM./day. To the extent that excretion exceeds intake, a negative balance of sodium obtains and this may be expected to be accompanied by a loss of water in proportion to the salt loss. It is not uncommon, therefore, to note significant lessening of the quantity of edema with the simple restriction of dietary sodium. This may be even more profound if rest in the recumbent position is included in the regimen.

(b) *Cation Exchange Resins.*[407-409] The ingestion of cation exchange resins, which release one cation (such as hydrogen or ammonium ion) in exchange for one sodium ion within the gastrointestinal tract, may be of some value in the management of patients with edema. The "efficiency" of the resins varies but is approximately 1 mM. of sodium exchanged per gram of resin. Hence, the ingestion of approximately 85 grams of resin would be necessary to remove 5 grams of dietary salt. It was anticipated that this method of treatment might be a valuable substitution for rigid salt restriction. The patient may decide, however, that the ingestion of this quantity of resin may be more unpleasant than the rigid regimen of dietary restriction. In addition, the development of a significant metabolic acidosis is one of the hazards of this therapy.

(c) *Restriction or Excesses of Water.* Under usual circumstances water is not retained in excess of sodium so that if attention is directed to the quantity of salt in the diet there is little need to consider the volume of water that may be ingested. If the disorder is so grave that water is retained in excess of salt, the decision concerning the restriction of water depends primarily on the comfort of the patient. If a limitation of water intake to avoid chronic dilutional hyponatremia is such as to make the patient miserably thirsty, there would seem to be little value in this approach. On the other hand, there is equally little reason to encourage and promote a greater degree of dilutional hyponatremia than is necessary.

It has been suggested by others[410] that the ingestion or administration of very large loads of water would promote an increased rate of excretion of sodium and, hence, be of value in inducing a negative balance of salt and a delivery of some of the edema. This has not proved of value. In some instances the volume of water administered has been considerably in excess of the patient's ability to excrete urine and acute water intoxication has supervened. This technique should therefore be discouraged. In summary, it may be stated that in most instances the best guide to the daily volume of water appropriate for the patient is that which is dictated by his own sensation of thirst. There are few instances in the management of edema in which the restriction of water is indicated and none in which the intake of excessively large volumes of water should be encouraged.

(d) *Urea.* Urea has been used as a diuretic for many years in doses of 40 to 60 grams per day dispensed as a 40 per cent solution. The ingestion of urea in these quantities promotes a solute diuresis because of the augmented rate of excretion of urea. This may well lead to a negative balance of water but rarely promotes a significant excretion of sodium when given in these amounts to patients with edema. Thus, it would seem to have little value in patients with normal concentrations of sodium since the negative balance of water would induce hypernatremia and ultimately intolerable thirst. (It may possibly be of some value in patients who have edema with hyponatremia when the correction of the concentration of sodium in the serum seems desirable.) In addition, urea has a most unpleasant taste which is difficult to disguise even when it is admixed with pleasant tasting solutions and served cold.

(e) *Ammonium Chloride.*[275,411,412] This acidifying salt has been used for many years to promote an increased excretion of sodium in the urine. In essence, the ammonium chloride is converted to urea and hydrochloric acid, and the latter induces a metabolic acidosis with the displacement of bicarbonate to carbonic acid. The acidosis is compensated along the lines discussed in the section on acid-base balance. In a matter of four to five days the daily administration of ammonium chloride can usually be accounted for in equivalent amounts in the urine. Although the increased rate of excretion of ammonia begins immediately, the quantity is small in the first few days, and during this period the augmented excretion of chloride is accompanied by sodium and, to a lesser extent, potassium. Thus, a negative balance of sodium may be achieved and this will usually be accompanied by an equivalent loss of water. Since the kidneys are usually able to excrete all the ammonium chloride as such by the fourth to fifth day, no further loss of salt may be expected. For this reason, it is recommended that this agent be administered at intervals rather than continuously unless it is used in conjunction with an organic mercurial compound. In addition to its utility in promoting a negative balance of sodium, it seems to potentiate the action of organic mercurial diuretics and may be used successfully to combat the alkalosis that may supervene as the result of diuresis promoted by mercurials. There are circumstances wherein the use of ammonium chloride may lead to severe metabolic acidosis and caution must be exercised in its use. This is especially true in patients with primary renal disease whose ability to acidify the urine may be seriously impaired. However, if the drug is used over short intervals and appropriate observations are made of the patient and if chemical data are obtained at frequent intervals, a serious state of acidosis may be prevented. Some preparations of ammonium chloride are coated to prevent gastric irritation; the coating may be so successful that the ammonium chloride passes through the entire gastrointestinal tract without being absorbed.

(f) *Xanthine Compounds.*[361,412] These are not very potent diuretics in and of themselves, but they do tend to augment GFR and depress the renal tubular reabsorption of sodium to some extent. Thus, they may be of some value when used with other more potent preparations and may render the latter more effective.

(g) *Carbonic Anhydrase Inhibitors.*[279,413] Some discussion of the role of carbonic anhydrase in the renal tubular reabsorption of sodium and acidification of the urine has been presented in the section dealing with renal physiology. The mode of action of a carbonic anhydrase enzyme inhibitor may be readily inferred from that discussion. The consequences of the loss of sodium bicarbonate are an isosmotic loss of water, a contraction of the extracellular fluid volume, a decrease in the concentration of bicarbonate and an increase in the concentration of chloride in the serum. The diminished rate of excretion of hydrogen ions and these compositional changes promote a metabolic acidosis.

Carbonic anhydrase inhibitor has been a useful diuretic agent, although it has not been as effective or consistent as others. It has been found to be most effective in patients with cardiopulmonary disease. This may simply be a reflection of the fact that in such patients with respiratory acidosis the rate of secretion of hydrogen ions may be accelerated and, hence, carbonic anhydrase inhibition might be expected to be followed by a greater effect than when the rate of reabsorption of bicarbonate is more normal.

(h) *Organic Mercurial Diuretics.* These are the most potent and consistently effective diuretics available. The questions of the site within the renal tubule where they act, the manner in which they interfere with the reabsorption of ions, and whether their effect is on sodium or chloride are still all unanswered.[412,414,415] Some believe that the potency of the mercurial diuretic is associated with certain specific characteristics of the molecules, while others believe that they act by liberating inorganic mercury. Many think that the primary effect is on the reabsorption of chloride and that the excretion of sodium is a secondary consequence.

The net effect, at any rate, is the increased excretion of salt accompanied by an isosmotic loss of water. The concentrations of electrolytes in the urine reveals that chloride is excreted in quantities either equal to or in excess of sodium. In either event, the ratio of urinary chloride to sodium is in excess of that which characterizes the extracellular fluid.[359] Moreover, the excretion of potassium may be accelerated so that a deficit of this cation obtains and each of these contributes to an altered composition of the extracellular fluid characterized by an increase in the concentration of bicarbonate, a decrease in the concentration of chloride and an associated metabolic alkalosis. For reasons which are not clear, this may make further use of the organic mercurial compounds futile until the alkalosis has been corrected;[360,362] this can always be accomplished with ammonium chloride and sometimes with a carbonic anhydrase inhibitor. A metabolic alkalosis is certainly one of the most important reasons for a refractory state to the mercury compounds. Another condition which impairs the response to these agents is a depressed rate of filtration of sodium,[361] which, in turn, may be due to a decrease in filtration rate with normal concentrations of sodium in the serum, a decrease in the concentration of sodium in the serum and hence in the filtrate, or both. When the filtration rate is depressed but the concentration of sodium in the serum is normal, it may be possible to influence a successful diuresis with mercury by utilizing a xanthine drug about one to two hours after the administration of the mercurial. The xanthine may augment the filtration rate sufficiently at the time of the peak action of mercury on the renal tubules to allow an escape of salt into the urine.

These compounds may be administered orally,[416] subcutaneously, intramuscularly or by vein.[412] Daily administration by any route may entail some danger of a cumulative toxic effect. This is unlikely so long as the agent promotes significant diureses following parenteral administration; however, when it is given by mouth absorption may be erratic and delayed, and it is possible to have little absorption on one day and excessive absorption on another. Acute fatal reactions are not common but do occur on occasion when the drug is administered by the intravenous route in patients with cardiac failure. It is therefore wise to use the subcutaneous or intramuscular route and to begin with small doses. It is also desirable to administer the drug early in the morning so that the bulk of the ensuing diuresis will obtain prior to evening and will not interfere with the patient's rest.

Many feel that these agents should not be used when there is significant intrinsic renal disease, since further renal damage may be provoked. This statement should not be interpreted as inveighing against their use in patients with congestive heart failure who may have modestly elevated concentrations of blood urea nitrogen as a consequence of the diminished cardiac output and impaired perfusion of the kidneys. Their use should not be continued if there is clear evidence of a failure to respond. It is in such situations that renal damage may result from accumulation of the drug in the kidneys. If there is a failure to respond the patient should be carefully evaluated to see whether there are reasons for the refractory state that may be corrected or modified as discussed above.

The chemical data from an analysis of serum may be the same in a patient with a metabolic alkalosis as in one with a respiratory acidosis, and either of these conditions may be seen in patients with congestive heart failure. If one wishes to correct the former, but not the latter, with ammonium chloride, the two disorders must be discriminated by an estimation of the *p*H and total CO_2 content of the serum. If these techniques are not available one may obtain help from the history and other laboratory data. If the patient has received no mercury and there is no obvious source of loss of potassium, it would be unlikely that he is suffering with a metabolic alkalosis. The *p*H of the urine may be helpful if it is alkaline (and uninfected). However, as noted in the discussion of acid-base balance, an acid urine does not exclude the possibility of a metabolic alkalosis. The concentration of potassium in the serum may be of some help if it is clearly depressed since this would be more suggestive of a metabolic alkalosis than of a respiratory acidosis.

2. Specific Measures. It is not within the scope of this discussion to present in any detail the more specific methods of treatment of the different types of edema. Digitalization, rest and salt restriction are still the most important measures in the management of con-

gestive heart failure. Analyses of myocardial tissue suggest no alteration in composition characterized by an increased content of sodium and a diminished quantity of potassium, and there are other data which suggest that digitalis tends to restore these changes toward normal.[417] This may represent an important clue concerning the manner in which the digitalis drugs improve myocardial function, since normal concentrations of potassium are apparently necessary for proper polarization across the cell membrane and may also be important for the most efficient utilization of metabolites. Potassium depletion should be carefully avoided in patients with congestive heart failure, since it may provoke serious evidences of digitalis intoxication[418–422] with doses of these drugs that are ordinarily tolerated quite well. Furthermore, a deficit of potassium may induce a metabolic alkalosis and a refractory state to the organic mercurial diuretics, and, lastly, potassium depletion may be associated with frank histologic lesions in the myocardium.

The management of the nephrotic syndrome[423–425] includes the use of adrenal cortical steroids or ACTH as well as the less specific measures which have already been noted. There seems to be good evidence that the adrenal cortical hormones (other than aldosterone) promote some favorable effect on the basic pathophysiology of the disease in addition to the probability that the discontinuous use of the steroids may lead to some "withdrawal" diureses. The exhibition of these agents has been accompanied by increases in glomerular filtration rate and diminution in proteinuria, and may be followed by substantial remissions. There is much controversy concerning the dose and duration of steroid therapy, although the majority of clinicians who have had considerable experience with this disease recommend a longer period than the 10 to 14 days that was formerly used. The current controversy is concerned with whether continuous treatment over many months has any advantage over treatment for a period of 4 to 6 weeks.

The treatment of patients with cirrhosis and ascites still does not involve measures which are known specifically to alter the basic pathology of the disease except for rest (which presumably increases hepatic blood flow), adequate diet and vitamins. Furthermore, it is certainly not clear how these measures tend to improve the level of circulating albumin and the resorption of edema and ascites when it occurs. The direct removal of ascitic fluid is frequently necessary in the interests of comfort and improvement of the patient's ability to eat a nourishing diet. However, paracenteses also remove albumin from the body and may have other undesirable complications if appropriate precautions are not taken (see section to follow on edema with hyponatremia).

Some brief mention should be made of the simple techniques that may be employed to follow the course of a patient with edema so that the therapy may be evaluated and complications avoided.[24] A daily record of intake and output is very useful, but it is everyone's experience that this information is extremely difficult to obtain in an accurate and consistent fashion on a busy hospital ward. Perhaps these data might be obtained with more success if they were requested only in carefully selected instances. A more simple technique to provide information concerning acute gains or losses of fluid is the daily measurement of weight. This requires considerably less time and should be an accurate estimate if reasonable care is taken to make the observations at approximately the same time of day (e.g., before breakfast), with the same amount of clothes, etc. A special stretcher scale is necessary for patients who are too ill to stand; since it is frequently in these patients that the data may be most critical to proper evaluation and management, it is certainly desirable to have such a scale available.

More elegant techniques involve the actual estimate of a "balance" of salt and water. For this, one must have information concerning the intake of fluid and sodium, an accurate collection of the daily 24-hour urine, analysis of this urine for its content of sodium, accurate daily weights and analyses of serum at intervals for electrolyte concentration. This estimate requires considerable time and care in the collection of the specimen and is difficult to achieve for the reasons already listed. Useful information concerning the balance may be had even if the sodium intake can only be approximated if one can be reasonably certain that the urine collection represents a full 24-hour period. The determination of chloride in the urine will suffice as a crude substitute for sodium determination so long as the patient is not receiving medications which contain chloride such as potassium chloride, ammonium chloride, etc.

The need for objective evaluation of therapy is obvious. The extent to which the physician may attempt to collect these data must be dictated by the available tools and the nature of the special problem at hand. Certainly detailed and expensive balance data are not necessary for the evaluation and management of most patients with edema. However, there certainly are some instances in which this information can be critical in the formulation of a therapeutic program. The vast majority of patients can be reasonably well followed with daily weights, analyses of serum at intervals and occasional examinations of 24-hour urine for sodium and other electrolytes.

The Significance of Hyponatremia

Although certain instances of the pathogenesis and management of hyponatremia have been discussed in earlier sections of this chapter, it may be worthwhile to try to integrate in a summary fashion some of the particular aspects of clinical disorders complicated by hyponatremia. This condition is observed fairly frequently in hospital practice, and there are many diverse avenues by which it may develop. Many instances are very poorly understood, and they may present difficult therapeutic dilemmas. Despite this lack of knowledge and understanding, there is a way to examine these problems which may be helpful in elucidating the particular pathogenesis in a given patient and this, in turn, will usually serve as the basis for a reasonable therapeutic approach. This discussion will be concerned only with those instances in which the hyponatremia may be considered to represent a diminution in the effective osmolality of the body fluids. This restriction excludes those circumstances wherein hyponatremia is associated with significant hyperglycemia[58] to account for the depressed concentration of sodium and the few instances of extreme hyperlipemia[59] in which the concentration of sodium is normal in terms of the *water* of serum but depressed when the concentration is referred to a liter of serum.

It must be re-emphasized that the *concentration* of sodium in the serum (and extracellular fluid) is simply a statement concerning the quantity of sodium in a particular volume (usually a liter) of serum. It carries absolutely no implications concerning the total volume of body water, since hyponatremia may exist with dehydration, edema or apparently *normal* volumes of body fluids.

Asymptomatic Hyponatremia.[24,56] There is a group of patients who have hyponatremia of mild or severe degree who appear to have no disturbance in terms of the total body water or its distribution among the several compartments, and in whom there are no evidences of dehydration, edema, or specific symptoms that can be ascribed to the hyponatremia. Examples may be found among any group of patients with far advanced and debilitating disease such as metastatic carcinoma, severe advanced tuberculosis and other grave and preterminal disorders. These patients are frequently referred to as "salt-wasters" (e.g., "pulmonary" salt-wasters when the underlying disorder is a disease of the lungs) since they continue to excrete salt in the urine despite hyponatremia. However, they are able to respond normally in the sense that they will usually eliminate salt from the urine in 4 to 7 days after they have started on a rigid regimen of salt restriction. No aspect of their symptom complex is favorably modified by restoring the concentration of sodium in the serum to normal. If this is attempted they become thirsty, ingest large quantities of water and then excrete the extra salt and water. There is no evidence of disease of the adrenal cortex, and the renal tubules respond to salt-retaining hormones.

The basic defect in these patients is not understood, but it has been suggested that perhaps the underlying disorder is a primary alteration in the effective osmolality within the cell fluid and that the excretion of sodium is a response intended to reduce the effective osmolality in the extracellular fluid to match the new level within the cells. This would result in no net change in the total body water or the disposition between the intra- and extracellular fluids; it would be characterized simply by a new level of the effective osmolality of the body fluids. It has been inferred that these changes are somehow related to the breakdown of certain mechanisms in severely ill patients, and some have referred to this disorder as the "sick-cell syndrome." It must be differentiated from other causes of hyponatremia that may need specific correction, such as a variety of dehydrations in general and adrenal cortical insufficiency in particular. The differential diagnosis between asymptomatic hyponatremia and adrenal cortical insufficiency may present some difficulty since patients with the former are so ill from the underlying disease. However, careful evaluation of the total disease picture and the specific tests of adrenal cortical function will resolve the issue. Clues which immediately favor asymptomatic hyponatremia are the normal concentrations of potassium and urea nitrogen in the serum. However, these might be elevated for other reasons and the problem made more difficult to unravel. If there is any uncertainty, the hyponatremia should be corrected and other appropriate remedies instituted.

Lastly, it must be emphasized that patients with asymptomatic hyponatremia are not immune to the common disorders of hydration and may develop dehydration or edema. In such instances, the hyponatremic feature of the disorder may be difficult to understand until the dehydration or edema is corrected and the true significance of the concentrations of electrolytes in the serum is unmasked.

Hyponatremia with Dehydration. This was discussed in some detail in the section on dehydration. Reference to this earlier presentation will help to emphasize the general pathways by which this type of dehydration may supervene, its significance with respect to the disposition of fluid between the extra- and intracellular compartments, and the implications with respect to the intensity of the dehydration. The principle of management and the alternative techniques of administering isotonic or hypertonic solutions of salt were also presented. In most instances the author would prefer to use a hypertonic solution since this helps to correct two aspects of the dehydration most quickly, restoration of tonicity as well as volume, and it does not depend on normal renal responses to effect this increase in tonicity. However, many others have had considerable success in treating such patients with isotonic solutions of sodium salts. It is probable that the use of a hypertonic solution is most valuable in selected instances in which normal renal function cannot be anticipated.

Hyponatremia with Edema.[84,160,323,393] This group of patients usually presents the most difficult problems with respect to choice of management. The most important consideration in arriving at a decision is the specific pathway by which the particular patient developed the dilutional hyponatremia. In general it may be stated that if hyponatremia develops in a patient with edema as some natural consequence of the underlying disease process and was not induced as a by-product of the physician's actions, it is unrealistic to expect that restoration of the concentration of serum sodium will improve the patient or be more than transient in duration. In contrast, if the development of hyponatremia can be traced to a sequence of events initiated by something that was done to the patient, it is probable that this complication can be corrected and that such correction will restore the patient to the status he enjoyed prior to the development of the hyponatremia. For purposes of this discussion one may classify edema with hyponatremia into three categories in terms of pathogenesis, namely, (1) chronic dilutional hyponatremia, (2) acute dilutional hyponatremia due to excessive administration of water with no antecedent loss of volume and (3) acute dilutional hyponatremia due to the retention of water precipitated by an acute loss of volume.

(1) CHRONIC DILUTIONAL HYPONATREMIA. This, the most common type of hyponatremia associated with edema, is due to some intense stimulus to the retention of water induced by some aspect of the underlying disease process. It may be due to a nonosmotic stimulus to the secretion of ADH[189] owing, perhaps, to some reduction in "volume" in some critical area of the circulation; or it may be due to the fact that the increased renal tubular reabsorption of sodium is such that it is virtually all accomplished at a site within the nephron (the proximal tubule), where an isosmotic reabsorption of water is mandatory even in the complete absence of ADH. Such a situation would make it quite difficult to excrete "free water," since this latter is dependent on the abstraction of solutes (predominantly sodium chloride) from the urine at a site where this can be accomplished without concomitant isosmotic reabsorption of water. It is probable that in many instances both these mechanisms are operative. More precise information on this problem is not available, but it is implicit that there must be an unusually intense stimulus to thirst as well as a limitation on the excretion of water by the kidneys. If the latter were the only abnormality, a normal concentration of sodium in the serum would be maintained by a corresponding decrease in the volume of water that was voluntarily ingested. The stimulus to thirst must obviously be something other than the primary one of an increase in the effective osmolality of the body fluids. This may well be a response to a volume deficit.

The most significant feature of this type of hyponatremia with edema is that it develops as part of the natural progression of the pathophysiology of the underlying disease, and, hence, it is most unlikely that the restoration of the concentration of serum sodium is desirable. Such attempts are usually followed by intense thirst, the administration or ingestion and retention of water and a consequent redilution. One of the interesting aspects of this sequence is the close identity between the initial and final concentrations of sodium in the serum.

Lastly, it is possible that patients with edema may develop "asymptomatic hyponatremia."[56] In these instances, however, they would reduce the effective osmolality of the body water commensurate with the presumed primary decrease within the cells by the ingestion and retention of water, since the underlying disturbance makes it impossible for them to excrete sodium in the urine. It would obviously be impossible to discriminate between such patients and those with chronic dilutional hyponatremia as previously described. However, the implications of the significance of the hyponatremia and its management are the same in each instance.

2. ACUTE DILUTIONAL HYPONATREMIA. (a) *Due to Excessive Administration of Water with No Antecedent Loss of Volume*. There are always limits to the rate of excretion of water which are determined by the filtration rate, the volume of isosmotic fluid that gains access to the distal tubule and the degree of antidiuretic activity. In the absence of ADH the rate of excretion of water is largely conditioned by the rate of excretion of

solutes. Patients who excrete little or no salt because of dietary restriction or increased renal tubular reabsorption, and who may excrete smaller loads of urea and other solutes because of diminished nitrogen turnover or depressed filtration rate or both, may have very serious limitations imposed on the maximum rate of excretion of water. Usually they develop no positive balance of water because their thirst mechanism operates to maintain a normal value of the effective osmolality of the body fluids. However, if such patients are urged to drink beyond the dictates of thirst or if they are unconscious and decisions concerning the volume of water to be administered are poorly reasoned and they receive larger volumes than they can excrete, they may develop *acute dilutional hyponatremia.* The symptoms are those of water intoxication,[426,427] which involve the central nervous system primarily and may culminate in seizures. It is quite possible that other visceral functions are unfavorably modified but there are less data on these points. However, to the extent that the acute water intoxication is responsible for untoward effects, it would be desirable to restore the concentration of sodium in the serum to normal. This could be accomplished by the administration of hypertonic saline, the restriction of water or the administration of some substance that will increase the rate of excretion of solutes and, hence, of water as well.

If acute water intoxication develops in a patient who is already edematous, it would be more desirable to rid the body of the excess water than to resort to the administration of hypertonic saline since the latter will result in a larger accumulation of edema. Nevertheless, if the effects of the water intoxication are extreme, this may be a necessary and appropriate price to pay for the correction. However, there are obvious advantages in attempting to effect a loss of the excess water if the situation is not extreme and a delay can be tolerated. A program of water restriction and the administration of urea will promote a negative balance of water. The urea may be given by mouth if the patient is conscious, or by gavage, and some have recommended its intravenous administration.[428] In the latter instance it should be included in a solution of dextrose and water to avoid hemolysis.

(b) *Due to Retention of Water Precipitated by an Acute Loss of Volume.* Patients with edema may develop *acute dilutional hyponatremia* which has some of the features of dehydration with hyponatremia. Improvement of these features may be expected to follow correction of the sodium deficiency. These acute episodes usually follow some sudden loss of volume such as in severe vomiting and diarrhea, an unusually brisk diuresis from an organic mercurial compound,[429–431] or the removal of a large collection of ascitic fluid.[323,432]

The course of events in this type of complication is best illustrated by the observations that may be recorded following the removal of a large volume of ascitic fluid, which include evidences of an increased rate of transudation into the peritoneal space accompanied by hemoconcentration as attested to by a rapid and significant rise in the value for the packed cell volume. These events are accompanied by thirst and oliguria so that ingested or administered water is retained and the patient develops an acute dilutional hyponatremia. These patients have the signs and symptoms of water intoxication and impaired peripheral blood flow. The clinical picture can be reversed by the restoration of the concentration of sodium to normal by the administration of a hypertonic solution of sodium salts.

More important is the fact that these complications are largely preventable. It is safer to limit the volume of a paracentesis to a few liters and repeat the procedure at intervals rather than to remove a large volume at a single time. The support of blood volume at the time of the procedure may prevent or modify the severity of the complication. Diuretics should be used in small doses at first to facilitate observation of the intensity of the diuresis and the patient's response to it.

Thus, it would appear that if one had the necessary data to ascertain the circumstances responsible for a particular instance of hyponatremia with edema, one would be in a position to reach a reasonable conclusion concerning the need for correction. Unfortunately, patients are seen quite frequently under circumstances in which it is impossible to tell whether the hyponatremia is of the chronic or acute dilutional type. Since more may be lost by not treating an instance of acute dilutional hyponatremia following a loss of volume than by unnecessarily correcting the hyponatremia of the chronic dilutional type, the author recommends that when there is doubt concerning the pathogenesis of the hyponatremia it should be properly corrected at least once. The fact that a normal concentration of sodium in the serum has been achieved should be demonstrated by analysis, and it should be maintained for at least six to twelve hours by the restriction of water. If it is chronic dilutional hyponatremia, the patient will develop thirst and redilute; the issue is then clear and the patient should not be treated with hypertonic saline again. There is admittedly some risk in this procedure, as there is with so many therapeutic techniques that are useful in seriously ill patients. However, appropriate sedation and the very slow administration of the saline under constant professional supervision will help to minimize the hazards.

Laragh[433,434] has reported an increase in the concentration of sodium in the serum of hyponatremic patients and in dogs when they were given KCl. The increased concentration of serum sodium could not be explained by a negative balance of water, an intercompartmental redisposition of water or a positive balance of sodium. It was therefore concluded that there had been an accession of sodium to the extracellular space from some other source, which may have been cells or bone. The increased concentration of sodium was not maintained for long after the administration of KCl was discontinued and seemed to have no significant beneficial effects.

Acute Renal Insufficiency[435–439]

Acute deterioration in renal function with oliguria or anuria may be transient and due solely to the consequences of dehydration with hypovolemia and impaired renal perfusion, or to obstruction of the lower urinary tract or, less commonly, to bilateral ureteral obstruction. These disorders may be quickly corrected by restoration of the volume and tonicity of the body fluids in the case of dehydration or relief of the obstruction when this is the basis for the reduced renal function. Other instances of acute renal insufficiency result from a variety of primary and severe insults to the kidneys and may be due to acute glomerulonephritis, necrotizing papillitis,[440–442] renal cortical necrosis, infarctions of the kidney, and—most commonly—*acute tubular necrosis.* Although this discussion will be based on acute tubular necrosis, the general management of acute renal insufficiency from the other causes is similar. In any instance, it is imperative that the clinician distinguish between dehydration or obstruction as opposed to these other disorders.

Etiology and Pathology.[435–439,443,448] Acute tubular necrosis may be induced by a variety of drugs and poisons, heavy metals, the products of hemolysis, or a period of shock with inadequate perfusion of the kidneys leading to hypoxia and necrosis of kidney substance. These disorders may occur in patients with previously normal kidneys or may be superimposed on chronic renal disease. Oliver and his associates[449] have evaluated the structural alterations in great detail, utilizing the technique of microdissection of whole nephrons as well as the more conventional tools of pathology. They described two types of lesions: (1) necrosis of the epithelium of the proximal tubular cells without alteration of the basement membrane, and (2) a more severe lesion scattered throughout the nephron in which epithelial necrosis was accompanied by disruption of the basement membrane. From a correlation of the lesions with the nature of the clinical or experimental circumstances in which they developed, these investigators concluded that the lesion confined to the proximal portion of the tubule was a result of contact with some specific nephrotoxin, whereas the more severe but less localized lesions were the consequence of impaired blood flow and renal ischemia.

Dehydration with hypovolemia is frequently associated with a diminution in visceral blood flow. Moreover, it must be emphasized that this may occur despite normal levels of blood pressure, since it is the vasoconstriction which supports the blood pressure that is responsible for the impaired perfusion of tissues. The renal vasculature participates in the vasoconstrictive response, and this plus some decrease in perfusion pressure may readily lead to renal ischemia of a degree sufficient to promote acute tubular necrosis in itself. In addition, a decrease in renal plasma flow and glomerular filtration rate would be associated with the reabsorption of a larger fraction of filtered solutes and water; this, in turn, might tend to increase the concentration of some noxious agent that had gained access to the luminal fluid. Thus, dehydration with or without the addition of some renal poison serves as a situation in which acute tubular necrosis may readily occur. To the extent that appropriate hydration may modify these factors, acute tubular necrosis may be prevented or at least the severity of the disorder may be modified. There is ample clinical and experimental evidence to support this contention.

A clinical problem which is frequently presented to the physician is one of oliguria which develops in a situation which *may* have induced acute tubular necrosis but which *may* be due solely to the consequences of dehydration. Too often the assumption is made that the patient has, in fact, developed acute tubular necrosis, and treatment is directed toward the prevention of overexpansion of the body fluids to the neglect of other factors of more immediate concern. The danger of this response is that some instances of oliguria due to dehydration may be allowed to persist long enough actually to develop acute tubular necrosis, whereas the judicious replacement of deficits could have prevented or modified the severity of this complication. It seems unnecessary and inappropriate to have to choose between two extremes of management. It is submitted that dehydration can be corrected without overexpansion of the body fluid, and to the extent that restoration of volume and tonicity can promote a flow of urine, this can be achieved without the formation of edema. On the other hand, it should be emphasized that severe oliguria and an impoverished renal blood flow do not result from *mild* dehydration so that there are little value and some admitted risks in forcing treatment to the point where the body fluids are significantly expanded. In general, it may be stated that the diagnosis of acute tubular necrosis should not be accepted until elements of dehydration have been corrected, the possibility of lower urinary tract obstruction has been eliminated by catheterization of the bladder, and any reasonable doubt concerning bilateral ureteral (or unilateral in the rare case of a single kidney) obstruction has been dissipated. A careful evaluation of the sequence of events leading to the oliguria will be most helpful in the differential diagnosis. Specific information must be obtained concerning any medication and drugs the patient may have ingested, the intensity and duration of dehydration, and any information concerning an episode of peripheral vascular collapse. It has been suggested that a careful examination of the urinary sediment may reveal the presence of sheets of epithelial cells in acute tubular necrosis.[450] Finally, there are data which imply that the concentration of sodium in the urine in the early oliguric phase of acute tubular necrosis may be high (about 80 to 110 mM./L).[451] In contrast, in severe dehydration one might anticipate that the urinary concentration of sodium would be low, and this may turn out to be a useful and discriminating datum. However, more information must be collected on this point before it can be used with any security in differential diagnosis.

Pathophysiology. The mechanism of the oliguria and anuria in acute tubular necrosis has been argued for many years. It should be pointed out initially that precise data concerning filtration rate and renal plasma flow are difficult or impossible to obtain in acute tubular necrosis. Estimation of renal plasma flow requires information concerning the extraction ratio of the test substance. In the diseased kidney a value cannot be assumed but must be determined in each instance by renal vein catheterization. Furthermore, the estimation of the rate of filtration at the glomeruli depends on the use of a substance which is filtered *but is not reabsorbed.* Since there are good reasons to believe that the functional as well as the anatomic integrity of the renal tubular cells is destroyed in acute tubular necrosis, the assumption that substances such as inulin do not cross the diseased tubular membrane is not valid in these disorders. Despite these objections, it is probably fair to state that a diminution in filtration rate contributes to the oliguria in acute tubular necrosis. However, in addition it appears quite likely that the renal tubular cells of many nephrons no longer serve as discriminating membranes. In this sense, the luminal fluid may be considered part of the renal interstitial space and, hence, subject to the forces that govern the exchange of fluid across the capillary endothelial membrane between the vascular and interstitial fluid phases of the kidney. The colloid osmotic pressure of the plasma would be expected to promote the reabsorption of a large bulk of any filtrate formed. The origin of the small quantities of urine that gain access to the bladder is not clear. Some have suggested, on the basis of data which indicated that the urine closely resembled filtrate, that this resulted from escape of filtered fluid. However, Meroney and Rubini[451] have pointed out that if one follows the characteristics of the composition of urine during the first week of the oliguric phase of acute tubular necrosis, one notes a steady decline in the concentration of sodium and an increase in the concentration of potassium, which certainly suggests that the bladder urine is considerably modified from filtrate. They offer the reasonable hypothesis that a good deal of the urine that gains access to the bladder has been processed by a small number of nephrons which have suffered little or no damage and that in acute tubular necrosis one may expect an entire series of gradations of severity from little to virtually complete involvement of every nephron. In addition to the diminished filtration rate and back-diffusion as the causes of the oliguria, some continue to suggest that obstruction of nephrons by casts composed of pigment, protein and cellular debris is an important feature. It is difficult to evaluate this possibility with any confidence at this time. It has also been suggested that an increase in renal interstitial pressure might compress and obstruct nephrons and contribute to the oliguria in this fashion. This may be dismissed, since measurements of renal interstitial pressure in clinical and experimental acute tubular necrosis have been made and were found to be normal.[452,453]

Acute tubular necrosis is a self-terminating and reversible disease process. The aim of therapy during the period of oliguria is to maintain the internal environment as near normal as is possible by the least hazardous methods and to prevent or treat complications as they may arise. The problems involved will be better understood if the consequences of the virtually total renal insufficiency are first examined.

Since the loss of fluid by way of the kidneys is no longer possible during the oliguric phase, water and ions which are ingested or administered in excess of those lost by extra-renal routes will accumulate within the body. If water is ingested or administered in excess, it will be distributed throughout the total body water, there will be a dilutional hyponatremia, and the signs and symptoms of water intoxication may supervene. If salt intake exceeds extrarenal loss, it will induce hypernatremia and thirst which will necessitate ingestion or administration of water and will lead to an approximately isotonic expansion of the body fluid. Since this latter represents an expansion of the extracellular space, it is a major hazard in terms of inducing or contributing to the frequent complication of heart failure.

The concentrations of urea and other nonprotein nitrogenous end-products of metabolism increase. There is no evidence that urea per se is harmful, but it is clear that other materials which accumulate as a consequence of the catabolism of protein do contribute to significant distortions of the internal environment and represent hazards in terms of visceral functions and may contribute to mortality. Some of these materials include acids whose anions are phosphate, sulfate, etc., potassium, and, perhaps, other unidentified substances which may be responsible for some of the manifestations of the "uremic state." The rapidity with which these materials accumulate is related to the rate of catabolism of cell proteins and will be conditioned by the extent of direct tissue damage the patient may have sustained,[286,288] the presence of infection,[289] the severity of the "injury reaction," the antecedent status of body protein stores and the availability of carbohydrate.

The accumulation of the acids of phosphate and sulfate (and ketones as well if carbohydrate starvation is allowed) and the inability to excrete hydrogen ions or to alter the composition of the extracellular fluids lead to a progressively severe metabolic acidosis with its attendant manifestations.[105,116,117,120] In addition, the hyperphosphatemia induces hypocalcemia. The precise mechanism for the depressed concentration of calcium in the serum is not clear, but it is apparent that calcium will be lost to traumatized tissue and that this route of loss is markedly increased when there is severely impaired renal function.[454] Hypocalcemia may be severe enough even in the presence of acidosis to give rise to neuromuscular irritability and frank carpopedal spasm.[455]

The increased concentration of potassium represents one of the most severe hazards during the oliguric phase of acute tubular necrosis. The intensity of the hyperkalemia is conditioned in part by the status of the body stores of this cation prior to the development of acute tubular necrosis and by the amount of potassium that may be lost with vomiting and diarrhea that may also be associated with the events that lead to the renal disorder. In some instances an increase in potassium is never a problem. In contrast, the levels of potassium may reach striking proportions[436-439,456] and induce marked changes in the electrocardiogram characterized by an increase in the amplitude and peaking of the T waves, depression of the ST segment, reduction in the amplitude of the R wave, widening of the QRS complex, prolongation of the P-R interval, a decrease in the amplitude and, finally, disappearance of the P wave, idioventricular rhythms, ventricular tachycardia, ventricular fibrillation and death. It is also possible that these patients develop acute marked elevations of the concentration of serum potassium because of hypoxia and the muscular effort which accompany vomiting and convulsive seizures. Acute hyperkalemia (or other associated changes in electrolyte composition of the serum[457]) can induce acute cardiac arrhythmias which may be responsible for sudden death. The deleterious effects of hyperpotassemia on the electrocardiogram are augmented by hypocalcemia and hyponatremia.

Hyponatremia is a frequent complication of the early course of this disorder and may be due to dilution caused by excessive administration of water or to the loss of sodium-containing fluids which are replaced by water alone. Occasional instances of hyponatremia have been noted in patients in whom the loss of sodium or the excessive administration of water could not be indicted as the cause. These have been associated with a sudden increase in the rate of rise of the concentration of urea nitrogen and potassium in the serum, suggesting an increased rate of catabolism and the release of water from cells.

Hypertension is very common, and necrotizing vascular disease[458] of major proportions may also complicate the clinical picture. Pericarditis, ulcerations of the gastrointestinal tract, hemorrhages and exudate in the fundi, cardiac failure and convulsions are all common events during the course of the oliguric phase of acute renal insufficiency. A normochromic normocytic anemia is also frequently noted.[459-461] The precise mechanisms responsible for these complications are unknown.

Management. Many of the consequences of acute renal insufficiency listed above may be prevented, modified or combated. The excess accumulation of fluid can be prevented by administration of no more fluid than is dissipated each day. In the absence of urine and gastrointestinal losses a volume of about 500 ml. of water per day may be quite adequate to replace the insensible loss that is not replaced by the metabolic production of endogenous water. The reasonableness of this figure can be checked by frequent determinations of the concentration of sodium in the serum and by daily observations of the body weight. If no salt is lost, a decrease or an increase in the concentration of sodium in the serum suggests too much or inadequate replacement of the daily water loss. Since adequate calories are not usually supplied from an exogenous source, one may anticipate a daily weight loss averaging about ½ pound.[462] Failure to lose this much weight suggests expansion of the body fluids. Weight loss in excess of this may provide a clue to the development of dehydration. The administered water should contain sufficient glucose to provide at least 100 grams of carbohydrate per day. In general, the 500 ml. of water may be administered as a solution of 20 to 25 per cent dextrose in a very slow drip by vein through a plastic catheter which is passed far into a large vein to avoid trauma. Sodium salts should be administered if they are lost in the gastrointestinal fluids, and hyponatremia should be corrected if it is presumed to be due to a *loss* of salt. In contrast, if a depressed concentration of sodium in the serum results from the administration of too much water, it is more desirable to restore the concentration of sodium by more drastic restriction of water intake. If sodium salts are to be administered and there is an associated acidosis, they might as well be given, in part at least, as sodium bicarbonate. Urine loss should be replaced, and in the absence of an actual estimate of the urine concentration of sodium, it may be replaced by an equivalent volume of a solution composed of equal parts of dextrose in water and an isotonic solution of sodium salts.

The hypocalcemia may be modified by the intravenous administration of a solution of calcium gluconate. This is especially indicated if there are electrocardiographic alterations due to hyperkalemia. In fact, it is desirable to administer calcium when the ECG abnormalities due to hyperkalemia supervene even if the concentration of calcium in the serum is not significantly depressed. The administration of calcium appears to have a specific effect in counteracting the noxious influences of hyperkalemia as these may be reflected in the ECG. It is well to administer the calcium gluconate slowly by vein and to monitor the electrocardiogram as this is being done. Initially it has sometimes been found necessary and desirable to administer as much as 50 ml. of a 10 per cent solution of calcium gluconate and then to follow this with a more dilute solution of calcium incorporated in the daily fluid volume, with frequent checks of the electrocardiogram to make sure that an excess is not administered. In addition, the effects of hyperkalemia may be favorably influenced by digitalization; this is recommended when there is life-threatening hyperkalemia even if heart failure is not yet a complication. The degree of the hyperkalemia may be modified by the use of cation exchange resins which may be given orally or instilled as an enema.[463-465] The oral route is frequently proscribed because of associated nausea and vomiting. The resin may be easily administered as a 10 to 15 per cent suspension in 200 ml. of water per rectum two to three times a day. When resins are administered by enema, the suspending fluid is frequently absorbed from the large bowel, and this volume of fluid must be considered as part of the total daily allotment. On occasion, it becomes quite difficult to restrict the daily fluid intake to 500 ml. and still treat the patient with enema resins and have sufficient leeway to administer 100 grams of carbohydrate by vein. In such instances a larger volume of water may have to be administered for a few days in the interests of combating the more serious immediate hazard of hyperkalemia. The cation exchange resins which are used for the purpose of removing potassium are either ammonium or sodium resins, and in either instance there may be untoward consequences from their use. If the resin is in the ammonium cycle, the exchange with potassium may exaggerate the metabolic acidosis; if the resin is in the sodium cycle, a slight excess of sodium may be accumulated as the potassium is exchanged. However, these are minor considerations when compared with the complication which is being treated.

Insulin may be administered along with glucose to reduce the concentration of potassium in the serum. The only criticism of this technique is the fact that it has a rather transient effect. Nevertheless, there are occasions when the reduction of the concentration of potassium in the serum to a lower level even for a few hours while other measures are prepared might conceivably be lifesaving. It is usually recommended that about one unit of regular insulin be administered for every 2 to 3 grams of glucose.

The role of dialysis in the management of acute renal insufficiency has become better defined in recent years through the accumulation of valuable experience and data by several groups of investigators in both civilian and military practice.[436-438] There is no doubt that many instances of acute tubular necrosis can be properly managed by the measures which have been mentioned briefly in the foregoing discussion. However, there are occasions when, despite careful and meticulous attention to details, the level of potassium in the serum reaches cardiotoxic levels. There is no doubt that the use of a dialysis technique may be lifesaving in such patients. However, other indications have been suggested for the use of dialysis, including a level of urea nitrogen in the blood in excess of 150 mg. per cent, a bicarbonate concentration of less than 12 mM./L., progressive mental deterioration, pulmonary edema, and abdominal distention and vomiting.[466] Merrill[438] emphasizes the use of dialysis to promote a generally improved clinical status which may make the patient better able to tolerate other complications such as infection and, hence, to cut down the mortality in this fashion. There is a fair unanimity among those who have had the most experience with dialysis that the procedure is indicated for reasons other than hyperkalemia and that the clinical status is frequently considerably improved beyond the point which one might justifiably anticipate simply from reduction of a level of potassium in the serum and an increase in the concentration of bicarbonate. The implication is that substances are dialyzed which are responsible for some of the striking clinical features of uremia. In the absence of proper controls to furnish data concerning morbidity and mortality with and without the use of artificial dialysis, it is certainly difficult to take a firm stand on the utility of dialysis for indications other than hyperkalemia. The reader is referred to the literature for more detailed presentation of the several points of view.

The dialysis techniques include intestinal and peritoneal lavage and the use of an extracorporeal procedure referred to as the artificial kidney. Intestinal lavage is not highly efficient, and one runs the risk of having the patient absorb a large fraction of the dialyzing fluid. Intermittent peritoneal lavage is much less likely to be complicated by peritonitis than continuous lavage. It is a simple technique available to everyone, and although it is not highly efficient, one can certainly reduce the concentration of potassium to normal levels and effect a significant improvement in acid-base equilibrium. The details of its use are described in Grollman's monograph.[437] Descriptions of the several extracorporeal techniques are presented by Merrill, and the advantages and disadvantages of each are evaluated. The reader is referred to these documents for further details. The use of extracorporeal dialysis necessitates heparinization so that the technique is contraindicated when there is bleeding from the gastrointestinal tract or into the central nervous system. In addition, the cardiac output is frequently increased during dialysis; hence, it is contraindicated in instances of tubular necrosis which follow acute myocardial infarction.

The diuretic phase of acute tubular necrosis is characterized by excretion of large volumes of urine whose composition reflects some continued loss of discriminatory function on the part of the renal tubules. If there is expansion of the body fluids, the replacement of salt and water may lag behind the losses of these materials until the edema has been dissipated. However, care must be taken to avoid significant dehydration since this will delay recovery. To be certain of the quantity of sodium loss in the urine, daily analyses must be made; if this is not possible, one may assume that the concentration of sodium in the urine is likely to be between 60 and 90 mM./L. and may be replaced with equal parts of dextrose and water and an isotonic solution of sodium salts. Since metabolic acidosis continues for some time, a portion of the sodium may as well be administered as bicarbonate. Considerable potassium may be swept out into the urine in this phase, and significant deficits of this cation have been known to develop. Repeated chemical analyses of the serum will make one aware of the early stage of deficiency, and this can be modified by appropriate replacement. Renal function improves rapidly, but it may take many months before completely normal function has been restored.

Another condition which mimics the diuretic phase of acute tubular necrosis is seen in association with the relief of obstruction to the urinary tract.[467] The pathogenesis of this disorder is not clear other than that it occasionally complicates obstructive uropathy. It has been noted following relief of prostatic obstruction and obstruction to ureters due to involvement with carcinoma. The patient excretes large volumes of urine whose composition is similar to that in the diuretic phase of acute tubular necrosis. The longer duration of this condition may, in part, be due to more permanent underlying renal disease. The unanticipated losses of water and ions that may develop following relief of the obstruction may not be recognized until the patient has developed a severe degree of dehydration. It is therefore important to anticipate this possible complication of obstructive uropathy and to be alert to its presence in the interest of avoiding serious and life-threatening dehydration.

Chronic Renal Insufficiency

Most of the considerations of the management of chronic renal insufficiency which are relevant to this discussion have been presented in earlier sections dealing with renal physiology, disorders of hydration and acid-base equilibrium, and in the foregoing discussion of acute renal insufficiency.

The problem of the management of patients with the terminal phase of chronic renal insufficiency parallels many of the problems and approaches which have just been described. The physician must first make certain that there is no element of the clinical picture which he may reverse such as dehydration, obstruction or infection. Once these elements have been evaluated and corrective measures taken, if necessary, the problem is one of maintaining the patient in a fashion which will allow him to survive long enough to reap the benefits of some "spontaneous" reversal of his underlying disease process. Supportive measures include all of those described for acute renal insufficiency aimed at modifying the hyperkalemia, the acidosis, the anemia, heart failure, the seizures, etc. Recently some groups have been evaluating the role of artificial dialysis in the management of such patients. Thus far it has not been very promising, but it deserves more careful consideration and evaluation since it is quite possible that many episodes of acute deterioration in the course of chronic renal failure may be partially reversible if sufficient time is allowed. This possibility may be realized only if patients are allowed to live longer during these acute episodes.

References

1. Edelman, I. S., Olney, J. M., James, A. H., Brooks, L., and Moore, F. D.: Science, *115:*447, 1952.
2. Edelman, I. S., Haley, H. B., Schloerb, P. R., Sheldon, D. B., Friis-Hansen, B. J., Stoll, G., and Moore, F. D.: Surg. Gynec. & Obst., *95:*1, 1952.
3. Friis-Hansen, B. J., Holliday, M., Stapleton, T., and Wallace, W. M.: Pediatrics, *7:*321, 1951.
4. London, I. M. and Rittenberg, D.: J. Biol. Chem., *184:*687, 1950.
5. Pinson, E. A.: Physiol. Rev., *32:*123, 1952.
6. Prentice, T. C., Siri, W., Berlin, N. I., Hyde, G. M., Parsons, R. J., Joiner, E. E., and Lawrence, J. H.: J. Clin. Invest., *31:*412, 1952.
7. Brodie, B. B., Axelrod, J., Soberman, R., and Levy, B. B.: J. Biol. Chem., *179:*25, 1949.
8. Soberman, R., Brodie, B. B., Levy, B. B., Axelrod, J., Hollander, V., and Steele, J. M.: J. Biol. Chem., *179:*31, 1949.
9. Brodie, B. B., Berger, E. Y., Axelrod, J., Dunning, M. F., Porosowska, Y., and Steele, J. M.: Proc. Soc. Exper. Biol. & Med., *77:*794, 1951.
10. Deane, N., Schreiner, G. E., and Robertson, J. S.: J. Clin. Invest., *30:*1463, 1951.
11. Raisz, L. G., Young, M. K., Jr., and Stinson, I. T.: Am. J. Physiol., *174:*72, 1953.
12. Cotlove, E.: Am. J. Physiol., *176:*396, 1954.
13. Deane, N. and Smith, H. W.: J. Clin. Invest., *34:*681, 1955.
14. Walser, M., Seldin, D. W., and Grollman, A.: J. Clin. Invest., *32:*299, 1953.
15. Walser, M., Seldin, D. W., and Grollman, A.: Am. J. Physiol., *176:*322, 1954.
16. Cardozo, R. H. and Edelman, I. S.: J. Clin. Invest., *31:*280, 1952.
17. Kowalski, H. J. and Rutstein, D. D.: J. Clin. Invest., *31:*370, 1952.
18. Last, J. H., McDonald, G. O., Jones, R. A., and Bond, E. E.: Proc. Soc. Exper. Biol. & Med., *79:*99, 1952.
19. Gamble, J. L., Jr., Robertson, J. S., Hannigan, C. A., Foster, C. G., and Farr, L. E.: J. Clin. Invest., *32:*483, 1953.
20. Epstein, F. H., Kleeman, C. R., Rubini, M. E., and Lamdin, E.: Am. J. Physiol., *182:*553, 1955.
21. Kleeman, C. R., Epstein. F. H., Rubini, M. E., and Lamdin, E.: Am. J. Physiol., *182:*548, 1955.
22. Gamble, J. L.: Chemical Anatomy, Physiology, and Pathology of Extracellular Fluid. Cambridge, Mass., Harvard University Press, 1950.
23. Manery, J. F.: Physiol. Rev., *34:*334, 1954.
24. Welt, L. G.: Clinical Disorders of Hydration and Acid-Base Equilibrium. Boston, Little, Brown and Co., 1955.
25. Elkinton, J. R. and Danowski, T. S.: The Body Fluids, Basic Physiology and Practical Therapeutics. Baltimore, Williams and Wilkins Co., 1955.
26. Citron, L., Exley, D., and Hallpike, C. S.: Brit. M. Bull., *12:*101, 1956.
27. Harrison, H. E., Darrow, D. C., and Yannet, H.: J. Biol. Chem., *113:*515, 1936.
28. Hastings, A. B. and Eichelberger, L.: J. Biol. Chem., *117:*73, 1937.
29. Wallace, W. M. and Hastings, A. B.: J. Biol. Chem., *144:*637, 1942.
30. Elkinton, J. R. and Taffel, M.: J. Clin. Invest., *21:*787, 1942.
31. Lillienthal, J. L., Jr., Zierler, K. L., Folk, B. P., Buka, R., and Riley, M. J.: J. Biol. Chem., *182:*501, 1950.
32. Elkinton, J. R., Winkler, A. W., and Danowski, T. S.: Yale J. Biol. & Med., *17:*383, 1944.
33. Nichols, G., Jr., Nichols, N., Weil, W. B., and Wallace, W. M.: J. Clin. Invest., *32:*1299, 1953.
34. Cheek, D. B., West, C. D., and Golden, C. C.: J. Clin. Invest., *36:*340, 1957.
35. Eisenman, A. J., Mackenzie, L. B., and Peters, J. P.: J. Biol. Chem., *116:*33, 1936.
36. Hopper, J., Jr., Tabor, H., and Winkler, A. W.: J. Clin. Invest., *23:*628, 1944.
37. Hopper, J., Jr., Winkler, A. W., and Elkinton, J. R.: J. Clin. Invest., *23:*636, 1944.
38. Freinkel, N., Schreiner, G. E., and Athens, J. W.: J. Clin. Invest., *32:*138, 1953.
39. Gibson, J. G., II, Weiss, S., Evans, R. D., Peacock, W. C., Irvine, J. W., Jr.,

Good, W. M., and Kip, A. F.: J. Clin. Invest., *25:*616, 1946.

40. Hevesy, G., Koster, K. H., Sorensen, G., Warburg, E., and Zerahn, K.: Acta med. scandinav., *116:*561, 1944.
41. Berson, S. A. and Yalow, R. S.: J. Clin. Invest., *31:*572, 1952.
42. Sterling, K. and Gray, S. J.: J. Clin. Invest., *29:*1614, 1950.
43. Gray, S. J. and Sterling, K.: J. Clin. Invest., *29:*1604, 1950.
44. Clark, W. M.: Topics in Physical Chemistry. 2nd ed. Baltimore, Williams and Wilkins, 1952, Ch. 8.
45. Chinard, F. P.: J. Chem. Ed., *31:*66, 1954.
46. Chinard, F. P.: J. Chem. Ed., *32:*377, 1955.
47. Robinson, J. R. and McCance, R. A.: Ann. Rev. Physiol., *14:*115, 1952.
48. Opie, E. L.: Harvey Lectures, *50:*292, 1954–55.
49. Brodsky, W. A., Appelboom, J. W., Dennis, W. H., Rehm, W. S., Miley, J. F., and Diamond, I.: J. Gen. Physiol., *40:*183, 1956.
50. Leaf, A.: Biochem. J., *62:*241, 1956.
51. Conway, E. J. and McCormack, J. I.: J. Physiol., *120:*1, 1953.
52. Appelboom, J. W. and Brodsky, W. A.: J. Clin. Invest., *36:*869, 1957.
53. Leaf, A., Chatillon, J. Y., Wrong, O., and Tuttle, E. P., Jr.: J. Clin. Invest., *33:*1261, 1954.
54. McDowell, M. E., Wolf, A. V., and Steer, A.: Am. J. Physiol., *180:*545, 1955.
55. Welt, L. G., Orloff, J., Kydd, D. M., and Oltman, J. E.: J. Clin. Invest., *29:*935, 1950.
56. Sims, E. A. H., Welt, L. G., Orloff, J., and Needham, J. W.: J. Clin. Invest., *29:*1545, 1950.
57. Darrow, D. C. and Yannet, H.: J. Clin. Invest., *14:*266, 1935.
58. Albrink, M. J., Hold, P. M., Man, E. B., and Peters, J. P.: J. Clin. Invest., *34:*1483, 1955.
59. Seldin, D. W. and Tarail, R.: Am. J. Physiol., *159:*160, 1949.
60. Krogh, A., Landis, E. M., and Turner, A. H.: J. Clin. Invest., *11:*63, 1932.
61. Teorell, T.: Ann. Rev. Physiol., *11:*545, 1949.
62. Beyer, K. H.: J. Pharmacol. & Exper. Therap., *99:*227, 1950.
63. Steinbach, H. B.: Ann. Rev. Physiol., *8:*21, 1951.
64. Davson, H. and Danielli, J. F.: The Permeability of Natural Membranes. Cambridge, England, Cambridge University Press, 1952.
65. Robinson, J. R.: Biol. Rev., *28:*158, 1953.
66. Ussing, H. H.: Ann. Rev. Physiol., *15:*1, 1953.
67. Clarke, H. T. (ed.): Ion Transport Across Membranes. New York, Academic Press, Inc., 1954.
68. Kitching, J. A. (ed.): Recent Developments in Cell Physiology. New York, Academic Press, Inc., 1954.
69. Symposia of the Society for Exper. Biol., VIII. Active Transport and Secretion. New York, Academic Press, Inc., 1954.
70. Wilde, W. S.: Ann. Rev. Physiol., *17:*17, 1955.
71. Shanes, A. M. (ed.): Electrolytes in Biological Systems. Washington, D. C., Am. Physiol. Soc., 1955.
72. Harris, E. J.: Transport and Accumulation in Biological Systems. New York, Academic Press, Inc., 1956.
73. Solomon, A. K., Lionetti, F., and Curran, P. F.: Nature, *178:*582, 1956.
74. Edelman, I. S., James, A. H., Baden, H., and Moore, F. D.: J. Clin. Invest., *33:*122, 1954.
75. Bergstrom, W. H.: Metabolism, *5:*433, 1956.
76. Nichols, G., Jr. and Nichols, N.: Metabolism, *5:*438, 1956.
77. Levitt, M., Turner, L. B., Sweet, A. Y., and Pandire, D.: J. Clin. Invest., *35:*98, 1956.
78. Willbanks, O. L., Jr. and Seldin, D. W.: Clin. Res. Proc., *4:*36, 1956.
79. McCance, R. A.: Lancet, *1:*643, 704, 765, 823, 1936.
80. Rosenbaum, J. D.: Yale J. Biol. & Med., *29:*263, 1956.
81. Strauss, M. B.: Body Water in Man. Boston, Little, Brown and Co., 1957.
82. Gilman, A.: Am. J. Physiol., *120:*323, 1937.
83. Peters, J. P.: J. Mt. Sinai Hosp., *17:*159, 1950.
84. Welt, L. G.: Clinical Physiology. New York, McGraw-Hill Book Co., 1957, Ch. 23.
85. Wolf, A. V.: Am. J. Physiol., *161:*75, 1950.
86. Cizek, L. J., Semple, R. E., Huang, K. C., and Gregersen, M. I.: Am. J. Physiol., *164:*415, 1951.
87. Stevenson, J. A. F., Welt, L. G., and Orloff, J.: Am. J. Physiol., *161:*35, 1950.
88. Andersson, B.: Acta physiol. scandinav., *28:*188, 1953.
89. Greer, M. A.: Proc. Soc. Exper. Biol. & Med., *89:*59, 1955.
90. Towbin, E. J.: Am. J. Physiol., *159:*533, 1949.
91. Welt, L. G., Seldin, D. W., Nelson, W. P., III, German, W. J., and Peters, J. P.: Arch. Int. Med., *90:*355, 1952.
92. Gilman, A. and Barbour, H. G.: Am. J. Physiol., *104:*392, 1933.
93. Amatruda, T. T. and Welt, L. G.: J. Appl. Physiol., *5:*759, 1953.

94. Robinson, S. and Robinson, A. H.: Physiol. Rev., *34:*202, 1954.
95. Kuno, Y.: Human Perspiration. Springfield, Ill., Charles C Thomas, 1956.
96. Conn, J. W.: The mechanism of acclimatization to heat. Advances in Internal Medicine, vol. 3. New York, Interscience Publishers, 1949, p. 373.
97. di Sant'Agnese, P. A.: Am. J. Med., *21:*406, 1956.
98. White, A. G., Entmacher, P. S., Rubin, G., and Leiter, L.: J. Clin. Invest., *34:*246, 1955.
99. Thull, N. B. and Rehm, W. S.: Am. J. Physiol., *185:*317, 1956.
100. D'Agostius, A., Leadbetter, W. F., and Schwartz, W. B.: J. Clin. Invest., *32:*444, 1953.
101. Edelman, I. S. and Sweet, N. J.: J. Clin. Invest., *35:*502, 1956.
102. Sweet, N. J. and Edelman, I. S.: J. Clin. Invest., *35:*512, 1956.
103. Sweet, N. J., Nadell, J., and Edelman, I. S.: J. Clin. Invest., *36:*279, 1957.
104. Gotch, F., Nadell, J., and Edelman, I. S.: J. Clin. Invest., *36:*289, 1957.
105. Davenport, H. W.: The ABC of Acid-Base Chemistry. Ann Arbor, Mich., Edwards Brothers, 1947.
106. Van Slyke, D. D. and Sendroy, J., Jr.: J. Biol. Chem., *79:*781, 1928.
107. Severinghaus, J. W., Stupfel, M., and Bradley, A. F.: J. App. Physiol., *9:*197, 1956.
108. Severinghaus, J. W., Stupfel, M., and Bradley, A. F.: J. App. Physiol., *9:*189, 1956.
109. Singer, R. B. and Hastings, A. B.: Medicine, *27:*223, 1948.
110. Rosenbaum, J. D.: J. Clin. Invest., *21:*735, 1942.
111. Elkinton, J. R., Squires, R. D., and Crosley, A. P. Jr.: J. Clin. Invest. *30:*369, 1951.
112. Cotlove, E., Holliday, M. A., Schwartz, R., and Wallace, W. M.: Am. J. Physiol., *167:*665, 1951.
113. Pitts, R. F.: Arch. Int. Med., *89:*864, 1952.
114. Pitts, R. F.: Harvey Lectures, *48:*172, 1952–53.
115. Orloff, J., Kennedy, T. J., Jr., and Berliner, R. W.: J. Clin. Invest., *32:*538, 1953.
116. Swan, R. C. and Pitts, R. F.: J. Clin. Invest., *34:*205, 1955.
117. Giebisch, G., Bergen, L., and Pitts, R. F.: J. Clin. Invest., *34:*231, 1955.
118. Scribner, B. H., Freemont-Smith, K., and Burnell, J. M.: J. Clin. Invest., *34:*1276, 1955.
119. Swan, R. C., Axelrod, D. R., Seip, M., and Pitts, R. F.: J. Clin. Invest., *34:*1795, 1955.
120. Elkinton, J. R.: Yale J. Biol. & Med., *29:*191, 1956.
121. Schwartz, W. B., Orning, K. J., and Porter, R.: J. Clin. Invest., *36:*373, 1957.
122. Elkinton, J. R.: Clin. Chem., *3:*319, 1957.
123. Gray, J. S.: Pulmonary Ventilation and Its Physiological Regulation. Springfield. Ill., Charles C Thomas, 1950.
124. Comroe, J. H., Jr., Forster, R. E., II, Dubois, A. B., Briscoe, W. A., and Carlsen, E.: The Lung, Clinical Physiology and Pulmonary Function Tests. Chicago, Year Book Publishers, Inc., 1955.
125. Brown, E. B., Jr.: Physiol. Rev., *33:*445, 1953.
126. Fishman, A. P., Samet, P., and Cournand, A.: Am. J. Med., *19:*533, 1955.
127. Alexander, J. K., West, J. R., Wood, J. A., and Richards, D. W.: J. Clin. Invest., *34:*511, 1955.
128. Winters, R. W., Lowder, J. A., and Ordway, N. K.: Am. J. Med., *22:*978, 1957.
129. Roberts, K. E., Poppell, J. W., Vanamee, P., Beals, R., and Randall, H. T.: J. Clin. Invest., *35:*261, 1956.
130. Wolf, A. V.: The Urinary Function of the Kidney. New York, Grune and Stratton, 1950.
131. Smith, H. W.: The Kidney: Structure and Function in Health and Disease. New York, Oxford University Press, 1951.
132. Robinson, J. R.: Reflections on Renal Function. Springfield, Ill., Charles C Thomas, 1954, pp. 83–90.
133. Smith, H. W.: Principles of Renal Physiology. New York, Oxford University Press, 1956.
134. Winton, F. R.: Modern Views on the Secretion of Urine. Boston, Little, Brown and Co., 1956.
135. Grollman, A.: Clinical Physiology. New York, Blakiston Division, McGraw-Hill Book Co., 1957.
136. Welt, L. G. (ed.): Essays in Metabolism. Boston, Little, Brown and Co., 1957.
137. Smith, H. W.: From Fish to Philosopher. Boston, Little, Brown and Co., 1953.
138. Pappenheimer, J. R. and Kinter, W. B.: Am. J. Physiol., *185:*377, 1956.
139. Kinter, W. B. and Pappenheimer, J. R.: Am. J. Physiol., *185:*391, 1956.
140. Kinter, W. B. and Pappenheimer, J. R.: Am. J. Physiol., *185:*399, 1956.
141. Mudge, G. H., Foulks, J., and Gilman, A.: Proc. Soc. Exper. Biol. & Med., *76:*545, 1948.
142. Mudge, G. H., Foulks, J., and Gilman, A.: Am. J. Physiol., *161:*159, 1950.
143. Berliner, R. W., Kennedy, T. J., Jr., and Orloff, J.: Am. J. Med., *11:*274, 1951.
144. Schmidt-Nielsen, B.: Physiol. Rev., *38:* 1958.
145. Trueta, J., Barclay, A. E., Daniel, P. M., Franklin, K. J., and Prichard, M. M. L.: Studies of the Renal Circulation. Springfield, Ill., Charles C Thomas, 1947.

146. Shannon, J. A., Farber, S., and Troast, L.: Am. J. Physiol., *133:*752, 1941.
147. Richards, A. N. and Walker, A. M.: Am. J. Physiol., *118:*111, 1937.
148. Walker, A. M., Hudson, C. L., Findley, T. Jr., and Richards, A. N.: Am. J. Physiol., *118:*121, 1937.
149. Walker, A. M., Bott, P. A., Oliver, J., and MacDowell, M. C.: Am. J. Physiol., *134:*580, 1941.
150. Wirz, H.: The Kidney. Boston, Little, Brown and Co., 1954, p. 38.
151. Wirz, H.: Internat. Physiol. Cong., *20:* 972, 1956.
152. Wirz, H.: Helvet. physiol. acta, *14:*353, 1956.
153. Wirz, H.: Colston Papers, *8:*157, 1956.
154. Gottschalk, C.: Personal communication.
155. Wesson, L. G., Jr. and Anslow, W. P., Jr.: Am. J. Physiol., *153:*465, 1948.
156. Wesson, L. G., Jr. and Anslow, W. P., Jr.: Am. J. Physiol., *170:*255, 1952.
157. Lewis, A. A. G.: Ann. Roy. Coll. Surg. Eng., *13:*36, 1952.
158. Zak, G. A., Brun, C., and Smith, H. W.: J. Clin. Invest. *33:*1064, 1954.
159. Welt, L. G.: Metabolism, *5:*395, 1956.
160. Welt, L. G.: Yale J. Biol. & Med., *29:*299, 1956.
161. Hollander, W., Jr., Winters, R. W., Williams, T. F., Bradley, J., Oliver, J., and Welt, L. G.: Am. J. Physiol., *189:*557, 1957.
162. Oliver, J., MacDowell, M., Welt, L. G., Holliday, M. A., Hollander, W., Jr., Winters, R. W., Williams, T. F., and Segar, W. E.: J. Exper. Med., *106:*563, 1957.
163. Shannon, J. A.: J. Exper. Med., *76:*371, 1942.
164. Berliner, R. W. and Davidson, D. G.: J. Clin. Invest., *35:*690, 1956.
165. Berliner, R. W.: Personal communication.
166. Ullrich, K. J., Dreuckhahn, F. O., and Jarausch, K. H.: Pflügers Arch. ges. Physiol., *261:*62, 1955.
167. Ullrich, K. J., Jarausch, K. H., and Overbeck, W.: Ber. ges. Physiol., *180:*131, 1956.
168. Welt, L. G., Young, D. T., Thorup, O. A., Jr., and Burnett, C. H.: Am. J. Med., *16:*612, 1954.
169. De Wardener, H. E. and Del Greco, F.: Clin. Sc., *14:*715, 1955.
170. Orloff, J. and Walser, M.: Clin. Res. Proc., *4:*136, 1956.
171. Scholandeo, P. F.: Scient. Am., *196:*97, 1957.
172. Rapoport, S., Brodsky, W. A., West, C. D., and Mackler, B.: Am. J. Physiol., *156:* 433, 1949.
173. Rapoport, S., Brodsky, W. A., and West, C. D.: Am. J. Physiol., *157:*357, 1949.
174. Rapoport, S., West, C. D., and Brodsky, W. A.: Am. J. Physiol., *157:*363, 1949.
175. Mudge, G. H., Foulks, J., and Gilman, A.: Am. J. Physiol., *158:*218, 1949.
176. Levy, M. N. and Ankeney, J. L.: Proc. Soc. Exper. Biol. & Med., *79:*491, 1952.
177. Kleeman, C. R., Epstein, F. H., and White, C.: J. Clin. Invest. *35:*749, 1956.
178. Verney, E. B.: Proc. Roy. Soc. London s.B., *135:*25, 1947.
179. Gilman, A. and Goodman, L.: J. Physiol., *90:*113, 1937.
180. O'Connor, W. J.: Biol. Rev., *22:*30, 1947.
181. Harris, G. W.: Physiol. Rev., *28:*139, 1948.
182. Von Euler, C.: Acta physiol. Scandinav., *29:*133, 1953.
183. Scharrer, E. and Scharrer, B.: Recent Progr. Horm. Res., *10:*183, 1954.
184. Martin, S. J., Herrlich, H. C., and Fazekas, J. F.: Am. J. Physiol., *127:*51, 1939.
185. Brun, C., Knudsen, E. O. E., and Raaschou, F.: Acta med. scandinav., *122:* 315, 1945.
186. Welt, L. G. and Orloff, J.: J. Clin. Invest., *30:*751, 1951.
187. Strauss, M. B., Davis, R. K., Rosenbaum, J. D., and Rossmeisl, E. C.: J. Clin. Invest., *30:*862, 1951.
188. Leaf, A. and Mamby, A. R.: J. Clin. Invest., *31:*60, 1952.
189. Strauss, M. B., Birchard, W. H., and Saxon, L.: Tran. A. Am. Physicians, *69:*222, 1956.
190. Rydin, H. and Verney, E. B.: Quart. J. Exper. Physiol., *27:*343, 1938.
191. Mirsky, I. A., Stein, M., and Pavlisch, G.: Endocrinology, *54:*491, 1954.
192. Mirsky, I. A., Stein, M., and Pavlisch, G.: Endocrinology, *55:*28, 1954.
193. Chalmers, T. M. and Lewis, A. A. G.: Clin. Sc., *10:*127, 1951.
194. Lewis, A. A. G. and Chalmers, T. M.: Clin. Sc., *10:*137, 1951.
195. Pickford, M.: Pharmacol. Rev., *4:*254, 1952.
196. Blackmore, W. P. and Cherry, G. R.: Am. J. Physiol., *180:*596, 1955.
197. Strauss, M. B., Rosenbaum, J. D., Nelson, W. P., III: J. Clin. Invest. *29:*1053, 1950.
198. Rubini, M. E., Kleeman, C. R., and Lamdin, E.: J. Clin. Invest., *34:*439, 1955.
199. Kleeman, C. R., Rubini, M. E., Lamdin, E., and Epstein, F. H.: J. Clin. Invest., *34:*448, 1955.
200. du Vigneaud, V.: Harvey Lectures, *50:*1, 1954–55.
201. du Vigneaud, V., Lawler, H. C., and Popenoe, E. A.: J. Am. Chem. Soc., *75:*4880, 1953.
202. du Vigneaud, V. Ressler, C., Swan, J. M., Roberts, C. W., Katsoyannis, P. G., and Gordon, S.: J. Am. Chem. Soc., *75:* 4879, 1953.
203. Koefoed-Johnsen, V. and Ussing, H. H.: Acta physiol. scandinav., *28:*60, 1953.

204. Hollander, W., Jr., Williams, T. F., Fordham, C. C., III, and Welt, L. G.: J. Clin. Invest., *36:*1059, 1957.
205. Van Dyke, H. B., Adamsons, K., Jr., and Engel, S. L.: Recent Progr. Horm. Res., *11:*1, 1955.
206. Thorn, N. A. and Silver, L.: J. Exper. Med., *105:*575, 1957.
207. Gaunt, R., Birnie, J. H., and Eversole, W. J.: Physiol. Rev., *29:*281, 1949.
208. Leaf, A., Mamby, A. R., Rasmussen, H., and Marasco, J. P.: J. Clin. Invest., *31:*914, 1952.
209. Raisz, L. G., McNeely, W. F., Saxon, L., and Rosenbaum, J. D.: J. Clin. Invest., *36:*767, 1957.
210. Demunbrun, T. W., Keller, A. D., Levkoff, A. H., and Purser, R. M., Jr.: Am. J. Physiol., *179:*429, 1954.
211. Selkurt, E. E.: Physiol. Rev., *34:*287, 1954.
212. Mueller, C. B., Surtshin, A., Carlin, M. R., and White, H. L.: Am. J. Physiol., *165:*411, 1951.
213. Darragh, J. H., Welt, L. G., Goodyer, A. V. N., and Abele, W. A.: J. Appl. Physiol., *5:*658, 1953.
214. Epstein, F. H.: Yale J. Biol. & Med., *29:*282, 1956.
215. Wrong, O.: Brit. M. Bull., *13:*10, 1957.
216. Epstein, F. H., Goodyer, A. V. N., Lawrason, F. D., and Relman, A. S.: J. Clin. Invest., *30:*63, 1951.
217. Goodyer, A. V. N. and Seldin, D. W.: J. Clin. Invest., *32:*242, 1953.
218. Strauss, M. B., Davis, R. K., Rosenbaum, J. D., and Rossmeisl, E. C.: J. Clin. Invest., *31:*80, 1952.
219. Epstein, F. H., Post, R. S., and McDowell, M.: J. Clin. Invest., *32:*233, 1953.
220. Gauer, O. H., Henry, J. P., Sieker, H. O., and Wendt, W. E.: J. Clin. Invest., *33:*287, 1954.
221. Henry, J. P. and Pearce, J. W.: J. Physiol., *131:*572, 1956.
222. Goodyer, A. V. N.., Peterson, E. R., and Relman, A. S.: J. Appl. Physiol., *1:*671, 1949.
223. Petersdorf, R. G., and Welt, L. G.: J. Clin. Invest., *32:*283, 1953.
224. Jungmann, P. and Meyer, E.: Arch. f. exper. Path. u. Pharmakol., *73:*49, 1913.
225. Marshall, E. K., Jr. and Kolls, A. C.: Am. J. Physiol., *49:*302, 1919.
226. Marshall, E. K., Jr. and Kolls, A. C.: Am. J. Physiol., *49:*317, 1919.
227. Marshall, E. K., Jr. and Kolls, A. C.: Am. J. Physiol., *49:*335, 1919.
228. Marshall, E. K., Jr. and Kolls, A. C.: Am. J. Physiol., *49:*339, 1919.
229. Kriss, J. P., Futcher, P. H., and Goldman, M. L.: Am. J. Physiol., *154:*229, 1948.
230. Kaplan, S. A. and Rapoport, S.: Am. J. Physiol., *164:*175, 1951.
231. Kaplan, S. A., Fomon, S. J., and Rapoport, S.: Am. J. Physiol., *166:*641, 1951.
232. Page, L. B., Baxter, C. F., Reem, G. H., Scott-Baker, J. C., and Smith, H. W.: Am. J. Physiol., *177:*194, 1954.
233. Sartorius, O. W. and Burlington, H.: Am. J. Physiol., *185:*407, 1956.
234. Surtshin, A. and Schmandt, W. P.: Am. J. Physiol., *185:*418, 1956.
235. Keeler, R. J.: J. Physiol., *130:*9P, 1955.
236. Peters, J. P., Welt, L. G., Sims, E. A. H., Orloff, J., and Needham, J.: Tr. A. Am. Physicians, *63:*57, 1950.
237. Cort, J. H.: Lancet, *1:*752, 1954.
238. Farrell, G., Rauschkalb, E. W., Fleming, R. B., and Yatsu, F. M.: Endoc. Soc. Abstract, 1957, p. 32.
239. Rauschkalb, E. W. and Farrell, G. L.: Endocrinology, *59:*526, 1956.
240. Simpson, S. A. and Tait, J. F.: Recent Progr. Horm. Res., *11:*183, 1955.
241. Luetscher, J. A., Jr. and Curtis, R. H.: Ann. Int. Med., *43:*658, 1955.
242. Beck, J. C., Dyrenfurth, I., Giroud, C., and Venning, E. H.: A.M.A. Arch. Int. Med., *96:*463, 1955.
243. Luetscher, J. A., Jr.: Advances Int. Med., *8:*155, 1956.
244. Farrell, G. L., Rosnagle, R. S., and Rauschkalb, E. W.: Fed. Proc., *15:*60, 1956.
245. Duncan, L. E., Jr., Liddle, G. W., and Bartter, F. C.: J. Clin. Invest., *35:*1299, 1956.
246. Bartter, F. C., Liddle, G. W., Duncan, L. E., Jr., Barber, J. K., and Delea, C.: J. Clin. Invest., *35:*1306, 1956.
247. Liddle, G. W., Duncan, L. E., Jr., and Bartter, F. C.: Am. J. Med., *21:*320, 1956.
248. Johnson, B. B., Lieberman, A. H., and Mulrow, P. J.: J. Clin. Invest., *36:*757, 1957.
249. Leaf, A., Bartter, F. C., Santos, R. F., and Wrong, O.: J. Clin. Invest., *32:*868, 1953.
250. Thompson, D. D. and Barrett, M. J.: Am. J. Physiol., *176:*33, 1954.
251. Williams, T. F., Hollander, W., Jr., Strauss, M. B., Rossmeisl, E. C., and McLean, R.: J. Clin. Invest., *34:*595, 1955.
252. Tarail, R., Seldin, D. W., and Goodyer, A. V. N.: J. Clin. Invest., *30:*1111, 1951.
253. Berliner, R. W. and Kennedy, T. J., Jr.: Proc. Soc. Exper. Biol. & Med., *67:*542, 1948.
254. Mudge, G. H.: Tr. 4th Conf. on Renal Function, New York, Josiah Macy, Jr. Foundation, 1952, p. 56.
255. Seldin, D. W., Welt, L. G., and Cort, J. H.: Yale J. Biol. & Med., *29:*229, 1956.

256. McCance, R. A. and Widdowson, E. M.: Proc. Roy. Soc. London, *120:*228, 1936.
257. Gilman, A. and Brazeau, P.: Am. J. Med., *15:*765, 1955.
258. Berliner, R. W. and Orloff, J.: Pharmacol. Rev., *8:*137, 1956.
259. Orloff, J.: Yale J. Biol. & Med., *29:*211, 1956.
260. Menaker, W.: Am. J. Physiol., *154:*174, 1948.
261. Pitts, R. F. and Alexander, R. S.: Am. J. Physiol., *144:*239, 1945.
262. Pitts, R. F., Ayer, J. L., and Schiess, W. A.: J. Clin. Invest., *28:*35, 1949.
263. Davenport, H. W.: Physiol. Rev., *26:*560, 1946.
264. Van Goor, H.: Enzymology, *13:*73, 1948–49.
265. Kennedy, T. J., Jr., Orloff, J., and Berliner, R. W.: Am. J. Physiol., *169:*596, 1952.
266. Ochwadt, B. K. and Pitts, R. F.: Am. J. Physiol., *185:*426, 1956.
267. Brazeau, P. and Gilman, A.: Am. J. Physiol., *175:*33, 1953.
268. Relman, A. S., Etsen, B., and Schwartz, W. B.: J. Clin. Invest., *32:*972, 1953.
269. Schwartz, W. B., Jenson, R. L., and Relman, A. S.: J. Clin. Invest., *34:*673, 1955.
270. Mudge, G. H.: Am. J. Physiol., *165:*113, 1951.
271. Roberts, K. E., Randall, H. T., Sanders, H. L., and Hood, M.: J. Clin. Invest., *34:*666, 1955.
272. Anderson, H. M. and Mudge, G. H.: J. Clin. Invest., *34:*1691, 1955.
273. Roberts, K. E., Randall, H. T., Vanamee, P., and Poppell, J. W.: Metabolism, *5:*404, 1956.
274. Van Slyke, D. D., Phillips, R. A., Hamilton, P. B., Archibald, R. M., Futcher, P. H., and Hiller, A.: J. Biol. Chem., *150:*481, 1943.
275. Sartorius, O. W., Roemmelt, J. C., and Pitts, R. F.: J. Clin. Invest., *28:*423, 1949.
276. Leonard, E. and Orloff, J.: Am. J. Physiol., *182:*131, 1955.
277. Rector, F. C., Seldin, D. W., and Copenhaver, J. H.: J. Clin. Invest., *34:*20, 1955.
278. Orloff, J. and Berliner, R. W.: J. Clin. Invest., *35:*223, 1956.
279. Leaf, A., Schwartz, W. B., and Relman, A. S.: New England J. Med., *250:*759, 1954.
280. Montgomery, H. and Pierce, J. A.: Am. J. Physiol., *118:*144, 1937.
281. Sartorius, O. W., Calhoon, D., and Pitts, R. F.: Endocrinology, *51:*444, 1952.
282. Sartorius, O. W., Calhoon, D., and Pitts, R. F.: Endocrinology, *52:*256, 1953.
283. Holliday, M. A. and Segar, W. E.: Parenteral Fluid Therapy. Indianapolis, Indiana University Medical Center, 1956.
284. Gamble, J. L.: Harvey Lectures, *42:*247, 1946–47.
285. Engel, F. L. and Jaeger, C.: Am. J. Med., *17:*196, 1954.
286. Cuthbertson, D. P.: Quart. J. Med., *1:*233, 1932.
287. Peters, J. P.: Ann. New York Acad. Sc., *47:*327, 1946.
288. Peters, J. P.: Am. J. Med., *5:*100, 1948.
289. Grossman, C. M., Sappington, T. S., Burrows, B. A., Lavietes, P. H., and Peters, J. P.: J. Clin. Invest., *24:*523, 1945.
290. Le Quesne, L. P.: Fluid Balance in Surgical Practice. Chicago, Year Book Publishers, Inc., 1955.
291. Butler, J. J.: New England J. Med., *249:* 988, 1953.
292. Danowski, T. S., Winkler, A. W., and Elkinton, J. R.: J. Clin. Invest., *26:*887, 1947.
293. Tucker, G. R., Jr., Blythe, G. N., and Welt, L. G.: Unpublished observations.
294. Seldin, D. W. and Tarail, R.: J. Clin. Invest., *29:*552, 1950.
295. MacCarty, C. S. and Cooper, I. S.: Proc. Staff Meet., Mayo Clin., *26:*185, 1951.
296. Cooper, I. S. and MacCarty, C. S.: Proc. Staff Meet., Mayo Clin., *26:*354, 1951.
297. Blotner, H.: Diabetes Insipidus. In Oxford Medicine, vol. 4, ch. 6. New York, Oxford University Press, 1949.
298. Cannon, J. F.: Arch. Int. Med., *96:*215, 1955.
299. White, A. G.: J. Mt. Sinai Hosp., *22:*15, 1955.
300. Williams, R. H. and Henry, C.: Ann. Int. Med., *27:*84, 1947.
301. Roussak, N. J. and Oleesky, S.: Quart. J. Med., *23:*147, 1954.
302. Darmady, E. M.: The Kidney. Boston, Little, Brown and Company, 1954, p. 27.
303. Earley, L. E.: New England J. Med., *255:*600, 1956.
304. Schwartz, W. B.: New England J. Med., *253:*601, 1955.
305. Relman, A. S. and Schwartz, W. B.: J. Clin. Invest., *34:*959, 1955.
306. Relman, A. S. and Schwartz, W. B.: New England J. Med., *255:*195, 1956.
307. Milne, M. D., Muehrcke, R. C., and Heard, B. E.: Brit. M. Bull., *13:*15, 1957.
308. Loeb, R. F.: Proc. Soc. Exper. Biol. & Med., *30:*808, 1933.
309. Thorn, G. W., Forsham, P. H., and Emerson, K., Jr.: The Diagnosis and Treatment of Adrenal Insufficiency. Springfield, Ill., Charles C Thomas, 1949.
310. Knowlton, A. I.: M. Clin. North America, *36:*721, 1952.

311. Knowlton, A. I.: Am. J. Med., *15:*771, 1953.
312. Overman, R. R.: Physiol. Rev., *31:*285, 1951.
313. Stern, T. N., Cole, V. V., Bass, A. C., and Overman, R. R.: Am. J. Physiol., *164:* 437, 1951.
314. Hills, A. G., Chalmers, T. M., Werster, G. D., Jr., and Rosenthal, O.: J. Clin. Invest., *32:*1236, 1953.
315. Peters, J. P., Wakeman, A. M., and Lee, C.: J. Clin. Invest., *6:*551, 1928–29.
316. Thorn, G. W., Koepf, G. F., and Clinton, M., Jr.: New England J. Med., *231:*76, 1944.
317. Sawyer, W. H. and Solez, C.: New England J. Med., *240:*210, 1949.
318. Hayman, J. M., Jr., Shumway, N. P., Dumke, P., and Miller, M.: J. Clin. Invest., *18:*195, 1939.
319. Platt, R.: Lancet, *1:*1239, 1951.
320. Platt, R., Roscoe, M. H., and Smith, F. W.: Clin. Sc., *11:*217, 1952.
321. Platt, R.: Brit. M. J., *1:*1313, 1372, 1952.
322. Nowaczyuski, W., Sander, T., Koiw, E., and Genest, J.: Endoc. Soc. Abstract, 1957, p. 17.
323. Welt, L. G.: Arch. Int. Med., *89:*931, 1952.
324. Fishman, A. P., Turino, G. M., and Bergofsky, E. H.: Am. J. Med., *23:*333, 1957.
325. Elkinton, J. R., Singer, R. B., Barker, E. S., and Clark, J. K.: Fed. Proc., *12:*120, 1953.
326. Dorman, P. J., Sullivan, W. J., and Pitts, R. F.: J. Clin. Invest., *33:*82, 1954.
327. Sullivan, W. J. and Dorman, P. J.: J. Clin. Invest., *34:*268, 1955.
328. Lovejoy, F. W., Yu, P. N. G., Nye, R. E., Jr., Joos, H. A., and Simpson, J. H.: Am. J. Med., *16:*4, 1954.
329. Westlake, E. K., Simpson, T., and Kaye, M.: Quart. J. Med., *24:*155, 1955.
330. Sieker, H. O. and Hickam, J. B.: Medicine, *35:*389, 1956.
331. Boutourline-Young, H. J. and Whittenberger, J. L.: J. Clin. Invest., *30:*838, 1951.
332. Galdston, M.: Am. J. Med., *19:*516, 1955.
333. Alexander, J. K., Spatter, H. F., and West, J. R.: J. Clin. Invest., *34:*533, 1955.
334. Tenney, S. M. and Miller, R. M.: Am. J. Med., *19:*498, 1955.
335. Wegria, R., Capeci, N., Kiss, G., Glaviano, V. V., Keating, J. H., and Hilton, J. G.: Am. J. Med., *19:*509, 1955.
336. Goldman, R. and Bassett, S. H.: J. Clin. Invest., *33:*1623, 1954.
337. Albright, F., Burnett, C. H., Parson, W., Reifenstein, E. C., Jr., and Roos, A.: Medicine, *25:*399, 1946.
338. Pines, K. L. and Mudge, G. H.: Am. J. Med., *11:*302, 1951.
339. Foss, G. L., Perry, C. B., and Wood, F. J. Y.: Quart. J. Med., *25:*185, 1956.
340. Wilansky, D. L. and Schneiderman, C.: New England J. Med., *257:*399, 1957.
341. Mahler, R. F. and Stanbury, S. W.: Quart. J. Med., *25:*21, 1956.
342. Conn, J. W.: J. Lab. & Clin. Med., *45:*6, 1955.
343. Conn, J. W.: Arch. Int. Med., *97:*135, 1956.
344. Hewlett, J. S., McCullagh, E. P., Farrell, G. L., Duston, H. P., Poutasse, E. F., and Proudfit, W. L.: J.A.M.A., *164:*719, 1957.
345. Vanamee, P., Poppell, J. W., Glicksman, A. S., Randall, H. T., and Roberts, K. E.: Arch. Int. Med., *97:*762, 1956.
346. Lewis, B. I.: Ann. Int. Med., *38:*918, 1953.
347. Rice, R. L.: Am. J. Med., *8:*691, 1950.
348. Sanderson, P. H.: The Kidney. In Ciba Foundation Symposium. Boston, Little, Brown and Company, 1954, p. 165.
349. Singer, R. B., Deering, R. C., and Clark, J. K.: J. Clin. Invest., *35:*245, 1956.
350. Holliday, M. A.: J. Clin. Invest., *34:*428, 1955.
351. Darrow, D. C.: J. Clin. Invest., *25:*324, 1946.
352. Cooke, R. E., Segar, W. E., Cheek, D. B., Coville, F. E., and Darrow, D. C.: J. Clin. Invest., *31:*798, 1952.
353. Cooke, R. E. and Segar, W. E.: Yale J. Biol. & Med., *25:*83, 1952–53.
354. Scribner, B. H. and Burnell, J. M.: Metabolism, *5:*468, 1956.
355. Gamble, J. L. and Ross, S. G.: J. Clin. Invest., *1:*403, 1924–25.
356. Burnett, C. H., Burrows, B. A., and Commons, R. R.: J. Clin. Invest., *29:*169, 1950.
357. Burnett, C. H., Burrows, B. A., Commons, R. R., and Towery, B. T.: J. Clin. Invest., *29:*175, 1950.
358. Van Slyke, K. K. and Evans, E. I.: Ann. Surg., *126:*545, 1947.
359. Schwartz, W. B. and Wallace, W. M.: J. Clin. Invest., *30:*1089, 1951.
360. Axelrod, D. R. and Pitts, R. F.: J. Clin. Invest., *31:*171, 1952.
361. Weston, R. E., Escher, D. J. W., Grossman, J., and Leiter, L.: J. Clin. Invest., *31:*901, 1952.
362. Mudge, G. H. and Hardin, B.: J. Clin. Invest., *35:*155, 1956.
363. Schwartz, W. B. and Relman, A. S.: J. Clin. Invest., *32:*258, 1953.
364. Earle, D. P., Sherry, S., Eichna, L. W., and Conan, N. J.: Am. J. Med., *11:*283, 1951.
365. Seldin, D. W., Rector, F. C., Jr., Carter, N., and Copenhaver, J.: J. Clin. Invest., *33:*965, 1954.
366. Teabeaut, R., Engel, F. L., and Taylor, H.: J. Clin. Endocrinol., *10:*399, 1950.

367. Follis, R. H., Jr., Orent-Keiles, E., and McCollum, E. V.: Am. J. Path., *18:*29, 1942.
368. Darrow, D. C. and Miller, H. C.: J. Clin. Invest., *21:*601, 1942.
369. Kornberg, A. and Endicott, K. M.: Am. J. Physiol., *145:*291, 1946.
370. Gamble, A. H., Wiese, H. F., and Hansen, A. E.: Pediatrics, *1:*58, 1948.
371. Webster, D. R., Henriksen, H. W., and Currie, D. J.: Ann. Surg., *123:*779, 1950.
372. Smith, S. G., Black-Schaffer, B., and Lasater, T. E.: Arch. Path., *49:*185, 1950.
373. Levine, H. D., Merrill, J. P., and Somerville, W.: Circulation, *3:*889, 1951.
374. Henrikson, H. W.: Am. J. Physiol., *164:* 263, 1951.
375. Fuhrman, F. A.: Am. J. Physiol., *167:*314, 1951.
376. Streeten, D. H. P. and Williams, E. M. V.: J. Physiol., *118:*149, 1952.
377. Cohen, J., Schwartz, R., and Wallace, W. M.: Arch. Path., *54:*119, 1952.
378. Carone, F. A. and Cooke, R. E.: Am. J. Physiol., *172:*684, 1953.
379. Schwartz, W. B., Levine, H. D., and Relman, A. S.: Am. J. Med., *16:*395, 1954.
380. Fourman, P., McCance, R. A., and Parker, R. A.: Brit. J. Exper. Path., *37:*40, 1956.
381. Danowski, T. S., Elkinton, J. R., Burrows, B. A., and Winkler, A. W.: J. Clin. Invest., *27:*65, 1948.
382. Gass, H., Cherkasky, M., and Savitsky, N.: Medicine, *27:*105, 1948.
383. Ziegler, M. R. and McQuarrie, I.: Metabolism, *1:*116, 1952.
384. McArdle, B.: Brit. M. Bull., *12:*226, 1956.
385. Zierler, K. L. and Andres, R.: J. Clin. Invest., *36:*730, 1957.
386. Linden, M. A.: Ann. Int. Med., *43:*241, 1955.
387. Conn, J. W., Fajans, S. S., Louis, L. H., Streeten, D. H. P., and Johnson, R. D.: Lancet, *1:*802, 1957.
388. Preedy, J. R. K. and Aitken, E. H.: J. Clin. Invest., *35:*423, 430, 443, 1956.
389. Bartter, F. C.: Metabolism, *5:*369, 1956.
390. Eder, H. A., Lauson, H. D., Chinard, F. P., Grief, R. L., Cotzias, G. C., and Van Slyke, D. D.: J. Clin. Invest., *33:* 636, 1954.
391. Orloff, J., Welt, L. G., and Stowe, L.: J. Clin. Invest., *29:*770, 1950.
392. Peters, J. P.: New England J. Med., *239:* 353, 1948.
393. Edelman, I. S.: Metabolism, *5:*500, 1956.
394. Ralli, E. P., Robson, S. S., Clarke, D., and Hoagland, C. L.: J. Clin. Invest., *24:*316, 1945.
395. Chart, J. J., Gordon, E. S., Helmer, P., and LeSher, M.: J. Clin.: Invest., *35:* 254, 1956.
396. Crosby, R. C. and Cooney, E. A.: New England J. Med. *235:*581, 1946.
397. Parker, M. L. and Breckler, I. A.: J.A.M.A., *144:*1091, 1950.
398. Laragh, J. H., Van Dyke, H. B., Jacobson, J., Adamsons, K., Jr., and Engel, L.: J. Clin. Invest., *35:*897, 1956.
399. Prentice, T. C., Berlin, N. I., Hyde, G. M., Parsons, R. J., Lawrence, J. H., and Port, S.: J. Clin. Invest., *30:*1471, 1951.
400. Schreiber, S. S., Bauman, A., Yalow, R. S., and Berson, S. A.: J. Clin. Invest., *33:*578, 1954.
401. Samet, P., Fritts, H. W., Jr., Fishman, A. P., and Cournand, A.: Medicine, *36:*211, 1957.
402. Merrill, A. J.: Am. J. Med., *6:*357, 1949.
403. Stead, E. A., Jr.: Circulation, *3:*294, 1951.
404. Peters, J. P.: Am. J. Med., *12:*66, 1952.
405. Barger, A. C.: Metabolism, *5:*480, 1956.
406. Eichna, L. W., Farber, S. J., Berger, A. R., Earle, D. P., Rader, B., Pellegrino, E., Albert, R. E., Alexander, J. D., Taube, H., and Youngwirth, S.: J. Clin. Invest., *30:*1250, 1951.
407. Greenman, L., Peters, J. H., Mateer, F. M., and Danowski, T. S.: J. Clin. Invest., *30:*1027, 1951.
408. Danowski, T. S., Greenman, L., Peters, J. H., Mateer, F. M., Weigand, F. A., and Tarail, R.: Ann. Int. Med., *35:*529, 1951.
409. Callahan, E. J., III, Frank, N. R., Kraus, H., and Ellis, L. B.: Am. J. M. Sc., *223:*117, 1952.
410. Shemm, F. R.: Ann. Int. Med., *17:*952, 1942.
411. Gamble, J. L., Blackfan, K. D., and Hamilton, B.: J. Clin. Invest., *1:*359, 1924–25.
412. Pitts, R. F. and Sartorius, O. W.: J. Pharmacol. & Exper. Therap., *98:*161, 1950.
413. Relman, A. S., Leaf, A., and Schwartz, W. B.: New England J. Med., *250:* 800, 1954.
414. Ray, C. T. and Burch, G. E.: Circulation, *3:*926, 1951.
415. Brodsky, W. A. and Graubarth, H. N.: Am. J. Physiol., *172:*67, 1953.
416. Bresnick, E. and Abramson, J.: New England J. Med., *249:*681, 1953.
417. Calhoun, J. A. and Harrison, T. R.: J. Clin. Invest., *10:*139, 1931.
418. Burstein, S. G., Bennett, L. L., Payne, F. E., and Hopper, J., Jr.: Fed. Proc., *8:*20, 1949.
419. Cohen, B. M.: New England J. Med., *246:*225, 1952.
420. Zeeman, S., Hirsch, S., and Bellett, S.: Am. J. M. Sc., *227:*65, 1954.
421. Holland, W. C., Greig, M. E., and Dunn, C. E.: Am. J. Physiol., *176:*227, 1954.
422. Lown, B.: Advances Int. Med., *8:*125, 1956.

423. Luetscher, J. A., Deming, Q. B., Johnson, B. B., and Piel, C. F.: J.A.M.A., *153:*1236, 1953.
424. Lauson, H. D., Forman, C. W., McNamara, H., Mattar, G., and Barnett, H.: J. Clin. Invest., *33:*657, 1954.
425. Squire, J. R., Blainey, J. D., and Hardwicke, J.: Brit. M. Bull., *13:*43, 1957.
426. Wynn, V. and Rob, C. G.: Lancet, *1:*587, 1954.
427. Wynn, V.: Metabolism, *5:*490, 1956.
428. Javid, M., Settlage, P., and Monfore, T.: Surg. Forum, *7*, 1957.
429. Soloff, L. A. and Zatuchni, J.: J.A.M.A., *139:*1136, 1949.
430. Jaffe, H. L., Master, A. M., and Dorrance, W.: Am. J. M. Sc., *220:*60, 1950.
431. McLester, J. S. and Holley, H. L.: Ann. Int. Med., *36:*562, 1952.
432. Nelson, W. P., III, Rosenbaum, J. D., and Strauss, M. B.: J. Clin. Invest., *30:*738, 1951.
433. Laragh, J. H.: J. Clin. Invest., *33:*807, 1954.
434. Laragh, J. H. and Capeci, N. E.: Am. J. Physiol., *180:*539, 1955.
435. Peters, J. P., Eisenman, A. J., and Kydd, D. M.: Am. J. M. Sc., *185:*149, 1933.
436. Meroney, W. H. and Herndon, R. F.: J.A.M.A., *155:*877, 1954.
437. Grollman, A.: Acute Renal Failure. Springfield, Ill., Charles C Thomas, 1954.
438. Merrill, J. P.: The Treatment of Renal Failure. New York, Grune and Stratton, 1955.
439. Strauss, M. B. and Raisz, L. G.: Clinical Management of Renal Failure. American Lecture Series No. 284. Springfield, Ill., Charles C Thomas, 1956.
440. Robbins, E. D. and Angrist, A.: Ann. Int. Med., *31:*773, 1949.
441. Mandel, E. E. and Popper, H.: Arch. Path, *52:*1, 1951.
442. Mandel, E. E.: Am. J. Med., *13:*322, 1952.
443. Lauson, H. D., Bradley, S. E., and Cournand, A.: J. Clin. Invest., *23:*381, 1944.
444. Van Slyke, D. D.: Ann. Int. Med., *28:*701, 1948.
445. Maluf, N. S. R.: Ann. Surg., *130:*49, 1949.
446. Remington, J. W., Hamilton, W. F., Caddell, H. M., Boyd, G. H., Jr., and Hamilton, W. F., Jr.: Am. J. Physiol., *161:*106, 1950.
447. Remington, J. W., Hamilton, W. F., Boyd, G. H., Jr., Hamilton, W. F., Jr., and Caddell, H. M.: Am. J. Physiol., *161:*116, 1950.
448. Remington, J. W., Remington, R. E., and Caddell, H. M.: Am. J. Physiol., *170:*564, 1952.
449. Oliver, J., MacDowell, M., and Tracy, A.: J. Clin. Invest., *30:*1307, 1951.
450. Seldin, D. W.: Personal communication.
451. Meroney, W. H. and Rubini, M.: Personal communication.
452. de Wardener, H. E.: Lancet, *1:*580, 1955.
453. Brun, C., Crone, C., Davidsen, H. G., Fabricius, J., Hansen, A. T., Lassen, N. A., and Munck, O.: Proc. Soc. Exper. Biol. & Med., *91:*199, 1956.
454. Meroney, W. H., Arney, G. K., Segar, W. E., and Balch, H. H.: J. Clin. Invest., *36:*825, 1957.
455. McLean, F. C. and Hastings, A. B.: J. Biol. Chem., *108:*285, 1935.
456. Hopper, J., Jr., O'Connell, B. P., and Fluss, H. R.: Ann. Int. Med., *38:*935, 1953.
457. Harris, J. S., Young, W. G., Jr., and Sealy, W. C.: Am. J. Med., *16:*595, 1954.
458. Muirhead, E. E. and Grollman, A.: Am. J. Med., *10:*780, 1951.
459. Emerson, C. P.: Blood, *3:*363, 1948.
460. Loge, J. P., Lange, R. D., and Moore, C. V.: J. Clin. Invest., *29:*830, 1950.
461. Muirhead, E. E., Jones, F., Stirman, J. A., and Lesch, W.: Am. J. Physiol., *173:*371, 1953.
462. Bluemle, L. W., Jr., Potter, H. P., and Elkinton, J. R.: J. Clin. Invest., *35:*1094, 1956.
463. Elkinton, J. R., Clark, J. K., Squires, R. D., Bluemle, L. W., and Crosley, A. P.: Am. J. M. Sc., *220:*547, 1950.
464. Knowles, H. C., Jr. and Kaplan, S. A.: Arch. Int. Med., *92:*189, 1953.
465. Martin, G. J.: Ion Exchange and Absorption Agents in Medicine. Boston, Little, Brown and Co., 1955.
466. Kolff, W. J.: Arch. Int. Med., *94:*142, 1954.
467. Wilson, B., Reisman, D. D., and Moyer, C. A.: J. Urol., *66:*805, 1951.

CHAPTER 6

By TOM D. SPIES, ROBERT W. HILLMAN, SIDNEY Q. COHLAN, BENJAMIN KRAMER, ABRAM KANOF

Vitamins and Avitaminoses

INTRODUCTION

The achievements in the young and vigorous science of nutrition are among the most significant that have been made in modern medical science. We could not hope to list, let alone properly describe, the ramifications of recent knowledge about vitamins. Thirty years ago the picture was vastly different. Since then, dozens of vitamins have been identified, isolated, synthesized and manufactured. Vitamins are organic food substances which, in small quantities, are necessary for maintaining proper growth and continued health of the body. The amounts required are so ridiculously small that it is thought that vitamins act as catalysts or as building blocks to form catalysts in the body. Already a number have been shown to be essential in the systems that govern oxidation of carbohydrates, proteins and fats. The vitamins are frequently termed accessory food factors. In many instances they differ widely from one another in their chemical structure. The body cannot make these substances, yet it must have them. The word "vitamin" has reference to the fact that they are essential to life. The authors consider that every living cell requires these substances. We should be concerned with the day-to-day relation of these nutrients to the dynamics of the healthy cell.

In the specific treatment directed against vitamin deficiency diseases the changes effected following the administration of the indicated vitamin or vitamins are miraculous and their judicious use in practice has revolutionized medicine. Much less dramatic, but probably more widely indicated, would be the application of the principles of nutrition toward the prevention of deficiency diseases. No longer are there millions of persons who are ill and eventually die because of an insufficiency of vitamins, but continued prophylaxis requires determination and perseverance. The vitamins are necessary for health and vigor, and they have interrelationships with the minerals and other important elements of the dietary which are described in other sections of this book.

Following what has been learned about diet over the last twenty-five or thirty years, nutritionists have developed strains of rats which are in many ways superior to their ancestors; they are longer lived, heavier, more fertile and more energetic. Livestock producers have made practical application of this knowledge and now produce animals and fowls suitable for marketing in much shorter time than formerly was required. Many fathers and mothers are aware that the health and well being of their children have been greatly benefited by improved diets. The modern science of nutrition promises a great deal but it offers no hope of an elixir of life and no panacea. Because it is a fruitful science, it already constitutes one of the most fascinating chapters in the history of the practice of medicine and promises even more far-reaching results in the future. It is making many practitioners more receptive to lessons that come from other sciences as they watch patients near death become restored to health. In the day-to-day practice of medicine, not only do the patients given adequate nutritive therapy under controlled observation have a greatly shortened period of convalescence, but the response of the patient is equally dramatic when he is treated in the office or in the home.

In many instances we can attain and maintain a perfectly functioning body with the proper diet, but it is a fallacy to think that all patients can be treated by diet alone. The synthetic vitamins and other nutrients have a necessary place, too. Some contemporaries worry that these synthetic substances will lead to economic disturbances and agricultural problems and thus will affect health adversely. The concern should be that there are substances yet to be isolated and that better methods of synthesis are yet to be perfected.

There is a logical basis for including adequate amounts of a variety of vitamins in a single therapeutic or preventive preparation, and there is an underlying unity of purpose in so doing. The vitamins occur together in varying amounts in nature, and the progress of medicine will advance significantly as more physicians realize that deficiency diseases occur as mixtures or complexities and not as single entities. Clinical, laboratory and dietary studies all indicate that the specific deficiency syndromes are interrelated and associated with a disturbance of general biochemical systems of our bodies. We do not recommend the treatment of a patient with a vitamin deficiency disease by means of a single chemical substance. Figure 1 gives some of the interrelationships between the vitamins; it should be helpful in indicating that it is humanly impossible to get a patient well when he is not given those necessary substances for his cellular life. So far as is feasible, we have written about the various vitamins in this chapter as separate units. We do this for ease of description only. Theories have been discussed with as little prejudice as strong personal opinion allows.

VITAMIN E

When compared to the other vitamins, vitamin E assumes a rather unimportant position since it has never been demonstrated that a deficiency of this substance occurs in man. As early as 1922 the necessity for this factor (then called "factor X") was recognized in animals, and in spite of a host of brilliant chemical and physiologic discoveries, attempts at clinical application of this knowledge have resulted only in controversy.

Chemistry

The formula for *alpha tocopherol* was proposed by Fernholz on the basis of oxidative degradation with chromic acid. Synthesis was later accomplished independently in three laboratories. At the present time three antisterility factors have been isolated from natural material, namely, alpha, beta and gamma tocopherols (Fig. 2).

Beta tocopherol and gamma tocopherol, which are homologues of the natural substance, have almost identical properties but slightly less biologic activity. These substances are readily soluble in lipid solvents but only slightly soluble in water. Although stable at high temperature (200° C.) they rapidly lose their activity in the presence of ultraviolet light or mild oxidizing agents. The long recognized resistance to rancidity of vegetable oil that contains vitamin E might be cited as an everyday example of its oxidation inhibiting quality. The antioxidation activity of vitamin E is perhaps one of its most striking chemical properties. It has been shown that body fat from the carcasses of vitamin E-deficient rats is abnormally susceptible to oxidation, and that the fat can be stabilized by doses of tocopherol. Stemming from this, another action of

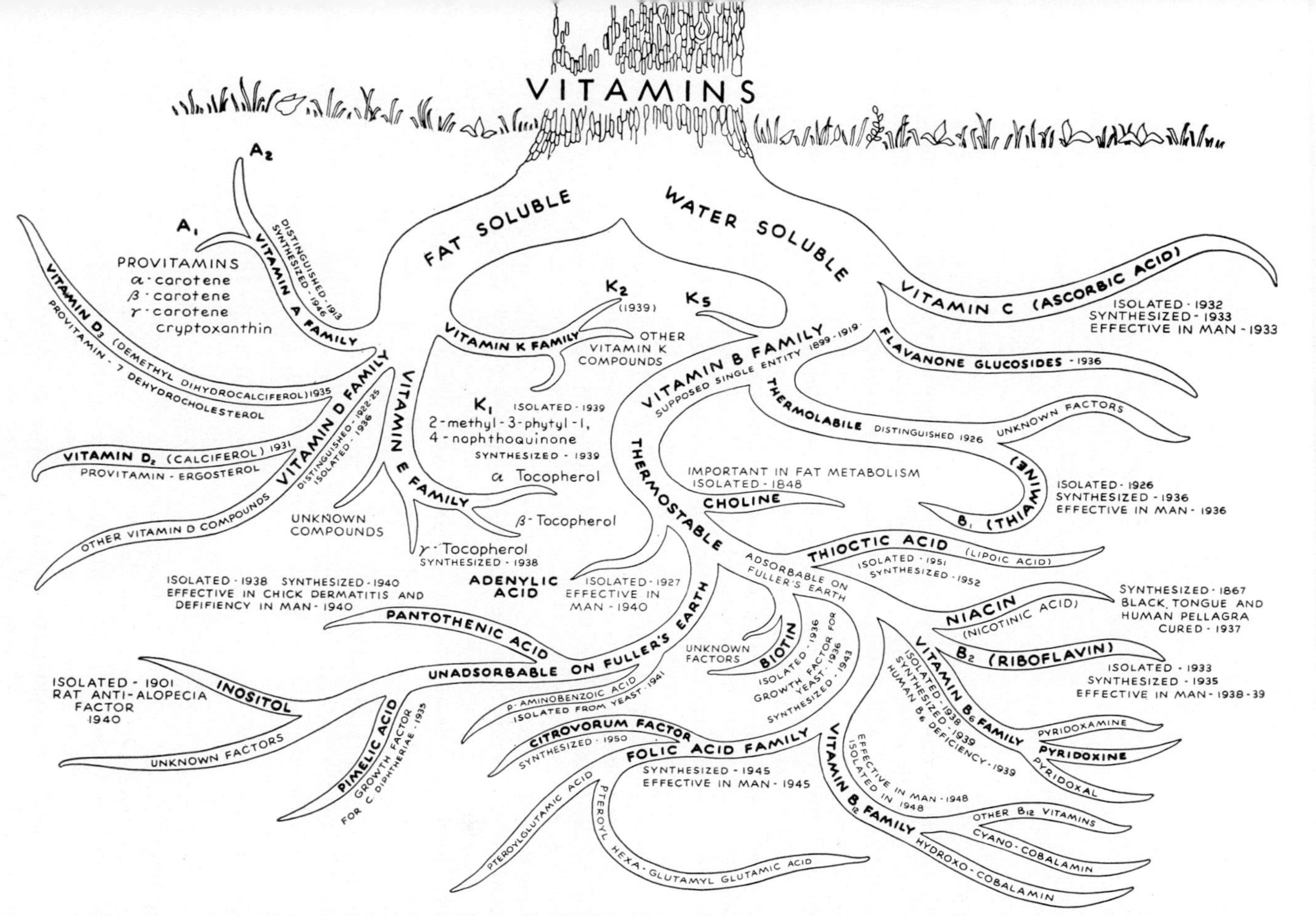

FIG. 1. This diagram portrays most of the known vitamins and many of the undifferentiated compounds with vitamin-like activities. They have, in this diagram, been separated rather arbitrarily on the basis of physiologic, physical and chemical properties. Most of the formulas of the compounds are shown in the text.

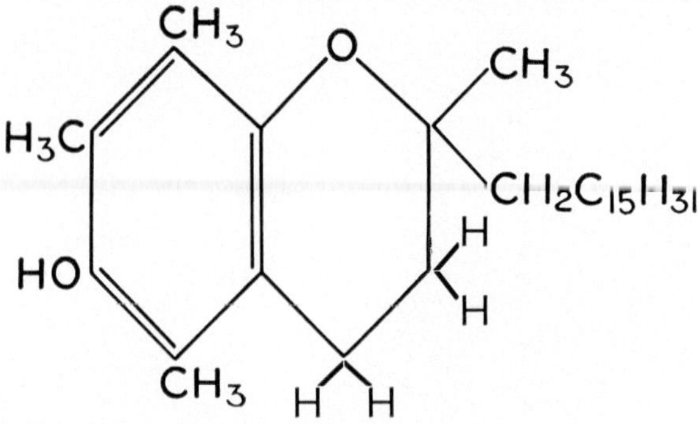

FIG. 2. Structural formula of alpha tocopherol.

vitamin E seems to be its protection of vitamin A and carotene from oxidation, in both the alimentary tract and the cells. It is likewise this antioxidation activity which has led investigators to postulate the possible role of vitamin E as a *respiratory enzyme* in the living organism.

Whereas most vitamins require a rather specific structure for their activity, of the 130 compounds tested, more than forty exhibit vitamin E activity but they do so in limited fashion when compared to tocopherol. The tocopherols themselves have a certain structural specificity and the removal of a methyl group from the aromatic nucleus or the aliphatic side chain greatly diminishes the E activity of these substances. The acetate of tocopherol is equal in biologic activity and possesses the added advantage of increased stability over tocopherol. Several methods exist for the chemical and biologic estimation of vitamin E but these are of little importance to the clinician.

Physiology and Pathology

In animals a lack of vitamin E manifests itself chiefly by changes in the reproductive mechanism; it was from this observation that the terms "antisterility vitamin" and "reproductive vitamin" were derived. This would appear to be a rather unfortunate choice since vitamin E has never been shown to bring about reproductive ability in cases of primary sterility. In the presence of vitamin E deficiency, conception occurs in the female rat but it is followed by "resorptive sterility." In the male rat degeneration of the germinal epithelium and spermatozoa develops to the point of complete loss of reproductive power.

In the absence of vitamin E in the diet of animals, muscular dystrophy and a characteristic paralysis of the hind quarters have been shown to develop. The relation of these disorders to human muscular dystrophy is by no means clear although some investigators claim that the microscopic changes in the muscles are indistinguishable in the two conditions. Vitamin E appears to be intimately related to growth, but to advance a theory for a vitamin as a growth factor has become almost trite. The possible relation of vitamin E to the glands of internal secretion has stimulated a great amount of experimental work but results are completely controversial. This is likewise the state of our knowledge regarding vitamin E in the occurrence and growth of tumors.

Clinical Use

One is impressed with the almost complete futility of attempting to arrive at any justifiable recommendations as to the effect of vitamin E on habitual abortions, abruptio placenta and other diseases of the reproductive system. Likewise, a cursory appraisal of the literature may lead some physicians to believe that vitamin E is useful in the treatment of myoneurogenic and cardiac disorders, but these recommendations are confusing and do not stand up well when rigid experimental conditions obtain.

A recent statement concerning the clinical manifestations of vitamin E deficiency in man and lower animals has been summarized by the Food and Nutrition Board of the National Research Council as follows:

"Tocopherol deficiency produces a variety of pathological findings in laboratory animals, including the Rhesus monkey, and in domesticated animals. Many of the effects, including inhibition of unsaturated fatty acid oxidation, are attributed to its properties as an intracellular anti-oxidant. A more specific action may exist, as for example in the enzymatic reduction of cytochrome c by reduced diphosphopyridine-nucleotide.

"Low tocopherol concentrations in tissues and blood and increased susceptibility of erythrocytes to hemolysis by hydrogen peroxide indicate the presence of a "physiologic" E deficiency state in newborn infants and a "conditioned" deficiency in infants, children, and adults with defective absorption of fat. The deficiency in newborn infants is self-limited, since breast feeding leads to a prompt rise in serum tocopherol and a reversal of the in vitro hemolysis. Artificial feeding with cow's milk is less effective, because of its lower tocopherol concentration. In physically normal adults, appreciable degrees of erythrocyte hemolysis and depression of plasma tocopherol have occurred only after 12 to 22 months on a daily diet containing approximately 2 milligrams d-alpha tocopherol daily. Tissue tocopherol levels are appreciably lower in children, adolescents, and young adults succumbing to various illnesses than in those whose deaths are accidental. The estimated daily adult per capita consumption of vitamin E has been estimated for one population group in the U.S.A. as 14 milligrams of d-alpha tocopherol.

"Although no clinical or physiologic correlates of the low levels of serum tocopherol in humans have been reported, the reversal of creatinuria following tocopherol administration to patients with absorptive defects and the finding of lesions similar to those of nutritional muscular dystrophy and of ceroid pigment in such patients suggest that vitamin E probably plays a role in human nutrition. However, no recommended allowances can be made from present information."

Requirements and Sources

As might be construed from what has already been observed in regard to vitamin E, the human requirements are unknown. Apparently vitamin E occurs in most foods; it is noteworthy that one of the greatest obstacles which investigators encountered was in obtaining a diet deficient in this vitamin. Wheat-germ oil is the richest source of vitamin E but it also is found in considerable amounts in cotton seed oil, lettuce oil, rice-germ oil and other seed-germ oils.

Various authors have used wheat-germ oil in doses varying from 0.25 to 6 cc. daily, and it may be of significance that any apparent success was the same in spite of any variation in dose. No toxic reactions have been reported in cases in which small doses were administered, and large doses of wheat-germ oil have given rise to only minor symptoms. The danger of production of neoplasms appears to be nonexistent.

References

American Medical Association Council on Pharmacy and Chemistry: The Treatment of Habitual Abortion with Vitamin E: J. A. M. A., *114:*2213–2218, 1940.

Dam, H.: Pharmacol. Rev., *9:*1, 1957.

Dinning, J. S. and Day, P. L.: J. Exper. Med., *105:*395, 1957.

Evans, H. M.: The William Henry Welch lectures, I. New Light on the Biological Role of Vitamin E.: J. Mt. Sinai Hosp., *6:*233–244, 1940.

György, P., Cogan, C. and Rose, C. S.: Proc. Soc. Exper. Biol. & Med., *81:*536, 1956.

Harris, P. L., Quaife, M. L. and O'Grady, P.: J. Nutrition, *46:*459, 1952.

Howritt, M. K., Harvey, C. C., Duncan, G. D., and Wilson, W. C.: Am. J. Clin. Nutrition, *4:*408, 1956.

MacKenzie, G.: In Herriott, R. M. (editor): Symposium on Nutrition. Baltimore, Johns Hopkins Press, 1953, p. 136.

Nason, A. and Lehman, I. R.: J. Biol. Chem., *222:*511, 1956.

National Research Council Publications: Nutrient Requirements for Domestic Animals, No. I (Poultry), III (Dairy Cattle), V (Sheep), VII (Foxes and Minks), VIII (Dogs), and IX (Rabbits).

Nitowsky, H. M., Cornblath, M. and Gordon, H. H.: Am. J. Dis Child., *92*:164, 1956.

Smith, L. I.: The Chemistry of Vitamin E.: Chem. Rev. *27*:287–329, 1940.

VITAMIN K

To observe certain patients bleed to death in spite of all known forms of treatment has been the unhappy experience of physicians and surgeons for many generations. This experience in the past was most common among patients who had jaundice and who underwent some surgical operation. It was fairly common, however, among patients who had surgical treatment for various intestinal disorders, and fatal hemorrhage in the newborn infant has been a sad experience of many physicians from time immemorial. All these instances of death were unusually shocking because the physician had no satisfactory form of treatment—the cause was unknown. It is pleasant and gratifying to know that most of these perplexing problems have been solved. These advances have been brought about by the isolation, synthesis and clinical application of vitamin K.

The introduction of vitamin K in clinical medicine came as a result of the observation of Dam and his associates of Copenhagen, Denmark. They showed that a deficiency disease could be produced in chicks by a diet washed in ether and could be cured by the administration of an antihemorrhagic material present in hog liver fat, hemp seed, and certain cereals and vegetables. It was shown by these investigators that deficiency in this dietary factor resulted in diminution in the amount of prothrombin in the circulating blood which led to a fatal hemorrhagic diathesis. The term vitamin K was proposed by Dam as an abbreviation of the name "Koagulations vitamin" to apply to the substance that was necessary for the prevention of a nutritional deficiency disease in chicks. Soon it was suggested by Quick of this country that deficiency in vitamin K might be present in patients who had obstructive jaundice, and it was demonstrated by Butt and his associates that a deficiency of prothrombin did exist in the blood of patients who had obstructive jaundice. These suggestions have now been amply confirmed and extended, and within a relatively short time various workers in this country and abroad have demonstrated that vitamin K under most circumstances is a specific remedy for deficiency of prothrombin.

Chemistry

In early attempts at isolation of vitamin K, concentrates of alfalfa, rich in the vitamin, were employed. Several attempts were made to crystallize the vitamin from these potent but impure concentrates but it was not until the spring of 1939 that it became apparent that more than one compound possesses vitamin K activity. From alfalfa was isolated a compound called vitamin K_1, and from putrefied fish meal a compound called vitamin K_2.

It was suggested by MacCorquodale and McKee that vitamin K_1 has a quinoid structure. For the final isolation and synthesis of vitamin K_1, Doisy and his associates, Almquist and Klose, and Fieser and his associates are responsible. Experiments from their laboratories demonstrated conclusively that the structure of vitamin K_1 is represented correctly by the formula 2-methyl-3-phytyl-1,4-naphthoquinone (Fig. 3). This vitamin is identical with 2-methyl-1,4-naphthoquinone with the exception that vitamin K_1 has a phytyl side chain in the three position; the synthetic product also is identical with natural vitamin K_1 which is obtained from alfalfa. Exposure to sunlight destroys the vitamin activity of alfalfa within several hours, although if artificial light is used little destruction is observed within twenty-four hours. The pure preparations, however, are destroyed by both sunlight and artificial light. A large part of the activity of concentrates of vitamin K is destroyed by alkali, by strong acids and by aluminum chloride. The vitamin is fat soluble and at low temperatures forms yellow crystals.

Vitamin K_2 was first isolated from putrefied fish meal. The empiric formula, $C_{41}H_{60}O_2$, has been proposed to represent its structure. Available data indicate that the structure may be 2,3-difarnesyl-1,4-naphthoquinone. This compound is also oil-soluble and has been obtained as light yellow, crystalline flakes. Its potency is found to be about 60 per cent of that of vitamin K_1.

After it was demonstrated that vitamin K is of a quinoid structure a large number of investigators began to study the known substances which possess a quinoid nucleus. It was first reported by Almquist and Klose that *phthiocol* (2-methyl-3-hydroxy-1,4-naphthoquinone) possesses physical and chemical properties similar to those of pure vitamin K and also possesses marked antihemorrhagic activity. Phthiocol is the yellow pigment found in the human tubercle bacillus. Many other derivatives of naphthoquinone have since been investigated and of all of these studied *2-methyl-1,4-naphthoquinone* has proved to possess the most marked antihemorrhagic activity. It is thought that this synthetic compound is even more active than vitamin K_1 itself. This material is very slightly soluble in water. In solution its activity is impaired by sterilization with steam; therefore, it is rather unstable unless special precautions are taken. This compound is so active that several investigators have suggested that it be adopted as a basic standard for assay of vitamin K. Total synthesis of vitamin K_1 through condensation of 2-methyl-1,4-naphthohydroquinone with synthetic isophytol in the presence of boron trifluoride-diethyl ether has been achieved by Isler and Doebel. Identity with the natural product in chemical configuration and biologic activity was adequately demonstrated.

Many other compounds have been tested for vitamin K activity. Most of those which have such activity are basically 1,4-naphthoquinone or the corresponding hydroquinone; a few, however, are not. The compounds, 4-amino-2-methyl-1-naphthol hydrochloride and 2-methyl-1,4-naphthohydroquinone-3-sodium sulfonate, are both water soluble and, therefore, have proved of considerable use clinically. These compounds are not as active as 2-methyl-1,4-naphthoquinone but they are active enough to produce desired clinical results. Both of these compounds, are now available commercially.

Recently, Isler and associates reported on the synthesis and action of 24 compounds related to vitamin K_1 against coumarin derivatives. These compounds were similar in structure except for the nature of the substituent in position three. Activity was measured by prothrombin time and rat survival time. The activity varied with the type of animal and coumarin derivative. Methyl branching and double bonds in the side chain promoted activity but were not essential. Derivatives with less than eight carbon atoms in the side chain were inactive. Vitamin K_1 showed full activity in all tests.

Physiology

Pure vitamin K has not been available long enough to allow complete knowledge of its physiologic action to be collected. Unlike some of the water soluble

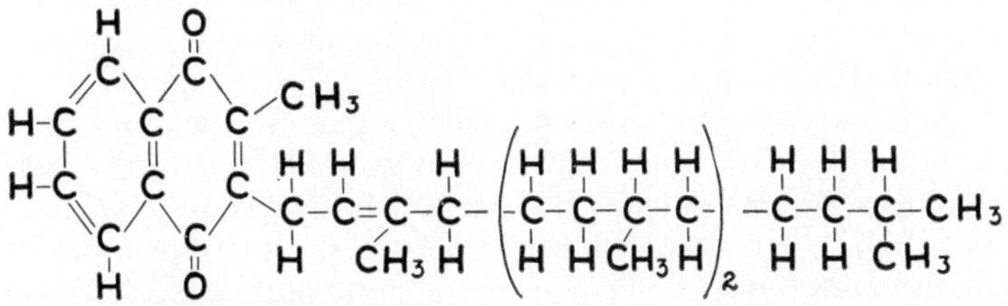

FIG. 3. The structural formula of vitamin K_1 (2-methyl-3-phytyl-1,4-naphthoquinone).

vitamins, little is known of the relation of vitamin K to the enzyme systems or to cell respiration, but it is known that it is associated intimately in some way with the integrity of the hepatic parenchyma and with the metabolism of prothrombin.

Absorption. Many investigators have shown that the presence of bile in the intestinal tract is essential for proper absorption of the fat soluble vitamin K, and there is furthermore some evidence to suggest that these fat soluble compounds are absorbed better if other fats are present in the intestinal tract. Clinically it is well established that the presence of bile, or more correctly the presence of adequate amounts of bile salts, is required for the proper absorption of vitamin K. The exact point of absorption in the intestinal tract is not known, but our own experience indicates that concentrates of vitamin K are not absorbed through the colon or upper part of the ileum but they are absorbed readily through the upper part of the small intestine.

Storage. The vitamin is not stored readily in the body, but it has been found in the livers of lower animals in relatively small amounts. Greaves has shown that in the liver of the rat vitamin K is not stored in appreciable quantities. In studies of the fate of vitamin K_1 injected as an aqueous dispersion into chicks and rats, Dam and associates found that approximately 70 per cent was recoverable in the liver and spleen and 1 per cent in the kidneys and lungs. None was found in the bile. Only traces were still in the blood 14 hours after intravenous injection. Ingestion of coumachlor, an anticoagulant, did not appear to affect the deposition of vitamin K. Only small amounts were found in the organs after oral or intramuscular administration. Partial blockage of the reticulo-endothelial system in chicks by India ink decreased the deposition of injected vitamin K_1 in the liver with a concurrent increase in the spleen. No vitamin K was found in the placenta, fetus or newborn young when a massive dose was injected intravenously in pregnant rats. Clinical work would indicate that the same observations are applicable in the human being.

Excretion. Insofar as is known vitamin K is not present in the urine. In 1954 it was reported that 2-methyl-C^{14}-1,4-naphthoquinone given in doses up to 11 mg. per Kg. to rats and guinea pigs is excreted in the urine chiefly as the diglucuronide, partly as the monosulfate, and also as an unidentified derivative. It can be demonstrated in the feces but whether it is there because the feces hold the organisms which are known to contain vitamin K or whether the presence of the vitamin in feces is referable to real excretion of vitamin K remains to be established. The vitamin is not present in human bile collected under sterile conditions. In chicks on a normal diet the spleen, red muscle, gizzard, bone marrow, and pancreas were found to contain relatively large amounts of vitamin K while the liver and lungs were found to contain somewhat less.

Metabolism. Little is really known of the metabolism of vitamin K but it might be assumed that it is absorbed as a bile acid compound. What happens when it enters the blood stream is not yet known. Some have suggested that the compound is carried as a prosthetic group with the prothrombin molecule and others have suggested that vitamin K acts in some capacity in the formation of prothrombin, but all of this is hypothetical. That proper response to vitamin K depends upon the integrity of the hepatic parenchyma is now a well established fact. More recently, Henrik Dam and Quick and their associates have extended studies which show more clearly the role of vitamin K in blood coagulation. This is a complicated subject, and the reader is referred to a clinical review of the problem in the *Nutrition Reviews,* vol. 9, February, 1951.

Insofar as is known at the present time, vitamin K has no relation to immunity, infection, pregnancy and lactation, the nervous system, gastrointestinal tract, or cardiovascular system, but it is intimately associated with normal physiologic function of the liver and with proper coagulation of the blood. Its exact role in blood coagulation is not known. It is known to be necessary for proper formation of prothrombin, but in what manner this is accomplished remains to be determined. A deficiency of vitamin K from any cause produces a deficiency of prothrombin in the circulating blood, and in all instances except those in which there is severe hepatic damage this deficiency of prothrombin can be corrected by the proper administration of vitamin K.

Effect of Deficiency of Vitamin K

In Animals. In chicks fed on a diet deficient in vitamin K there develop subcutaneous, intramuscular and internal hemorrhages, profuse bleeding from minor abrasions, and a delayed clotting time associated with a low level of plasma prothrombin. Injuries in a wide sense may determine the occurrence and severity of these hemorrhages. Studies of the plasma prothrombin level in hemorrhagic chick disease by many investigators show that hemorrhages do not occur until the level of prothrombin has declined to about 10 to 15 per cent of normal. It has been indicated that the clotting time is delayed only if the prothrombin level has declined to less than 30 to 40 per cent of normal. Thus, early in the course of the disease when deficiency of the vitamin is less severe, the level of plasma prothrombin may be reduced considerably and yet the clotting time will remain normal. This is extremely important as a clinical factor. Determinations of the plasma prothrombin are essential if any but the more severe grades of deficiency are to be detected. Deficiency of prothrombin has also been produced in rats, mice, ducklings, young geese, pigeons, canaries and rabbits that were fed diets deficient in vitamin K.

It has been long known that in dogs which have biliary fistulas, in addition to many pathologic complications, an abnormal tendency to bleed also develops. Furthermore, it has been pointed out that continuous subsequent feeding of bile to such animals will correct this abnormality. This tendency of dogs which have biliary fistulas toward bleeding was shown later to be caused by deficiency of prothrombin which could be corrected by the administration of vitamin K. In rats which have renal biliary fistulas there is likewise a diminution in the circulating prothrombin which can be corrected by the administration of vitamin K.

In Man. Inadequate Diet. The production of a diminished level of prothrombin in the circulating blood of man resulting from inadequate intake of vitamin K has never been accomplished. However, several cases of scurvy, chronic alcoholism, pellagra or a combination of the three have been reported in which there was a significant decrease in the level of plasma prothrombin. It is assumed that this resulted from the simple nutritional deficiency of vitamin K. These decreased levels of prothrombin were increased following the administration of vitamin K. This work remains to be adequately confirmed.

Biliary Fistula. Clinically it is well known that among patients who have chronic biliary fistulas an abnormal tendency to bleed sometimes develops. It has been demonstrated that in these instances there is an associated deficiency of prothrombin in the circulating blood which can be corrected by the administration of vitamin K.

Obstructive Jaundice. It is now well established that the absence of bile from the intestinal tract of man from any cause is capable of producing a deficiency of prothrombin in the circulating blood which is corrected by the administration of vitamin K, provided that there is an intact hepatic parenchyma. This work also has been confirmed adequately by experiments on animals.

Intestinal Lesions. It is obvious that normal absorption of a fat soluble material from the intestine cannot take place unless an adequate and physiologically intact intestinal surface is available, that an adequate dietary intake of vitamin K and the presence of bile in

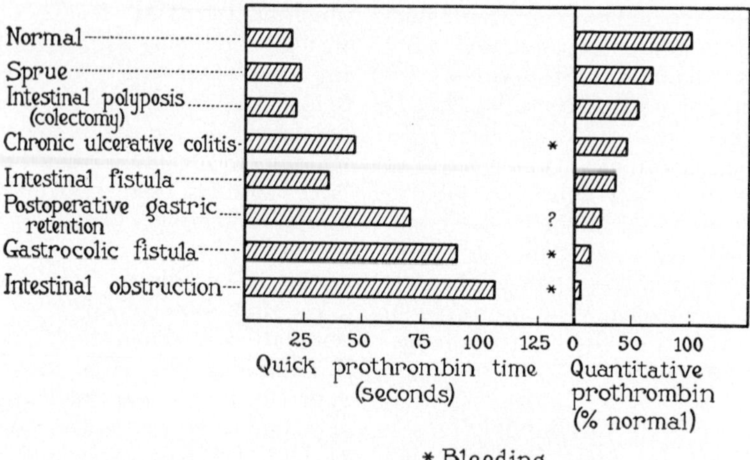

FIG. 4. The various intestinal disorders with which may be associated a deficiency of prothrombin which is readily corrected by the proper administration of compounds with vitamin K activity. (Butt and Snell, *Vitamin K.*)

the intestinal tract are prerequisites to the proper metabolism of vitamin K, and that both factors may be altered seriously by various intestinal disorders. Many persons, because of the disease from which they suffer, have been compelled to remain on limited diets. For others it is necessary to withhold food and to establish intestinal intubation in order to control symptoms of obstruction. Profuse discharge from ileac stomas further complicates the situation in many other cases. All patients, however, may be affected by both morphologic and functional disturbances involving the small intestine. However, a number of patients who have had anorexia and nervous vomiting have been studied and the plasma was not strikingly deficient in prothrombin. A previously deficient diet, continued vomiting or diarrhea, however, may lay the groundwork for a deficiency state in respect to vitamin K, but some other factor such as an abdominal operation may be required for its precipitation. Under such circumstances adequate amounts of vitamin K may not be absorbed, and in various intestinal disorders, such as sprue, chronic diarrhea, short-circuiting operation of the small and large intestine, and intestinal obstruction, deficiency of vitamin K and subsequent development of deficiency of prothrombin may ensue (Fig. 4).

NEWBORN INFANTS. During the first few days of an infant's life some deficiency of prothrombin in the circulating blood apparently exists. The cause of this deficiency is debated. It has been suggested by many that lack of a reserve of prothrombin in the blood of the newborn infant is the result of a deficiency of vitamin K, since a normal level of prothrombin can be restored by the parenteral administration to the infant of a concentrate of the vitamin or by the oral administration of this accessory food substance. Others believe that in the blood of the normal infant a moderate deficiency of vitamin K develops during the first few days of life and that it arises from an insufficient supply of vitamin K from the intestine (Fig. 5). To explain the return of the value of prothrombin to normal by the end of the third day it must be assumed that the infant after birth receives a supply of vitamin K which was not present at birth.

It has been suggested that as soon as the presence of bacterial flora of the intestinal tract is established the infant is capable of synthesizing vitamin K, a fact which is well proved experimentally. This explanation, however, does not explain the delay of four days in the return to normal of the value for prothrombin, a delay which occurs in many infants. A normal value is reached usually by the fifth day. To explain this phenomenon it must be recalled that the liver of the newborn infant is unable to secrete sufficient bile, that absorption of fat is very limited and that gastrointestinal hypermotility is the rule. Thus, even though vitamin K is present proper absorption of the vitamin is unlikely until the digestive function approaches normal. This occurs on about the third or fourth day of life. To support the suggestion that the presence of bacterial flora in the intestinal tract is intimately connected with the return of the value for prothrombin to normal at the end of the third day, some investigators have shown that extra feeding, started within two hours after delivery of the infant, can prevent the subsequent development of hypoprothrombinemia.

Hepatic Injury. By injury to the hepatic parenchyma, deficiency of prothrombin can be produced in both man and animal in the presence of adequate amounts of vitamin K. This result must be considered not as a deficiency of vitamin K but rather as a disruption of the organ which is responsible for proper metabolism of the substance known as prothrombin. Intoxication with chloroform produces in animals a marked deficiency of prothrombin and results in hemorrhagic diathesis. It has also been shown that injury of the liver by carbon tetrachloride produces a tendency to bleed and that this tendency is not corrected by the administration of vitamin K if hepatic damage has been too great. All these experimental facts have been well established clinically.

To recapitulate, it appears now well established that a deficiency of prothrombin can occur if certain animals are sustained on diets which are lacking in certain fat soluble substances, and that such a deficiency can occur in experimental animals which have external or renal biliary fistulas and in dogs of which the livers have been injured by chloroform. All these conditions are associated with a well-marked hemorrhagic tendency and it is interesting that in each, one or a combination of these conditions may exist: bile is excluded from the bowel, the liver is injured by toxic substances, or a state of nutritional deficiency exists. The probable relationship of a deficiency of vitamin K to a deficiency of prothrombin in

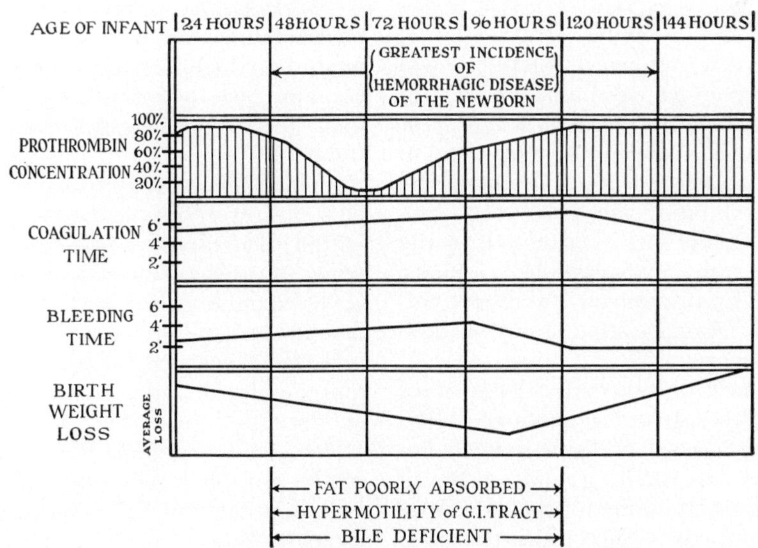

Fig. 5. A composite chart taken from the work of Grossman which shows the level of prothrombin in the circulating blood at birth and during the subsequent six days of life.

the plasma of dogs which have biliary fistulas or obstructive jaundice, or the plasma of human beings who have these conditions is reasonably clear, since bile acids are required for the normal absorption of fat soluble substances from the bowel and since, in the conditions mentioned, bile usually is excluded completely from the bowel. Two factors, therefore, the presence of bile in the bowel, and vitamin K, are known to be of importance in the maintenance of a normal concentration of prothrombin. A third and equally important factor is the liver; its importance in the synthesis of prothrombin already has been mentioned.

An important development associated with increased understanding of blood coagulation mechanism is the demonstration that the principal action of vitamin K and of anticoagulants is on the blood concentration of factor VII (proconvertin) rather than on that of prothrombin. Vitamin K has been found to have a beneficial effect on the blood concentration of factor VII in the newborn and in patients with obstructive jaundice. Details of the relation of vitamin K to the physiology, pharmacology and clinical significance of blood coagulation are given in the excellent papers of Koller and Jurgens.

Toxicity

Few serious untoward reactions have been observed in the human being receiving reasonable therapeutic doses of either natural concentrates of vitamin K, synthetic vitamin K_1 or quinone derivatives exhibiting antihemorrhagic activity. No effect has been noted on the blood pressure, respiration, capillary permeability or urinary excretion following the administration of any of these compounds.

It has been observed that large doses of 2-methyl-1,4-naphthoquinone (180 mg.) administered orally to human beings result in vomiting and porphyrinuria. A dose of 30 mg. of the substance per kg. of body weight injected intramuscularly into a dog caused vomiting, porphyrinuria and albuminuria. Others have noted that large doses of this compound administered to rats produced a decrease in the number of erythrocytes and in the quantity of hemoglobin. These doses, however, are obviously greater than those employed for therapeutic use in man, and to date no one has noted any untoward reaction in man after administration of reasonable therapeutic doses of any of these compounds.

Human Requirements

Distribution. Vitamin K is distributed widely in nature; among its richest sources are *green leaves* of different kinds. Alfalfa and spinach are very rich in it and cabbage, cauliflower, kale, carrot tops, chestnut leaves, soybean oil and seaweed are all good sources of this vitamin. Less potent are tomatoes, orange peel and hemp seed. Seeds, fruits and roots contain in general considerably less vitamin K than do green leaves of different kinds. The parts of the plant which contain chlorophyl usually have the largest amounts of vitamin K and because of this it was postulated early that vitamin K_1, like chlorophyl, probably would contain a phytyl group.

Vitamin K is found also in a number of *bacteria*. Apparently during the growth of the bacteria the vitamin K is synthesized and is retained within the bacteria since the filtrate of the culture medium which is free of the bacteria contains none of the vitamin. Dried human feces, both normal and acholic stools, are also rich in the vitamin but the vitamin K activity of feces undoubtedly results from the bacterial content within them. It is surprising that chicks when germ-free have been found to recover spontaneously from a vitamin K deficiency.

Nothing is known of the minimal requirements of vitamin K for infant, child, mother, or normal adult. This lack of knowledge undoubtedly will be corrected as soon as methods are developed by which vitamin K can be measured in biologic fluids.

Although minimal requirements for the normal person in respect to vitamin

K are still unknown, it is known that pure vitamin K_1 or synthetic compounds exhibiting vitamin K activity in doses of 1 to 2 mg. are capable of correcting deficiency of vitamin K in most instances. However, apparently depending on the degree of hepatic damage, this dose may have to be increased considerably in order to produce the desired result. It is known that diarrhea and inadequate intestinal absorptive surface will increase the need for vitamin K. Similar increased requirements are found in such diseases as sprue and celiac disease.

Assay Methods and Unitage

Like every new vitamin, vitamin K possesses numerous methods of assay and standards of unitage. There are primarily two methods of assay which have been employed to measure the antihemorrhagic activity of a given material. One method is known as the *preventive method.* In this, foodstuffs are assayed by rearing chicks for a month on a diet deficient in vitamin K and rearing other chicks for a like period on a diet in which test material has been incorporated. A protective action which these materials afforded is determined by measurement of the coagulation time of the blood of the chick. If the coagulation time of the blood of chicks fed the diet containing the test material is found to be shorter than that of the controls which had received unsupplemented rations the material assayed is said to contain vitamin K.

One of the other most favored methods, known as the *curative method,* is based on the observation that animals which suffer from deficiency of vitamin K become normal with reference to the clotting time of their blood within three days of their beginning to ingest sufficient food containing vitamin K. Other reliable assays have since been developed and with each new assay there has developed a standard of unitage. The subject of the correct unit to use is still controversial. Obviously there is considerable disagreement among the various investigators working in the same field as to the exact definition of a unit and the best method of assay. It has been suggested that 2-methyl-1,4-naphthoquinone be adopted as a standard of reference for vitamin K. Obviously this would greatly simplify the various and diversified systems now employed. One of the most commonly used unit systems at the present time is that developed by Thayer and his associates, in which 1 mg. of pure vitamin K_1 contains 1000 Thayer-Doisy units.

Methods of Measuring Deficiency of Prothrombin

To have a proper evaluation of hemorrhagic diatheses the reader must be conversant with at least the fundamental properties of blood and also with the current hypothesis by means of which attempts are made to explain the normal coagulation of blood. Suffice it to say here that present evidence indicates that the phenomenon of coagulation of blood involves two consecutive reactions: (1) the interaction of calcium, prothrombin and platelet (or tissue extract) to form thrombin and (2) the reaction of fibrinogen with thrombin to form fibrin.

Methods designed in the past for the measurement of the tendency of a jaundiced patient to bleed have been almost as uncertain as have been the conclusions derived from some of the older studies on the mechanism of bleeding. Most determinations of coagulation time and of bleeding time are of little or no value for determination of the potential danger of hemorrhages afflicting a patient who has jaundice. The usual methods employed for measurement of the ability of the blood to coagulate give little evidence of deviation from the normal until the patient is on the verge of experiencing hemorrhage. Several excellent methods for measuring deficiency of prothrombin in the blood of man have been described but the method developed by Quick and his associates has been found well adapted for general use in the clinical laboratory. This method as modified by Magath has proved in our hands to be very satisfactory. When the expressions "prothrombin time" or "prothrombin clotting time" are used subsequently they will refer to the clotting time of recalcified plasma to which optimal amounts of thromboplastin have been added as determined by the *method of Quick*. This method requires as much as 4.5 cc. of venous blood of the patient. The necessity of obtaining this much blood, particularly among premature infants, often is a real obstacle, especially if the tests are to be repeated at frequent intervals upon the same patient. For this reason several micromethods for the determination of prothrombin have been suggested.

It must be admitted that all the current methods for the estimation of prothrombin are of necessity indirect. However, certain of these methods of measuring prothrombin are the most nearly accurate methods available at present for estimation of a patient's tendency to bleed in the presence of a suspected deficiency of prothrombin. The information afforded by the measurement of prothrombin in the circulating blood is much more nearly accurate in the prediction of the tendency of a patient to bleed than is the measurement of the coagulation or bleeding time as formerly used in the consideration of such a tendency.

Diagnosis

Incidence and Manner of Bleeding. IN JAUNDICE. The bleeding of patients who have jaundice occurs most frequently after surgical intervention which was calculated to relieve biliary obstruction. Hemorrhage usually is noted between the first and fourth postoperative days but it may appear as late as the twelfth to eighteenth day after operation. As is well known, cholemic bleeding ordinarily begins as a slow oozing from the operative incision, from the gums or nose, or from the gastrointestinal tract. Often, however, the first evidence of hemorrhage is afforded by the appearance of severe hematemesis or melena. Such bleeding often is controlled temporarily by transfusions of whole blood, but all too frequently even repeated transfusions fail to control the hemorrhagic diathesis. Bleeding of this type apparently is invariably associated with prolongation of the prothrombin clotting time.

As is well known, bleeding of patients suffering from jaundice occurs most often in the presence of those conditions in which bile is excluded completely from the gastrointestinal tract. Those types of biliary obstruction in hepatic disease most commonly responsible for serious hemorrhage long have been familiar to the clinician and surgeon. Complete biliary obstruction produced by neoplasm of the pancreas, ampulla or gallbladder heads the list. Postoperative stricture of the common bile duct is accompanied perhaps by the second highest incidence of bleeding, and intermittent obstruction caused by the presence of stones comes third. Complete external fistulas are relatively rare but often are associated with bleeding. Bleeding is more likely to occur in those cases in which bile is excluded completely from the intestine, yet the physician must not overlook the fact that bleeding also can occur in the absence of jaundice if the liver has been injured considerably as the result of chronic cholecystic disease. Although the foregoing facts are somewhat useful for predicting whether or not a patient will bleed, the exceptions are so frequent that rigid clinical rules cannot be devised.

IN SEVERE HEPATIC DAMAGE. It has been well demonstrated experimentally that if the hepatic parenchyma is injured the amount of prothrombin in the circulating blood decreases. It has been further demonstrated by Warner and his associates and by Bollman and his associates that if the hepatic damage in these animals is too severe the level of prothrombin in the circulating blood does not rise after administration of vitamin K. It has been likewise well demonstrated clinically that patients who have severe hepatic damage have a decrease in the prothrombin in the circulating blood and that occasionally they will not respond to the administration of vitamin K.

Severe hepatic damage can occur in any disease in which the liver might be involved but most frequently it is seen in cases of cirrhosis of the liver, in those in which obstruction or stricture of the common duct has existed over long periods and in those in which there is acute or subacute atrophy of the liver resulting from some primary disease or associated with cholecystitis. Although this group of cases is somewhat small, it is well to remember that it does exist. It is true that, frequently, repeated doses of vitamin K are necessary in order to produce the desired effect, but when one has doubled or tripled the usual therapeutic dose of vitamin K without producing desired effects one can be fairly certain that, regardless of the amounts of vitamin K administered, there will be little elevation of the prothrombin in the circulating blood.

IN VARIOUS INTESTINAL DISORDERS. A deficiency of prothrombin as the cause of bleeding in patients who have various intestinal disorders is something new in clinical medicine, and although instances of deficiency of prothrombin referable to the effects of intestinal absorption are not often encountered, they do comprise a rather distinct group and one which bears further investigation. The pathologic physiology concerned in such cases has been described under the section on pathology. When patients who have extensive disease of the intestine, such as sprue, celiac disease, chronic ulcerative colitis, intestinal obstruction, multiple short-circuiting operations on the intestinal tract, ileitis, and so forth, experience hemorrhage, either before or after surgical treatment, deficiency in prothrombin should be recognized and corrected before other forms of treatment are instituted. The most important point in diagnosis of these conditions is for the surgeon and clinician to follow the prothrombin coagulation time closely in all cases of abnormalities of the intestinal mucosa or of interference with the continuity of the gastrointestinal tract and in cases in which the postoperative condition requires continued aspiration of gas and secretions from the intestinal tract. This practice has solved the mystery of obscure intestinal bleeding, which occurs frequently in such cases, and definitely has reduced postoperative morbidity and mortality.

OF INFANTS. The entire subject of bleeding in the newborn infant has been in a confused state chiefly because of the difficulty in a given situation of determining what is and what is not a real state of hemorrhagic diathesis. It is now well known that a deficiency of prothrombin in the circulating blood of infants is usually a physiologic occurrence. Many instances now have been reported of hemorrhagic disease of the newborn in which there was a deficiency of prothrombin and in which the bleeding was alleviated promptly by oral or parenteral administration of vitamin K. It also has been suggested that a deficiency of prothrombin existing at birth might account in many instances for those intracranial hemorrhages which frequently are associated with labor.

Value of the Prothrombin Clotting Time. Obviously, knowledge of the conditions in which deficiency of prothrombin may occur is fundamental for correct diagnosis of possible deficiency of vitamin K. Although the possibility of hemorrhagic diathesis may be suspected in a particular case, the measurement of the prothrombin content of the circulating blood is necessary for accurate diagnosis as well as to evaluate proper treatment. Present methods for measurement of the content of prothrombin in the circulating blood of patients are subject to considerable error. The decrease in the concentration of prothrombin in the circulating blood of man seems to depend on certain unknown individual factors. Although in certain instances the concentration of prothrombin in the blood apparently depends on the degree of hepatic injury, it certainly does not have any constant relationship to the type of hepatic or biliary disease present.

On the basis of the various studies of Smith and his associates it would appear

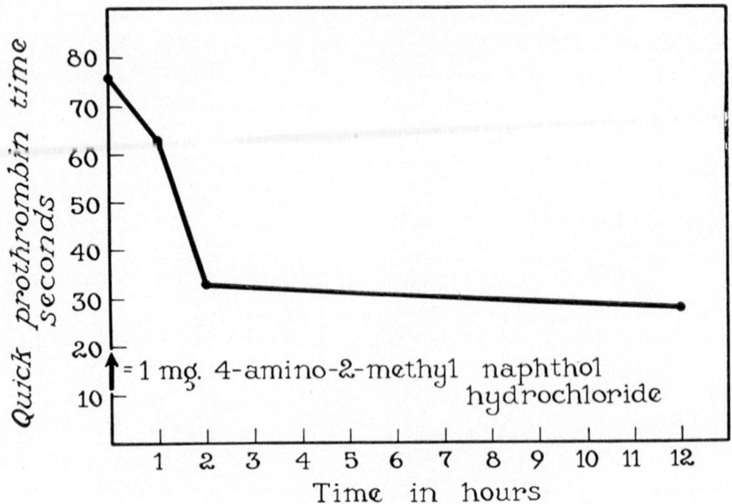

FIG. 6. The effect of the intravenous injection of 1 mg. of 4-amino-2-methyl-1-naphthol hydrochloride on the elevated prothrombin clotting time of a patient who had obstructive jaundice. (Butt and Snell, *Vitamin K.*)

that bleeding among animals in the experimental laboratory occurs when the value for prothrombin becomes less than 20 or 25 per cent of normal and that conversely so long as the value remains at about 20 or 25 per cent bleeding does not occur. If this conception is understood it is easy to see why in certain cases bleeding in man may occur postoperatively with little warning. Loss of blood, surgical trauma and the effects of anesthesia may reduce an already depleted supply of prothrombin to a dangerously low value; of these factors mechanical trauma is thought to be the most important. The prothrombin clotting time may and frequently does increase with no apparent reason within six to eight hours, and with this increase free bleeding may occur without warning and apparently normal, coagulable blood may become virtually incoagulable.

INDICATION FOR TREATMENT WITH VITAMIN K. The prothrombin clotting time of the blood of patients who have *jaundice* usually increases to some extent for the first three or four days after surgical operation but it may increase rapidly even as late as the eighteenth postoperative day. For this reason the prothrombin clotting time should be determined daily for the first four days after operation and then every other day for at least eight or ten days longer. Any increase in the prothrombin clotting time should constitute an indication for the immediate oral or intravenous administration of vitamin K. In patients whose prothrombin clotting time is high before surgical treatment, it is perhaps wise to administer vitamin K daily for several days after surgical operation even though their prothrombin clotting time has become normal. A patient whose blood gives a prothrombin clotting time of more than thirty seconds should be prepared with particular care, and one whose blood gives a prothrombin clotting time of more than forty-five seconds must be considered to be a potential bleeder and treated as such.

The same important diagnostic points are also applicable to those cases of various intestinal lesions in which a deficiency of prothrombin in the circulating blood may develop.

It is equally important to follow if possible the prothrombin clotting time of newborn infants, although it is well known that during the first few days there is a physiologic deficiency of prothrombin. This caution is particularly important if any surgical procedure is contemplated during this period of life.

Unfortunately, the measure of prothrombin in the circulating blood does not always give the exact index of the tendency of the patient to bleed. Like any laboratory method, this method may not give the clinical information which is always desirable. For these reasons prophylactic treatment is much better than treatment after bleeding occurs.

Treatment

It is well to remember that no single specific remedy for the prevention and control of all instances of bleeding resulting from deficiency of prothrombin yet has been discovered. Proper administration of vitamin K or related compounds in most instances will be effective but, in addition, to obtain the best results all procedures which are known to be of value in the maintenance of adequate hepatic function must be employed. Obviously the *first objective* in treatment of the jaundiced patient who has a tendency to bleed is to restore continuity of the biliary passages and protection of the hepatic parenchyma. The latter objective still requires injections of glucose and a diet high in carbohydrates and proteins, as has been necessary in the past.

Since the synthetic preparations which possess vitamin K activity have appeared on the market we have discontinued the use of naturally occurring concentrates of vitamin K. Details of the use of these concentrates can be found in the older work in the literature which appears in the references.

For purposes of routine *preoperative treatment,* patients who have jaundice are divided into three groups: (1) those whose blood gives a normal prothrombin clotting time; (2) those whose blood gives a prolonged prothrombin clotting time although active bleeding is not present and (3) those whose blood gives a prolonged prothrombin clotting time, active bleeding being present.

Those jaundiced patients of the first group, the prothrombin clotting time of whose blood is normal, receive prophylactic treatment for from two to five days before surgical intervention is undertaken. Usually 1 to 2 mg. daily of one of the synthetic products that have vitamin K activity given orally constitutes an adequate daily dose. This should be given together with from 1 to 3 gm. of animal bile salts. Almost any type of animal bile salts can be used; bile of man obtained from a biliary fistula or T tube can be employed.

Patients who have jaundice and the prothrombin time of whose blood is prolonged constitute a potential or real emergency. Patients whose blood gives a prothrombin clotting time of from thirty to forty-five seconds will respond well to the plan of prophylactic treatment for patients of the first group previously mentioned, but if the prothrombin clotting time is longer than forty-five or fifty seconds it has been thought advisable to administer vitamin K intramuscularly or intravenously. In such instances one of the water soluble synthetic compounds that have vitamin K activity is administered in doses of 1 to 2 mg. by the intramuscular or intravenous route. One such dose as a rule will bring the prothrombin clotting time to normal (Fig. 6), but in an exceptional instance it has been necessary to repeat this procedure once or more than once.

The problem of treating patients who are bleeding actively (patients of group 3) is difficult, but not nearly so difficult since the availability of synthetic products with vitamin K activity which can be administered by the intravenous route. A transfusion of blood often is necessary to aid in combating the shock produced by hemorrhage and to provide a temporary supply of prothrombin. As a rule, transfusion will control bleeding only so long as the added supply of prothrombin lasts, a matter of from six to twelve hours. In such instances the intravenous administration of synthetic compounds possessing vitamin K activity in doses of 1 to 4 mg. often will control the hemorrhagic diathesis (Fig. 7), but not infrequently repeated doses of the same magnitude must be administered. The value of preoperative treatment cannot be overemphasized and when bleeding occurs which is the result of hypoprothrom-

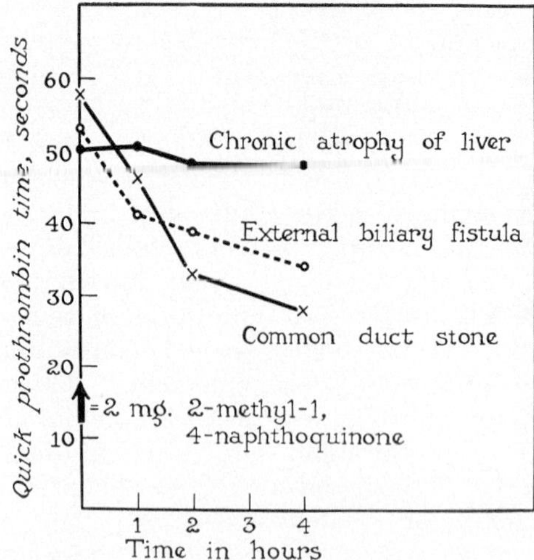

FIG. 7. The effect and rapidity of action of the intravenous injection of 2 mg. of 2-methyl-1,4-naphthoquinone in a case of external biliary fistula and in one of calculus of the common duct. The figure also shows the failure of this compound to reduce the elevated prothrombin clotting time in a case of chronic atrophy of the liver. (Butt and Snell, *Vitamin K.*)

binemia the condition in most instances has not been well managed.

Severe Hepatic Damage. Although hepatic damage occasionally will not respond to the administration of vitamin K, this does not mean that vitamin K should not be administered to these patients. It has been our experience that although there is little or no response to vitamin K in such instances, the patient to whom vitamin K is administered, in spite of severe hepatic damage and an elevated prothrombin clotting time, rarely dies of hemorrhagic diathesis resulting from a deficiency of prothrombin (Fig. 8). In most instances we have administered as much as 3 to 5 mg. daily of one of the synthetic compounds exhibiting antihemorrhagic activity.

Intestinal Diseases. In this group of cases treatment depends upon the fundamental facts already outlined for cases of obstructive jaundice and biliary fistula. Here again early recognition of possible instances in which hypoprothrombinemia may occur is all-important in treatment. The same dosage of the same compounds can also be employed here.

The Newborn Infant. It appears that a dose of from 1 to 5 mg. of 2-methyl-1,4-naphthoquinone or any of the other synthetic quinone compounds available commercially is sufficient in most instances to control hemorrhagic disease of the newborn and that, if it is administered at the time of birth, it will prevent *transitory hypoprothrombinemia.* Failures can occur in treatment of infants if sufficient hepatic damage has occurred. It has also been demonstrated that the same dose of vitamin K as given to the newborn infant, when administered to the mother twelve to twenty-four hours prior to delivery, results in the birth of a baby who has a higher value for prothrombin in the blood than is normally present. These synthetic compounds apparently are effective when administered either orally or parenterally. Toxic effects have not been noted in the examination of either the mother or the infant.

There would seem to be some surgical significance to these observations, and it perhaps would be wise to administer vitamin K before a contemplated surgical operation is undertaken at this age. Such a simple precaution might greatly lessen the chance of unpleasant and serious bleeding at the time of and after operation. We would suggest that for the pregnant mother vitamin K be administered as 2-methy-1,4,naphthoquinone, 2 mg. daily for one week prior to delivery and that, if necessity demands, the form of this compound prepared for intravenous use could be administered in the same dose at the time of labor. For the infant we suggest that 3.2 mg. of 2-methyl-1,4-naphthohydroquinone-3-sodium sulfonate or any other water soluble compound that has equal vitamin K activity be given intramuscularly immediately after birth. This, in almost all instances, will prevent the occurrence of hemorrhagic diathesis resulting from a deficiency of prothrombin.

Use of Vitamin K in Dicumarol Therapy. A compound called "Dicumarol," 3,3′-methylenebis (4-hydroxycoumarin) when administered to man results in a decrease of prothrombin in the circulating blood. The mechanism through which the prothrombin is reduced is still obscure. Dicumarol usually is administered to patients who have thrombophlebitis or pulmonary embolism or who, before operation, give a history of these difficulties. In some individuals the ingestion of Dicumarol is followed by an excessive decrease in the level of prothrombin and in these instances bleeding may occur. Miller and his associates have shown that water-soluble K preparations have little predictable effect in correcting the excessive prothrombin deficiencies sometimes produced by the ingestion of Dicumarol, whereas vitamin K and vitamin K_1 oxide were effective in decreasing the prothrombin time. It is, therefore, strongly recommended that either vitamin K, or its oxide or blood

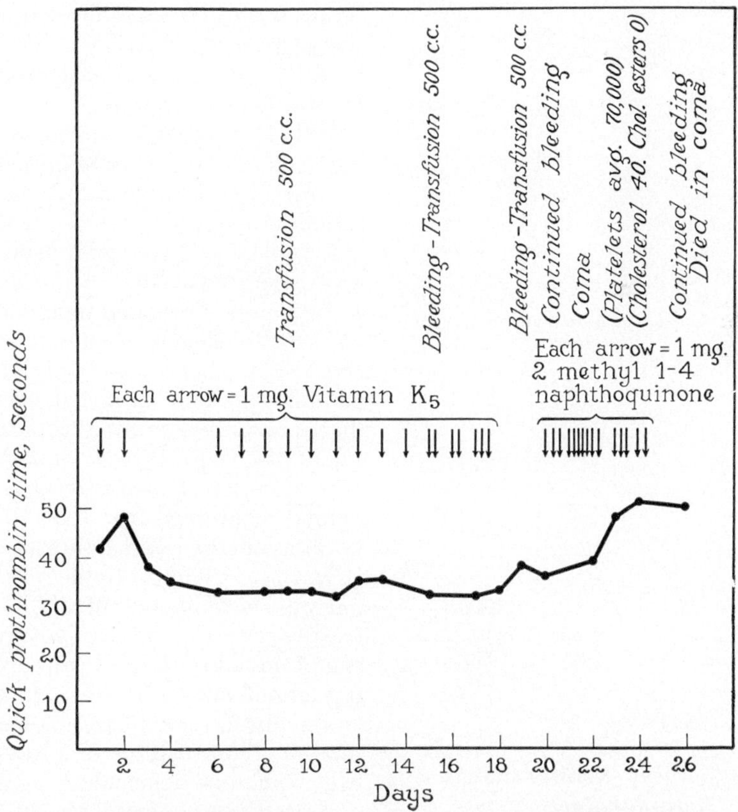

FIG. 8. The prothrombin clotting time of a patient who had severe cirrhosis of the liver and who received over a long period various synthetic preparations possessing marked antihemorrhagic activity. In spite of these materials the prothrombin clotting time remained elevated. This type of case constitutes a failure of vitamin K to correct an elevated prothrombin clotting time. (Butt and Snell, *Vitamin K.*)

be administered in the treatment of hemorrhage following use of Dicumarol.

Preparations of Vitamin K Available Commercially. SYNTHETIC COMPOUNDS. 2-methyl-1,4-naphthoquinone possesses marked antihemorrhagic activity. It is available commercially for both oral and intravenous administration. For simple deficiencies of vitamin K, the water soluble analogs are generally preferred, such as menadione sodium bisulfite, 4-amino-2-methylnaphthol HCl or 2-methyl-1,4-naphthohydroquinone diphosphate tetra sodium (a menadiol derivative). In the complicated vitamin K deficiencies, menadione has been found to be the strongest corrective analog.

References

Brinkhous, K. M.: Plasma Prothrombin—Vitamin K. Medicine, *19:*329–416, 1940.
Butt, H. R. and Snell, A. M.: Vitamin K. Philadelphia, W. B. Saunders Company, 1941.
Collentine, G. E. and Quick, A. J.: Am. J. M. Sc., *222:*7, 1951.
Cromer, H. E., Jr. and Barker, N. W.: Proc. Staff Meet., Mayo Clin., *19:*217, 1944.
Dam, H., Prange, I. and Sondergaard, E.: Acta pharmacol. et toxicol., *10:*58, 1954.
Dam, H., Prange, I. and Sondergaard, E.: Acta pharmacol. et toxicol., *11:*90, 1955.
Glander, R. and Landbeck, G.: Ztschr. Kinderh., *75:*392, 1954.
Hoskin, F. C. G., Spinks, J. W. T. and Jacques, L. B.: Canad. J. Biochem. & Physiol., *32:*240, 1954.
Isler, O. and Doebel, K.: Helvet. chim. acta, *37:*225, 1954.
Isler, O., Rüegg, R., Studer, A. and Jurgens, K.: Ztschr. physiol. Chem., *295:*290, 1953.
Jurgens, K.: Arch. exper. Path. u. Pharmakol., *222:*107, 1954.
Koller, F.: Arch. exper. Path. u. Pharmakol., *222:*89, 1954.
Luckey, T. D., Pleasants, J. R. and Reyniers, J. A.: J. Nutrition, *55:*105, 1955.
Marx, R.: Med. Monatsschr., *9:*371, 1955.
Miller, R., Harvey, W. P. and Finch, C. A.: New England J. Med., *242:*211, 1950.

VITAMIN A

Night Blindness, Keratomalacia, Xerophthalmia

It is difficult historically to trace the effects of deficiency of vitamin A, but even as long as sixty or seventy years ago there were several definite medical reports about occurrence of grave epidemics of xerophthalmia and keratomalacia. It was noted then that this disease appeared chiefly in children whose food was principally of vegetable origin, whereas among the children of the coast, whose diets consisted principally of fish, the disease was rarely seen. It was noted also that this disease was eminently improved by ingestion of chicken liver, veal fat or cod liver oil. These clinical observations were then followed by many experimental studies which suggested strongly that there was present in certain foodstuffs a fat soluble compound which was essential for normal growth. It was not, however, until 1913 that McCollum and Davis reported the occurrence in certain foods of a compound termed *"fat soluble A."* These authors later reported that severe spontaneous infection developed in rats suffering from deficiency of vitamin A, and although in this earlier work the diets used had been often deficient in vitamin D as well as in vitamin A, in 1922 it was shown clearly that the antixerophthalmic factor in cod liver oil could be destroyed by oxidation without destroying the antirachitic factor.

In these early experiments it was noted that a swelling of the lids of one or both eyes developed in animals (rats) on a diet deficient in vitamin A, following which there commonly developed an inflamed and catarrhal condition of the conjunctiva with a bloody or purulent discharge. It was noted that if this eye condition was not treated and the animal continued to live, the cornea became affected and blindness resulted. It was also significantly noted that without any local treatment, if the eye disease were not too far advanced, the symptoms disappeared rapidly following administration to the animal of food containing an adequate amount of vitamin A. This relation of disease of the eye to dietary deficiency was also demonstrated experimentally in other species as well as rats, and it was shown in these studies that certain diseases of the eye of man might be the result of deficiency of vitamin A; and soon it was reported that xerophthalmia in man could be prevented or cured by the administration of food rich in the A vitamin.

Chemistry

Although vitamin A was the first vitamin to be described, it was not until many years later that it was isolated and its definite function in the metabolism established. The structural formula of vitamin A_1 is as shown in Figure 9.

This primary alcoholic structure of vitamin A is important in that it allows for esterification and, therefore, the formation of compounds of vitamin A with protein, bile acids and fatty acids. These compounds of vitamin A are decomposed with liberation of the vitamin by such hydrolytic processes as occur in saponification. The vitamin is an alcohol; hence, it is not itself saponifiable. Vitamin A is a hydrogen acceptor probably because of its unsaturated form. There is some evidence to indicate that the substance readily absorbs oxygen in solution and is markedly pro-oxygenic when undergoing oxidation. However, highly oxidized vitamin A has no biologic activity.

Other known vitamin A substances are structurally related either as a stereoisomer such as neovitamin A or as oxidation-reduction or dehydration products such as vitamin A aldehyde (retinene) and vitamin A_2 respectively. Vitamin A aldehyde (retinene) is essential for retinal metabolism and will be briefly discussed in reference to the rhodopsin cycle. Vitamin A_2, biologically similar to vitamin A_1 present in salt water fish, is found predominantly in fresh water fish.

Vitamin A occurs naturally as the ester, a more stable form than the alcohol. The acetate has been adopted by the World Health Organization as the international standard. The absorption curve of the blue color produced by the reaction of vitamin A with antimony trichloride in chloroform (Price-Carr reaction) is commonly used as the standard assay method. A broad absorption band in the ultraviolet region of the spectrum is the basis for the direct spectrophotometric quantitative estimation of vitamin A.

Most of the vitamin A available to man in his diet is in the form of its precursors, the yellow and red carotenoid pigments (*provitamins*). For this reason the chemical properties of these compounds are rather important. Of this large group of pigments, only four substances are known at present from which animals can form vitamin A: alpha, beta, and gamma carotene and a related substance, cryptoxanthin, are all capable of yielding vitamin A. Of this group, however, the beta form yields two molecules of the vitamin, whereas each of the others produces only one molecule. This can be seen easily in the formula of beta carotene shown in Figure 10. Theoretically, if the splitting occurs in the middle, one molecule may give rise to two molecules of vitamin A. It was the ingenious research of Karrer which first proved that beta carotene contains two beta-ionone rings. It was also shown by these investigations that the beta-ionone ring is an essential component of the molecular structure of vitamin A. All the carotenoids that yield vitamin A exhibit characteristic absorp-

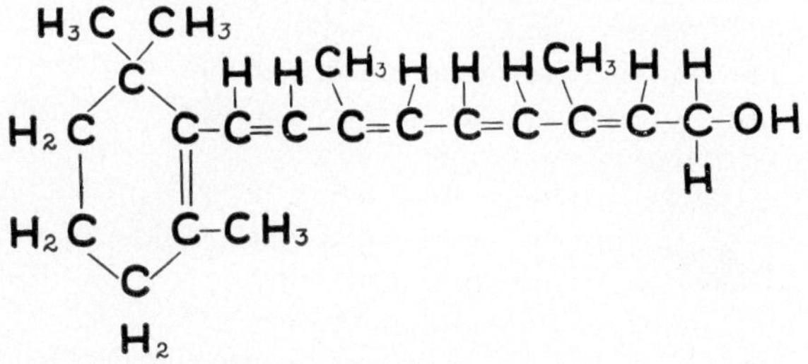

FIG. 9. The structural formula of vitamin A_1

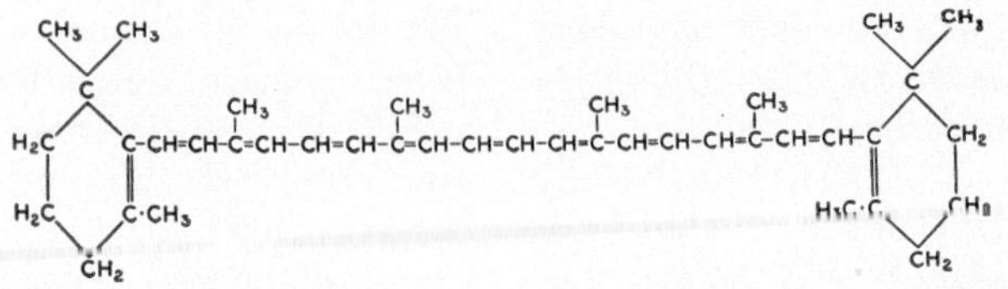

FIG. 10. The structural formula of beta carotene, showing that, if the splitting occurs in the middle, one molecule may give rise to two molecules of vitamin A.

tion bands in the visible region of the spectrum.

Although its exact function is unknown, *carotene* obviously is of great importance in the physiologic processes of plants. It is a family associated closely with chlorophyll although it is not lost when the chlorophyll disappears at the time of the yellowing of the leaves. However, it is destroyed completely in dry dead leaves. Rapid drying by artificial heat also destroys the provitamin. All these facts are important because carotene of green leaves is brought indirectly into human nutrition through milk and eggs.

Physiology

Absorption. CAROTENE. It had been believed previously that the conversion of carotene to vitamin A took place in the liver with the aid of a hypothetical enzyme, carotenase; however, Glover and others have clearly demonstrated in animals, that the conversion takes place in the wall of the small intestine and not in the liver. The carotene value of a foodstuff is not synonymous with its biologic vitamin A effectiveness in human nutrition since carotene is poorly absorbed, not completely converted, and a large percentage of intake is excreted or destroyed.

The normal absorption of dietary fat is necessary for optimum carotene absorption; however, abnormal increases in fat intake do not enhance carotene absorption. Adequate intestinal bile and lipase activity are essential for carotene utilization; where these enzymes are deficient, replacement therapy is indicated. Carotene absorption is impaired in disorders of intestinal digestion and motility such as chronic diarrhea, pancreatic disease, celiac syndrome, sprue, giardiasis and colitis. The administration of liquid paraffin or mineral oil seriously interferes with carotene absorption by dissolving it from the food in the intestine. Absorption of carotene normally reaches maximal levels in the blood in from six to eight hours after administration and, since fecal excretion accounts for only a small amount of the unutilized excess, it is presumably destroyed in the intestine.

VITAMIN A. The absorption of vitamin A, a fat soluble compound, is enhanced or impaired by the same factors which similarly affect fat absorption. The naturally occurring vitamin A esters are first hydrolyzed to the alcoholic form, cross the intestinal wall as the alcohol, and are esterified again before entering the lacteals for transport to the liver for storage. Absorption of vitamin A as judged by blood levels reaches its maximum at three to six hours following administration. The ester and alcohol form both appear in the blood; the latter is believed to be the active form comprising 80 per cent, while the former, serving as transport from intestine to liver, comprises about 20 per cent.

In disease, particularly where intestinal digestion of fat is impaired, emulsification and "aqueous" dispersion of vitamin A increases its effectiveness by allowing direct absorption of the chemically unchanged, finely dispersed vitamin particle. The differential absorption of "aqueous" and oily preparations of vitamin A as well as the differential existing between the vitamin ester and the alcohol or aldehyde may be a useful diagnostic tool in disorders of fat absorption, particularly in distinguishing between celiac disease and cystic fibrosis of the pancreas.

Storage. Liver storage in man ranges normally from an average of 50 I.U. per gram of liver in the neonatal period to 350 I.U. in the adult. Individual variations are very great, ranging from 14 to 134 I.U. in the infant and child, while in the adult the spread in liver storage has varied from 50 to 2,000 units. There is still no definitive knowledge as to the precise mechanism of liver storage and mobilization of vitamin A. Popper, utilizing fluorescence microscopy, finds that both the hepatic and Kupffer cells store vitamin A and that the Kupffer cell is the last to release and the first to replenish its store of vitamin A. Others believe that only the hepatic cell is active in the release of stored vitamin A, the Kupffer cell storing the inactive excess. Liver regulation of vitamin A metabolism tends to stabilize individual blood levels, so that within 24 hours of a single large dose of vitamin A, normal levels prevail. Similarly, there is little change in blood levels for many months during volunteer depletion experiments. It is noteworthy that, in the rat, vitamin E has been shown to spare hepatic stores of vitamin A.

It has been estimated that 90 to 95 per cent of the body store of vitamin A is concentrated in the liver; the remainder is found in minimal amounts in the kidney, adrenals, testes and lactating breast. Vitamin A storage in the healthy person is so protective that Mason states it would take two or three years of deprivation to induce pathognomonic symptoms of deficiency. Avitaminosis A alone, therefore, occurs rarely in adult man; it is usually a phase of a multiple deficiency associated with generalized malnutrition.

Excretion and Destruction. Vitamin A is not excreted in the urine except in certain diseases such as pneumonia, chronic nephritis and obstructive jaundice; minimal spillage has been reported in rheumatic fever, diabetes and infectious hepatitis. Urinary vitamin A is always associated with proteinuria. Relatively small amounts of vitamin A or carotene are normally found in the stool. The unaccounted for excess is presumed to be destroyed in an unknown fashion.

Human milk contains both carotene and vitamin A. The colostrum from the human breast has from two to three times the biologic vitamin A activity of early milk, and early human milk has from five to ten times the biologic vitamin A activity of cow's milk. It is interesting that this biologic vitamin A activity of early human milk is not increased by feeding supplements of cod liver oil to the mother. Late human milk contains about the same amount of carotene and vitamin A as cow's milk.

Relation of Vitamin A to Specific Body Function and Specific Organs. Relation to Infection. Since McCollum in 1917 first pointed out that severe spontaneous infection develops in rats suffering from deficiency of vitamin A, there has been a bulk of literature on this subject. Undoubtedly, severe deficiency of vitamin A in man will lower the resistance to infection; yet administration of vitamin A during the course of an infection apparently does not have any beneficial effect on the outcome of the infection unless a severe deficiency of vitamin A also is present. Certainly there is enough evidence to indicate that there are many other factors of equal or greater influence on infection than is vitamin A and that there is no justification for calling vitamin A "the anti-infective vitamin."

Reproductive System. Nothing is known of the effect of deficiency of vitamin A on the fertility of man nor of the importance of moderate deficiencies in either men or women. It is of experimental import, however, that in the rat fetal resorption and predictable congenital malformations can be produced by either maternal vitamin A deficiency or excess.

Central Nervous System. Vitamin A deficiency has not been shown to exert any definite effect on the central nervous system in adult man. However, a perplexing syndrome in infants characterized by irritability, low grade fever and a marked bulging of the fontanelle with increased intracranial pressure has been attributed to vitamin A deficiency. Several cases resulted from prolonged feedings of soy bean formulas without vitamin additive, and the symptoms rapidly disappeared following vitamin A administration. Experimentally, congenital hydrocephalus, believed due to excessive production of cerebrospinal fluid, has been produced in rabbits born of vitamin A deficient mothers. The extensive studies of Wolbach and Bessey and of Fell and Mellanby have shown that the pathologic changes in the central nervous system of the growing vitamin A deficient laboratory animal are secondary to a profound growth disturbance of the bones of the skull.

EYE. Decreased facility for *dark adaptation* is one of the earliest functional changes associated with deficiency of vitamin A. Evidence has been reported which suggests that the visual purple of the retina is a conjugated protein in which vitamin A aldehyde is a prosthetic group. With exposure to light, the visual purple (rhodopsin) enters a reversible cycle, breaking down to a yellow compound, retinene (vitamin A aldehyde), and a retinal protein, opsin. Visual purple is then resynthesized from these two substances. During the reaction some retinene is lost and must be replaced by vitamin A from either the retina, blood or tissue stores. When these stores are deficient, visual purple will be inadequate and impaired dark adaptation will ensue. The selection of color and other visual functions depends on light of high intensity associated with the cones of the retina, whereas the rods are sensitive only to light and are especially adapted to function in dim light. Visual purple is found only in the rods and apparently serves to transform the energy of dim light into nerve impulses which within limits vary with intensity of the light. Although it was believed formerly that the cone played no part in vitamin A metabolism, it has been demonstrated recently that formation of visual violet or iodopsin in the cone takes place in much the same manner as does formation of visual purple in the rods.

EPITHELIUM. Since the malnourished person with avitaminosis A presents a complex of disordered physiology, and since dermatologic nomenclature is often vague and nonspecific, a multitude of skin eruptions has been attributed to vitamin A deficiency, and inordinate amounts of vitamin A preparations, local and systemic, have been used for a variety of unrelated skin disorders. The skin lesion considered specific for vitamin A deficiency is follicular hyperkeratosis (toad skin, phrynoderma), which is characterized by a dry, scaly skin with spinous papules appearing at the sites of hair follicles and distributed usually at the extensor surfaces of both upper and lower extremities, the shoulders and the lower part of the abdomen, and to a less extent on the chest, back and buttocks. These papules vary in diameter up to 5 mm., are hard and deeply pigmented and have a surrounding area of depigmentation. In the center is an epithelial plug which when expressed leaves a crater. An acne-like eruption of the face has also been described, differing from acne vulgaris in its lack of pustulation and dryness of the skin. Microscopically there are epithelial keratinization, mechanical occlusion of the hair follicles and sweat ducts, and secondary degeneration of the sebaceous and sweat glands. The skin lesion of vitamin A deficiency in infants and children is described as a moderately severe xerosis. Vitamin A toxicity has been reported in adults following prolonged massive therapy for skin lesions often only superficially similar clinically and probably unrelated to vitamin deficiency.

URINARY SYSTEM. Some experimental evidence seems to suggest that calculi of the urinary tract may result from a diet deficient in vitamin A, but this never has been definitely established in man and certainly further studies are required before the results can be applied to man.

THYROID. The relationship of the thyroid to vitamin A metabolism has intrigued many investigators, but the diversity of observations does not allow an integrated explanation. Laboratory and clinical observations relevant to this problem include: (1) Milk from thyroidectomized goats is yellow, instead of the normal pure white. This is attributed to the failure of conversion of carotene to vitamin A in the absence of thyroxine. (2) Cretins are reported to have a relatively low blood level of vitamin A and a relatively high concentration of carotene. (3) Poor dark adaptation has been reported in myxedema. (4) The thyroid affects carotene metabolism by increasing its absorption from the gut into the gut wall and is *not* involved in the conversion mechanism. (5) Vitamin A may decrease the effect of thyroxine in stimulating metabolism.

LIVER. Since it is no longer believed that the liver converts carotene to vitamin A, the effects of liver disease on vitamin A metabolism are now related to its maintenance of adequate storage and its ability to transform stored vitamin A ester to the alcoholic form needed in tissue metabolism.

Pathology

Effect of Deficiency of Vitamin A in Animals. EYE. In the experimental animal, as in man, pathologic changes in the eye occur late. Changes in both animals and man are essentially the same. Metaplasia of the epithelium of the conjunctiva and cornea is the earliest change, followed by vascularization of the cornea with edema and perhaps necrosis. Accumulation of keratin itself favors infection of the cornea, which may ultimately lead to ulceration and hypopyon.

EPITHELIUM. In deficiency of vitamin A, certain specific pathologic changes are observed in many epithelial structures. There usually is atrophy of the epithelium concerned, as well as a gradual proliferation of basal cells and differentiation of the new product into a stratified keratinized epithelium. The replacement of epithelium is identical with epidermis. Accumulation of keratinized epithelial cells may give rise to many striking gross pathologic features. This may lead to the occlusion of the bronchi and subsequent atelectasis.

MISCELLANEOUS ORGANS. In growing animals, retardation of skeletal growth occurs early with characteristic cessation of remodelling sequences. Compact bone formation is arrested while appositional bone formation continues, resulting in greater thickness and alterations in contours.

Atrophy and metaplasia of the enamel organs take place in rats. Enamel formation ceases and tooth deformities commonly result from defective formation of dentine.

In the genitourinary tract of rats, the ureters and renal tubules may be completely obstructed owing to accumulation of keratinized cells. Atrophy of the testis in the male and retardation of growth and death of fetuses in the female may occur.

Degeneration of cells of the superior ganglion and of the ophthalmic division of the fifth nerve in rabbits, dogs and rats on diets deficient in vitamin A has been reported by Mellanby. These observations want confirmation; most investigators believe that deficiency of this vitamin in animals results in few if any definite nerve lesions and that abnormalities noted in this system are largely secondary to pressure effects from bone changes.

Effect of Deficiency of Vitamin A in Man. EYE. The loss of visual acuity in dim light is one of the first symptoms of vitamin A deficiency in man. However, definite pathologic changes in the eye occur late in man on diets deficient in vitamin A. The early pathologic changes are the same as those described previously for animals. In this country xerophthalmia is an extremely rare disease. Although it is most common in infancy it may be seen at all ages. *Night blindness* usually develops in adults before any ophthalmias develop but usually the disease is ushered in by small triangular white patches on the outer and inner sides of the cornea covered by white, foam-like spots consisting of corneal epithelium, which has been shed and accumulates in this position (*Bitot's* *spots*). Photophobia and conjunctivitis appear early followed by a light brown pigmentation of the conjunctiva. The keratinization of the cunjunctiva may extend to the cornea and lead to extreme softness and degeneration of the cornea and to ulceration, perforation and total destruction of the eye (*keratomalacia*). This disease may destroy the eye rapidly and its prompt recognition therefore is very important.

For a number of years, Spies and associates have studied the ocular symptoms occurring from malnutrition in human beings. Ascher and Spies have observed that Bitot spots are frequent findings in these patients and disappear soon after large doses of vitamin A. Follicular conjunctivitis is a frequent finding, particularly in children, and it also often disappears following the administration of large amounts of vitamin A.

EPITHELIUM. In the human infant, Wolbach and his associates have observed keratinizing metaplasia appearing earliest and most often in the trachea and bronchi and in the pelvis of the kidney. It was observed also in the conjunctiva, cornea, accessory sinuses, salivary glands, ureter, uterus and perisalivary glands. In these cases no cutaneous condition which could be attributed soley to deficiency of vitamin A was observed. However, cutaneous lesions associated with deficiency of vitamin A and analogous to those occurring in other epithelial structures have been reported by several investigators. These changes have been discussed already under the heading "Relation of Vitamin A to Specific Body Functions and Specific Organs." Recently an excellent experimental study of deprivation of vitamin A in man was reported by the Vitamin A Subcommittee of the Medical Research Council of Great Britain. Of the sixteen subjects receiving a diet containing about 70 international units of carotene and negligible amounts of vitamin A for eleven to twenty-five months, only three displayed unmistakable signs of deficiency.

Toxicity

Carotenemia, or more properly, carotenosis, sometimes develops in patients with disorders such as diabetes and myxedema. It is characterized by an excess of this substance in the blood and by its accumulation in the skin in sufficient amounts to cause a yellow pigmentation (xanthosis cuti). The syndrome, which has been reported also in apparently normal persons, has been ascribed to the ingestion of foods containing an excess of carotene. Since it does not always disappear readily when their intake is restricted, however, mechanisms regulating utilization and/or destruction also appear to be implicated. Carotenemia has been induced experimentally by administration of large quantities of concentrated preparations over a short period and seems to reflect in part a wide variation in individual susceptibility. Carotenemia per se appears generally compatible with good health.

Reports of hypervitaminosis A are becoming more numerous. Adults as well as children have been affected, although it has occurred predominantly in the younger group, to whom excessive amounts of fish liver oil concentrates are not uncommonly administered. Acute vitamin A poisoning classically has been described following ingestion of polar bear liver by Arctic explorers. Most clinical cases, however, are of the chronic type. As with carotene, there appears to be a wide difference in susceptibility between individuals and, as noted in the experimental induction of hypervitaminosis A, even in the same individual at different times. Many persons have undoubtedly consumed, without apparent ill effect, quantities of this substance in excess of amounts producing symptoms in more susceptible individuals. The type of preparation as well as the dose and duration of intake is important, although a daily consumption of not more than 50,000 units is generally considered safe.

Acute toxicity is characterized usually by a short, severe reaction with vomiting and prostration followed by generalized desquamation and a rapid recovery. The clinical picture of chronic poisoning varies greatly, especially with the age of the patient. Changes in the long bones, with localized swelling, pain and tenderness, and roentgen evidence of thickening and subperiosteal elevation occur typically in children, as does hepatomegaly. Other common manifestations include general weakness and fatigability, irritability, severe headache, dizziness, anorexia, diarrhea, epistaxis, cheilosis with splitting of the lips, arthralgia, and a widespread pruritic dermatitis with folliculosis and keratinization. Remissions may occur without consistent relationship to the usually greatly elevated blood vitamin A concentration. Numerous other abnormal laboratory findings have been described but not regularly demonstrated. When vitamin A is withheld, the blood level returns rapidly to normal and complete clinical recovery is usual, even after prolonged disability.

Sources and Human Requirements

Food Sources. Vitamin A is widespread in nature in the form of its precursors, the yellow and red carotenoid pigments (*provitamins*). These pigments are found in the plant world, being distributed from bacteria to garden fruits and vegetables. The pigments are found chiefly in association with chlorophyll and in the green leaves of plants but this is not invariably true, since carrots and sweet potatoes with their yellow color also are rich in these substances. Since most of our vitamin A is obtained in the form of its precursors, the plant pigments, the distribution of vitamin A will be discussed in terms of the distribution of the carotenoid pigments in nature.

There apparently is a direct parallel between greenness (chlorophyll content) and vitamin A activity in foods of plant origin. Among the best sources of vitamin A are thin green leaves. The exact relation between the degree of greenness and vitamin A activity is not understood but it is well known that the outer green leaves of iceberg lettuce or cabbage are much more potent in vitamin A than are the inner leaves. Peas, green beans, green peppers, parsley stocks, asparagus and green celery are all known to have high vitamin A content. Carrots, sweet potatoes, apricots, yellow peaches, bananas, and yellow tomatoes, all of which possess a yellowish color, are rich sources of vitamin A. Nuts and cereal grains, with the exception of those having considerable green and yellow color, are very poor sources of vitamin A. Yellow corn is the most important vitamin A food in this group.

Whole milk, eggs, and milk products are perhaps the most important sources of vitamin A of animal origin.

Vitamin A is fairly stable to heat and not appreciably soluble in water; it is, however, destroyed by oxidation, and foods that are heated for long periods show appreciable loss of vitamin A potency. Since the vitamin activity is not affected at the temperature of boiling water, foods cooked in this manner retain their vitamin A potency. Canned foods have practically the same vitamin A value as the corresponding fresh foods, and foods that are stored in the frozen state maintain their maximal vitamin A value, but dried and dehydrated foods show considerable loss of vitamin A content.

Requirements. The Recommended Daily Dietary Allowances of the Food and Nutrition Board, National Research Council (1953 revision) are predicated on the assumption that two-thirds of the vitamin A intake is in the form of its carotene precursor. A margin of safety is provided above estimated average needs, but larger doses may be required where absorption or utilization of vitamin A is impaired. It has been postulated that optimum amounts conducive to improved over-all health may be considerably in excess of vitamin A intakes required to protect against manifest deficiency.

Infants. It is believed that approximately 1500 I.U. is the minimal vitamin A requirement of most infants. The diets, however, of young infants usually contain more milk than the diets of adults and also their diets usually are supplemented with some kind of fish liver oil so that most infants obtain ten to twelve times as many units of vitamin A as those usually considered to be minimal requirements. It must be remembered that in the presence of diarrhea or jaundice larger doses of vitamin A must be administered. It may be necessary in such conditions to administer the material, if available, by the parenteral route.

CHILDREN. For children one to three years of age, the daily requirement is 2000 I.U.; from four to six years, 2500 I.U.; from seven to nine years, 3500 I.U.; from ten to twelve years, 4500 I.U.; and from thirteen to nineteen years it is 5000 I.U. This is provided with about 1 quart (1 liter) of milk in addition to an egg, servings of green leafy vegetables and butter, and 3 gm. of cod liver oil daily as the main sources of protective foods rich in vitamin A. In growing children as well as infants, diarrhea and so forth may result in increased requirements of vitamin A, which at times must be administered parenterally.

ADULTS. The National Research Council recommendation is 5000 I.U. daily for both men and women, except during pregnancy (6000 I.U.) and lactation (8000 I.U.). No additional allowance is usually indicated for strenuous physical activity. The average adult should meet his vitamin A needs through the daily consumption of one egg, two portions of a leafy green or deep yellow vegetable, yellow fruits, three teaspoons of butter or margarine and frequent servings of milk and liver. One or more liters of milk and an extra serving of the leafy green or yellow vegetables should satisfy the added requirements of pregnancy and lactation.

Diagnosis

Undoubtedly the incidence of marked vitamin A deficiency in the United States is very small. Of course, the supposition that states of partial deficiency may be common has received repeated emphasis but as yet no definite methods have been developed by which these subnutritional states can be diagnosed.

Night Blindness. The first symptom of this syndrome is a loss of visual acuity in dim light. This particular symptom may occur in various diseases of the eye, such as toxic amblyopia, detachment of the retina or retinitis pigmentosa, but these conditions usually are excluded easily. The patient may complain of dancing lights before his eyes or similar visual disturbance and, of course, by means of dark adaptation he will show a pathologic condition. This condition must be suspected in cirrhosis of the liver, instances of severe and prolonged pyloric obstruction, severe chronic diarrhea and any other condition which may produce a generalized nutritional deficiency.

The dark adaptation test classically confirms the visual impairment in dim light. This procedure has definite limitations, however. Reproducibility is difficult to achieve, and different conclusions commonly derive from differences in instrumentation and methodology. Measurement of dark adaptation is time consuming and not practically adaptable to routine clinical procedure. Results of this test often correlate poorly with impressions provided by other phases of the clinical examination.

Eye Lesions. Thickening of the conjunctiva, with or without Bitot's spots, and follicular conjunctivitis may suggest the possibility of vitamin A deficiency before the more pathognomonic signs of xerophthalmia or keratomalacia appear.

Skin Lesions. Follicular hyperkeratosis, xerosis and related manifestations with horny keratin obstruction of sebaceous ducts may occur, especially during the winter months, involving notably the lateral surfaces of arms and thighs and the buttocks (Figure 11). Therapeutic trial is the principal means of distinguishing lesions due to vitamin A deficiency from seemingly identical patterns of other, usually unknown, etiology.

Blood Levels. The plasma concentration of vitamin A questionably reflects the over-all intake of this substance; it may remain within the normal range throughout more than a year of drastic deprivation. The carotene level is usually a more sensitive index of early deficiency. Since both of these levels are readily, if temporarily, affected by conditions other than the nutritional state (acute infections, physical stress, etc.), single determinations are much inferior to repeated measurements in the same subject. Similarly, plasma concentrations are more meaningful in population studies than in the evaluation of individual patients. No correlation between the blood vitamin A content and biophotometric readings has been observed. The generally accepted normal range for the plasma vitamin A level is 30 to 65 micrograms per 100 ml.; a concentration below 20 micrograms is definitely abnormal. The carotene content usually falls between 60 and 240 micrograms per 100 ml. In general, vitamin A levels are slightly higher in men than in women; carotene levels are slightly higher in women.

Subclinical Form. It is practically impossible to diagnose clinically subnutrition of vitamin A. However, these forms probably are frequent and must be considered under various conditions in which one would suspect inability for proper absorption or proper intake or utilization of vitamin A.

Differential Diagnosis. Although various laboratory procedures such as measurement of vitamin A in the blood and urine and the measurement of dark adaptation may be in time very helpful in diagnosis of vitamin A deficiency, the best method of differential diagnosis still depends on close clinical observation. Night blindness, xerophthalmia and keratomalacia are not confused easily with any other conditions and should be recognized readily. Treatment should be instituted at once.

Treatment

The use of vitamin A in treatment is indicated in those syndromes which result from deficiency of vitamin A in the diet or from deficiency of vitamin A resulting from improper absorption or utilization. The best treatment with vitamin A still involves prophylactic therapy. In general, the response to treatment with vitamin A of specific syndromes resulting from the deficiency is prompt and effective. Moreover, a good diet rich not only in vitamin A but in all essential nutrients is a sine qua

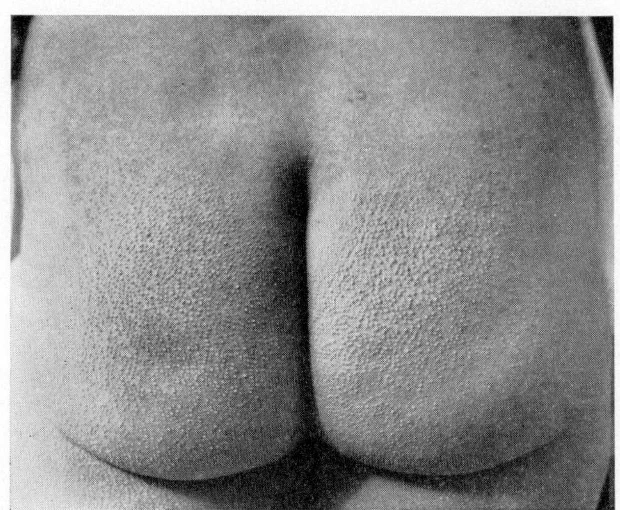

FIG. 11. Photograph of the buttocks showing follicular hyperkeratosis which is associated with a deficiency of vitamin A. (Reproduced by courtesy of Section of Dermatology and Syphilology, Mayo Clinic.)

non for any therapeutic regimen. Where supplementary vitamin A is prescribed, a multivitamin preparation containing 1 to 2 times the National Research Council recommendations should also be administered.

Night Blindness. Persons who possess normal powers of absorption of carotene and vitamin A and who have night blindness may be treated by diet alone or diet plus vitamin A supplement. Following the administration of 1,000 units of vitamin A in the form of potent fish liver oil, an improvement in dark adaptation may be demonstrable within normal limits. In those cases in which night blindness results from faulty absorption, such as is caused by gastrocolic fistula, gastrointestinal continuity first must be established before treatment unless the compounds are administered intramuscularly.

Xerophthalmia and Keratomalacia. These conditions require the same treatment as night blindness, but it is perhaps wise to give doses of from 50,000 to 100,000 units in the form of potent fish liver oil by the oral or parenteral route.

Skin Lesions. In this condition the best results have been obtained from doses of 100,000 to 300,000 international units of vitamin A given daily over a period of from two to three months. Results from treatment of skin lesions require periods of from two to three months, and one should not become discouraged because there is not a dramatic response such as occurs in the treatment of night blindness resulting from deficiency of vitamin A. Favorable responses do occur even in occasional instances of long standing, apparently familial dermatoses such as ichthyosis. Doses of 50,000 to 200,000 I.U. daily are sometimes required for short periods during which evidence of hypervitaminosis must be watched for. In contrast to that noted in eye abnormalities, improvement is commonly slow, requiring weeks or months.

Gastrointestinal Diseases. Patients who have chronic diarrhea require more vitamin A than is necessary for normal persons. Patients who have hepatic disease likewise require a rather large dose. In such instances from 10,000 to 20,000 international units of vitamin A daily are considered an adequate dose. A person from whose intestinal tract bile is excluded completely or partially should be given supplements of bile salts with vitamin A supplement.

Obviously in the treatment of any of these conditions, *diets* rich in vitamin A and its precursors should be prescribed in addition to the potent supplement containing vitamin A. Both oily and aqueous preparations of vitamin A are now available some of which are listed herewith:

1. *Carotene:* carotene in oil is on the market. It has a vitamin A content of not less than 7,500 units per gram. (The potency of any preparation always appears on the label.) Combinations of carotene with vitamin D concentrate are available in various brands. Fish liver oil is the most common form of prescribing vitamin A.
2. *Cod liver oil* (U.S.P.) has a minimum vitamin content of 600 A and 250 D per gram. The U.S.P. dose is: infants 4 cc., adults 8 cc. There is little danger of overdosage, the main objection being taste.
3. *Cod liver oil obtainable in capsules* of 0.62 cc. (10 minims), 1.25 cc. (20 minims) or even larger.
4. *Cod liver oil reinforced with viosterol* is available in potency up to 60,000 A and 8,500 D per gram. This is also marketed in capsules containing more than 10,000 A and approximately 1,500 D each or in tablets containing more than 2,000 A and 300 D.
5. *Halibut liver oil* (N.N.R.) containing 44,800 A and 540 D per gram. It is obtainable in capsules containing 10,000 A and 170 D.
6. *Percomorph liver oil* (N.N.R.) has a maximal content of 60,000 A and 8,500 D per gram. In capsules as much as 13,300 A and 1,800 D are available
7. *Natural vitamin A oil preparations* contain natural alcohols and esters, 25,000 to 50,000 units of A per capsule.
8. *Synthetic vitamin A preparations*

contain the acetate or palmitate ester, 25,000 to 100,000 units of A per capsule.

9. *Water dispersible vitamin A preparations* contain natural alcohols and esters or synthetic esters, in drops, 50,000 units of A per cc., and capsules, 25,000 to 100,000 units.

10. *Parenteral vitamin A preparations* contain water dispersible natural vitamin A, 50,000 units per 2 cc. ampule.

References

Caffey, John: Pediatrics, *5:*672, 1950.

Cohlan, S. Q.: Science, *117:*535, 1953.

Hillman, R. W.: Am. J. Clin. Nutrition, *6:*603, 1956.

Hume, E. M. and Krebs, H. A.: Medical Research Council Special Report Series. London, His Majesty's Stationery Office, 1949, vol. 264, p. 7.

Lewis, J. M. and Cohlan, S. Q.: M. Clin. North America, *34:*413, 1950.

Moore, Thomas: Vitamin A and Carotene: XIII. The Vitamin A Reserve of the Adult Human Being in Health and Disease. Biochem. J., *31:*155–164, 1937.

Sulzberger, M. B. and Lazar, M. P.: J.A.M.A., *146:*788, 1951.

The Vitamins, published by the American Medical Association, under the auspices of the Council on Pharmacy and Chemistry and the Council on Foods, 1939.

Wolbach, S. B.: The Pathologic Changes Resulting from Vitamin Deficiency. J.A.M.A., *108:*7–13, (Jan. 2) 1937.

DEFICIENCY OF VITAMIN D (RICKETS AND OSTEOMALACIA)

Introduction

An attempt to trace the history of rickets through the ages is not a particularly satisfactory task. Medical historians have found in ancient writings many descriptions of a disease which they believed to be rickets. Such interpretations, however, are subject to doubt when one realizes that rickets is almost strictly a disease of the temperate zone, whereas ancient civilization was cradled chiefly in tropical or subtropical areas. It is also true that Hippocrates is credited with a description of this disorder, but this has been true of almost every other disease, and the description by Hippocrates would seem to fit more closely what is recognized today as tuberculous spondylitis. Since the birth of Christ, however, there have been numerous descriptions of undoubted rickets, and there can be no denying that it has been a very prevalent disorder for many centuries. Like many other diseases, its form has seemed to change as time advances, and even in the last few decades physicians have noted that the characteristic deformities are not so common as they were formerly. Physicians seem to be dealing today with a milder form than that with which their fathers were familiar, but equally serious since it has become more difficult to recognize.

The evolution of the etiology and specific treatment of rickets is an outstanding example of the value of the basic sciences to clinical medicine, since there are few instances in which biology, inorganic and organic chemistry, and physics have made such contributions to the understanding of a disease.

In rickets, the pathogenesis lies in the condition of the Ca^{++} and PO_4^{---} in the blood serum. Further investigation led to the discovery of a relation between the sun's rays and the blood phosphate, namely, that the concentration of phosphate in the blood was higher in the summer than it was in the winter. It then followed for the physicist to segregate the rays of the solar spectrum and discover that the antirachitic properties of sunlight were attributable to the ultraviolet rays.

Chemistry

The term vitamin D is generally applied to two antirachitic substances, vitamin D_2 (calciferol) and vitamin D_3 (activated 7-dehydrocholesterol). These vitamins are derived by irradiation of provitamins: D_2 by irradiation of ergosterol, and D_3 by irradiation of dehydrocholesterol. The provitamins belong to the group of substances called sterols. The sterol skeleton is a perhydro-1, 2-cyclopentenophenanthrene ring system with 2 methyl groups and a side chain. It occurs not only in the common sterols but also in the sex and adrenal cortical hormones, in bile acids, cardiac glucosides, and in some carcinogens. The pro-

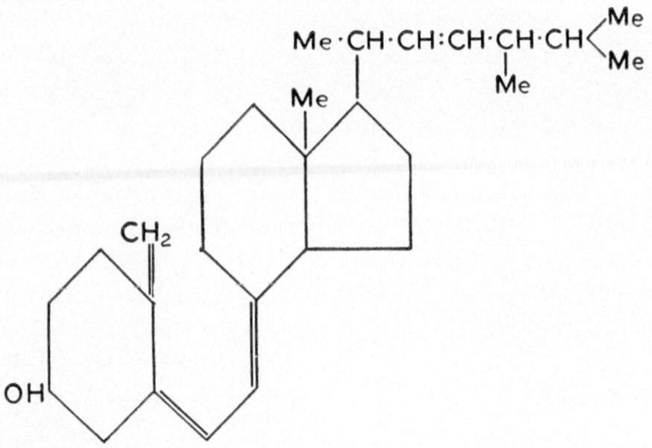

FIG. 12. The structural formula for calciferol (vitamin D_2).

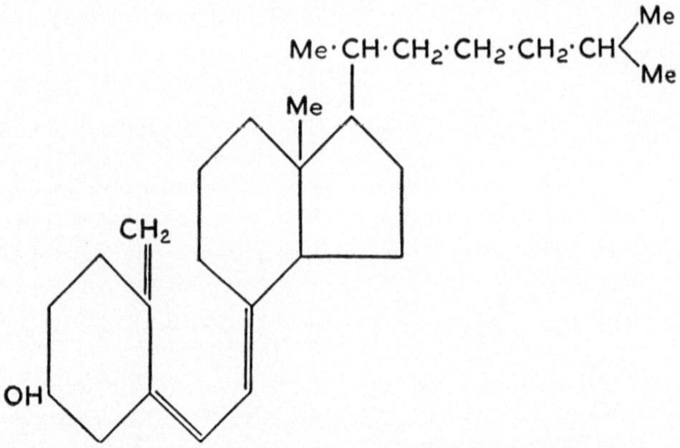

FIG. 13. The structural formula for activated 7-dehydrocholesterol (vitamin D_3).

vitamin D type of sterol compounds from which the vitamins D_2 and D_3 are derived differs from others in that there are two double bonds in the ring system, always at C-5 and C-7.

Much study has gone into the nature of the process by which the provitamin type of sterol is activated by irradiation into active vitamin D. It has been adequately proved that the process is photochemical, not chemical, in nature and that there is no change in the structure of the molecules.

The most important provitamin, ergosterol, was discovered by Tanret in ergot, but the ergosterol of commerce is now usually obtained from baker's yeast. Ergosterol has also been isolated from several species of Penicillium, but the yield is too low to make this a practical source. 7-dehydrocholesterol is found naturally in mammals but there are no good commercial sources. Vitamin D activity may be generated in lard, butter, chicken fat and in skin by activation of the 7-dehydrocholesterol in these substances through irradiation with ultraviolet rays of appropriate wave length.

Active vitamin D occurs in small amounts in nature. The most important source of active vitamin D is fish oils. The principle storage depots in fish are the muscle tissues and liver; for commercial purposes the liver oil of tuna, cod and halibut are the most important. Two or three eggs daily will provide enough vitamin D to cure most cases of infantile rickets.

The quantitative determination of vitamin D is based on biologic methods. Biologically rats or chicks show measurable responses to vitamin D in their diets even if it is present in minute amounts, and it requires gross contamination with disturbing substances such as phosphate to interfere with its action. In the completely rachitic rat, calcium phosphate is completely absent from the zone of primary calcification. After a small dose of vitamin D is administered, calcification is resumed as a line across the provisional zone where it would have occurred had there been no rickets. Thus a vertical section of long bone such as the tibia shows a clear area of cartilage, then a line of calcium phosphate stained with silver nitrate to give silver phosphate which darkens on exposure to ultraviolet light, then another clear area (the rachitic metaphysis) and finally the shaft or diaphysis. The test can be so standardized that one unit of vitamin D produces a complete line in a given number of days. The official method of estimating vitamin D in pharmaceutical preparations is a seven day test of its curative power, observations being made by the line test on a rat previously rendered rachitic.* The present international standard for vitamin D is pure vitamin D_3. The vitamin D unit is defined as the vitamin D activity of 0.025 gamma of this standard. (1 mg. of calciferol equals 40,000 units of vitamin D.)

Physiology

The physiologic activity of vitamin D is directed to promoting calcification and preventing the development of rickets. In the last analysis, prevention of rickets depends upon the maintenance of a normal concentration of calcium and inorganic phosphorus in the plasma and tissue fluids, thus insuring a constant and adequate supply of these elements for mineralization of newly formed cartilage matrix and osteoid. To understand the mechanism of rickets prevention, therefore, involves an understanding of calcium and inorganic phosphorus homeostasis. There are four facets to this problem: (1) the mechanism of absorption of calcium and inorganic phosphorus from the gastrointestinal tract, (2) the factors determining the level of these elements in the blood, (3) the role of the kidneys in this process, and (4) the factors which determine deposition of calcium salts in the cartilage and osteoid (the local factor).

Just how calcium is absorbed from the gastrointestinal tract is unknown. We know that soluble calcium salts are more easily absorbed than insoluble salts and that an acid *p*H of the intestinal contents aids this process. The presence of large amounts of fat gives rise to highly insoluble calcium salts, while an excess of carbohydrate, by increasing fermentation, shifts the *p*H of the intestinal contents to the acid side and may give rise to the more volatile and more soluble lower fatty acids. We know, however, that the presence of vitamin D promotes absorption. In the absence of vitamin D, less than 20 per cent of ingested calcium is absorbed from the gastrointestinal tract; if there is an adequate vitamin D intake, 50 to 90 per cent may be absorbed.

The absorption of phosphorus from the gut is in large measure independent of vitamin D intake, and the inefficiency of absorption observed in rickets is secondary to the failure of calcium absorption, while improvement of phosphorus absorption obtained by feeding vitamin D to the rachitic patient results from improvement of calcium absorption.

The level of calcium and phosphorus in the blood is not entirely dependent upon the amount absorbed from the gut. Physiochemical and endocrine factors play their part, and both help to determine the individual's saturation level and consequently his solubility product. The attainment of a normal saturation level in the normal person depends chiefly on an adequate intake of vitamin D. In the serum of normal children the concentration of calcium is remarkably constant at about 10 plus or minus 1.5

* Other active sterols have been produced by irradiation. However, only one of these is of clinical importance, namely A.T. 10 (dehydrotachysterol). It is very useful in the treatment of idiopathic hypoparathyroidism and, as will be shown later, in chronic glomerulotubular disease complicated by nephrocalcinosis and hyperparathyroidism.

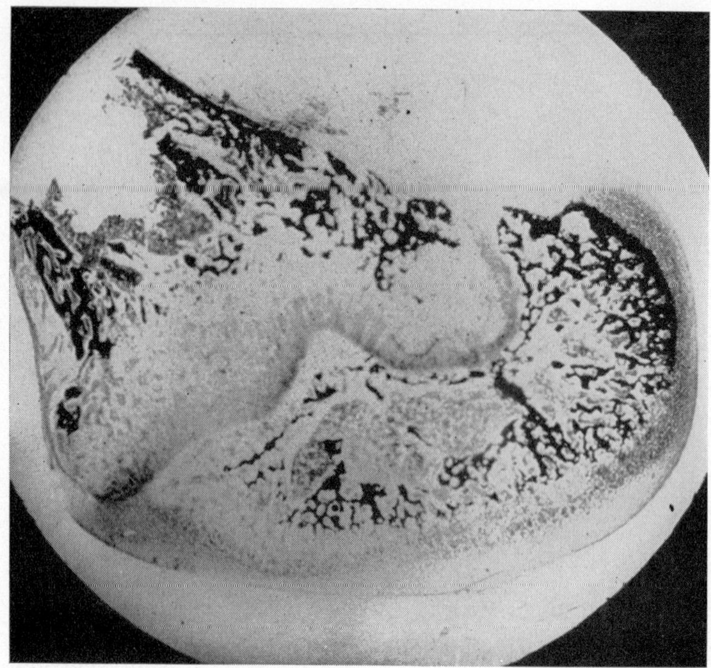

FIG. 14. Vertical section of the femoral head of a rachitic rat, showing irregular calcification of the femoral epiphysis, complete absence of calcium salts in the cartilage and metaphysis.

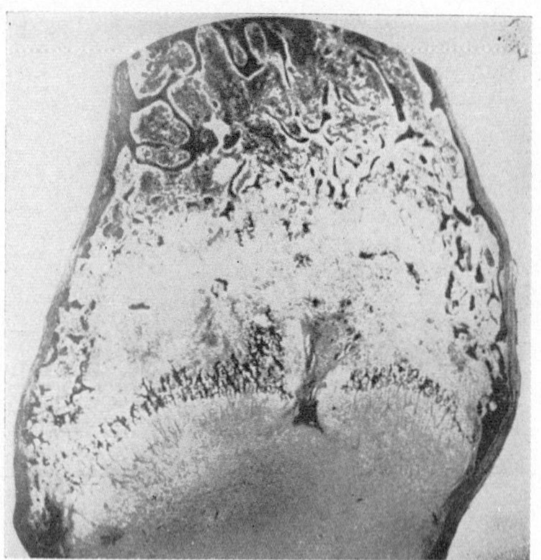

FIG. 15. The line of fresh calcium phosphate deposition in the provisional zone of calcification. Cross section of a costochondral junction.

mg. per cent. The inorganic phosphorus content of the serum is also fairly constant at about 6 plus or minus 1 mg. per cent. These values are slightly lower after 3 years of age, and still lower in adults. Howland and Kramer developed a mathematical formula which represents one of the chemical requirements for normal bone mineral deposition. They found that in most cases of uncomplicated rickets, the product of calcium concentration in milligrams per cent and the inorganic phosphorus concentration in milligrams per cent is 30 or less; if it is above 40, rickets is not present or is healing.

Park has pointed out that growth plays an important role in this equation. With cessation of growth, osteoporosis rather than rickets develops, while occasionally when organic bone growth is very rapid in the newly or prematurely born infant rickets may develop even in the presence of a normal plasma calcium and inorganic phosphorus. Rachitic cartilage will calcify when placed in an artificial serum solution containing calcium and inorganic phosphorus with a product of 40 or more. The effective product level will vary with such conditions as the *p*H of the solution, the total ionic strength, etc. Rachitic cartilage will calcify in normal serum but will not do so in rachitic serum. Damage to the cartilage itself will affect its ability to calcify.*

In the rachitic child with hypocalcemia the administration of soluble calcium salts in the absence of vitamin D will restore the normal serum calcium level, but there will follow a simultaneous drop in inorganic phosphorus concentration. In the presence of adequate vitamin D intake, normal calcium level is restored while normal inorganic phosphorus remains unchanged, thus establishing a higher calcium-phosphorus product.

In the normal child, vitamin D therefore influences the concentration of calcium in at least two ways: by increasing absorption from the gastrointestinal tract, and by regulating renal loss of calcium and phosphate either directly or through the parathyroid glands, thereby raising the solubility product of calcium phosphate in the plasma. The mechanism seems to be as follows: Vitamin D produces a rise in the serum calcium, which in turn depresses parathyroid activity. Since the action of the parathyroids is to diminish the renal threshold for phosphorus and to decrease P(Tm), their suppression raises the threshold and elevates the serum phosphorus level. Parathyroid secretion prevents reabsorption of phosphate from the renal tubules. Inhibition by vitamin D of parathyroid function favors such reabsorption and enables the organism to maintain a normal serum inorganic phosphorus level. It has been suggested that parathyroid hormone also affects glomerular filtration rate.

To summarize, the action of vitamin D in the rachitic child is fourfold: (1) It increases the absorption of calcium from the gastrointestinal tract. (2) It improves phosphorus absorption. (3) It increases urinary phosphorus excretion, although phosphorus clearance actually is decreased because of increased tubular resorption. This is accomplished presumably by the inhibitory effect of increased plasma calcium upon parathyroid hormone secretion. In the absence of the parathyroids, phosphorus clearance is actually increased by vitamin D intake. (4) It restores the ability of cartilage and osteoid to take up calcium phosphate in the form of hydroxy apatite and stops the random proliferation of cartilage and osteoid.

Etiology

Rickets in the human results from a deficiency of vitamin D. Normally this vitamin is supplied to a small extent by the ingestion of the preformed vitamin, but largely through the ingestion of a provitamin which is transformed by the action of ultraviolet rays of the sun into the vitamin. The wave length of the active sun rays is between 313 and 230 mu. Their availability varies with the season, time of day, location, whether radiation is direct or diffuse, and the interposition of glass and clothes. In our civilization chance is eliminated by the regular administration of vitamin D.

The dependence of the human on the sun for the elaboration of the vitamin makes it obvious that the disease will occur more frequently in the winter and spring and in shut-ins at any season. There are also other predisposing factors. Rapid growth, pregnancy and lactation, with their need for increased amounts of calcium, are such factors. A diet deficient in calcium or phospho-

* Citrate plays a unique but not well understood role in this process. Although it interferes with in vitro calcification, it facilitates the in vivo healing.

rus, or containing these elements in improper combinations or proportions, predisposes to rickets. In this respect, cow's milk, in contrast to human milk, predisposes to the disease. The superiority of mother's milk in the prevention of rickets cannot be explained on the basis of any known factor. Age is a factor—the full term newborn baby even on a poor diet will stave off rickets for a length of time depending on how much calcium and phosphorus he has been able to store from his mother's reserves. Prematurity predisposes to rickets on a multiple basis, namely rapidity of growth, insufficient time to acquire material from maternal reserves and defective absorption of fats and fat soluble vitamins. Finally, there is some evidence that heredity plays a part in the varying susceptibility of different babies and in many forms of refractory rickets and osteomalacia.

The relation of vitamin D to parathyroid function requires clarification. As shown above, vitamin D favors the absorption of calcium and secondarily of phosphate from the gastrointestinal tract. By facilitating the resorption of phosphorus from the renal tubules, it maintains a more nearly normal calcium-phosphorus product and restores the deposition of hydroxy apatite crystals in the cartilage matrix and osteoid. Parathyroid extract, on the other hand, has no effect upon the resorption of calcium and phosphorus from the gastrointestinal tract but mobilizes these elements from the bones, thus maintaining a normal or abnormally high serum calcium level. It interferes with the normal resorption of phosphate from the renal tubules and thereby produces a hypophosphatemia. Bone resorption produced by parathyroid extract affects both organic matrix as well as minerals, and the space thus left is filled with connective tissue. Parathyroid glands hypertrophy when serum calcium is low or serum phosphorus level is abnormally high. After parathyroidectomy, serum calcium level drops; when blood is removed and decalcified and returned to the circulation, bone calcium is mobilized and the pre-existing low level is restored, whereas a similar procedure in a normal animal restores the calcium to a normal level. Thus, rapid mobilization of calcium from bone can occur even in the absence of the parathyroids but not to the same degree. Animals whose parathyroids have been removed may show a progressively rising serum phosphorus level when fed a phosphorus-rich diet until they die in convulsions. Infants fed a high phosphorus diet may show parathyroid hyperplasia. Toxic doses of vitamin D mobilize calcium phosphate from bone without connective tissue replacement. Parathyroid hormone affects the metabolism of both calcium and phosphorus. The drop in serum calcium level is not necessarily dependent upon a rise in inorganic phosphorus level. It is this independence of the two phenomena, namely the rise in serum calcium following the injection of parathormone without a compensating drop in serum phosphorus, and vice versa, that has suggested the existence of two parathyroid hormones, one affecting calcium metabolism, the other phosphorus metabolism.

The Human Requirement

In general terms, the amount of vitamin D required is the amount needed to permit normal growth and mineralization of the bones and teeth during infancy and childhood and to maintain these structures during later life, as well as to meet the increased demands of infection, pregnancy and lactation. Specifically, the determining factors for vitamin D requirement in the individual are: the varying capacity of people of various ages to absorb and retain calcium, the rate of growth of the individual, the adequacy of the diet as regards the absolute amounts of calcium and inorganic phosphorus as well as the ratio of these elements to each other, and the amount of vitamin D received inadvertently in their diet or the amount of chance irradiation.

Roughly, the daily need for calcium is 0.6 to 1.0 gram through infancy, 1.0 to 1.2 grams during childhood, and 1.3 to

1.4 grams during adolescence. The actual amount will depend on the rate of growth; hence, the increased tendency of the rapidly growing infant to develop rickets. The premature infant, born with a minimal store of calcium and phosphorus and subject to an increased rate of growth, thus suffers from a double handicap and is very susceptible to rickets.

For the prevention of rickets the average normal infant needs 1000 units of vitamin D daily given orally either as a concentrated fish oil or as vitamin D dispersed in water. Vitamin D-enriched milk containing 400 U.S.P. units per liter is also effective and is now widely used with fresh cow's milk, evaporated or dried milk. The advantage of vitamin D-enriched milk is that calcium and phosphorus are ingested simultaneously and in a fixed ratio to each other and to vitamin D. Occasionally, as in premature infants, larger doses are required. The actual amounts may have to be determined by the method of trial and error, controlled with serial x-rays of the extremities and repeated determinations of plasma calcium, inorganic phosphorus and alkaline phosphatase. When concentrated forms of vitamin D are indicated they should be given in water-dispersed form in doses of 3000 units per day to obviate possible defects in the absorption of fat soluble vitamins.

Prophylaxis should be continued throughout the year. When mothers cannot be trusted to continue this medication, where conditions exist that make adequate medical supervision impossible, or in the presence of prolonged infection, a large single dose of 600,000 units every 6 months apparently may be used with favorable results. There is little risk of hypervitaminosis with such therapy.

For the treatment of rickets in the otherwise normal child, smaller doses will suffice. Vitamin D highly dispersed in milk or in water seems to be more effective than when administered as a concentrated fish oil. As little as 400 units of vitamin D in milk will, in due time, cure the majority of rachitic children. When administered as vitamin D in oil, 1000 units daily is usually required. It is important that the diet contain adequate amounts of calcium and phosphorus, preferably in a 2:1 ratio, as well as a mixture of good proteins.

Although the practice of discontinuing the prophylactic use of the vitamin after the age of two, when a mixed diet is ingested, is widespread, Park's studies have demonstrated histologic evidence of rickets in children even up to 14 years. This would indicate the need for the continuance of supplementary vitamin D up to that age, in doses about half that for infants. Normal adults may rely on sunshine and incidental ingestion of the vitamin, but women during pregnancy and lactation require about 1000 units daily to avoid the deleterious effects of vitamin D deficiency. To insure an adequate dose of all known vitamins for children fed processed milk, evaporated dried and various artificial milk substitutes, mixtures of vitamins A, D, C and B complex, including B_1, riboflavin, niacinamide, B_6 and B_{12}, etc., are being used. These usually contain 5000 to 10,000 units of vitamin A, 1000 units of vitamin D and variable amounts of all the other vitamins, usually stated on the label, in 0.6 cc. of fluid.

All the oily concentrates of vitamin D usually contain about 220 units of the vitamin per drop, or about 10,000 units per gm. of oily material, such as cod, halibut or percomorph oil. All milks fortified with vitamin D contain 400 units per liter, while evaporated and dried milks contain an equal amount of vitamin D when reconstituted to correspond to whole milk.

Although oily preparations may be used for normal newborns and older children, the water dispersed preparations are to be preferred for prematures and for children suffering from some form of malabsorption, celiac disease, sprue, cystic fibrosis of the pancreas, intestinal shunts, parasitic infestation, etc. The use of oily preparations should be avoided in children who vomit. Aspiration of this material and the develop-

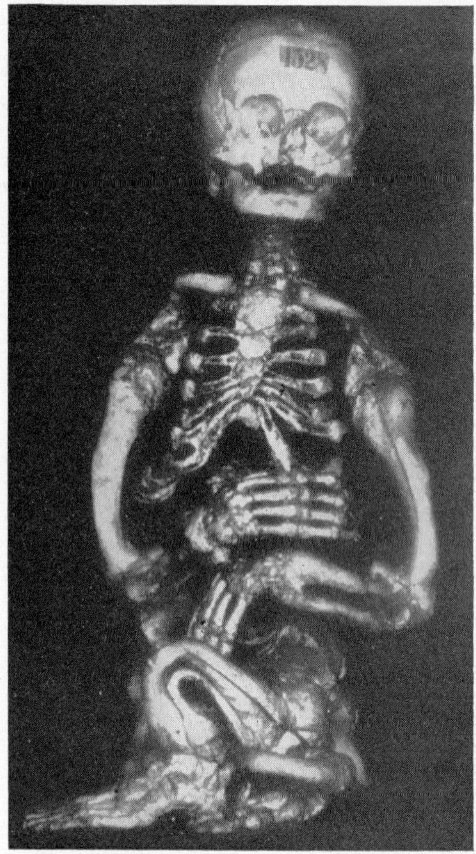

FIG. 16. Gross deformities produced by severe rickets.

ment of lipoid pneumonia may thus be avoided. Pure vitamin D_2 calciferol and vitamin D_3 7-dehydrocholesterol contain 40,000 units per 1 mg. of material. All dosage should be determined in units of vitamin D.

Pathology of Deficiency of Vitamin D

The pathologic changes resulting from a deficiency of vitamin D are almost entirely confined to the skeleton.* There develops a distortion of bone growth which gives rise to the clinical picture of rickets. The primary disturbance responsible for this distortion is a failure to mineralize newly formed osteoid tissue and cartilage matrix. Hence, the unusual softness of the bone which under the stress and strain of weight bearing and locomotion gives rise to the characteristic deformities of the disease.

To understand the bony changes which occur in deficiency of vitamin D, a review of the normal sequence of events in the growth of bones is pertinent. Long bones increase in length by endochondral bone formation. The narrow plate of epiphyseal cartilage is supported by bone on the epiphyseal surface and its diaphyseal side is uniformly penetrated by capillaries. During growth, a continuous proliferation of cartilage cells occurs on the epiphyseal side and there is degeneration of matured cells on the diaphyseal surface. These degenerating cells are replaced by capillaries and osteoblasts, which affect the deposition of bony matrix. Wolbach said that the growth of bone by endochondral bone formation is achieved by a continuously retreating

* Amino aciduria has been described in ordinary vitamin D deficiency rickets in children, indicating a disturbance in intermediary metabolism of protein or a defect in renal tubular reabsorption of amino acids.

gap in the continuity of tissues, maintained on the epiphyseal side of continuous renewal of cartilage cells and on the diaphyseal side repaired by vascular outgrowth comparable to repair of any defect of tissues by the process of organization or granulation tissue formation. In normal growth there presents on the diaphyseal side of the narrow cartilage a continuous layer of clear or empty cartilage cells forming an almost straight line.

In the development of rickets the first change is the cessation of this degenerative process in the mature cartilage cells and, consequently, there is no ingrowth of capillaries and osteoblasts. The epiphyseal cartilage increases in width because of continued proliferative activity; this thickening is irregular since the cessation of degeneration does not occur simultaneously in all portions of the plate.

In the absence of the ingrowth of capillaries and osteoblasts, there is a failure of calcification of the cartilaginous matrix, and newly formed bones during the active stage of the disease have an osteoid structure. The basic structural alteration in rickets is not the failure of formation of bone but the failure of calcification.

The disturbance manifests itself most markedly where the most rapid growth occurs, for example, at the lower epiphysis of the femur. Longitudinal sections of a rachitic bone will reveal a wide, irregular zone of ossification at the junction of the epiphysis and diaphysis. This region is known as the rachitic zone. Microscopically, a large amount of osteoid tissue is found adjacent to the shaft, and irregular columns of cartilage cells project into this osteoid tissue. Growth of the bone is delayed or stopped completely, in proportion to the severity of the process. On microscopic examination of sections of the shaft, osteoid lamellae are found under the periosteum and lining the Haversian canals and marrow spaces. The structural changes in the bone are not identical in every case. In one type of the disease there is a large medullary cavity with a thin, porous cortex—a form approaching osteomalacia; in another type, the cortex is thick but porous and the medullary cavity is small.

Elongation of the bone takes place at

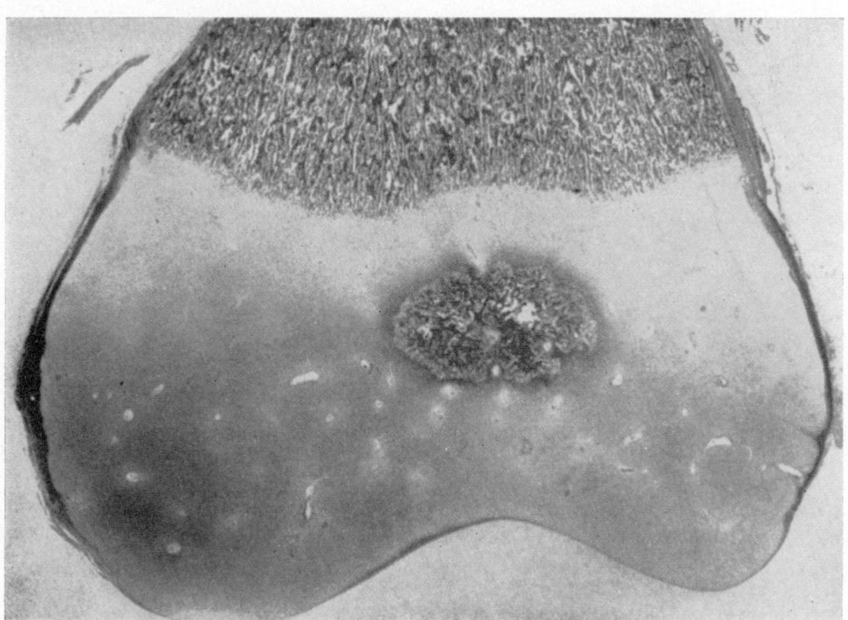

FIG. 17. Vertical section of a tibia, showing the center of ossification, the cartilaginous epiphysis and the chondro-osseous junction.

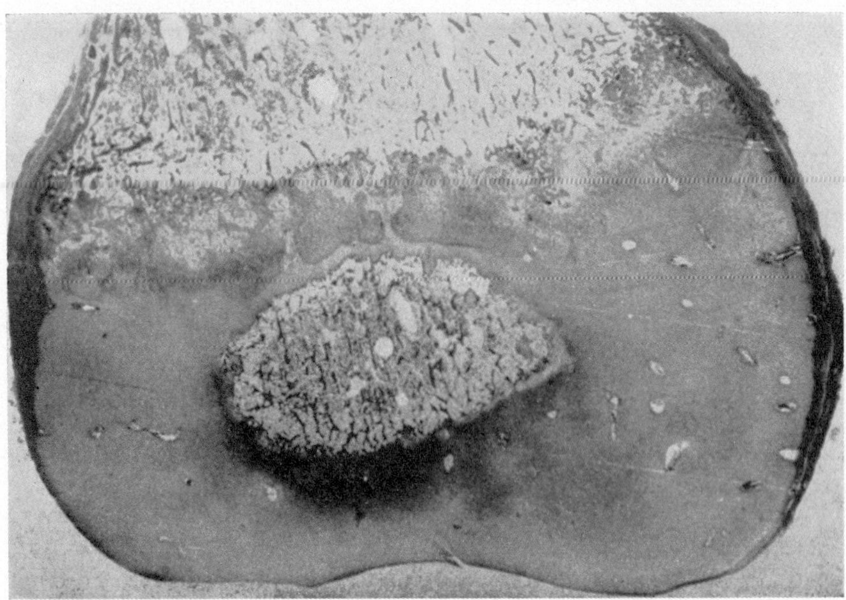

FIG. 18. Vertical section of a tibia, showing severe rachitic changes at the chondro-osseous junction.

its ends, where the condensation of mesenchymal cells has resulted in the formation of a cartilaginous plate which during childhood remains distinct from the shaft and is called the epiphysis. The flattened cells in this plate are normally arranged in columns, each cell separated from its fellow by a thin bridge of matrix.

The cells most distant from the shaft (zone of resting cartilage) consist of individual large cartilage cells surrounded by a uniform matrix. As we proceed in the direction of the shaft or diaphysis toward the second layer, the cells are arranged in columns and begin to show evidence of degeneration. In the third layer, the zone of preparatory calcification, the process of cell disintegration is almost complete. Here, if there are adequate concentrations of calcium and phosphate, there is a precipitation of calcium salts in the matrix but not in the cells themselves which results in calcification. Immediately to the shaft side of this area of preparatory calcification, the final stage of actual ossification takes place. The cell columns are invaded by loops of blood vessels and the cartilage cells seem to disappear, leaving the calcified matrix, blood vessels and connective tissue.

An adequate concentration of calcium and inorganic phosphorus both in the bone matrix and the tissue fluid is essential for this process, but the exact level at which calcification occurs is as yet poorly defined, and the mechanism itself is not clear. The metabolism of the hydroxy apatite crystals with reference to the collagen fibers of the matrix has been studied intensively by Robinson and others. These studies have thrown new light on the composition of the matrix. This material has been shown to be made up of collagen fibers and a ground substance containing a number of mucopolysaccharides. Under certain conditions collagen fibers acquire the capacity to take up calcium and inorganic phosphorus in the form of hydroxy apatite crystals. This work has cast doubt upon the crucial importance of alkaline phosphatase in the calcifying process and promises to throw light upon the nature of the so-called "local factor."

The chief consequence of vitamin D deficiency is the disruption of the orderly processes of bone formation and the production instead of an excessive amount of uncalcified bone, called osteoid, which is both soft and radiolucent. The amount of osteoid laid down varies at different points, increasing at areas of stress and strain, but decreasing at points of tension. When this soft bone is subjected to various stresses and pressures such as those that occur in walking and sitting, many types of deformities result. The deformities depend on the severity and extent of the disease process, its duration, the age of the child and the stresses and strains to which the bones are subject. Changes in the skull are among the earliest manifestations of rickets. There are flattening of the occipital bones from the pull of gravity and lack of calcification in circumscribed areas of the skull (craniotabes). Multiple fractures may add to the bizarre deformities.

Deformities of the chest and consequent physiologic inadequacy of the respiratory organs represent some of the most dramatic and serious consequences of severe rickets. In the advanced case, as the child lies in bed, the front of the chest is seen as a blunt wedge protruding forward, the sternum and adjacent ends of the ribs resembling the prow of a ship. The anterolateral portions of the ribs, corresponding to the costochondral junctions, have sunk inward, producing depressions running the vertical length

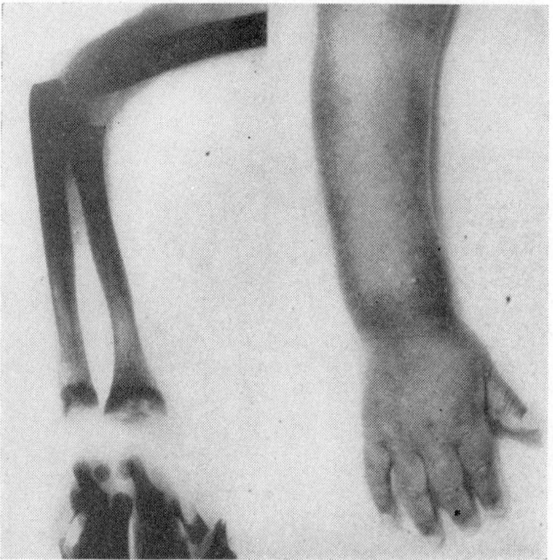

FIG. 19. Wrist of a rachitic child, showing the reason for the swelling—spreading of the distal end of the radius and ulna with swelling of the epiphyseal cartilage.

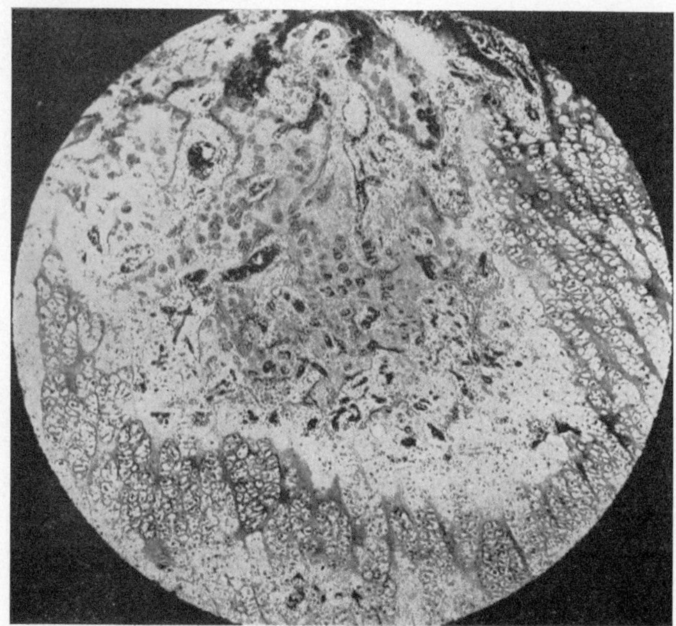

FIG. 20. Histopathology of severe rickets, showing a large capillary tuft replacing the cartilage columns, with scattered calcium deposits in the osteoid tissue and degenerative changes in adjacent cartilage cells.

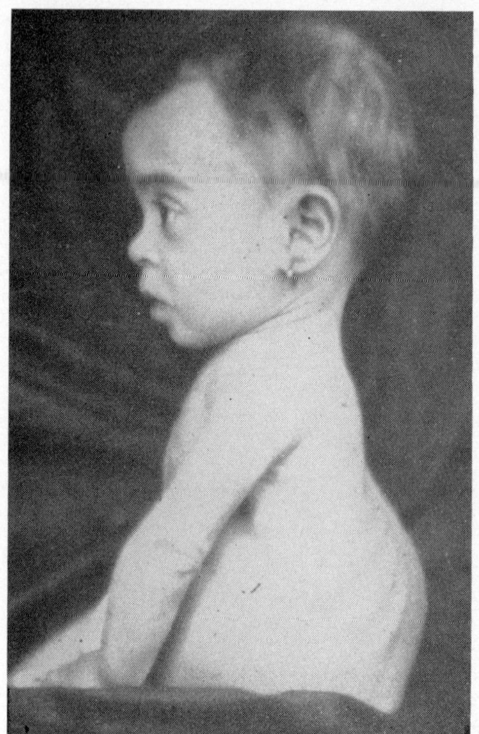

FIG. 21. Dorsolumbar kyphosis in a rachitic child.

of the chest. The essential difficulty physiologically is the loss of thoracic rigidity. As this process progresses, the linear depressions which at first were present only during inspiration tend to persist in expiration. As the efficiency of each respiration is diminished by collapse of the chest and the intrusion of the costochondral junctions and the rib ends into the chest cavity, pressure atelectasis of the lung is produced, with compensating emphysema of adjacent lung areas. The margin between vital capacity and tidal air volume decreases until the former is actually smaller than the latter and persistent cyanosis and dyspnea result. Such patients require intensive treatment with large doses of vitamin D to impart quickly the necessary rigidity to the chest by rapid mineralization of the organic bone tissue.

In infantile rickets, the pelvis becomes flattened by the pull of gravity on the soft structures. After a few months, when the child begins to sit, the pelvis must now support the weight of the head and trunk; as a result of this new stress and relaxation of ligaments a dorsal kyphosis appears when the child sits up and disappears when he lies down. When the child stands up, and later when he begins to walk, the strain on the spine changes again. Now the dorsal kyphosis changes to a sharp lumbar lordosis, thus further decreasing the antero-posterior diameter of the pelvis by anterior displacement of the sacral promontory. In the most severe cases, the head of the femur may push up the acetabulum, thus further encroaching upon the pelvic space. Pressure upon the sacrum from above increases the forward position of the sacral promontory, thereby narrowing the antero-posterior measurement of the pelvic

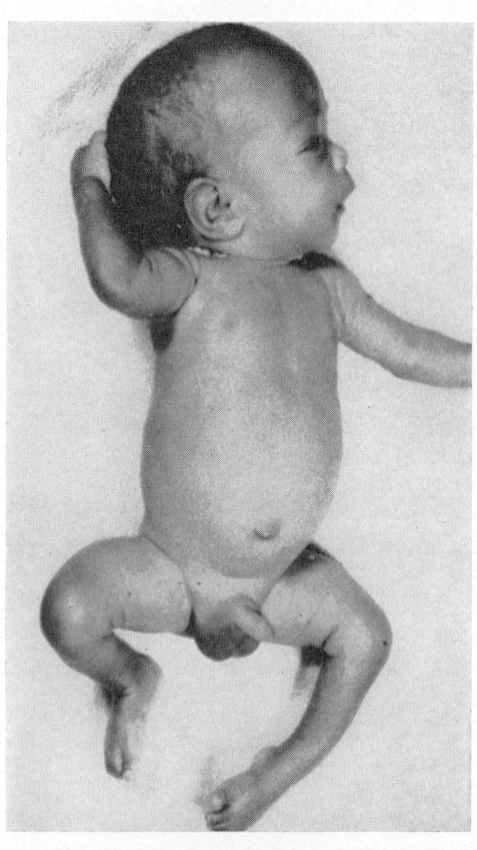

FIG. 22. A severely rachitic, prematurely born infant, showing severe rachitic changes in all the bones, marked craniotabes at 6 weeks of age and only slight deformities (some bowing) of the legs and thighs.

inlet while pressure on the lower sacrum and coccyx narrows the outlet; later, in the female, this makes the delivery of the product of conception difficult if not impossible during normal labor.

In the period during which the child begins to sit up, various deformities of the long bones may develop. The severely rachitic child sits cross-legged and supports the weight of his body with his hands. The upper of the two crossed legs is bent by gravity as it extends over the lower shin, which acts as a fulcrum. At the same time the wrists against which the weight of the body rests may also bend. Bending deformities may also be due to fractures which occur in the more severe forms of the disease. In addition to the actual bone involvement, there is great relaxation of the ligaments and traction on the bone by the tendons at their attachment which seems to initiate or accentuate many of the deformities.

Since endochondral ossification ceases with the closure of the epiphyses, deficiency of vitamin D in older people results only in shaft or diaphyseal changes; the disease thus produced is called osteomalacia. Pathologically we see only the superabundance of osteoid around the trabeculae and beneath the periosteum and a certain amount of osteoporosis. Linear fractures occur in which the fragments are held together by newly formed osteoid (Milkman's disease). All the complications of bone softening can then occur.

Severe osteomalacia occurs rarely in the Western world except during exceptional times of great stress. It has been reported in India, in Japan and in northern China among women during prolonged lactation with its drain on the calcium reserves. It also occurs among women of the higher classes in India who practice purdah and are therefore confined indoors away from the sun. Rickets and osteomalacia may vary in severity from a mere increase in the width of the osteoid seam in the shaft demonstrable only histologically to the most bizarre and crippling deformities.

Pathology of Hypervitaminosis D

The pathologic effects of overdosage with vitamin D have been studied chiefly in persons who have received massive doses of calciferol in the treatment of arthritis. In children additional cases have been reported as a side effect of vitamin D treatment for tuberculosis or after administration of imperfectly irradiated ergosterol preparations containing large amounts of toxic intermediates (vigantol). The basic pathologic effect is the precipitation of calcium in various tissues. Sometimes, withdrawal of large amounts of calcium into these abnormal foci may result in demineralization of bone.

The gross and histologic findings have been frequently reported and are similar in both children and adults, although fatalities seem to occur more frequently in the young. There is diffuse calcinosis affecting the joints, synovial membranes, kidneys, myocardium, pulmonary alveoli, parathyroid glands, pancreas, skin, lymph glands, large and medium-sized arteries, the conjunctivae and cornea, and the acid-secreting portion of the stomach. The abnormal calcification can be seen grossly as a whitish, chalky material. The bones in the early stages may show accelerated calcification of the provisional zone of calcification with thickening of the periosteum. In more advanced cases, however, there is interference with cartilage growth, and several authors have demonstrated diffuse demineralization of the bones. Shelling and Asher pointed out that osteoporosis produced by hypervitaminosis differs from that produced by parathormone in that the resorbed areas are not replaced by fibrous tissue. The most serious involvement is that of the kidneys, and most of the fatal cases terminate in uremia. The best evidence seems to indicate that the initial kidney damage is due to deposition of calcium in areas of degeneration, and later there is complete obstruction of renal tubules by calcium salts. As a result of the obstruction several nephrons at first dilate and then atrophy. The kidney damage in turn is responsible for such pathology as hypertension, hypertensive retinopathy and chemical evidence of renal insufficiency.

The dosages administered before evidence of intoxication appears vary tremendously. As little as 400 units daily seems to have produced fatal pathology in one instance. The shortest length of time over which the vitamin has been given before demonstrable calcification was produced was 14 days. Albright and Reifenstein ascribed all the manifestations of hypervitaminosis D to an exaggeration of the normal action of the vitamin: (a) to an increase in the absorption of calcium from the gastrointestinal tract, and (b) to an increase in the urinary excretion of phosphorus.

Clinical symptoms in nonfatal cases are anorexia, nausea, vomiting, diarrhea, polyuria, weakness, lassitude, headache, hyperesthesia, the appearance of areas of brown pigmentation over the skin and evidence of renal insufficiency.

*Rachitic Tetany**

Tetany is a disease characterized by convulsions and hyperirritability of the nervous system due to a low level of calcium in the blood. Since we have already noted that the serum calcium depends to an extent on the intake of vitamin D, we should expect some relationship between vitamin D deficiency, rickets and tetany. Actually, since the development of rickets depends on the lowering of the calcium-phosphorus product in the blood, the disease may result from insufficiency of either element. Most cases of rickets are due to a low phosphate in the blood, and these patients will not suffer from tetany. In the infrequent instances of low calcium rickets, tetany is a concurrent condition.

The symptoms of tetany are convulsions, carpopedal spasm, occasional laryngospasm and the objective findings of Chvostek's sign, Trousseau's phenomenon and anodal reversal on galvanic stimulation and an anodal opening reaction with a stimulus of less than 5 ma. The diagnosis is confirmed by the finding of a blood calcium of 7 mg./100 cc. of serum or less in the presence of a normal plasma protein level.

Prevention depends upon proper diet and the administration of an adequate amount of vitamin D. Treatment during a convulsive attack should be with intravenous calcium solution, i.e., 10 per cent calcium gluconate or lactate (1.0 cc./Kg.) intravenously, followed by adequate dosage of vitamins as well as oral calcium chloride (1.0 gm. in a concentration not to exceed 2 per cent, i.e., 50 cc. 3 times a day). A daily dose of 100,000 units of vitamin D for 3 days followed by the usual 400 units daily will stop further convulsions and quickly restore a safe serum calcium level.

* Other forms of tetany may or may not be associated with hypocalcemia. These do not concern us, since they have no relation to vitamin D deficiency.

Diagnosis of Rickets

The diagnosis of rickets is easy when the disease is advanced, but the chief challenge occurs in the early stages of the disease. In advanced cases the presence of craniotabes, bossing of the cranial vault due to periosteal thickening, persistence of a large open fontanel, enlargement of the epiphyses at the wrists and ankles and of the costochondral junctions of the ribs, the presence of the characteristic deformity of the chest, curvature of the spine, deformity of the pelvis, fractures and curvatures of the long bones, knock knees, coxa vara and delayed dentition make the diagnosis simple.

In less advanced cases the most delicate criteria of rickets are the calcium and inorganic phosphorus concentrations in the serum, characteristic x-ray findings of the extremities, especially the wrists, and the serum alkaline phosphatase level. The blood calcium level in normal children varies between 9.5 and 11 mg. per cent. The phosphorus level is much less constant, but 5 mg. per cent is average. The product of serum calcium and phosphorus should exceed 40; if it is 30 or less, rickets probably exists. While rickets may occur with either a low serum calcium or a low phosphorus, it is usually the latter which is reduced, usually to 2 to 4 mg. per cent, but sometimes as low as 0.5 mg. per 100 cc. of plasma.

Following treatment, blood serum calcium and inorganic phosphorus usually return to a normal level in 3 to 4 weeks. At this time, or soon after, the first evidence of healing is demonstrable in the x-rays of the long bones. The alkaline phosphatase level which in untreated cases may be 15 to 40 units (Bodansky), drops to a lower level but remains abnormally high long after the blood calcium and inorganic phosphorus are normal and bone healing is well advanced. A normal alkaline phosphatase level is usually not attained until healing is almost complete. During the active rachitic process the ratio of fecal calcium to urinary calcium or the similar phosphorus ratio is high. As healing progresses these ratios drop, and in the case of phosphorus the ratio may actually be reversed. Actual retention of these elements increases markedly during healing.

Examination of the lower end of the radius and ulna are most useful for roentgenologic diagnosis of this disease. The characteristic changes are found at the cartilage-shaft junction: cupping, spreading, spur formation, fringing and stippling. Cupping refers to a concavity of the distal ends of the radius and ulna, replacing the usual sharp delineation of the end of the bone. In severe rickets the cupping may not be manifest until healing begins. Cupping may be seen in scurvy and may also be found in the chondrodystrophies, and so it is not in itself diagnostic of rickets. Spreading of the end of the shaft may occur in any of the long bones. This too is often seen in scurvy. Spurs are elongated shadows which are prolongations of the cortex along the sides of the epiphyseal cartilage. They are composed of tissues containing lime salt. Irregularities in the laying down of calcium salts gives rise to fraying and stippling. Fraying consists of thread-like shadows extending from the ends of the shaft into the transparent cartilage. They may be long and coarse, as in advanced rickets, or they may be short and thin, as in early cases. Stippling is present when the outline of the end of the shaft has an irregular appearance. It may appear early but is more often found late, and this appearance is also due to irregular deposition of lime salts. It should be emphasized again that spreading, cupping, spur formation and stippling are not by themselves diagnostic of rickets. Ossification centers are often delayed in their appearance or, if present, are so poorly calcified that their margins merge imperceptibly with the surrounding cartilage. The area between the shaft and the epiphysis is of varying width in rickets, depending upon the severity and duration of the process, and narrows with healing. Distinct trabeculation is seen in the shafts of the long bones; the cortex is thin and may be reduplicated because of deposition of repeated layers of osteoid tissue. This may not be visible until healing has begun.

The first evidence of recovery from rickets consists of a deposit of lime salt at the cartilage-shaft junction in the zone of preparatory calcification. Roentgenologically this is visualized as a linear shadow between the epiphysis and shaft or metaphysis at right angle to the shaft. As healing progresses, the space between shaft and line of initial calcification becomes narrower until they unite. Early calcification of the metaphysis may give a homogeneous shadow which later undergoes rebuilding into normal bone architecture.

Differential Diagnosis

Scurvy frequently has to be differentiated from rickets. Tenderness and pain exceeds that found in rickets. If teeth have erupted there is bluish discoloration of the gums. The crowns of the teeth are partly or completely covered by the swollen, bleeding gums. Evidence of a hemorrhagic tendency may be seen in other parts of the body. Conjunctival and retro-orbital hemorrhage and subperiosteal bleeding give a characteristic picture, and the associated pain compels the child to hold the extremities immobile, suggesting a pseudoparalysis. Conjunctival hemorrhages are usually seen in the bulbar conjunctiva, and retro-orbital bleeding may cause unilateral proptosis. Subperiostal hemorrhage causes local swelling with marked tenderness and may be mistaken clinically for osteomyelitis. An incision into such a mass may be fatal. Blood ascorbic acid level is low or absent, and loading tests reveal a marked depletion of tissue ascorbic acid. The roentgenologic picture in scurvy is usually readily distinguishable from that in rickets. Epiphyseal separations, which are common in scurvy, seldom occur in rickets. The differential diagnosis can be established by a consideration of the clinical course and careful survey of the x-rays and the blood chemistry, but it should be pointed out that scurvy and rickets frequently occur simultaneously. In uncomplicated scurvy serum calcium and phosphorus are normal, while alkaline phosphatase may be decreased.

Chondrodystrophy is fully developed at birth, and the patient has the characteristic dwarf stature, abnormally shaped head, abnormal facies, and usually an abnormal gait due to unusually short extremities. X-ray examination may reveal cupping at the bone ends but the bones are otherwise well calcified and may even be broader than normal. Fraying may be present in one form of this disease. Serum calcium, inorganic phosphorus and alkaline phosphatase are all normal.

Osteogenesis imperfecta in infants may be associated with craniotabes; in fact, most of the skull may be membranous. The disease is present at birth, and it is associated with blue sclerae and multiple fractures. X-rays show no evidence of rickets but very delicate bones with multiple fractures, most of which show callus formation often with gross deformities. The blood calcium and phosphorus are normal.

Refractory Rickets

In his Harvey Lectures on the "Etiology and Pathogenesis of Rickets" (The Harvey Lectures, 1922–23), Dr. Howland in a prophetic mood concluded, "Rickets has had its day. It will be stamped out." He then cautiously added, "Or at least reduced to insignificant proportions." That prophecy has been realized. Vitamin D deficiency rickets has practically disappeared. However, this has brought into focus a group of cases due not to a deficiency of vitamin D but to some metabolic defect in the patient. Though few in number, their importance is great because of the light which they throw on the nature of the rachitic process. These cases have been called endogenous rickets, in contrast to vitamin D deficiency rickets, known as exogenous rickets. The English authors have preferred to characterize the first as rickets due to nature, the second as rickets due to nurture.

Endogenous rickets may be divided into three types depending upon the organ involved. In Type 1, the abnormality is due mainly to intestinal dysfunction. In Type 2, the disease is primarily renal. In Type 3 (and this is the least certain), it is hepatic. Type 1 is a form of rickets due for the most part to malabsorption from the gastrointestinal tract. This may involve calcium, phosphorus or vitamin D, or all three. The result is a deficiency of vitamin D and a metabolic disturbance identical with that seen in vitamin D deficiency rickets, namely, deficient absorption of calcium primarily, impairment in the absorption of phosphorus secondarily, and impairment in vitamin D absorption which is probably responsible for the first two. This condition occurs to some extent in the premature and to a greater degree in the celiac syndrome, cystic fibrosis of the pancreas, idiopathic steatorrhea, sprue, etc. In these cases there are likely to be a low blood serum calcium, normal or low blood serum phosphorus, defective absorption of both of these elements from the intestines and a high ratio of stool to urine calcium and phosphorus. A large dose of vitamin D given in a water dispersed medium or by parenteral administration will usually correct this defect. The renal lesion is

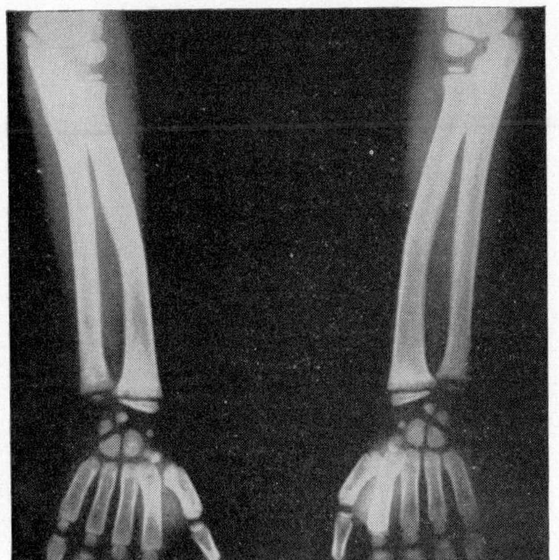

FIG. 23. X-rays of an infant with active rickets, showing thinning of the cortex, spur formation and diffuseness of the ends of the bones with cupping.

essentially the same as that seen in ordinary vitamin D deficiency rickets.

Hepatic disease may interfere with the storage of vitamin D and in some as yet unknown manner may decrease the calcifying properties of the vitamin, giving rise to a rachitic picture. Such cases are very rare.

Harrison and Harrison have shown that, in the absence of vitamin D, inorganic phosphorus clearance by the kidneys is increased, or rather, resorption of phosphorus from the renal tubules is diminished so that the inorganic phosphorus level in the blood plasma is low, and that if this persists for a sufficient length of time, rickets develops. When vitamin D is administered, resorption of phosphorus from the renal tubules is improved. The level of inorganic phosphorus in the blood rises and the rickets heals. Vitamin D improves the absorption of phosphorus from the gastrointestinal tract; increased amounts of phosphorus appear in the urine, and this masks the improvement in phosphorus reabsorption from the tubules. It has been postulated that this function is mediated through the parathyroid glands; that is, the improved absorption of calcium caused by vitamin D tends to raise the calcium level in the blood plasma. This in turn inhibits parathyroid function, resulting in decreased clearance of phosphorus by the kidneys and the re-establishment of a normal inorganic phosphorus in the blood plasma.

It is obvious, therefore, that any condition which affects renal function in such a way as to interfere with the resorption of inorganic phosphorus and with the role of the kidneys in calcium and phosphorus homeostasis may give rise to rickets. A number of such cases have been reported. It is now clear that there are different degrees of renal tubule involvement giving rise to excessive losses of various materials, inorganic phosphorus, glucose, amino acids, water and potassium on the positive side, while on the negative side, the tubules

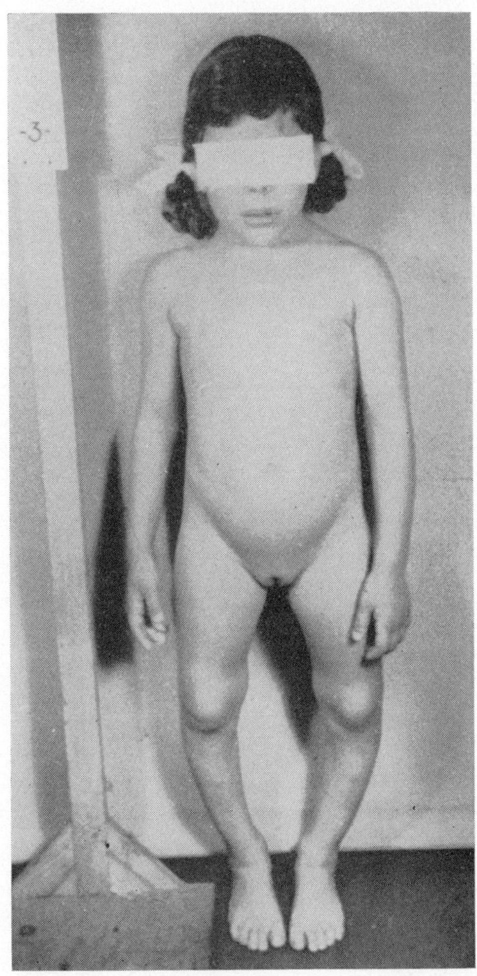

FIG. 24. Refractory rickets with dwarfism, bow legs and swelling of the ankles.

TABLE 1. RICKETS OR OSTEOMALACIA ASSOCIATED WITH DEFECTS OF TUBULE FUNCTION (AND SOMETIMES WITH OTHER METABOLIC DEFECTS)

TYPE	TUBULE REABSORPTION DEFECT					TUBULE FUNCTION DEFECT		NAMES USED IN LITERATURE TO DESCRIBE THESE SYNDROMES
1	Phosphate							Resistant (or refractory) rickets, raised late rickets resistance to vitamin D(RRD) essential hypophosphataemic rickets, idiopathic osteomalacia, Milkman's syndrome.
2	Phosphate	Glucose						
3	Phosphate	Glucose	Amino-acids	Water*				Fanconi syndrome, Debre-deToni-Fanconi syndrome, Lignac's disease, cystine rickets, cystinosis, rickets with cystinuria, amindiabetes, diabetes aminicus et acidaminicus, "renal rickets," (?) hepatic rickets, hypophosphataemic glycosuric rickets.
4	Phosphate	Glucose	Amino-acids	Water*	Potassium*	Urine Acidification		
5	Phosphate				Potassium*	Urine Acidification		Nephrocalcinosis with renal rickets and dwarfism, hyperchloraemic nephrocalcinosis, Butler-Albright syndrome, renal tubular acidosis.
6	Phosphate				Potassium*	Urine Acidification	Ammonia formation	

* Defect not always conspicuous. (*Courtesy of C. E. Dent.*)

seem at times incapable of performing certain normal functions such as urine acidification through the exchange of hydrogen in the blood for sodium in the urine or an inability of the tubular cells to form ammonia.

In all of these forms of rickets, with the exception of the glomerular tubular disease associated with osseous dystrophy, nephrocalcinosis, dwarfism, hyperchloruria, hypercalcinuria and elevation of blood urea nitrogen originally described by Butler and Albright, there are a hypophosphatemia, a normal or moderately low calcium and, in some instances, an increased excretion of amino acids and other organic acids in the urine. Severe polyuria may be present with or without glycosuria. Increased excretion of potassium may give rise to the clinical syndrome of hypopotassemia with muscular weakness, pseudoparalysis and an abnormal electrocardiogram reflecting the severe electrolyte imbalance. The inability of the tubular cells to exchange hydrogen for sodium may give rise to a slightly acid or an alkaline urine and a chronic renal acidosis with a loss of calcium to supply the necessary fixed base needed to neutralize urine acidity in the absence of adequate ammonia formation. This may lead to excessive excretion of calcium in the urine and nephrocalcinosis. In one form of refractory rickets, excessive amounts of glycine alone appear in the urine. In another, cystine constitutes the major portion of the organic acid fraction. Cystine crystals may be present not only in the urine but also in the various tissues, including the liver, spleen and the kidneys, and even in the eyes, where they can be detected with the slit lamp. The cystine crystal deposits in the viscera may give rise to splenohepatomegaly. The nature of the agent which produces the injury to the renal tubular mechanism is not clear, but it must be some cytotoxic agent as indicated by the fact that in lead poisoning, a clinical syndrome simulating the so-called Fanconi syndrome of phosphaturia, hypophosphatemia, glucosuria and amino aciduria with rickets may appear and may be cured with calcium and E.D.T.A. A similar condition, except for the bone changes, can be produced in rats by the intraperitoneal injection of malic acid. In cases where polyuria is present, marked dehydration may be a very disturbing symptom. In the type of renal rickets in which there is advanced glomerular tubular disease as described by Butler and Albright, serum calcium is low or only slightly decreased, serum chloride is increased, and inorganic phosphorus is normal or increased. Calcification of the kidneys may be demonstrated by plain x-ray of the abdomen. Harrison has shown that this may be due to diminished excretion of citric acid in the urine. The renal involvement in glomerular tubular disease often leads to parathyroid hyperplasia, and evidences of secondary hyperparathyroidism can be seen along with typical rachitic changes in the x-rays of the bones. Dent has recently reported consistent healing of both the rachitic and hyperparathyroid bone lesions through the use of 5 to 15 mg. of A.T. 10 (dihydrotachysterol) given over a period of months. (This corresponds to 200,000 to 600,000 units of vitamin D.)

Differences in the susceptibility of children and even of animals to vitamin D deficiency rickets suggests that heredity may play a part. In cases of refractory rickets that simulate vitamin D deficiency disease but require large doses of vitamin D, the disease is apparently inherited as an autosomal dominant. The diagnosis of rickets in the child leads to an examination of parents and siblings. Some may have gross rachitic deformities with dwarfism, others may show hypophosphatemia, while still others may have defective absorption of calcium and phosphorus with minimal amounts of calcium in the urine and no rachitic changes in the bones. In other forms of refractory rickets the disease is inherited as a recessive. In these patients the rickets is usually not severe. It is associated with some degree of dwarfism with characteristic deformities of the extremities, a low inorganic phosphorus in the blood serum, a normal calcium and a high alkaline phosphatase level. Muscular development is good and activity and vigor are unimpaired. However, characteristic x-rays, blood chemical studies, metabolic studies on calcium and phosphorus and the response to vitamin D therapy leave no doubt as to the diagnosis.

Treatment. Treatment of refractory rickets is based upon a careful analysis of the clinical symptoms, the chemical pathology and the x-ray findings.

In all cases, large doses of vitamin D, beginning with 20,000 units and increasing at monthly intervals, if necessary, up to 500,000 units daily are indicated. This is given preferably orally in water dispersion. Increase in dosage is stopped when the urine shows a more positive Sulkowitch test or the x-rays reveal evidence of healing, the blood inorganic phosphorus exceeds 2.5 mg./100 ml. of plasma and the calcium attains a level of 10 to 11 mg./100 ml. of plasma. The dose is then gradually reduced until the minimal effective dose is reached.

In patients who have chronic renal acidosis, sodium bicarbonate 5 to 10 grams daily or a mixture of sodium citrate-citric acid* 5 to 10 cc. daily should

* Citric acid crystals contain ½ molecule of water to each molecule of citric acid. To prepare a molar solution of this acid, use 200 gm. of citric acid to 1 liter of water. Sodium citrate crystals may contain either 5½ molecules of water or 2 molecules of water in each molecule of sodium citrate; hence in the first case, 357 gm. of sodium citrate per liter of water will make up a molar solution. In the second case, 294 gm. per liter will be required. The dose is 40 cc. of citric acid solution to 20 cc. of molar citrate daily.

be given in addition to vitamin D. In patients with potassium deficiency, potassium chloride or bicarbonate 5 to 10 grams is indicated, to be administered daily by mouth and to be followed with repeated electrocardiograms and plasma potassium determinations. In patients suffering from glomerulonephritis with renal rickets, with or without hyperparathyroidism or with nephrocalcinosis, A.T. 10 (dihydrotachysterol) 5 to 15 mg. daily or 200,000 to 1 million units of vitamin D daily with 5 to 10 cc. of citrate mixture is recommended. In any case, vitamin D medication should be stopped or reduced when nausea, vomiting and polyuria appear, or when the Sulkowitch reaction becomes strongly positive. In advanced renal disease the Sulkowitch may not be reliable because of decreased calcium excretory capacity of the kidneys. In some cases the progress of the renal lesion may be temporarily arrested. In others the renal lesion is progressive and uremia may supervene in spite of definite improvement of the bone lesions.

OSTEOMALACIA

Although osteomalacia is a rare disease in the United States, it is important enough to merit some mention. It is generally agreed that in cases of rickets or osteomalacia the essential abnormality is the same, namely, a deficient calcification of the osteoid tissue. The term "osteomalacia" is often erroneously used to designate the existence of any skeletal disease characterized by "bone softness."

Numerous causative factors are usually operative in any single case of osteomalacia. Cases may be roughly divided into those due to a deficiency of vitamin D and those due to defective intestinal or renal function. In most of the cases of osteomalacia observed in the United States the condition is associated with chronic steatorrhea. As a result of the faulty digestion and absorption of fat, insoluble calcium salts are formed and the fat soluble vitamin D is excreted in the excess fat. The increased demands of pregnancy and lactation often intensify the symptoms.

In the mild form of osteomalacia the patient may complain only of weakness and pains in the bones of the legs or in the lower part of the back or other parts of the body while standing or walking. These symptoms may precede by months or even by years the appearance of characteristic x-ray findings in the bones. In cases of severe osteomalacia the patient may seek medical aid because of the distressing symptoms of severe tetany. Another patient may suffer from crushed vertebrae resulting from moderate lifting or a minor fall. In cases of advanced disease, severe backache is a common symptom. This pain often is generalized and is worse in the winter when there is greater deficiency of vitamin D. Muscular weakness may be marked, and a waddling gait is not uncommon. There is often marked sensitivity of the bones, including the ribs, the hips and the thighs, to light pressure. Skeletal deformities may develop. In the roentgenogram one finds generalized thinning of the bones with distinct trabeculation, thinning of the cortices, bowing, fractures and deformities of various types.

The diagnosis of osteomalacia may be difficult because of the insidious onset of the disease and the absence of characteristic x-ray findings early in its course. The administration of vitamin D at this stage often relieves the subjective symptoms and thereby points to the underlying nature of the disease. Tetany occurring during pregnancy or lactation or in association with chronic steatorrhea should suggest osteomalacia. Any skeletal disease characterized by generalized decalcification, such as the osteoporotic forms of hyperparathyroidism, senile osteoporosis, the osteoporosis of hyperthyroidism, bone changes due to basophilic adenoma of the pituitary body or suprarenal cortical tumor, occasionally multiple myeloma, disuse atrophy and the adult form of osteogenesis imperfecta may be mistaken for osteomalacia. It is obvious, therefore, that no final diagnosis should be made until an exhaustive study of the patient's condition has been made. Osteomalacia in the adult may also be caused by the same metabolic abnormalities that are responsible for the various forms of refractory rickets in the child and requires the same therapy.

HYPOPHOSPHATASIA

The role of alkaline phosphatase in the calcifying mechanism is not clear. Immature cartilage matrix lacks phosphatase and does not calcify. As it matures it acquires phosphatase and calcifies. After conversion into mature bone, alkaline phosphatase disappears. It is therefore not surprising to find that a marked depression of alkaline phosphatase in blood and bone is associated with a gross defect in bone formation. The condition known as hypophosphatasia or osteoblastic dysplasia first described by Rathbyn (1948) is characterized by a marked decrease of alkaline phosphatase in blood and bone as well as in the kidney, liver and other tissues associated with a rachitic-like bone change, namely, marked osteoporosis with irregular calcification of the ends of the long bones as well as the epiphyses. Flat bones of the skull also show irregular calcification with osteoporosis. The anterior fontanel is large and bulging, suggesting an increase of intracranial pressure. This bulge remains after closure of the fontanel. Craniosynostosis may be present.

Chemical findings in addition to hypophosphatasia are hypercalcemia 12 to 15 mg., normal or slightly decreased inorganic phosphorus, normal bicarbonate. There is no amino aciduria or hypercalcinuria. In the patients studied, calcium and phosphorus retention was good, although it is not clear at which stage of the disease.

Clinically the condition may be present at birth or may develop after several months or years. In infancy the symptoms are anorexia, vomiting, failure to gain weight in the absence of infection, failure to grow normally and periods of unexplained fever. Bulging of the anterior fontanel suggests increased intracranial pressure and often leads to lumbar puncture in infants and trephine of the skull in the older child. In either case, the cerebrospinal fluid is normal. The burr holes heal slowly and tend to enlarge. Rachitic-like swelling of the wrists, ankles and costochondral junctions is present.

Radiologically there are some significant differences. The ends of the femora show marked osteoporosis but maintain normal contour, and the fine fringing seen in rickets may be replaced by coarse irregularity with some spreading. The shafts are very osteoporotic; the cortices are thin but may be normal and areas of osteosclerosis may be present. The condition is often fatal in infancy but may go on to spontaneous recovery. Normal doses of vitamin D are ineffective, but large doses may bring about improvement. A markedly positive Sulkowitch reaction is an indication for reduction of vitamin D dosage. Impairment of renal function is indicated by increased blood urea nitrogen and decreased urea clearance as well as decreased excretion of phenolsulphonphthalein. Hypophosphatasia persists even after healing of the bone lesion. Vitamin D therapy improves not only the bone anomaly but the patient's general condition. Pains disappear, appetite returns, weight gain is accelerated and there is striking improvement in the sense of well-being.

References

Albright, F., Butler, A. M. and Bloomberg, E.: Am. J. Dis. Child., *54:*529, 1937.

Albright, F. and Drake, T. G.: Bull. Johns Hopkins Hosp., *60:*377, 1937.

Albright, F.: J.A.M.A., *112:*2592, 1937.

Albright, F. and Bloomberg, E.: Tr. Am. A. Genito-Urin. Surgeons, *27:*195, 1934.

Bills, C. E.: Physiol. Rev. *15:*1–97, 1935.

Chisholm, J. J. and Harrison, H. E.: J. Clin. Invest., *35:*1131, 1956.

Dent, C. E.: J. Bone & Joint Surg., *34B*, p. 266, May 1952.

Dent, C. E. and Harris, H.: J. Bone & Joint Surg., *38B:*204, 1956.

Dent, C. E.: Paper presented before the Gordon Research Conference on Bones and Teeth, 1957. Personal communication.

Eliot, M. M. and Park, E. A.: Rickets. In Brenneman and McQuarrie: Practice of Pediatrics. Hagerstown, Md., W. F. Prior Company, 1954, vol. 1, chap. 36, page 10.

Harrison, H. E.: Pediatrics, *14:*285–295, 1954. 1954.

Harrison, H. E. and Harrison, H. C.: J. Clin. Invest., *34:*1662, 1955.

Howland, J.: Harvey Lect., *18*:189, 1922–23.
Howland, J. and Kramer, B.: Monatsschr. Kinderh., *25*:279, 1923.
Kramer, B. and Kanof, A.: Vitamin D in Pathology of human Beings. In Sebrell and Harris: The Vitamins, vol. II. New York, Academic Press, Inc., 1954.
Kyle, L. H., Meroney, W. H. and Freeman, M. E.: J. Clin. Endocrinol., *14*:365, 1954.
Lowe, C. U., Terry M. and MacLachlan, E. A.: Am. J. Dis. Child., *83*:164, 1952.
Rathbun, J. C.: Am. J. Dis. Child., *75*:822, 1948.
Schlesinger, B., Luder, J. and Bodian, M.: Arch. Dis. Childhood, *30*:265, 1955.
Shelling, D. H., Asher, D. E. and Jackson, D. A.: Bull. Johns Hopkins Hosp., *53*:348, 1933.
Sobel, E. H., Clark, L. C., Fox, R. P. and Robinow, M.: Pediatrics, *11*:309, 1953.

THIAMINE DEFICIENCY (BERIBERI)

The achievement of the Americans in the Philippines, of the English in India and the Malay States, of the Dutch in the East Indies, and of the Japanese in their own country has inspired intense study of deficiency diseases throughout the western world. To mention the names of all who participated in the discovery and application of thiamine would be to list some 50 per cent of the mature biochemists of the world of today. It is doubtful that any substance ever isolated by biochemical means has cost so much in labor. The first gram of pure thiamine must have cost considerably more than several hundred thousand dollars. With quantity production now at hand, and with the ever-increasing knowledge of thiamine, a gift arising from a disease in the Orient is bringing relief to persons all over the world. For many it has banished ill health, making it possible for them to return to work; to others it has given rest and freedom from the pain that arises from nutritional neuritis. It has returned to normal persons with anxiety states that have been attended by unreasonable apprehension, fear and rage.

The vast expense of maintaining armies and missionaries in the Orient since the time of Columbus has been a heavy drain on the western world. It is regrettable that relatively insignificant expenditures have been devoted to scientific enterprise during this period. Certainly it is fair to say that the West and the East have profited little in the exchange of various infectious diseases with one another, but they have profited much from the benefits derived from the exchange of ideas. Throughout the scientific world, the names of Takaki, Eijkman, Funk, Vedder, Grijns, Williams, Peters, Westenbrink, Jansen, Seidell, Sinclair, Waterman, and many others are held in high esteem.

A disease affecting the teeming millions of the Orient incited and maintained the interest of scientists of the Occident until at last thiamine is relieving persons whose diet is deficient in this vitamin not only in the East but also in the western world.

Biochemistry and Physiology

Thiamine functions in a wide variety of microorganisms, in lower and higher plants, in insects, and in all higher animals. In the higher forms of life it performs a fundamental role in the physiology and chemistry of the cells. Thiamine is a colorless, basic organic compound, composed of a thiazole and a pyrimidine ring. The pyrimidine ring occurs in many physiologic substances, whereas the thiazole ring is rare in nature. The ease with which the connecting valence bond is broken between these two rings affects the stability of the compound. Any alkali cleaves it, and at room temperature sodium sulfite cleaves the bond so that the whole molecule is destroyed. The most widely used chemical test for thiamine depends upon the thiochrome reaction. It involves the use in acid solution of oxidizing agents, such as potassium ferricyanide, hydrogen peroxide and potassium permanganate. The amino group on the pyrimidine ring is oxidized and unites with the carbon in the thiazole ring. The resulting product, termed *thiochrome,* is an unsaturated three-ring structure. It has an intense blue fluorescence which can be measured quantitatively.

Any discussion of the physiology or biochemistry of thiamine must, for purposes of brevity, be limited to a survey of the present knowledge concerning its relationship to the various functions of the body. Although the final answer is not known, the volume of relevant literature thus far accumulated is so enormous as to make a thorough review of it impossible at this time.

Absorption. Thiamine is readily absorbed from both the small and the large intestine, but individuals vary with respect to the efficiency of absorption. Thiamine is not readily eluted from a fuller's earth absorbate (such as the present international B_1 standard) in the large intestine. Such a product is therefore less effective than those which contain the vitamin already dissolved in a suitable aqueous medium. Dann and Cowgill found experimentally that diarrhea causes a failure of absorption of an appreciable fraction of the ingested vitamin; it does not cause an excretion of thiamine from the organism through the intestinal wall into the lumen of the intestine.

Storage and Excretion. The various tissues of experimental animals contain thiamine in greater or lesser amounts, depending upon the thiamine content of the diets to which the animals have been subjected. The muscles, liver, heart, kidney and brain are rich in thiamine; the blood, spleen and lungs contain only traces. Westenbrink concluded that the liver and heart lose about four fifths of their thiamine content during a single week of deficiency and that the loss thereafter proceeds more slowly. The brain is best able to conserve its thiamine supply. In general, the amounts stored decline rapidly at first, then more slowly, the last minimal amount being retained persistently. Of all tissues, the muscle is first and most nearly depleted. In birds and mammals a depletion period is necessary before thiamine deficiency becomes apparent. This is strong evidence of the capacity for temporary storage.

Fecal excretion of thiamine is small and substantially constant over the usual range of intakes. The feces contain unabsorbed thiamine. Synthesis of thiamine by the intestinal flora does not take place in human beings. Thiamine is excreted mainly by the kidneys. The proportion that is excreted or destroyed by metabolic processes is not established, but changes in the intake are promptly reflected by the urinary output. In work on the metabolism of S^{35} labeled thiamine and 2-C^{14} thiazole labeled thiamine, it was determined that the urine was the principal excretory pathway. Only small amounts of expired $C^{14}O_2$ were obtained and only small quantities of radioactivity appeared in the feces. By paper chromatography of the urine of rats receiving C^{14} labeled thiamine, sixteen different compounds were separated. In addition to traces of phosphorylated forms of thiamine and larger amounts of thiazole derivatives, eight gave a positive thiamine response with *Lactobacillus fermenti.* It would appear that these compounds are mixed disulfides of thiamine being excreted by the body. In addition, thiamine has also been found to be excreted in sweat in small amounts comprising about 1 microgram per milliliter. It is clear that during periods of plentiful supply, the body stores thiamine; the excess is largely excreted. This limited capacity for storage requires that an adequate intake of thiamine be maintained.

Thiamine and Metabolism. An increase in the total body metabolism raises the requirement for thiamine. The precise chemical processes in which the vitamin participates are not clearly understood, but it is known that thiamine is intimately concerned in intermediary carbohydrate metabolism and in biologic oxidative reactions.

One function has been fairly well established. Thiamine in its biologically active form, the pyrophosphate, is a coenzyme which, in combination with a specific protein, acts as a catalyst in the removal of pyruvic acid derived from lactic acid in normal carbohydrate metabolism. A secondary consequence of this removal is the dissipation of lactic acid, the dehydrogenation of which is inhibited by excess pyruvate. This phenomenon is accompanied by an increase in carbon dioxide and often by an increased oxygen uptake. The relative predominance of the two varies from one tissue to another.

In beriberi there is an accumulation of bisulfite-binding substances (chiefly pyruvic acid) in the blood, urine and cerebrospinal fluid. Although a return to normal respiration and blood pyruvate concentration can be induced by thiamine or thiamine pyrophosphate, many investigators do not believe that the amount of bisulfite-binding substances in the blood is a specific test for thiamine deficiency. They point out that a similar increase occurs in other conditions, such as diabetes mellitus, in certain infectious diseases, and in severe congestive failure caused by organic heart disease. They state that any compound containing a carbonyl radical will give this reaction. There is much evidence to indicate that an accumulation of blood pyruvates does not cause the symptoms of beriberi.

Methyl glyoxal has been found in the urine of thiamine deficient rats. This compound is not present in the urine of normal rats. The apparent reason for the accumulation of methyl glyoxal in thiamine deficiency is the marked reduction in liver glyoxalase.

It is conceded that thiamine pyrophosphate serves in the disposal of pyruvic acid, but the method of disposal is subject to much disagreement. Peters and his associates favor the pyruvate oxidase theory; Lohman believes that it acts as a cocarboxylase; others regard it as a coenzyme for a dehydrogenase-carboxylase; and it has been suggested that by its action pyruvic acid is used in the synthesis of fat.

Peters and his associates look upon the process as an oxidation of pyruvic acid with the formation of acetic acid and carbon dioxide, and it is a fact that a large increase in oxygen uptake accompanies the removal of pyruvic acid from the brain and other tissues. In 1937 Lohman and Schuster isolated from yeast a pyrophosphoric ester of thiamine which appears to act as part of a decarboxylating enzyme system. They attribute to it the power to dispose of pyruvic acid by a simple decarboxylation with the formation of acetaldehyde and carbon dioxide. They state that cocarboxylase is synthesized from free thiamine by brain tissues. A combined oxidative and decarboxylating effect is favored by Lipman, who believes that thiamine pyrophosphate functions as a coenzyme for a certain pyruvic acid dehydrogenase. He concludes that there is simultaneous loosening of hydrogen atoms as decarboxylation occurs in a single reaction:

$$CH_3COCOOH \longrightarrow CH_3COOH + CO_2$$

Cocarboxylase, when used to refer to thiamine pyrophosphate, is objectionable in that it emphasizes only one aspect of its physiologic activity.

A fourth role of thiamine has been suggested. McHenry has proposed the hypothesis that fat is synthesized in the presence of thiamine, utilizing pyruvic acid as the intermediate. This hypothesis offers a concrete idea of the mechanism of the thiamine-sparing action of fat. Minz has reported an entirely different function of thiamine. He concludes that thiamine intensifies the action of acetylcholine, and that phosphorylated thiamine acts as a coferment with acetylcholine in the humoral stimulation of the nervous system. Birch and Mapson state that thiamine causes the deaminization of adenine nucleotides.

All tissue respiration experiments, by virtue of their complicated nature, necessitate a great deal of interpretation by inference. We are compelled, by a consideration of the enzyme studies carried out to date, to suppose that thiamine has many functions as a coenzyme in nature. The best established ones are the two known reactions of its pyrophosphate which, in association with a protein of yeast, can bring about a pure decarboxylation of pyruvic acid, or, in association with other proteins, can act to promote a simultaneous dehydrogenation and decarboxylation of pyruvic acid to form acetic acid and carbon dioxide. The other functions mentioned are less thoroughly established. Some of these reactions may predominate in one tissue; others, in another tissue. It is not unreasonable to suppose that thiamine, in the form of its pyrophosphoric ester, acts as a coenzyme for several enzymic systems. The outstanding fact is that the metabolic processes concerned take place not in the individual organ as a whole or in specialized tissues, but in the cells themselves. Thiaminase, an enzyme isolated from raw fish muscle, destroys thiamine. In man the availability of thiamine is reduced approximately 50 per cent by the ingestion of raw clams, probably because of their thiaminase content. There is also a synthetic analogue of thiamine called pyrithiamin, in which the sulfur atom in the thiazole ring is replaced by —c=c—. This compound has antithiamine properties in microorganisms and mice and presumably would have an effect in human beings if it were administered in sufficient amounts. This, like the other so-called antivitamins, is believed to act by entering into some part of the essential cellular reaction because of the similarity of the structure of the compound and the vitamin. It is most important to keep in mind that sufficient concentration of the vitamin will suffice to overcome the effect of the antimetabolite.

Thiamine and the Nervous System. The exact role of thiamine in the nervous system is not known. It is known, however, that brain tissue depends predominantly upon combustion of carbohydrate. Himwich et al., found an average glucose utilization of 14.6 mg. per 100 cc. in normal persons; in contrast, pellagrins who also had beriberi had an average value of 6.4 mg. per 100 cc. and a subnormal oxygen utilization. The diminished cerebral metabolism offers an explanation for the mental changes observed in persons with thiamine deficiency.

In some cases, thiamine deficiency has been associated with the etiology of Wernicke's disease (acute hemorrhagic polioencephalopathy). Clinically, the disease is characterized by vertigo, headache, nystagmus, photophobia, optic neuropathy, clouding of consciousness, oculomotor dysfunction, ataxia and bulbar paralyses. The syndrome is seen most frequently in chronic alcoholic addiction but has been reported in nonalcoholics as well. The neuropathology is variable but may consist of more or less symmetrical hemorrhagic degeneration of the gray matter around the third ventricle and aqueduct extending from the thalamic and lenticular nuclei down through the medullary nuclei. Occasionally, the mammillary bodies are also involved. Microscopically there are varicose dilatation and endothelial and perithelial hyperplasia of the small blood vessels. The nerve cells and parenchyma show nonspecific degenerative changes with foci of necrosis and reactive gliosis. There may be some fibrous thickening of the leptomeninges along with a minimal leukocytic infiltration. The lesions are similar to, if not identical with, those found in experimental thiamine deficiency.

Thiamine and the Heart. Aalsmeer and Wenckebach stress that the cardiac enlargement of beriberi is due essentially to edema of the muscle tissue. Certainly the change is not a hypertrophy, because the administration of thiamine causes the edema to disappear rapidly. Hastings found that the auricle is more sensitive to thiamine shortage than the ventricle and therefore loses tone and becomes distended. It is difficult to state what part the peripheral dilation and increased capillary pressure may play in leading to right-sided dilatation of the heart. Weiss has reported that peripheral arteriolar dilation may predispose to circulatory shock and the formation of edema. Keefer emphasizes the fact that muscular exercise plays a tremendous role in the course of the disease. If the patient is not disabled by polyneuritis and is able to do muscular work, cardiac insufficiency tends to result; if painful polyneuritis prohibits muscular activity, the myocardium is protected and cardiac failure does not occur. The heart lesions and edema have not been produced experimentally as a result of increased blood pyruvate concentration. It is known that the carbohydrate metabolism of the heart tissues is affected by thiamine deprivation, but this does not explain the predominance of right-sided failure. Although thiamine deficiency may result in left-sided enlargement or enlargement of the entire heart, the prevalent opinion concerning Oriental beriberi is that the picture is chiefly one of right-sided enlargement. Further work is necessary to prove the mechanism and the chemical changes through which this is brought about.

Thiamine and the Gastrointestinal Tract. It is well known that animals and human beings with thiamine deficiency have symptoms arising from the gastrointestinal tract. Loss of appetite has long been regarded as a prominent feature of this deficiency state, yet no specific cellular changes have been demonstrated to account for any of these symptoms. Our observations indicate that the symptoms of so-called "indigestion" and severe constipation in malnourished persons are frequently relieved by the administration of crystalline thiamine. Cowgill and his associates, and Fitts, have reported anorexia associated with gastric atony, spastic colon and hypochlorhydria in thiamine-deficient persons. It should be emphasized that thiamine plays a most important role in all the cells of the body and that alterations in the cells ultimately produce symptoms which disappear following therapy.

Pathology

Pertinent information with regard to the underlying pathologic changes of thiamine deficiency in human beings is more restricted than one would expect after many years of study. The ordinary methods of studying such changes have shown little concerning mild thiamine deficiency, yet one must assume that the minute biochemical changes have already occurred in the cells even though the crude methods of staining and microscopic examination do not detect them. The discussion which follows will deal with the findings of advanced thiamine deficiency, primarily with the accepted postmortem studies of typical cases of Oriental beriberi. These findings vary tremendously from patient to patient; for convenience, they will be discussed under three major headings.

The Nervous System. The most constant and striking findings of thiamine deficiency arise from chemical alterations which lead ultimately to degenerative changes in the nervous system. Many pathologists have reported congestion and edema of the brain and spinal cord in beriberi, but reports of microscopic studies of the central nervous system are relatively rare. Changes in the posterior spinal ganglion and anterior horn cells, as well as in the ganglion cells of the medulla and pons, have been noted. These cells may show chromatolysis and sometimes swollen and dislocated nuclei. These changes, in most instances, do not mean death of the cell, but indicate severe involvement. Degeneration of the medullary sheaths has been demonstrated in scattered fibers in all tracts of the cord, but especially in the posterior columns.

The pathologic changes in the peripheral nerves resulting from protracted deficiency of thiamine are indistinguishable, whether the person had uncomplicated beriberi or thiamine deficiency associated with conditions such as chronic alcoholic addiction, Korsakoff's syndrome, pellagra, sprue, pernicious anemia, pregnancy, diabetes, tuberculosis, colitis, senility, malignancy or cirrhosis of the liver. Hence, the authors regard the polyneuritis arising from a deficiency of thiamine as beriberi, irrespective of any other condition present.

Degeneration is most severe in the sciatic nerve and its branches, but degenerative changes may be found in any of the peripheral nerves. Characteristically, the distal portions of the nerves are first and most seriously affected. In the average case, early degeneration occurs in the brachial nerves at about the same time that late changes appear in the sciatic nerves. Changes often may be found in the phrenic, the recurrent laryngeal and the cranial nerves, particularly the vagi. Degenerative changes of the branches of the cardiac plexus, the splanchnic nerves and branches of the solar and renal plexuses have been described.

Degeneration of the myelin sheath is

constant and affects the majority of the fibers. Observations from the Nutrition Clinic of the Hillman Hospital, Birmingham, Alabama, show that counts done on biopsies of terminal portions of the anterior tibial nerves of patients with thiamine deficiency show fewer myelin sheaths in a given area than are normally present. It has been stated that the axis cylinders may show fragmentation and atrophy, but except in more chronic and advanced beriberi the majority of the axis cylinders appear normal. In the cases studied at the Nutrition Clinic, the axis cylinders were involved in the degenerative process usually in the same severity as the myelin sheaths (see Figs. 25 and 26).

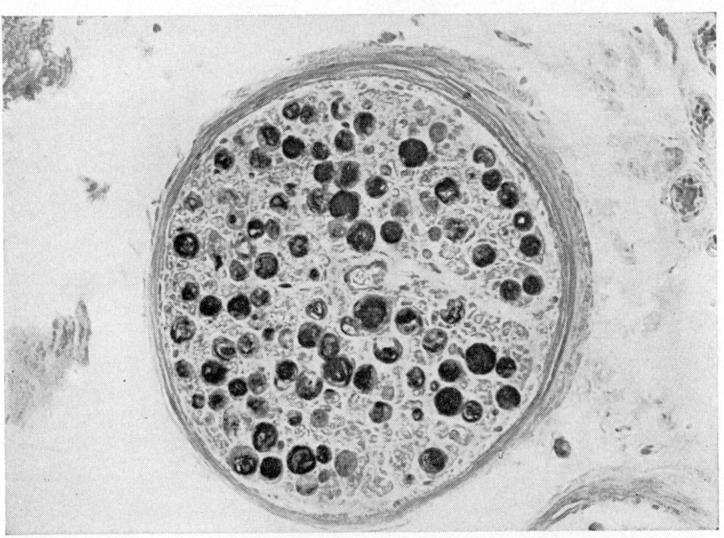

FIG. 25. Cross section of the terminal portion of the internal branch of the anterior tibial nerve in neuritis due to thiamine deficiency, stained with osmic acid (× 350). The myelin sheath count in this nerve is 2674/sq. mm. There are many large sheaths whose centers are filled with black-stained material. (This may represent swelling in a degenerating nerve.)

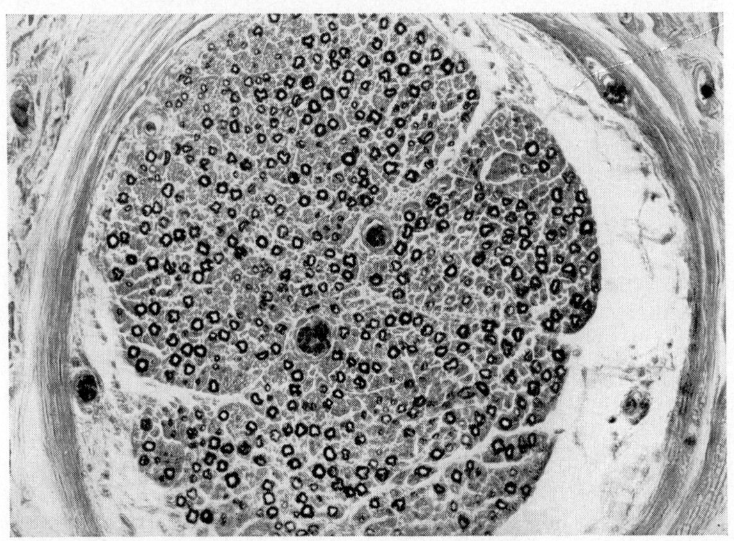

FIG. 26. Cross section of a normal nerve (terminal portion of the internal branch of the anterior tibial nerve), stained with osmic acid (× 350). The myelin sheath count in this nerve is 6836/sq. mm. (normal 5000 to 10,000/sq. mm.). The myelin sheaths stain black with clear centers and are uniform in size.

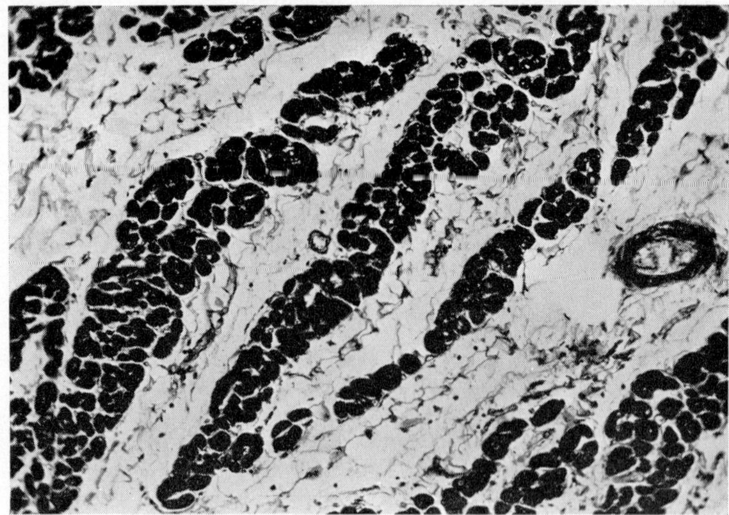

FIG. 27. Microphotograph of a section taken from the heart of a patient with the clinical picture of wet beriberi. The interstitial spaces are widened by edema and a moderate increase of collagenous tissue. The muscle bundles are swollen and show vacuolization (× 175).

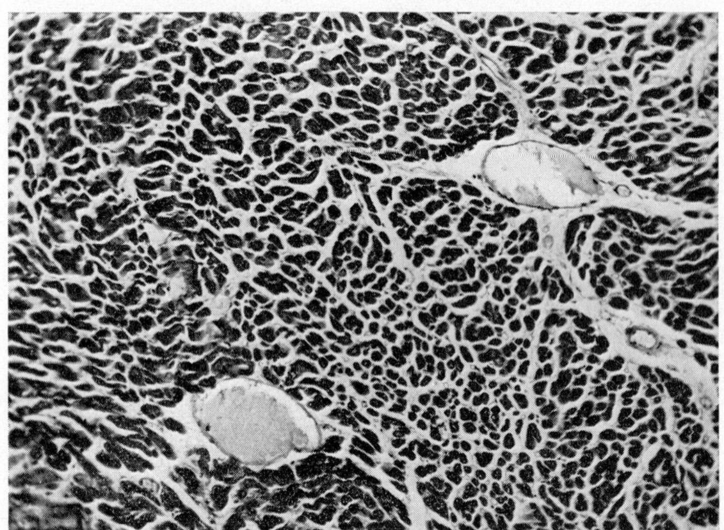

FIG. 28. Microphotograph of a section of normal heart muscle (× 175).

The Heart. In acute beriberi the heart is dilated and enlarged. Ellis found that the average weight of the hearts in 125 necropsies of beriberi was 379 gm. while the average weight of the hearts of 204 patients dying of other diseases was 255 gm. Japanese investigators also reported that the average weight of the hearts of patients with beriberi is above the maximum weight of the normal heart. In Oriental beriberi the enlargement is most pronounced in the right heart where the muscle is coarse and firm and the trabeculate and papillary muscles are especially prominent. The right auricle may be huge, with a "paper-thin" wall, through which dark blood is visible. The valves are normal. Some cases with sudden circulatory collapse and death show hydropic degeneration of the cardiac musculature and pronounced edema (see Figs. 27 and 28).

Weiss and Wilkins have reported that persons with thiamine deficiency in the

United States may have small hearts, less right- than left-sided failure, or left-sided failure alone. Since these findings differ strikingly from the classic picture of Oriental beriberi, could it not be that cases with small hearts also exist frequently in the Orient?

Edema and Serous Effusions. Edema and serous effusions are common in adults or in infants with acute beriberi. The edema may be confined to the legs and thighs, or it may be generalized, but the tissues of the face are rarely involved. Following postmortem incision, large amounts of serous fluid pour from the subcutaneous tissue. This edema is frequently associated with serous effusions which occur most often in the following sequence: hydrops of the pericardium, pulmonary edema, hydrothorax and ascites. The fluid is clear and greenish-yellow in color and often occurs in quantities of 50 to 500 cc. in the pericardium and 50 to 2000 cc. in the pleural spaces. Ascites is seldom severe.

Other Pathologic Observations. There is a loss of the subcutaneous, retroperitoneal and epicardial fat in persons having chronic beriberi. The muscles supplied by the diseased nerves, particularly those of the leg and thigh, are atrophied. Histologic studies show loss of cross striation and shrinkage of the sarcoplasm, often associated with cloudy swelling or fatty degeneration. Chronic passive congestion of the liver, spleen, kidneys and intestines is usually present. Punctate hemorrhages are often found subpleurally and in the walls of the stomach and intestines.

Infantile Beriberi. McLaughlin and Andrews have described postmortem findings in infantile beriberi similar to those found in adults dying of "acute cardiac beriberi." In their cases, the body appeared plump and well nourished, the skin was usually pale and anemic, and the flesh of the thighs and legs was often soft and flabby and, as a rule, pitted on pressure. The subcutaneous fat was grayish-white and moist; the edema tended to mask the actual loss of fat and the muscle atrophy. The changes in the heart were the same as those described in the adult. The hearts of the infants who died of beriberi had an average weight of 34.1 gm., while those of infants of comparable ages, who died of other conditions, weighed 20 gm. The lungs, abdominal organs, brain and other tissues were congested and edematous, and frequently showed petechial hemorrhages. The central and peripheral nervous systems in infants are less severely affected by thiamine deficiency than are those of adults. Although much has been learned from animal experimentation concerning the etiology of beriberi, the pathology of human beriberi must not be confused with that of birds and animals. The histopathologic findings, however, are similar in experimental and human beriberi, and in both, the functional disturbances precede any anatomic changes.

Symptomatology

Beriberi is characterized by multiple neuritis, often associated with congestive failure, generalized edema and serous effusions, and sudden death. Because these manifestations vary greatly in type, number, severity, and order of appearance, beriberi in the adult has been classified in three clinical types: (1) *dry* beriberi, in which degeneration of the nervous system, chiefly a multiple peripheral neuritis, is the chief manifestation; (2) *wet* beriberi, in which serous effusions and edema are the outstanding features; (3) *fulminating*, acute or pernicious beriberi, in which acute cardiovascular symptoms predominate. A combination of two or more of these types is often referred to as *mixed* beriberi.

Study of many persons developing beriberi shows that they have a long prodromal period of ill health. Observations by Spies et al. show that some impairment of intellectual and cognitive functions, exemplified by difficulties in concentration, attention and comprehension, and probably slight memory defects, may occur before any evidence of peripheral neuritis. These changes are usually accompanied by emotional disturbances, such as fear, apprehension, irritability, anger, hostility, depression, extreme sensitivity and general emotional instability. Because these symptoms are relieved by the administration of thiamine, it seems evident that they constitute an important feature of thiamine deficiency disease.

Loss of weight, strength and appetite precede diagnostic evidence of neuritis. For weeks or years the patient may complain of fatigue, of sensations of heaviness and a stiffness of the legs, and of inability to walk long distances. Other ill-defined disturbances, such as headache, insomnia, vertigo, dyspnea, dyspepsia, tachycardia, burning sensations in various parts of the body, and cramping and tenderness of the muscles, particularly in the lower extremities, may be present. If subclinical beriberi is not treated appropriately, eventually the full clinical syndrome will develop.

Nervous System. The symptoms arising from involvement of the nervous system are predominantly those of an ascending symmetrical, peripheral neuritis, of which the initial symptoms are pain, weakness and cramps in the legs. Heaviness of the legs and tenderness to pressure of the calf muscles are noted. Weakness is often followed by burning and numbness of the ankles and feet, and impairment of dorsiflexion of the toes. The Achilles and patellar reflexes may be increased, later diminished, and finally absent. The weakness spreads upward, involving first the extensors and flexors of the leg; at this time toe and foot drop may be demonstrated. The muscles of the arms may be affected similarly, but motor symptoms do not usually appear in the muscles of the upper extremities until the symptoms of the lower extremities have become severe. The upper extremities, however, may be affected first, particularly in persons who use their hands a great deal more than their legs.

Sensory disturbances may appear first and may be more prominent than the motor changes. Loss of sensation is greatest in the distal parts, but there may be no sharp distinction between the areas containing normal and diminished sensation. Appreciation of vibration is diminished or lost. Hyperesthesia spreads over the lower extremities in a socklike distribution, with anesthesia following in its wake.

Beriberi strikingly affects the vagi and occasionally other cranial nerves. Phrenic or recurrent laryngeal nerve involvement may occur. In severe cases, the musculature of the trunk and abdomen is affected. In most instances, the sphincter muscles are not involved until the late stages of the disease. When muscular degeneration is severe, the gait usually becomes altered; there may be ataxia and incoordination. Contractures are common when paralysis is long standing. The patient may become bedridden, suffer pain from the pressure of the bedding, and tend to develop decubitus ulcers.

Cardiorespiratory System. The cardiac type of adult beriberi is relatively infrequent in the western world. The manifestations most commonly seen are dyspnea and palpitation on exertion, tachycardia and edema. In the case uncomplicated by failure, the arterial blood pressure is usually normal or low, often with an increased pulse pressure. On palpation of the larger arteries, a bounding quality is noted and "pistol shots" may be heard on auscultation. The venous pressure is generally increased but may be normal. Electrocardiographic changes, chiefly of the T wave and QT interval, have been reported. The skin is usually warm and of normal color. At any time during the course of the disease, more severe cardiac symptoms may develop. Without previous warning to the physician, acute cardiac failure may occur abruptly, with paroxysmal onset of dyspnea, cyanosis, increased venous pressure, tachycardia, precordial pain and a small thready pulse. The heart generally shows striking enlargement, associated with pulmonary congestion. The speed of circulation is increased in the cardiovascular type of beriberi, whereas in other congestive failure, except that due to hyperthyroidism, there is usually a conspicuous slowing of the circulation.

Edema and Serous Effusions. Edema,

the most outstanding feature of "wet" beriberi, begins in the feet and legs, and may be mild or extreme. It frequently conceals the underlying muscular atrophy. Hydropericardium, hydrothorax and ascites are frequently associated with a generalized edema. Edema of the lungs occurs in at least 50 per cent of the acute cases.

Observations on the children of several hundred families having pellagra, beriberi or riboflavin deficiency show that many develop early clinical signs of thiamine deficiency. The early symptoms are similar to those of pellagra, but these children, if untreated, eventually develop other evidence of beriberi.

Infantile Beriberi. Three clinical forms of infantile beriberi have been described—the aphonic, the pseudomeningitic and the cardiac. The cardiac type is the most common and occurs most frequently during the first three months of life, although cases of four, five, six and even ten months of age have been noted. It affects chiefly breast-fed infants whose mothers have latent or manifest thiamine deficiency.

The onset of symptoms is insidious. The infant is nearly always plump, apparently well-nourished, good-natured and playful. The face is full, sometimes presenting a swollen appearance. Frequently edema of the lower extremities may be demonstrated. Somewhat later there is cyanosis, slight dyspnea, periodic restlessness and moaning, disturbed sleep and occasional vomiting. There may be a slight cough and a peculiar shrill whining cry. Aphonia may be present for several weeks or it may occur only later in the disease. Constipation is the rule; diarrhea may occur, but in some cases the bowels are normal. Oliguria is a later symptom. The temperature tends to be subnormal. The skin is pale, soft and velvety. The pulse is normal or slightly increased in rate, irregular and of fair volume. The heart is grossly enlarged. The second pulmonic sound is accentuated. The apex beat may be clear or muffled. Later in the course of the disease, acute attacks of dyspnea appear. Eventually, if untreated, the infant dies of cardiac failure.

Diagnosis

The physician must bear in mind that thiamine deficiency occurs particularly among the following groups:

1. The indigent and persons who have faulty dietary habits and idiosyncrasies. Such persons usually subsist on a diet abundant in overmilled rice, wheat or corn. Their diets are high in carbohydrates and relatively low in protein, minerals and vitamins.

2. Patients who have organic diseases or other conditions which may affect their appetites or the assimilation and utilization of the essential food substances. Beriberi is associated particularly with functional and organic gastrointestinal diseases, chronic debilitating diseases, pernicious vomiting of pregnancy, chronic alcoholic addiction, diabetes and pellagra.

3. Persons in whom the thiamine requirement is distinctly above the average because of rapid growth, the increased metabolic demands of pregnancy and lactation, febrile diseases, hyperthyroidism or hard physical exertion.

The following procedures suggested by Vedder often aid in the diagnosis of mild cases of thiamine deficiency: Squeeze the muscles of the calf to detect *muscular hyperesthesia;* test the anterior surface of the leg with a pin for *anesthesia;* test the *ankle jerk* (any modification is to be suspected); have the patient perform the *squatting test,* squatting upon his heels in the Oriental manner of sitting (in the patient with beriberi this may cause pain and he may be unable to rise except by using his hands).

There is no satisfactory diagnostic test for thiamine deficiency suitable for the clinical laboratory or for the doctor in general practice, but the response to an adequately controlled therapeutic test is pathognomonic of thiamine deficiency. The patient should be given 50 mg. of thiamine hydrochloride in physiologic saline intravenously for several days. In making a diagnosis of uncomplicated beriberi, other causes of peripheral neuritis, organic heart disease and nephritis must be excluded. It is well to keep in mind, however, that beriberi may occur along with other organic diseases.

Course and Prognosis

Beriberi in the adult, whether endemic or associated with other diseases, is generally insidious in onset and chronic in course, except in cases of acute cardiac beriberi. Since most patients suffer from a partial deficiency of the vitamin, they may continue for long periods without further progression of their disease. Acute attacks may be precipitated by infections or excessive physical activity.

A favorable course depends upon an early diagnosis and intensive and persistent therapy. In acute beriberi of infants or adults, recovery is nearly always prompt and complete if proper treatment is given; chronic beriberi responds less rapidly and completely.

Treatment with Thiamine

Chemical Description. Thiamine is a white crystalline compound which is prepared synthetically as the hydrochloride. It is a combination of a pyrimidine and a thiazole ring (see Fig. 29).

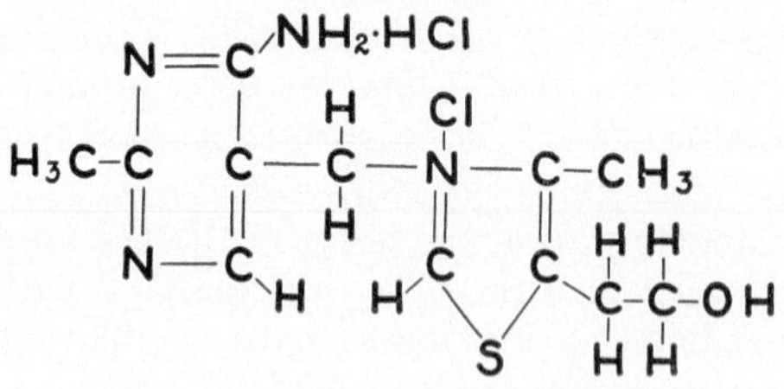

FIG. 29. Thiamine hydrochloride.

Because it contains sulfur, it is unique among the vitamins. The properties of the natural and the synthetic compounds are identical. The hydrochloride melts at 248 to 250° C. and is extremely soluble in water. It is stable at 100° C. in acid solution but is destroyed at 100° C. in neutral or alkaline solution.

Method of Administration. Oral administration is the procedure of choice for the average ambulatory patient, although its effect is slower and much less certain. For the severely ill person with neuritis, edema or cardiovascular involvement, the use of the parenteral route is imperative. This method is also indicated in persons with intrinsic disease of the gastrointestinal tract or in those recovering from major abdominal operations. Excretion is very rapid following parenteral administration, making frequent injections necessary to maintain a high blood thiamine concentration. The authors prefer the intravenous to the intramuscular route, since the devitalized tissues of persons with nutritional deficiency diseases are prone to infection and abscess formation following repeated intramuscular injections. Thiamine, dissolved in physiologic salt solution or in 5 per cent glucose in physiologic saline, may be given by slow infusion. Since this vitamin is heat-labile, it cannot be autoclaved for sterilization.

In adults, mild thiamine deficiency may be treated by the oral administration of 10 mg. three times daily; for more severe cases, 25 mg. twice daily should be given parenterally. Mild cases in children respond to 5 mg. orally; for severely ill infants and children, the intravenous administration of 10 mg. twice daily is recommended. Thiamine administered to the nursing mother will increase the amount contained in the milk, and thus the breast-fed infant will benefit indirectly.

No toxic symptoms in man follow the ingestion of 25,000 times the maintenance dose of thiamine, and no untoward results complicate the intravenous therapy of deficient persons with massive doses of the vitamin (500 mg.).

Response to Thiamine. The parenteral administration of 50 mg. of thiamine to persons with thiamine deficiency is followed by rapid improvement of the initial nervous syndrome of thiamine deficiency; relief of pain and paresthesia due to peripheral neuritis, within twenty-four hours; disappearance of cardiac signs and symptoms, within twenty-four to thirty-six hours; and decrease or loss of edema, within twenty-four to forty-eight hours. Spies, Knott and Hamilton, in some carefully selected cases with thiamine deficiency, observed a striking change in the electroencephalogram soon after the intravenous administration of 50 mg. thiamine hydrochloride. Motor weakness and other manifestations of neuritis improve less dramatically, and two or three months of continuous thiamine administration may be required before any motor power returns. A person with thiamine deficiency should be treated with the idea of improving his general nutritive state.

Toxicity

Thiamine is a very safe therapeutic remedy, but thiamine shock has been described in a few laboratories in various parts of the world. The mechanism of the toxicity has been generally ascribed to anaphylaxis. Evidence is emerging that the reaction may be attributable to ganglionic blockage in highly susceptible organisms.

References

Aring, C. D. and Spies, T. D.: J. Neurol. & Psychiat., *2:*335, 1939.

Aring, C. D., Evans, J. P. and Spies, T. D.: J.A.M.A., *113:*2105, 1939.

Barbieri, L. L., Franco, T. and Parenti, C.: Acta Vitaminol., *8:*65, 1954.

Blankenhourn, M. A. and Spies, T. D.: Tr. A. Am. Physicians, *50:*164, 1935.

Iacono, J. M., Wolf, G. and Johnson, B. C.: Fed. Proc., *12:*223, 1953.

Lugg, J. W. and Ellis, F. P.: Brit. J. Nutrition, *8:*71, 1954.

McCarthy, P. T., Cerecedo, L. H. and Brown, E. V.: J. Biol. Chem. *209:*611, 1954.

Spies, T. D. and Aring, C. D.: J.A.M.A., *110:* 1081, 1942.

Williams, R. R. and Spies, T. D.: Vitamin B_1 and Its Use in Medicine. New York, The Macmillan Company, 1938.

NICOTINIC ACID AMIDE DEFICIENCY (PELLAGRA)

Millions of persons have died from the lack of nicotinic acid while bottles containing it have gathered dust on the shelves of chemical laboratories and warehouses. But how could Huber, the German chemist who first derived it from nicotine in 1867, understand that this laboratory product was a vitamin essential to life? Seventy years were to pass before it was shown to be a specific therapeutic agent in the relief of canine black tongue and pellagra in human beings. These observations gave a focal point for more vigorous investigation in the fields of biology, chemistry, physiology, pharmacology and medicine. The rapid advances are astounding. It seems wise to limit this discussion to that which is fully accepted and to accentuate the underlying principles concerned, with special emphasis on practical application to the health and vigor of human beings.

Many studies indicate that nicotinic acid or its amide is an essential factor in promoting certain physiologic processes in a great variety of living organisms. Since the authors are concerned chiefly with the early symptoms that arise in human beings from a deficiency of this material in their diet, let us consider the clinical findings after a discussion of the underlying physiology and chemistry.

Pathologic Physiology

The antiquity of pellagra is a subject of considerable dispute, but any theory which attempts to explain the pathogenesis of this disease must harmonize some apparently contradictory facts and explain the complicated interrelationship of symptoms. Perhaps no single factor has so retarded the comprehension of this syndrome as the overemphasis placed upon the skin lesions. It is now agreed that pellagra is a systemic or general disease, affecting all the cells of the body. We must look to a disturbance in the cells and the fluids of the body for an understanding of the symptoms arising from a deficiency of nicotinic acid. This will be more fully discussed in considering the relationship between coenzymes and nicotinic acid amide deficiency.

Relationship Between Coenzymes I and II and Nicotinic Acid Amide Deficiency Disease. The spectacular clinical improvement following the administration of nicotinic acid or nicotinic acid amide to pellagrins has led to increased interest in the respiratory coenzymes I and II, cozymase and coferment, respectively, which are known to contain nicotinic acid amide. By definition these coenzymes are relatively heat-stable, dialyzable organic catalysts which retain activity even when separated from the living cell. They are necessary for the function of specific protein enzymes. Each is produced by living cells from a combination of nicotinic acid amide, ribose, adenylic acid and phosphoric acid. The present knowledge of the chemical constitution of coenzymes I and II indicates that they are similar in that both are pyridine nucleotides, differing only in their content of phosphoric acid. Position 4 of the pyridine ring is the site of enzymic hydrogen transfer. These transfers are stereospecific. The authors consider that the formation of enzymes governing respiration and growth of cells involves the synthesis of complex substances from simple compounds.

The methods for studying these enzymes are not satisfactory for the practicing physician, but nevertheless they offer important information concerning certain aspects of the pathogenesis of pellagra and other diseases. The concentration of coenzymes I and II in the whole blood of persons with deficiency diseases is lower than in normal persons on optimal diets. Low values for the coenzyme concentration of whole blood may be observed also in persons with diabetes mellitus, roentgen sickness, leukemia and pneumococcal pneumonia. Infections, fever, and excessive physical exercise tend to lower the concentration in the blood, whereas rest in bed and increased intake of nicotinic acid or related pyridine compounds tend to increase the concentration.

The coenzyme I content of the erythrocyte does not decrease as much in human pellagra as does the content of striated muscle. The very ill pellagrin may have only 60 per cent of the normal concentration of coenzyme I in his muscles. This offers a marvelous explanation of the long lingering weakness which characterizes the period of development of dietary deficiency. Spies, von Euler, Vilter, Bean and Schlenk have shown that the intravenous injection of from 10 to 50 mg. of coenzyme I of the highest activity is followed by dramatic clinical improvement in acute pellagrous manifestations. This amount when distributed throughout the body is not detectable by our highly sensitive laboratory methods.

These observations lead to an *hypothesis* which may be stated as follows: When the available nicotinic acid amide or compounds with similar functions are not adequate to supply the needs of the body for reasons of decreased supply, inadequate assimilation, increased demand or increased loss, a disorder in respiratory enzyme systems occurs. As a result a state of generalized reduction in normal cellular respiration supervenes. When this biochemical lesion is severe enough, or has existed long enough, it is translated into functional disturbances in various organ systems of the body. Vasomotor instability in the skin and functional disorders of the alimentary canal, the nervous system and the circulatory system may occur. It is probable that the most readily affected systems are those weakened by hereditary predisposition or trauma in the wear and tear of everyday life. This may explain the infinite variety of the clinical picture. Finally, severe or persisting alterations in physiology lead to structural changes in various tissues which ultimately present the diagnostic lesions of pellagra.

That such an hypothesis is not established is indicated by the fact that pyrazine monocarboxylic acid and the diethyl amide of nicotinic acid (coramine) may relieve the symptoms of pellagra without any observable changes in the coenzyme factors so far studied. It may be that there are many respiratory ferments not yet known and some of these may explain apparent gaps in the chain of evidence pointing to a disorder of the pyridine coenzyme system as the basis of the pathogenesis of pellagra.

Antimetabolites for nicotinic acid have been synthesized and are of great interest from a scientific point of view. The interrelationship of the vitamins, which we have always stressed, is shown to some extent by tuberculous patients who, when given isonicotinic acid hydrazide, sometimes develop symptoms which can be relieved by pyridoxine.

Progress has been made in elucidating mechanisms of isonicotinic acid hydrazide detoxication. In addition to the transformation into analogues of nicotinic acid-containing coenzymes, isonicotinic acid hydrazide is hydrolyzed to isonicotinic acid. It is conjugated with glycine or acetic acid forming 1-isonicotinyl-2-acetyl hydrazine and 1-isonicotinyl-2-glycyl hydrazine and also forms isonicotinic acid hydrazones of pyruvic acid and ketoglutaric acid. These compounds have been identified in the urines of rats and man.

General Clinical Considerations

Pellagra is a noncontagious, nonhereditary clinical syndrome which may occur in persons of any age, of either sex and of every stratum of society. It occurs most commonly among the poorer classes, following a prolonged dietary inadequacy of nicotinic acid and substances physiologically similar. The lack of nicotinic acid affects every cell in the body, though the diagnostic signs and symptoms arise predominantly from involvement of the skin, alimentary tract and nervous system. The incidence of the disease is greatest during the spring and summer, and it characteristically recurs at those times unless proper measures are rigidly and persistently applied.

The accumulated clinical information indicates that pellagra is caused primarily by a nutritional deficiency. The factors that operate to produce a nutritional deficiency are an inadequate intake, increased requirement, diminished absorption or utilization, or increased destruction or excretion of essential nutritional substances.

Pellagra as a widespread problem in the southeastern part of the United States has disappeared. The authors, who formerly saw thousands of cases each year, have not seen a typical, uncomplicated case of endemic pellagra for six years.

Diathesis. Pellagra, like most deficiency states, is particularly prevalent among the following groups:

1. The poor and ignorant who live on an unbalanced diet, usually rich in carbohydrates and fats but low in proteins, minerals and vitamins. This is called *endemic pellagra.*

2. Persons who, because of organic disease, have difficulty in ingesting, assimilating or utilizing nicotinic acid compounds. Within this group we include persons who have lost teeth, those with disorders and diseases of the alimentary tract, or those who have surgical operations. This type is frequently called *pellagra secondary to organic disease.*

3. Persons with alcohol addiction who subsist mainly on calories derived from alcohol and whose appetites have decreased to such an extent that they eat little. These persons do not ingest sufficient nicotinic acid or substances acting similarly, and when they develop pellagra it is frequently called *alcoholic pellagra* or "pseudopellagra."

4. Food faddists and other persons with capricious appetites who tend to eat little food containing antipellagric materials. Some of these patients are on diets prescribed by physicians for the treatment of certain diseases and develop pellagra because the prescribed diet contains little of the antipellagric factor.

5. Persons whose requirements for antipellagric substances are greatly increased. Pregnancy, lactation, unusual growth, hyperthyroidism, infections, increased physical exercise all greatly increase the daily requirement for nicotinic acid.

Prodromal Symptoms. This period may be of long duration with insidiously advancing symptoms, trivial in nature but gaining importance by their persistence rather than by their severity. Before diagnostic lesions of the mucous membranes or skin appear, there is loss

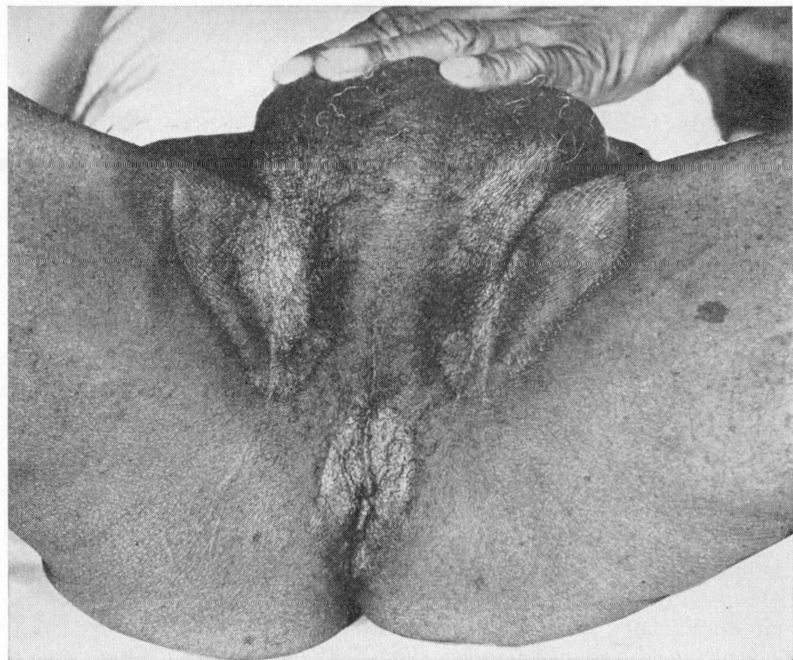

FIG. 30. Typical perineal lesions in a 47-year-old colored male pellagrin. There was also dermatitis of the hands and feet. The symmetry, lines of demarcation, and general distribution are typical. Severe vomiting, diarrhea, glossitis, fever, tachycardia and psychosis promptly improved following the administration of nicotinic acid.

of appetite which is at least in part responsible for weight loss. Ill defined disturbances of the alimentary tract, including "indigestion," and changes in bowel function occur. General muscular weakness, lassitude, irritability, depression, memory loss, headache and insomnia develop without obvious reason. Inability to work, abdominal pain, burning sensations in various parts of the body, vertigo, numbness, nervousness, palpitation, distractability, flights of ideas, apprehension, morbid fears, mental confusion and forgetfulness frequently occur. There may be intermittent diarrhea and constipation. There is much that obviously is abnormal at this stage, but nothing that is pathognomonic. Since the entire syndrome often appears without objective cause, a diagnosis of neurasthenia, anxiety state, malingering or neurosis is usually entertained.

After a long period of ill health which might properly be termed the deficiency development time, outstanding clinical lesions may arise in the skin, alimentary tract or the nervous system. These symptoms are not invariably involved nor are they affected in any regular order, nor with the same degree of severity from case to case. Out of many thousands of cases studied, we have not seen two which are identical. The individual case, however, usually repeats with each recurrence the same order of development of symptoms.

Pellagra in Infancy and Childhood. Spies, Walker and Woods have shown that early clinical signs of endemic pellagra are prone to develop in infants and children in "pellagra families." The identity of pellagra in the infant and in the adult is thoroughly established, but differences between the symptoms found in the two age groups make it advisable to consider them separately. These distinctions are due largely to the fact that in the adult deficiencies affect mature tissues, whereas in the infant or child they are engrafted upon tissues which are in the process of rapid growth and development. The symptomatology is also influenced by the striking difference in environment, the infant leading a sheltered existence compared with the active and exposed life of the adult. For purposes of clarity, infantile pellagra will be considered separately, but it should be borne in mind that from etiologic and pathologic points of view such a distinction is artificial.

A careful history usually shows that the diet of the mother during pregnancy and lactation was inadequate and that her breast milk was therefore lacking in quantity and quality. The infant was accordingly weaned soon after birth and was given a type of food which was inadequate for good nutrition. At a very early age, these children show poor appetites and usually eat irregularly. Most of them prefer carbohydrate foods and refuse most of the other foods offered. The parents seldom make any attempt to correct the food habits of such children even if a good diet becomes available.

The parents state that these children are irritable, easily frightened, apprehensive and fretful. They cry a great deal and are listless, apathetic and tired. They do not show the normal interests of childhood, and if they have developed special interests before the onset of their illness, they soon lose them. They are too tired to play and too fretful to rest; they sleep poorly and frequently awake crying. They gain weight slowly, or if they have been more robust before their illness, often lose weight rapidly. Most of these children

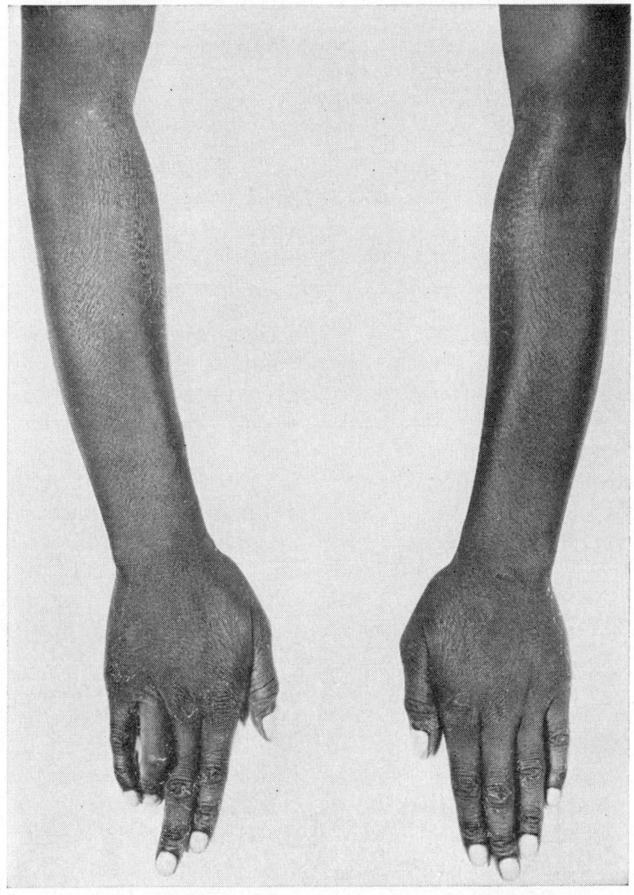

FIG. 31. Stages in dermatitis of pellagra. I. Early phase showing changes a few days after the erythema has faded, leaving pigmented, roughened skin and early desquamation. The hands show only very slight changes. Note the line of demarcation above the elbow and wrinkling of the skin of the hands.

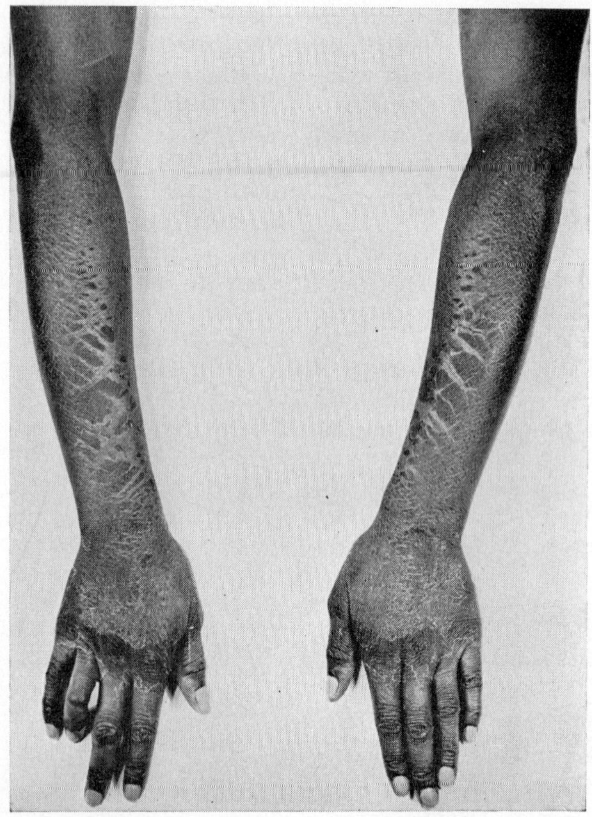

FIG. 32. Stages in dermatitis of pellagra. II. Stage of desquamation. Large flakes may be pulled from dark areas over the surface, leaving tender new skin. There is relatively little involvement of the fingers. (Taken ten days after the first picture.)

complain of soreness of the tongue or lips and of burning and pain in the abdomen, or of cramps and burning sensations in the legs. Vomiting and "indigestion" are common. Frequently they suffer from constipation, but occasionally they have bouts of diarrhea, especially during the spring and summer months. Their symptoms wax and wane but tend to increase in severity with advancing years if adequate treatment is not instituted. As time passes, such children become increasingly subnormal in height and weight; they find it difficult to concentrate and make poor progress in school.

Physical examination shows that these children are undernourished and underdeveloped for their age. They obviously are in ill health. Their skin is dry and atrophic, and they look like nothing so much as sad little old men and women. They may or may not have the typical dermal and alimentary tract lesions described in adult pellagrins; indeed, such diagnostic lesions frequently do not appear, but very ill children showing none of the typical lesions have been brought from the verge of death by prompt and intensive treatment with nicotinic acid or nicotinic acid amide.

A history of prolonged subsistence on an inadequate diet, plus the presence of pellagra in one or more members of the family, should lead one to suspect the diagnosis of pellagra in ill infants and children even in the absence of pathognomonic lesions. When there is doubt, the patient should be given the benefit of a controlled therapeutic test, since it is known that such children will show rapid improvement following specific therapy if early pellagra is present.

Diagnosis. The clinical diagnosis of pellagra in adults or children depends upon identifying typical dermal lesions or characteristic mucous membrane lesions, or both. Typical dermal lesions are pathognomonic, and it is from them that the disease derived its name (*pelle* meaning skin, and *agra* meaning rough). Characteristic *skin lesions* may appear symmetrically placed on any part of the body. They are most frequently observed over sites of irritation, such as the dorsum of the hands, wrists, elbows, face, neck, knees, feet, under the breasts and in the perineal region (see Fig. 30). In most instances, the area of dermatitis is separated sharply from the normal skin. The lesions are never static; they either advance or regress. Typical changes are well portrayed in Figures 31, 32 and 33. Bean and Spies have found that a considerable number of patients have skin lesions in atypical distribution, particularly around areas of old scars or on sites where the irritation is greatest. It should be emphasized that in many cases skin lesions never appear; these cases are termed "pellagra sine pellagra." The mucous membrane le-

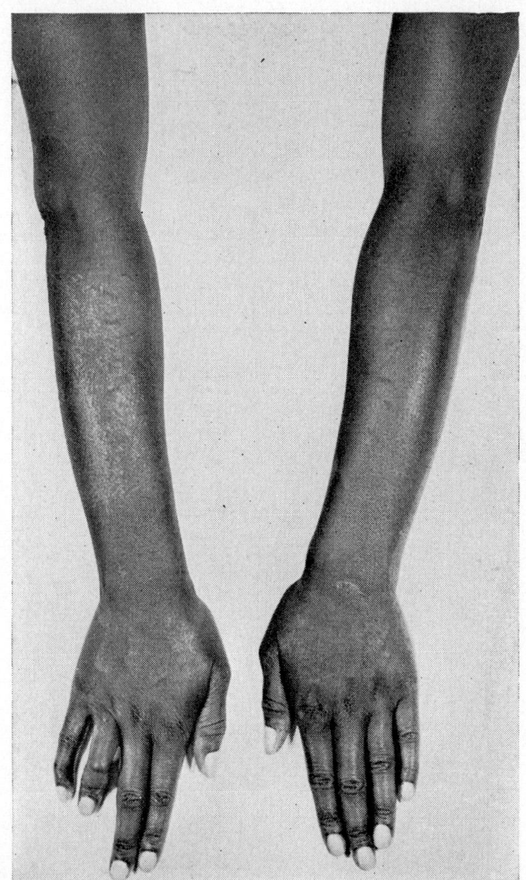

FIG. 33. Stages of dermatitis of pellagra. III. Stage of healing. The process of desquamation is complete and new tender skin has replaced that involved in the dermatitis. It is smooth, not wrinkled. Streaks of pigmentation remain. (Taken thirty days after the first picture.)

FIG. 34. Nicotinic acid (3-pyridine carboxyl acid).

	Structural Formula	Melting Point Centigrade	BLACKTONGUE-Dogs Dose Milligrams	BLACKTONGUE-Dogs Change in Symptoms	PELLAGRA Dose Milligrams	PELLAGRA Change in Symptoms	Staph. Aureus Concentration	Staph. Aureus Change in Growth	Dysentery B. Concentration	Dysentery B. Change in Growth	Flushing	Dinitrochlorobenzene Test Color
Nicotinic Acid	COOH, N	230°	60	Rapid Improvement		R.I.		+	MX10^{-7}	+	+	+
Sodium Nicotinate	COONa, N					R.I.		+			+	
Ammonium Nicotinate	$COONH_4$, N											
Methyl Nicotinate	$COOCH_3$, N							+	MX10^{-7}	+		
Ethyl Nicotinate	$COOC_2H_5$, N	129						0	MX10^{-6}	+		
Nicotinic Acid Amide	$CONH_2$, N					R.I.		+	MX10^{-7}	+	0	+
Nicotinamide HCl	$CONH_2$, H-N-Cl	121	50	R.I.								
Nicotinamide Methochloride	$CONH_2$, CH_3-N-Cl	235										
Nicotinamide Glucosido-Iodide	$CONH_2$, I-N-$CH(CHOH)_3CHCH_2OH$ (O bridge)		334	R.I.								
Nicotinic Acid N-Methyl Amide	$CONHCH_3$, N	104-5	110	R.I.					MX10^{-5}	+		
Nicotinic Acid N-Diethyl Amide	$CON(C_2H_5)_2$, N	liquid	140	R.I.		R.I.		0			0	+
Nicotinuric Acid	$CONHCH_2COOH$, N	ca240	147	R.I.				0	MX10^{-6}	+		
Trigonellin Chloride	COOH, CH_3-N-Cl	258				No I.						0
Trigonellin Methyl Sulfate	COOH, CH_3-N-SO_4CH_3											0
Trigonellin Amide	$CONH_2$, CH_3-N-OH								MX10^{-6}	+		
6-Methyl Nicotinic Acid	COOH, CH_3, N	206-7	168	No Improvement						0	0	0
β-Acetyl Pyridine HCl	$COCH_3$, H-N-Cl	174	193	Worse								
Isonicotinic Acid	COOH, N	310-3	100	W.				0		0		

	Structural Formula	Melting Point Centigrade	BLACKTONGUE-Dogs Dose Milligrams	Change in Symptoms	PELLAGRA Dose Milligrams	Change in Symptoms	Staph. Aureus Concentration	Change in Growth	Dysentery B. Concentration	Change in Growth	Flushing	Dinitrochlorobenzene Test Color
Picolinic Acid	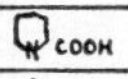 COOH					Toxic		0	$M \times 10^4$	Some		0
Picolinic Acid HCl	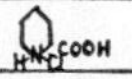 HCl COOH	214	260	W.								
Quinolinic Acid	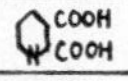 COOH COOH		50	W.				0	$M \times 10^4$	Some		+
Dinicotinic Acid	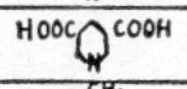 HOOC COOH					R.I.						0
2-4 Dimethyl Pyridine 3-5 Dicarboxylic A.	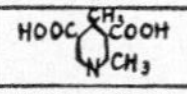 HOOC CH_3 COOH CH_3							0				
2-6 Dimethyl Pyridine 3-5 Dicarboxylic A.	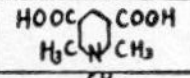 HOOC COOH H_3C CH_3										0	+
2-4-6 Trimethyl Pyridine 3-5 Dicarboxylic A.	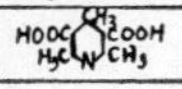 HOOC CH_3 COOH H_3C CH_3							0				
Pyridine		liquid	100							0		+
β-Picoline	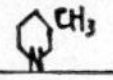 CH_3	140-3	50 200	W. R.I.		±		0		0		+
α-Picoline	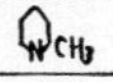 CH_3											
Nicotinonitrile	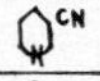 CN	50	150	No I.				0	$M \times 10^4$	+		
3-Amino Pyridine	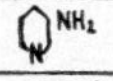 NH_2										0	
Pyridine β-Sulfonic Acid	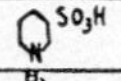 SO_3H		200	Dogs died 2-3 days						0		
Nipicotic Acid HCl	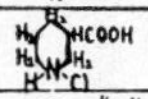 HCOOH HCl	237-9	130	No I.						0		
Nicotine	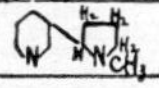 NCH_3	liquid						0				+

FIG. 35. Some chemical, physiologic and bacteriologic attributes of various pyridine compounds which bear some relation to nicotinic acid.

sions affecting the tongue, oral cavity and vagina are usually the earliest lesions diagnostic of the disease. The central nervous system frequently is affected, and the *mental symptoms* have been emphasized as a part of the pellagra syndrome for years. The patient may present a train of symptoms characteristic of neurasthenia, anxiety state or other neuroses. In later stages, there are loss of memory, excitement, mania, delirium, hallucinations and dementia.

In the past, many cases of pellagra were designated "pseudopellagra," "pellagra sine pellagra," "postalcoholic dermatitis," "secondary pellagra" or "alcoholic pellagra." Such terms are confusing and should be abandoned. The disease is or is not pellagra and should be so designated and treated.

Treatment with Nicotinic Acid

Nicotinic acid may be prepared in several ways, one of which is the strong acid oxidation of nicotine. It was from this method of preparation that the acid received its name, but its properties differ widely from those of the parent compound. Nicotinic acid is a white, crystalline compound (see Figs. 34 and 35) which melts at 230 to 232° C. and is moderately soluble in hot water but only slightly soluble in cold water. The sodium salt and the amide are more soluble; hence, some commercial concerns prepare these in sterile physiologic solution of sodium chloride for intravenous or intramuscular use. For parenteral administration, the amide (see Fig. 36) is

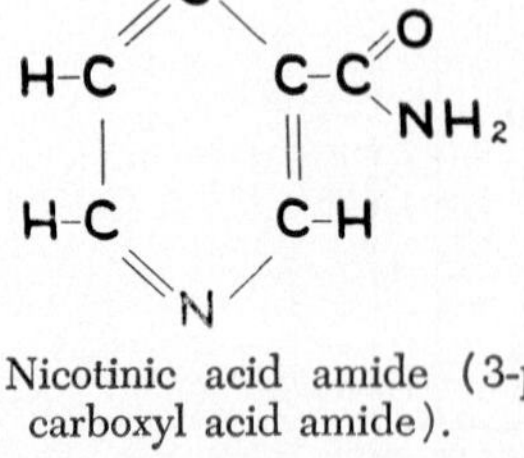

FIG. 36. Nicotinic acid amide (3-pyridine carboxyl acid amide).

preferable since it does not cause the flushing produced by nicotinic acid.

Clinical Pharmacology. 1. ABSORPTION. Observations on skin temperature have shown that following oral administration, nicotinic acid is absorbed fairly rapidly from the stomach and small intestine. Absorption is more rapid from an empty stomach than it is after meals (see Fig. 37).

Bean, Dexter and Spies, using skin temperature studies and bacteriologic assays of nicotinic acid concentration in the blood, showed that nicotinic acid is absorbed from the small and large bowel, as well as from the lower sigmoid and rectum.

2. STORAGE AND EXCRETION. Excretion is more rapid when the material is administered parenterally than when it is given orally, but regardless of the mode of administration, a large part of the total dose is soon excreted. A considerable amount appears in the urine as N′-methylnicotinamide and the 6-pyridone of N′-methylnicotinamide, some as free nicotinic acid, and the remainder in some unidentified form.

Nicotinic acid compounds have been found in all animal tissue. In general, the concentration is highest in tissues in which the metabolism is high. In human beings with severe nicotinic acid deficiency, the content of the nicotinic-acid-amide-containing substance, coenzyme I, is decreased as much as 60 per cent in striated muscle and may be somewhat decreased in the erythrocytes. Likewise, in this deficiency, the content of the nicotinic acid derivatives is below normal in whole blood and urine. When such patients are treated with nicotinic acid, the content of the nicotinic-acid-containing compounds in the muscle, blood and urine increases.

A knowledge of the level of nicotinic acid in the body tissues and excretions of pellagrins sometimes contributes valuable information concerning the degree of nicotinic acid deficiency. It is also useful in following the rate of recovery after nicotinic acid therapy has been initiated. Several methods, both chemical and microbiologic, for the determination of nicotinic acid in micro quantities have therefore been introduced. We are using the microbiologic techniques in the study of biologically derived specimens since they possess extreme sensitivity, permitting the determination of nicotinic acid in amounts as small as a few hundredths of a microgram, and may be used in analyzing for nicotinic acid in the presence of large amounts of foreign material even if this be pigmented or in a solid state.

The microbiologic method of Snell and Wright depends upon the estimation of the amount of growth of *Lactobacillus arabinosus* in a synthetic medium containing all of the essential nutrients for this organism with the exception of nicotinic acid. Any nicotinic acid supplied to the organisms therefore comes from the specimen being tested, which is added to the culture in known small amount. Since this amount of growth of the organisms in the lower range is proportional to the limiting nutrient, nicotinic acid, the measurement of the extent of growth by titration of the lactic acid produced by the Lactobacillus also affords an estimate of the amount of nicotinic acid present. Absolute values for nicotinic acid in samples may then be determined by reference to the amount of growth produced in a set of standards containing graduated amounts of nicotinic acid. This method has been used successfully in determining minute quantities of nicotinic acid in blood, urine, feces, saliva, fresh tissues and foods.

Using the above method, Gross, Swain and Spies have found that the average person with pellagra retains more of a 100-mg. test dose of nicotinic acid than the average person of similar size, injected under the same conditions, but having no evidence of pellagra.

The determination of nicotinic acid by a modified König reaction using sulfanilic acid for color development has been proposed recently as the Official Method of the Association of Agricultural Chemists.

3. TOXICITY. Nicotinic acid, in the amounts recommended for therapy, is not toxic although it and all related compounds containing the free

O
C
O—
N

radical produce vasodilation in the skin and an increase in skin temperatures. Over 80 per cent of the persons to whom 100 to 300 mg. of nicotinic acid are administered orally feel temporary

SKIN TEMPERATURE RISE AFTER NICOTINIC ACID

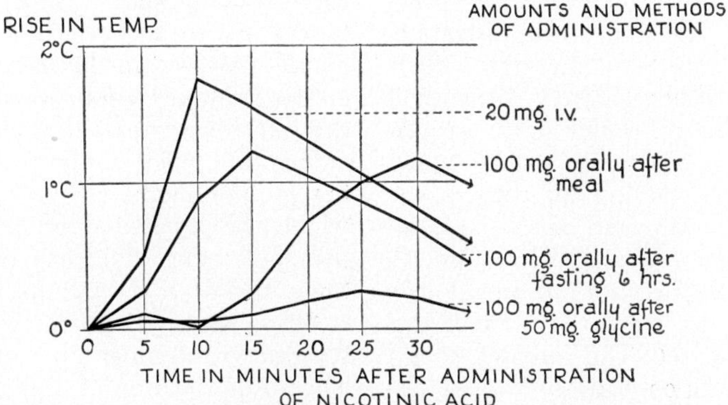

FIG. 37. This figure gives the changes in skin temperature obtained on an individual who had been kept in a constant temperature room (20° C.) for one hour before the various tests were made with nicotinic acid. Skin temperature was measured on fifteen spots on the head and neck using the Taylor Dermatherm. It can be seen that intravenous injection produces much more rapid rise in temperature than oral ingestion and that in addition the material is absorbed much more slowly in an individual when it is administered after a meal. In some instances, glycerine prevents the rise in skin temperature when given shortly before an oral dose of nicotinic acid.

prickly or burning sensations. A few persons complain of nausea and cramping pains in the stomach. These symptoms are transient and are not associated with change in general body temperature, pulse, respiration, or blood pressure. All persons to whom 20 mg. of nicotinic acid are administered intravenously have transitory vasodilation. It should be remembered, however, that nicotinic acid amide, which is also antipellagric, is the physiologic form of the compound and does not produce these vasodilating reactions.

The administration of quinine nicotinate (New York Quinine and Chemical Works) in sufficient amounts is followed by the vasodilator reaction. Quinine nicotinate is very effective in treating persons with malaria, as would be expected, and it is also effective in the treatment of persons with pellagra. Our experience is too small to warrant saying that it is better in the cerebral type of malaria than quinine per se, but we have seen spectacular results. On theoretical grounds, it might be said that quinine nicotinate dilates the blood vessels of the brain, thus allowing freer passage of blood and quinine.

Further studies on ferrous nicotinate, quinine nicotinate and glutamine nicotinate have shown that all produce the same vasodilatation as that which occurs from other sources of nicotinate.

Indications for Oral Administration. Oral administration of nicotinic acid is preferable to other methods because it is absorbed more slowly and an elevated blood concentration is maintained over a longer period of time. The amount of nicotinic acid or similar compounds necessary for a therapeutic response in pellagra varies tremendously from patient to patient. No arbitrary dosage can be set. The amount necessary depends upon the severity of the disease, the nature and severity of complications, and the condition of the alimentary tract. We have observed one person with long-standing pellagra who failed to respond to oral doses of nicotinic acid as high as 1500 mg. per day, but who improved rapidly following the intravenous administration of 50 mg. of nicotinic acid six times a day. For the average pellagrin, we recommend 50 mg. nicotinic acid, orally, ten times a day.

Indications for Parenteral Administration. Parenteral therapy should be used wherever a high blood concentration is desired within a short space of time and wherever gastrointestinal absorption is inadequate. For *intravenous* administration, nicotinic acid amide is preferred because it is not attended by a flushing reaction. In most cases, 100 mg. per day is sufficient. As in oral administration, small doses at frequent intervals are desirable in order to keep the blood concentration at a high level. It should be administered in 25-mg. doses four times a day, and injected slowly. In acutely ill patients, when parenteral administration of saline or glucose is indicated, the vitamin can be dissolved in a physiologic solution of saline or 5 per cent glucose and administered by a slow drip.

Nicotinic acid can be given *intramuscularly* in the same dosage as that suggested for intravenous injection. However, intramuscular therapy in persons with deficiency diseases is *not recommended* because it is attended by some risk of abscess formation in devitalized tissues.

Administration to Infants and Children. For infants a satisfactory daily dose is 50 to 100 mg. of nicotinic acid amide dissolved in the feeding. For parenteral administration, we suggest 5 mg. three to four times a day. Nicotinic acid or nicotinic acid amide given to a nursing mother increases the nicotinic acid which the breast-fed infant receives in the milk. For children, two or three times the dose for infants is suggested.

Response to Nicotinic Acid and Substances with Similar Physiologic Action. The administration of adequate doses of nicotinic acid or similar substances to a pellagrin will: cause fading of the fiery redness of the mucous membrane lesions and disappearance of the associated Vincent's organisms; cause disappearance of the acute mental symptoms of pellagra, such as delirium, hallucinations and mental confusion; relieve him of symptoms such as diarrhea, vomiting and cramping which arise from alterations in alimentary function; cause fading of the dermal erythema; increase his strength and feeling of well-being; cause the disappearance of ether soluble red pigments from the urine; increase the coenzyme I and II concentration in whole blood and urine; and, when therapy is prolonged, increase the coenzyme content of the muscle. The pellagrin and *not his disease* should be treated, as outlined in the section on general management (p. 495).

Under certain conditions the amino acid tryptophan may reduce the amount of niacin required in the diet of man and lower animals. As compared to nicotinic acid, large amounts of tryptophan per unit of weight are required in order to have a specific effect against the pellagrous lesions. The authors' early description of nicotinic acid therapy stressed the need that it be given along with a diet high in protein. In recent years it has been shown by Bean and others that tryptophan can be used successfully in the treatment of pellagra without the administration of niacin.

In recent years there has been great interest in the metabolic interrelationship between the amino acid tryptophan and the vitamin nicotinic acid. Studies with Neurospora, rats, dogs, cattle and horses indicate that the conversion of tryptophan to nicotinic acid proceeds through a series of intermediate compounds which include kynurenine, 3-hydroxykynurenine, 3-hydroxyanthranilic acid and quinolinic acid. Knowledge of the manner in which this conversion occurs in man is as yet sketchy. The process at best is an inefficient one. Yet it serves to explain to some extent the historical association between endemic pellagra and the corn eating populations of the world, for although corn contains some nicotinic acid, it is lacking in tryptophan.

References

Hughes, H. B.: J. Pharmacol. & Exper. Therap., *109:*444, 1953.

Makino, K., Kinoshita, T. and Itoh, T.: Nature, *173:*36, 1954.

Spies, T. D.: Proc. Soc. Exper. Biol. & Med., *29:*83, 1931.

Spies, T. D.: J. Clin. Invest., *13:*807, 1934.

Spies, T. D., Chinn, A. and McLester, J. B.: South. M. J., *30:*18, 1937.

Spies, T. D. and Cooper, C.: Internat. Clin., *4:*1, 1937.

Spies, T. D., Aring, C. D., Gelpern, J. and Bean, W. B.: Am. J. M. Sc., *196:*461, 1938.

RIBOFLAVIN DEFICIENCY (ARIBOFLAVINOSIS)

Little could Blythe, the brilliant English chemist who first obtained a yellow-green pigment from milk in 1879, have realized that he possessed a chemical compound necessary for the health and well-being of animals and human beings. The world paid scant attention to his discovery, for the time was not yet ripe for its significance to be appreciated. The undernourished millions of the East had no thought that chemistry might ever benefit them. America was busy healing the scars of the Civil War and extending the western frontier. Even the scientists of Europe were but slightly interested in his announcement, for they were engaged in heated argument concerning the germ theory of disease. Eighty years later we see that there has been a slow evolution of the scientist's thinking about his great natural enemies, pathogenic micro-organisms. Today, the germ theory is fully accepted and its application has been of immeasurable benefit to mankind. Yellow fever, smallpox, diphtheria, plague and many other infectious diseases are no longer rampant. Man is much concerned with the wide variety of maladies which threaten his health and life, and during the past twenty years the science of nutrition has developed vigorously. Studies in nutrition are steadily aiding in advancing the scientific aspects of medicine, with the result that certainty is replacing the art of speculation in the diagnosis and treatment of diseases of nutritional origin. During recent years, the science of nutrition has threatened to outstrip the worthwhile contributions to the well-being of the human race which resulted from the application of

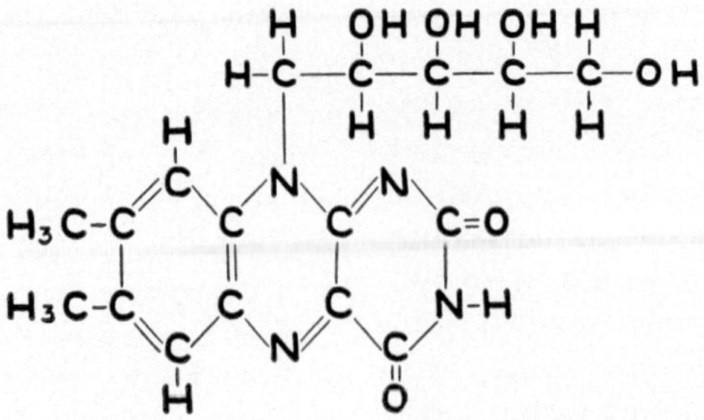

```
              H   OH OH OH H
              |   |  |  |  |
            H-C---C--C--C--C-OH
              |   |  |  |  |
      H       |   H  H  H  H
      |       |
     /C\     /N\    /N\
H3C-C    C       C     C=O
    |    ||      |     |
H3C-C    C       C     N-H
     \C/   \N//   \C/
      |            ||
      H            O
```

FIG. 38. d-Riboflavin (6,7-dimethyl-9-(1′-d-ribityl)-isoalloxazine).

the germ theory of disease. It seems to be leading the scientific medicine of the future to heights as yet undreamed. What price we have paid in lives and funds for our existing knowledge concerning nutrition no one could or would venture to guess. That this knowledge has advanced our civilization and restored the health and well-being of countless numbers, we cannot gainsay. Each year, more tools are becoming available for work. Blythe's insignificant appearing yellow-green pigment has come into its own. Its isolation and synthesis were contributions of far-reaching importance for they made possible studies on plants, animals and human beings which show that it is practically indispensable for all forms of life. It is becoming increasingly evident that riboflavin will be an important aid in building a stronger and more vigorous civilization. Before proceeding to the incidence, diagnosis, and therapy of the syndrome resulting from a deficiency of riboflavin in the diet of human beings, we shall discuss those aspects of biochemistry and physiology which have a practical application to medicine and to the science of nutrition.

Biochemistry and Physiology

Riboflavin was considered of no biologic importance until Warburg and Christian discovered it to be an important constituent of a cellular respiratory enzyme system. It was first isolated in 1933 and artificially synthesized in 1935. The structural formula is shown in Figure 38. It is now identified as a combination of d-ribose and isoalloxazine. It is a freely dialyzable, intensely yellow, water soluble pigment which exhibits a characteristic green fluorescence under ultraviolet rays. It is irreversibly inactivated by either visible or ultraviolet light in acid or alkaline solutions. The phosphoric acid ester of riboflavin, believed to have the structure shown in Figure 39, unites with a specific nonactive bearer protein to form the yellow enzyme.

In the presence of an "activating enzyme" from yeast (*Zwischenferment*) and a thermostable coenzyme (since identified as coenzyme II—triphosphopyridine nucleotide), the yellow enzyme is capable of oxidizing Robison's hexose monophosphoric ester. The scheme as represented in [A] below has been postulated for the action of this system.

This system, in contrast to other well-known oxidation-reduction systems, is not poisoned by hydrocyanic acid or carbon monoxide. Since the coenzyme is alternately reduced and oxidized by the yellow enzyme and the yellow enzyme itself is reversibly oxidized and reduced, only a very small amount of both these

---

[A]

(1) Coenzyme + hexose monophosphoric acid $\xrightarrow{\textit{Zwischenferment}}$ reduced coenzyme + phosphohexonic acid.

(2) Reduced coenzyme + yellow enzyme $\longrightarrow$ coenzyme + reduced yellow enzyme.

(3) Reduced yellow enzyme + molecular oxygen $\longrightarrow$ H_2O_2 + yellow enzyme.

substances is required for the reaction to proceed.

Studies on similar enzyme systems have shown that there exists in nature a whole class of similar compounds (alloxazine proteids) differing in the constitution of the prosthetic group and in the structure of the bearer protein. Among such flavoproteins are d-amino acid oxidase, xanthine oxidase, and a flavoprotein recently isolated from heart muscle.

The yellow enzyme is present in all types of living cells, where it functions as an oxygen carrier between molecular oxygen and the substrate in association with other oxidative systems. The indispensability of riboflavin in the diet probably is due to the fact that it is an essential constituent of this yellow enzyme. When the identity of riboflavin and vitamin B_2 (G) was established, a rational approach to certain problems in vitamin research was possible.

Riboflavin has been demonstrated to be essential in the diet of the rat, chick, dog, pig and man. A deficiency of this vitamin in the rat produces dermatitis, a marked decrease in the rate of growth and cataract. If daily supplements of riboflavin are added to the diet when the first signs of lens opacity are noted, the cataract can be cured or its progress arrested. Riboflavin deficiency in the dog gives rise to vomiting and diarrhea, marked spasticity and muscular weakness with fatal termination, preceded by coma, fall in temperature and respiratory rate, and collapse. Death apparently is caused by cellular asphyxiation brought about by the lack of the oxidation catalyst.

Several investigators have reported the yellow color and fatty appearance of livers of riboflavin-deficient dogs, fowls and rats. The experimental work of Lepkovsky, Jukes, Norris, Engel and others has shown that riboflavin is indispensable for the nutrition of the chick and is required for a normal rate of hatching and viability.

Occurrence. Flavins have been isolated from many natural sources, including egg white, milk, liver, kidney, barley malt, dandelion blossoms, grasses, egg yolk, yeast, the retina of fish eyes and urine. (It should be emphasized that riboflavin deteriorates when exposed to sunlight, so that milk and other natural sources exposed even for relatively short periods of time may lose a high percentage of their initial store.) It was formerly believed that these compounds were different chemical substances, but further study has indicated that all are identical with riboflavin.

Absorption. Riboflavin is readily absorbed from the alimentary canal. Phosphorylation occurs in the intestinal wall and other tissues throughout the body. Thus, it exerts its normal effect regardless of the way in which it is administered.

Storage and Excretion. The flavin content of the body organs cannot be increased above a certain level even by forced feeding. The heart, liver, and kidneys of rats which have died of riboflavin deficiency contain one third of their normal riboflavin content. Sherman demonstrated that the optimum intake of riboflavin in the rat is much greater than the minimum requirement. He concluded that the enrichment with

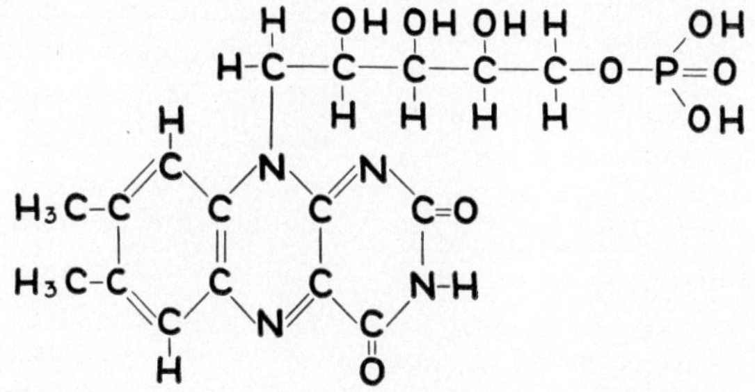

FIG. 39. Riboflavin 5′-phosphoric acid ester (6, 7-dimethyl-9-(1′-d-ribityl)-isoalloxazine-5′-phosphoric acid).

riboflavin of an already adequate diet produced a healthier race. The blood content of riboflavin may range from 0.28 to 0.55 gamma per cc. of whole blood. There appears to be little correlation between the amount of riboflavin in the blood and the clinical symptoms of riboflavin deficiency.

Riboflavin is a normal constituent of the urine. Although assays in persons suffering from clinical riboflavin deficiency have shown that there is no significant alteration of the blood riboflavin, a decreased urinary excretion is generally the rule. When the dietary intake is very low, the excretion may for a time exceed the intake and, conversely, when the intake is high, the excretion may lag behind. The daily urinary loss of the normal adult on an adequate diet varies from 750 to 1250 gamma. Saturation tests, similar to those used to detect thiamine deficiency, have not proved effective for the diagnosis of riboflavin deficiency. The rate of destruction of riboflavin in the body is not known, but adults need about 3 mg. per day.

In exophthalmic goiter very little riboflavin is excreted in the urine. When riboflavin is given either orally or by injection it is very rapidly excreted and the urine after 8 hours falls to the previous low level. The high excretion in such cases apparently does not indicate saturated body stores but metabolic failure in riboflavin utilization.

An increased consumption of riboflavin causes an increase in the flavin content of breast milk of lactating women. Work on the riboflavin requirement of women during pregnancy indicates a need of about 2 mg. per day based on the intake required to bring the urinary excretion in pregnancy up to that of nonpregnant women. In pregnancy the placenta maintains a concentration four times that of maternal fetal blood by splitting flavine-adenine-dinucleotide built from maternal blood riboflavin.

Toxicity. Riboflavin is nontoxic in amounts which far exceed therapeutic dosage.

General Clinical Considerations

Riboflavin deficiency is a noncontagious, nonhereditary clinical syndrome. It occurs in any race and affects both males and females at any time from infancy to old age. It is more common in women than in men. The incidence tends to be higher in the spring and summer than at any other season of the year. Unless the diet becomes adequate or riboflavin or substances containing it are administered, relapses are likely to occur from time to time throughout the year.

Twenty years ago the clinical syndrome of riboflavin deficiency was not recognized in human beings. From the observations of Sebrell, Spies, Sydenstricker and their associates, certain symptoms and signs have been pieced together and correlated, and we now have sufficient knowledge of the disease to be able to diagnose and treat it. Studies by the authors have led them to conclude that it is the most common vitamin deficiency disease in the United States. It probably affects several million people in this country, and reaches even into the very highest stratum of society. Although it occurs in association with a variety of conditions, it is very common among persons with pellagra, beriberi or other deficiency diseases, and may appear before, during or after the development of diagnostic lesions of these diseases. The concurrence of riboflavin deficiency and deficiencies of other B-complex vitamins is due to the impossibility of eating a diet of natural foods deficient in only one of these vitamins. Diagnosis depends not only on the recognition of the usual clinical manifestations of the disease, but also on watching carefully for them under circumstances in which they are likely to appear. Only by these means can early changes be detected and early therapy initiated. The available laboratory tests, although precise, are not suitable for the use of the practitioner. Accordingly, diagnosis must depend upon the recognition of characteristic lesions and therapeutic tests with riboflavin.

Etiologic Factors. The many factors which either singly or in combination give rise to or precipitate the appearance of clinical symptoms of the disease will be discussed briefly.

1. Inadequate Food Intake. Among all strata of society there are persons who consume inadequate diets, but among the indigent and poor this is the most common cause of riboflavin deficiency. Others whose diets are frequently inadequate are food faddists, persons with idiosyncrasies of taste and appetite, and those who follow overconscientiously dietary regimens prescribed for allergy, diabetes, peptic ulcer, obesity, hypertension and many other conditions. Such diets often fail to supply adequate amounts of riboflavin. Riboflavin deficiency is found frequently in nursing infants whose mothers during pregnancy and lactation have had clinical or subclinical riboflavin deficiency. Lack of milk in the daily diet leaves many people on the borderline of a deficiency state.

2. Faulty Absorption or Utilization of Food. Interference with the absorption of food predisposes to the development of riboflavin deficiency. Disorders of the alimentary canal, congestive heart failure, cirrhosis and nephritis frequently interfere with proper absorption or utilization.

3. Increased Requirement. Several factors may increase the requirement for vitamins. During periods of rapid growth in children, the amount of riboflavin required increases and if it is not met, riboflavin deficiency develops. The requirement during pregnancy and lactation is increased, and the clinical syndrome frequently appears in the later months of pregnancy. Hyperthyroidism and fevers increase metabolic needs and lead to a disparity between the intake and the need. In infections, especially chronic ones, there often is a combination of increased need to satisfy accelerated metabolism and loss of appetite which precludes filling this need. In diabetes mellitus, abrupt increments in carbohydrate intake and insulin may precipitate the deficiency syndrome.

4. Increased Excretion. Although it is not known that an increased loss of riboflavin may occur in conditions in which there is an abnormally high excretion in the urine, this possibility should be kept in mind as a complicating factor in patients with diabetes insipidus or in persons undergoing diuresis of any sort.

5. Chronic Alcoholic Addiction. Persons who regularly consume large amounts of alcohol usually fail to eat sufficient food to satisfy their nutritional requirements. In addition, alcoholic gastritis probably interferes with proper alimentation, and a certain number of persons addicted to alcohol develop liver disease which may interfere with the intermediary metabolism of riboflavin.

Prodromal Symptoms. It is important to emphasize that a long period of ill health with symptoms of a vague, nondescriptive character usually precedes the appearance of diagnostic lesions. Because deficiencies of the B-complex vitamins tend to occur as complexities rather than as single entities, it is impossible to separate the premonitory symptoms of spontaneous riboflavin deficiency from those of pellagra or beriberi. Prominent among such symptoms are anorexia, weight loss, weakness and inability to perform mental work. Digestive disturbances, nervousness, vague pains in various parts of the body, burning sensations of the skin, eyes and corners of the mouth, as well as soreness at the corners of the mouth, pain in the eyes and visual disturbances, headaches, dizziness, mental depression, insomnia, forgetfulness and mild states of confusion are common complaints. Frequently none of the symptoms are objective, and there are no signs indicating that any specific system in the body is primarily affected. Such symptoms may persist for a long time after diagnostic lesions appear, and in some persons they remain constant while the specific lesions wax and wane. The physician who is unfamiliar with deficiency diseases may interpret these prodromal symptoms as being functional in origin. They should, however, lead him to consider the possibility of an inadequate food intake or the faulty utilization of food playing a role in their development. Even though persons with such symptoms have no diagnostic signs of a deficiency disease, they should be observed repeatedly over a long period of time for, in many cases, diagnostic lesions eventually appear. From the knowledge gained from such retrospective studies, it is now possible to recognize many early cases and institute treatment when it is most valuable.

Special Lesions. A. CHEILOSIS. The most characteristic clinical sign in riboflavin deficiency is an angular stomatitis and an involvement of the lips in a process that is variously called cheilosis or cheilitis. Such lesions had long been observed in association with pellagra and it was known that they responded to treatment with yeast. Not until Sebrell and Butler reported the results of their classic investigations on riboflavin deficiency, however, was the significance of these lesions appreciated. The earlier changes occur as a paleness in the lips, particularly at the angles, but not the moist area of the buccal mucosa. The pallor usually continues for days and is followed by maceration and piling up of whitish tissue on a pink background. Superficial fissures may invade the site of natural wrinkles at the corners of the mouth. These fissures may be single or multiple and usually appear on both sides. Subsequently the macerated lesions become dry, and a yellowish crust which forms at the angles may be removed without bleeding. The lips are usually red and there is likely to be an increase in the transverse markings, particularly on the lower lip. Inspection of the tongue indicates that there are changes in the superficial epithelium, in the capillaries, or distortion of the normal papillae. In some cases the tongue has a magenta hue which is similar to, but can be distinguished from, that seen in cyanosis. As the disease progresses, the fissures in the corners of the mouth tend to become deeper and extend on to the cheek. They may extend within the mouth so that the constantly irritated angles become raw, bleeding areas with crusts or scabs. Such lesions are sometimes very painful in the acute stage, and occasionally are painful throughout the course of the disease. If the lesions recur frequently a cicatrix may be formed, giving the affected area an atrophic appearance. Hemolytic streptococci, hemolytic staphylococci and, in some cases, various yeasts and fungi have been obtained in cultures from acute lesions. Presumably these are secondary infections since the organisms disappear following adequate treatment with riboflavin. It is possible that the morphology of the lesions is altered to some extent by these secondary invaders. Bilateral angular cheilosis is a nonspecific lesion. There are factors other than riboflavin deficiency which are responsible for the appearance of such lesions. Older persons with artificial dentures in which the vertical dimension is greatly decreased are particularly prone to have this type of nonspecific cheilitis, as has been shown by Dreizen, Mann and Spies.

B. OCULAR SYMPTOMS. Spies and his associates first showed that riboflavin is an important factor in the relief of certain ocular disturbances. These disturbances disappear after riboflavin is given and return when therapy is discontinued. In many persons with ocular symptoms, vitamin A also is of specific value in relieving certain symptoms which persist after riboflavin therapy. Conversely, it has been found that when vitamin A is given before treatment with riboflavin, the addition of the latter produces further improvement. The disturbances include conjunctivitis (particularly of the lower palpebral and bulbar conjunctiva), itching, burning, photophobia, and the sensation of having sand or cinders in the eyes. Important observations by Sydenstricker, Sebrell, Cleckley and Kruse with the slit lamp indicate that many of these symptoms are associated with a superficial and interstitial keratitis. The earlier changes are described as an invasion of the cornea by the capillaries arising from the circumcorneal region. Anastomoses of the capillaries from different areas occur and from these, small branching capillaries appear to invade the cornea in the centripetal direction. Circumcorneal injection is usually obvious to the naked eye at such a stage. Later, interstitial infiltration with exudation may give rise to opacites either punctate or generalized. In some cases, there is also involvement of the iris. The characteristic changes occurring in such conditions as well as their treatment have been described in detail by Sydenstricker and his coworkers. Similar findings in rosacea keratitis have been reported by Johnson and Eckhardt.

C. Unilateral Lesions. It should be emphasized that lesions sometimes occur on one side of the mouth only, and occasionally only one eye is involved. Furthermore, there are frequently differences in the severity of the lesions at the two angles of the mouth, and we have seen patients in whom the lesions at one angle progressed while the other regressed. We have seen at least one woman in whom the lesion appeared only at the right angle of the mouth, through four periods of relapse and remission. Some of the remissions were induced and others occurred spontaneously.

D. The Skin. There may be a fine, scaly, slightly crusty desquamation on a mildly erythematous base in the nasolabial folds, on the alae nasi, within the nostrils, and on and about the ears. Very firm filiform excrescences may occur in a butterfly distribution across the nose and cheeks. A fine, scaly dermatitis of the hands, and areas of dermatitis around the vulva, anus, and perineum have been observed to heal along with the remission of the mouth lesions following the administration of riboflavin.

We are at a loss to explain the irregular sequence in which the lesions of the mouth, skin and eyes occur in different persons. In some there is a tendency for the conjunctival and corneal lesions to appear first and to be followed by the development of the oral and skin lesions. In others, lesions at the angles of the mouth occur before any of the specific eye symptoms appear. Changes in the skin, particularly over the bridge of the nose, over the cheek bones, and in the area where the nose joins the upper lip or cheek, in some cases, appear before the oral or ocular lesions. In still others, the mouth, eyes and skin are affected at approximately the same time and to the same degree of severity.

Riboflavin Deficiency in Infants and Children. In our experience we have found that riboflavin deficiency is particularly common among children and that diagnostic lesions frequently appear even when there is no evidence of a deficiency of any other factor of the vitamin B complex. From the study of a large number of children we have learned that long periods of ill health associated with poor nutrition precede the appearance of diagnostic lesions. The lesions in children are similar to those seen in the adult (Fig. 40). We

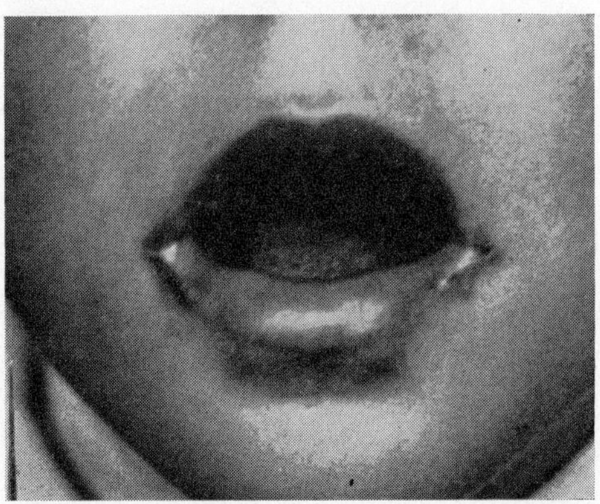

FIG. 40. Bilateral cheilosis in a young boy who was stunted and who had a diet very low in riboflavin. The lesions healed after 5 mg. twice a day was given for a period of several weeks.

have noticed particularly that the younger children in a large family are more likely to develop the disease. One possible explanation for this is that in large families in which the mother has had an almost continuous round of pregnancies alternating with lactation, or occasionally the two simultaneously, these children may begin vitamin deficiencies while still in utero. In many children general ill health and inability to make normal progress in school or to take part in the activities of childhood have been considered characteristic of poor racial stock. We believe that often they may be caused by a deficiency of vitamins rather than a deficiency in germ plasm. The evidence for this rests in the fact that children in families in which any of the members have riboflavin deficiency often are benefited spectacularly by dietary supplements of riboflavin even though they have no diagnostic evidence of riboflavin deficiency.

Recurrence. Manifestations of riboflavin deficiency, particularly the changes that occur in the lips, at the angles of the mouth and in the eyes, tend to undergo irregular cyclic variations in that the lesions wax and wane, sometimes clearing up completely, sometimes advancing to extreme severity over periods of weeks or months. The severity of the disease tends to be greatest during the spring and occasionally in the fall. Furthermore, in some patients these relapses occur without obvious relation to season. Usually, the feeling of ill health among persons with riboflavin deficiency is most intense during the time the lesions are increasing in severity and as they clear up, general health improves. This is especially true when the lesions heal in association with the administration of riboflavin. There is evidence that infections are sometimes associated with a relapse of the lesions and that periods of improved diet tend to be followed by remission.

Diagnosis

The diagnosis of riboflavin deficiency is not difficult when lesions characteristic of the disease are present. During the prodromal period, it is not easy. The physician should suspect riboflavin deficiency in persons who subsist on poorly balanced diets containing little milk, meat and green vegetables, in those who have diseases which interfere with the utilization and absorption of food, and in those whose requirements might for any reason be increased.

The diagnosis of riboflavin deficiency depends upon the observation of one or more of the following: angular stomatitis and cheilosis; ocular disturbances with inflammation of the conjunctival vessels, and growth of vessels into the cornea; seborrheic changes in the skin of the face, particularly of the nose and adjacent regions; "magenta tongue," which includes changes in the papillae and in the capillaries. The beneficial response of the patient to the administration of riboflavin is the most important criterion for establishing a diagnosis in subclinical cases. If the patients improve regularly following the administration of riboflavin and relapse when it is discontinued, it is likely that they have a deficiency of this substance. There is no satisfactory clinical laboratory test for the diagnosis of riboflavin deficiency. When such a deficiency is suspected, the diagnosis can best be made by careful interpretation of an accurate history and physical examination, aided by a well-controlled therapeutic test.

Chemisty of Riboflavin

Riboflavin is an orange crystalline compound which is sparingly soluble in water. The crystals have no sharp melting point but darken at 240° C. and decompose between 274 and 282° C. It possesses a characteristic yellow-green fluorescence in aqueous solution. Riboflavin is stable to heat and acids, but is readily destroyed by strong alkali and by exposure to ultraviolet or visible light. It is a complex organic molecule composed of isoalloxazine and d-ribose, and is identical with the naturally occurring flavins.

Mode of Administration

Riboflavin is well tolerated when administered orally, intravenously or intramuscularly. Oral administration is the method of choice, since riboflavin is readily absorbed from the normal gastrointestinal tract. Some difficulty is encountered in preparing solutions of the vitamin for intravenous administration because of its low solubility in water, physiologic saline or glucose. Sterile solutions of riboflavin can be obtained from reputable pharmaceutical concerns or can be prepared and autoclaved with safety. In treating nearly a thousand cases of riboflavin deficiency, we have encountered no acute emergencies requiring parenteral therapy to save life.

The dose of riboflavin for adults is 2 mg. three times a day for several weeks. Children showing signs of riboflavin deficiency should be given 1 mg. three times a day for a similar period. Riboflavin may be administered to infants by adding 0.5 mg. twice daily in the prepared food. If the infant is being nursed, riboflavin administered to the mother in sufficient amounts will relieve the child's symptoms.

In order to avoid any anxiety on the part of the patient taking riboflavin, he should be informed that the compound will color the urine bright yellow. Intravenous or intramuscular administration may be used in all persons who for any reason cannot take the vitamin by mouth. The dose is 2 mg., dissolved in 10 cc. of sterile physiologic saline, three times a day. Following the intravenous administration, a considerable portion is excreted in the urine. Persons receiving frequent intravenous injections of physiologic salt solution may be given the vitamin dissolved in this solution.

A preparation of riboflavin which has been lyophilized so that it is very soluble is on the market. It is readily used in parenteral therapy.

Response to Riboflavin. The administration of sufficient amounts of riboflavin, or substances acting similarly, to persons with clinical evidence of riboflavin deficiency induces a prompt increase in the amount excreted in the urine and a general rise in the blood content, striking increase in strength and sense of well-being within twelve to twenty-four hours, and gradual healing of the cheilosis, conjunctivitis and keratitis so characteristic of the disease. Just as we have seen pellagrins restricted to a deficient diet relapse while receiving large doses of nicotinic acid, so have we seen persons with riboflavin deficiency eating a restricted diet relapse in the face of taking large doses of riboflavin. Thus, the administration of a well-balanced diet is indicated. Patients with riboflavin deficiency should be considered as having a general nutritive failure, and the application of the principles outlined in the section on general management is recommended.

References

Lust, J. E., Hagerman, D. D. and Villee, C. A.: J. Clin. Invest., *33:*38, 1954.

Shapiro, Y. E.: Terap. Arkh., *25:*48, 1953.

Spies, T. D.: Am. J. M. Sc., *198:*40, 1039.

Spies, T. D., Vilter, R. W. and Ashe, W. F.: J.A.M.A., *113:*931, 1939.

Spies, T. D., Bean, W. B., Vilter, R. W. and Huff, N. E.: Am. J. M. Sc., *200:*697, 1940.

VITAMINS AND BLOOD REGENERATION

Until thirty-two years ago a diagnosis of pernicious anemia meant almost certain death. Then Minot and Murphy reported that patients with pernicious anemia could be relieved of many of their symptoms by eating large amounts of whole liver. The blood levels of these patients were increased and could be maintained at a satisfactory level if they continued to eat sufficient liver. Many patients would not eat adequate amounts of liver, and through the efforts of many investigators, eventually the excellent liver extracts were developed.

In the making of the refined liver extracts vitamin B_{12} was being concentrated, whereas the folic acid normally present in liver tended to be discarded. Following the synthesis of folic acid, the chemical era in the treatment of certain types of macrocytic anemia was initiated by Spies et al. when they showed that a single synthetic compound of known molecular structure was capable of promoting hemopoiesis in persons with certain types of macrocytic anemia. Within a year from the time folic acid was shown to produce blood regeneration in persons with pernicious anemia, nutritional macrocytic anemia, the macrocytic anemia of pregnancy, the macrocytic anemia of tropical sprue, and the megaloblastic anemia of infancy, Spies and his associates reported its failure to protect or to cure the symptoms arising from acute degeneration of the spinal cord frequently associated with pernicious anemia; folic acid was not a complete therapeutic agent for the treatment of pernicious anemia. Un-

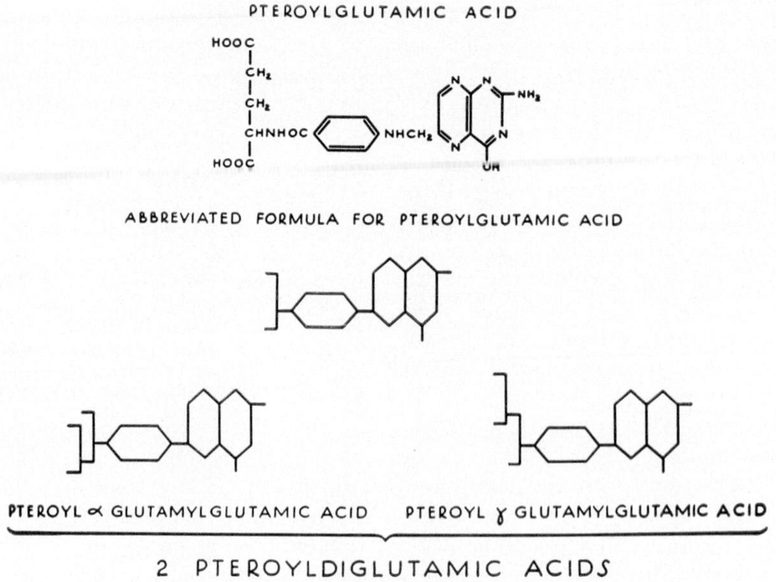

PTEROYLGLUTAMIC ACID

ABBREVIATED FORMULA FOR PTEROYLGLUTAMIC ACID

PTEROYL α GLUTAMYLGLUTAMIC ACID PTEROYL γ GLUTAMYLGLUTAMIC ACID

2 PTEROYLDIGLUTAMIC ACIDS

FIG. 41.

equivocal evidence that folic acid neither causes nor relieves the neural degeneration soon became available, however. It is now known that in certain types of anemia it is an essential therapeutic agent.

Since liver extracts were known to contain little, if any, folic acid and since they also protected against neural degeneration while folic acid did not, it was obvious that liver contained some other antianemic factor or factors. Since macrocytic anemias occur throughout the world and since certain types are found more frequently in some areas than in others, it was decided that these diseases should be studied simultaneously in the temperate zones and in the tropics. Accordingly, centers were established in Birmingham, Alabama, Havana, Cuba and San Juan, Puerto Rico, where the same criteria for selecting patients could be used and the same chemical compounds could be tested under the same controlled conditions.

Within a relatively short time after folic acid was shown to have antianemic properties, it was demonstrated that the following distinct chemical molecules produce blood regeneration by their specific effect on the bone marrow: thymine, the vitamin B_{12} family and the citrovorum family. Folinic acid and leucovorin have been synthesized and have what is termed citrovorum activity. Considering the difference in chemical structure of these compounds, it is surprising that they all induce blood regeneration. (There probably are still other substances in liver and yeast capable of producing blood regeneration which as yet have not been isolated and synthesized.)

These nutrients, which have been identified as specific chemical substances, will be discussed in some detail and in the order in which they first came into clinical usefulness.

FOLIC ACID

Folic acid is a vitamin essential for life. It is widely distributed in nature and it is particularly plentiful in green leaves, liver and yeast. Meats in general are only fair sources, and milk is uniquely low in folic acid content. It is a most important member of the B group of vitamins, and now it is recognized as a chief factor in the family of biologically active substances called "pteroylglutamates." The pteroylglutamates differ from each other in the number of glutamic acid radicals in the side chain. Folic acid is essential to all forms of bacterial life, and the indispensability of this substance for the growth of *Lac-*

tobacillus casei and *Streptococcus lactis R* led to the discovery of these substances. Bacteria which do not require a supply of it furnished to them apparently can synthesize it in sufficient amount. Folic acid exists in nature not only free but in conjugated forms, and it is now known that much of the early difficulty in interpreting properly certain growth factors for bacteria and animals was due to the fact that these substances exhibit similar biologic activity, although each has its own chemical and bacteriologic properties. Folic acid, or the *L. casei* factor, was synthesized in 1945.

As can be seen in the formula (Fig. 41), the folic acid molecule contains a pteridine ring, one molecule of glutamic acid and one molecule of para-amino benzoic acid. At the top of the figure is shown the abbreviated formula for folic acid. In Figure 42 the same simplified form for the folic acid formula is used to present the formula for 5-pteroyltriglutamic acids. Pteroic acid differs from folic acid in the absence of one molecule of glutamic acid. Folic acid, which is composed of a glutamic acid residue and pteroic acid (Figs. 43 and 44) must be prefabricated before it can be used by the higher forms of life. Pteroic acid and glutamic acid show no hemopoietic activity in man when administered either separately or together. The folic acid crystals are bright yellow in color

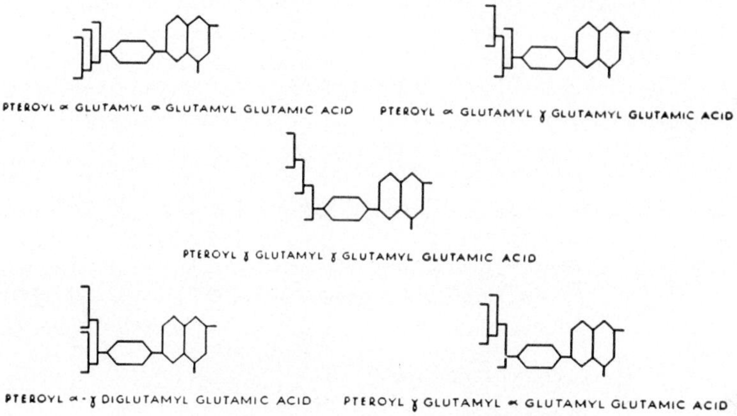

FIG. 42.

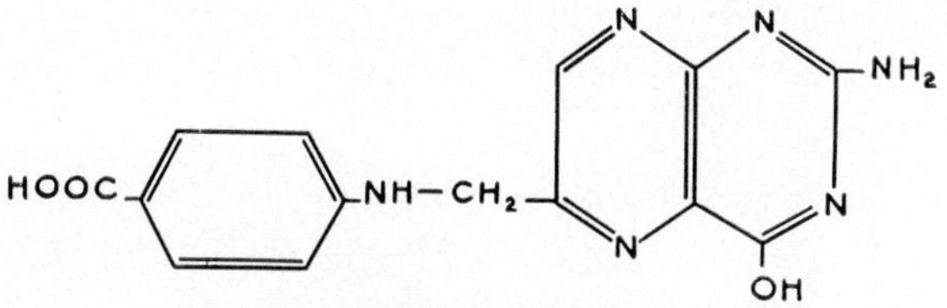

FIG. 43. Pteroic acid.

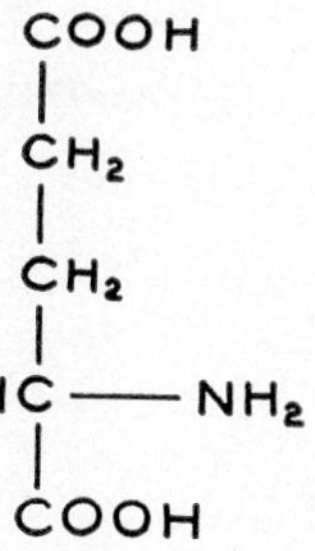

FIG. 44. Glutamic acid.

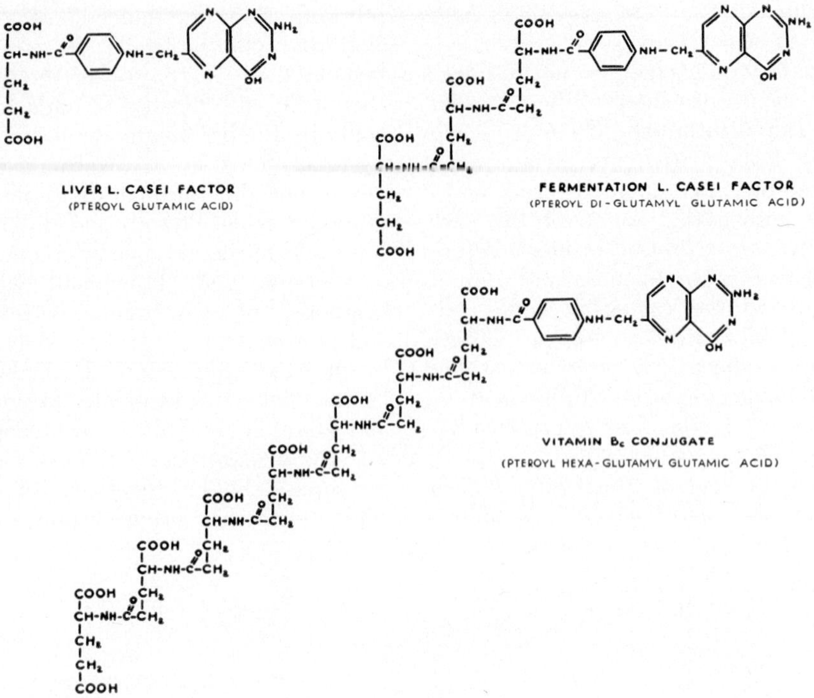

LIVER L. CASEI FACTOR
(PTEROYL GLUTAMIC ACID)

FERMENTATION L. CASEI FACTOR
(PTEROYL DI-GLUTAMYL GLUTAMIC ACID)

VITAMIN B_c CONJUGATE
(PTEROYL HEXA-GLUTAMYL GLUTAMIC ACID)

FIG. 45.

"FOLIC ACID" CONTENT OF FOODS

HIGH
- Fresh dark green leafy vegetables
- Liver
- Cauliflower
- Kidney

MEDIUM
- Beef
- Veal
- Dry wheat breakfast cereals

LOW
- Root vegetables
- Tomatoes, Bananas
- Milk, Cheese
- Pork, Ham, Lamb
- Rice, Corn meal, Sweet potato

FIG. 46.

and are destroyed fairly rapidly by heating with dilute mineral acids. As shown in Figure 45, this substance occurs in nature as a part of various complexes and most commonly in yeast and liver as the vitamin B_c conjugate which contains seven molecules of glutamic acid and is termed pteroylheptaglutamic acid. This figure shows some of the naturally-occurring forms of the folic acid compound and how the molecules of glutamic acid are linked together.

Although not present in high concentration, this substance tends to be widely distributed throughout plants and animal tissues. The table shown in Figure 46, prepared from observations by Olsen and his associates, shows the relative concentration of folic acid in a number of foods.

The so-called folic acid antagonists are of great interest and considerable work has been done with some, such as methylfolic acid. The synthesis of 4-amino-pteroylglutamic acid initiated the discovery of a new series of potent antagonists. A newly discovered factor, sometimes called folinic acid, the citrovorum factor or leucovorin has been shown to reverse the effects of this 4-amino-pteroylglutamic acid. These effects serve to emphasize the essential nature of folic acid in the biochemical processes. Although the chemistry of many different forms of folic acid has been thoroughly studied, as yet it is not entirely clear which form or forms occur in cells and tissues and serve as coenzymes in the enzymatic processes. For a time it was generally believed that the citrovorum factor, N[5]-formyl-tetra-hydro-pteroylglutamic acid served invariably as the coenzyme, but in the past few years a great deal of evidence has been presented against this concept. In addition to the citrovorum factor, other forms of folic acid which have been suggested as serving

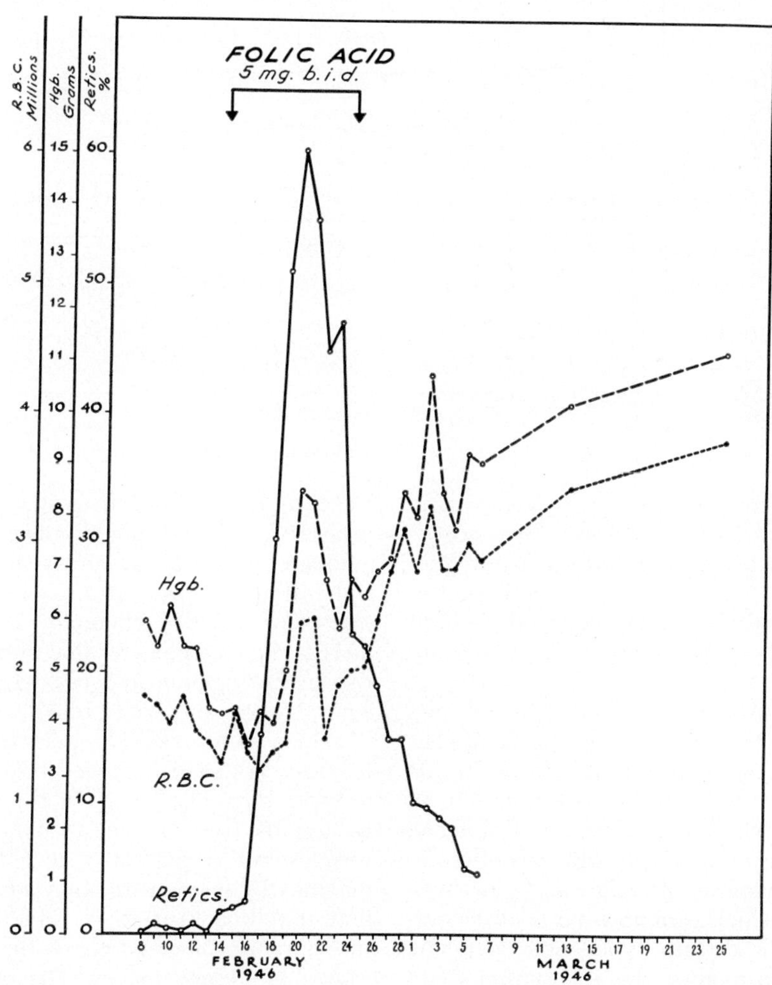

FIG. 47. E.G.S. Case of nutritional macrocytic anemia—folic acid therapy.

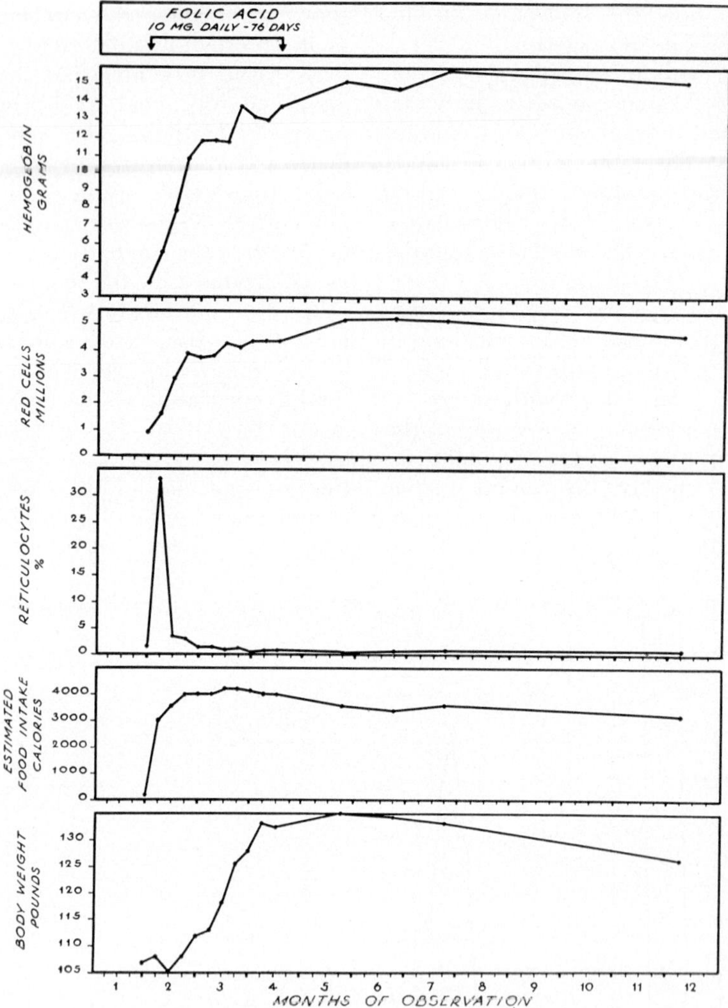

FIG. 48. Response of a case of sprue to folic acid.

as a coenzyme in certain enzymatic processes have included N[10]-formylpteroylglutamic acid, tetrahydro-pteroylglutamic acid, N[5]-hydroxymethyl-tetrahydro-pteroylglutamic acid and perhaps other folic acid compounds as yet unknown.

No satisfactory over-all clinical picture of the effect of folic acid has emerged; it is still best known for its influence upon blood regeneration in persons with certain types of anemia. Following the administration of sufficient amounts of folic acid, or substances which contain folic acid, to persons with certain types of macrocytic anemia in relapse, there is, within six to ten hours, an increase in reticulocytes in the bone marrow, the number of megaloblasts in the bone marrow decreases progressively, and the number of normoblasts increases. Changes in the peripheral blood occur after several days of treatment and are characterized by an increase in reticulocytes and subsequent rise in hemoglobin and red blood cells. The platelets and white blood cells tend to return to normal. The peak of reticulocytosis is usually reached on the sixth to tenth day. The height of the rise varies greatly from patient to patient. The response of a patient with nutritional macrocytic anemia to the administration of folic acid is shown in Figure 47; the response of a patient with sprue is shown in Figure 48; and the responses of a case of macrocytic anemia of pregnancy and of a case of the megaloblastic

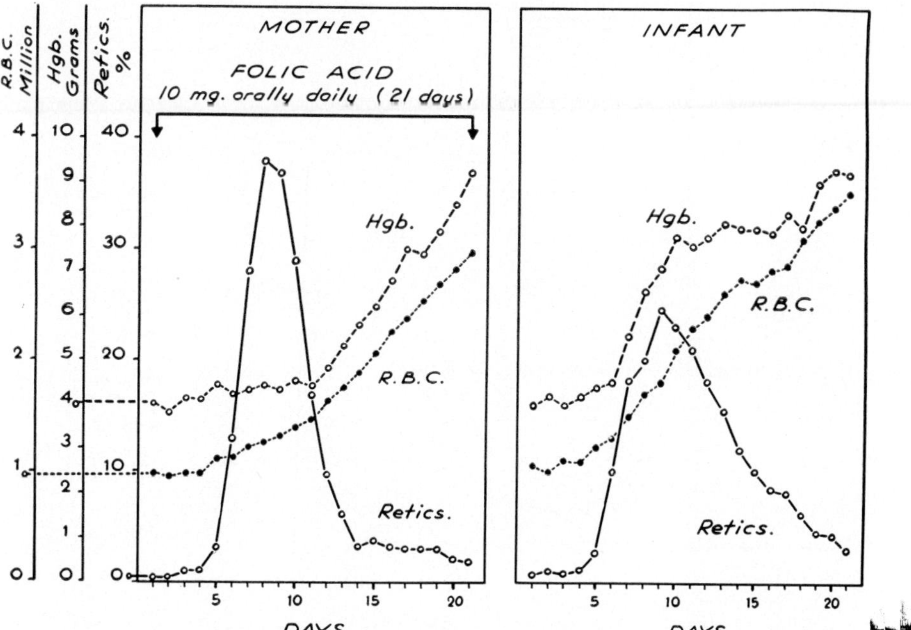

FIG. 49. Hemopoietic response of a woman with macrocytic anemia and her eight week old infant with macrocytic anemia following administration of folic acid to the mother.

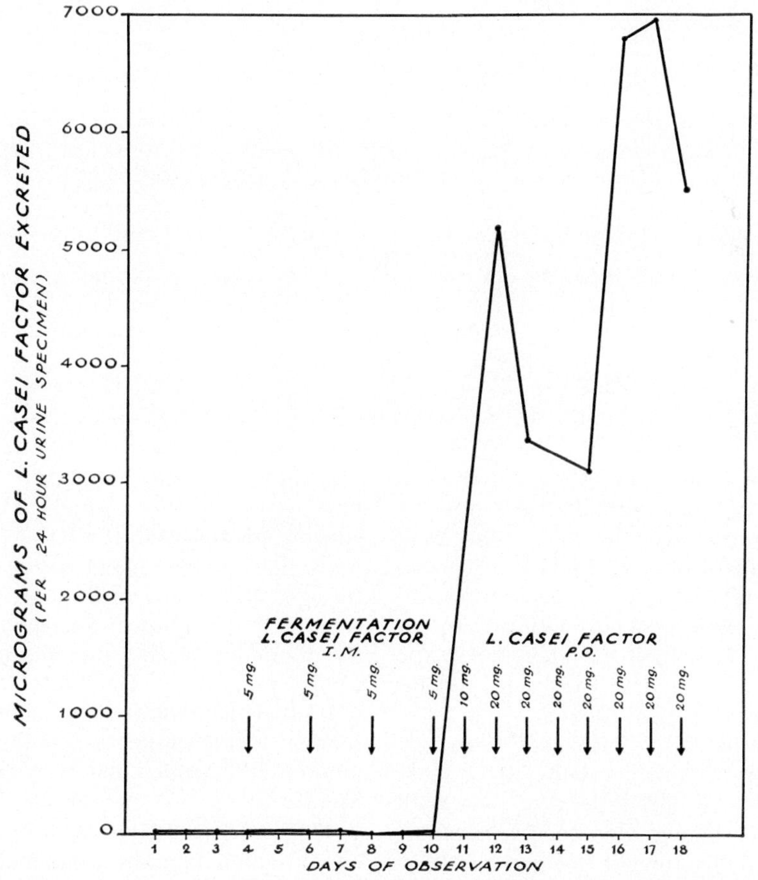

FIG. 50. W.L. Macrocytic anemia. Urinary excretion of *L. casei* factor.

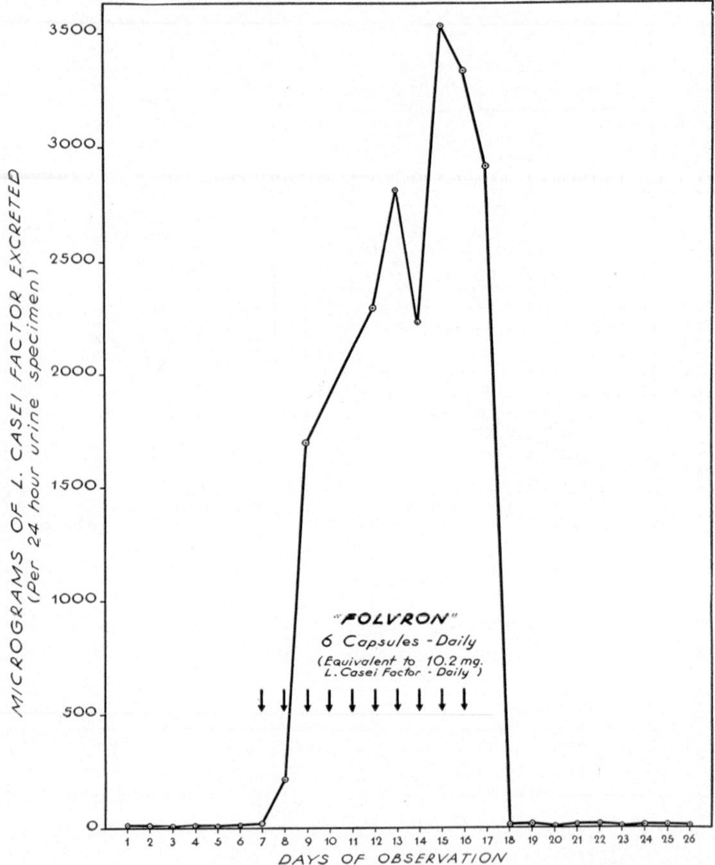

FIG. 51. M.P. Macrocytic anemia with iron deficiency urinary excretion of *L. casei* factor.

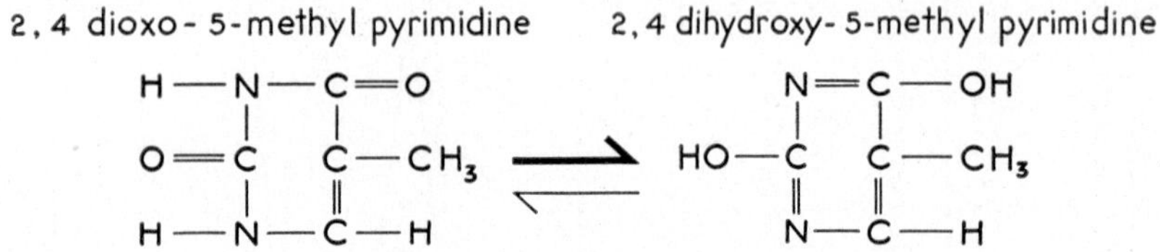

2,4 dioxo-5-methyl pyrimidine ⇌ 2,4 dihydroxy-5-methyl pyrimidine

```
H—N—C=O              N=C—OH
  |  |               |  |
O=C  C—CH3    ⇌   HO—C  C—CH3
  |  ||              ||  ||
H—N—C—H              N—C—H
```

FIG. 52. Methyl uracil (thymine).

anemia of infancy are shown in Figure 49. As shown in Figure 48, following the administration of folic acid, there is a great increase in food intake and gain in body weight. Under controlled conditions this patient, who continued to eat the diet on which he developed the anemia, responded to folic acid and his condition improved.

The hematologic responses shown in these figures were paralleled by a striking increase in strength, vigor and feeling of well-being. This occurs, irrespective of whether or not the patients have parasites or irrespective of the diets they have eaten or are eating. There is a specific, definite effect of the folic acid molecule on the megaloblasts and on the general tissues cells, which is evidenced by the clinical improvement and the tendency of the alimentary tract to return to normal. The diets of persons with these anemias were comprised of foods containing relatively small amounts of folic acid (Angulo and Spies).

The administration of folic acid, or foods which contain folic acid, to ex-

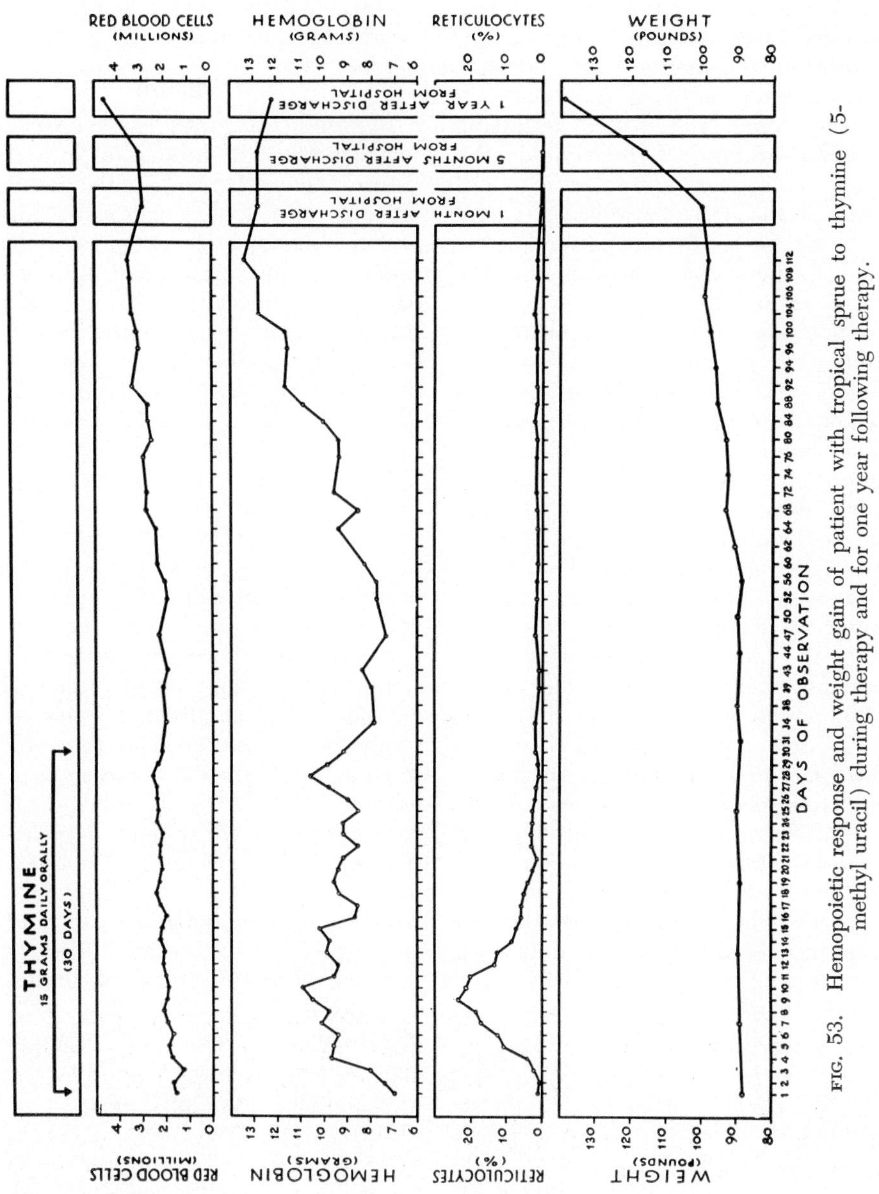

FIG. 53. Hemopoietic response and weight gain of patient with tropical sprue to thymine (5-methyl uracil) during therapy and for one year following therapy.

pectant mothers whose diets are low in folic acid is mandatory. The megaloblastic anemia of pregnancy, infancy and early childhood can be prevented by treating the mother in the later stages of pregnancy with either folic acid or substances which contain it. It is recommended that at least 2 mg. be administered to the mother each day during the latter months of pregnancy. It has been demonstrated that following the administration of folic acid, the mother can concentrate folic acid and transmit it through her milk to the infant so as to produce what might be termed a therapeutic response in the infant. (See Fig. 49.)

As shown in Figure 50, the utilization of folic acid by the body is not well understood. The *L. casei* factor produces a hemopoietic and clinical response in persons with certain types of anemia but in some instances the body enzymes cannot liberate excess residues of glutamic acid and change it into the free form (*L. casei* factor). In all instances the conjugated forms are therapeutically effective. Figure 50 shows that following the administration of such a compound, there is a slight lag before the compound is excreted in the urine in large amounts. The addition of iron to folic acid does not prevent the therapeutic usefulness nor the urinary excretion of folic acid (Fig. 51).

Soon after folic acid was administered to patients with pernicious anemia, it was learned that the folic acid did not prevent nor heal the neural degeneration associated with this disease. Later, when the authors found that synthetic 5-methyl uracil (Fig. 52) produced hemopoiesis and a clinical response similar to that of folic acid (Fig. 53), it was determined that this substance likewise neither prevented nor relieved the symptoms of neural degeneration associated with pernicious anemia. Hence, 5-methyl uracil and folic acid therapies are incomplete for pernicious anemia. (5-methyl uracil has no specificity in hemopoiesis. Many structures related to it are not effective in promoting either a clinical response or blood regeneration.) The required dosage of 5-methyl uracil is so large, it is impractical for everyday practice. However, folic acid is a most important therapeutic agent, not only in some cases of pernicious anemia but in a number of types of macrocytic anemias which are not associated with neural degeneration.

Diagnosis

A precise diagnosis is the essence of successful use of folic acid as a therapeutic agent. Persons with pernicious anemia, nutritional macrocytic anemia and the macrocytic anemia of pellagra, pregnancy and sprue have prompt clinical improvement and blood regeneration following its administration. *Folic acid is not useful in the treatment of nerve degeneration associated with pernicious anemia or in the treatment of leukemia, aplastic anemia or iron deficiency anemia.*

Treatment

Folic acid is effective when given orally or parenterally. The precise dosage cannot be stated, since there is considerable variation from patient to patient. We give the average patient about 10 mg. a day in divided doses, either orally or parenterally, until a full remission is obtained; in most cases oral administration is the method of choice. Many patients will respond to as little as 0.5 mg. a day. Others will not respond at all to 2 or 3 mg. a day. The dramatic response in the bone marrow and peripheral blood is associated with a great increase in desire for food; frequently patients begin to eat 3000 or 4000 calories a day, whereas prior to treatment they had eaten little or nothing. The severe diarrhea associated with these syndromes tends to subside rapidly. The stools become more normal in frequency, color and volume (Figures 54 and 55), and this is associated with a striking effect on the gastrointestinal tract. The abnormal dilatation and spasms tend to disappear and a barium column becomes continuous following the administration of folic acid (Figures 56 and 57).

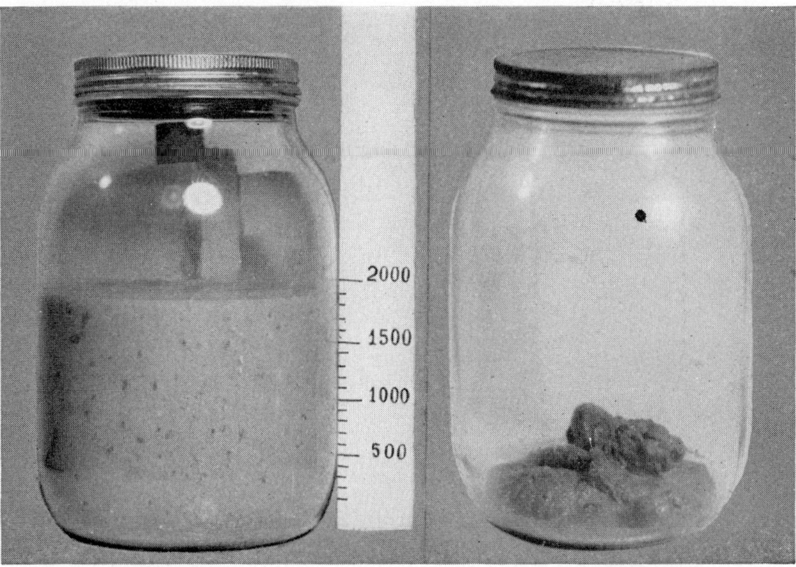

FIG. 54. FIG. 55.

FIG. 54. Stools passed in a twenty-four hour period the day preceding the initiation of folic acid therapy.

FIG. 55. Stools passed in a twenty-four hour period after two days on folic acid therapy.

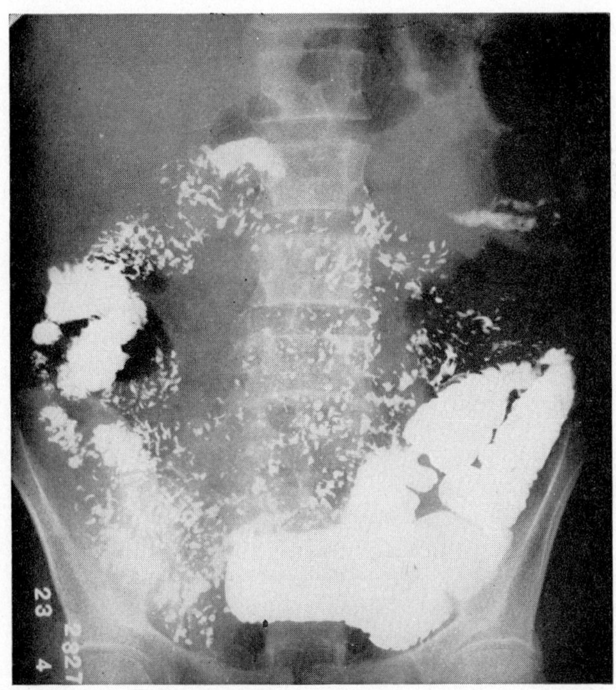

FIG. 56. Film made during gastrointestinal studies before folic acid therapy. It should be noted that the diarrhea was so profound that nearly all the barium column had been passed out of the body. There are isolated areas showing evidence of spasms and abnormal dilatations, and one notices a somewhat moulage effect.

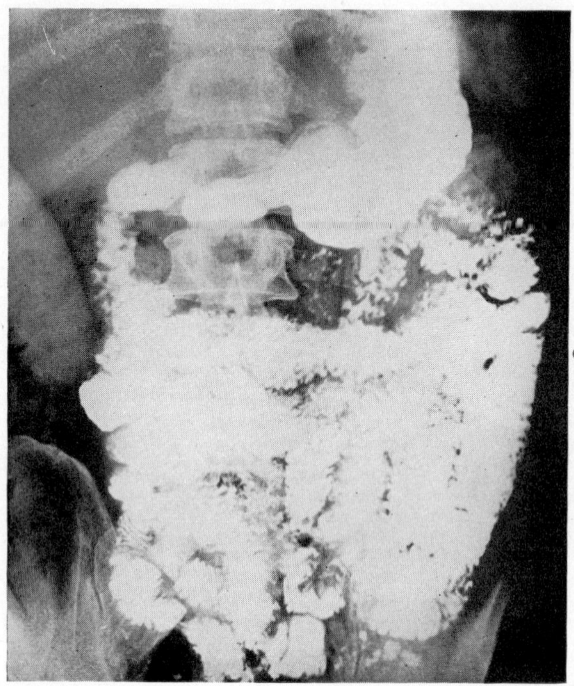

FIG. 57. Film made during gastrointestinal studies after 18 days on folic acid shows a continuous barium column and no evidence of spasm or abnormal dilatation.

Toxicity

We have given as much as 400 mg. daily for a period of five months and 10 mg. a day for a period of five years and in no instance did any untoward symptoms develop.

THE CITROVORUM FAMILY

Folinic acid and leucovorin are synthetic compounds which have citrovorum factor activity. The identification of other new but related compounds may be expected. Some of these compounds occur naturally and they have been made synthetically, and in a number of ways they are closely related to folic acid. The structural formula and the crystalline structure are shown in Figure 58. They may have folic acid activity in microorganisms and in man, but in some instances they are more effective in reversing the effects of folic acid inhibitors than folic acid, per se. The prevention and reversing of these toxic reactions in man hold promise as a tool for research, pointing toward indirect therapy in the treatment of leukemia.

In 1948 Sauberlich and Baumann found that the organism *Leuconostoc citrovorum* would not grow on the customary synthetic medium which was used; however, it would grow on the medium when certain extracts of liver were added. This organism could be used successfully for an assay of alanine and other amino acids. Other uses of this organism as a growth factor soon were determined, and it was learned that the response of the organism to liver extract could not be attributed to its folic acid, vitamin B_{12} or thymine content. Shive and his associates isolated a crystalline factor which was functionally related to folic acid. They reported that methyl folic acid (a folic acid antagonist) interfered with the growth of certain microorganisms and that this toxicity was overcome more effectively by thymidine (Fig. 59) than by folic acid itself. By this time it had occurred to those studying the literature as well as the primary investigators, such as Shive's group, Baumann's group and Broquist's group, that the *citrovorum factor* was related to folic acid in some way because: (1) the administration of large supplements of folic acid resulted in an increased excretion of the citrovorum factor in the urine; (2) when large amounts of folic acid were added to the medium, folic acid would partially replace a factor in liver, not vitamin B_{12}, which caused the growth of the L. citrovorum factor; and (3) the citrovorum factor was much more effective against folic acid antagonists than folic acid itself.

Nichol and Welch showed that slices of rat livers could convert folic acid to the citrovorum factor. Working independently, Bond et al. demonstrated that there was a substance in liver which was much more active than folic acid and which would reverse the toxicity of the antimetabolite, methylfolic acid (for the organism *L. casei*). This material was concentrated and found to have a structural and functional relationship to folic acid and was called *folinic acid.*

Broquist, Stokstad and Jukes found that folinic acid was similar to the citrovorum factor in its growth promoting properties for the *L. citrovorum.* Shive et al. reported that the synthesis of a factor from folic acid through the intermediate synthesis of formylfolic acid had physiologic properties similar to the naturally-occurring folic acid concentrate derived from liver. Brockman and his group reported on the synthesis of a material which was active for the *L. citrovorum* and as a growth factor for chicks, and which was also effective in reversing the toxicity of the folic acid antagonists.

A number of years prior to this work, the group working on anemias at the Nutrition Clinic, Hillman Hospital in Birmingham, Alabama, used as its working hypothesis that there was an interrelationship between the vitamins and the nucleic acids. From 1945 to 1950 this group studied the response of persons with anemia to the administration of folic acid compounds, 5-methyl uracil and related compounds, and the vitamin B_{12} family. It seemed important to study this new group of vitamins. Accordingly, Spies, Garcia Lopez, Milanes, Lopez Toca, Reboredo and Stone determined that when a synthetic substance termed folinic acid and another termed the citrovum factor (leucovorin) were administered to persons with per-

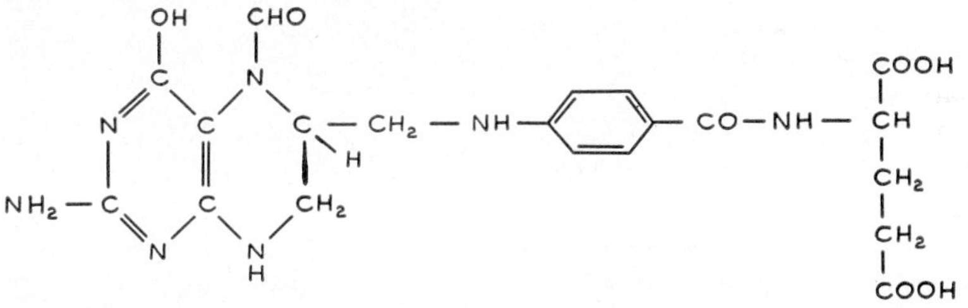

FIG. 58. 5-Formyl-5,6,7,8-tetrahydropteroylglutamic acid (leucovorin).

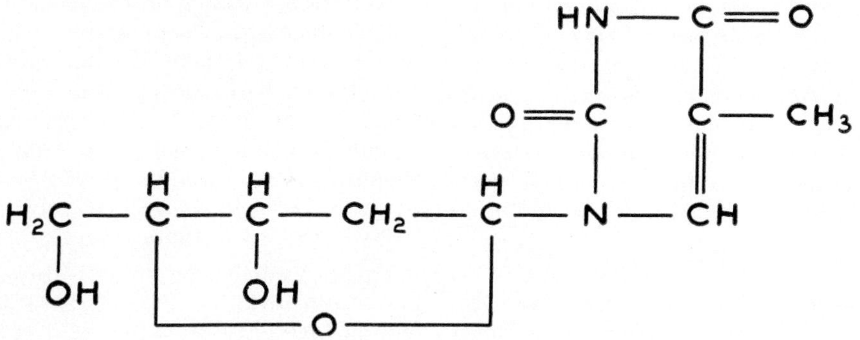

FIG. 59. Thymidine (thymine desoxyriboside).

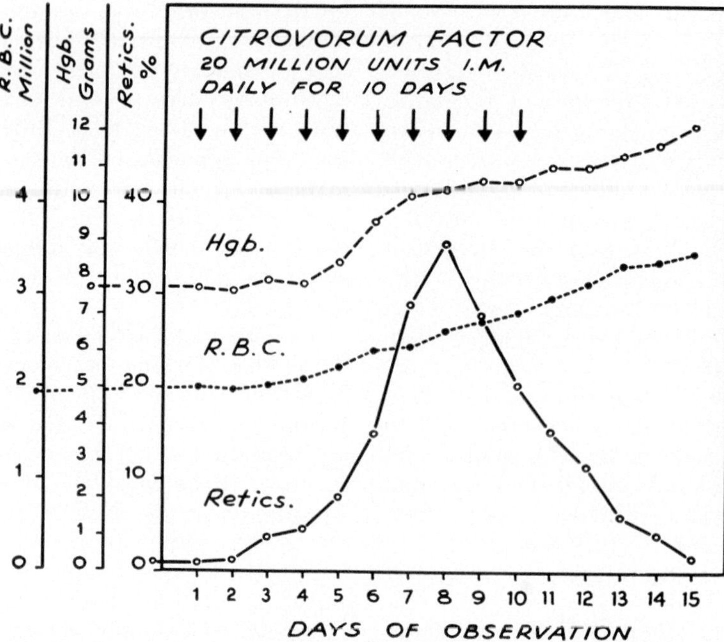

FIG. 60. Hemopoietic response of a patient with pernicious anemia to citrovorum factor.

nicious anemia, nutritional macrocytic anemia and tropical sprue in relapse, clinical and hemopoietic responses followed. Since these patients were carefully controlled and were not allowed to eat meat, meat products, milk or any substance capable of promoting blood regeneration, it was clear that the substances had a specific effect on the megaloblasts of the bone marrow. By using various dosage levels it was determined that this new compound had little or no more activity per unit of weight than free folic acid. Figure 60 shows the response to the citrovorum factor (leucovorin). These factors apparently have the same therapeutic indications as folic acid, per se. They do not protect against the neural degeneration associated with pernicious anemia and for that reason are not complete treatments for pernicious anemia. It appears that the field of greatest therapeutic usefulness for these substances is as effective countermeasures against folic acid antagonists.

Symptomatology

The diseases which are relieved by these substances are the same as those relieved by folic acid.

Diagnosis

Patients with pernicious anemia, nutritional macrocytic anemia and macrocytic anemia of pellagra, pregnancy and sprue in relapse have both clinical improvement and blood regeneration following the administration of any one of these substances in adequate amounts. The specific usefulness is in persons with symptoms arising from massive doses of antifolic acid compounds.

Treatment

These substances are effective when given orally or parenterally. However, when administered orally to persons having free hydrochloric acid in their gastric juice they seem to be changed promptly to folic acid, per se. The precise dosage varies from patient to patient but in general, about the same amount per unit of weight as folic acid should be administered.

Toxicity

Large amounts of these substances have been given over a period of eight months. Patients receiving 4 or 5 mg. several times a week during this period did not develop any untoward signs or symptoms.

VITAMIN B_{12}

Pernicious anemia has been recognized as a clinical entity for more than 100 years. Substances of vitamin B_{12} activity are widely scattered in nature and have existed for eons of time. However, the ingestion of ordinary foods which contain small quantities of substances exhibiting vitamin B_{12} does not produce beneficial effects in persons with pernicious anemia. The role of liver as a therapeutic agent has been known for 32 years and resulted from the discovery that the administration of massive doses of this substance to patients with pernicious anemia in relapse produced a favorable hemopoietic and clinical response.

While liver contains relatively little vitamin B_{12}, nevertheless it is one of the most highly concentrated of the natural sources of vitamin B_{12}; hence, it is most logical that the pharmaceutical industry should make highly refined liver extracts. In 1948 Rickes et al. isolated from liver a crystalline compound which they called vitamin B_{12}. Working independently, Smith noted the presence of more than one pink hemopoietically active substance in liver extract. Kaczka, Wolf and Folkers produced a crystalline product of vitamin B_{12} by means of a catalytic reaction with hydrogen. Since the original product had been termed vitamin B_{12}, they designated this new product vitamin B_{12} . Pierce et al. separated from a vitamin B_{12} concentrate a crystalline material which had a different absorption spectrum from vitamin B_{12}. They showed that these crystals were active in chick assay and in assay with *L. leichmannii* 212 and suggested the term vitamin B_{12_b}. Spies and associates showed that these various compounds and vitamin B_{12}, per se, produced similar, if not identical, clinical and hematologic responses.

West, using vitamin B_{12}, first reported a positive hemopoietic response in three patients with pernicious anemia following the injection of 3, 6, and 150 micrograms of vitamin B_{12} respectively. Spies, Stone and Aramburu reported favorable clinical and hematologic responses following the administration of vitamin B_{12} in two cases of pernicious anemia, two cases of nutritional macrocytic anemia and one case of nontropical sprue; Spies and co-workers reported a similar response in two cases of tropical sprue in Cuba; Suarez et al. reported the response in a case of tropical sprue in Puerto Rico. Stone and Spies showed the specific effect of vitamin B_{12} on the neurologic symptoms of patients with pernicious anemia and in relieving lesions of the mucous membrane. Berk et al. independently demonstrated its effect on patients with the degeneration of the nervous system.

Vitamin B_{12} should be regarded as a family of vitamins, some members of which are not yet identified. All members are of great interest in human nutrition and, like other compounds previously discussed in this section, promote blood regeneration in certain types of anemia (Figs. 61 and 62). A few pertinent points are summarized briefly in Figure 63.

As far as the authors have been able to ascertain, all members of this family of vitamins contain 5,6-dimethylbenzimidazole (Fig. 64). The vitamin B_{12} compound, containing about 4 per cent cobalt and phosphorus, is a cobalt complex and is easily destroyed by excessive light.

Cannon, Johnson and Todd isolated a red crystalline hexacarboxylic acid following treatment of vitamin B_{12} with 30 per cent sodium hydroxide at 150° C. Amorphous tetra- and pentacarboxylic acids were obtained in a lesser yield. All were nucleotide free. The hexacarboxylic acid $C_{46}H_{60}O_{13}N_6CoCl \cdot 2H_2O$ crystallized as needles and dimorphic prisms, the latter being suitable for single crystal study. X-ray analysis of this acid in conjunction with comparative results on vitamin B_{12} provided evidence for the presence around the cobalt atom of a porphyrin-like cyclic structure minus one methine carbone bridge. Hodgkin and associates identified the projected

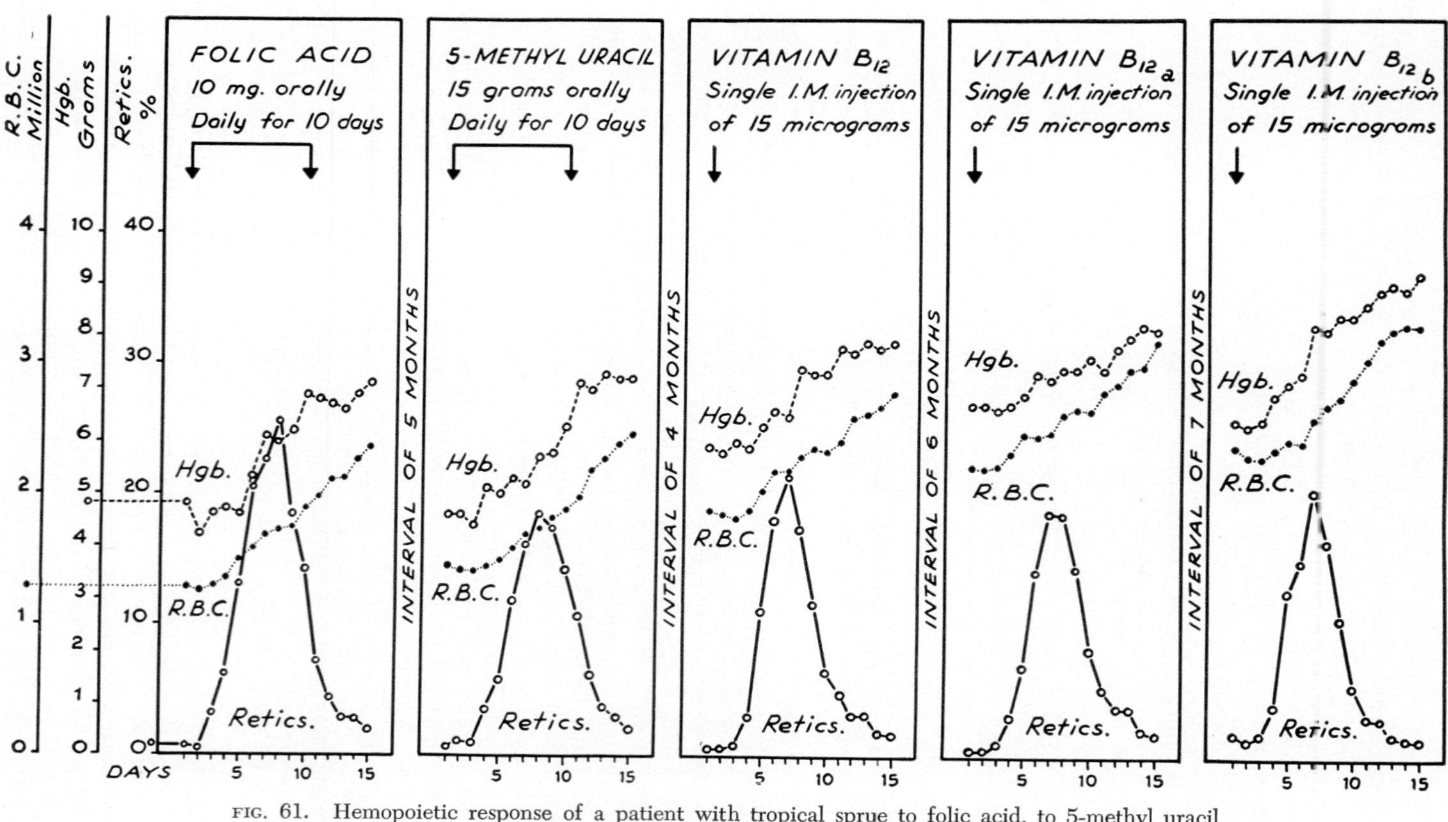

FIG. 61. Hemopoietic response of a patient with tropical sprue to folic acid, to 5-methyl uracil to vitamin B_{12}, to vitamin B_{12a} and to vitamin B_{12b}.

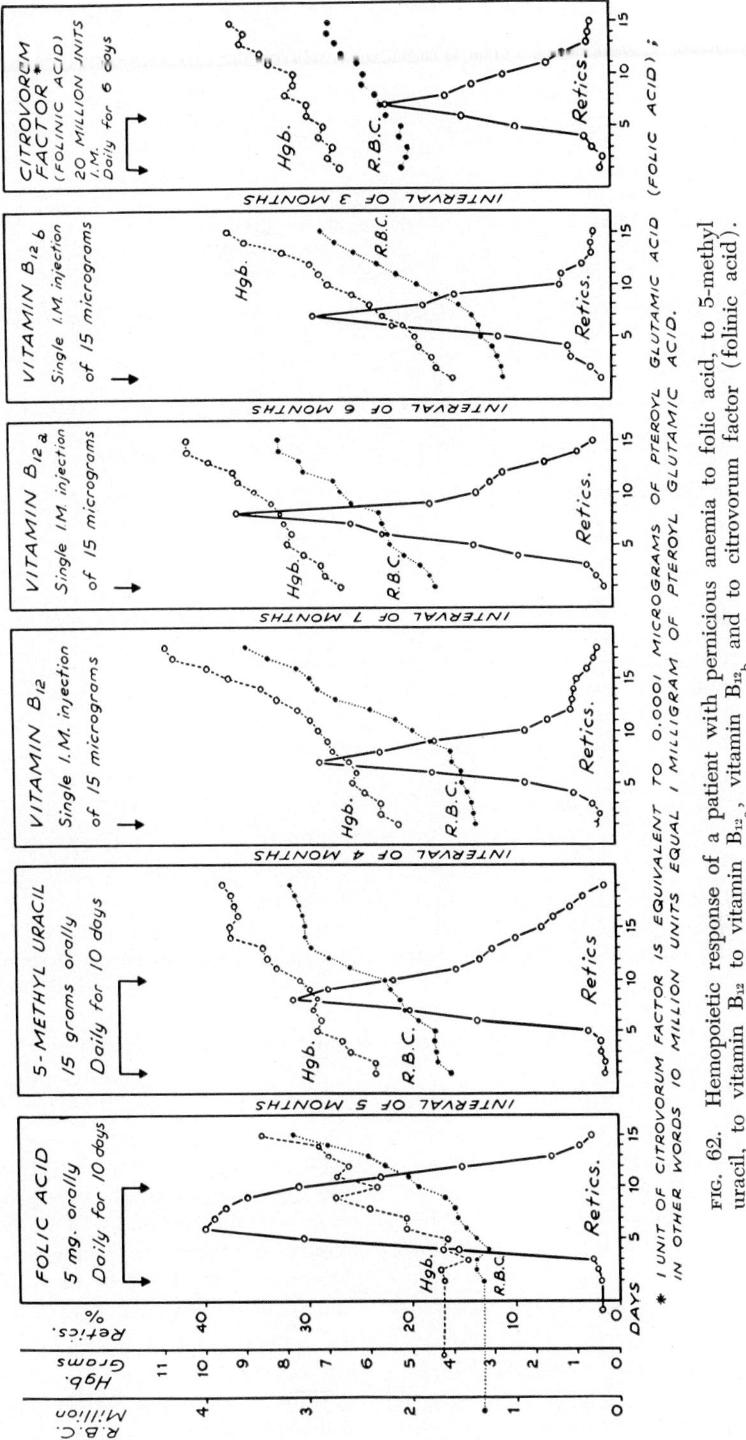

FIG. 62. Hemopoietic response of a patient with pernicious anemia to folic acid, to 5-methyl uracil, to vitamin B_{12} to vitamin B_{12_a}, vitamin B_{12_b} and to citrovorum factor (folinic acid).

1. Vitamin B_{12a} and vitamin B_{12b} are identical.
2. Vitamin B_{12} contains a cyano group which is not present in vitamin B_{12a}.
3. The cyano group is present in the vitamin B_{12} cobalt coordination complex.
4. Cobalamin designates all the vitamin B_{12} molecules except the cyano group. Vitamin B_{12} can then be termed cyano-cobalamin and vitamin B_{12a} termed hydroxo-cobalamin.
5. Both have been found active by parenteral injection in producing clinical and hemopoietic improvement in persons with pernicious anemia, nutritional macrocytic anemia and tropical sprue.

FIG. 63.

atomic positions of 62 atoms out of about 70, not counting hydrogen. The structure of vitamin B_{12} ($C_{63}H_{90}O_{14}N_{14}$-PCo) (Fig. 64) was then proposed by Hodgkin's and Todd's groups. The five-membered lactam ring fused to ring B in the hexacarboxylic acid arises presumably from closure of the ring following hydroxylation of ring B during hydrolysis of vitamin B_{12} in strong alkali. A number of features of this structure are admittedly not yet proved, but the proposed structure is in agreement with all presently available physical and chemical evidence.

Vitamin B_{12} is unique in being the only vitamin that contains cobalt, a metal, as an integral part of its structure. This "red" vitamin is one of the most potent of all catalysts. A relatively few molecules are sufficient to maintain life. Boger, Bayne, Strickland and Wright recently have shown that the circulating concentration of vitamin B_{12} is lower in older persons and still lower in pregnant women. Higher than normal concentration of vitamin B_{12} occurs in healthy newborn infants and in myelogenous leukemia.

Today vitamin B_{12} is available in ample amounts for clinical and scientific use as a result of its commercial production from Streptomyces fermentations. Ox liver usually contains less than one part in a million of the vitamin B_{12} family. This vitamin is loosely bound to protein. Liver is an uneconomic source of material for the commercial production of vitamin B_{12}. Sewage sludge contains a considerable amount of vitamin B_{12} and some of its analogues. Certainly the best commercial source for pharmaceutical use is to recover it from streptomycin or Aureomycin manufacture or by special fermentations. It it important to select species that make vitamin B_{12} exclusively. Some manufacturers were led astray by organisms that gave high yields of pseudo vitamin B_{12}. This vitamin tends to be concentrated largely in the cells. The vitamin B_{12} molecule is moderately large as can be seen from its structural formula (Figure 64). There are few rich sources of vitamin B_{12} in nature. It is a fundamental nutrient for a wide variety of living organisms and man depends on an exogenous supply.

While vitamin B_{12} appears in foods of animal origin, it should be kept in mind that certain herbivorous animals obtain their vitamin B_{12} from bacteria in their rumen through synthesis. Bacterial synthesis of vitamin B_{12} in man occurs in the colon. Patients with pernicious anemia in relapse have large amounts of this vitamin in their feces. The colon of man, however, does not absorb much of this vitamin under ordinary circumstances.

The importance of vitamin B_{12} in animal metabolism is well established. In chicks its lack causes kidney damage and perosis. In rats a high mortality occurs soon after weaning and various abnormal hematologic findings appear. This vitamin influences the metabolism of protein, carbohydrate and fat. It seems that vitamin B_{12} is necessary for the biosynthesis of labile methyl groups and in the reduction of thiole compounds.

The human body is capable of storing large amounts of vitamin B_{12}; thus, clinical manifestations or abnormal laboratory findings may be delayed for a long time after the body's external supply has been restricted. Because of our prolonged ignorance of the fact that the intrinsic factor in the gastric juice is required for the proper absorption of ingested vitamin B_{12}, we have not understood much of the physiology. It appears to the authors that vitamin B_{12} deficiency in man may occur as a result of at least four different mechanisms:

1. A deficiency of intrinsic factor in the gastric juice,
2. Bacterial or parasitic interference of the normal absorption of vitamin B_{12} in the alimentary tract,
3. Defects in the capacity of the intestines properly to absorb this substance,
4. An inadequate dietary intake of vitamin B_{12} or substances that may act similarly.

Vitamin B_{12} is necessary for every cell in the body, but in its protracted absence the presenting symptoms tend to arise from the hemopoietic system, the nervous system or the alimentary tract. Glossitis, stomatitis and pharyngitis are frequent symptoms in persons with pernicious anemia in relapse, sprue, nutritional macrocytic anemia and the macrocytic anemia of pregnancy. In some instances the mucous membrane lesions are relieved by the administration of folic acid; at other times they are only partially relieved by its administration. However, when the diagnosis is precise, these lesions are always relieved by adequate dosage of vitamin B_{12} administered parenterally.

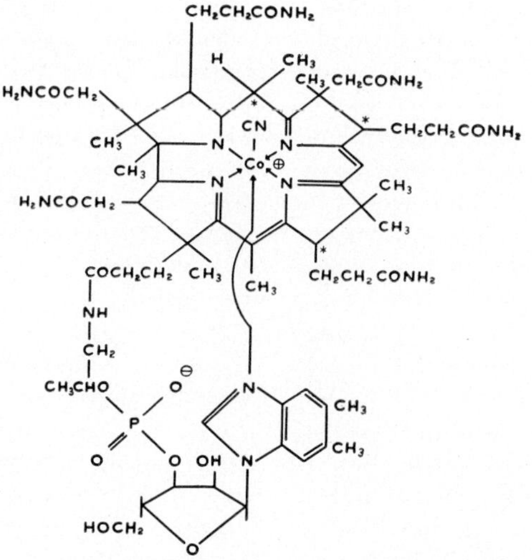

VITAMIN B_{12} $C_{63}H_{90}O_{14}N_{14}PCo$

FIG. 64.

The introduction of radioactive B_{12} has somewhat simplified the diagnosis of pernicious anemia. In some medical centers the existence of vitamin B_{12} deficiency may be suspected from poor absorption with radioactive B_{12}, and additional evidence is the finding that body fluids are low in this vitamin. This type of study should supplement, not replace, time-honored methods of evaluation.

Relationship of Vitamin B_{12} to as Yet Unidentified Factor in Gastric Juice

Prolonged deficiencies of B complex vitamins which affect other organs and systems so dramatically often leave characteristic changes in the cellular elements of bone marrow and blood. Castle's classic experiments on the etiology of macrocytic anemia showed that an extrinsic factor (the food factor) and an intrinsic factor (the stomach factor) were essential to proper maturation of erythrocytes. Without the erythrocyte maturation factor, formed from the intrinsic and extrinsic factors and stored in the liver, the red cells in the bone marrow are arrested at the megaloblast stage and a macrocytic anemia occurs. It was considered probable that a deficiency of either the extrinsic or the intrinsic factor could bring about macrocytic anemia, and Castle concluded from his studies that Addisonian pernicious anemia was due to the intrinsic factor deficiency.

Several observers have noted and reported isolated cases of macrocytic anemia occurring in persons on grossly deficient diets. Spies and Chinn were able to produce such an anemia in two epileptics who were maintained on a diet deficient in B complex vitamins for several months (see Fig. 65). A high protein diet restored the red blood cells to normal. Spies and Payne, and Sydenstricker, Schmidt, Geeslin and Weaver recognized the frequent association of macrocytic anemia and pellagra, and independently demonstrated the presence of intrinsic factor in the gastric juice of these pellagrins (see Fig. 66). These demonstrations eliminated intrinsic factor deficiency as the cause of these macrocytic anemias. Wills has indicated that a food factor other than the "extrinsic factor" may also be necessary for the maturation of red blood cells. She demonstrated that persons with nutritional macrocytic anemia in India did not respond to treatment with highly concentrated liver extracts which contained large amounts of the erythrocyte maturation factor, but did respond with characteristic reticulocytosis when given crude liver extract or yeast products.

Moore, Vilter and Spies analyzed the cellular elements of the blood and bone marrow in ten persons with severe macrocytic anemias, coexisting with nicotinic acid, thiamine or riboflavin deficiency states. These studies showed that macrocytic anemia of all degrees may be encountered in persons who subsist on grossly deficient diets. It may rival neglected pernicious anemia in severity. They found erythrocyte counts as low as 1,000,000, with the hemoglobin high in comparison and a color index above 1. The mean corpuscular volume, mean corpuscular hemoglobin and mean corpuscular hemoglobin concentration per unit of cell indicated that the cells were large and well-filled with hemoglobin. Blood smears showed variations in size and shape of red cells with the large cells predominating. The white blood counts were usually low or low normal; the platelets were reduced in number; a relative lymphocytosis was present frequently; and the polymorphonuclear leukocytes were hypersegmented. The degree of reticulocytosis (less than 1 per cent to 10 per cent) seemed to depend upon whether or not the diet of the patient had improved recently.

The bone marrow biopsies taken from these patients were indistinguishable from those found in Addisonian pernicious anemia. Megaloblasts and early erythroblasts predominated and there was a general decrease in activity of the myeloid series of cells and of the megakarocytes.

The gastric juice contained small amounts of free hydrochloric acid following histamine, except in two cases where there was a total achlorhydria. Intrinsic factor was present as was demonstrated by incubation of the gastric juice with raw ground beef and feeding the mixture to known cases of pernicious anemia with subsequent characteristic reticulocytosis.

These patients responded with a significant reticulocytosis and a rise in the red blood count when one-half pound of raw beef was added to their deficient diets for ten days, or when reticulogen (concentrated liver extract) was administered intravenously. The studies suggest that an extrinsic factor deficiency was responsible for the anemia which did not improve following the administration of nicotonic acid, thiamine, riboflavin, pyridoxine or pantothenic acid.

Moore, Vilter, Minnich and Spies showed that the oral administration of a 70 per cent alcoholic solution of beef, in amounts of a few cubic centimeters each day for ten days, to persons with nutritional macrocytic anemia results in an increase in reticulocytes up to 25 per cent, followed by a rise of hemoglobin and red cells.

When vitamin B_{12} is incubated with normal human gastric juice its effect, when administered orally to persons with

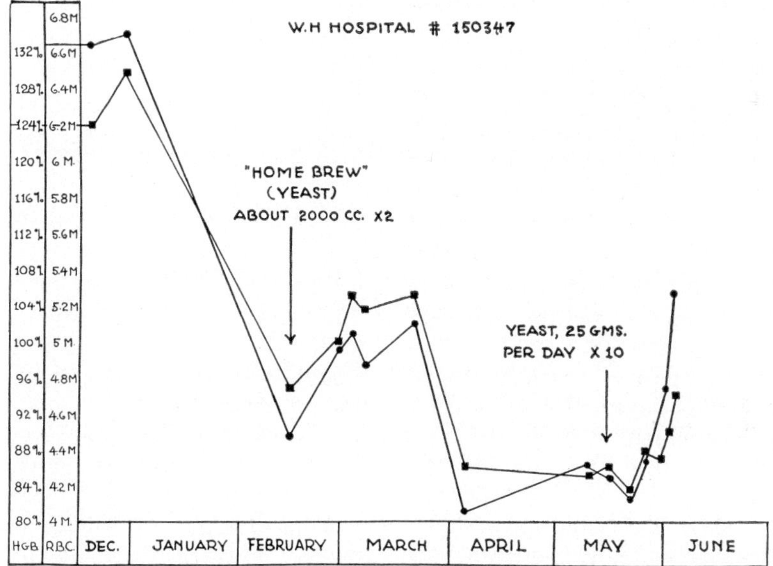

FIG. 65. Figure shows the fall in red count and hemoglobin in an epileptic on a vitamin B deficient diet, and the response to the administration of yeast on two occasions.

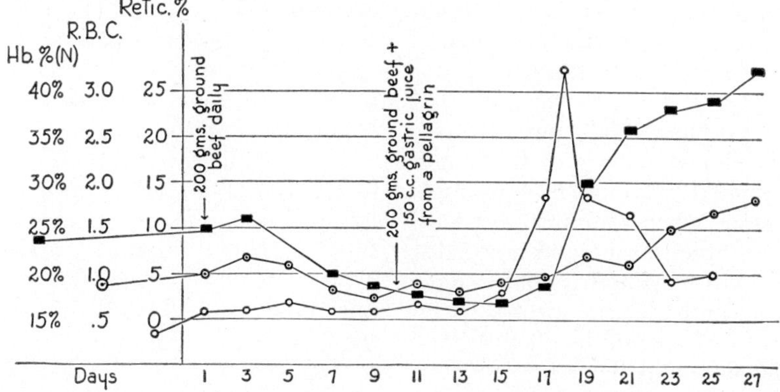

FIG. 66. Hematopoietic response of patient with pernicious anemia to beef incubated with gastric juice from a pellagrin.

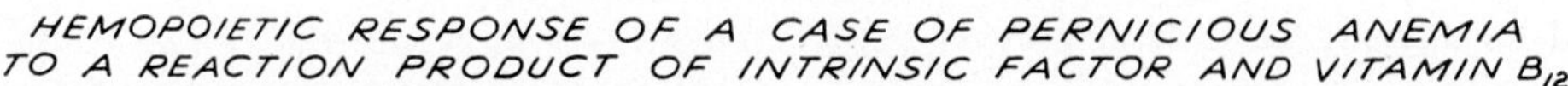

HEMOPOIETIC RESPONSE OF A CASE OF PERNICIOUS ANEMIA
TO A REACTION PRODUCT OF INTRINSIC FACTOR AND VITAMIN B12

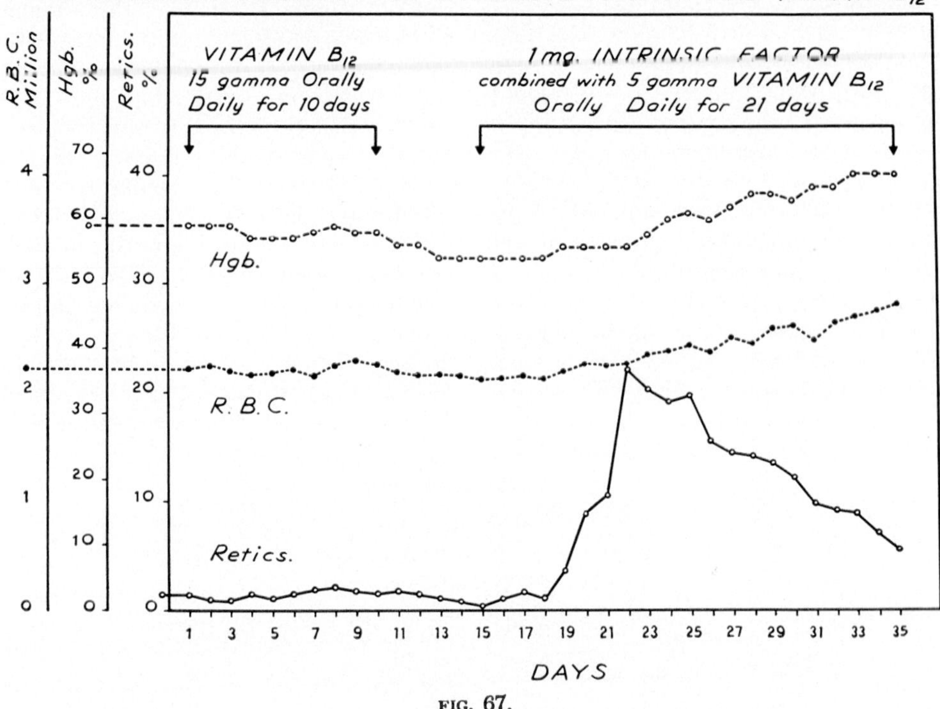

FIG. 67.

macrocytic anemia, is greatly increased. Berk et al. suggested that the food factor previously termed extrinsic factor might be identical with the anti-anemic factor in liver which, in itself, was very similar or identical to vitamin B_{12}. Bethell et al., Hall, et al., and Spies and Stone and their associates have shown that normal gastric juice aids the absorption of this vitamin or protects it from destruction in the upper gastrointestinal tract, Bethell and his group found a large fecal excretion of vitamin B_{12} in persons with pernicious anemia in relapse, thus demonstrating the problem of getting it through the gut wall and into the tissues. Hall and his associates have shown that both the crude and the refined vitamin B_{12} products have an effect when administered with gastric juice. Spies, Stone and associates in similar studies on nutritional macrocytic anemia and tropical sprue as well as on pernicious anemia in relapse have shown that vitamin B_{12} can be "activated" or "potentiated" by the administration of gastric juice.

Remarkably little is known about the mode of action of intrinsic factor, although it is concerned with the absorption of vitamin B_{12} through the intestine. How this is done is a mystery, although many people are guessing.

Comparative studies of severe cases of tropical sprue, nutritional macrocytic anemia and pernicious anemia in relapse show that the average person with tropical sprue has a greater deficiency of intrinsic factor than the average case of pernicious anemia. The intrinsic factor is a polypeptide that can give a full response in amounts as small as 1 mg. per day when administered with vitamin B_{12} orally (Fig. 67).

The chemical structure of the intrinsic factor is not known. There have been isolated a number of chemical substances which various groups have claimed would activate the food factor, but more critical study has eliminated them from consideration. Until more information is available, it is impossible to consider vitamin B_{12} a universal oral therapeutic agent for persons with macrocytic anemia. Cases vary a great deal; one patient may respond to as little as 5 micrograms daily for ten days, whereas another may not respond on ten times this dosage. A substantial number of cases have responded when 3 milligrams was administered orally. This response, however, while satisfactory, was not as good as when 30 micrograms were administered intramuscularly to the same patient.

Vitamin B_{12} (Neural Involvement)

For years physicians have recognized that patients with pernicious anemia have an imperfect secretion of gastric juice, the cause of which is not clear, although it is known that it tends to run in families and usually occurs late in life. As early as 1884 it was shown that patients with pernicious anemia have neural degeneration. The anemia usually precedes the neural disturbances, although such disturbances may occur without any blood changes and the extent of the involvement is not directly dependent on the degree of anemia.

When there is an inadequate amount of vitamin B_{12} in the nerve tissues, pain, numbness and tingling of the fingers and toes and stiffness of the extremities develop. The peripheral reflexes become hyperactive and the severity of all the symptoms may rather steadily increase. In some instances, however, when the onset is very acute the patient may first note paralysis of the extremities or parts thereof. It has been known for some time that all these neurologic symptoms of pernicious anemia could be prevented by the injection of adequate amounts of liver extract. Spies and Stone reported the first group of patients in whom relief of the symptoms arising from nerve degeneration followed the administration of vitamin B_{12}. This report was followed by a report of three more cases and one case reported by Castle. Hall, Campbell and many others in the United States have confirmed these observations and Ungley has made most important contributions in Great Britain.

It is now accepted that symptoms arising from combined system disease can be ameliorated by the injection of vitamin B_{12} provided that the patient is treated during the acute phase of the disease. It also is accepted that there comes a time when, if the patient is not properly treated, the disease may become chronic, and such symptoms are irreversible. Recently the authors have had occasion to study patients who have developed neural disturbances as the first symptom of pernicious anemia and who were treated with vitamin B_{12}; the symptoms arising from nerve involvement disappeared and the anemia so characteristic of the disease did not develop. Many younger clinicians have not paid adequate attention to such cases in which nerve degeneration is the only presenting symptom and for this reason they have not treated them early. The essence of the best treatment of pernicious anemia is dependent on an early diagnosis. When mental impairment, paresthesias, loss of vibratory sense, loss of position sense, ataxia and hyperactivity of the reflexes are the results of an acute involvement of nerve tissue, there is a prompt and definite disappearance of these symptoms following the administration of vitamin B_{12} (see Fig. 68). This might be termed the neurologic response to vitamin B_{12} also observed in correcting diabetic neuropathies (Duncan).

It has been shown that persons with pernicious anemia who are treated with folic acid may develop nerve degeneration, but it also has been shown that folic acid does not act as a neurotoxin. Persons who develop this type of nerve degeneration need a member of the vitamin B_{12} family; no other vitamin will take its place. Spies and his group have administered folic acid in doses ranging from 1 to 10 mg. daily to eighty patients with pernicious anemia for a period of from four to five years. These patients also have had frequent injections of either liver extract or vitamin B_{12} or both. None of them has developed neural degeneration, indicating that in the presence of vitamin B_{12} or substances containing vitamin B_{12}, such

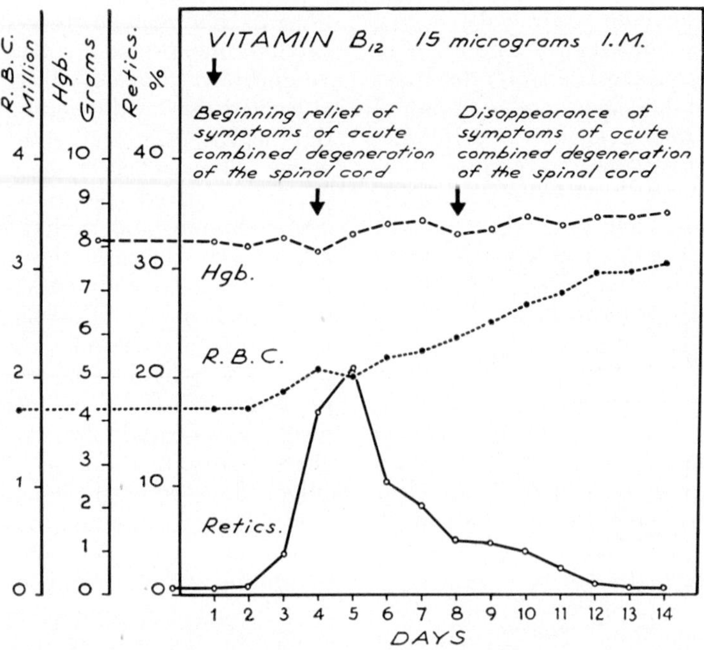

FIG. 68. Hemopoietic response of a patient (J.J.) with pernicious anemia to vitamin B_{12}.

as refined liver extract, folic acid in no way adversely affects the nerve tissue.

Some 50,000 persons in the United States have pernicious anemia. Many of them are being satisfactorily maintained by repeated injections of liver extract or vitamin B_{12} or by the oral administration of ventriculin. There are some who maintain themselves by eating large amounts of whole liver daily although this is an arduous task for most of them. Liver is, nevertheless, a most satisfactory therapeutic agent in other respects and presumably contains a number of important nutrients not as yet isolated and identified.

The Effects of Vitamin B_{12} upon the Megaloblasts of the Bone Marrow

For reasons not clearly understood, some persons are unable to produce sufficient blood. Gradually they become weaker, their red blood cells decrease in number, and eventually they develop clinical syndromes.

Some persons with anemia do not fit into an exact classification, and frequently highly trained physicians differ as to the classification of the type of anemia.

From a physiologic point of view, the bone marrow attempts to make blood, but lacking an essential substance, it is unable to complete the process. Then another megaloblast is formed and this new parent cell, lacking the same chemical substance or substances, likewise is unable to produce cells. Eventually, because of this fundamental lack, the person develops a severe anemia in spite of the fact that there is a great excess of parent cells in the bone marrow. If, however, a substance such as vitamin B_{12} is supplied, the whole mechanism begins to function properly, and within six to twelve hours the megaloblasts can be seen to produce offspring. Could this not mean that these megaloblasts probably need, say, a molecule of vitamin B_{12} to put into each cell that is made?

At any rate, the mechanism is beautifully and delicately balanced. If too much vitamin B_{12} is administered, the excess is excreted in the urine. If too little is administered, the body uses in the megaloblasts all that can be obtained. An amount hardly visible to the naked eye can cause a profound effect. Within a few hours after the institution of this specific therapy, depending upon the amount administered and the response of the patient, the megaloblastic arrest of the bone marrow begins to decrease. The bone marrow changes from what is called a megaloblastic marrow to a normoblastic marrow. The changes in the peripheral blood also are specific and definite. First, young red blood cells (reticulocytes) pour out into the blood. The peak of reticulocytosis is reached on the third to eighth day of therapy,

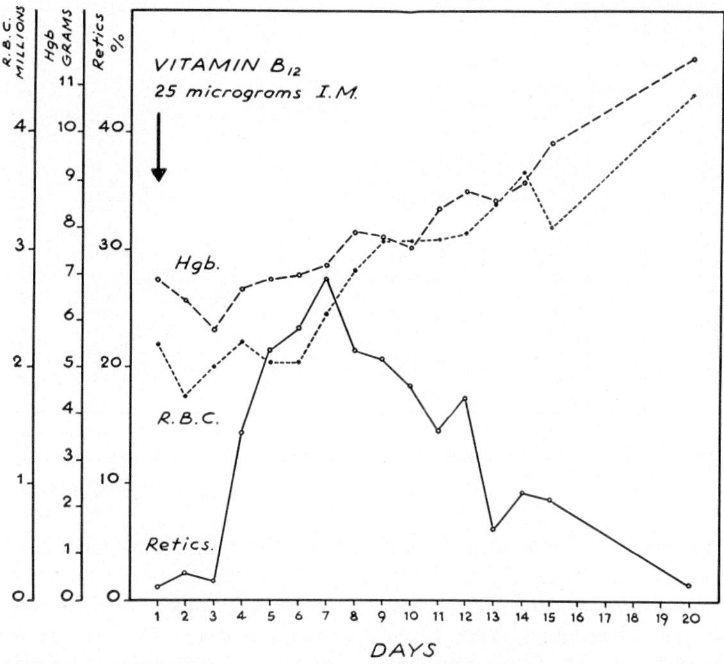

FIG. 69. Hemopoietic response of a patient (W.K.) with pernicious anemia to vitamin B_{12}.

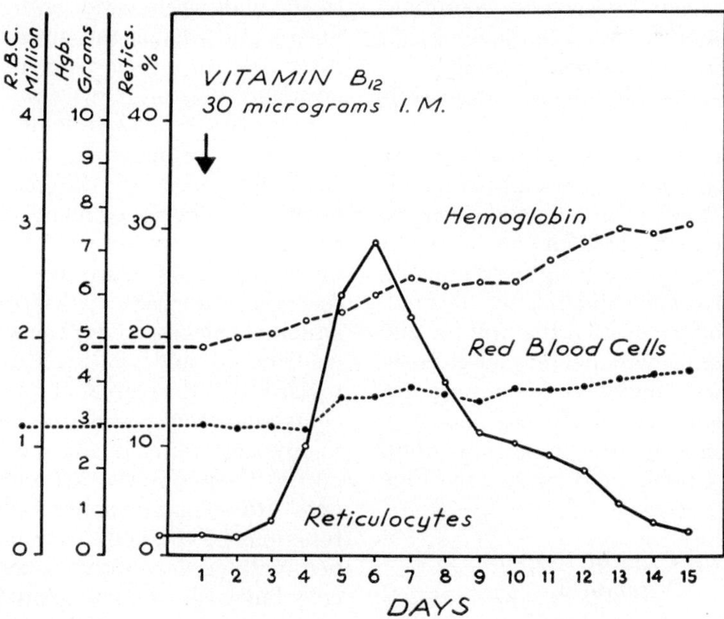

FIG. 70. Hemopoietic response of a patient (J.A.) with nutritional macrocytic anemia to vitamin B_{12}.

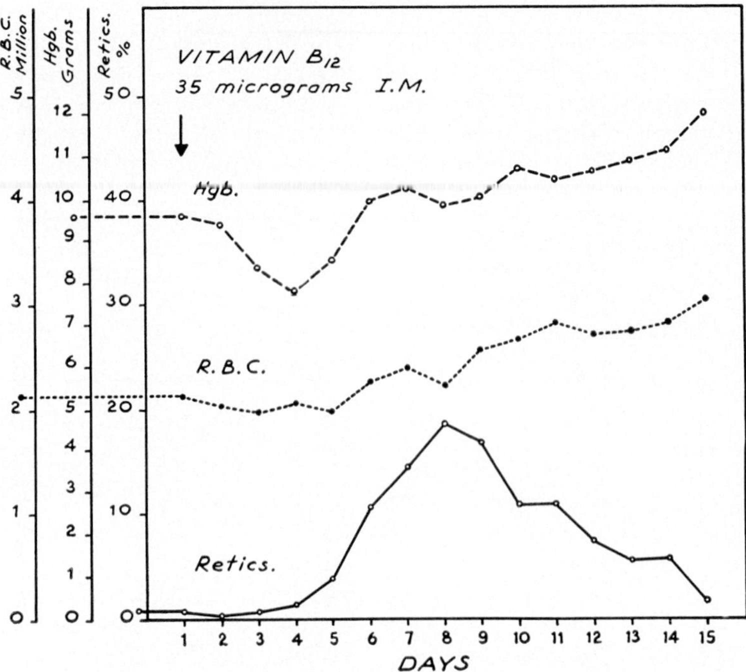

FIG. 71. Hemopoietic response of a patient (A.M.) with tropical sprue to vitamin B_{12}.

depending upon the patient and dosage of vitamin B_{12}. Following the reticulocyte response, there is an increase in the number of circulating red blood cells and in the amount of hemoglobin. The leukopenia and neutropenia so frequently associated with these conditions tend to disappear. Each patient has his own pattern of response, and there tends to be considerable variation from one to the other.

It is arbitrarily accepted that 1 microgram of vitamin B_{12} is approximately equivalent to 1 U.S.P. unit of liver extract, which in itself is an arbitrary standard. Per unit of weight vitamin B_{12} is the most potent antianemic substance known. It offers specific therapy for pernicious anemia whether or not it is associated with nerve degeneration and mucous membrane changes, and it is useful in the treatment of nutritional macrocytic anemia and sprue (see Figs. 69, 70, 71).

General Clinical Response to Vitamin B_{12}

A striking clinical response parallels the hemopoietic response. About the time the reticulocytes begin to increase, the patients volunteer that they feel stronger. Those whose appetites have failed have a sudden desire for food (see Fig. 73). The severe glossitis present in some cases heals spectacularly. In patients with sprue and with nutritional macrocytic anemia the number of stools decreases and they tend to return to normal.

Relatively few crystals of vitamin B_{12} or one of the members of the vitamin B_{12} family mean the difference between health and illness in many of these patients. These vitamins that promote blood regeneration are like yeast cells in that they are basic, versatile nutrients which are necessary for man. They have contributed and will contribute much toward the development of basic concepts concerning enzymes, genetics, cytology and perhaps all scientific disciplines. They may give us impetus in our effort to explain some of the specific functions of the cells. We are not satisfied with a descriptive account of the cells but wish to know about their function in terms of physiology and chemistry.

As an example, for a number of years we have been trying to learn of the functions of the nucleic acids but so far we have not succeeded in answering many questions. We have learned that nucleic acids and these vitamins which produce blood regeneration are intimately concerned with the basic phenomena of life. How can we as investigators determine their full potential on growth, reproduction, and heredity? Following the brilliant researches of Kossel delineating the early chemistry of the nucleic acids, there was rather a long lag period. A few years ago it was shown that thymine (5-methyl uracil) could promote blood regeneration. The substance used was prepared synthetically but is identical with an integral part of nucleic acid. (Other integral parts of nucleic acid do not have this property.) We think it likely that nucleic acids are strongly linked with blood cell synthesis and the formation of hemoglobin and that these vitamins are keys to physiology and reproduction; hence, is it any surprise that when the body for any reason has an inadequate amount of these materials, ill health eventually results?

There have been a number of reports proclaiming the human growth promoting properties of vitamin B_{12}. Spies, Dreizen, Currie and Buehl found that in the absence of definite clinical indications of megaloblastic anemia and in the presence of a limited food intake, vitamin B_{12} does not increase the efficiency of utilization of substandard diets.

Dosage

The authors know of no disease in which dosage varies so much from patient to patient and from time to time. Each patient should be treated in the manner best suited to him and macrocytic anemia should be considered merely as a symptom. Irrespective of what therapeutic agents are administered individually or as mixtures, they must be given in excess of the amount necessary to maintain the blood values of the patient at normal levels. Such patients should have a diet rich in animal protein and should have all coexisting diseases treated. As can be seen from the blood responses shown in Figures 70, 71 and 72, vitamin B_{12} is very effective per unit of weight when it is administered parenterally, and it may be very effective when taken by mouth. We recommend parenteral administration in persons with pernicious anemia.

Toxicity

We have given as much as 1 milligram of vitamin B_{12} intramuscularly daily for ten days and as much as 1 mg. intravenously daily for three days without untoward symptoms developing. At this dosage level 98 per cent or more of the material can be recovered in the urine within from twenty-four to forty-eight hours. We have given daily injections of from 10 to 15 micrograms for months without the development of untoward symptoms. This substance must be considered innocuous at the dosage level effective for human beings.

Because of our interest in the relationship between better food and health, the authors always have sought an explanation of why people did not get enough of the various essential nutrients from their usual diets. Now that we know which foods contain the largest amounts of folic acid it is difficult to understand why people do not eat such foods. As yet some hematologists apparently do not appreciate that folic acid is a vitamin of great importance and that the dramatic relief of megaloblastic arrest of the bone marrow is only one of its many cellular functions. It is difficult to understand why they are not impressed by the fact that vitamin B_{12}, folic acid, thiamine and riboflavin all occur naturally in liver. Blunders concerning the medical use of all the vitamins including folic acid and vitamin B_{12} and other essential nutrients as therapeutic agents are becoming difficult to find. It is with the prevention of disease that the authors are concerned, and it is in the maintenance of good health that these essential factors have the greatest usefulness. Because of the use of

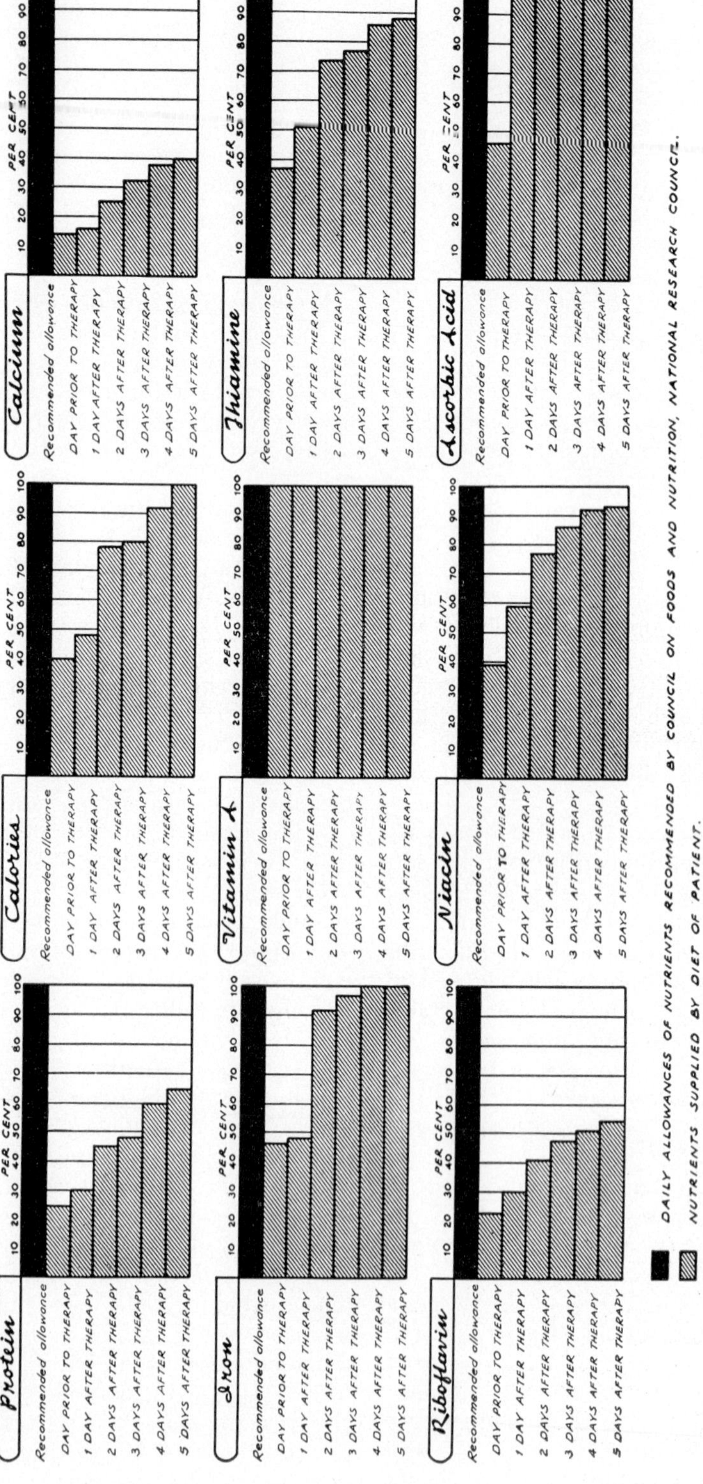

FIG. 72. Case of a tropical sprue. Nutrients ingested by a patient (M.D.) before and after vitamin B_{12} therapy.

synthetic folic acid, folic acid in food and substances that act similarly, severe cases of tropical sprue are virtually nonexistent in Cuba and Puerto Rico, whereas they were at one time rampant. For the same reasons, severe cases of nutritional macrocytic anemia, macrocytic anemia of pregnancy and megaloblastic anemia of infancy have almost disappeared in the severe forms from the southern part of the United States, Puerto Rico and Cuba. Only by continued interest in supplying these necessary materials will the gains we have made be sustained. Some of the less experienced clinical investigators in this field are inclined to think these diseases have "changed their form." Of course, such diseases have not changed their form. It is just that these physicians are looking for classic lesions, and the cases with the atypical lesions are the ones now most prevalent, although they, too, are rare.

References

Angier, R. B., Boothe, J. H., Hutchings, B. L., Mowat, J. H., Semb, J., Stokstad, E. L. R., Subbarrow, Y., Waller, C. W., Cosulich, D. B., Fahrenbach, M. J., Hultquist, M. F., Kuh, E., Northey, E. H., Seeger, D. R., Sickels, J. P. and Smith, J. M., Jr.: Synthesis of a Compound Identical with the L. Casei Factor Isolated from Liver. Science, *102:*227, 1945.

Angulo, J. J. and Spies, T. D.: The Determination of the Folic Acid Content of Foods Usually Consumed by Patients with Tropical Sprue. Am. J. Trop. Med., *27:*317, 1947.

Berk, L., Castle, W. B., Welch, A. D., Heinle, R. W., Anker, R. and Epstein, M.: Observations on the Etiologic Relationship of Achylia Gastrica to Pernicious Anemia: Activity of Vitamin B_{12} as Food (Extrinsic Factor). New England J. Med., *238:*911, 1948.

Berk, L., Denny-Brown, D., Finland, M. and Castle, W. B.: Effectiveness of Vitamin B_{12} in Combined System Disease. New England J. Med., *239:*328, 1948.

Bethell, H., Swendseid, M. E., Bird, O. D., Meyers, M. C., Andrews, G. A. and Brown, A. A.: Observations on the Utilization of Folic Acid (Vitamin B_c) and Vitamin B_c Conjugate by Persons with Pernicious Anemia and Macrocytic Anemia Following Gastrectomy. Univ. Hosp. Bull., Ann Arbor, *12:*42, 1946.

Bethell, F. H., Swendseid, M. E., Meyers, M. C., Neligh, R. B. and Richards, H. G.: Observations on the Hemopoietic Factors in Hog Stomach and Duodenum, and the Treatment of Pernicious Anemia by Orally Administered Vitamin B_{12} in Combination with Extracts of Duodenal Mucosa. Univ. Hosp. Bull., Ann Arbor, *15:*50, 1949.

Boger, W. P., Bayne, G. M., Strickland, S. C. and Wright, L. D.: Studies of Serum B_{12} Concentrations in Man. Norristown State Hospital, Department of Research Therapeutics, Norristown, Pennsylvania, 1957.

Bond, T. J., Bardos, T. J., Sibley, M. and Shive, W.: The Folinic Acid Group, a Series of New Vitamins Related to Folic Acid. J. Am. Chem. Soc., *71:*3852, 1949.

Bonnett, R., Cannon, J. R., Johnson, A. W., Sutherland, I., Todd, A. R. and Smith, E. L.: Nature, *176:*328, 1955.

Brockman, J. A., Jr., Roth, B., Broquist, H. P., Hultquist, M. E., Smith, J. M., Jr., Fahrenbach, M. J., Cosulich, D. B., Parker, R. P., Stokstad, E. L. R. and Jukes, T. H.: Synthesis and Isolation of a Crystalline Substance with the Properties of a New B Vitamin. J. Am. Chem. Soc., *72:*4325, 1950.

Broquist, H. P., Stokstad, E. L. R., and Jukes, T. H.: Some Biological and Chemical Properties of the Citrovorum Factor. J. Biol. Chem., *158:*399, 1950.

Cannon, J. R., Johnson, A. W. and Todd, A. R.: Nature, *174:*1169, 1954.

Castle, W. B., Minot, G. R. and Christian, H. A.: Pathological Physiology and Clinical Description of the Anemias. Oxford University Press, 1936.

Castle, W. B. and Townsend, W. C.: Observations on the Etiologic Relationship of Achylia Gastrica to Pernicious Anemia; the Effect of the Administration to Patients with Pernicious Anemia of Beef Muscle after the Incubation with Normal Human Gastric Juice. Am. J. M. Sc., *178:*764, 1929.

Darby, W. J. and Jones, E.: Treatment of Sprue with Synthetic L. Casei Factor (Folic Acid, Vitamin M). Proc. Soc. Exper. Biol. & Med., *60:*259, 1945.

Doan, C. A., Wilson, H. E., Jr., and Wright, C. S.: Folic Acid (L. Casei Factor), an Essential Pan-Hematopoietic Factor; Experimental and Clinical Studies. Ohio State M. J., *42:*139, 1946.

Hall, B. E. and Campbell, D. C.: Vitamin B_{12} Therapy in Pernicious Anemia; Effect on the General Clinical and Neurologic Manifestations: Preliminary Report. Proc. Staff Meet., Mayo Clin., *23:*591, 1948.

Hodgkin, D. C., Pickworth, J., Robertson, J. H., Trueblood, K. N., Prosen, R. J. and White, J. G.: Nature, *176:*325, 1955.

Kaczka, E., Wolf, D. E. and Folkers, K.: Vitamin B_{12}. V. Identification of Crystalline Vitamin B_{12a}. J. Am. Chem. Soc., *17:*1514, 1949.

Kossel, A.: Ueber das Nuclein der Hefe. Ztschr. f. physiol. Chemie., *3:*284, 1879.

Minot, G. R. and Murphy, W. P.: Treatment of Pernicious Anemia by a Special Diet. J.A.M.A., *87:*470, 1926.

Moore, C. V., Bierbaum, O. S., Welch, A. D. and Wright, L. D.: The Activity of Synthetic Lactobacillus Casei Factor ("Folic Acid") as an Antipernicious Anemia Substance. J. Lab. & Clin. Med., *30:*1056, 1945.

Moore, C. V., Doan, C. A. and Arrowsmith, W. R.: Studies in Iron Transportation and Metabolism; Mechanism of Iron Transportation: Its Significance in Iron Utilization in Anemic States of Varied Etiology. J. Clin. Investigation, *16:*627, 1937.

Moore, C. V., Vilter, R. W., Minnich, V. and Spies, T. D.: Nutritional Macrocytic Anemia in Patients with Pellagra or Deficiency of the Vitamin B Complex. J. Lab. & Clin. Med., *29:*1226, 1944.

Nichol, C. A. and Welch, A. D.: Synthesis of Citrovorum Factor from Folic Acid by Liver Slices; Augmentation by Ascorbic Acid. Proc. Soc. Exper. Biol. & Med., *74:*52, 1950.

Olson, O. E., Burris, R. H. and Elvehjem, C. A.: A Preliminary Report of the "Folic Acid" Content of Certain Foods. J. Am. Dietet. A., *23:*200, 1947.

Pierce, J. V., Page, A. C., Jr., Stokstad, E. L. R. and Jukes, T. H.: Crystallization of Vitamin B_{12b}. J. Am. Chem. Soc., *71:*2952, 1949.

Rickes, E. L., Brink, N. G., Koniuszy, F. R., Wood, T. R. and Folkers, K.: Crystalline Vitamin B_{12}. Science, *107:*496, 1948.

Sauberlich, H. E. and Baumann, C. A.: A Factor Required for the Growth of Leuconostoc citrovorum. J. Biol. Chem., *176:*165, 1948.

Schilling, R. F.: J. Lab. & Clin. Med., *42:* 860, 1953.

Shive, W., Bardos, T. J., Bond, T. J. and Rogers, L. L.: Synthetic Members of the Folinic Acid Group. J. Am. Chem. Soc., *72:*2817, 1950.

Smith, E. L.: Purification of Anti-Pernicious Anaemia Factors from Liver. Nature, *161:* 638, 1948.

Spies, T. D.: Experiences with Folic Acid. Year Book Publishers, Inc., Chicago, 1947.

Spies, T. D.: Nutrition and Disease. Postgraduate Medicine, *17:*1–96, 1957.

Spies, T. D. and Butt, H. R.: Vitamins and Vitamin Deficiencies. Oxford Medicine, Oxford University Press, 1948.

Spies, T. D. and Chinn, A. B.: Studies on the Anemia of Pellagra. J. Clin. Investigation, *14:*941, 1935.

Spies, T. D., Dreizen, S., Currie, C. and Buehl, C. C.: Ztschr. f. Vitaminforsch., *23:*414, 1952.

Spies, T. D., Garcia Lopez, G., Milanes, F., Lopez Toca, R. and Culver, B.: Observations on the Hemopoietic Response of Persons with Tropical Sprue to Vitamin B_{12}. South. M. J., *41:*523, 1948.

Spies, T. D., Garcia Lopez, G., Milanes, F., Lopez Toca, R. and Reboredo, A.: Antianemic Properties of a Reaction Product of Vitamin B_{12} and the Intrinsic Factor. South. M. J., *43:*206, 1950.

Spies, T. D., Garcia Lopez, G., Milanes, F., Lopez Toca, R., Reboredo, A. and Stone, R. E.: The Response of Patients with Pernicious Anemia, with Nutritional Macrocytic Anemia and with Tropical Sprue to Folinic Acid or Citrovorum Factor. South. M. J., *43:*1076, 1950.

Spies, T. D. and Stone, R. E.: Liver Extract, Folic Acid and Thymine in Pernicious Anemia and Acute Combined Degeneration. The Lancet (Feb. 1), p. 174, 1947.

Spies, T. D. and Stone, R. E.: Some Recent Experiences with Vitamins and Vitamin Deficiencies. South. M. J., *40:*46, 1947.

Spies, T. D., Stone, R. E. and Aramburu, T.: Observations on the Antianemia Properties of Vitamin B_{12}. South. M. J., *41:*522, 1948.

Spies, T. D., Stone, R. E., Garcia Lopez, G., Lopez Toca, R. and Reboredo, A.: Therapeutic Indications for Vitamins in Mixtures, Postgraduate Medicine, *10:*269, 1951.

Spies, T. D., Stone, R. E., Koch, M. B., Grant, H. M. and Moore, M. M.: The Hemopoietic Response of Patients with Pernicious Anemia to Crystalline Vitamin B_{12b}. South. M. J., *43:* 50, 1950.

Spies, T. D., Suarez, R. M., Garcia Lopez, G., Milanes, F., Stone, R. E., Lopez Toca, R., Aramburu, T. and Kartus, S.: Tentative Appraisal of Vitamin B_{12} as a Therapeutic Agent. J.A.M.A., *139:*521, 1949.

Spies, T. D., Vilter, C. F., Cline, J. K. and Frommeyer, W. B., Jr.: The Substitution of Thymine for Folic Acid in the Treatment of Macrocytic Anemias in Relapse. South. M. J., *39:*269, 1946.

Spies, T. D., Vilter, C. F., Koch, M. B. and Caldwell, M. H.: Observations on the Antianemic Properties of Synthetic Folic Acid. South. M. J., *38:*707, 1945.

Stone, R. E. and Spies, T. D.: Vitamin B_{12} and Subacute Combined Degeneration of the Spinal Cord. Tirage a part de la Revue Internationale de Vitaminologie, Tome XX Cahier 1/3, 1948.

Suarez, R. M., Spies, T. D., Hernandez-Morales, F. and Perez, E.: A Note on the Effectiveness of Vitamin B_{12} in the Treatment of Tropical Sprue in Relapse. Blood, *4:*1124, 1949.

Ungley, C. C.: Vitamin B_{12} in Pernicious Anemia; Parenteral Administration. Brit. Med. J., *2:*1370, 1949.

Vilter, C. F., Vilter, R. W. and Spies, T. D.: The Treatment of Pernicious and Related Anemias with Synthetic Folic Acid. I. Observations on the Maintenance of a Normal Hematologic Status and on the Occurrence of Combined System Disease at the End of One Year. J. Lab. & Clin. Med., *32:*262, 1947.

West, R.: Activity of Vitamin B_{12} in Addisonian Pernicious Anemia. Science, *107:*398, 1948.

Wills, L. and Mehta, M. M.: Studies in "Pernicious Anemia" of Pregnancy; Preliminary Report. Indian J. M. Research, *17:*777, 1930.

Wills, L. and Bilimoria, H. S.: Studies in Pernicious Anemia of Pregnancy; Production of Macrocytic Anemia in Monkeys by Deficient Feeding. Indian J. M. Research, *20:* 391, 1932.

Zuelzer, W. W. and Ogden, F. N.: Folic Acid Therapy in Macrocytic Anemias of Infancy. Proc. Soc. Exper. Biol. & Med., *61:*176, 1946.

ASCORBIC ACID DEFICIENCY (SCURVY)

In the eighteenth century James Lind, a famous surgeon in the British Navy, demonstrated that citrus fruit juices will prevent and cure scurvy. Unfortunately, Lind did not live to see scurvy disappear from the British Navy, as the Admiralty waited until the year after his death to apply his findings rigidly and stamp out the disease. Sailors in other countries taunted the British tar by calling him "limey," an epithet which is inaccurate because the citrus fruit which was used to prevent scurvy was not the lime, which actually contains little ascorbic acid, but the lemon.

The authors are unable to explain the great interest of western scientists of that period in the beriberi of the far-off Orient, in contrast with their meager attention to scurvy, which they recognized in their midst. Perhaps they were troubled by the apparent incongruity of deficiency diseases existing in a land of plenty and chose to think of them as affecting people in distant places. No country is free of scurvy, although it is usually most prevalent where vegetation is scarce. For hundreds of years there were epidemics in Europe among soldiers, sailors, and inmates of prisons, insane asylums and poorhouses. Infantile scurvy was described in England in 1668, but it was almost entirely overlooked for two hundred years. Eventually, however, it was recognized that the disease affects many children in England and in America, where there is extensive use of artificial and processed foods.

It is one thing to know that citrus fruit juice will prevent or cure scurvy and another to identify the constituent responsible for this remarkable property. To Theobald Smith we owe the first description of experimentally induced scurvy. Some fifty years ago, according to Sibyl L. Smith, Theobald Smith wrote as follows: "The death of No. 254 was undoubtedly due to the absence of such (green) food as the attendant had neglected to provide it after the disappearance of grass in the fall of the year. . . . When guinea pigs are fed with cereals (bran and oats mixed) without any grass, clover or succulent vegetables such as cabbage a peculiar disease, chiefly recognizable by subcutaneous extravasation of blood (that is, hemorrhages under the skin), carries them off in four to eight weeks." Smith did not associate this disease of improperly fed guinea pigs with human scurvy as his work was concerned primarily with the study of poultry, swine and cattle. More than a decade later, Holst and Frölich demonstrated that the symptoms of scurvy induced in guinea pigs are identical with those of scurvy in man. Twenty-five years were to pass before the substance responsible for its prevention and cure was identified and synthesized, and even now twenty-six years after this discovery there is much uncertainty as to human requirements for ascorbic acid and its mode of action in the body.

Biochemistry and Physiology

The isolation and identification of vitamin C by King and others in 1932 was followed by its synthesis in 1933 by Reichstein, Grussner and Oppenauer. Ascorbic acid is related to the sugars, being an enediol-lactone of an acid similar in configuration to L-gulose. The formula for it appears below with that of the vitamin.

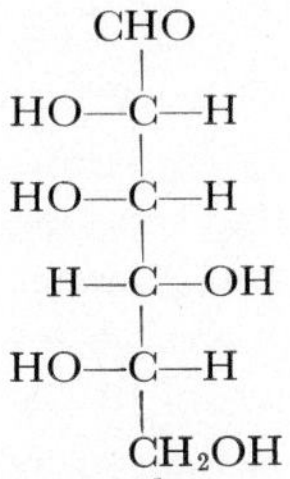

```
     CHO                     O=C———┐
      |                        |    |
 HO—C—H                    HO—C    |
      |                        ||   O
 HO—C—H                    HO—C    |
      |                        |    |
  H—C—OH                    H—C———┘
      |                        |
 HO—C—H                    HO—C—H
      |                        |
    CH2OH                    CH2OH
  L-gulose          Vitamin C (L-ascorbic acid)
```

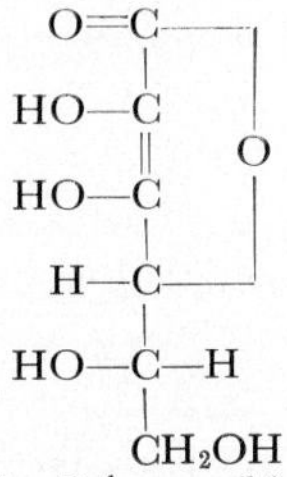

Several other synthetic substances have antiscorbutic activity, but to a lesser degree. D-Ascorbic acid will not protect against scurvy. Below a *p*H of 7.6 the vitamin in solution is not oxidized by exposure to air unless traces of copper or other catalysts are present. Methylene blue, quinones and certain other organic compounds have the ability to bring about the oxidation, which is reversible below *p*H 4. At more alkaline reactions the process becomes irreversible, the first product, dehydroascorbic acid, giving rise to another strongly reducing substance of unknown structure which is in turn oxidized to oxalic and l-threonic acids.

Dry crystals of the vitamin do not decompose even when exposed to air and sunlight at room temperature for several years. The rate of aerobic oxidation in aqueous solution is greatly increased by exposure to light, especially in the presence of flavin.

Of the large number of species which have been examined, only man, the other primates and guinea pigs lack the ability to synthesize ascorbic acid. The evidence which is frequently cited to prove its synthesis in infants, placental tissues or any of the tissues of the animals named can better be interpreted as a selective conservation of vitamin in vital organs. The concentration of vitamin C in the tissues parallels roughly their metabolic activity. The following list approximates the concentration of ascorbic acid in descending order: the pituitary body, corpus luteum, adrenal cortex, young thymus, liver, brain, testes, ovaries, spleen, thyroid, pancreas, salivary glands, lung, kidney, intestinal wall, heart, muscle, spinal fluid and blood.

Normal human *blood plasma* contains about 1.2 mg. ascorbic acid per 100 cc. When there is no dietary intake this value rapidly falls to zero, but apparently there is no direct correlation between plasma levels and the state of nutrition. While a plasma concentration below 0.5 mg. per 100 cc. may not be dangerously low, such a finding indicates a dietary paucity of vitamin C. Crandon and Lund showed that the vitamin C content of the plasma may remain at zero for as long as three months before the appearance of clinical scurvy. They suggest that the concentration in the white cell-platelet layer of centrifuged blood is a much better index of a vitamin C deficiency since this value fell to zero shortly before the subject developed typical scorbutic lesions.

Normal *human milk* contains four to five times as much vitamin C as cow's milk. If the mother's diet is deficient in antiscorbutic foods, the vitamin C concentration in the milk may fall below that of cow's milk; when the dietary deficiency is corrected the amount rises to normal levels. The pasteurization of milk destroys much, if not all, of the ascorbic acid.

Vitamin C is normally found in the urine, but when there is no dietary intake the excretion gradually diminishes as the tissues become depleted. Restoration of a normal ascorbic acid intake replenishes the tissues and is followed by a resumption of excretion. In the normal state of saturation, the amount taken in exceeds that excreted by 50 mg. or more daily. The amount of the vitamin required to induce saturation appears to be a very rough measure of the state of vitamin C nutrition. In man, guinea pigs and rats part of labeled ascorbic-1-C^{14} acid appears in respired CO_2 and part in the urine as free ascorbic acid, 2,3-diketogulonic acid and as an oxalate.

Ascorbic acid is essential for the maintenance of normal intercellular material of connective tissue, bones, teeth and perhaps blood vessels. The fibrils in loose connective tissue normally are cemented together by a translucent matrix of collagen, but in vitamin C deficient animals fibrils and collagen are absent. The formation of osteoid tissue and dentin is similarly dependent upon a supply of vitamin C. It is not known whether lack of vitamin C directly affects the intercellular colloids or the fibroblasts.

Sensitivity to injections of bacterial toxins, lowered metabolic activity, and lowered resistance to infection are some of the early changes in vitamin C deficient animals. A close relationship exists between vitamin C and guinea-pig blood complement. Normal activity of complement is dependent upon its being in the reduced state, and ascorbic acid was found to be the most important reducing agent in blood plasma in this connection. No positive identification of vitamin C with enzymatic processes in normal animal tissues has been made, but many in vitro experiments suggest such a relation. The catalyst often called "ascorbic acid oxidase" is a protein combined with copper but is probably not specific for vitamin C as a substrate. The cytochrome-indophenol oxidase system has been shown to act as a catalyst for the aerobic oxidation of ascorbic acid, and the reducing power of plasma on dichlorophenolindophenol has been used in the clinical laboratory as a test for vitamin C.

Apparently ascorbic acid works specifically in the hydroxylation of p-hydroxyphenylpyruvic acid to homogentistic acid. The renal enzyme catalyzing this reaction requires small amounts of ascorbate. Although it may be premature to call ascorbic acid a coenzyme for this reaction, it probably represents one specific site of ascorbate function.

Pathologic Physiology

The primary effect of vitamin C deficiency is reflected in the intercellular substance of the connective tissue. Eventually this results in weakening of the periosteum, diminished muscular power, defective osteoid and dentin formation, and hemorrhage.

The changes in the *long bones* constitute one of the most uniform findings in vitamin C deficiency. Lesions are widely distributed throughout the skeleton but are most pronounced where growth is normally most rapid. The costochondral junction, the distal end of the femur, the proximal end of the humerus, both ends of the tibia and fibula, and the distal end of the radius and ulna are involved in approximately the order given.

In the affected regions enchondral bone growth ceases and the existing osseous bone becomes rarefied, widened and conical. Microscopic sections of the cartilage-shaft junction show a collection of columns, larger and less numerous than in normal bone, separated by an irregular mass of matrix. The calcified matrix contains numerous fractures. In severe scurvy, no conversion of matrix into bone occurs. Trabeculae previously formed are separated from the calcified matrix by a zone devoid of newly formed trabeculae—the "zone of destruction" or "zone of rarefaction" visible in the roentgenogram. Throughout the entire bone the osseous framework becomes attenuated. The carpal and tarsal bones and the centers of the ossification of the long bones show changes of a similar nature but less pronounced degree.

Normal marrow at the epiphyseal ends of the bone is replaced by loose fibrous tissue, the so-called framework marrow or "*Gerüstmark*" which occupies the width of the shaft, forming a band which includes the zone of destruction. This abnormal marrow extends into the shaft for a variable distance, depending upon the duration and severity of the deficiency. The periosteum strips readily from the underlying bone, but invariably remains adherent at its junction with the perichondrium. Subperiosteal hemorrhages are common, and may be confined to the ends of the shaft, or may elevate the entire length of the periosteum.

In the *teeth* of adults with scurvy the dentin is resorbed and porotic, and the little replacement dentin that is formed is of inferior quality. In the pulp, chiefly around the vessels, atrophy, hyperemia, degeneration of odontoblasts and the formation of small cysts and foci of calcification occur. Boyle was unable to find any specific changes in the teeth of children with infantile scurvy on microscopic examination of ground sections, but in the rapidly growing teeth of the guinea pig early and extensive changes occur in the dentin, enamel and cementum. Involvement of the gingiva is most frequent and severe when the teeth are erupted, particularly if they are deformed and broken. The lesions begin on the papillae as a hyperemia; destruction of epithelium follows. Infection, with ulceration, granulation and even gangrene may occur. Rarefaction of the alveolar bone results in loosening of the teeth.

The *skin* commonly shows petechiae of various sizes, particularly on the trunk and lower extremities. In adults they are often perifollicular. Ecchymoses are common and are most frequent about the knees and ankles but may appear anywhere. In severe scurvy, particularly in adults, changes occur in the muscles; fragmentation of the striated fibers, multiplication of the sarcolemma, and, in prolonged cases, replacement by connective tissue poor in collagen. Moderate effusions, often blood-tinged, may occur in the pericardial, pleural and peritoneal cavities. Hemorrhage may be found anywhere in the body.

Symptomatology

Because the tissues of the infant are in the process of rapid growth and development, there are certain differences in the symptomatology of scurvy in the adult and in the infant. For the purpose of clarity, the two conditions will be discussed separately, although from the viewpoint of etiology and general pathology this distinction is arbitrary.

Infantile Scurvy. This disease occurs most commonly in artificially-fed infants; it develops in breast-fed infants only when the mother's diet is unusually limited in vitamin C. Restriction of the mother's diet during pregnancy seems to lead more often to deficiency in the mother than to deprivation of the fetus. The ability of the human breast to excrete milk with a higher concentration of ascorbic acid than is found in the maternal blood is a protection for the breast-fed infant.

In the majority of cases, symptoms of manifest scurvy appear between the ages of eight and thirteen months. Symptoms of mild vitamin C deficiency begin insidiously. The patient may show vague digestive disturbances—loss of appetite, irregular diarrhea and failure to gain weight—associated with pallor, apathy, irritability and possibly an increased susceptibility to infection. These symptoms disappear following adequate treatment with vitamin C, but if no therapy is given the full syndrome of manifest scurvy (severe vitamin C deficiency) develops, often with alarming abruptness.

Manifest scurvy is not rare among infants and, like the subclinical form of the disease, occurs more frequently than is recognized. The infant appears pale, listless and unhappy. He may have a peculiarly alert and worried expression, and cries when approached. He makes no effort to kick or play. Growth may be mildly retarded; weight is usually even more abnormal, often 10 to 20 per cent below average, but it may be spuriously high due to the presence of edema. The soft tissues are flabby and muscle tone is decreased.

Swelling of the extremities, due to subperiosteal hemorrhage, is a common finding. It appears suddenly, frequently at the lower end of the femur, and is produced by trauma which is often so mild as to be unrecognized. Pain and tenderness may be localized at the swelling or may extend over the entire extremity. The position assumed by the infant often bears a close relationship to the site involved: infants with subperiosteal hemorrhages in both thighs and legs generally assume the "pithed frog" position, with thighs semiflexed and externally rotated, and the legs semiflexed at the knee joints. The fingers, wrists, toes and, less often, the ankles may be moved spontaneously even when the rest of the extremity exhibits a pseudo-paralysis. At the costochondral junctions scurvy produces a chain of tender enlargements. These swellings may be rounded, or they may exhibit a sharp ridge where the cartilage and bone meet. In extreme cases, the entire sternochondral plate is often displaced posteriorly. Submetaphyseal infractions, the so-called "epiphyseal separations," are common in severe cases. They may be shown by crepitus or by roentgen examination, but should be suspected clinically by the persistence of localized tenderness after treatment has relieved the generalized tenderness.

Lesions of the gums are characteristic of scurvy. The gums appear swollen, congested and dark red or purple. With moderate swelling the surface is smooth and glistening, but later it becomes irregular and friable and hemorrhage occurs readily. In some cases, the swelling is so extensive as to bury the teeth. The breath is fetid and Vincent's infection is common. Frequently there is no clinical evidence of lesions in edentulous people.

Hemorrhage may occur anywhere in the body, giving rise to epistaxis, vomiting of blood, bloody stools, or when it occurs in the brain or abdominal organs, very alarming and confusing symptoms. Orbital hemorrhage, usually unilateral but occasionally bilateral, may cause proptosis. Ecchymoses of the eyelids are common and may be associated with edema. Subconjunctival hemorrhage is rare; the eyeball is usually not affected.

Petechiae and *ecchymoses* of varying size may appear anywhere in the skin, but they are most common where the hydrostatic pressure of the capillaries is elevated or where trauma has been inflicted: the lower extremities, the lower half of the trunk, forearms, face and neck. The miliaria seen in vitamin C deficiency is not specific and its pathogenesis is not known. Although some of the macules are hemorrhagic, the majority are not.

Fever and *increased pulse and respiratory rates* are common in infants with manifest scurvy. Rapid, shallow breathing, out of proportion to the fever and pulse rate, may be due to painfulness of the ribs and costochondral junctions. Hypochromic anemia, unassociated with blood loss, is a common finding. In uncomplicated scurvy the leukocyte and differential counts are normal. The number of platelets is not decreased; bleeding and coagulation times are usually normal, but in severe cases prolongation of either or both may occur. There may be changes in the serum calcium and inorganic phosphorus, but these changes are not constant. Hematuria occurs with great frequency; oliguria is common. Hyalin or granular casts, sometimes blood casts, and pyuria may be found.

Adult Scurvy. The scurvy of the clipper ship era so vividly described by Hakluyt and Lind is now an infrequent disease. Even now, however, a large general hospital will admit some cases each year and the disease may be endemic in prison camps and homes for the indigent.

Characteristic is the long period (perhaps three months) during which total lack of vitamin C may produce no symptoms other than lassitude, weakness, irritability and an insidious loss of weight. During this time, intercurrent infections or metabolic disorders may precipitate the classic picture, the largest part of which is the result of capillary hemorrhage and anemia. Signs first seen are a sallow complexion and bloating of the face, especially a swelling of the pinnae which may extend into the scalp. Aching pains appear in the muscles at points of stress (usually the calves) and may be followed by painful swelling of the knees and edema of the ankles. Changes in the gums, similar to those seen in severe infantile scurvy, take place, particularly around broken and carious teeth.

Hemorrhages predominate in the general picture, appearing at points of mild trauma and sites of stress. Those in the muscles cause brawny induration and tenderness. Hemorrhages into the muscles are more common in adults than in infants and may extend into the skin causing wide areas of lividity. Petechiae and ecchymoses occur as in infantile scurvy (see Figs. 73 and 74). Less frequently there are epistaxis, conjunctival, retinal and cerebral hemorrhages. Convulsions and paralyses may result from intracranial extravasation of blood. Bleeding from the gastrointestinal and genitourinary tracts is rare except in severe cases. Palpitation, dyspnea and cardiac dilatation may be noted. Vasomotor collapse has been described. Changes in the blood and urine do not differ significantly from those seen in infantile scurvy.

It should be emphasized that scurvy in the infant and in the adult is not a self-limiting disease. If untreated, it will progress to a fatal outcome.

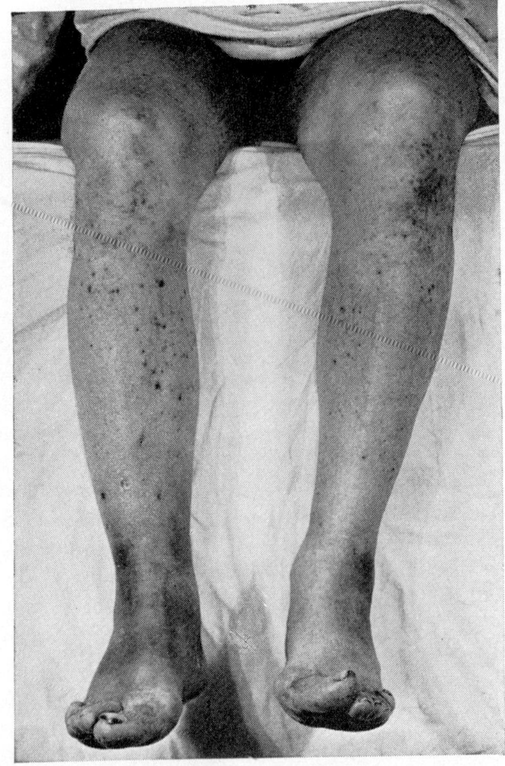

FIG. 73. Adult scurvy, showing typical distribution of hemorrhagic skin lesions. The purpuric areas vary greatly in size and large ecchymoses are present over sites particularly subject to trauma.

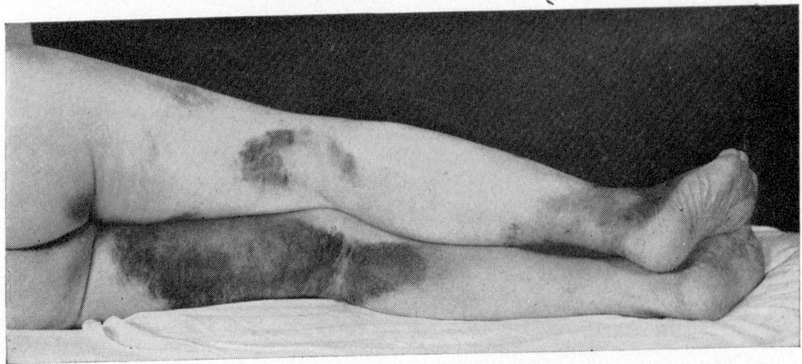

FIG. 74. Same patient as shown in Figure 73. Note extensive ecchymoses over the lower extremities and buttocks.

Diagnosis

The diagnosis of manifest scurvy is not difficult. A careful physical examination and a history of inadequate intake of vitamin C may be helpful in making the diagnosis of mild deficiency. Characteristic roentgenologic changes add confirmatory evidence. A positive capillary resistance test suggests depletion of vitamin C, but false positives frequently occur in the presence of severe anemia or blood dyscrasia. Even in severe scurvy, a negative capillary test often occurs. It was thought that plasma levels of ascorbic acid below 0.3 mg. per cent gives presumptive evidence of scurvy. Recently, however, it has been indicated that the ascorbic acid content of the white cell-platelet layer of centrifuged blood is much more accurate. When depletion has been severe or long-continued, very little vitamin C is eliminated in the urine and most of a test dose is retained. If the diagnosis is in doubt a therapeutic test is recommended: 250 mg. of ascorbic acid should be given parenterally; the patient should be kept on his usual routine, and should be watched carefully for alteration of symptoms.

Treatment with Ascorbic Acid

Chemistry. Ascorbic acid is a crystalline, colorless, water-soluble compound which melts at 192° C. Its structural formula is shown in Figure 75. The substance is fairly stable in acidic water solutions which are not exposed to air or contaminating metallic radicals.

```
 O
  \\
    C──────┐
    |      |
 HO-C      O
    ||     |
 HO-C      |
    |      |
  H-C──────┘
    |
 HO-C-H
    |
  H-C-OH
    |
    H
```

FIG. 75. Ascorbic acid (1-2,3-enediol-gluconic acid lactone).

Methods of Administration. Ascorbic acid may be administered orally, intravenously or intramuscularly. Parenteral injection is about twice as effective as oral administration. No difficulty is experienced in bringing ascorbic acid into solution in physiologic saline or 5 per cent glucose. Since the solution is strongly acid, the suggestion has been made that it be partially neutralized with sterile sodium bicarbonate for parenteral injection.

IN PREVENTION. Beginning in the second or third week of life, the infant should be given 1 to 2 teaspoonfuls of fresh orange juice daily. The amount should be increased to 2 ounces by three months of age and to 3 ounces by five months. Other citrus fruit juices may be substituted, but when tomato juice is used, larger amounts must be given. If fruit juices are not tolerated, 25 to 50 mg. of ascorbic acid should be given daily. At least 3 ounces of orange juice, or comparable amounts of citrus fruits or tomato juice, should be taken daily by the average adult (or 50 to 100 mg. of ascorbic acid). Larger amounts are indicated during pregnancy and lactation.

IN TREATMENT. For infants, 50 mg. of ascorbic acid four times a day orally or 25 mg. twice daily intravenously or intramuscularly should be given. For older children or adults, the recommended amount is 100 mg. three to five times a day orally, or 100 mg. twice a day parenterally. In all cases ascorbic acid therapy should be supplemented by the addition of orange juice, other citrus fruits or tomato juice.

Ascorbic acid has a very low toxicity. Six grams have been given orally, and massive doses of 500 to 1000 mg. have been given intravenously without ill effects. (Vagotonic effects, such as bradycardia, increased peristalsis and erythema, have been described in children but are attributed to idiosyncrasy to ascorbic acid and not to hypervitaminosis.)

The present knowledge is so meager that a precise statement of what constitutes proper dosage is not practicable. To commemorate the two hundredth anniversary of the publication of Lind's "Treatise of the Scurvy," a symposium was held at the University of Edinburgh at which a careful investigation of the vitamin C requirements of man was summarized by Krebs. Less than 10 mg. of ascorbic acid per day was found sufficient to prevent or cure scurvy in young adult volunteers on an otherwise complete diet. This figure is of little practical aid. The problem of scurvy is in the young and the old. It is difficult, indeed, to find any critical evidence in a young adult even though he is ill, whereas notoriously the infant and the elderly are afflicted. Since vitamin C deficiency is frequently a part of mixed

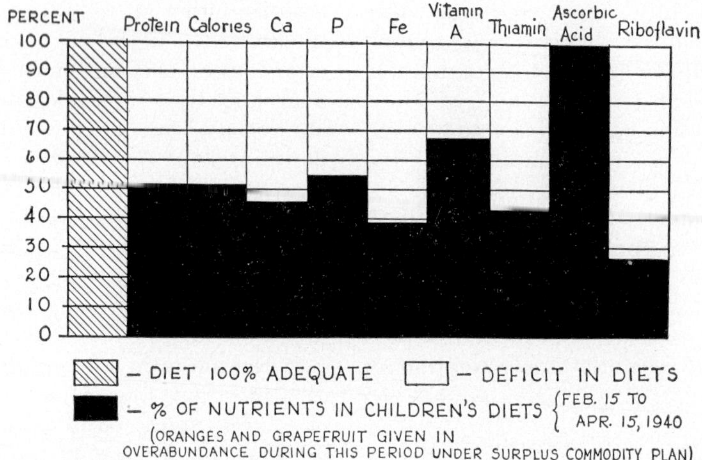

FIG. 76. The dietaries of fifty children with deficiency diseases compared with an adequate diet.

deficiency diseases, it is not enough to insure an adequate intake of vitamin C alone. Figure 76 illustrates the degree of deficiency of other essential nutrients which may remain after vitamin C deficiency is corrected.

Response to Adequate Therapy with Ascorbic Acid. Bone tenderness decreases, purpura begins to fade, gums improve, appetite increases, and loss of apprehension occurs within twenty-four hours after adequate parenteral injection of ascorbic acid is given. The general treatment should aim at restoring the patient to a state of perfect nutrition.

References

Hellman, L. and Burns, J. J.: Fed. Proc., *14:*225, 1955.

Krebs, H. A.: Roy. Nutrition Soc. (Engl. and Scot.), *12:*237, 1953.

CLINICALLY LESS WELL KNOWN VITAMINS

Throughout the vast literature on biology, organic substances are described as being essential to certain species. We know that vitamins are concerned not only with the nutrition of human beings but also with that of lower animals, birds and many other species. One can not argue a priori that a deficiency of vitamins will produce certain effects in human beings merely because such a deficiency has produced an effect in animals, nor can one say that organic compounds which are necessary for some lower animal will not prove to be of great importance in understanding the physiology of the higher species. Nevertheless, studies of animals, plants, insects and bacteria are adding to our understanding of the various factors concerned with human nutrition.

The literature is so filled with ill-defined, often still unnamed vitamins that we cannot list them. Considering the difficult technique used in the isolation of new factors, the progress is rapid indeed. Conservative investigators are of the opinion that the chemical structure of most, if not all, vitamins soon will be known and that many, if not all, will be synthesized. Many investigators are concentrating their efforts on the isolation, identification, and synthesis of the various members of the vitamin B complex, and it is in this field that we may expect the most rapid strides. Perhaps the simplest definition of the vitamin B complex is a composite of all the water-soluble vitamins found in yeast and liver, exclusive of ascorbic acid. They are concerned with oxidation and reduction in the cells and with many other biochemical processes. Vitamin B_1 (thiamine), vitamin B_2 (riboflavin), nicotinic acid, folic acid, the vitamin B_{12} family and citrovorum factor have been discussed in preceding sections. Indications of the existence of many other members of the vitamin B complex are too numerous to list but we will discuss those which are more definitely established.

Vitamin B_6 Family (Pyridoxine, Pyridoxal, Pyridoxamine)

Vitamin B_6 occurs in nature in three forms: pyridoxine, which is most plentiful in plants, and pyridoxal and pyridoxamine, which predominate in animal tissues. Pyridoxine, pyridoxal and pyridoxamine (Fig. 77) and their respective phosphates owe their vitamin activity to the ability of the organism to convert them into the enzymatically active form, pyridoxal-5-phosphate.

The average human adult intake of pyridoxine has been estimated to be 2 to 3 mg. daily; 0.8 mg. is excreted in the feces, 3 to 5 mg. in the urine mainly as 4-pyridoxic acid, and 0.2 mg. in the circulating blood. Excretion exceeds dietary intake, at least at low levels of intake, an observation noted by many investigators. The vitamin has widespread metabolic activity, being concerned in decarboxylation, transamination, desulfuration, racemization of amino acids and facilitation of the conversion of tryptophan to N_1-methylnicotinamide.

Pyridoxine was synthesized by Harris and Folkers in 1939. It is crystallized usually as the hydrochloride, melts at 204 to 206° C., is extremely soluble in water and when dissolved has a *p*H of 2.3.

The signs of dietary deficiency of vitamin B_6 vary in different species. Acrodynia, which develops regularly in the rat, is not encountered in monkeys or dogs maintained on a vitamin B_6 deficient diet. The microcytic anemia seen in vitamin B_6 deficient dogs is not found uniformly in the monkey and not at all in the rat. It is interesting that an alteration of the tryptophan load test occurs in practically all species. In rats and monkeys there is a prompt and sudden loss of appetite, followed by a tremendous loss of body weight. In vitamin B_6 deficient monkeys, degenerative vascular lesions have been described by Rinehart and Greenberg. The findings have been amply confirmed in this species and similar lesions have been induced in dogs. The lesions bear a very close similarity to spontaneously occurring arteriosclerosis in man.

Clinically, vitamin B_6 has come of age. Synthetic pyridoxine was first administered to human beings by Spies, Bean and Ashe, who showed that patients on inadequate diets who develop deficiencies of niacin, riboflavin and thiamine were also somewhat deficient in pyridoxine. They stressed that after the deficiencies of niacin, riboflavin and thiamine were corrected and the patients were still restricted to their former deficient diets, pyridoxine produced additional improvement. In following this work and in discussing it, Elvehjem stated in 1952 that dogs on a diet which induced a niacin deficiency responded well to niacin therapy unless the treat-

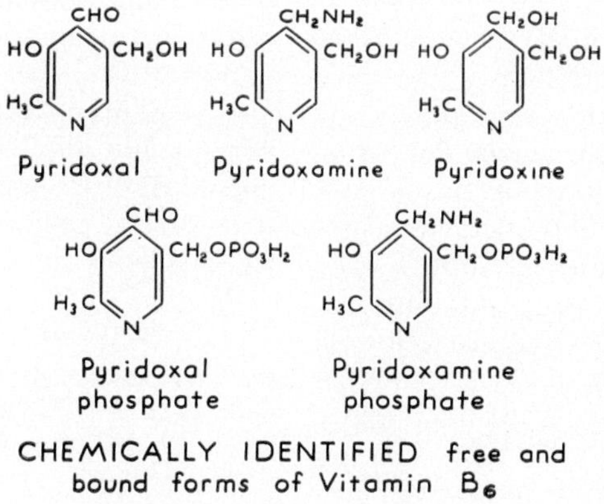

CHEMICALLY IDENTIFIED free and bound forms of Vitamin B_6

FIG. 77.

ment was repeated too many times. He then found that tryptophan could replace niacin in alleviating these deficiencies. Elvehjem and associates showed that there was an interrelationship between tryptophan metabolism and pyridoxine in animals. A straightforward, uncomplicated vitamin B_6 deficiency had not been induced in adult human beings, although it was attempted by several workers. Spies and associates and others recommended the use of this vitamin in the treatment of the nausea of pregnancy.

The clinical appearance of a vitamin B_6 deficiency in man was first described by Mueller and Vilter in 1949. The deficiency was induced by the administration of desoxypyridoxine, a metabolic antagonist of pyridoxine. The most common lesion was a dermatitis characterized by itching erythema and greasy yellow scales. Lesions developed in the nasolabial folds, eyebrows and behind the ears and spread in some cases over various parts of the face and scalp. Hyperpigmented scaly lesions resembling pellagrous dermatitis occurred over the elbows, forearms, thighs and neck. Other findings included glossitis, stomatitis, conjunctivitis, angular cheilosis and peripheral neuritis. Weight loss, anorexia, weakness, lassitude and depression were observed. The most notable change in the peripheral blood was a lymphocytopenia. Biochemical alterations included elevated blood urea nitrogen and increased xanthurenic acid excretion in the urine following the administration of a test dose of tryptophan.

A widespread outbreak of convulsive seizures in the United States between 1951 and 1953 provided evidence of an essential dietary requirement for vitamin B_6 in infancy. The clinical observations made by many physicians in various parts of our country fit into a uniform pattern. While the symptoms observed varied in degree of severity, it soon became obvious that the convulsions were unassociated with other signs of illness, and no physical findings or laboratory abnormalities indicated any known etiologic factor. In all instances the infants had developed normally until they were at least some 18 weeks of age. The onset of the convulsions was sudden. Invariably the infant had been fed a commercial liquid synthetic milk formula containing defatted cow's milk, vegetable and animal fats, vitamins and iron. Infants receiving the same formula in powdered form did not develop hyperirritability and convulsions. The difference in response to the two forms was rapidly traced to the loss of pyridoxine during the processing of the liquid preparation. The administration by certain physicians of pyridoxine either orally or by injection was followed by prompt disappearance of the convulsions, and convulsions did not occur as long as the supplement of pyridoxine was continued, even though the diet remained constant. When the company which made this formula removed the deficient material from the market, the seizures promptly disappeared as suddenly as they had occurred.

The relationship between a lack of pyridoxine and convulsive seizures in rats, chicks and pigs had been demonstrated many years previously. The important members of the B complex group of vitamins are necessary for proper nerve metabolism of human beings and vitamin B_6 is no exception. The neuritis induced by isonicotinic acid hydrazide in the treatment of tuberculosis has been treated successfully with pyridoxine. Administration of pyridoxine in intravenous doses of 200 to 400 mg. is effective in preventing and controlling such manifestations. It is not certain whether this represents an actual poisoning of the nerve cells by the isonicotinic acid hydrazide or a secondary effect of rapid depletion of available pyridoxine through its chemical combination with the hydrazide to form a hydrazone which cannot be used and is excreted.

References

Birch, T. W., Gyorgy, P. and Harris, L. J.: Biochem. J., *29*:2830, 1935.

Chick, H., MacRae, T. F., Martin, A. J. P. and Martin, C.: Biochem. J., *32*:2207, 1938.

Coursin, D. B.: J.A.M.A., *154*:406, 1954.

Elvehjem, C. A., Madden, R. J., Strong, F. M.

and Woolley, D. W.: J. Am. Chem. Soc., *59:*1767, 1937.
Fouts, P. J., Helmer, O. M., Lepkovsky, S. and Jukes, T. H.: J. Nutrition, *16:*197, 1938.
Harris, S. A. and Folkers, K.: J. Am. Chem. Soc., *61:*1245, 1939.
Jukes, T. H. and Lepkovsky, S.: J. Biol. Chem. *114:*117, 1936.
May, C. D.: Pediatrics, *14:*269, 1954.
Mushett, C. W. and Emerson, G.: Fed. Proc., *15:*526, 1956.
Rinehart, J. F. and Greenberg, L. D.: Am. J. Path., *25:*481, 1949.
Snyderman, S. E., Carretero, R. and Holt, L. E., Jr.: Fed. Proc., *9:*371, 1950.
Vilter, R. W., Mueller, J. F., Glazer, H. S., Jarrold, T., Abraham, J., Thompson, C. and Hawkins, V. R.: J. Lab. & Clin. Med., *42:* 335, 1953.

Pantothenic Acid

d-Pantothenic acid is a pale yellow viscous oil that is difficult to purify. The active material is prepared for commercial use in the form of the water soluble calcium salt which is stable in solution and has a *p*H of approximately 8. The formula of the d-acid is seen in Figure 78. Pantothenic acid is present in

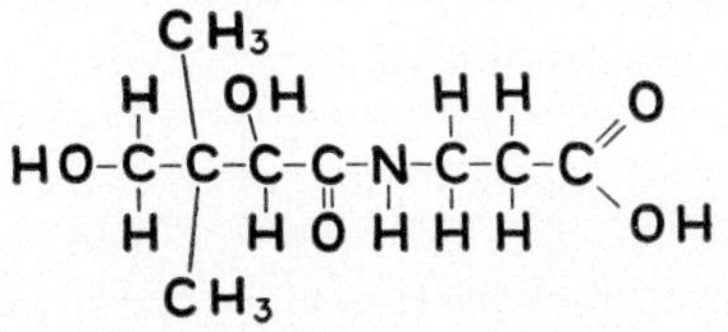

FIG. 78. Pantothenic acid (N-(α,γ-dihydroxy-β,β-dimethylbutyryl)-β-alanine).

all plant and animal tissue, and it was from its universal occurrence that it received its name.

Pantothenic acid is an integral part of coenzyme A, as seen in Figure 79. As

COENZYME A

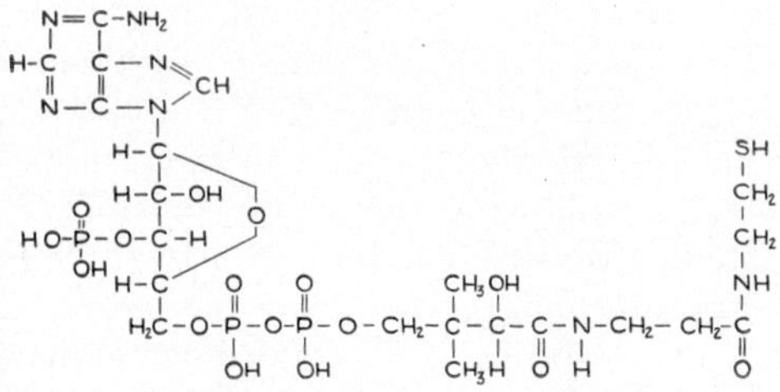

FIG. 79.

such it is relatively abundant in all living cells, the liver containing up to 400 mg. per kilogram. Coenzyme A is essential for a large number of metabolic processes. In carbohydrate metabolism it functions in citric acid synthesis and ketoglutarate and pyruvate oxidation. This coenzyme is involved in the synthesis of amino acids from carbohydrate sources. Through succinyl transfer it is concerned in the synthesis of the pyrrole ring in the heme molecule. Coenzyme A is essential in acetoacetate synthesis and in the transfer of acetyl groups. It is involved in fatty acid and cholesterol synthesis, thus playing an important role in fat and steroid metabolism. It is a normal constituent of the blood and urine. Studies by Spies, Stanbery, Williams, Jukes and Babcock on pantothenic acid in the blood of patients with multiple B complex deficiencies reveal a 25 to 50 per cent reduction from normal. These patients also show a lower urinary excretion. The excretion of pantothenic acid is increased temporarily after parenteral injection or oral administration of the vitamin. The increased concentration in the blood is not sustained for long, except in persons whose initial concentration is low. We have given a large series of persons from 50 to 100 mg. of pantothenic acid daily for more than a month without any evidence of toxicity.

Stanbery and Spies showed that under similar conditions of study, normal persons excrete a higher percentage of a standard dose of dextrorotatory calcium pantothenate than do persons having typical lesions of nicotinic acid deficiency, thiamine deficiency or riboflavin deficiency. The procedure on the normals and persons with deficient diets was as follows: A one-hour urine specimen was taken following which 50 mg. of dextrorotatory calcium pantothenate (Merck), dissolved in 5 cc. of sterile distilled water, were injected intravenously. The entire urinary output for the following 24 hours was collected. These urine specimens were assayed for pantothenic acid by means of the microbiologic method. (The error in this method is approximately 10 per cent.) Since the hour-to-hour variation in pantothenic acid excretion has not been determined, we arbitrarily multiplied the amount excreted in the preinjection sample by four and subtracted this quantity from the amount found in the four-hour postinjection sample. The result was expressed as per cent of the 50 mg. which were excreted. The average excretion of persons with vitamin deficiency was 19 per cent, whereas the average excretion of controls was 102 per cent.

Pantothenic acid is present in such quantities in common foods that a naturally occurring specific deficiency of this vitamin has not yet been described in man. Bean and his associates induced a pantothenic acid deficiency in human volunteers by administering the pantothenic acid antagonist omega-methylpantothenic acid along with a highly purified diet "devoid" of pantothenic acid. The clinical signs and metabolic abnormalities which developed in these subjects consisted of an illness characterized by torpor, apathy and depression; cardiovascular instability, especially in the erect position; a neuromuscular disorder with paresthesias, burning sensations and muscle weakness; abdominal pains and disturbances of alimentary function; and frequent respiratory infections. Biochemical alterations included an inconstant reduction in the percentage of p-aminobenzoic acid excreted in the urine in the acetylated form; irregularities in glucose tolerance and increased sensitivity to insulin; a failure of ACTH to induce eosinopenia; an irregular reduction in 17-ketosteroid excretion; and the development of a histamine refractory achlorhydria without any disturbance in gastric motility. The severity of the symptoms required cortisone, a rich diet and added vitamins for correction. In a subsequent study using an improved experimental design, Bean and co-workers extended and confirmed their previous observations. A clinical state of lethargy, weakness, burning paresthesias and cramps with signs of tetany was noted. Low serum potassium was suspected as causing many of the clinical findings. In addition, hypokalemia, hypochloremia, hypochlorhydria, metabolic alkalosis and a defect in carbohydrate metabolism were encountered in the subjects exposed to the experimental regimen. The failure to elicit a completely favorable response by the administration of large amounts of pantothenic acid raises some doubt as to whether the syndrome is representative of a pure pantothenic acid deficiency or is due in part to the toxicity of omega-methylpantothenic acid, which acts as a general protoplasmic poison; some unrecognized deficiency in the experimental diet; and irreversible tissue changes. The changes suggestive of disturbed adrenal function are particularly interesting in view of the demonstration that pantothenic acid deficiencies in rats produce gross structural alterations in the adrenal gland which affect its function.

Pantothenic acid has been reported as the anti-gray hair factor for certain animals under experimental conditions. Stanbery and Spies have administered it over a period of four to six months to six persons with gray hair. In no case did the hair change to its original color. Occasionally, in giving liver extract or yeast, or one of the specific chemical vitamins, such as nicotinic acid, along with an improved diet, we have noticed a great change in the hair. It has appeared younger in texture and in rare instances has returned to its original pigment content. Such cases showing changes, however, are extremely rare; we have seen only a few among several hundred treated and observed. It would seem unwarranted to allow claims for any of these substances as being a specific therapeutic agent for the treatment of gray hair. In certain persons with macrocytic anemia in relapse, it is observed that the pigment of the hair may be increased following the administration of vitamin B_{12} or folic acid. However, this response is unpredictable.

The "burning feet" syndrome, a disabling disease of nutritional origin, was relatively unknown in America prior to World War II. Its common occurrence among prisoners of war in the Asiatic-Pacific area drew widespread attention.

The symptoms consisted of a gradual onset of bilateral numbness and tingling of the toes. The paresthesias were succeeded by burning pains radiating from the dorsa of the feet up to the legs. The pains were most severe at night and were relieved somewhat by immersing the feet in cold water. The symptoms were exclusively sensory in nature, the reflexes and motor function being preserved. Sleep was disturbed and walking was extremely difficult, the gait assuming a characteristic flat-footed quality to avoid use of the oversensitive toes. Glusman noted that when the pain was very severe the patients would sit in their beds cross-legged holding their feet in their hands and rocking rhythmically back and forth with pain, an attitude which he regarded as pathognomonic of the disease.

The syndrome has been known and described under a variety of names in the Orient for more than a hundred years. Gopalan working in southern India found the incidence most frequent among the poorer classes whose diet consisted mainly of rice gruel and cheap vegetables. Administration of nicotinic acid, thiamine and riboflavin improved the nutritional status of both the Indian patients and prisoners of war but failed to afford complete relief from the burning feet. In the Indian series, the symptoms disappeared only after the administration of 20 to 40 mg. per day of calcium pantothenate intramuscularly. The burning and hyperhidrosis were relieved first, the pins and needles sensation later. Spies and associates have shown that injections of riboflavin and biotin produce an elevation of the pantothenic acid level in the blood. This may account for the moderate improvement noted following administration of some of the other B vitamins. It would appear that the syndrome is essentially a pantothenic acid deficiency with an overlay of deficiencies of other members of the B group of vitamins.

References

Bean, W. B. and Hodges, R. E.: Proc. Soc. Exper. Biol. & Med., *86*:693, 1954.

Glusman, M.: Am. J. Med., *3*:211, 1947.

Gopalan, C.: Indian Med. Gaz., *81*:22, 1946.

Lubin, R., Daum, K. A. and Bean, W. B.: Am. J. Clin. Nutrition, *4*:420, 1956.

Spies, T. D., Stanbery, S. R., Williams, R. J., Jukes, T. H. and Babcock, S. H.: J.A.M.A., *115*:523, 1940.

Inositol

Inositol is a colorless, water-soluble crystalline solid that melts at 247° C. It is a saturated cyclic compound with some carbohydrate properties, but without the reducing power of a sugar. Its formula is found in Figure 80.

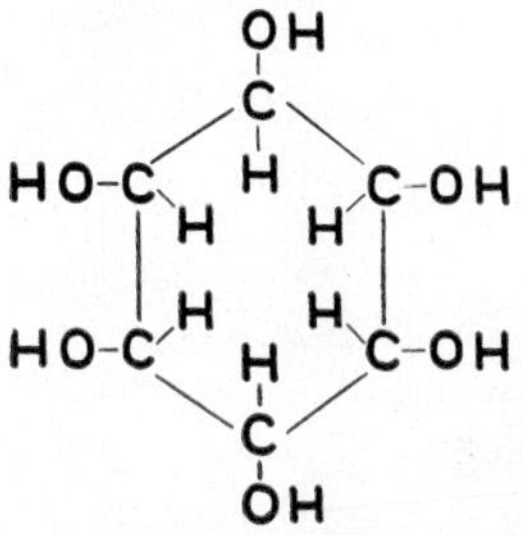

FIG. 80. Inositol (hexahydroxycyclohexane).

The different tests for inositol have not had wide application, and therefore very little is known of its place in plant and animal physiology. The content of inositol and its phosphoric acid ester, phytin, is high in the average diet, but normally most of it is oxidized or otherwise destroyed in the body and only a small part is excreted in the kidneys. Inositol is present in blood, muscle, heart and liver, and probably in other tissues. Its toxicity is apparently very low, since it has been reported that no harmful effects followed the ingestion of a dose as large as 50 gm. Woolley has found this substance curative in mouse alopecia. Its role in human physiology is not known. We have given 50 mg. of inositol a day for a week to normal adults and pellagrins without evidence of toxic symptoms. We have observed no specific syndrome of man which is relieved by inositol.

Biotin

Biotin, a growth-stimulating substance, has been separated from the bios complex of vitamin-like growth factors. Its physiologic activity has been investigated in lower forms of plant and animal life, and its occurrence in mammalian tissue forecasts wide importance. Recently, biotin has been shown to possess the biologic activity previously ascribed to vitamin H (the egg-white injury factor), and coenzyme R. Williams and associates, and Dreizen, Mosny, Gilley and Spies have demonstrated an interrelationship between biotin and oleic acid in the metabolism of bacteria producing lactic acid.

The chemical properties of biotin were first described by Kögl who crystallized small quantities of it from egg yolk. According to this investigator, it has a basic nitrogen, a carboxyl group, and is amphoteric. Analysis of the compound has given the following empirical formula: $C_{11}H_{18}O_3N_2S$. The methyl ester crystallizes readily, melts at 148° C. and is physiologically active. Biotin is destroyed by benzoylation and acetylation, but not by methylation or by boiling with acid or alkali. Nitrous acid destroys the compound at the same rate as it does alpha amino acids.

When rats are kept on diets containing uncooked egg-white, they develop a characteristic syndrome known as *egg-white injury*. Continued feeding of this diet ultimately results in the death of the animal. It has been demonstrated that the injuries produced by such diets are not due to any direct toxic action of the egg white, but result from an interaction of a specific protein, avidin, present in the egg white with the biotin of the diet. As a result, the biotin is rendered unavailable to the animal and a biotin deficiency develops, producing the typical "egg-white injury" syndrome. Highly concentrated preparations of avidin are just as effective as the original egg white in producing the biotin deficiency.

Spies and Eakin have found subnormal biotin levels for the bloods of some patients who have been living on diets very poor in the B vitamins, but no clinical symptoms have been found which can definitely be associated with these low biotin values. They have also found that the urinary biotin excretion drops when patients are placed on diets containing raw egg white. The biotin output of one patient who was kept on such a diet for a month was less than one tenth the base-line value but no symptoms developed.

Biotin is a normal component of human tissue and excretory products. It is present in beef liver in a combined form from which it can be released by hydrolysis. Its function in human nutrition is unknown.

References

Williams, W. L., Broquist, H. P. and Snell, E. E.: J. Biol. Chem., *170*:619, 1947.

Dreizen, S., Mosny, J. J., Gilley, E. J. and Spies, T. D.: Ztschr. f. Vitaminforsch., *26*: 257, 1955.

Thioctic Acid (α-Lipoic Acid)

Thioctic acid (Fig. 81) has been isolated and has been shown to be a

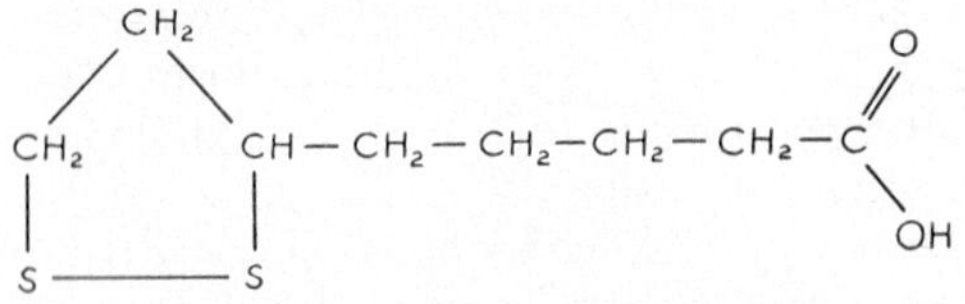

```
        CH2                                      O
       /   \                                    //
   CH2      CH — CH2 — CH2 — CH2 — CH2 — C
    |        |                             \
    S ————— S                              OH
```

(Synthetic) 6,8 - thioctic acid

FIG. 81.

bacterial growth factor and an important factor in certain enzyme systems which activate acetate. It has not as yet been shown to be important in either human or animal nutrition.

Gibberellic Acid

Within the past two years, gibberellic acid has gained prominence as a plant growth factor. It has been shown to stimulate stem and leaf elongation in a number of plants. The specific genetic constitution of a strain or variety appears to determine whether it will respond to applied gibberellic acid by increased shoot growth. Thus far, the most notable results have been obtained with dwarf types. Its role in animal and human metabolism is unknown.

Reference

Whaley, W. G. and Kephart, J.: Science, *125:* 234, 1957.

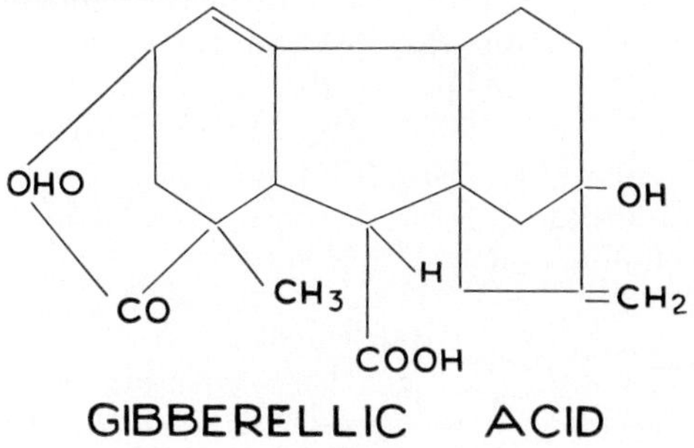

GIBBERELLIC ACID

FIG. 82.

Mevalonic Acid Lactone

Mevalonic acid has been produced but has not yet been shown to have any function in either animals or man.

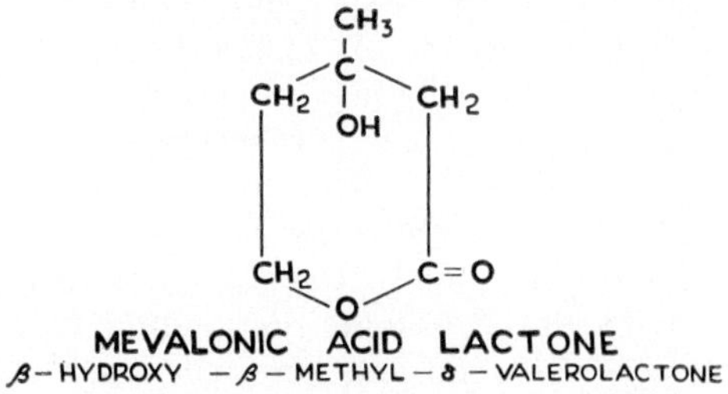

MEVALONIC ACID LACTONE
β-HYDROXY -β-METHYL-δ-VALEROLACTONE

FIG. 83.

Vitamin B_t

Vitamin B_t, described by Fraenkel and associates, is a growth factor for the mealworm, *Tenebrio molitor,* and some other beetle larvae. Chemically it has been identified as carnitine, the betaine of beta-hydroxy-gamma amino butyric acid. Carnitine is widely distributed in animal tissues, particularly in muscle. From experiments with germ-free chickens it is evident that carnitine is synthesized in human and animal tissues, but neither the mechanism nor its function is known. In man carnitine is excreted in the urine in amounts depending on the nature of the diet. Excretion is highest following a heavy meat meal and after a 3-day period of starvation. Low amounts are excreted when the diet contains mainly fruits and vegetables.

Reference

Fraenkel, G., Blewett, M. and Coles, M.: Nature, *161:*981, 1948.

Vitamin T

Vitamin T, described by Goetsch as an insect growth factor, should not be confused with vitamin B_t. Vitamin T is found in various kinds of yeasts, particularly the genus *Torula,* and in ascomycetes such as *Penicillium.* The vitamin is soluble in water and ethyl alcohol and is resistant to heat. It is too early to determine whether it has a specific function in human beings, though it has been clearly demonstrated to affect the size and habits of fruit flies and ants.

The work with vitamin T is an example of the special problems of invertebrate nutrition. To the familiar aspects of growth, reproduction and maintenance are added those of drastic alterations of forms and modes of life. These metamorphoses are probably associated with changes in nutritional requirements. Studies of these variations may clarify not only problems of insect biology, but also many general and fundamental aspects of vertebrate metabolism.

Reference

Goetsch, W.: Oesterr. Ztschr. f. Zool., *1:*193, 1947.

Choline

Choline is a colorless base (see Fig. 84) which is usually crystallized as the

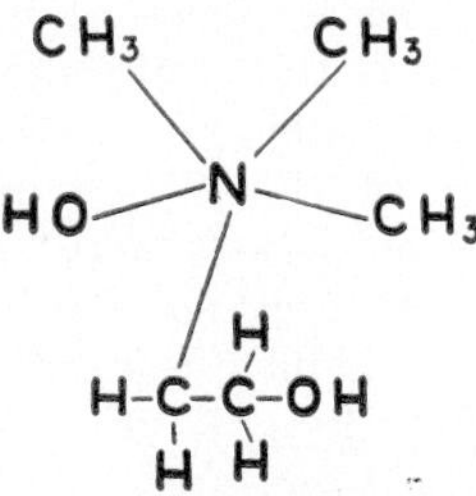

FIG. 84. Choline (trimethyl-β-hydroxyethyl ammonium hydroxide).

hydrochloride. It is water soluble and stable in acid solution, but is split by strong alkali. The free base is strongly alkaline, absorbing carbon dioxide readily from the air. Choline is present in large quantities in the animal body as a constituent of the phospholipid, lecithin, and of acetylcholine. In addition to serving as a precursor of these compounds, choline functions as a donor of labile methyl groups in transmethylation reactions. These reactions which involve the transfer of a methyl group from one substance to another occur in the metabolism of nitrogen, sulfur, proteins, fats and carbohydrates. A well balanced diet contains substances which can supply methyl groups for transmethylation. In animal experiments it has been shown that if these substances are omitted from the diet growth ceases, the liver becomes infiltrated with fat, there is hemorrhage into the renal tubules and death ensues. When methyl donors, such as choline, betaine or methionine, are added to the diet, these disturbances are prevented or corrected. Demonstration of the transfer of methyl groups in animal tissues by isotope experiments is largely the work of du Vigneaud and associates.

The pharmacologic actions of choline and its more powerful derivative, acetylcholine, have been exhaustively investigated. These compounds are vasodilators; they cause a fall in blood pressure and have a profound secretagogue effect. This effect does not seem to be exhausted by continuous functioning, because choline can be perfused through an isolated stomach and will stimulate steady secretion.

There is no evidence of toxic symptoms following the administration of 50 mg. choline daily for a week. When large doses of choline are ingested by normal persons, about 50 per cent is decomposed by intestinal bacteria to trimethylamine, which is excreted in the urine. This decomposition has been shown to be suppressed in man by the oral administration of certain antibiotics or by feeding a lactobacillus culture.

In dogs and rats, choline deficiency causes the development of fatty livers, and choline is said to prevent the excessive deposition of neutral fats and to aid in the synthesis of the phosphatides in the livers of these animals. Absorbable broad spectrum antibodies added to the daily diet of rats delays the development of cirrhosis for 100 days or more when they are restricted to a choline-deficient diet. Nonabsorbable antibiotics added to the daily diet prevent the development of cirrhosis in the rats for as long as 750 days. This suggests that intestinal bacteria are largely, if not entirely, responsible for the cirrhosis in rats on a choline-deficient diet.

References

du Vigneaud, V.: Biol. Symposia, *5*:234, 1941.

Rutenberg, A. M., Sonnenblick, E., Koven, I., Aprahamian, H. A., Reiner, L. and Fine, J.: J. Exper. Med., *106*:1, 1957.

Para-aminobenzoic Acid

Para-aminobenzoic acid is another vitamin of the B complex. It is a constituent of yeast and of liver, and is a growth factor for chicks and certain organisms. It appears to nullify the bacteriostatic effect of chemotherapeutic agents of the sulfanilamide group. It has some anti-gray hair potency in the nutritional achromotrichia of the mouse and rat, and there is one report that the human is affected by the oral administration of this substance. Para-amino-benzoic acid has no anti-gray hair effect in the human in the opinion of the authors.

THE HUMAN DIET AND MIXED DEFICIENCY DISEASES

For the student who would understand some of the problems facing the physician who must treat patients with mixed deficiency diseases, it is essential that he think in terms of a new field of medicine, the science of nutrition. It is a field concerned primarily with the proper nourishment of the individual cells. Because it is growing rapidly, information is often sketchy and uncertain; it lacks stability in nomenclature, and many of the problems concerned are still in dispute. Accordingly, we shall not touch on the alarming number of conflicting hypotheses, but will discuss the problems which invite the physician's study because of their practical value.

The respiration and growth of cells involve the synthesis of complex substances from simpler chemical compounds. By means of substances called *enzymes,* the cells are able to perform these functions without increased temperature and pressure. Enzymes are catalysts produced by living cells from combinations of organic substances, including the vitamins. These enzymes retain activity even when separated from the living cell. When a dietary deficiency of vitamins has existed over a long period of time, a biochemical lesion develops in the cell, often severe enough to cause functional disturbances. If the deficiency is not corrected, these disturbances become more widespread and eventually give rise to an infinite variety of symptoms forming a complex clinical picture. Finally, severe or persistent alterations lead to structural changes in the tissue, and ultimately the diagnostic lesions of a deficiency disease are likely to appear. The complexity of the subject is greatly increased by the fact that the several groups of the various vitamins usually occur together in nature, and the failure to provide one usually results in failure to provide many. Then, one has arising from a dietary fault innumerable vague, indefinite symptoms coming from cells affected because a number of catalysts are not working efficiently.

Often isolation and synthesis of a new vitamin shake the whole structure of medical theory to its foundation, and usually bring new hope to the sick and afflicted. Unfortunately, the application of these findings with vigor and enthusiasm has led to thinking too much in terms of isolated vitamin deficiencies, although *every method of study has indicated the predominance of mixed rather than single deficiency* of elements essential for life and well-being. So great has been the interest aroused by the recent discoveries among the laity and physicians alike that today everyone knows something about the vitamins. Investigation of the diets of large groups of people correlated with laboratory studies and direct experimentation has led to the startling observation that the margin of safety against deficiency disease is narrow rather than broad, that the presence of nutritional inadequacy is widespread and not limited to the lower economic group. As information is increasing, it is found that relatively few people in the United States consistently eat diets that are adequate in all respects.

Primary Etiology

Studies of the food consumed by families in various sections of the country show that the chief difference between the better diets and the poor diets lies in the amount of milk, lean meat, fresh vegetables and fruit included. Table 2, showing the results of an analysis of diets eaten by persons with varying degrees of deficiency diseases, indicates how truly serious the deficiency states may be in some areas of the country. Table 3 impresses one even more with a comparison of the amounts of nutrients supplied to the same individuals and the estimated normal adequate diet. As reflected in Table 2, we have analyzed the diets of a group of persons with deficiency diseases who have come under

TABLE 2. FOODS CONSUMED BY PERSONS ON DEFICIENT DIETS IN CONTRAST TO RECOMMENDED LOW COST DIET

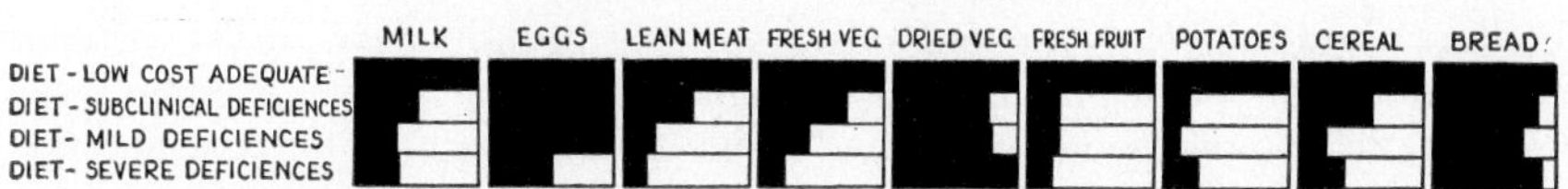

*Adequate diet: Stiebeling, Hazel K., and Clark, Faith: Good Diets at Low and Moderate Costs. Food and Life, Yearbook of Agriculture, 1939, p. 332.

■ – In the low cost diet, this represents the amount of each food recommended. In the diets of persons with deficiency diseases it represents the fractions of these amounts actually consumed.

□ – This represents the difference between the food theoretically needed and that actually consumed by persons with deficiency diseases.

TABLE 3. AVERAGE DIETARIES OF FAMILIES WITH DEFICIENCY DISEASES COMPARED WITH AN ADEQUATE DIET

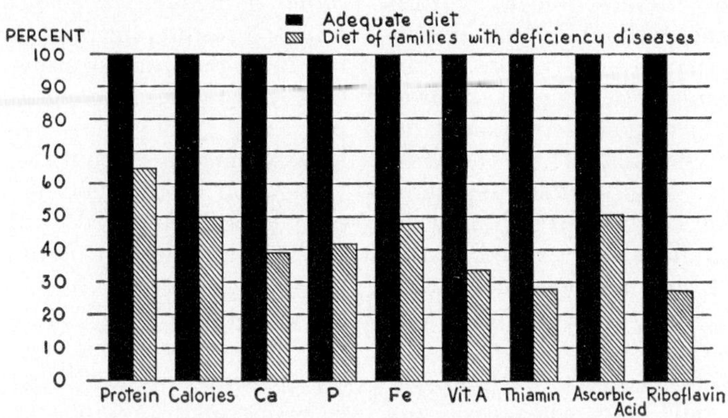

The degree of nicotinic acid deficiency in the dietaries cannot be evaluated from the data on the nicotinic acid content of food available at the present time.

The majority of persons in these twenty families had clinical symptoms of pellagra, beriberi, scurvy, riboflavin deficiency or vitamin A deficiency.

our observation. It is obvious that although these people may have had one outstanding deficiency disease syndrome, they actually were suffering from mixed deficiency diseases operating simultaneously. The average dietary of this group, classed as consuming poor diets, furnished only 50 per cent of their estimated energy requirement. Assuming 0.5 gm. protein per kilogram per day to be the maintenance requirement, their intake was only 35 per cent of this amount. Although the average person received 0.68 gm. protein per kilogram of body weight, an amount above the theoretical maintenance requirement, only 5 per cent of the group had an optimum intake of 1 gm. per kilogram. The total protein intake in at least 35 per cent of the cases studied was too low to maintain nitrogen equilibrium. Whether this results in a specific or general amino acid deficiency is uncertain, but it should be corrected if health is to be restored. Nearly all of these persons received substandard amounts of calcium, phosphorus and iron, and none obtained adequate amounts of all three elements.

The vitamin deficiencies in these dietaries were, on the whole, greater than those of other nutrients and the degree of the deficiency in the B complex vitamins was greater than that of any other vitamins. The thiamine and riboflavin intakes were only 28 per cent and 27 per cent, respectively, of the suggested standards. The pyridoxine content of a dietary cannot be estimated from the data available and man's requirement for it is not definitely known. Since the factors of the B complex are closely associated in natural foodstuffs, it is reasonable to assume that they, too, were present in amounts considerably below those required. The vitamin A content of the dietaries was 33 per cent of the requirement suggested for this vitamin. The deficiency of vitamin C, which was 53 per cent of standard, appears to be less severe than in the case of other vitamins. However, these figures represent the average intake of a group of fifty patients. Several persons consumed diets in which there were no vitamin C-containing foods.

Why should this country, called by poets and statesmen "a land of plenty," provide a daily fare that is often inadequate for poor and rich alike? The average person fails to appreciate the relation of food to health. Some diets become deficient through habit. In many instances, the knowledge of food values in relation to food cost is erroneous and the nutritive return on the money spent is paltry. On the other hand, the pauper's income, if any, provides the pauper's diet which, no matter how carefully it may be chosen, cannot supply the minimum food requirements. We are convinced that this last factor is an important cause of deficiency diseases among persons living in areas in which these diseases are endemic.

To take the passive stand that these people must continue to have deficiency diseases until there is a revolution in economic affairs is of course a counsel of despair—a socialist's nightmare. It is not too much to expect, however, that changes in the processing of foodstuffs or even the addition of essential elements as a nutritional subsidy may do much toward alleviating this burden of civilization. A noteworthy paper by Baker, Wright and Drummond traces the increasing use of white flour to the introduction of silk bolting cloth in 1840 and of roller mills in 1870 to satisfy greater demand. They estimate that "the best fed members of the population today are getting twice as much vitamin B_1 as people on a low income level, yet consume less vitamin B_1 than the parish poor of the eighteenth and early nineteenth centuries." We are realizing more and more that decortification of grain is dangerous, that there must be some change in milling methods. Greater care in guarding against loss of vitamins and minerals through processing, marketing and storing of foods would undoubtedly improve the quality of many diets. Among low income groups especially, education is necessary in respect to the use of evaporated and dried milk, and in the use of larger quantities of the less expensive green and yellow vegetables, fruits, tomatoes, potatoes, legumes and nuts—foods that yield excellent returns at a relatively low cost.

Secondary Etiology

The primary etiology of deficiency states occurring in the average person has already been discussed. This is to be modified by the knowledge that individual requirements for vitamins and minerals vary greatly. It is known that under altered environment or increased activity there may be increased need and more rapid destruction, diminished absorption and impaired utilization of the protective materials. Thus, a period of rest in bed without change in diet has caused the remission of symptoms in many pellagrins, symptoms which recur with resumption of normal activity.

A consideration of the changes in requirements wrought by altered environ-

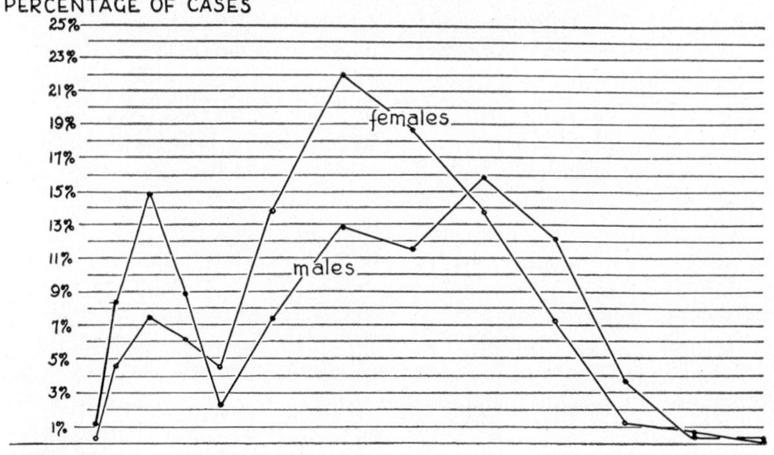

FIG. 85.

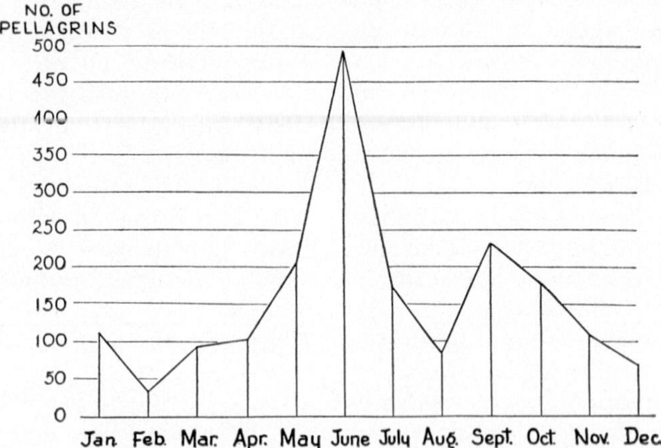

FIG. 86. This figure shows the monthly incidence of pellagra. This curve is essentially the same for all deficiency diseases arising from lack of the water-soluble vitamins. Note the high peak in summer and the secondary peak in the fall. Early symptoms of deficiency disease appear months before the average patient seeks a doctor. If the doctor would treat malnourished persons throughout the year rather than await the appearance of the full-blown clinical syndrome in the summer and fall, such peaks would tend to disappear.

ment introduces the secondary causes of nutritional deficiency. Because of the narrow margin of safety these may appear rapidly under the burden of acute or chronic infection, not only through infection per se but also as a result of the regimen to which the patient is subjected. Observations by Bean and Spies have shown that in an area where pellagra is endemic, approximately 10 per cent of the patients with clinical evidence of deficiency disease had some form of chronic diarrhea, including cases with partial intestinal obstruction, carcinoma of the rectum, colon or stomach, stricture of lymphopathia, bacillary dysentery, sprue, ulcerative colitis, intestinal tuberculosis, and gastrocolic fistula.

Extensive studies of nonalcoholic and nonendemic cases of pellagra in Cleveland and Cincinnati have indicated that many diseases predispose to or precipitate this syndrome. This isolated observation merely confirms the long-established belief that a number of factors are usually involved in the production of clinical vitamin deficiency diseases. In eighty-five such cases in which alcoholism and deficient diets were excluded as the primary factors leading to pellagra, we found twenty-eight cases secondary to acute or chronic infection with organic lesions of the alimentary canal, eighteen associated with congestive heart failure, ten with hyperthyroidism, diabetes mellitus, and other metabolic disorders, and ten with miscellaneous diseases. We have not included patients in whom lactation and pregnancy were possible factors.

Therapeutic diets, like many drugs, are fine for the disease, faulty for the patient. Reducing diets, diets given to patients with alimentary tract disease, allergy, hypertension, nephritis, or heart disease frequently tend insidiously to produce deficiency diseases. Too often the patient is told what he must *not* eat but not what he *may* eat and, as a result, he chooses a grossly inadequate diet.

In summary, pellagra or other vitamin deficiency states may follow those conditions which prevent the normal intake, digestion, absorption, storage or utilization of vitamins. On the other hand, these states may succeed conditions associated with an elevated metabolic level and an unsatisfied increase in the vitamin requirements of the body. These factors may operate singly or in combination, and may be enhanced by the restricted regimen prescribed by the physician for the patient.

Clinical Features

The clinical picture presented by deficiency diseases is extremely complex. The ill informed might contend that persons who do not have pellagra, beriberi or scurvy have an adequate amount of nicotinic acid, thiamine and ascorbic acid. However, investigators in the field of nutrition have incontrovertible evidence that there is a wide gap between the amount of these substances needed to prevent the well defined, usually terminal clinical signs of deficiency, and the optimum amount necessary to insure full health and vigor. It may well be said that subnormal or borderline nutritional states are those which occur most frequently and are least frequently recognized.

These early symptoms and signs are not well defined and have been constantly attributed to a deficiency of one or another of the individual vitamins. Deficiency symptoms may not appear for several months or a year after deprivation has started or they may appear after only a few weeks, particularly if some precipitating factor arises. The intensity of each likewise is variable. The *prodromal symptoms* common to many of the vitamin deficiencies, and hence to mixed deficiency, are loss of weight and strength, insomnia, depressed mental states and lassitude, nervousness and irritability, headaches, diarrhea, abdominal cramps, anorexia, indigestion, heartburn and vague paresthesias. It is to be noted that these symptoms have been ascribed individually at various times to a deficiency of vitamin B_1, nicotinic acid, vitamin B_6, riboflavin, vitamin C and vitamin E.

A most important aid in discovering mixed deficiency is the constant suspicion that where there are clear evidences of one deficiency there must certainly be some signs, perhaps veiled, of other specific deficiency states. It must be stated repeatedly that pure clinical pictures produced by the lack of a single vitamin rarely exist (except perhaps vitamins D and K). The classic pictures of beriberi, of pellagra, of scurvy have always been described as separate entities for the purposes of recognition and of specific therapy.

Diagnosis

Because deficiency diseases are progressive rather than self-limited and because we possess specific remedies for their prevention, the importance of early diagnosis and therapy cannot be overemphasized. Recognition generally is not difficult for those who have seen cases, but it is not easy for one who has gleaned the symptomatology from textbooks. It is our experience that the physician conversant with the literature from a theoretical standpoint frequently fails to diagnose a case, even a typical case, presented to him in the clinic. Where the classic signs are absent and the diagnosis uncertain, the most important aid is a precise knowledge of previous diet, accurate history and physical examinations, and observation of the response of the patient to specific therapy. These diagnostic points of necessity must be kept in mind in relation to the discussions which follow.

Deficiency diseases in adults and in *infants and children* are similar, but naturally differ in the interpretation of subjective symptoms according to the mental age of the individual. An adult with scurvy complains of pains in various parts of the body and bleeding gums. The infant is irritable, refuses to eat and cries when touched at the tender areas over the bones. The dermatitis, diarrhea and dementia of the adult pellagrin are characteristic, but the listless infant with enteritis who has failed to gain weight is a familiar problem to the pediatrician and may represent many conditions other than nicotinic acid deficiency. Once again, only a careful dietary analysis of the nursing mother, including knowledge of the diet prior to and during pregnancy, will give a hint as to the nature of the disease. In addition, should her diet be inadequate, one should suspect either an iron deficiency or a deficiency of the entire B complex or both. The fact that rickets and vitamin A deficiency and scurvy are less frequently seen even in areas where B deficiency diseases are endemic bears testimony to the benefits derived from the education of parents to the use of cod liver oil and orange juice in infants' diets.

All possible combinations of vitamin and mineral deficiency cannot be described for they are innumerable and vary with the individual. We have seen patients suspected of having only two or three deficiencies who showed improvement only up to a certain point when given the two or three specific vitamins. In such cases, residual burning of the mouth or paresthesias of the extremities may be relieved by adenylic acid; or refractory nervousness, abdominal cramps and muscular rigidity may respond to vitamin B_6; again, insomnia, tinnitus and neuromuscular symptoms may cease only upon the administration of alpha-tocopherol.

The following representative history of Mr. and Mrs. Z. and family with clinically associated deficiency diseases is rather typical of affected families living in the rural areas in which these diseases are endemic. The studies extended through the calendar years of 1939 and 1940.

METHOD OF STUDY

Since all members of a family living together tend to eat a similar diet, a number of years ago we adopted the policy of studying an entire family. All members of the family were asked to report to the hospital at least once a month, and those in ill health were urged to come more frequently. Repeated clinical and laboratory examinations were made both in the home and in the clinic, or when the patient was severely ill, in the hospital ward. The dietary surveys included visits to the home, where the methods of food preparation and the types of food used were observed. A record of the actual food intake of each member of the family was kept for a period of one week. Special chemical, physiologic and bacteriologic tests were done on the blood and urine, and sometimes nerves and muscles were biopsied before, during and after therapy. Even though we had excellent laboratory facilities available and experts in various fields collaborated with us to aid in interpreting our findings, we placed ourselves in the position of the general practitioner and studied our patients as they came to us. Whenever a diagnosis of a deficiency disease was made on any one patient, our studies were extended to include his family as a whole.

ECONOMIC STATUS

M. Z., a thirty-year-old white man, his wife, twenty-eight years old, and four children, one, three, four, and five years of age, lived on a ten-acre farm which he owned. Approximately one-half the land was planted in cotton, two acres in corn, and the rest in pasture and garden. They had one cow, one mule, two hogs, two dogs, and a cat. Their cash income for the year was seldom more than $12 from their cotton crop. They lived in a two-room cabin. In the kitchen a small wood stove used for cooking was the only source of heat. Fuel was scarce. In the winter the walls were covered with newspapers to keep out the wind. In the room used as a bedroom the three oldest children slept in a single bed and the parents and baby in a double bed. A dilapidated table and three old chairs were the only other pieces of furniture in the two rooms.

DIETARY HISTORY

As nearly as could be ascertained this dietary history is typical of their habits for at least the past six years: During the summer they ate green vegetables from the garden, but before fall the garden was usually "burned out." Mrs. Z. canned about two dozen quart jars of vegetables each year but could not can more as she had no more jars and could not afford to buy more. The supply of canned vegetables never lasted beyond Christmas. During the winter they lived on black-eyed peas and dried beans which they grew, cornmeal, wheat flour, part of the meat from one hog they slaughtered, and sorghum syrup for which they traded the rest of their meat. The cow went dry a month or so after the calf was born, and the family had no milk the rest of the year. The two dogs and cat ate scraps from the family meals and rustled what they could. The children were very fond of candy and ate as much of it as possible. The parents dipped snuff whenever they could get a few pennies to buy it.

HISTORY OF ILLNESS (MRS. Z.)

One of the neighbors, who had been insane from pellagra and had returned home from a mental hospital after we treated her with nicotinic acid, told Mrs. Z. that she too had pellagra, and suggested that she come to us for treatment. At first, she was afraid to come. She was ashamed to think she might have a disease which in her neighborhood was considered a disgrace. Finally, early in April, her husband persuaded her to come to us. By this time, she said she was crazy and that she would "kill the kids if she could find them." She could not remember where they were.

In January or February of each year for several years, Mrs. Z. began to feel badly and each year felt a little worse than the previous year. By March, she began to have trouble with her stomach. Everything she ate caused pain and burning. She felt that she could drink milk, but they had no milk and could not afford to buy it. She lost all desire for food and could "scarcely stand to smell it cooking." Her tongue began to "burn" and became increasingly worse until it felt as if it had been scalded with boiling water and "nearly killed her" when she tried to eat. She lost weight and strength. Although she felt tired all the time, she could not rest. She worried constantly about her husband and children, and was afraid something was going to happen to them. She was irritable and cross, and although she loved her husband and children they "got on her nerves" and she felt as if she would have to run away. She could not stand having people around, yet when she was alone she wished she were dead. Her head ached terribly all day, and she felt dizzy and confused. It seemed to her that the harder she worked, the less she accomplished. Often when she tried to make bread she could not remember whether or not she had included all the ingredients. Even when it was cold she could not keep the bed covers on her feet because they "burned like fire." She had to get up and walk around frequently, trying to get the cramps out of her feet and legs, but most of the time she just lay in bed and cried with pain.

By March her tongue was red and sore, and the corners of her mouth began to macerate, crack, itch and burn. Some time before, the light began to hurt her eyes so much that she had to keep the shades down all day. When the light first struck her eyes as she walked outdoors, she cried out with pain. The skin on her whole body itched and burned, and she felt as though insects were crawling over it continuously. The skin on her forearms, neck, and ankles became red and sore "like sunburn," although she seldom exposed herself to the sun because she thought it made her worse. During all these months, she had been constipated but by the middle of March began having diarrhea, her bowels moving every hour or so. The soreness of her mouth and tongue became so severe that she could eat very little food. Finally, she became so weak she could scarcely get out of bed.

LABORATORY FINDINGS

Myriads of hemolytic Streptococci and Staphylococci, and Vincent's organisms were identified in the smears taken from the mucous membrane lesions in the oral cavity and in the vagina of this patient. *Streptococcus hemolyticus* and hemolytic strains of *Staphylococcus aureus* were isolated in pure culture from the cheilotic lesions and from some of the ocular lesions. Following the administration of nicotinic acid, which healed the mucous membrane lesions, and the administration of riboflavin, which healed the cheilosis and ocular lesions, the organisms disappeared rapidly.

Red cell and white cell counts, hemoglobin and hematocrit determinations showed that this patient had a macrocytic anemia. The red cell count was 2.8 million; white cell count, 4200; hemoglobin, 11.6 grams (75 per cent); hematocrit, 34. Sedimentation was faster than normal. Blood smears showed variations in the size and shape of the erythrocytes. This type of macrocytic nutritional anemia, which is not unusual in pellagra, has been studied extensively by the authors. It responds to long-continued dietary treatment, to persistent yeast or liver therapy, or to the oral administration of beef. Apparently it is due to a lack of the extrinsic factor from the diet.

The concentration of *coenzymes* I and II in whole blood was determined, using the biologic method of Vilter, Vilter and Spies, which depends upon the specific requirement of *H. influenzae* for these coenzymes. The coenzymes I and II concentration of the whole blood of this patient, in terms of coenzymase equivalents, was 14 gamma/cc. of blood, which is lower than the normal average of 31 gamma/cc. Following bed rest and the administration of nicotinic acid, the blood coenzyme values became normal. The coenzyme I content of the erythrocytes was determined, using the Barcroft apparatus. There was a tendency for the coenzyme I content to be slightly lower than the normal, but not strikingly so.

The *plasma prothrombin* level in this patient was normal, whereas in an occasional patient in the clinic, particularly one who has inadequate absorption from the intestine because of diarrhea, there is a slight lowering of the plasma prothrombin level.

Comparative determinations for *oxygen, glucose,* and *lactic acid* were made on the blood from the femoral artery and from the internal jugular vein. The average A:V difference for oxygen was 5.8 per cent, compared with 7.43 per cent in normal subjects. The average difference in the glucose content of the blood from artery and vein was 7.6 mg. per 100 cc. compared to the arterial-venous difference of 14.6 mg. of glucose per 100 cc. in normal persons. There was no difference in the lactic acid content of the arterial and venous blood. These findings suggest a diminished cerebral carbohydrate metabolism and might offer a partial explanation for the mental changes observed.

The concentration of *nicotinic acid* in the blood was studied, using Koch's modification of the Koser and Saunders method, which depends upon the fact that the dysentery bacillus requires for growth nicotinic acid or a compound which acts similarly. At the time this patient had pellagra, repeated daily tests showed that her blood supported growth for the Hiss dysentery bacillus in dilution of 1:160, which is equivalent to a content of about 0.48 mg. per cent of nicotinic acid or compounds which are physiologically similar. The blood concentration of nicotinic acid in normal persons is about 2 to 3 mg. per cent. Within twenty-four hours following the oral administration of 1000 mg. nicotinic acid, in divided doses, her blood supported growth of the Hiss dysentery in dilution of 1:320, which is equivalent to about 0.96 mg. per cent of nicotinic acid. After seven days of nicotinic acid therapy, her blood contained 1.92 mg. per cent nicotinic acid. She remained on her usual deficient diet and one month later, the nicotinic acid content of her blood had dropped to 0.96 mg. per cent. This test is not of diagnostic value, but it does give some idea as to blood level of nicotinic acid in pellagra during relapse and subsequent to nicotinic acid therapy.

The blood concentration of *riboflavin* was determined by a biologic method, using the growth of the *Lactobacillus casei* as an indicator. This patient had a value of 0.48 gamma riboflavin per cc. of whole blood. This method is very accurate, but the test is of no diagnostic value so far as the clinician is concerned, for the blood concentration of riboflavin in persons with a deficiency of this substance shows no significant variation from normal. Pantothenic acid was determined with a modified procedure, for the same strain of *L. casei* requires both pantothenic acid and riboflavin for growth. The method has been reported in detail by Pennington, Snell and Williams, and we have modified it so that it can be used in the clinic as a test for the blood pantothenic acid concentration. We have found that a high percentage of persons with beriberi, pellagra or riboflavin deficiency have a low level of pantothenic acid in the blood. The blood *pantothenic acid* for this patient was 0.19 gamma/cc., whereas that of a normal person is 0.23 gamma/cc. Tests were done for *biotin*, but the results were inconclusive.

The whole blood and plasma *ascorbic acid* concentrations were studied, and were found to be considerably lower than normal, in fact, so low as to suggest that the depletion was advanced. Repeated blood samples showed values within the normal range for calcium, phosphorus and phosphatase.

Serum protein determinations showed a 30 per cent reduction from normal. Many patients in the clinic used as controls did not show this degree of low serum protein. Serum iron determinations were slightly lower than normal. The serum colloid osmotic pressure was variable but appeared to be less than one would anticipate from the serum protein level.

Tests for *albumin and sugar in the urine* were negative. The specific gravity was 1.020. Studies of urinary pigments by the B.E.S. technique revealed ether-soluble red pigments both before and after the addition of nitrites. There was an increase over the normal amount of indican excreted in the urine. These abnormal pigments disappeared or returned to normal levels following treatment with nicotinic acid. Determination of the coenzyme content of the urine revealed an excretion of 0 to 3 gamma/hour (normal, 3 to 10 gamma/hr.).

Nicotinic acid was excreted in considerably less than normal amounts, when tested by either bacteriologic or biochemical methods, although the exact amount is difficult to determine. Thiamine excretion revealed a figure slightly lower than normal for the twenty-four-hour period. The urinary excretion of riboflavin amounted to approximately 1 gamma per hour (normal, 2 to 5 gamma/hr), and of pantothenic acid, 0.5 gamma per hour which was considerably lower than the normal excretion of 25 gamma per hour. Pyridoxine (vitamin B_6) was excreted in small quantities for the twenty-four-hour period. (Within the first hour following the injection of 50 mg. pyridoxine, only 0.5 per cent was excreted, whereas in normal persons between 6 and 10 per cent is excreted.) The urinary excretion of each of the vitamins was lower than normal before treatment but increased following therapy with each specific crystalline vitamin.

Biopsy sections of muscle were studied for such evidence of *vitamin E* deficiency as defective striation, swelling of the fibers, and infiltration. The coenzyme I content of muscle was decreased 30 per cent.

Neurologic examination, including chromaximetric determinations, showed that there was considerable polyneuropathy of the motor and sensory nerves. Within one to four hours following the injection of 50 mg. thiamine, there was quantitative improvement in the electrical excitability of the muscles and in sensitivity to touch and pin prick. This improvement was maintained from one to five days, but the patient slowly regressed and eventually returned to the condition preceding thiamine therapy. Microscopic examination of biopsied peripheral nerves in this patient revealed a marked degeneration and loss of myelin sheaths. The axis cylinders were involved in the degenerative process, to the same degree of severity as the myelin sheaths.

Skin biopsies showed advanced hyperkeratosis with formation of verrucae (see Figs. 87 and 88). There was a focal atrophy of the epidermis, edema of the upper part of the corium, and atrophy of the sebaceous glands. Hyalinization and mucoid degeneration were present in the connective tissue of the deeper corium. The skin all over the body, irrespective of whether it was in the lesion, showed changes.

Gastric analyses were done before and after histamine injections. No free HCl, pepsinogen or rennin were found. The presence of the intrinsic factor of Castle was demonstrated by incubating raw beef with the gastric juice from this patient and giving the mixture for ten consecutive days to a patient with pernicious anemia. (The patient with pernicious anemia had a characteristic reticulocyte response, indicating that the intrinsic factor was present in the gastric juice of the pellagrin.)

The *eyes* were examined by the physicians who made the routine examination in the clinic, and since abnormalities were found, further studies were made, with particular reference to the lesions of the conjunctiva. In addition, ophthalmoscopic studies were made, and the corneal lesions were followed by repeated examination under the slit lamp. Biophotometer and adaptometer tests for vitamin A deficiency were not made.

HOME HISTORY

When Mr. Z. brought his wife to the Nutrition Clinic he, too, was examined. For some time he had been unable to do much work. He complained of loss of appetite, weakness, indigestion, headache and insomnia. He was worried, apprehensive and depressed. When asked about the children, he said he knew they were not well because they were cross, irritable, ate very little food, and refused to play. Both he and the mother noticed that the nursing infant and the three-year-old child had cracking at the corners of their mouths which their mother thought had been "caught" from her. We suggested that they bring all the

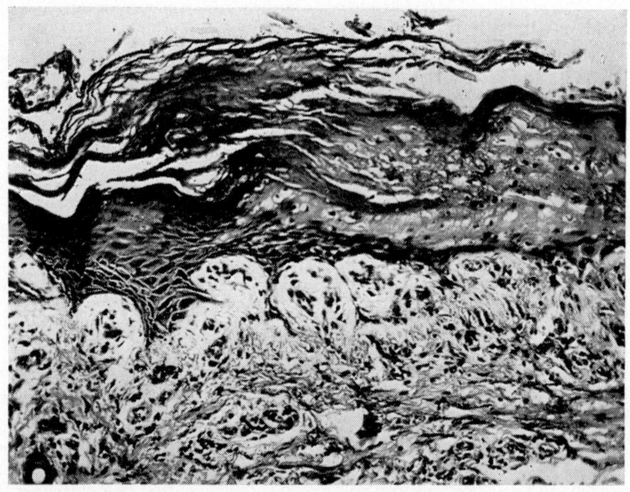

FIG. 87. Figure shows area in skin in which desquamation has taken place, with the separation of the superficial layer of the epidermis from the underlying tissue. The horny layer of the skin shows marked hyperkeratosis. There is deformity of the papillary layer of the skin.

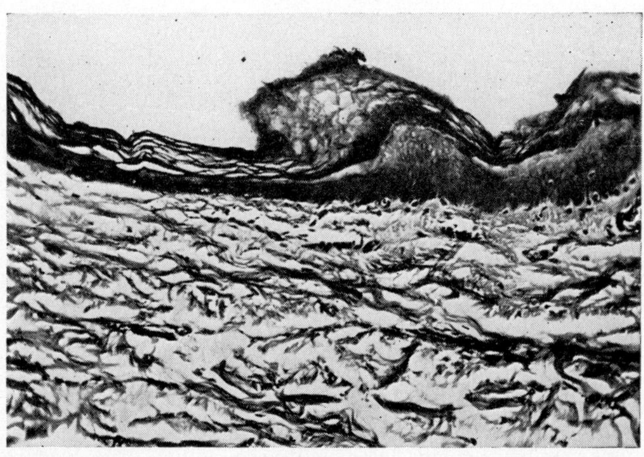

FIG. 88. This figure shows the same changes as in Fig. 87 in the superficial layer of the skin, with areas of hyperkeratosis and formatioin the skin, with the exception of the superficia has not yet become detached from the underlying skin. There is extensive atrophy of all layers in the skin, with the exception of the superficial horny area. Edema may be seen in the interstitial areas of the subcutaneous tissue, and there is atrophy of the glandular elements.

children in for examination, but Mrs. Z. refused to let them come because she thought we might "experiment on them." A few days later we visited the home to obtain a dietary history and find out something of the family background. While there, we noticed an emaciated, dejected looking dog, its head hanging low, saliva drooling from its mouth, and so weak that it could not stand up. Mr. Z. said it had been having diarrhea for several days. Examination of the mouth showed redness along the gum margins and the back of the tongue, and ulcerated areas which were sharply demarcated from the surrounding zones of healthy tissue. The ulcers were filled with Vincent's organisms. The cat also appeared sluggish and apathetic. It made no effort to move when touched and offered no resistance when an examination of the oral cavity was made. Thick, foul smelling saliva drooled from its mouth; there was an ulcerated reddish margin in the upper part of the palate close to the midline, and the tongue was very red over the terminal portion. Mr. Z. said both animals "got to feeling bad like that every year." They both lived on scraps from the family's meals. The dog was given 50 mg. nicotinic acid three times a day, and the cat, 40 mg. three times a day for two days. At the end of forty-eight hours, they had both improved remarkably.

Mrs. Z. was so impressed by what seemed to her the magic recovery of the dog and cat that she agreed to let Mr. Z. bring the children to the clinic. Examinations showed that the two youngest children had cheilosis and injection of the conjunctivae, lesions characteristic of riboflavin deficiency. Pellagrous glossitis and stomatitis were present in all the children but were more severe in the oldest child who also had the typical erythematous dermal lesions of pellagra on her hands and ankles. The father said they had had intermittent diarrhea for the past month. All the children cried when one touched their legs, but the four-year-old child's legs hurt her so much that she cried almost constantly and screamed when she thought anyone was going to touch them.

RESPONSE TO ORAL TREATMENT

We gave Mrs. Z. 2 mg. of riboflavin three times a day which, in a few days, healed not only her lesions but those of the breast-fed infant. We then gave her nicotinic acid, in doses of 50 mg. ten times daily, and her diarrhea as well as the diarrhea of the infant ceased. Within two days following the administration of 1000 mg. nicotinic acid, her mental symptoms had disappeared, her appetite improved, and she became strong enough to stay up most of the day. The burning in her feet and cramping in her legs and feet continued until she was given intravenous injections, 10 mg. each, of thiamine daily for three days.

Mr. Z. was given 50 mg. of nicotinic acid four times a day, and the following day he felt strong enough to do his farm work again. Soon after this, he obtained part-time work in a nearby mine and was able to provide a better diet for the family.

The children were treated individually, each child being given specific vitamin therapy for his outstanding deficiency disease. The oldest child, who had the dermal lesions, stomatitis and glossitis of pellagra, was given nicotinic acid amide, 50 mg. three times a day, for four days. The four-year-old, who had the severe thiamine deficiency, was given thiamine, 5 mg. three times a day, for a week, and the two-year-old, in whom the riboflavin deficiency was most severe, was given riboflavin, 2 mg. twice daily, for a week. As has been pointed out, the breast-fed infant was treated by giving the mother appropriate therapy. In each case, the symptoms for which these substances are specific improved rapidly. After the father was able to provide an improved diet, all their other symptoms disappeared slowly.

In all the members of the family who were given nicotinic acid, the B.E.S. test on their urine, which had been positive before treatment, became negative following therapy with nicotinic acid. An interesting observation was that while pellagra in man and blacktongue in animals respond to the same therapy, urine from the dog with blacktongue did not give a positive B.E.S. test.

Mrs. Z. improved remarkably following treatment and soon began to do her own housework again. Her diet did not improve, however, for although Mr. Z. was earning a little money she gave the additional food it provided to her husband and children while she continued to eat much the same food she had had all winter, except that her appetite improved and she ate more. She was kept under observation by weekly visits to the clinic and frequent visits to her home. Three weeks from the time treatment was discontinued, she began to complain of extreme nervousness, insomnia, irritability, difficulty in walking and pain in her abdomen. She became progressively worse until, at the end of four weeks, she was so weak she was unable to take more than a few steps. We had observed these symptoms in other patients who had been treated with nicotinic acid, riboflavin and thiamine, but who continued to eat their customary inadequate diets and had obtained a beneficial response to pyridoxine. Accordingly, Mrs. Z. was given 50 mg. of pyridoxine, in sterile physiologic solution of sodium chloride, intravenously, and within twenty-four hours her symptoms had disappeared and her strength had increased so much that she walked well. She was urged to eat a more varied and liberal diet and has, to a certain extent, done so. When she was last seen, two months after treatment, she felt well.

Summary of Family and Case History

Observations of such persons over a long period of time has convinced the authors that the onset of various deficiency diseases is slow, insidious and difficult to recognize. Long before nutritional failure has developed to a degree where one can diagnose beriberi, pellagra, riboflavin deficiency, scurvy or other well-defined syndromes, the persons have had months and years of ill health characterized by many vague symptoms and inability to work. The rapidity of the response to therapy is astounding and leaves no doubt that the tissues which contain insufficient amounts of these chemical substances are allowed to function at a higher and more normal level as soon as they are supplied. This case and others like it indicate that such persons, when studied over a long period of time, have malnutrition with many vitamin deficiency diseases rather than a single clinical entity. The whole matter is very complex, and the presentation of today must be greatly altered because of the extraordinary speed with which new discoveries are being made. The most notable advances are resulting from the collaboration of biologists, chemists, physiologists and clinicians, and as can be seen in this attempt at study, we have tried to intensify this cooperative effort. With all this available information coming from a large group of recognized specialists and advisors in the field, we suspect there is much more to learn than we have learned about Mrs. Z. and her family. Yet Mrs. Z. and her family are representative of a large group of persons who present themselves to the practising physician, and he with all his manifold duties and lack of trained specialists to assist him is expected to understand the numerous ramifications of their disease.

For 20 years we have observed from time to time the Z. family and their progeny. We have been impressed with the over-all improvement in the general physical and mental well-being of the parents. Even more impressive is the change for the better in outlook and physical and mental well-being of the children. During this period of time the children have matured and some of them now have children and homes of their own. It is interesting to see the over-all improvement in this new generation of children relative to the generation which we studied and described above.

THE TREATMENT OF DIETARY DEFICIENCY DISEASES

In the preceding sections we have seen that the common dietary deficiency diseases arise from a simultaneous deficiency of many factors. We have described patients with mixed deficiencies and the resultant complex clinical manifestations. We have pointed out that improper diet is not the sole cause of dietary deficiency diseases, but that impaired absorption from the alimentary tract, failure of utilization by the tissues, and inadequate storage may be contributing factors. Frequently, increased metabolism due to rapid growth, hyperthyroidism, exercise, infectious diseases and pregnancy and lactation may predispose to the development of clinical deficiency states. We have stressed particularly that the problems presented by patients with deficiency diseases vary greatly from one to another, and that it is essential for the physician to give careful consideration to the problems presented by each patient and to prescribe the type of therapy best suited to his needs. The following general principles of therapy, however, are applicable for all deficiency diseases: (1) the administration of a well-balanced, high protein diet, (2) the administration of specific therapeutic agents as supplements to the diet, (3) the elimination of coexisting conditions causing excess requirement for the vitamins, (4) symptomatic treatment.

General Management

The object of treatment is to restore the patient to health as quickly as possible and to prevent recurrences. Whether the most prominent clinical syndrome arises from a lack of the water-soluble or fat-soluble vitamins, or both, a deficiency of many of the essential nutrients is likely to exist, even though symptoms are not apparent. The therapeutic agents prescribed depend upon the symptoms presented by each case under consideration, but of prime importance in every case are the ingestion and retention of a diet which will meet the body's requirements for calories, protein, minerals and vitamins. The diet must be one that the patient can eat, digest and assimilate. It must be remembered, however, that complete reliance on dietary therapy is inadvisable as well as impractical. In the first place, deprivation of these substances may have existed for years and consequently the deficiency is advanced. Many of the nutrients are present in foods in only trivial amounts and it is impossible for the patient to eat enough food to supply the amount necessary to restore his health quickly. Even the most carefully planned diets offer only slightly above the daily maintenance requirement of certain vitamins, and recovery from a nutritional deficiency is usually retarded if one depends only upon the vitamins supplied in food. The indications and limitations of dietetic measures in general will be discussed in detail under the section on dietotherapy. The advances in our knowledge of dietary therapy during the past few years have been spectacular and far-reaching in their importance to human nutrition.

The more accurate the initial diagnosis of a deficiency of one or more of the water-soluble or fat-soluble vitamins, or any combination of them, the more likely is the physician to avoid futile treatment with unnecessary preparations. Where the diagnosis is clear-cut, the problem is one of administering adequate amounts of the deficient substance or substances in a way that will insure satisfactory utilization. The amount necessary varies considerably from one patient to another and even in the same patient at different times. Since the minimal, maximal and optimal doses of the specific therapeutic agents are not known, no definite routine of treatment can be followed satisfactorily. It is better to prescribe too much than too little, too soon rather than too late. Irrespective of whether the manifestations of deficiency disease are mild or severe, the patient should have rest until convalescence is well established. It is advisable to hospitalize the more severely ill patients in order that they be under constant supervision of physician, nurse and dietitian. Every possible effort must be made to eliminate the conditions which give rise to the disease. Where there is defective absorption or poor utilization, therapeutic substances should be administered parenterally to assure immediate availability in the systemic circulation. Patients with increased requirement should be given additional amounts of the materials to meet the increased demand. In all cases, the proper utilization of the required amount of the essential vitamin or vitamins is necessary for the cure of deficiency diseases. Failing in that, all therapy fails.

The Proper Use of Vitamins in Mixtures

It is apparent from the previous chapters that prolonged deprivation of vitamins produces a variety of diseases. The symptoms associated with these diseases are seldom well-defined and rarely appear uncomplicated. The resulting clinical picture is a complex one, and the physician frequently recognizes a number of distinct deficiency diseases in the same patient. While the functions of the individual vitamins, whether members of the fat-soluble or the water-soluble group, vary, they do tend to occur together in nature to some extent, and they are used customarily for therapeutic purposes as mixtures in the form of such preparations as cod liver oil, oleum percomorphum, yeast, liver extract, wheat germ, etc. Vitamin mixtures, whether natural or artificial, should not supplant all preventive and therapeutic measures but should supplement them.

We all deplore polypharmacy and the so-called "shotgun" prescriptions, given in the hope that if one ingredient doesn't hit, another will. Our studies have shown that there is considerable logic, however, in including some of the vitamins together. The patients fare much better when diseases are treated simultaneously, and the physician is not confused by the necessity of prescribing six or seven different preparations. Our clinical experience during the past thirty years in the treatment of many thousands of patients with deficiency diseases has shown that convalescence is delayed when one gives only one vitamin at a time in contrast to giving a number at once.

Spies, Stone, Garcia Lopez, Lopez Toca and Reboredo summarized the therapeutic indications for vitamins in mixtures and stressed the principles in the treatment of nutritive failure based on their own work as follows:

"By nutritive failure we mean a clinical condition which connotes the failure of an adequate supply of specific nutrients. It would appear that all tissues, and indeed all living things, require these nutrients for their normal functioning. As they function in our tissues, these vitamins are important in aiding the processes of repair so that those of decay may be overcome or retarded. Persons whose eating habits are poor are apt to have trouble. The burdens of motherhood and of hard labor increase the need for these materials, and thus predispose to critical shortages. In the practice of medicine, mixed vitamin therapy has a definite, well earned and useful place.

"How to use the vitamins to replenish the tissues is the physician's problem. We know these nutrients must be supplied to the body from the outside. If he has made a precise diagnosis and prescribed judicially, even a short, intensive period of therapy will convince the most skeptical physician. It is our observation that large doses of materials should be prescribed at first, and that they should be prescribed by mouth, unless, for some reason, parenteral administration is necessary, as it sometimes is. Certainly the patient with pernicious anemia can be more surely protected if vitamin B_{12} is administered by injection rather than by mouth.

"A freshly prepared sterile solution containing 15 micrograms of vitamin B_{12} concentrate and 5 mg. of folic acid in distilled water has been administered intramuscularly daily for ten days to each of five patients with the following types of anemia in relapse: pernicious anemia with acute neural degeneration, nutritional macrocytic anemia, the macrocytic anemia of pregnancy, the macrocytic anemia of tropical sprue and the megaloblastic anemia of infancy. In each instance there was a prompt hemopoietic and clinical response. Except in the macrocytic anemia of pregnancy this response could have been produced by either the vitamin B_{12} or the folic acid in the preparation.

"It has been shown repeatedly, however, that the macrocytic anemia of pregnancy is not relieved by vitamin B_{12} so that the response of the patients with this type of anemia should be attributed to the folic acid. The preparation was effective in relieving the symptoms arising from the nerve degeneration and the acute glossitis of pernicious anemia. Since it has been shown that such symptoms cannot be relieved by folic acid, their relief obviously was effected by the vitamin B_{12}.

"Since 1945 we have been administering folic acid to patients with pernicious anemia and, since 1946, when we started a large series of patients on folic acid, a total of eighty patients has had folic acid for four or five years in doses ranging from 1 to 10 mg. each day. They also have had frequent injections of either liver extract or vitamin B_{12}, or both. None of these patients has developed neural degeneration, thus indicating that in the presence of vitamin B_{12} or substances containing vitamin B_{12}, such as refined liver extract, folic acid has in no way adversely affected the nerve tissue. It is well known that neural degeneration is an integral part of the pernicious anemia syndrome and that folic acid will not prevent its occurrence. It also has been demonstrated conclusively by our group and by other investigators that folic acid and vitamin B_{12} are essential in the treatment of certain types of anemia. They occur together in liver and some other natural foods, and it is well to prescribe them together in suitable doses. All patients with pernicious anemia should have parenteral injections of either vitamin B_{12} or liver extract. It is likely that liver extract and yeast contain many important nutrients not now identified.

"We have stressed that vitamin therapy alone is not sufficient. The vitamins, however necessary, cannot take the place of a well balanced diet in restoring the tissues of a malnourished person. In the present practice of medicine the newer vitamins, which we have discussed at some length, play a most important role in blood-building. These vitamins, folic acid, vitamin B_{12} and its family, and the citrovorum factor, should be considered as nutritional factors as well as antianemic substances. The four principles of therapy which we have used so successfully in the rehabilitation of persons with various types of nutritional failure are:

1. Conditions causing excessive requirements for nutrients were removed or relieved whenever possible.
2. Symptomatic treatment and treatment for coexisting diseases were given.
3. It was made certain that the patient daily ate a diet which supplied 3000 to 4000 calories, 120 to 150 gm. of protein, and liberal amounts of minerals and vitamins.
4. Therapeutic substances, such as dried brewers' yeast powder, liver extract, or vitamins in the form of synthetic substances, were administered in sufficient amounts to correct the deficiency.

"It cannot be expected that these four principles will be effective if the diagnosis is not precise or if they are not applied persistently."

Summary of Treatment

We owe much of our freedom from infectious diseases to those who have applied effective control measures on a wide scale. Unfortunately, many of those working in the interest of public health attempt to apply the same formula to the problem of eradicating deficiency diseases as they apply to preventing infectious diseases. It is hoped that they will soon reach the point of view that vitamins are necessary to the body and that they tend gradually to be lost from it, whereas pathogenic micro-organisms are foreign to the body and tend to multiply in it. It is vain to hope that attempts to prevent and treat deficiency diseases will be very successful until the general health of the people is considered rather than the eradication of a single deficiency disease.

The problem of increasing the well-being of all people by means of better diet depends upon the continued collaborative effort of physicians, nutritionists and groups concerned primarily with public health. Each must share in the responsibility of teaching the public the importance of good nutrition and the simple dietary rules for achieving it. The physician and nutritionist can aid by supporting important changes, such as the enrichment of flour with vitamins, fortification of oleomargarine with vitamin A, and the dissemination of a good grade of dried brewers yeast and peanut butter mixture where indicated.

Without the full support of the physician, prevention and treatment of deficiency diseases are impossible. He not only is of aid in supporting the measures directed toward improving the nutrition of the whole population and in making specific recommendations in his own community, but he, more than any other, can assess the dietaries of persons in general. By recognizing malnutrition in the early stages, he can prevent years of illness. He and he alone can tell in any specific case whether a deficiency disease is likely to develop because of an inadequate diet or because of the presence of a disease which may interfere with proper nutrition.

The means of treating deficiency diseases at the disposal of the physician today are so great that all the therapeutic preparations available cannot even be catalogued. The physician and the patient naturally wish to use the simplest, cheapest, most effective and most easily administered therapy, but the wealth of effective compounds makes it impossible to be didactic in the choice of a therapeutic agent. Treatment must be adapted to the individual case. Accordingly, we have indicated only in general the principles of treatment, the management of the patient, the indications for the various types of therapy and the judicious use of vitamin mixtures.

Diagnosis must be stressed as the foundation upon which to build proper vitamin therapy. It is not uncommon for a patient with ill-defined symptoms arising from a deficiency of vitamins to undergo many tests and to seek advice from many physicians before a diagnosis is made and effective treatment is applied. Such cases are often said to be atypical and rare, whereas our experience has shown that they are far more common than the "textbook picture." We have found it wise to make a tentative diagnosis based on careful study of the patient and to verify or disprove it by subsequent effort. The reduction in morbidity and mortality among persons with deficiency diseases proves that modern therapy is effective in saving lives, but it is also altering and improving the practice of medicine and nursing, as well as reducing the time the patient spends in the hospital, the cost of his treatment, the length of his convalescence and, thus, the time he loses from work.

RECAPITULATION

In the preceding text an effort has been made to describe a scientific basis for coordinating action in effecting better nutrition of the people. In order to have good health, the factors which operate to disturb the balance of the vitamins in the tissues must be equalized or overcome by factors which operate to maintain it. The most frequent cause of nutritional deficiency disease is a decreased intake of vitamins, though many persons develop deficiency diseases because of faulty assimilation or because of an abnormally high requirement. Excessive exercise precipitates clinical manifestations of deficiency diseases, and acute infections and fever place a still greater demand for vitamins upon the body. The homeostatic equilibrium is preserved in many ways. Long before the etiology of deficiency diseases was in any way understood, rest was advocated as a good method of treatment for the disease. The processes carry on for the benefit of some organs at the expense of others, but the maintenance of equilibrium becomes more and more difficult as the stores of these substances are depleted so that eventually they must be replenished. We have seen how these various deficiency diseases are characterized by a great diversity of disturbances. It is clear now that scientists in the past have placed too narrow significance on the role of the vitamins in the general physiologic processes. It would be far wiser to consider that all tissues need the vitamins for performance of their natural functions and that certain tissues, perhaps because they are more highly organized and more delicately balanced so far as specific requirement is concerned, become sufficiently altered after long deprivation as to give rise to clinical signs. For reasons which we do not fully comprehend at present, these clinical signs, which are most conspicuous in the late stages of deficiency diseases, arise predominantly from certain systems of the body.

The confusing and contradictory state of our present knowledge is due in the main to the fact that what we once supposed to be a single substance and glibly termed vitamin B, has turned out to be some fifteen separate entities. It would be stupid to suppose that we have safely passed all these pitfalls. The self-respecting physician will justifiably extend his clinical experimentation with the vitamins, for they appear harmless, but he should wisely exercise the greatest skepticism regarding how much may be attributed to their therapeutic effect. We have noted particularly that clinical deficiency diseases can be corrected by therapy directed along three lines: (1) the administration of the substances in adequate amounts to correct the deficiencies, (2) the elimination of conditions necessitating excess requirement for the vitamins, (3) the treatment of coexisting diseases. Although a dramatic therapeutic response follows the administration of synthetic vitamins, they cannot replace a well balanced diet and should be recommended as supplements to the diet of persons with nutritional deficiency diseases only until an adequate and well balanced diet can be procured.

The science of nutrition is making advances each year. Vitamins should not be regarded as curiosities of long-haired research workers but should be considered matters of life and death to every individual and to all nations. The life-giving substances come, directly or indirectly, from the soil. Primitive man had the advantage of natural whole foods, whereas comparatively few people today live on natural foods. The vitamins are often lessened or lost in the harvesting, the distribution, the processing and the cooking; hence, tradition and food habits are not safe guides to the selection of foods.

People must be properly fed if the best is to be expected of them. Through plant and animal life the vitamins come from the soil and on decay they or their constituents must return to the soil, with the result, it seems, that the vitamin content of the soil might affect the vitamin content of the growing plant, which in turn would affect the animal or man feeding on the plant. It is appalling that agricultural people who should "feast on the fruits of the earth" should be suffering from protracted vitamin deficiencies.

References

Annual Review of Biochemistry, Vol. IX, 1940.

Annual Review of Physiology, Vol. II, 1940.

Cowgill, G. R.: The Vitamin B Requirement of Man. New Haven, Yale University Press, 1934.

Food and Life (Yearbook of Agriculture). United States Department of Agriculture, 1939.

Matthews, A. P.: Physiological Chemistry. Baltimore, The Williams and Wilkins Company, 1939.

McLester, J. S. and Darby, W. J.: Nutrition and Diet in Health and Disease. Philadelphia, W. B. Saunders Company, Ed. 6, 1952.

Modern Medical Therapy in General Practice (Edited by Dr. D. P. Barr), Section on Deficiency Diseases. Baltimore, The Williams and Wilkins Company, 1940.

The Vitamins, Published by the American Medical Association, under the auspices of the Council on Pharmacy and Chemistry and the Council on Foods, 1939.

Williams, R. R. and Spies, T. D.: Vitamin B_1 and Its Use in Medicine. New York, The Macmillan Company, 1938.

CHAPTER 7

By ANCEL KEYS, PH.D.

Undernutrition

GENERAL CONSIDERATIONS

Theoretically, the number of varieties of undernutrition is as great as the number of possible permutations and combinations of deficiencies of essential nutrients. Since the human body must obtain from food at least 35 different amino acids, minerals and vitamins besides calories, "essential" fatty acid and a minimal amount of carbohydrate, so the number of possible combinations of deficiencies of individual nutrients is of astronomical order. Considering 10 amino acids alone, all other nutrients being in adequate supply, there could be, theoretically, 1024 deficiency disorders. Add only combinations with deficiencies of calories or one essential amino acid, making 12 nutrients in all, and there are conceivably 4096 kinds of deficiency in nutrients. Now add all combinations with one or more of only 2 or 3 vitamins . . . and consider that there are still some 18 more vitamins and 10 minerals . . . !

Fortunately, only very few foods are limited to single chemical entities. Sugar and corn starch provide only carbohydrate (and calories), table salt provides only sodium and chlorine, refined oils provide linoleic acid (i.e. "essential" fatty acid) and fat calories, but practically all other foods are mixtures of many nutrients. Moreover, besides the fact that people eat foods, not nutrients, they tend to eat groups of foods as dietary constellations and eat a considerable number of kinds of foods, even on the most monotonous diets. As a result, only a minute fraction of all conceivable nutritional deficiencies have any significant statistical probability of representation in man and fewer still occur often enough to be recognizable.

Nutritional deficiencies, like nutrients, generally occur in constellations. Even the classic vitamin and mineral deficiencies probably involve a multiplicity of nutrients. Beriberi, scurvy and pellagra may be dominated by thiamine, ascorbic acid and nicotinic acid or tryptophane deficiencies, respectively, but we doubt that these classic deficiency diseases represent *only* deficiencies of the corresponding vitamins.

Broadly, human undernutrition may be classified as starvation (calorie deficiency), avitaminoses, protein or amino acid deficiency and mineral deficiency. Elsewhere in this book there are discussions of protein metabolism and deficiency (Chapter 1), avitaminoses (Chapter 6) and mineral deficiencies (Chapter 4). The present chapter deals with starvation and general undernutrition in which calorie deficiency is a major factor in producing the disability and disease picture.

General undernutrition is probably the most common metabolic abnormality or defect in hospital patients everywhere and in the entire populations of many parts of the world. By general undernutrition we mean a condition in which there is no dominant single nutrient deficiency except that of calories. Frequently, general undernutrition tends to involve primary or secondary protein deficiency. Subordinate deficiencies of other nutrients—notably water-soluble vitamins and iron—are not infrequent. General undernutrition arises because ordinary foods have been supplied in insufficient amount or because the major nutrients in them have been denied to the tissues by faulty digestion or absorption, vomiting or faults in the tissues themselves.

Almost every serious illness or injury tends to produce general undernutrition by interfering with appetite or assimilation of food, by increasing catabolism, or both. Moreover, in the United States, where food is abundant, every community has its quota of semistarvation among recluses, psychoneurotics and cases of anorexia nervosa. Finally, it should be observed that war invariably produces starvation and that the modern complexity of food production and distribution makes for increasing vulnerability of the populations, both civilian and military, which are dependent on the orderly operation of this complexity. These arguments for the importance of general undernutrition need emphasis because concentration on the developments in the fields of the vitamins and minerals and on the prevalence of obesity leads to neglect of the more homely problems of inadequate calories.

THE CAUSES OF GENERAL UNDERNUTRITION

Historically, by far the most common cause of general undernutrition is simple inability to obtain food. This situation is still lamentably common in many parts of Asia, Latin America and Africa and becomes common in other parts of the world in time of war or political chaos. In the United States a political or economic basis for general undernutrition is rare indeed, but the condition itself, that is, undernutrition, has other origins. The factors which can produce undernutrition are very numerous. The summary of these factors given in previous editions of this book continues to be inclusive and is reproduced here as Table 1 (p. 503).

Ordinarily, the appetite does an amazing job of regulating the calorie intake to match the requirements of the body, but the incidence of imperfection in this regulation is not small, as is evident from the frequency with which we see excessively thin or fat people who appear to be normal otherwise. Appetite regulation has recently been ascribed to the "appestat," a physiologic mechanism, or complex of mechanisms, which adjusts to the correct demands of the body. But psychologic interference with the effective operation of this appestat is common and may almost completely inactivate it as a purely physiologic mechanism. When there is severe appetite failure without discoverable physical basis it is customary to speak of anorexia nervosa. It might be suggested that "anorexia idiopathica" would be a better term, but the designation "nervosa" has a long history of use and some other justifications. The fact is that in many of these patients it is readily possible to discern a psychologic or "nervous" basis which is of real importance in treatment and it may be suspected that such psychologic factors are involved but are not revealed in other patients. But the physical changes in anorexia nervosa are the same as seen in starvation from other causes.[4,5]

It is probable that only a very small percentage of persons afflicted with anorexia nervosa ever receive that designation. The majority do not seek medical advice or, if they do, they may not complain of lack of appetite. The usual patient with anorexia nervosa reaches a physician only under family compulsion or personally seeks help because of the effects of starvation on strength or other functions, including personal appearance.

Appetite failure from disease of the pituitary gland or hypophysis may be difficult to differentiate from anorexia nervosa, and the resulting emaciation is similar. Simmonds' disease, or hypophyseal cachexia, has a voluminous literature,[26] but is by no means common. Sheehan's disease[77,78] is apparently still more rare; it involves necrosis of the pituitary gland. In both of these conditions the presenting complaint is usually appetite failure and emaciation. The precise mechanism of interference with appetite is unknown in these diseases; indeed the general mechanism of appetite regulation is still shrouded in obscurity.

Appetite failure may be induced by malnutrition, particularly by thiamine deficiency. A diet really devoid of thiamine produces severe anorexia, usually accompanied by nausea. Anorexia is so prominent after a few weeks on a diet which is very markedly deficient in thiamine that caloric and protein deficiencies—that is, general undernutrition—readily develop. But it is unjustifiable to assume, therefore, that thiamine deficiency explains more than a minute fraction of the cases when anorexia is a complaint or is obviously involved. Actually, in the great majority of patients of all types in whom appetite is depressed, the administration of thiamine has no effect whatever.

Appetite failure of some degree is commonly produced by a great variety of diseases and injuries, and it is probable that most patients who have been seriously ill for more than a few days are undernourished for this reason. Such a temporary state of negative caloric balance should occasion no concern for many patients and, indeed, may be beneficial. At least there is no theoretical reason why a brief departure from exact calorie equilibrium is undesirable in previously well-nourished persons. Natural selection in human evolution has resulted in a very considerable margin of safety which assures homeostasis to the cells in the face of calorie deficits or excesses of the order of a thousand calories a day for some days or even weeks. In obese people the physiologic tolerance of calorie deficiency is proportionately greater.

Besides appetite failure, another reason why general undernutrition is so common in hospitals is the fact that many diseases and injuries result in elevated nutritional requirements. This may result from increased energy dissipation, as in fever or restlessness, or from decreased energy intake, as in anorexia nervosa, or from poor food energy absorption, as in dysentery and

TABLE 1. FACTORS WHICH CAN PRODUCE UNDERNUTRITION

A. *By Interference with Food Consumption*
   1. Impaired appetite—infectious disease, cardiac disease, surgery and anesthesia, pain and drugs used in its treatment, thiamine deficiency, alcohol
   2. Gastrointestinal disease—peptic ulcer, diarrheas, biliary and liver disease, acute gastroenteritis, obstructive lesions
   3. Traumatic and neurologic disorders interfering with self-feeding
   4. Neuropsychiatric disorders—neurosis, psychosis, migraine
   5. Oral disease—sore mouth, loss of teeth, painful dentures
   6. Pregnancy anorexia and vomiting
   7. Food allergy
   8. Therapy—drugs which cause anorexia, diet restricting essential foods

B. *By Increasing Destruction*
   1. In gastrointestinal tract—achlorhydria, alkali therapy
   2. After absorption—heavy metals, trinitrotoluene, sulfonamides

C. *By Interference with Absorption*
   1. Absence of normal digestive secretions—achlorhydria, obstructive jaundice, pancreatic achylia, gastric resection
   2. Intestinal hypermotility—ulcerative colitis, bacillary and amebic dysentery, other diarrheal diseases
   3. Reduction of effective absorbing surface—intestinal resections, short-circuiting operations, small bowel disease
   4. Impairment of intrinsic mechanism of absorption—sprue, vitamin deficiencies
   5. Drugs preventing absorption—mineral oil, drastic cathartics, colloidal absorbents

D. *By Interfering with Utilization or Storage*
   1. Impaired liver function—in hepatitis, cirrhosis, uncontrolled diabetes, alcoholism
   2. Hypothyroidism
   3. Neoplasm of gastrointestinal tract
   4. Therapy—sulfonamide, roentgen therapy

E. *By Increasing Excretion or Loss*
   1. Lactation
   2. Loss in serous exudates, as in severe burns
   3. Glycosuria and albuminuria
   4. Acute or chronic blood loss

F. *By Increasing Nutritive Requirements*
   1. Increased physical activity—strenuous exertion, delirium, certain psychoses
   2. Periods of rapid growth
   3. Pregnancy and lactation
   4. Fever
   5. Hyperthyroidism
   6. Treatment—thyroid medication, fever therapy, high carbohydrate diets, insulin, parenteral dextrose administration

other gastrointestinal disorders. The combination of appetite failure with increased calorie needs is common in hospital patients and, indeed, among all patients who exhibit marked and progressive emaciation. Both correction or inadequate intake and of excessive loss of calories should be considered in the treatment of all such patients.

The febrile patient uses energy at an excessive rate in basal metabolism and often accentuates his calorie needs further by physical restlessness. According to DuBois and others, a rise in body temperature of one degree Centigrade results in an increase of about 13 per cent in the basal metabolic rate (BMR). Accordingly, the average patient with a body temperature of 102° F. may be expected to have a BMR of about + 25 per cent if his BMR were exactly 100 per cent with a body temperature of 98.6° F. If the patient is restless and "toxic" as well, another 10 to 30 per cent of extra caloric needs will arise, so the result is that the febrile patient may have a requirement for calories of some 30 to 50 per cent above the expectation for a quiet, nonfebrile bed patient. A diet which does not allow for this fact will rapidly produce a state of undernutrition, of course.

Persistent proteinuria obviously requires an increased protein intake to maintain balance, as does injury resulting in large exudation and weeping from the surface of the body. The protein losses in the exudate from burned surfaces may reach tremendous amounts, frequently as much as 10 gm. a day and in some cases as much as 50 gm. a day. These direct losses, added to the pyrexia and anorexia often present, make it clear that burned patients may easily become seriously undernourished with regard to proteins and may have some added requirements for calories also. Similar factors operate in patterns with copiously draining infections. With all patients in whom excessive nitrogen loss is known or suspected, care must be taken to supply an abundance of calories as well as to provide more than usual amounts of proteins in the diet or by parenteral means. If the total calories supplied are deficient, some of the protein given to counteract the excessive loss of nitrogen or protein from the body will be burnt simply for calories.

One of the most frequent contributing causes to nutritional deficiency is diarrhea.[57] Normally, about 95 per cent of all the calories ingested are utilized by the body, but in sprue, ulcerative colitis, steatorrhea and the dysenteries there is great waste and even large intakes of food may be insufficient to prevent undernutrition. A vicious cycle can occur in severe cachexia and is often seen in famine victims in whom greater calorie deficiency, usually associated with protein deficiency as well, may produce copious and almost continuous diarrhea, sometimes bloody. The loss of nutrients in this way adds further to the calorie deficit. This phenomenon tends to be a late development in prolonged starvation and carries a bad prognosis. Examination of the intestines in such patients reveals such advanced atrophy of the mucosa that this alone might suffice to explain the diarrhea.[35] Vitamin deficiency has been suggested as a cause, but vitamin administration was without effect in famine victims.[52,85]

Mechanical interference with the ingestion or digestion of food is, of course, a frequent cause of undernutrition in surgical patients. Some of the most obvious cases of starvation seen in hospitals are patients with esophageal stricture and with neoplasms of the gastrointestinal tract. The prevention of general undernutrition is often a problem in patients who have undergone subtotal gastrectomy for peptic ulcer. Edentulous patients or persons who have oral disease such as Vincent's angina have problems of eating which can lead to general undernutrition or to specific deficiencies.

Finally, among the causes of general undernutrition, mention must be made of the catabolic phase of metabolism in severe injury or illness. Though the mechanism remains obscure as yet, it seems clear that many diseases and apparently all serious injuries tend to produce a state in which, for a time at least, there is a great tendency to negative nitrogen balance, even though the calorie and protein intakes seem reasonably good. The resulting protein deficiency may produce anorexia, and general undernutrition may ensue.

The influence of the state of the water balance on the recognition and evaluation of general undernutrition must be mentioned here to emphasize that edema may mask an underlying serious degree of emaciation and that dehydration may produce a picture superficially resembling that resulting from serious calorie shortage. These factors must be ruled out before deciding that the state of calorie nutrition of a patient is actually good or that a cause for apparent emaciation must be sought in the calorie intake or loss.

THE PICTURE OF UNDERNUTRITION

Serious states of undernutrition are easily recognized, unless there is massive edema, by the low body weight and by the signs of emaciation—prominent cheekbones and ribs, "winged" scapulae, deep suprasternal notch, sharply outlined pelvis and generally "bony" appearance. In the presence of edema, both general appearance and body weight are misleading so that the extent of undernutrition is not easily appreciated, but if the patient can be kept seated upright for several hours the underlying emaciation will become visible in the upper part of the body and the face.

The body weight is an obvious guide which is, however, of limited value unless the patient's previous "normal" weight is known and there is no, or at least no great amount of, edema. A simple and perhaps more reliable indicator of the extent of undernutrition is the thickness of the skin folds on the trunk and on the backs of the upper arms. A little experience with normally nourished people will allow a rough estimate of the degree of wasting if it is realized that the thickness of the skin fold is contributed mainly by subcutaneous fat[9] and that differences in the thickness of skin folds are direct measures of fatness.[8a]

The presence of unexplained edema is in itself an indicator of undernutrition which will be discussed below. Other characteristics associated with starvation may be confused by the presence of concurrent disease, but the picture of uncomplicated severe undernutrition includes hypotension, bradycardia, pallor, weakness, apathy and depression. The skin is dry, cold and "dead" to the touch. Folliculosis and "permanent goose flesh" may be evident, especially on the thighs and the backs of the upper arms. A patchy, dirty-appearing pigmentation is not uncommon. Faint cyanosis is common in the lips and nail beds, especially in cold weather. The body temperature is usually subnormal.

In simple starvation the mind is clear until near extremis and there is no loss of visual or auditory acuity. An impression of mental dullness and stupidity may be given, however, by apathy and reluctance to engage in any activity, including talking, and indifference to personal appearance and cleanliness. In contrast to the loss in strength, coordination for small movements is usually not greatly diminished. Fainting and giddiness on suddenly arising or on prolonged standing are common, but syncope is usually only momentary. Tendon reflexes tend to be diminished or absent. If major sensory or neurologic disturbances are observed in the cachectic patient, the cause for these should be sought elsewhere than in the simple cachexia itself.

LABORATORY FINDINGS IN UNDERNUTRITION

Knowledge of the laboratory findings in uncomplicated undernutrition helps to understand the picture presented by the patient in whom starvation is secondary or is associated with other disease or injury. The blood chemistry is not remarkable, though the blood sugar and serum cholesterol values tend to be low. The plasma or serum protein concentration is usually only slightly low

TABLE 2. THE PLASMA PROTEINS

Before and After Six Months of Severe Undernutrition, as Determined by Electrophoresis in Two Typical Young Men. "Conc." = Concentration in gm. per 100 ml. of Serum. "Total" = Total Circulating Protein in gm.*

ITEM	SUBJECT 122				SUBJECT 123			
	Conc.		Total		Conc.		Total	
	C	S 24	C	S 24	C	S 24	C	S 24
Total Prot.	6.89	6.88	189	220	6.99	6.16	214	210
Albumin	4.33	4.33	119	139	4.45	4.03	136	137
Glob. α_1	0.34	0.32	9	10	0.31	0.20	10	7
" α_2	0.58	0.67	16	22	0.53	0.46	16	16
" β	0.81	0.89	22	29	0.78	0.84	24	29
" γ	0.83	0.67	23	22	0.92	0.63	28	21

* Cf. Taylor, Mickelsen and Keys, 1949; Keys et al.,[48] 1950, Chap. 20.

unless there has been specific protein deficiency as well as general undernutrition. The hemoglobin, hematocrit and red cell count indicate moderate macrocytic anemia, while the white count merely shows an inconstant tendency toward leukopenia. The sedimentation rate is within the normal range. The urine is typically pale, clear and dilute. Departures from the foregoing picture are cause to look for complications or other associated disorders in addition to cachexia.

It is widely taught and believed that hypoproteinemia, generally with a reduced ratio of albumin to globulin, is the hallmark of starvation. Although this may be true in Oriental famine and in some diseases, including hepatic and renal disease, it is not the typical picture in European famine or in simple starvation.

In many studies in Europe, as well as in controlled laboratory experiments, the typical picture is one of only small changes in the plasma proteins. It is clear that the plasma proteins are relatively well maintained, both in concentration and in total circulating quantity, in simple undernutrition, at least for periods of many months. Representative findings on young men are given in Table 2.

In Table 2 it will be observed that not only concentrations, but also the total amounts of circulating proteins are well retained. In these same men, however, there was a considerable loss of tissue protein—of the order of 2 to 3 kg. per man—so it is obvious that the examination of the serum is not very revealing in such cases.

THE BASAL METABOLISM IN UNDERNUTRITION

One of the most constant and important facts in the starved person is a remarkably low basal metabolic rate (BMR). In terms of the usual standards, based on the oxygen consumption per square meter of body surface, the rate is from —10 to —50 per cent, most severely undernourished persons having rates of the order of —30 to —40 per cent. The basal metabolism per unit of body weight, however, is less severely depressed, and the rate per unit of calculated fat-free tissue is only slightly lowered. In other words, the rate of oxygen consumption per unit mass of surviving metabolizing tissue is not seriously reduced, but the total basal metabolism of the individual may be only half of the amount in the normal, prestarvation state.

TABLE 3. MEAN CHANGE IN BASAL METABOLIC RATE (BMR), EXPRESSED AS PERCENTAGE OF PRE-STARVATION VALUE, IN 32 YOUNG MEN SUBSISTING ON A EUROPEAN TYPE OF FAMINE DIET FOR 6 MONTHS

Δ Body Weight	−24.2%
Δ BMR, Cal./hr. per man	−38.9%
" " " " " kg. Wt.	−19.5%
" " " " " kg. "Cells"	−15.5%

(Data from Keys et al.[48])

These facts are illustrated in Table 3 for 32 men not previously overweight, who lost an average of 24.2 per cent of their body weight in a six-months experiment on a European type of famine diet. The decline in basal oxygen consumption per man of 38.9 per cent from the prestarvation level is much greater than would be expected from the change in body surface. The BMR per unit of body surface fell by an average of 31.3 per cent. When the results are expressed per unit of body weight the decline is less startling, but a fall of 19.5 per cent is still very substantial. Similar changes take place in famine victims.[2,89] In this series it was possible to estimate the "cells" mass or "active tissue" mass from body density and extracellular fluid measurements. The basal oxygen consumption per kg. of "cells," which fell by 15.5 per cent, is the best expression of the decline in fundamental metabolic activity induced by the undernutrition in these men.

TABLE 4. MEAN CHANGE IN BASAL METABOLIC RATE (BMR), EXPRESSED AS PERCENTAGE OF PRESTARVATION RATE FOR THE BODY AND PER KG. OF "CELLS," FOR SOLDIERS WORKING ON A DIET OF 1000 CAL. PER DAY WITH ZERO PROTEIN INTAKE

EXPT. YEAR	NO. OF MEN	DAYS ON DIET	% CHANGES		
			BODY WT., KG.	BMR PER MAN	BMR/KG "CELLS"
1954	13	24	−9.8%	−17.1%	−11.8%
1955	12	16	−8.4%	−21.3%	−16.6%

(From Grande, F., Anderson, J. T. and Keys, A.[34])

Similar changes result from shorter periods of time with greater daily calorie deficits, as is evident from Table 4. Detailed computations from all of these experiments show that most of the change in the BMR per unit mass of "cells" takes place by the time 10 per cent of the body weight is lost. The explanation seems to be that a large part of the total BMR is accounted for by the liver, and depression of the liver oxygen metabolism is an early response to undernutrition.[34]

X-RAY AND ELECTROCARDIOGRAPHIC FINDINGS

Typically, the only characteristic roentgenographic features of the starved person are a small heart and a stomach very low in the abdomen. Infrequently the picture of hunger osteopathology may be seen—spontaneous fractures and "pseudo fractures" of weight-bearing bones and areas of rarefaction and decalcification. Often, but not always, there are complaints of pain in these cases.

The electrocardiogram in starvation normally shows sinus bradycardia and small voltages in all deflections.[79] Nodal rhythm develops in a few instances. In basal rest the rate may be as low as 30 beats per minute, and even under less relaxed conditions the heart rate is frequently between 40 and 50 beats per minute.

EDEMA IN UNDERNUTRITION

Nutritional edema may be of either, or both, of two kinds.[48,49,80,82,89] Where there is protracted protein deficiency, the resulting decline in the concentration of proteins in the blood plasma is sufficient to produce the edema of hypoproteinemia; the colloid osmotic pressure is not enough to prevent a net differential filtration of blood water (and electrolytes) into the tissue spaces. Plasma protein concentrations of the order of 5 gm. or less per 100 cc., with low albumin/globulin ratios, are observed in this situation and the edema may be of any grade, including ascites and anasarca. In very severe cachexia, notably in moribund famine victims, it may be observed that the plasma protein concentration and the albumin/globulin ratio are very low, yet there is no edema.[1,52] These patients are usually in a state of severe dehydration, in some cases induced by persistent diarrhea. If rehydration can be accomplished, edema promptly appears.

On the other hand, simple calorie deficiency, which results when a European type of famine diet is used or when an ordinary diet is merely reduced in amount, does not produce marked hypoproteinemia, yet there is edema.[1,48,49,60] This edema is of the soft, dependent type and is rarely more than moderate in amount on clinical grading unless there are complicating factors. The edema fluid itself is very low in protein, and no peculiarity of capillary permeability is indicated. Finally, there are no signs of cardiac failure, and the venous pressure is unusually low in the typical patient.

The explanation of this true hunger edema, which is characteristic of prolonged subsistence on inadequate amounts of western, i.e., European and United States, diets, raises difficult questions. It should be noted, however, that this edema is remarkable in that it does not represent, as do other edemas, an excess *accumulation* of fluid but merely the retention of the prestarvation level of extracellular fluid. The tissues become "watery" because there is a diminution of cellular substance—fat and protein—and not an accretion of new fluid. Measurements of the thiocyanate space, for example, show this to be substantially unchanged in this type of undernutrition; only the *proportion* of this fluid to the total body mass changes radically. In a sense, then, there is no real edema problem at all, since it is unnecessary to suggest any altered fluid exchanges at the capillary wall. A tendency toward a small decrease in plasma colloid osmotic pressure is offset by a fall in intracapillary pressure so there is no net change.

In the ordinary sense, however, there is edema, and its magnitude may be estimated by the thiocyanate (SCN) space. In the well-nourished young man the SCN space represents about 23.5 per cent of the body weight. When such young men are severely starved and have lost a fourth of their original body weight, the SCN space represents 30 to 40 per cent of the body weight. One interesting finding in such studies is the fact that minimal clinical edema is not recorded until the proportion of body weight included in the SCN space is of the order of 30 per cent. In the average adult this means that some 10 to 15 pounds of "edema fluid" must be present before it can be discerned as "minimal pitting edema, grade I." A similar situation apparently exists in simple fasting; the SCN space tends to remain constant while the cellular mass shrinks.[84]

It is sometimes stated that hunger edema does not appear in anorexia nervosa. This is incorrect. Definite edema does indeed occur in this condition, though with less frequency than in famine victims.[5] The reason for the difference in incidence is probably the fact that anorexia nervosa patients are often almost as reluctant to drink water as they are to eat and thus tend to keep themselves relatively dehydrated.

CALORIE REQUIREMENTS

The Problem. Every dietary prescription and every analysis of a dietary history should start with an appraisal of the nutritional requirements of the individual, and this must be in quantitative terms to have any practical value. In the case of the vitamins and minerals it may be good enough to make sure only that the requirements, whatever they may be, are more than covered by the diet to be supplied. But this approach is worse than wasteful in the case of calories. It is certainly undesirable to force consumption of more food than is needed, and it is dangerous folly to suppose that obesity is tolerable while emaciation is not. For calories, at least, the problem of actual requirements must be faced.[44]

The first question is: What is meant by requirement? Requirement for what? The simplest answer is to define the calorie requirement as that intake which will just balance the energy expenditure. This is suitable for the adult patient who is already at the desired level of fatness, but it is by no means the answer for the thin or the fat patient; the provision of the balance requirement would simply perpetuate whatever fault of emaciation or obesity is already present.

In the present chapter we are concerned primarily with undernutrition, so the requirement question is directed in large part toward the prevention of undernutrition and the restoration of the undernourished person to a more nearly normal state. How much emaciation corresponds to or may result from a given low level of feeding? How much food should be supplied to rehabilitate a given emaciated person? The problem must be examined in its details for each individual, so no precise formulae can be given for general application. The items for consideration are discussed below. It must be emphasized, however, that even when all details are considered for an individual, the resulting estimate should be considered as only a rough guide for a dietary prescription which should be adjusted and corrected according to the results of subsistence on the diet.

Basal Metabolism. All estimations of calorie requirements must begin with the energy expenditure for balance, and the first item is the basal metabolism. For most patients, particularly those requiring hospitalization, the basal metabolic rate is the largest item of energy expenditure; fortunately, it may be measured easily. For relatively normal persons, the basal metabolism may be predicted from tables such as those of the Mayo Clinic.[6] Such estimates are entirely satisfactory for predicting the calorie requirements for the BMR portion of total expenditure by groups of people if a deduction of about 10 per cent is made.[42] But such average values are not reliable for individuals, even though they are well nourished; for undernourished persons the standard tables are grossly incorrect.

Where BMR measurements cannot be made, a crude estimate of the BMR is possible for persons who were formerly well nourished (but not fat) and who have lost much weight in the past year. From standard BMR tables, compute the normal 24-hour basal metabolism calories corresponding to the previous body weight and deduct 10 per cent. This yields an estimate of the 24-hour BMR for the person before he was undernourished. Now express the body weight loss as a percentage of the previous weight, multiply this by 1.5 and subtract the result from the BMR estimate. For example, consider a person weighing 120 pounds who weighed 150 pounds six months ago, at which time the tables indicate that his 24-hour BMR was 1500 Calories. The 10 per cent deduction yields 1350 Cal. as the estimated true basal metabolism prior to weight loss. But there has been a weight loss of 30 pounds or 20 per cent, and $1.5 \times 20 = 30$ per cent as the estimated reduction in basal metabolism. Then $0.30 \times 1350 = 405$, and $1350 - 405 = 945$ Cal.; this is the estimated 24-hour expenditure for basal metabolism at present.

Specific Dynamic Action. The processes of digestion and assimilation of food involve a special energy expenditure which is termed the specific dynamic action of food. This differs somewhat according to the character of the diet, but it is proportional to the amount of the diet. For most purposes it is accurate enough to allow 10 per cent of the dietary calories for specific dynamic action.[32,90] If the diet provides a total of 2000 Calories per day, there will be 200 Cal. devoted to specific dynamic action and 1800 Cal. will be available for all other purposes. It has long been known that feeding pure protein, carbohydrate or fat produces differing amounts of specific dynamic action, but many studies show that in mixed diets the proportions of these nutrients in the diet have very little effect on the total specific dynamic action.

Muscular Activity. Estimation of the energy requirement for muscular activity is particularly difficult because of the multitudinous muscular activities, many of them incapable of precise definition, which enter into the 24-hour total. Tables of the average estimated costs of various occupational activities are provided in textbooks of metabolism and nutrition, but these are highly unreliable for all individuals and particularly for undernourished patients. Some guidance may be afforded, however, by the fact that in many muscular activities the energy cost is proportional to the body weight; this is true because the cost of moving the body and its parts is a large part of the energy expenditure in many physical activities.[25,28]

Perhaps the most satisfactory way of discussing the cost of muscular activity is to express it as a multiple of the basal metabolic rate. In this way we may estimate that the cost of sleep, of sitting quietly reading or writing, and of walking slowly are, respectively, of the order of 0.9, 1.3 and 2.0 times the basal metabolic rate. The most severe forms of exercise, such as running up hill, may demand energy expenditure up to 10 or 15 times the BMR, but such efforts are possible only for the very fit young man and then only for brief spurts of activity. For the entire twenty-four hours, the cost of muscular activity is such that the total expenditure of healthy men at hard labor seldom exceeds 3 times the basal metabolism, and for men at light to moderate work the overall average is not far from 2 times the BMR. For sedentary persons—for example, office workers who have no hobbies or sports or other physical activities—an average of the order of 1.7 seems to apply, and 1.4 to 1.5 is the general range for placid patients confined to room rest. The strictly bed patient requires even less; an average factor of 1.2 times BMR is commonly applied. It must be realized, however, that differences in muscular tonus and of habit of movement and gesture make for larger individual differences than might be suspected otherwise and that some patients in bed may expend as much energy as when they are allowed room privileges.

The Total Energy Expenditures. Theoretically, of course, the total energy expenditure can be computed as the sum of all the factors which dissipate energy —basal metabolism, specific dynamic action and muscular activity of all kinds. In a few demonstrative researches it has been a nice exercise to show that indeed, the total is the sum of the parts. However, this factorial computation has little to recommend it in individual estimations for practical purposes. For practical work with patients, these elaborations are neither required nor, if they are made, are they very useful. Since the patient who is being re-fed from the undernourished state is changing from day to day, the daily corrections in the necessary calculations would be impracticable at best.

It must not be forgotten that there are large differences between individuals who are maintaining similar modes of existence. Newburgh and Robinson, in the second edition of this book (p. 512), remarked on two men, both engaged in relatively sedentary occupations and who had almost identical basal metabolic energy losses of 1640 and 1600 Cal., but whose total daily metabolic requirements were 2500 and 3570 Cal., respectively. Every investigator who has made such studies has had comparable experiences.

Unfortunately, there are great technical difficulties in the way of estimating total metabolism directly. It can be done, of course, with the patient maintained inside a calorimeter, but this is possible only in a few research demonstrations. The major use of direct calorimetry has been the demonstration that indirect methods are, in fact, accurate and reliable. Even the few research laboratories where direct calorimetry was formerly employed now seem to have abandoned the method in favor of far simpler indirect methods that are almost equally precise.

Newburgh and associates[40] devised a less precise but less cumbersome method in which the insensible water loss is estimated by weighing on sensitive scales. Even this simplified indirect method, however, will appear as more suitable for research than for general routine work. The basic data is that under certain specified conditions the vaporization of water as insensible perspiration accounts for a considerable and substantially constant fraction of the total heat dissipation from the body. Under comfortable conditions, that is, where the patient feels neither too warm nor too cool, it is estimated that about 25 per cent of the total heat loss of the body occurs through the vaporization of water. Although this method produced very useful results for the Michigan group, it never achieved any general popularity and is now mainly of historical interest.

In many practical situations, the only feasible way to estimate the energy expenditure is from the body weight and the energy intake. The energy intake is readily computed from precise measurement of the food intake, with translation to calories by the use of standard tables. This method is quite satisfactory, provided that: (1) food intake and energy expenditure are not far from the balance point, (2) the time period is not too short—several weeks, or more, are desirable and anything less than 1 week is certainly too short, (3) there is assurance that there are no substantial changes in body hydration.

Small changes in body weight may be allowed for on the basis that 1 kg. of body weight change represents about 5000 Calories. For example, suppose a man weighs 65.0 kg. initially and ten days later his weight is 65.5 kg. and that during these ten days his food intake amounted to 30,000 Calories. His mean daily energy expenditure is estimated as $\frac{1}{10} \times (30{,}000 - 2500) = 2750$ Cal.

This simple method can be very accurate when periods of several months are used if the food computations are precise and if there are no unusual losses in the excreta. If desired, the results can be checked by estimations of the mass of the gross body compartments, in which extracellular water is estimated as thiocyanate space and fat is estimated from specific gravity.

In recent years indirect calorimetry by measurement of oxygen consumption has been greatly facilitated by the development of a very light weight gas meter (the Michaelis-Kofranyi meter) which takes the place of the old bulky Douglas bag and allows much longer periods of measurement since it actually collects only a small fixed proportion of the expired air.[72] The simultaneous development of more rapid and convenient methods of gas analysis now makes the measurement of energy expenditure at work far more practicable than formerly.

Normal Standards. The "normal" calorie requirement may be considered the calorie intake which will cover all energy needs of a well nourished person without provoking either emaciation or obesity. In view of the phenomena considered below in regard to adaptation, it will be appreciated that the calorie requirement is not a fixed theoretic value; insofar as there is no theoretic perfect state of nutrition, so there can be no fixed and perfect theoretic calorie requirement. But general figures—estimated averages—for populations and for quick and rough guidance for individuals have practical justification. Many estimates of normal standards for calorie requirements have been proposed from time to time.[17,28,53,68] Experience shows that none of these is reliable for individuals, though they may be very valuable for population groups.

In the formulation of normal standards for calorie requirements several methods have been used. Attempts have been made to calculate the actual daily total energy expenditure of typical individuals by adding estimates of the calorie cost of so many hours of sleep, of work, of recreation, and so on. This factorial method, however, has been less used than estimates based on observations on actual food consumption of population groups; the assumption is made that the amount of food habitually consumed by healthy people living a normal life represents their requirement. Often both theoretic summations and observations of intake have been considered in constructing standards.

For many years the most widely used standards for calorie requirements were the "Recommended Dietary Allowances" of the National Research Council Food and Nutrition Board as revised from time to time.[68] These, like almost all such standards and recommendations, were devised for application to populations rather than to individuals, and the major concern was to assure that enough nutriment would be provided to cover all but the most extremely abnormal demands. Although this philosophy was perhaps justifiable in dealing with vitamins and minerals, it obviously could lead to absurdity with calories. The latest (1958) revision of the N.R.C. "Allowances"[68] attempted to treat calorie "requirements" more reasonably in view of the growing concern about obesity, and the results are more suitable for populations than previous versions but can not be applied to individuals with any security. Similar considerations apply to the standards adopted by the Canadian Council on Nutrition,[17] though these are based on a somewhat different approach to the problem.

CALORIE REQUIREMENTS—FAO STANDARDS

In 1949 the whole question of calorie requirement standards was carefully examined by a Committee convened by the Food and Agriculture Organization (FAO) of the United Nations. The Committee attempted to attack the question from a strictly physiologic approach and devised a system entirely novel in this field which was published in 1950.[28] A second session of the Committee in 1955 re-examined the matter and has recently (1957) published a revised report.[29]

Experience in the use of the FAO system as set forth in 1950 showed that it was both sound and practical, and the same system, with relatively minor alterations and additions, is incorporated in the 1957 Report. It is still true that even the latest FAO system of standards[29] is far more suitable for groups of people than for individuals.

The FAO approach is to set up defined reference standards and then to make extrapolations from these for departures in age, climate, body size and activity. The "reference man" is 25 years of age, weighs 65 kg. (143.3 lbs.), lives in a temperate zone (mean external temperature 10° C.), is healthy and well nourished, and is engaged in moderate activity. It is believed that the yearly average requirement for such a man is 3200 Calories daily. The counterpart "reference woman" is of the same age, weighs 55 kg. (121.3 lbs.) and is believed to have an average requirement of 2300 Calories daily.

The factor of body size for men otherwise conforming to the FAO references may be calculated from the equation: $E = 152(W)^{0.73}$, where E is the total daily calorie requirement and W is the weight in kg. For women the requirement is 81 per cent that of men, or it may be calculated directly: $E = 123.4 (W)^{0.73}$. Pregnant women are allocated an additional 40,000 Calories for the entire pregnancy. The standard allowance for lactation is 1000 Calories daily for six months. Table 5 summarizes the allowances for 25-year-old people engaged in moderate work and living in a climate like that of the reference, e.g., Boston or Indianapolis. Table 5 gives the recommendations for age 25.

TABLE 5. BODY WEIGHT AND CALORIC REQUIREMENTS OF 25-YEAR-OLD ADULTS ENGAGED IN MODERATE ACTIVITY IN A TEMPERATE CLIMATE*

WEIGHT (KG.)	MEN	WOMEN	LACTATING WOMEN
	Calories per day		
40		1823	2823
45	2447	1987	2987
50	2643	2146	3146
55	2833	2300	3300
60	3019	2451	3451
65	3200	2599	2599
70	3379	2743	3743
75	3553	—	—
80	3725	—	—

* (FAO,[29] 1957.)

It is commonly realized that, in general, the calorie expenditures, and therefore the requirements, of adults decrease with age. The first FAO Report[28] recommended a reduced calorie allowance of 7.5 per cent for each decade of age beyond 25 years. Although it still seems that this may be appropriate for a large part of the population in the United States, for the world as a whole the average decline in activity with age may be somewhat slower and the adjustment in calories should be less. The new FAO recommendation[29] is to provide a decrease of 3 per cent for each of the decades of 25 to 35 and 35 to 45 years. After age 45 the previous decrease of 7.5 per cent per decade has been retained. Table 6 provides the calorie allowances recommended by FAO for persons of differing ages.

TABLE 6. AGE AND DAILY CALORIE REQUIREMENTS OF ADULTS CORRESPONDING TO THE FAO REFERENCE MAN AND WOMAN (BODY WEIGHTS 65 AND 55 KG., OR 143 AND 121 POUNDS RESPECTIVELY)

AGE	PERCENTAGE OF REFERENCE	MEN	WOMEN
20 to 30	100.0	3200 Cal.	2300 Cal.
30 to 40	97.0	3104	2231
40 to 50	94.0	3008	2162
50 to 60	86.5	2768	1990
60 to 70	79.0	2528	1817

The factor of environmental temperature occupies a position similar to that of age; an effect on calorie needs, immensely related to the temperature, is obvious but it has been inadequately studied. Basal metabolic rates recorded in the tropics are usually somewhat lower than those recorded on persons of the same size, age and sex in temperate regions, and repeated measurements on individuals moving from one climate to another follow the same trend. Great effects on the calories devoted to physical activity are often seen; all activity may be shunned when the heat is excessive, whereas when it is very cold vigorous exercise is indulged in solely to keep warm. Even the energy cost of the same movements may be affected by the environmental temperature because clothing hobbles movements; in walking, for example, energy is spent in bending the trousers.

The FAO recommendation[29] is to increase the food allowance by 3 per cent for each 10 degrees Centigrade of external environmental temperature below 10° C., and to decrease in the same proportion for environments in which the mean annual temperature exceeds 10° C. The mean annual temperature of Boston is about 10° C. The range of such annual means in various parts of the United States is from about 5° to 25° C., so provision for the climatic effect at most is an increase of about 2 per cent for the coldest regions and a decrease of about 5 per cent in the food needed in our hottest regions. This adjustment allows for the fact that the actual environmental temperature in which men live is much moderated from that of the outside air.

The FAO calorie requirements for ages 1 to 19 are summarized in Table 7. It is judged that both sexes have the same calorie needs at all ages up to and including 12 years, but from age 13 on there is a progressive difference between the sexes. This reflects average activity habits. Also, it is to be noted that no provision is made for differences in body size in these requirements. Any other system would tend to penalize the previously underfed and stunted child by reducing the calories supplied in the diet.

ADAPTATION TO UNDERNUTRITION

It is not always appreciated that man has a large capacity for automatic adjustment to alterations in the calorie intake. This is fortunate, of course, for otherwise small systematic imperfections in the appetite regulation of intake would lead to fantastic excesses of emaciation or obesity. It is interesting to compute the conceivable result of eating an extra slice of bread a day: in twenty years the added 65 calories per day would add up to 474,500 Calories. In terms of adipose tissue, at 7650 Calories per kg., this would be the equivalent of 62 kg., or 137 lb. Actually, nothing remotely like this happens because, after a very limited weight gain, the energy expenditure will have risen to balance the excess food consumption. In the opposite situation, when the calorie intake is changed to be less than the energy "requirement" at the time, there is also adaptation which tends to bring intake and output in equality.

In the Minnesota experiment[48] it was possible to examine in detail the adaptation to undernutrition under controlled conditions.[86] The thirty-two young men subjects required, on the average, 3492 Calories daily to maintain

TABLE 7. FAO RECOMMENDATIONS FOR NORMAL BOYS AND GIRLS LIVING IN A TEMPERATE ENVIRONMENT

AGE IN YEARS	CALORIE REQUIREMENT		AGE GROUP IN YEARS	CALORIE REQUIREMENT	
1	1,150		1 to 3 inclusive	1,300	
2	1,300				
3	1,450		4 to 6 inclusive	1,700	
4	1,550				
5	1,700		7 to 9 inclusive	2,100	
6	1,850				
7	1,950		10 to 12 inclusive	2,500	
8	2,100				
9	2,250				
10	2,350				
11	2,500				
12	2,650				
	MALE	FEMALE		MALE	FEMALE
13	2,950	2,650			
14	3,100	2,600	13 to 15 inclusive	3,100	2,600
15	3,250	2,550			
16	3,450	2,450			
17	3,550	2,400	16 to 19 inclusive	3,600	2,400
18	3,650	2,400			
19	3,750	2,350			

balance before they were placed on a diet of 1570 Calories for six months. Throughout the "control" and the "semi-starvation" periods these men maintained the same general pattern of life—regular hours for study, housekeeping and laboratory chores, fixed outdoor walks, etc. There was an average loss of 24 per cent of the body weight, but this loss followed a parabolic course. At the end of six months the weight loss had ceased and the subjects were in substantial metabolic balance. An economy of 1922 Calories a day had been achieved. The gross picture of how this was achieved is given in Table 8.

TABLE 8. PARTITION OF THE TOTAL ENERGY EXPENDITURE, IN CAL./DAY, BEFORE AND AT THE END OF SIX MONTHS OF SEVERE UNDERNUTRITION: MEAN VALUES FOR 32 YOUNG MEN*

	BEFORE	AFTER	Δ
Basal metabolism	1576	962	− 614
Specific dynamic action	349	157	− 192
Physical activity	1567	451	−1116
Total	3492	1570	−1922

* Cf. Taylor and Keys, 1950,[86] p. 2.

The basal metabolism decreased by 39 per cent and the metabolic cost of physical activity decreased by 71 per cent. The specific dynamic action was reduced in proportion to the calorie intake, that is, by 55 per cent. Of the total saving of 1922 Calories, basal metabolism accounted for 32 per cent, activity for 58 per cent, and specific dynamic action for 10 per cent. Further examination of these changes is of interest. The change in specific dynamic action requires no special explanation, but the other two items each involve several considerations.

The changed cost of activity must be the result of changes either in the total physical tasks undertaken or in the cost of performing those tasks, or both. Since most of the cost of physical activity consists in moving the body and its parts, it is obvious that a change in body weight alone will produce an alteration in the cost of activity, even if the same frequency and extent of muscular movement are maintained, unless there is a change in efficiency. But the metabolic cost, that is, efficiency, of standard work does not change in simple undernutrition until weakness produces definite clumsiness.

Analysis of the data from the Minnesota experiment showed that 60 per cent of the observed total reduction in the cost of physical activity was due to decrease in the physical tasks undertaken and 40 per cent to a decrease in the cost of performing those tasks; the latter item was a direct reflection of the weight loss.

A decline in basal metabolism such as observed in the Minnesota experiment would be expected to follow from the fact that there was a very considerable reduction in body size. Using the common method of expressing basal metabolism per unit of body surface, it appears that there was a decline of 31.2 per cent in the BMR (cf. Keys et al., 1950,[48] Chap. 17). But it might seem more appropriate to express the metabolism in terms of the mass of "active tissue" of the body—the body weight less the estimated weights of fat, of extracellular water and of bone mineral. In these terms, the intensity of basal metabolism declined only about 15 per cent. The data indicate that the greater part of the decline in basal metabolism reflected the diminution of the metabolizing mass of tissue and that only about one third of the economy in basal metabolism should be ascribed to a decrease in the intensity of metabolism of the living cells.

It will be recalled that there is a distinct tendency toward hypothermia in starvation. In the Minnesota experiment the mean change in body temperature ranged from about −0.1° C. to more than −1.0° C. This will explain, of course, some decline in the intensity of the basal metabolism, since the rate of metabolic reactions in the human body varies according to the temperature, the relation being of the order of $Q_{10} = 2.3$. In the Minnesota experiment the body temperature effect accounted for about one third of the decreased intensity of basal metabolism.

The foregoing discussion on adaptation has been provided in some detail to show that the adjustment of energy expenditure to undernutrition is large and complex. For practical purposes, the important points are that the energy output tends to adjust to the intake level and that the extent to which this adjustment has been made can be estimated from the basal metabolism and the time course of weight change. Similar adjustments in the opposite direction occur when refeeding is undertaken.

In shorter periods of undernutrition than that of the Minnesota experiment, an important reduction in total calorie expenditure can take place. The reduction in basal metabolism that takes place in a few days of severe calorie deficit has been noted above. Often the circumstances of acquiring severe calorie deficits in a short time also involve a great reduction in physical activity so that the calorie needs to maintain equilibrium may be reduced to half the previous level in a week or two.

This is particularly common in persons who develop a severe illness accompanied by fever and anorexia or vomiting and are then hospitalized. If before the illness they needed 2500 Calories a day, they may well be gaining weight during recuperation on as little as 1600 to 1800 Calories a day.

COMPOSITION OF THE BODY

In recent years methods for estimating the gross composition of the body by indirect means have developed to the point of rather wide application in research, and the results provide new understanding about weight changes and the nutritional state.[46,58,81] Basically, these new indirect methods attempt to estimate body fat by taking advantage of the following facts:

1. The major variables that make up the gross body weight are fat, extracellular fluid, "cells" and bone mineral. Among these, fat is the most variable; water varies a great deal in some types of patients but the "cells" and bone mineral components are much more constant.

2. Body fat has a low density, averaging 0.9007 gm. per cc. (of pure ether

TABLE 9. MEAN VALUES FOR THE MAJOR COMPARTMENTS OF THE BODY IN THE MINNESOTA EXPERIMENT

"Cells" is the gross body weight less fat, SCN space and bone mineral. S12 and S24 indicate the weeks of semistarvation; R12, R20, etc., indicate weeks of rehabilitation.

PERIOD	BODY WT.		SCN SPACE		FAT		"CELLS"	
	Kg.	%	Kg.	%	Kg.	%	Kg.	%
Control	69.50	100	17.13	23.50	9.66	13.90	39.93	57.45
S 12	56.90	100	17.21	30.25	4.95	8.70	31.96	56.16
S 24	53.63	100	17.88	33.98	2.78	5.18	29.19	55.15
R 12	59.76	100	17.93	30.00	5.97	10.00	32.07	53.66
R 20	70.80	100	16.88	23.75	13.38	18.87	37.84	53.39
R 33	72.48	100	17.51	24.15	14.30	19.72	37.89	52.27
R 58	69.80	100	16.61	23.79	10.61	15.20	39.80	57.02

TABLE 10. GAINS IN BODY WEIGHT, FAT, EXTRACELLULAR FLUID ("EX. FL.") AND "CELLS" FROM 6 MONTHS' OVEREATING

SUBJECT NO. (Initial Weight)	TOTAL WT. GAIN		% OF GAIN ACCOUNTED FOR BY:		
	Kg.	Lbs.	Fat.	Ex. Fl.	Cells
1 (150 lbs.)	21.0	46.3	77%	11%	12%
2 (199 lbs.)	20.9	46.0	66%	16%	18%
1–10 (147 lbs.)	11.4	25.2	64%	14%	22%

extract) at normal body temperature, whereas the other body tissues are much more dense. Hence, the density of the whole body is inversely related to the proportion of the body weight represented by fat.

3. Normally, the concentration of water in the cells is very constant and the volume of extracellular fluid tends to be highly correlated with the mass of cells in the body. Hence, if body hydration is not deranged, a measurement of the total water in the body will allow an estimate of the combined cell mass and extracellular fluid and so, indirectly, of the body fat.

The density of the body may be estimated by weighing underwater, which is neither difficult (in the research laboratory), nor uncomfortable. The buoyant effect of the air enclosed in the lungs and respiratory passages at the time of weighing must be allowed for. For accurate results it is necessary to measure this residual air directly at the time of underwater weighing.[9a,46] This latter requirement is obviated when the body volume is estimated by air displacement, using the dilution of a known amount of helium in the air tank to estimate the air space not occupied by the body.[81] The general validity of densitometry for estimating body fat has been confirmed by several independent methods.[50,63]

Estimation of body fat from the total body water is relatively easy, using deuterium oxide ("heavy" water), tritium labelled water or possibly even urea.[58,59] The antipyrine dilution method is technically troublesome. The estimation of body fat from total body water involves many assumptions and it is obvious that it is inapplicable if there is even a moderate amount of edema or dehydration. Edema may not be clinically recognizable in undernourished people short of a body fluid excess of the order of 7 to 10 per cent of the gross body weight.[48] The combination of densitometry with measurements of total body water and extracellular fluid (e.g., by thiocyanate space), provides the most detailed and reliable estimation of body fat and the state of hydration.[48,81]

Results of the application of densitometry and estimation of the extracellular fluid space in semistarvation and recovery of young men are given in Table 9. It will be noted that in these severely

volved in violent crime but have no compunction about thievery, dishonesty or any immoral behavior that takes little effort and promises an immediate reward or satisfaction. The extent to which these changes develop is, in part, dependent on the degree of starvation, but the basic moral character of the individual has a powerful modifying influence.

INFECTIONS IN UNDERNUTRITION

The situations in nature which produce severe undernutrition are often such as to produce other stresses and hazards beyond those of the simple calorie deficit. In famine, that is, when whole populations are starving, it is understandable that elementary sanitation and public health measures are neglected and that the familiar historical association of famine and pestilence may occur. From experience in famine areas and in prison camps, it might appear that starving persons are peculiarly susceptible to many infections, notably tuberculosis, pyodermas and dysenteries. But the experience of World War II and after shows that when general sanitary measures and personal hygiene are well maintained the incidence of such infections is not necessarily high; critical factors seem to be more those of pure water, soap and decent housing than of lack of "resistance" or increased "susceptibility" (cf. Keys et al., 1950,[48] Chap. 46). The complexities of the general problem of the effects of nutrition on resistance to infection have been ably discussed by Schneider.[75,76]

Tuberculosis is rather a special case among infectious diseases in that there is a good deal of evidence which suggests strongly, though it may not actually prove, that undernutrition heightens susceptibility and lowers resistance (cf. Keys et al., 1950,[48] Chap. 47). The course of the disease in severe undernutrition, moreover, is often of a fulminating character, with frequent miliary spread.[36,38,52] Such patients may cause difficulties in diagnosis and evaluation because they may show little elevation of temperature above normal in cool or cold climates. It is interesting, also, that serologic tests may lose much of their value in severely undernourished people; positive reactions to the Pirquet and Mantoux tests are seldom elicited in a starving population, even when there is present a high incidence of active tuberculosis.[7]

The course of tuberculosis in severely undernourished patients may be surprisingly favorable if both dietary measures and general care are good.[38] Among 180 patients with severe, active tuberculosis who were freed from German prison camps, eleven died within a few days after hospitalization in Switzerland, but in the next eight months there were only four deaths and the great majority of the patients were obviously improving on conservative therapy.[51] In contrast, where there are serious shortages of both food and nursing service, starved persons with tuberculosis have an extremely bad prognosis.[19] In general, the experience with famine victims offers support to the customary practice of supplying abundant diets to all patients with tuberculosis.

All of the foregoing remarks have reference to simple undernutrition. Where there are specific deficiencies and qualitative as well as quantitative malnutrition the situation may be different but generalizations are impossible. In recent years the greatest emphasis has been placed on protein and amino acid deficiencies as possibly contributory to increased susceptibility and decreased resistance to infectious diseases. There has been rather undue haste to extrapolate to man from the results of animal experiments which involve extreme conditions. It is interesting and theoretically important that Cannon has demonstrated a reduced capacity to form antibodies in rabbits severely depleted of proteins,[92] but the practical application of these findings to natural situations in man is questionable. The few studies on antibody formation in semistarved man are not confirmatory,[31] probably because the degree of protein depletion involved in the animal experiments is seldom seen in man.

UNDERNUTRITION AND OTHER DISEASE OR INJURY

The patient who is severely undernourished presents some special problems when he is also suffering from other disease or injury. Apart from the effects of the other disease or injury on the production of undernutrition, which have been mentioned earlier in this chapter, there is the other aspect, namely, the effects of undernutrition on the character and course of concomitant disease. We have already mentioned infectious diseases, and it was apparent that scientific data are few and generalizations are unsafe. The same is true in regard to other diseases and injuries.

It is useful to re-emphasize the general characteristics of undernourished people which form a background and set of determinants to be considered in evaluating the patient. Among the more important points are the tendencies toward hypothermia, hypotension, bradycardia, anemia, apathy and lethargy, low muscular and tissue tension, edema and low metabolic rate. Where fever, tachycardia, hyperpnea and dyspnea are ordinarily expected, the undernourished patient will exhibit these in low degree or not at all. Complaints are apt to be less or at least less volubly expressed. Anemia, pallor, cyanosis and the appearance of prostration and weakness will be more marked in the undernourished than in the well fed patient.

An important characteristic of the severely undernourished body is a general state of unreactivity, particularly in regard to the autonomic nervous system. This fact tends to alter clinical phenomena as well as the effects of drugs. Responses to epinephrine, atropine, pilocarpine and insulin are diminished, and even large doses of these drugs may fail to elicit a prompt response of normal magnitude[30,74] (Keys et al., 1950,[48] p. 613). Some, but by no means all, of these peculiarities are related to the sluggish circulation in the starving patient.

The slow rate of circulation in the semistarved patient limits his reactivity and produces difficulties by itself (cf. Keys et al., 1950,[48] Chap. 38). Erythema is much reduced. There is a greatly increased tendency toward venous thrombosis.[1,52] The sequence of venous thrombosis (often in the femoral or iliac veins)–pulmonary embolism–pulmonary infarction with cavity formation, is not rare in extreme undernutrition, and this may produce a problem for consideration in the diagnosis of tuberculosis.[87] Starving children show a marked tendency to develop venous thrombi.[7]

Wound healing is generally considered to be retarded in undernourished patients, but there is relatively little detailed and objective evidence except in specific deficiencies, notably in ascorbic acid deficiency. The severely protein-depleted animal exhibits markedly unsatisfactory wound healing, and methionine administration may be helpful.[55] A protein-deficient diet (6 per cent casein) provided to wounded rats, previously well nourished, results in poor healing as compared with that obtained on a 20 per cent casein diet.[91]

Undernutrition does not have an unfavorable effect on the course of all diseases. Diabetes is an outstanding example: all evidence tends to show a distinctly favorable effect of general undernutrition and famine diets on both mortality and the clinical course of the disease (cf. Keys et al., 1950,[48] Chap. 48). This is particularly true of the adult, obese form of diabetes.

The effects of undernutrition on hypertension and cardiovascular disease are interesting[11,14] (Keys et al., 1950,[48] pp. 617–621). There is a tendency toward a beneficial effect in hypertension with accentuation of the disease in refeeding. During the starvation of the siege of Leningrad there seemed to be a definite reduction in coronary occlusions and myocardial infarctions but no great change in hypertension; in the refeeding period afterwards hypertension reached epidemic proportions and the disease assumed severe forms.

A large amount of experimental work

has proved that general undernutrition, if severe enough, has a marked effect on the incidence and growth, in rats and mice, of several neoplasms, including mammary carcinoma and Rous' sarcoma (cf. Keys et al., 1950,[48] Chap. 49). In such experiments, however, positive effects were obtained when the diet was maintained for a long time at a level low enough to impair the normal growth of the host tissue.[66]

The data on the effect of undernutrition on cancer in man are not better than suggestive but, so far as they go, they are interesting. Actuarial records on insured persons in the United States indicate some inverse relationship between eventual cancer mortality and the relative body weight at the time insurance was issued. In the records of 192,000 men 45 years old or older, Dublin[23] found 15 per cent lower cancer mortality among the men who were definitely underweight (15 to 50 per cent under standard average weight for height) than among men of average weight for height. Similar results emerged from later analyses of data of this type.[39] Changes in cancer mortality in populations subjected to prolonged major dietary changes tend to be in the same direction[16] (Keys et al., 1950,[48] p. 1053).

TREATMENT

General Considerations

Proper and effective treatment of undernutrition requires an accurate diagnosis of the degree and character of the undernutrition and an understanding of its cause. Merely prescribing an abundant diet of good quality will suffice in some cases, such as in many ambulant famine victims, but even in these patients the physician has a responsibility which cannot entirely be foisted onto the dietitian and nurse. In the majority of patients to be found in ordinary civil practice, the cause of the undernutrition is not simply previous inability to obtain food, so mere presentation of more food is by no means the answer for therapy. Obviously, every effort must be made to correct the basic cause which has produced the undernourished state. At the same time, however, the nutrient intake may be increased by special devices—tube feeding, parenteral administration, etc.—if this is warranted.

One general rule of importance is to initiate refeeding gradually; heroic efforts at rapid repletion are dangerous and are seldom justified. The metabolic and circulatory load imposed by doubling or tripling the previous calorie intake may cause bloating, diarrhea and other distress and can precipitate heart failure. Moderation should be the rule, particularly in the amount of food given at any one feeding and in the kinds of food provided. The patient who seems to be moribund, or nearly so, may be treated as a medical emergency for whom emergency measures—mainly supportive and to maintain and restore the circulation—apply. For the other patients, however, there is little or no danger in a thoroughly conservative approach. In any case, it is better that the first feedings in the treatment program underestimate rather than overestimate his ability to assimilate and utilize food.

The best guide to the feeding program for the first few days is probably the estimate of the dietary intake of the preceding few days. If this is considered to have been of the order of 1000 to 1500 Calories, it may be safe to increase this by 50 per cent. If the patient is extremely cachetic, even this modest amount should be provided in 5 or more daily feedings of highly digestible foods, chiefly liquid.

For the patient whose condition and history suggest that his diet immediately preceding has provided less than 1000 Calories daily, the first day's quota may be set at 1000 to 1500 Calories divided into 5 or more feedings of liquid, highly digestible food.

The whole feeding program should be devised to increase the nutrient intake as rapidly as is consistent with safety and comfort to reach the maximal rate at which the body can really utilize the food. Surpassing this rate means at best either gastrointestinal problems or excessive fat deposition or both. Unlimited crowding of either calories or proteins in the diet into the body does not necessarily mean any gain in tissues rebuilt or strength restored.

Liberal supplies of vitamins, in crude concentrates, and vitamin-rich foods as well as pure preparations, should be provided routinely in the first few days. This saves effort to establish a diagnosis about the vitamin status and will do no harm at worst. During this early period the salt intake should be restricted unless the patient is dehydrated.

After the first few days many immediate dangers and problems will have been surmounted, but the succeeding few weeks also bring difficulties. If the patient is responding properly he will clamor for more food, will be apt to complain about his treatment and may be as troublesome as his strength will allow. This is normal, and tact and firmness may be required to meet it. As a result of the loss of edema fluid the patient's weight may fall and his emaciation may seemingly fail to respond for some weeks. This tends to discourage both the patient and those who minister to him. But both may be assured that definite evidence of his improvement will come in a few weeks and that, actually, great improvement is shown by the loss of edema and the reduction in apathy.

During the first few weeks, however, recurrences of edema are not uncommon. They may be caused by overexercise, by excessive salt ingestion, by infection, or may seemingly arise without cause. In the latter case overeating, with a resultant tendency toward heart failure, may be suspected. If an elevated venous pressure confirms the suspicion of heart failure, this should be treated conservatively as such. A recurrence of edema calls for bed rest, salt restriction and dietary reduction, but not necessarily any alarm. Small amounts of diuretics may be given if the edema is persistent and marked.

The feeding program for the first few weeks should continue to be conservative. For a severely starved man whose normal body weight would be 65 kg., and who is ambulatory but not laboring or continuously active, an average intake of 3000 Cal. daily for the first month is probably ample and anything over 3500 Cal. is excessive. For women and for older men the diet should be correspondingly less.

If possible, it is desirable to continue the division of the daily diet into more than three meals. Midmorning, midafternoon and evening snacks will be helpful and are usually received with enthusiasm.

The character of the diet is not of critical importance in this period. It should, of course, be readily digestible and should contain a good provision of proteins and vitamins. A goal (which may be unduly luxurious) could be a daily average, for all persons beyond ten or twelve years of age, of 100 gm. of proteins, 2 mg. each of riboflavin and thiamine, 20 mg. of nicotinic acid and 100 mg. of ascorbic acid, together with 15 mg. of iron and 1 gm. of calcium. If the daily equivalent, in any form, of a quart of milk, two eggs and a large portion of meat, together with a variety of any other foods to make up the remaining calories, can be provided, there need be no concern about dietary adequacy.

During this period, that is, after one or two weeks, it is time to institute a cautious program of mild exercise for all patients for whom it seems safe to attempt it. *Feeding alone will not restore strength, and wasted muscles are not rebuilt without exercise.* Care is needed, however, because many patients may tend to overdo in their pleasure at the sense of returning strength.

After a month of such treatment, the most severely starved patients will still be extremely weak, definitely anemic and in no condition to do without much care, either in the hospital or in the hands of sympathetic relatives or friends. The less severely starved patients may be ready to care for themselves on an outpatient basis but should receive dietary and medical guidance and should be protected from heavy work or exposure to inclement weather. As a matter of fact, they will not be fully recovered for many months to come, during which time the program should continue to be one of good but not overly abundant diet, plenty of rest and regular but mild exercise. If the normal body weight of an adult is regained in less than five or six months, the body composition will be excessively high in fat; in no case can one expect complete restoration of proper body composition and function in less than this time or, indeed, short of eight or ten months. During all this time a relatively high intake of proteins, vitamins and minerals is advisable. The calories, however, should be reduced as the body weight approaches normal and should be sharply reduced if the weight tends to increase further.

Where the previous malnutrition involved specific deficiencies, the diet and adjuvants such as vitamin pills will have been adjusted accordingly. Otherwise, any good diet will suffice. In no case should there be allowed a high consumption of sweets or of fats.

Treatment of Anorexia Nervosa

Anorexia nervosa has, as the name suggests, no discoverable physical basis and is attributed to psychologic abnormality. It would be reasonable, then, to suggest that psychotherapy might be the treatment of choice. Actually, the physician who successfully treats anorexia nervosa always employs psychotherapy, though he might not label it as such. But the crux of the problem is to initiate weight gain. Once real weight gain has started, the subsequent management is often progressively easier. The mere fact of establishing a positive calorie and nitrogen balance for a few weeks tends to alter the basic attitude of the patient in a way which is difficult or impossible to achieve at the purely psychologic level of approach.

On the other hand, it should be recalled that relapses in anorexia nervosa are by no means rare. The patient with anorexia nervosa who has made substantial progress, as judged by simple body weight, is quite capable of relapsing to the former status, or worse, and this is generally the result when the weight gain has been brought about by forced feeding or its equivalent. If possible, the basic fears and anxieties should be unearthed and removed at the same time that every device of persuasion and ingenuity of food presentation is exploited to get maximal food consumption. Successful treatment demands great clinical skill and endless patience on the part of the physician. Administration of thiamine, insulin and thyroxine to stimulate appetite is not often useful.

Parenteral Feeding

Parenteral feeding should not be undertaken if it can be avoided because this procedure has special hazards for severely undernourished people. Fortunately, the great majority of patients suffering from severe undernutrition without other complications can be fed adequately by the oral route.[15] In the severely starved patient, parenteral feeding is attended by constant danger of circulatory embarrassment, pulmonary edema and sudden heart failure.

In general, all intravenous infusions given to starved patients should be administered much more slowly than to well nourished patients and should be discontinued at the first sign of circulatory embarrassment. Since the latter may develop and rapidly progress to a fatal outcome, constant observation is essential. Signs of venous engorgement, dyspnea, tachycardia or the appearance of irregularities in the heart rate are signals of danger. It should be noted that tachycardia is relative—a heart rate of eighty beats a minute is real tachycardia in a patient whose heart rate has been in the range of fifty or less.

The most useful agent for providing calories parenterally is still glucose. A major limitation is the amount of glucose that can be provided without flooding the body with an exorbitant volume of fluid. Glucose may be given in concentrations of 10 to 25 per cent, but concentrations of 20 per cent, or more, frequently produce venous thrombosis. Glycosuria usually results with an administration rate of more than 0.8 gm. per kg. of body weight per hour and may occur at lower rates in severely starved and debilitated persons. This means a maximum provision of the order of 200 Cal. per hour in the average adult. More rapid administration is possible if the body hydration is carefully controlled, since the major objection to glycosuria is the tendency to produce dehydration. The amount of glucose actually lost in glycosuria is not great so that a considerable gain in glucose retained can be achieved with rates of administration of 1.0 to 1.5 gm. per kg. per hour. The provision of the glucose in normal saline solution diminishes the dehydrating effect of the glucose alone.

The limitation to the number of calories that can be provided by intravenous glucose has led to the attempt to provide fat emulsions for intravenous use.[33,56,61,62,69] In spite of many improvements, problems still remain, and intravenous fat feeding has not become as safe and popular as the early enthusiasts had hoped. When more calories are needed and no other way of providing them seems feasible, fat emulsions for intravenous use may be tried, but caution should be exercised, especially at first. Some patients tolerate them very well for long periods.

A better use of fat in almost all patients is as emulsions for tube feedings. Large amounts of calories can be provided in this way with far greater safety and convenience than by the intravenous route (see the Symposium in Ann. New York Acad. Sc., Vol. 56, Article 1, 1952.

Protein nutrition may be aided by the parenteral route by the use of protein hydrolysates.[24] A variety of these are now available for intravenous use. The better preparations are made from casein, animal blood fibrin or animal blood plasma, by hydrolysis either with strong acid or with enzymes. In general, the acid hydrolysates are more completely hydrolyzed and produce fewer reactions. On the other hand, the acid hydrolysis destroys some of the amino acids so that the resulting product is deficient unless the acids are replaced from some other source.

Besides the dangers of infection and of pyrogens which attend any intravenous therapy, the protein hydrolysates, when used in sufficient quantity to have a real effect on the nitrogen balance of the patient, also tend to produce other undesirable reactions, notably anorexia, nausea, vomiting, venous thrombosis and, occasionally, antigenic phenomena. The incidence of anorexia, nausea and vomiting is reduced with very slow rates of infusion and is reported to be much lower in preparations which are low in, or free from, glutamic and aspartic acids.

The parenteral provision of whole blood, plasma and gelatin for the purpose of protein nutrition is entirely unjustifiable. The proteins in whole blood and in plasma are only very slowly made available for metabolism and tissue replacement. Gelatin is likewise only very slowly metabolized from the blood and, moreover, it is an incomplete protein. None of these materials can be given in amounts which are nutritionally important. These materials have, of course, a very important use for blood replacement and for osmotic effects, but their administration should be reserved strictly for these purposes.

For clinical use it is recommended that intravenous alimentation, where it is needed, be applied with caution, starting with 10 per cent glucose and allowing two hours or more for the intravenous infusion of one liter (providing 400 Cal.). If this is well tolerated, a more complete infusion can be attempted with a mixture of glucose and protein hydrolysate. With a 2-liter infusion flask, the following preparation of 1700 cc. may be given in two to four hours and will provide 1000 Cal. and 50 gm. of protein hydrolysate: 1 liter of 10 per cent glucose, 200 cc. of 50 per cent glucose, 500 cc. of 10 per cent protein hydrolysate. If it seems desirable to provide some salt, the total volume can be increased to 1800 cc. by the addition of

100 cc. of 5 per cent NaCl. It should be noted again that preparations containing salt should be given only under constant observation because of the danger of sudden pulmonary edema.

For patients who appear able to tolerate and to benefit from such treatment, a schedule of two infusions a day may be attempted. This should provide a reasonably satisfactory rate of initial repletion for the very emaciated patient. It should be noted that the energy expenditure of an adult patient of this type is generally less than 1500 Calories a day, with a basic endogenous loss of protein of less than 30 gm., so that an intake of 2000 Calories and 100 gm. of protein provides a very substantial allowance for repletion. Vitamins and minerals may be added to the infusion mixture, but it is usually simpler to give these separately by subcutaneous or intramuscular injection. With this type of feeding, a minimal vitamin provision per day might be considered to be 100 mg. of ascorbic acid, 2 mg. each of thiamine and riboflavin and 20 mg. of nicotinic acid amide. In some situations many physicians may wish to double or triple these allowances; where there is evidence of specific avitaminosis still larger dosages may be given.

Except in rare situations, it is to be expected that such intravenous feeding will not be continued more than a few days and that in the meantime oral feeding will be started and increased as rapidly as possible. As a rule, then, it is unnecessary to be concerned for this short period about the provision of all supplementary nutrients in the infusions and injections. The temporary deficiency of calcium, phosphorus, potassium, iodine, iron, biotin, choline, pantothenic acid, pyridoxine, inositol, folic acid and vitamin B_{12} may be accepted with equanimity; these nutrients will be supplied in the oral feeding soon to be provided.

As has been noted, blood transfusions are not justifiable for purely nutritive purposes. For the most severely starved patients, however, transfusions are often of very great value for the maintenance and restoration of the failing circulation and as a generally supportive measure.

Treatment of Vitamin Deficiencies

When vitamin deficiencies are of major importance in a person with general undernutrition, the treatment is, essentially, simply the addition of the appropriate vitamins to the treatment outlined above. When the patient is clearly undernourished in regard to calories but is weaker than would seem to be ascribable to the state of emaciation (allowing for the masking effect of edema, of course), and other contributing causes are not apparent, vitamin deficiencies should be suspected. Although it is desirable to make a positive differential diagnosis, the fact that excesses of most of the vitamins are innocuous allows them to be used at will, even in large amounts, on a purely trial basis.

It is now well known that many of the so-called signs of vitamin deficiencies are far from being pathognomonic. A condition of vitamin deficiency in the cachectic patient cannot safely be inferred from a dry skin, hyperkeratosis, "staring" hair, leg weakness or even some degree of angular stomatitis. But large (not massive) doses of multiple vitamin preparations may properly be given to such patients to be on the safe side.

The treatment of vitamin deficiencies is discussed in detail in Chapter 6. Here it may be useful to insist on three points: (1) Vitamin deficiencies seldom occur singly; hence, polyvitamin therapy is advisable in almost all cases, particularly when deficiencies of vitamins of the B complex are involved. (2) Pure vitamin and vitamin-concentrate preparations allow the administration of extremely large amounts, but heroic dosage is not necessarily desirable. The propaganda of commercial interests has, in general, succeeded in persuading both physicians and patients to use far larger dosages than are needed. (3) Oral therapy is entirely satisfactory for the great majority of patients who need supplementary vitamins.

Rehabilitation and Residues

The treatment of the undernourished patient should aim at complete rehabilitation; mere recovery of lost weight is not the end. In the severely undernourished person this means that muscle as well as fat must be built, and this requires a program of physical exercise. In starved young men, otherwise normal, body weight may be regained in a few months, but the early weight gain is largely fat. Full reconstitution of the body takes many months. In older people, or in patients who have had complications of other severe illness or injury, it may be expected that real recovery will be even slower. Constant advice and attention may be unnecessary after a few weeks or months, but the physician should realize, and should instruct his patient accordingly, that attention to diet, to exercise and to general hygiene should not be abandoned merely because the body weight approaches normality.

Follow-up studies on persons who have been subjected to prolonged periods of severe undernutrition have been carried out among former prisoners of war and inmates of concentration camps[20,36,60] as well as on the men starved in the Minnesota experiment.[48] In general, it appears that among persons clinically healthy and well nourished before a long period of undernutrition without concurrent infections or specific vitamin deficiencies, recuperation is slow but complete and residues are few. On the other hand, the kind of undernutrition that involves bad nutritional quality as well as quantity seems to have an effect in after years.

A follow-up study was made on behalf of the Veterans Administration on military personnel captured and imprisoned, and almost invariably undernourished in this process, in Europe and in the Far East during World War II.[6] "The European prisoners showed no measurable effect of their imprisonment, at least during the first 6 years after liberation. . . . For the Pacific prisoners the evidence is unequivocal that the effects of imprisonment resulted in a markedly reduced survival potential at liberation."[6]

Among the former prisoners in the Far East (i.e., the Western Pacific area) there was a markedly excessive death rate in the first 2 years after liberation, but mortality was excessive also during the succeeding 4 years. The principal causes of the excessive mortality have been tuberculosis and accidents. The high incidence of accidents is interesting and raises the question as to whether this is related to psychologic residues of the prolonged prison and starvation experience. Morbidity surveys of these former Far East prisoners showed an excessive frequency of psychoneuroses as well as of gastrointestinal disorders among them. The persistence of such results of vitamin malnutrition as optic atrophy, which developed in some of the Far East prison camps, was to be expected, of course.

References

1. Apfelbaum, E. (ed.): Maladie de famine. Recherches cliniques sur la famine executées dans le Ghetto de Varsovie en 1942. Warsaw, Am. Joint Distribution Committee, 1946.
2. Beatie, J., and Herbert, P. H.: Brit. J. Nutrition, *1:*185, 1947.
3. Behnke, A. R.: Ann. New York Acad. Sc., *56:*1095, 1953.
4. Berkman, J. M.: Postgrad. Med., *3:*237, 1948.
5. Berkman, J. M., Weir, J. F., and Kepler, E. J.: Gastroenterology, *9:*357, 1947.
6. Boothby, W. M., Berkson, J., and Dunn, H. L.: Am. J. Physiol., *116:*408, 1938.
7. Braude-Heller, A., Rotbalsam, J., and Elbinger, R.: Clinique de la famine chez les enfants. In Apfelbaum (ed.), op. cit., 1946, pp. 173–187.
8. Brozek, J.: J. Am. Dietet. A., *31:*703, 1955.
8a. Brozek, J.: Human Biology, *28:*124, 1956.
9. Brozek, J., and Keys, A.: Nutrition Abstr. & Rev., *20:*247, 1950.
9a. Brozek, J., Henschel, A., and Keys, A.: J. Appl. Physiol., *2:*240, 1949.
10. Brozek, J., and Keys, A.: Brit. J. Nutrition, *5:*194, 1951.
11. Brozek, J., Chapman, C. B., and Keys, A.: J.A.M.A., *137:*1569, 1948.
12. Brozek, J., and Grande, F.: Human Biology, *27:*22, 1955.
13. Brozek, J., Keys, A., et al.: J. Appl. Physiol., *10:*412, 1957.

14. Brozek, J., Wells, S., and Keys, A.: Am. Rev. Soviet Med., *4:*70, 1946.
15. Burger, G. C. E., Drummond, J. C., and Sandstead, H. R.: Malnutrition and Starvation in Western Netherlands, September 1944–July 1945. 2 vols. The Hague, General State Printing Office, 1948.
16. Burkard, O.: Wien. klin. Wchnschr., *53:* 65, 1940.
17. Canadian Council on Nutrition: Canadian Bulletin on Nutrition. A Dietary Standard for Canada Approved by the Canadian Council on Nutrition. Ottawa, King's Printer, 1950.
18. Charney, J., Williamson, M. B., and Bernhard, F. W.: Science, *105:*396, 1947.
19. Chortis, P.: Am. Rev. Tuberc., *54:*219, 1946.
20. Cohen, B. M., and Cooper, M. Z.: A Follow-Up Study of World War II Prisoners of War. Veterans Admin. Med. Monograph. Washington, D.C., 1954.
21. Da Costa, E., Krzywicki, H. J., Bell, J., Clayton, R., and Friedemann, T. E.: U. S. Army Med. Nutr. Lab. Rep. No. 133, 30 July, 1954.
22. Döbeln, W. von: Acta physiol. scandinav., *37:* Suppl. 126, 1956.
23. Dublin, L. I.: Bull. New York Acad. Med., *8:*687, 1932.
24. Elman, R. and Cannon, P. R.: Protein Malnutrition. In Jolliffe, Tisdall and Cannon (eds.): Clinical Nutrition. New York, Paul B. Hoeber, Inc., 1950, pp. 183–207.
25. Erickson, L., Simonson, E., Taylor, H. L., Alexander, H., and Keys, A.: Am. J. Physiol., *145:*391, 1946.
26. Escamilla, R. F., and Lisser, H.: J. Clin. Endocrinol., *2:*65, 1943.
27. Everitt, A. V., and Webb, C.: J. Gerontol., *12:*128, 1957.
28. Food and Agriculture Organization of the United Nations: Calorie Requirements. Report of the Committee on Calorie Requirements. F.A.O. Nutritional Studies No. 5. Washington, Food and Agric. Organ. U.N., 1950.
29. Food and Agriculture Organization of the United Nations: Calorie Requirements. Report of the Second Committee on Calorie Requirements. F.A.O. Nutritional Studies No. 15. Rome, Food and Agric. Organ. U.N., 1957.
30. Fliederbaum, J., et al.: Recherches cliniques et biochimiques sur les malades en famine. In Apfelbaum (ed.), op. cit., 1946, pp. 79–172.
31. Gell, P. C.: Proc. Roy. Soc. Med., *41:*323, 1948.
32. Glickman, N., Mitchell, H. H., Lambert, E. H., and Keeton, R. W.: J. Nutrition, *36:*41, 1948.
33. Gorens, S. W., Geyer, R. P., Matthews, L. W., and Stare, F. J.: J. Lab. & Clin. Med., *34:*1627, 1949.
34. Grande, F., Anderson, J. T., and Keys, A.: J. Appl. Physiol., *12:*230, 1958.
35. Grande, F., Anderson, J. T., and Taylor, H. L.: J. Appl. Physiol., *10:*430, 1957.
36. Helweg-Larsen, P., et al.: Famine Disease in German Concentration Camps; Complications and Sequels. Acta med. scandinav., Supp. 274, 1952.
37. Henschel, A., Mickelsen, O., Taylor, H. L., and Keys, A.: Am. J. Physiol., *150:*170, 1947.
38. Hottinger, A., Gsell, O., Uehlinger, E., Salzmann, C., and Labhart, A.: Hungerkrankheit, Hungerödem, Hungertuberkulose. Basel, Benno Schwalbe, 1948.
39. Hunter, A.: Tr. Actuarial Soc. Am., *40:* 394, 1939.
40. Johnston, M. W., and Newburgh, L. H.: J. Clin. Invest., *21:*357, 1942.
41. Jolliffe, N., Tisdall, F. F., and Cannon, P. R. (eds.): Clinical Nutrition. New York, Paul B. Hoeber, Inc., 1950.
42. Keys, A.: Nutrition Abst. Rev., *19:*1, 1949.
43. Keys, A.: Science, *112:*371, 1950.
44. Keys, A.: J.A.M.A., *142:*333, 1950.
45. Keys, A.: In Weight Control. Ames, Iowa, Iowa State College Press, p. 18.
46. Keys, A., and Brozek, J.: Physiol. Rev., *33:*245, 1953.
47. Keys, A., Anderson, J. T., and Brozek, J.: Metabolism, *4:*427, 1955.
48. Keys, A., Brozek, J., Henschel, A., Mickelsen, O., and Taylor, H. L., with Simonson, E., Skinner, A. S., and Wells, S. M.: The Biology of Human Starvation. Minneapolis, University of Minnesota Press, 1950.
49. Keys, A., Taylor, H. L., Mickelsen, O., and Henschel, A.: Science, *103:*669, 1946.
50. Kraybill, H. F., Hankins, O. G., and Bitter, H. L.: J. Applied Physiol., *3:*681, 1951.
51. Labhart, A.: Gestalt und Frühverlauf der Tuberkulose bei Patienten aus Konzentrationslagern. Hottinger et al., op. cit., 1948, pp. 247–97.
52. Lamy, M., Lamotte, M., and Lamotte-Barrillon, S.: La dénutrition: Clinique-biologie-thérapeutique. Paris, Doin, 1948.
53. League of Nations, Health Organization: Ser. League of Nat. Publ. III, Health, Sept. 8, 1937, pp. 65–77.
54. Lesser, G. T., Blumberg, A. G., and Steele, J. M.: Am. J. Physiol., *169:*545, 1952.
55. Localio, S. A., Morgan, M. E., and Hinton, J. W.: Surg. Gynec. & Obst., *86:* 582, 1948.
56. Mann, G. V., Geyer, R. P., Watkin, D. M., and Stare, F. J.: J. Lab. & Clin. Med., *34:*699, 1949.

57. Mann, G. V., and Stare, F. J.: Nutritional Needs in Illness and Disease. Handbook of Nutrition. 2d ed. A. M. A., Philadelphia, Blakiston, 1941, pp. 351–382.
58. McCance, R. A.: Lancet, *265:*739 (Oct. 10), 1953.
59. McCance, R. A., and Widdowson, E. M.: Proc. Roy. Soc. Med. (London) B, *138:* 115, 1951.
60. Members of the Department of Experimental Medicine, Cambridge, and Associated Workers: Studies of Undernutrition Wuppertal, 1946–9. Med. Res. Council Spec. Rep. Ser. No. 275. London, H. M. Stationery Office, 1951.
61. Meng, H. C.: J. Lab. & Clin. Med., *37:* 222, 1951.
62. Meng, H. C., and Early, F.: J. Lab. & Clin. Med., *34:*1121, 1949.
63. Messinger, W. J., and Steele, J. M.: Proc. Soc. Exper. Biol. & Med., *70:*316, 1949.
64. Miller, A. T., Jr., and Blyth, C. S.: J. Appl. Physiol., *5:*73, 1952.
65. Miller, A. T., Jr., and Blyth, C. S.: J. Appl. Physiol., *5:*311, 1953.
66. Morris, H. P.: Science, *101:*457, 1945.
67. Munro, H. N., and Chalmers, M. L.: Brit. J. Exper. Path., *26:*396, 1945.
68. National Research Council: Recommended Dietary Allowances. Revised 1958. National Academy of Sciences-National Research Council Publication 589, Washington, D.C., 1958.
69. Neptune, E. M., Geyer, R. P., Saslaw, I. M., and Stare, F. J.: Surg., Gynec. & Obst., *92:*365, 1951.
70. Pace, N., Kline, L., Schachman, H. K., and Harfenist, M.: J. Biol. Chem., *168:*459, 1947.
71. Pace, N., and Rathbun, E. N.: J. Biol. Chem., *158:*685, 1945.
72. Passmore, R., and Durnin, J. V.: Physiol. Rev., *35:*801, 1955.
73. Pett, L. B.: Am. J. Pub. Health, *45:*862, 1955.
74. Schittenhelm, A., and Schlecht, H.: Arch. f.d. ges. exp. Med., *9:*1, 1919.
75. Schneider, H. A.: Amer. J. Pub. Health, *39:*57, 1949.
76. Schneider, H. A.: Vitamins and Hormones, *4:35*, 1946.
77. Sheehan, H. L.: J. Path. Bact., *45:*189, 1937.
78. Sheehan, H. L., and Murdoch, R.: J. Obst. & Gynaec. Brit. Emp., *45:*456, 1938.
79. Simonson, E., Henschel, A., and Keys, A.: Am. Heart J., *35:*84, 1948.
80. Sinclair, H. M.: Proc. Roy. Soc. Med. (London), *41:*541, 1948.
81. Siri, W.: Advances Biol. & Med. Physics, *4:*239, 1956.
82. Smith, D. A., and Woodruff, M. F. Q.: Deficiency Diseases in Japanese Prison Camps. Med. Res. Council Spec. Rep. Ser. No. 274. London, H. M. Stationery Office, 1951.
83. Soberman, R. et al.: J. Biol. Chem., *179:* 31, 1949.
84. Sunderman, F. W.: Am. J. Clin. Path., *17:*169, 1947.
85. Spillane, J. D.: Nutritional Disorders of the Nervous System. Baltimore, Williams and Wilkins Co., 1947.
86. Taylor, H. L., and Keys, A.: Science, *112:*215, 1950.
87. Uehlinger, E.: Die pathologische Anatomie der Hungerkrankheit und des Hungerödems. In Hottinger et al., op. cit., 1948, p. 181–246.
88. Varco, R. L.: Surg., Gynec. & Obst., *84:* 611, 1947.
89. Venkatachalam, P. S., Srikantia, S. G., and Gopalan, C.: Metabolism, *3:*138, 1954.
90. Wachholder, K., and Franz, H.: Arch. f.d. ges. Physiol., *247:*632, 1944.
91. Williamson, M. B., McCarthy, T. H., and Fromm, H. J.: Proc. Soc. Exper. Biol. & Med., *77:*302, 1951.
92. Wissler, R. L.: Woolridge, R. L., Steffee, C. H., Jr., and Cannon, P. R.: J. Immunol., *53:*267, 1946.

CHAPTER 8

By JAMES M. STRANG, M.D.

Obesity

Obesity is a form of malnutrition characterized by excessive fat deposits. It may or may not be associated with other forms of malnutrition, especially protein deficiency, or it may be found in association with other disorders of the body or mind.

HISTORICAL NOTE

Hippocrates and later Celsus and Galen[1] wrote about obesity. Cullen[2] in his "First Lines of the Practice of Physic," Edinburgh, 1784, wrote: "This corpulency, or obesity, is in very different degrees in different persons, and is often considerable without being considered a disease. There is, however, a certain degree of it which will be generally allowed to be a disease; as, for example, when it renders persons, from a difficult respiration, uneasy in themselves, and, from the inability of exercise, unfit for discharging the duties of life to others." William Wadd in 1816 published a book entitled "Cursory Remarks on Corpulence: or Obesity Considered as a Disease." An appreciation of the relationship between fatty foods and obesity was expressed in "Domestic Medicine," London, 1826.[3] "Fat people should not eat freely of oily nourishing diet. They ought frequently to use radish, garlic, spices, or such things as are heating and promote perspiration and urine. Their drink should be water, coffee, tea, or the like; and they ought to take much exercise and little sleep."

Tanner in his "Practice of Medicine," 1867, devoted a chapter to obesity which contains many of the clinical observations found in modern texts. He stated that fat could be produced from high carbohydrate feeding, quoting animal experiments to this effect. Referring to the production of paté de fois gras, he remarked, "All the conditions for insuring obesity are resorted to, viz., external heat, obscurity, inactivity, and the cramming of the animals with nourishment." "The consequences of obesity are often more serious than is generally believed."[4] Paragraphs on the treatment of obesity enumerate a list of remedies which had been employed in earlier years. His statement, "For it must be remembered that, as physicians, we are called upon not only to prevent the increase of fat, but to diminish the redundant quantity which has already been formed without lessening the normal vigor of the system," cannot be improved upon today. Tanner's discussion of the Banting (1864) diet clearly separated the nitrogenous from the non-nitrogenous foods and indicated the proper nutritional function of each.

Duckworth in 1897[5] reviewed the subject of obesity indicating that: (1) a distinction can be made between fatty infiltration and fatty degeneration; (2) the liver becomes fatty when people eat fatty food or much carbohydrate material; (3) it is not sufficiently recognized that fat deposits are constantly undergoing change by decomposition and reformation; (4) fat may be formed from protein; (5) there is a relation of obesity to gout and diabetes; (6) the hazards of surgery are greater in obese patients; (7) obesity was recognized by life insurance companies as an added hazard requiring extra premiums; (8) a small proportion of both fat and carbohydrate must be combined with protein food to insure normal metabolism on a reduction diet; (9) the spa treatments were in great vogue at the time.

Many of the basic facts about obesity and of the principles of therapy which are accepted at present were available prior to 1900. Early in this century the study of nutrition in this country made great progress under the influence of Chittenden, Lusk and, later, Benedict.

IMPORTANCE OF THE PROBLEM

The importance of the problem of obesity in relation to the health of the individual and to the welfare of the populace as a whole is becoming increasingly apparent. Obesity is a disorder of prosperity. In times of plenty the average intake of food increases and in times of full employment, more money is available for both food and leisure. However, the influence of the resultant increase in over-all obesity upon the health of the nation has been regarded as abstract and impersonal.

Of recent years, because of the publicity given to the immediate personal risks, people are beginning to realize what it means to their own health and their probable longevity. Commercial interests have been quick to recognize the potentialities for gain and, in their exploitation of the subject, have helped to stir up popular interest. A recognition of the basic nature of the problem of obesity is slowly spreading. It is now somewhat appreciated that the types of feeding habits which were essential for people who did manual labor for long hours a day, who walked, who lived and worked in poorly heated buildings, are quite improper now. The fuel requirements of the working man today rarely approximate his needs fifty or even thirty years ago. The positive note in family nutrition is no longer the search for an evanescent food supply but the selection from or even the resistance to the constant and steady pressures from the food purveyors. It is therefore important that persons no longer confine their interests solely to the unusually severe grades of obesity. An increasing appreciation of the true significance of moderate or sometimes even mild grades of obesity is a hopeful sign. It is human nature, however, to search for the quick and painless method of reduction. This desire supports each new fad of either drug or diet. In so far as fat is removed from the body, any harmless procedure has certain merit. It is not always realized that loss of weight is not synonymous with loss of fat. Fortunately, fads in diets, as in other fields, are usually short-lived and the faddist jumps to a new panacea. Much harm may be done by improper procedures but national publicity, provided by profit-hungry magazines, for grossly inadequate reduction diets continues. Professional counter-propaganda[7] will perhaps have some balancing influence in time. It is not yet adequately appreciated that obesity is a form of malnutrition and that it frequently is associated with other forms of malnutrition, notably protein deficiency.

DIAGNOSIS

The diagnosis of gross obesity is simple, but the distinction between normal fat deposits and the early stages of obesity is not easily made. Tanner[4] stated, "A moderate amount of fat is a sign of good health; and physiologists generally allow that the tissue ought to form about the twentieth part of the weight of a man and the sixteenth of woman." Whether or not we accept this ratio, it is evident that a normal person may have substantial amounts of fat. "Adults of medium height and fair symmetry, who weigh over fifteen stones (210 lb.) may be considered moderately obese. A weight of twenty stones (280 lb.) and over constitutes a grave case. . . ."[5] The "sly and subtle onset"[6] of overweight is common experience, and a patient does not recollect when he first thought he was obese.[8]

Standards. It is a general practice to compare the weight of a patient with that of the average person of comparable age, sex and height as recorded in the statistical tables of life insurance companies (see appendix). This practice has the merit of simplicity and for clinical purposes is quite satisfactory. Body build, in addition to the above factors, has considerable influence on the proper weight of a person. "Yet it must be remembered that a man may be large, having the muscular system well developed, and the fat proportionately increased, without being obese"—Tanner, 1867. Weight tables often state a range of weights for height, thus permitting correction for body build. Another standard of reference for the diagnosis of obesity is that of Robinson and Brucer,[9] who use an index which includes height, weight and chest circumference, whereby the influence of build is incorporated in the index. For the purposes of clinical studies, this index has many advantages, but its need in medical practice has not been demonstrated. The standard tables are a sufficiently reliable measure of the degree of obesity for routine work, regardless of body type.[10,11]

These standards have been accepted by many,[11,12] and a person who weighs 10 per cent above his standard weight is considered to be "overweight"; if he weighs 20 per cent above standard, he is "obese." Since the variations in body weight due to build are not of the order of 20 per cent, complete neglect of this factor would not introduce any serious error in the analysis of a clinical problem. The use of standard height-weight tables merely indicates that many people, presumably normal, have been observed to weigh as stated. It is not known that a specified weight figure represents the "optimum" or "best possible" weight for an individual.

The reliability of the standards of reference has been repeatedly questioned, most recently by Keys and his associates.[13] The origin of the data on which the standards are based reflects a selection of individuals rather than a statistically valid sample of men and women of the ages and statures indicated. The composition of the body, the amounts of body water, bone, muscle and fat, varies with build. The correlation of the estimates of these substances by physical measurements with the chemical analysis of the cadaver, as in animal studies, presents practical difficulties in human beings. Such studies are few. In only a portion of these analyses was a normal distribution of tissues present. Thus, absolute standards of reference for man are lacking, but approximations by indirect methods have been made. Keys reviewed exhaustively the current methods for the estimation of (1) the mass of vital tissue, (2) the extracellular water, (3) the bone mass, and (4) the adipose tissue of persons. For our present purpose, it is sufficient to mention that adipose tissue in the human can be approximated by caliper, density and the extracellular water methods. The *caliper method* involves the measurement of the thickness of folds of the skin at stated areas of the body by means of a specially designed caliper. From these measurements the subcutaneous fat is estimated. The subcutaneous fat is assumed to be a fixed percentage of the total body fat. The body *density method* is based on the fact that fat has a low density in contrast to the rest of the body substances. If the density of the total body is determined by a water displacement technique, the percentage of fat can be estimated from the calculated bone mass, lean body mass and extracellular water. The *extracellular water method* is based upon the measurement of the total extracellular water by one of several current methods. Since the bone mass and lean body mass have a more or less constant relationship to the extracellular water, the body fat is obtained by subtracting the total of these three factors from the observed weight.

Although such methods for the determination of the amount of fat deposition in man are not of clinical importance, several points of practical value have been developed. With regard to basal metabolism, the main difference between men and women resides in the greater percentage of fat in women. This

TABLE 1. OBESITY BY AGE GROUPS. 1000 CASES[16]

AGE	0–20	21–30	31–40	41–50	51–60	61–70	71 AND OVER	TOTAL
Men	1	11	53	85	68	18	8	244
Women	7	65	178	238	196	62	10	756
Total	8	76	231	323	264	80	18	1000

fact is also reflected in the sex differences in the standard height-weight tables. The factors in body build which produce deviation from the weights of the standard tables have been more precisely defined. The clinical impression regarding the significance of the age factor in the weight tables has been confirmed. Efforts have been directed to determine the major groups of components and their variations in normal men. Fifteen per cent fat may be considered a normal amount for young men.[14] The observations which have been made on obese persons tend to demonstrate that the methods could be applied with perhaps comparable precision in these cases.

In practice we are usually dealing with masses of fat far beyond the range of the normal variations, so that even if precise methods of fat determination were readily available, their value might not be evident. With all their recognized faults, the standard height-weight tables provide the best tool, currently available, for the study of nutrition problems.

Incidence. The incidence of obesity varies with the definition of this disorder. Statistics are greatly influenced by the population sample which is analyzed, and since no broad census has ever been conducted, the figures which are sometimes quoted reflect the experience and opinions of the observer. Armstrong[12] stated that in this country at least one fifth of the population over 30 years of age, or about 15,000,000 people, are overweight, which is defined as 10 per cent above the standard. If 20 per cent above standard constitutes obesity, 5,000,000 adults of our population are obese. The stated incidence in any given community would, however, be affected by local customs and manner of living. Likewise, average age, sex and body build would have specific influences upon the apparent over-all incidence of obesity.

Age. There are no age limits for the occurrence of obesity; it has been reported at birth and at the upper limits of longevity. Definitions are important. In infancy and childhood, relatively large weight changes at irregular intervals are to be expected. The demonstration of excessive fat deposits at any given observation of a child may be quite difficult, and the tendency for many adolescents to store fat for relatively short periods is well recognized. In general, the period of early maturity, and incidentally, of greatest activity, which is usually placed around the twenty-fifth year, has perhaps the lowest incidence of obesity of any age group. There is a gradual increase in weight after age 30. This increase is probably due to augmented fat deposits resulting from the maintenance of the intake of youth associated with the lessened activities of increasing years. Clinically, the increases starting at 40 years appear to be of greatest significance for men, whereas in women obesity develops readily after the age of 30. The gradual increase in weight which is associated with age may not be entirely unfavorable, but a normal concomitant of a contented life.[15] Preble[16] showed the age distribution of 1000 cases of obesity (Table 1). It may be noted that relatively few cases occur before the age of 30 and that relatively few obese patients live beyond 60 years.

The greatest importance of the age factor for clinical practice is in the demonstration that the body composition changes with age.[14] Adults tend to increase the amount of fat in their bodies as they grow older, and often, in later years, do so at the expense of vital tissue. Hence, in obesity problems, the proper standard of reference for a given person is not the weight recorded for the observed age but the weight recorded for the age 30 to 35. In effect, this increases somewhat the estimated degree of obesity of an older person but, at the same time, more clearly indicates the amount of weight reduction to be desired.

Sex. Women normally have a higher content of fat in their bodies. Keys found that metabolically there is no difference between the sexes which is not accounted for by the increased proportion of fat in the female. There is, however, a greater incidence of obesity in women. The precise values of the increased percentages vary with the investigators. In some series obese women outnumbered obese men ten to one. However, Hunt[17] found little sex difference in his overweight children. Dublin and Lotka[18] stated that in one group of 60,000 applicants for insurance, 2.66 per cent were rejected because of obesity. The ratio was 2.1 per hundred for males and 4 per hundred for females. The older authors stress the frequency of obesity in single women, and especially after menopause.[1,4] Women are more likely to have the so-called "anemic" type of obesity, whereas men tend toward the "plethoric" form. This phenomenon is due to mode of life rather than sex per se.

Body Build. In a study of 3400 men and 2200 women, Robinson et al.[9] found that, if patients are grouped according to body build (slender to broad) and these groups are broken down by weight (light to heavy), there is a marked correlation between the build and the occurrence of obesity (Table 2).

Of the men, only 3 per cent of the slender group were overweight, whereas 37 per cent of the broad group were overweight. Five per cent of the slender group of women and 67 per cent of the broad group were obese. Body build is a fundamental property which facilitates the development of obesity and also of the degenerative disorders often attributed to obesity.[9] In view of the influence of body build on normal weight standards, this study suggests that the manner of life in early years, which resulted in "bigness," tends to resist the necessary disciplines of later life.

CHARACTERISTICS OF A BODY

One's attitude toward "body weight" is influenced by his concept of a human body. A living body has no fixity, in spite of its apparent uniformity from day to day. It represents the residuum of the excess of intake or output over the period of its existence. This residuum is not static. The particles which compose the organs and tissues are in a constant state of flux. Not just the body fluids or active tissues, but tissues commonly regarded as stable, such as bone or the central nervous system, are constantly changing their particles—but, of course, at rates of change which are characteristic of the tissues concerned. The magnitude of this activity varies, but the average over-all daily mass exchange is probably in the neighborhood of 5 per cent of the total body weight;[19] i.e., a person turns over each 20 days a mass

TABLE 2. THE INCIDENCE OF WEIGHT CLASSES IN BODY BUILD GROUPS IN 3436 MEN AND 2184 WOMEN[9]

	LINEAR BUILD (SLENDER)		LINEAR INTERMEDIATE		LATERAL INTERMEDIATE		LATERAL BUILD (BROAD)	
	Men	Women	Men	Women	Men	Women	Men	Women
Lightweight	267 (49%)	261 (40%)	311 (23%)	165 (21%)	117 (11%)	36 (8%)	8 (2%)	9 (3%)
Mediumweight	262 (48%)	355 (55%)	965 (71%)	498 (63%)	851 (75%)	252 (54%)	252 (61%)	83 (30%)
Heavyweight	15 (3%)	35 (5%)	75 (6%)	127 (16%)	163 (14%)	176 (38%)	150 (37%)	187 (67%)
Total	544	651	1351	790	1131	464	410	279

of material which approximates his average body weight. "It is not sufficiently recognized that fat deposits are constantly undergoing change by decomposition and reformation. As with all other tissues, intimate change proceeds even in the densest layers of fat; and in no part of the body does any fatty deposit lie out of the current of life and unaltered" (Duckworth).[5]

The demonstration of the phenomena of tissue change is possible by isotope tracer studies. Buchanan and Hastings[20] described some of the features of fat deposition. "Mice forming fat from carbohydrate will resynthesize one-half of the total fat deposits during a period of seven days. If the animal maintains a static weight for seven days, one-half of the original amount of fat in the deposit will have been degraded and contributed to the metabolic pool in the form of oxidizable intermediates." Hepatic fat is synthesized and degraded seven times faster than depot fat. Observations of the rates of turnover of the protein of the liver, of the lipids in the central nervous system, etc., have resulted in the generalizations such as Schoenheimer's theory of the dynamic state of body constituents, as stated by Clarke:[21] "As a result of Schoenheimer's investigations, there has emerged a concept of metabolic 'regeneration,' wherein the central idea is the continual release and uptake of the chemical substances by tissues to and from a circulating metabolic 'pool.' Coincident with these cyclic processes, there occur among the components of the pool multitudinous chemical reactions of which relatively few are concerned with elimination of waste products." This theory of dynamic equilibrium indicates the relation of structural and storage materials to the metabolic pool and how these body materials "reflect the composition of the metabolic pool from which they originate."[20]

In spite of such rates of change of body material, the body has a marked degree of average stability and appears much the same day after day. The organs and tissues maintain anatomically and physiologically about the same composition and function. This persistent average stability results from an intricate system of chemical reactions finely regulated by a group of endocrine and nervous regulators which is appreciated only in part.

This concept of the body as a residual mass in a constant state of flux requires a reexamination of certain terminology. Material streams into the body proper from the outside. The processes concerned with the *supply* of the necessary particles may be grouped under "nutrition" processes. They include the processes of ingestion, digestion and absorption of food. After absorption, particles undergo a variety of physical and chemical reactions which may be called "metabolism." These reactions are altered quantitatively, but not qualitatively, by the control of the rates of production of essential catalysts which is effected through "endocrine regulation" or "nerve regulation." The removal of the end products of metabolism is the role of the "excretory" systems. If we use these definitions, nutrition problems are supply problems. Malnutrition indicates a failure of proper supply of matter. It may be too little or too much. The adequacy of supply of material can be greatly influenced by true abnormalities of metabolism, of which very few have been found which are consistent with continued life; by disorders of the endocrine or nerve regulatory mechanisms, whereby the materials supplied are not efficiently utilized; or by disorders of excretion, whereby potential food is wasted by premature excretion. Likewise, abnormalities of supply can in turn materially influence the function of the other three areas. The further discussion of obesity is based on the idea that obesity is a nutrition problem primarily. No abnormalities of metabolism essential to obesity have been shown. Disturbances of endocrine and nerve regulation have been noted in association with and as a result of the obese state. However, if *supply* is not excessive, no amount of alteration in the other realms such as metabolism, regulation or excretion, can produce excessive deposition of fat.

Meaning of "Body Weight." The use of body weight as an index of nutritional status requires an examination of the term "true body weight." The concept of a dynamic equilibrium of the body focuses attention on the continuous change in its weight. Lusk[22] stated, "It was understood early in the history of physiology that the weight added by the ingestion of food and drink was lost in the urine, the feces, and the 'insensible perspiration.'" He described the experiments of Sanctorius in 1614 to determine the amount of insensible perspiration by means of a counterbalanced chair. The refined techniques of today indicate that in the basal state an insensible weight loss of one and one half to two ounces per hour is not unusual. However, the knowledge of the effects of food and water ingestion, of urination, of defecation and of sweating upon body weight is rarely applied to a specific observation of the weight of a patient. A "standard" weight observation should exclude, as far as possible, the controllable variables. Obtained under basal conditions at a fixed time, e.g., 7 A.M., after urination and before anything is ingested, such standard weights are suitable for comparison with other standard weights.

Even a "standard" weight varies from day to day under the most favorable conditions for the control of intake and output. This should be expected, and since the stream of intake varies independently from the stream of output, the residual mass, the body, must necessarily vary at any arbitrarily selected moment. How great this daily variation becomes must depend upon the uniformity of a person's daily activity. One experiment involved the detailed metabolic study of a normal girl for 37 days of continuous observation. This girl showed an average daily variation of her "standard" weight of 300 grams in a total weight of 62.0 kilograms. On only two occasions was an identical weight found on two successive mornings. The maximum difference on two successive days was 1.3 kilograms, which was accounted for by temporary storage of water and its overcorrection the following day. The significance of these data is accentuated in that her average daily intake by mouth for these 37 days was 3170 grams per day, or 10 times the average variation in her daily standard weight.[19] We have, then, a person with an average weight of 62.0 kilograms who turned over each day about 3.17 kilograms or 5 per cent of her mass, and, at the same time, had an average change in standard weight of only 300 grams or 0.5 per cent of her mass.

The demonstration that the total mass of the body is inconstant is further complicated by the fact that components of the total mass also vary considerably and independently. This truth is responsible for many of the difficulties in nutrition studies. A pound of water, of fat tissue and of protein tissue weigh the same, but the physiologic significance of a change in a pound of one is vastly different from that of a change in each of the others. Since water makes up approximately two thirds of the weight of a body, the shifting of water in or out of the body in response to the normal fluctuation of intake and output produces little stress. Hydration and dehydration effects of 2 to 5 pounds are frequent and silent physiologically. In contrast, a pound of fat tissue, allowing for 10 to 20 per cent associated water, represents a shift of about 3700 calories, and a movement of that magnitude is physiologically significant. In protein tissue, an ounce of dry protein usually binds about 3 ounces of water, so the movement of one pound of protein tissue involves not only a change of 4 ounces of active protein material with its caloric equivalent of around 450 calories, but also a large water shift. The importance of a recognition of these factors in the interpretation of therapeutic weight changes is apparent if we consider only the energy transfer in these three illustrations: one pound of water —no calories; one pound of protein tissue—450 calories; one pound of fat tissue—3700 calories.

The normal variations in the composition of the body, even in terms of large chemical groupings such as water, fat, protein and minerals, are not known. Much information is available from the many metabolic studies by "balance" technique regarding the daily turnover of material, and much is known about the intake and output of protein, as nitrogen, of carbohydrate, fat, water, minerals and, in fact, all of the important food groups. However, little is known about the amounts of these materials which remain in the body from day to day. The actual number of grams of sodium, of nitrogen or even of fat which are present at any moment cannot be determined. Consequently, although we can in many instances demonstrate the amount of change of a substance, we are not able to discuss the much more important physiologic problem of the relation of the stream to the residual mass, that is, the rate of change. With regard to lipid materials, 15 per cent fat may have been estimated as an average fat content for some bodies. That does not mean that other bodies must have this percentage to be normal, nor does it mean that this is the "optimum" or most desirable amount physiologically.

Keys has provided much information by dividing the body into four classes of substance (1) bone mineral, (2) cells or "active tissue," (3) extracellular water, and (4) fat. A normal young man might have 4 per cent of his body weight as bone mineral, 58 per cent as cells or "active tissue," 23 per cent as extracellular water, and 15 per cent as fat.[14] Other investigators have obtained different relationships; e.g., one study[23] indicated the total body water as 53 per cent of the body weight, with 16 per cent as extracellular and 37 per cent as intracellular water. It is obvious that the bone mineral will vary with the skeletal proportions. The active tissue factor would be greatly affected by the degree of muscular development. The extracellular water may vary considerably in various physiologic states, whereas fat tissue shows the greatest variability of all components. The influence of age and sex as additional factors causing variations was discussed above. The exact interpretation of a weight change is very complicated. It depends upon the correlation of water balance, nitrogen balance and energy balance studies, and particularly upon a method for approximating the total insensible weight loss.

The use of gross body weight as a standard of reference for nutritional work leaves much to be desired. The statistical "normal" tables are not altogether reliable. An observed weight represents a total mass at a given moment and may include factors not pertaining to the body proper, such as undigested food or urine in the bladder. Variations, slow or rapid, in the composition of the body may be considerable, but the fact remains that gross body weight, especially when taken under "standard" conditions, supplies a very good point of reference when one is dealing with changes in the nutritional status of a specific person. Under these conditions, it makes little difference whether the goal is described as "ideal weight," "normal weight," "optimum weight" or any other arbitrary standard. By noting successive body weights, an obese person, who is 20 or 200 pounds overweight, is provided with a reasonable measure of his problem and of his progress in the correction of obesity.

OBSERVATIONS ON THE OBESE STATE: CLINICAL

The Hazards of Obesity. The effect of gross obesity on health and life expectancy was noted by Tanner in 1867: "The consequences of obesity are often more serious than is generally believed. . . . It may be taken as a general rule that obesity does not conduce to longevity."[4] Duckworth stated,[5] "Obesity is recognized by medical officers for life-assurance as an indication of imperfect health. . . . Such cases are either "loaded" or declined as second or third class lives. . . . Obese persons bear accidents badly, are unsatisfactory subjects for surgical operations, and are apt to succumb to serious illnesses." Williams[6] wrote as follows: " . . . For obesity, even though it be not itself a disease (which in the view of many it is), is admittedly the most consistent confederate of all the deadly diseases, both microbic and metabolic, as well as the uncompromising enemy of recovery from accident and injury."

The experience of many life insurance companies provides the statistical basis for the statements that obesity increases mortality rates; that this increased death rate occurs at all age groups; and that, in a general way, the increase parallels the degree of obesity. These studies have been published from time to time over the past 30 to 40 years; hence, the basic data of one report do not necessarily correspond to those of others. The tables, in general, deal with selected groups of the population above average economically and possibly intellectually. No data are available for a statistical unit of the population at large. Likewise, the classification of applicants for insurance on a weight basis has been more closely observed by the companies in recent years because of their earlier experience; hence, the newer tables are more conservative.[12] In general, all reports agree on the increased hazard of obesity, which is shown best by illustrative tables.

Preble[16] presented data on 213,000 men and 50,000 women who were overweight. Table 3 shows the effect of weight per se in the normal death rate.

However, when the age factor is introduced, very little change is noted under 30 years of age, but a very significant rise is seen after 40 years (Table 4).

Table 5 expresses the experience of 32 life insurance companies with a group of men of average size.[12]

A study of 25,998 men and 24,901 women who were substandard risks because of obesity alone and who were followed for 25 years re-emphasized the familiar story of increased death rate among the obese and the variations with age and degree. When overweight

TABLE 3. ACTUAL DEATH RATE BY WEIGHT INCREMENTS OF OBESE MEN AND WOMEN EXPRESSED IN PER CENT OF EXPECTED DEATH RATE[16]

VARIATION FROM AVERAGE WEIGHT	RATIO TO NORMAL DEATH RATE
Men	
+10 Lbs.	97
+15–20 "	104
+25–30 "	113
+35–45 "	131
+50–60 "	144
+65–80 "	165
+85 and more Lbs.	223
Women	
+ 5–10 Lbs.	101
+15–20 "	114
+25–30 "	109
+35–45 "	122
+50–60 "	120
+65–80 "	157
+85 and more Lbs.	. . .

TABLE 4. ACTUAL DEATH RATE ACCORDING TO AGE AND DEGREE OF OBESITY EXPRESSED IN PER CENT OF EXPECTED DEATH RATE[16]

AGES AT ENTRY	VARIATION FROM AVERAGE WEIGHT IN POUNDS 5–10 Lbs. Overweight	15–20 Lbs. Overweight	25–45 Lbs. Overweight	50–80 Lbs. Overweight
20–24 years	96	96	101	103
25–29 years	93	90	112	117
30–34 years	99	86	119	134
35–39 years	100	101	131	155
40–44 years	94	110	140	175
45–49 years	103	109	131	151
50–56 years	102	121	124	149
57–62 years	102	125	112	138

TABLE 5. MORTALITY OF MEN ACCORDING TO BODY BUILD[12]

BODY-BUILD GROUP	PER CENT ACTUAL OF EXPECTED DEATHS* Ages 20 to 29	Ages 30 to 39	Ages 40 to 49	Ages 50 to 59
Underweight (%):				
15 or more	115	103	85	79
5 to 14	101	95	77	82
Average weight	93	84	86	93
Overweight (%):				
5 to 14	99	90	97	91
15 to 24	107	120	117	118
25 to 34	134	137	141	122
35 or more	163	137	141	143

* Death rate of all standard risks equals 100%. Experience of 32 life insurance companies, standard and substandard cases combined, 1909 to 1928, by ages at issue of insurance.

Note that these data relate to men 5 ft. 3 in. to 6 ft. 2 in. tall.

(*By permission of the authors, the American Medical Association and the Metropolitan Life Insurance Company.*)

TABLE 6. MORTALITY OF OVERWEIGHT MEN AND WOMEN[12]

AGE AT ISSUE	PER CENT ACTUAL OF EXPECTED DEATHS*	PER CENT ACTUAL OF EXPECTED DEATHS*
All Ages	150	147
20–29	180	134
30–39	169	152
40–49	152	150
50–64	131	138
Time Elapsed Since Examination (Yr.)		
Under 5	133	151
5–14	152	144
15–24	160	149
Degree of Overweight		
Moderate obesity	142	142
Marked obesity	179	161

* Men and women limited to substandard insurance because of overweight. Death rates of standard risks equals 100%. Separate mortality standards were used for men and for women. Experience of Metropolitan Life Insurance Company, Ordinary Department. Cases insured in 1925 to 1934 traced to 1950.

(*By permission of the authors, the American Medical Association and the Metropolitan Life Insurance Company.*)

men were divided into groups according to age at examination, the mortality relative to normal was greatest at the *younger* ages and least in the older ages. Thus, the 20 to 29 year group had 80 per cent more deaths than normal, whereas the 50 to 64 year group had only 31 per cent. This fact was not found among the women, who showed less fluctuation with age and a maximum rate of 52 per cent in the 30 to 39 year group.

Also elicited was the fact that deaths within 5 years of the initial examination were increased above normal, being 133 per cent for men and 151 per cent for women. As time progressed, the rate for men increased to a maximum of 160 per cent in the 15 to 24 year period, while the rate for women changed but slightly with increasing years. The summary figure of 150 per cent over-all increase in expected deaths for all ages and the figures of 142 per cent for moderate obesity and 161 to 179 per cent for marked obesity again emphasize that degree of obesity, per se, has a specific effect.

Obesity throws an excessive physiologic load on a person, and it is to be expected that the causes of death would be largely in the group of strain disorders such as cardiovascular disease and diabetes and the degenerative disorders such as arteriosclerosis. Statistics seem to confirm this opinion.[24] One possible reason for this increase in death rate from the degenerative disorders is gross overloading of the relatively normal amounts of active tissue of body which must deal continuously with the greatly increased mass and energy exchanges imposed on it by the excessive fat.

Among obese persons, the observed deaths from degenerative diseases of the heart, arteries and kidneys are about 70 per cent greater than expected. The increase is even greater, nearer 100 per cent, when these diseases occur in persons under 40 years of age.[12] Diabetes causes more than three times the expected rate. Likewise, gallbladder disease and cirrhosis of the liver contribute appreciably to the higher mortality rates. Table 7, adapted from Barr,[25] indicates the increased hazard of obesity for many common causes of death. The high rates associated with appendicitis and automobile accidents perhaps reflect the added surgical problems of obesity.

Table 8 depicts more specifically the increase in death rate for the several diseases with increasing degrees of obesity. The death rates are significantly increased in even the 15 per cent overweight group and become markedly altered in the "over 25 per cent" group. It is literally correct to state that obesity rarely kills anyone. However, the evidence available indicates that obesity increases one's chance of dying.[27]

TABLE 7. RATIO OF ACTUAL TO EXPECTED DEATHS BETWEEN OVERWEIGHT AND STANDARD RISKS[25]

CONDITION	MEN	WOMEN
Diabetes	383	372
Cirrhosis of Liver	249	147
Appendicitis	223	195
Biliary Calculi	206	284
Chronic Nephritis	191	212
Liver and Gallbladder Cancer	168	211
Cerebral Hemorrhage	159	162
Coronary Disease	142	175
Auto Accidents	131	120
Puerperal Conditions	...	162

(*By permission of The National Vitamin Foundation, Inc.*)

Clinical Classification. Clinically, obese patients may be roughly grouped into the plethoric and the anemic types. The descriptions used by Duckworth in 1897[5] do not differ materially from those of the more modern writers.[1,6]

The plethoric type of obesity, more common in the male, is associated with general overnutrition. It may appear in early life. The body is well developed, especially the skeletal and cardiac muscles. The blood count is normal or above. The complexion is florid, with often some congestion of the lips and ears. The neck is thick and the abdomen is prominent. These patients often stabilize at a moderate degree of obesity, but occasionally they become grotesquely

TABLE 8. STANDARDIZED DEATH RATES PER 100,000 FOR SPECIFIED CAUSES OF DEATH, ALL AGES COMBINED, BY WEIGHT CLASSES—BASED ON THE MORTALITY EXPERIENCE ON ABOUT 200,000 INSURED LIVES[26]

CAUSE OF DEATH	STANDARDIZED DEATH RATE PER 100,000							
	Underweight			Normal Weight	Overweight			
	Total	15–34%	5–14%		5–14%	15–24%	25%+	Total
All causes	848	913	833	844	1027	1215	1472	1111
Organic heart diseases	65	63	66	80	115	135	129	121
Angina pectoris	14	12	14	16	32	39	37	35
Disease of the arteries	17	15	17	23	34	46	41	38
Acute and chronic nephritis	63	56	64	82	108	202	224	141
Cerebral hemorrhage and apoplexy	49	46	50	70	101	115	170	110
Cancer	62	54	64	61	64	73	86	68
Diabetes	9	9	9	14	22	45	117	36
Pulmonary tuberculosis	115	166	103	57	28	21	*	26
Pneumonia (lobar and unspecified)	70	90	66	63	56	64	72	59
Influenza	20	29	18	20	29	24	*	28
Accidents	55	44	58	60	65	65	87	67
Suicides	27	33	25	24	31	29	42	31

* Not significant.

obese. They tend to develop cardiovascular degeneration with arteriosclerosis and the consequences thereof.

The anemic type of obesity is more frequent among women. "The obesity may be extreme; but the fatty masses are flabby, and the muscles are ill-developed and feeble. The heart partakes of this muscular inadequacy and acts feebly, the pulse being small. Some elevation of arterial pressure, due to peripheral resistance, may, however, be met with as in ordinary cases of anemia. In short, we have all the prominent features of anemia, together with excessive fatty deposition; the great incapacity for exertion, ready induction of palpitation and dyspnea, and the small appetite. These patients are neither gross feeders nor always large drinkers. They have often, indeed, an aversion from animal food, and prefer a dietary rich in carbohydrates. The deficiency in hemoglobin in the blood and the consequent inadequate oxidation maintain and increase the tendency to obesity. As already stated, women are common subjects of anemic obesity; and the disorder may be manifested before full growth of the body is established, namely before the age of twenty-two. Menstruation is generally disordered or absent. Menorrhagia, or losses of blood after child bearing, may lead subsequently to anemia and to obesity."[5]

This old classification has much merit. The varieties of physiologic weaknesses to be expected and the late prognosis are indicated. Of especial value is the information provided regarding the nature of the food intake which produced the obesity and the forms of associated malnutrition to be expected. The plethoric type ingests a great variety of foods. Rarely is deficiency in any food type present. The anemic type reflects the high carbohydrate, low protein intake of many young women. Inadequacy of meat and other iron-supplying foods results in the characteristic iron deficiency anemia. The poorly developed muscular system, including the uterine muscles, results in weakness and lack of stamina as well as dysmenorrhea. These patients are more seriously ill. They are much more difficult to treat, not only because of the obesity, per se, but because of the associated forms of malnutrition, especially iron and protein deficiency.

Symptoms. The symptoms which are associated with obesity, per se, are usually not oppressive except in the extreme cases, in which the mechanical problems associated with bulk may be troublesome. The presenting symptoms may be dyspnea, orthopnea and tachycardia on slight exertion. Edema may be present but difficult to identify. Flushing, excessive sweating and intolerance to heat reflect the difficulties in heat elimination. Headaches, instability or even dizziness from elevated blood pressure are common. Hyperacidity may develop. Irritability of the colon may be shown by constipation and, in some, by diarrhea. Flatulence and indigestion may indicate an embarrassed visceral circulation as well as the sequelae of too rapid food ingestion or the mechanical and chemical difficulties of handling the food load. Skin disorders—acne, intertrigo and pruritus—frequently occur, but usually the patient is so accustomed to them that they are ignored. The strain on the skeletal system may be shown in weakness of the knees and of the arches of the feet. Patients are prone to develop flat feet and degenerative changes in the knees. In general, however, the presenting symptoms, by the time a physician is consulted, are those of the complications found in association with the obese state.

A fundamental biologic principle, which truly applies in medical practice, is the tremendous capacity of an organism to adapt itself to its environment, and particularly to its nutritional environment. The phenomena concerned with the conservation of body water, of body protein, of body energy in times of deprivation have been well studied and documented. Also many of the capacities of the body to adjust from one food pattern to another are known, e.g., the ability to change from carbohydrate to protein or fat as a source of energy as the need requires. Likewise, there is a capacity to readjust to great variations in the average food need. Thus, the body mechanisms concerned with supply, with metabolism and with regulation can all adjust to the large mass and energy exchanges of the obese with an efficiency which minimizes symptoms. Patients rarely go to a doctor for a primary problem of food imbalance. They go because of unpleasant symptoms which represent the overstepping of the limits of the body to adapt itself to the load thrown upon it, and the presenting picture is that of the primary illness plus the features of the particular breakdown in adaptation.

Complications. Obesity increases morbidity, although this is not as clearly demonstrable statistically as is increased mortality. Obese persons tolerate illness less well than those of normal weight, and again the logical explanation seems to be that the physiologic strains of an illness are imposed upon a body already handicapped by the strains of the excess weight.

Malnutrition. Other forms of malnutrition are commonly associated with obesity. It is probable that some of the intangible problems of water balance and nerve irritability are related to the prolonged high carbohydrate, low thiamine intake of many obese patients. Protein deficiency states are often seen among young women, and the "anemic" type of obesity shows clearly the effect of a prolonged low protein, high carbohydrate diet. This description is typical of many young women who by careless eating in the late teens go on to a particularly difficult obesity problem at the age of 30 to 40 after marriage and one or more pregnancies. By this time, the over-all protein deficit, reflected in the weakness, languor, anemia and general hypofunction, is responsible for most of the symptoms, though the disabilities are aggravated by the physiologic load of twenty to fifty pounds of fat.

Liver and Gallbladder. Cirrhosis of the liver is reported to be more frequent in obese persons. The current opinion that cirrhosis results from prolonged malnutrition makes this increased incidence more understandable. It is probable that the long continued high carbohydrate, low thiamine, low protein diet which is so commonly encountered in obesity contributes largely to the liver damage which Zelman[28] noted in all of his obese patients. The development of cirrhosis after years of chronic hepatic injury is not surprising.

Gallstones occur with great frequency in the obese. Eighty-eight per cent of 215 patients operated upon for gallstones were overweight.[1] Fifty per cent of women and 40 per cent of men who had gallstones were obese.[24] Technical difficulties are increased in removing a gallbladder which lies beneath a layer of fat three to four inches deep, and postoperative complications, both abdominal and pulmonary, are more serious in the obese. The association of gallstones and obesity is significant with respect to incidence, morbidity and mortality.

Hypertension. A large literature is devoted to the relationship between obesity and hypertension. Hartman[29] arranged over 2000 patients in groups from 50 per cent underweight to 75 per cent overweight and found a steplike increase in systolic blood pressure with increasing weight but little effect on the diastolic pressure. Evans[30] found the systolic blood pressures of 100 consecutive cases taken without regard to age, sex and degree or duration of the obesity to be above 140 mm. Hg in 61 per cent. Eleven per cent of the total were above 180 mm. and 10 per cent above 200 mm. The diastolic pressures of these patients were above 100 mm. in 36 per cent, above 110 in 7 per cent and above 120 in 8 per cent. From another point of view, Palmer[31] found obesity to occur three times as often in 100 hypertensive patients as in 100 miscellaneous patients. Barr[25] stated that "the results [of studies quoted] have indicated that in every age and in both sexes a steady progression of blood pressure, both systolic and diastolic, occurs with each increase in body weight per height of the

TABLE 9. A. THE RELATIONSHIP OF OBESITY TO HYPERTENSION[9]

(The relative strength of expected trend with progression from lig ht to heavyweight in specific build groups. This table shows the inconstant effect of obesity on blood pressure.)

	LINEAR BUILD (SLENDER)		LINEAR INTERMEDIATE		LATERAL INTERMEDIATE		LATERAL BUILD (BROAD)	
	Men	Women	Men	Women	Men	Women	Men	Women
Mean systolic pressure	+	+	+	++	−−	+	0	−−
% low systolic pressure (under 110 mm.)	+	+	+	++	−	+	+	0
% high systolic pressure (120 mm. and over)	++	++	+	+	−	0	+	−
Mean diastolic pressure	+	0	+	+	+	0	++	0
% low diastolic pressure (under 65 mm.)	+	+	++	+	+	0	+	−
% high diastolic pressure (80 and over)	++	0	++	++	++	+	+	−

B. THE RELATION OF BODY BUILD TO HYPERTENSION

(The relative strength of expected trend with progression from linear to lateral build in specific weight groups. This table shows the marked constant effect of body build on blood pressure.)

	LIGHTWEIGHT		MEDIUMWEIGHT		HEAVYWEIGHT	
	Men	Women	Men	Women	Men	Women
Mean systolic pressure	+++	+++	+++	+++	+++	+++
% low systolic pressure (under 110 mm.)	+++	+++	+++	+++	+	+++
% high systolic pressure (120 mm. and over)	+++	+++	+++	+++	+++	+++
Mean diastolic pressure	+++	+++	+++	+++	+++	+++
% low diastolic pressure (under 65 mm.)	+++	+++	+	+++	+	+++
% high diastolic pressure (80 mm. and over)	+++	+++	+++	+++	+++	+++

+++ Marked correlation, ++ good correlation, + slight correlation, 0 no correlation, − slight reverse correlation, −− marked reverse correlation.

(*By permission of The American Journal of the Medical Sciences.*)

individual." Barr quoted Levy as having shown that sustained hypertension develops in the obese at a rate two and a half times as high as in those of normal weight. Wood and Cash[32] found, on fattening animals which had been made hypertensive by the Goldblatt technique, that obesity elevated the systolic but not the diastolic pressure and that the pressure increment dropped with reduction to previous weights. Robinson et al.,[33] in observing the blood pressure in relation to the weights of 7478 men and 3405 women who were clinically essentially normal, found that systolic hypertension was almost three times and diastolic hypertension four times as frequent in the obese men as compared with undernourished men and that both were six times as frequent in obese women as in undernourished women. Also, among obese men, high systolic and diastolic pressures were respectively two and one half and three times as frequent as low pressures. The figures for women were comparable.

Although such evidence indicates the apparent frequency of the association of obesity and hypertension, the significance of these observations is not entirely clear. Master and Joffe[34] found that, although hypertension is frequent in obese men, there is no exact relationship between high blood pressure and obesity, as they found that the same percentage of grossly obese patients had normal blood pressure as had high blood pressure.

Robinson et al.[9] observed hypertension to be related to body build as well as to obesity, and when the influence of these two factors was separated, the body build rather than the obesity correlated with the incidence of hypertension. The incidence of systolic hypertension rose with obesity in the slender build group but not in the heavy build. The incidence of diastolic hypertension showed more correlation with obesity in all groups. However, there was a marked correlation at all weights—light, medium and heavy—of the incidence of hypertension with the build of the patients, there being less than half the incidence of hypertension in the slender groups as compared with the heavy build groups. Similar results have been reported by others.[12]

Physicians who see large numbers of obese patients cannot fail to observe the difficulties encountered in determining blood pressures with the instruments usually available. Particularly questionable is the effectiveness of the ordinary wrap-around cuff in occluding the brachial artery. In many obese women the upper arm has a sharp cone shape, and in others the circumference is so great that the ordinary cuff can hardly be secured. It is also evident that, with the depths of tissue involved, the pressure in a cuff of standard width would of necessity be much increased in order effectively to occlude an artery far below the surface. This fact was demonstrated in the early studies of blood pressure in the leg.[35] In all probability, obesity has an influence on the incidence of hypertension, but it is perhaps not as great as is frequently supposed.[1,9,34,36]

CARDIAC DISEASE. An increased incidence of cardiac disease is to be expected in obesity—the result of the added load thrown upon the circulation by the transportation of the increased mass and by the elimination of the excess heat. Clinically, there is no doubt of the effect of excessive weight upon the incidence and the intensity of the signs and symptoms of a laboring circulation. Coronary disease is much more common among the obese than among controls, and obesity predisposes to both anginal pain and congestive failure.[34] Also, of 1000 men receiving periodic health examinations, 15 per cent of those who were more than 25 per cent overweight showed abnormal EKG changes as compared with 8.5 per cent of normal and 2 per cent of those who were underweight.[37]

ARTERIOSCLEROSIS. Arteriosclerosis is an important complication of obesity. A review of this subject by Wilens[38] was based on the study of 1250 autopsies, of which 250 subjects were obese. Though 23 per cent of obese men and 30 per cent of obese women had no arteriosclerosis, and 16 per cent of thin men and 18 per cent of thin women had advanced arteriosclerosis, there was a marked increase in the occurrence of severe arteriosclerosis in the obese as compared with the thin of both sexes. This increased incidence was noted in each decade, but "obesity accelerates the development of severe arteriosclerosis by about ten years."[38] Age, hypertension and obesity are considered to be independently associated with arteriosclerosis. When all three exist simultaneously, there is a high percentage of severe arteriosclerosis; 60 per cent of obese persons with high blood pressure were over 60 years of age. Only 10 per cent of this group had slight arteriosclerosis. Although poor nutrition retards arteriosclerosis in the old or the hypertensive, *obesity is relatively less important than either age or hypertension in its production.* Not only is arteriosclerosis rare in the obese under 35 years of age, but one fourth of the obese over 35 years of age have no arteriosclerosis. A relatively small amount of arteriosclerosis is found in patients dying of chronic wasting diseases. This suggests that arteriosclerosis is perhaps a reversible process and that the state of nutrition may influence its disappearance as well as its development.

It has been postulated that there is

an effect of the blood lipids on the development of arteriosclerosis. There is evidence that certain lipoprotein fractions may be altered disproportionately in persons with arteriosclerosis. However, the relation of the studies on lipoproteins to the problem of arteriosclerosis in obesity must depend upon the demonstration of a characteristic alteration of the blood lipids in obesity. Peters and Man[39] found great variability in the normal serum lipids. They found no differences between the obese and those of normal weight and no sex difference. Also, the obese and the normal have the same range of cholesterol variations. Moore[40] found no consistent relationship between obesity and any of the blood lipids, but Walker,[41] in a study of 1000 patients, reported a definite increase in the S_f 12–20 lipoprotein fraction with increasing overweight, especially in men. Changes in blood lipids characteristic of obesity have not uniformly been demonstrated.

Blood lipids may possibly be affected by the type of diet which produces obesity. However, a high fat diet caused only a slight rise in the blood cholesterol in 4 of 9 subjects, and there was a remarkable constancy of cholesterol over periods of months.[42] Hatch et al.,[43] in a report on the effect of high carbohydrate, low fat diets, found that marked restriction of dietary fat with the elimination of cholesterol did not reduce serum lipid or lipoprotein below normal in any patient and that the serum lipid pattern varied greatly. Certain patients gained weight because of the high caloric content of the diets. Walker[41] found a marked increase in the S_f 12–20 fraction of lipoproteins but an even greater increase in the S_f 35–100 fraction on high calorie low fat diets. This increase was due to the high calories rather than to the fat in the diet. Cholesterol levels were less affected. He concluded that, in many persons, the serum lipoprotein levels are very sensitive to the level of caloric intake. It is possible that high calorie diets which cause obesity may affect the blood lipids.

Clinically, arteriosclerotic obese patients, as do those with other nutritional states, manifest symptoms depending upon the regions of most advanced arteriosclerosis—usually the brain, the heart or the kidneys. Since obesity adds materially to the physiologic stresses and strains, it is not unexpected that arteriosclerotic degeneration should be accelerated. It is generally accepted that coronary disease is much more common in the obese. The increased oxygen consumption requires increased cardiac work, which predisposes to anginal pain or congestive failure. From the prognostic point of view, there is a low incidence of overweight among patients who have made long-lasting, complete functionary recovery from coronary occlusion.[34]

The hypothesis that obesity is unduly associated with or responsible for arteriosclerosis is not unequivocally established, even though there is an increased incidence of the sequelae of arteriosclerosis in the obese.

ENDOCRINE DISORDERS. It has been customary to discuss "endocrine obesity" as a form of obesity due to endocrine dysfunction. Such a diagnosis is untenable. There is no dispute about the coexistence of obesity and endocrine disorders. However, Nicholson[44] found no endocrine disorders among 88 obese patients except 2 patients with hyperinsulinism, whereas Greene[45] found no more obesity in a group having endocrine disorders than among normal persons. There is no evidence that obesity results from any endocrine disorder. Evidence indicates that any degree of malnutrition, either over normal or under normal, can be found with any of the endocrine disorders and that the state of nutrition is dependent upon the supply of food material rather than upon the regulation of the rates of distribution of the food substances after they have entered the body. This statement should not be interpreted to mean that endocrine regulation has nothing to do with the disposition of the excess intake, that is, the type and location of the fat deposits. On the other hand, the degree of nutrition, and especially of overnutrition, has a definite influence upon the function of certain endocrine glands.

Fat Distribution. Conn[46] observed that, with the development of certain endocrine disorders, the body fat *already present is redistributed* according to characteristic patterns and that any new increments of fat which are added as a result of overnutrition are deposited in the same manner. The addition of fat increments is not inseparable from the endocrine disorder. In fact, any of these patients may lose weight in the face of a negative caloric balance.[30,46] However, the typical distribution of the body fat remaining persists. The form of obesity sometimes seen in patients with pituitary disorders and hypogonadism and the distribution of body fat seen in disorders of the adrenal cortex are striking. The influence of the sex hormone on fat distribution is appreciated as a normal function. When abnormal amounts of sex hormones appear in a person of the opposite sex, their influence produces changes which are dramatic but nevertheless normal in character. The influence of long-standing tumors and the effects of their removal on the appearance of patients are well known. Similar effects on fat distribution are of regular occurrence as a result of our present-day therapeutics, e.g., the hormone treatment of certain cancers. As a rule, the dosage is not great and the duration of therapy is relatively short. Hence, the fat alteration is not always striking. However, a patient with cancer of the prostate who received moderate doses of an estrogen preparation for over three years showed in his last year unmistakable changes toward the female type of fat distribution. The fat distribution was more noticeable than usual because he was maintained in excellent nutritional balance.

Sex Organ Disorders. Concerning the fat young girl with menstrual disturbances, Tanner[4] observed, "In general . . . in fat women the menstrual flow is more scanty and irregular than in those whose organs are not so encumbered." Rogers et al.[47] found no convincing evidence that obesity and menstrual disturbances were causally related. Of 100 patients with menstrual disorders, 43 were obese; in the control group, which was comparable except for the absence of gynecologic problems, 13 per cent were obese. Of those with functional bleeding, 58 per cent were obese. In the age group of 16 to 29 years, which included 47 of the 60 with amenorrhea, 55 per cent were obese; in the age group of 30 to 40, 3 of 13 or 23 per cent were obese. Given[48] observed 50 patients who were around 25 years of age and who had absent or scanty menstruation. Forty per cent were overweight. A frequent association of the development of amenorrhea with a sudden gain in weight was noted, and a reduction in weight often led to spontaneous return of periods. The basal metabolic rate was above minus 16 per cent in most patients of Given's series, and only 12 per cent were below minus 20 per cent. These observations do not necessarily reflect the basal level of metabolism of these patients, especially those who are overweight, but they do reflect, fairly well, the state of protein nutrition. There is no evidence that the amenorrhea causes obesity, but there is much indirect evidence that the obesity may cause the amenorrhea.

Other forms of sex organ disorders are associated with obesity. The menopause, normal or artificial, is often followed by increase in weight. This is, however, not uniformly true. In the male, obesity sometimes but not always, or even usually, follows castration. An influence of impotence and the absence of the sex hormone on obesity, apart from its effect on general activity—that is, energy output—has not been shown.

Diabetes. Diabetes is common in the obese. This is especially true for diabetics over the age of 40. According to Joslin,[49] 70 to 85 per cent of persons with diabetes gave a history of obesity. Duckworth[5] noted the frequent association of glycosuria and obesity and that a true diabetes might develop in neglected patients. John[50] reported that, among 12 patients 29 to 115 per cent overweight, there were two diabetics and three mild or prediabetics. Newburgh and Conn[51] found that 49 per cent of 337 patients diagnosed as diabetic were obese. When the patients in the age group 30 to 65 were separated, it was found that of these 61 per cent were obese. The predisposition of obese patients to the development of diabetes was demonstrated by Beeler and Fitz,[52] who observed the glucose tolerance curves of 32 obese patients, some of them very obese, none of whom showed glycosuria before testing. Eight had glucose tolerance curves typical of diabetes. Ogilvie[53] observed that in the early stages of obesity, the glucose tolerance may be increased but that, in a high percentage of cases, after 8 or more years of obesity the tolerance was definitely impaired, and that after 18 years every patient in his series showed diminished carbohydrate tolerance. This evidence fits in with the experience of others that the duration of the obesity rather than its severity is the diabetogenic factor.

Pancreatic Islets. Prolonged overnutrition is undoubtedly responsible for progressive failure of islet function. However, the relation between an excessive function of the islets and obesity must be clarified. Insulin was at one time extensively used to promote temporary overnutrition. The weight increases which were obtained were always consistent with the increase in food intake which was secured. Insulin does affect appetite, but its variable effect on satiety may be the factor responsible for the lack of consistent weight gain with this therapy. A more dramatic form of hyperinsulinism is the spontaneous variety found in association with islet cell tumors. When such a patient becomes obese, the obesity is related to his excessive intake of food, especially carbohydrate, which he has found will give relief from the symptoms of hypoglycemia. A patient with the same disorder who does not eat excessively does not become fat.

Thyroid. The effect of hyperthyroidism on the reduction of body weight when the intake is not forced up to parallel the excessive energy output suggests that hypothyroidism might be related to obesity. In the extreme degrees of myxedema, the weight changes are not due to increase in fat. For the less severe levels of postulated hypofunction, much has been claimed. The fallacy in the logic, which presumes a positive caloric balance as a result of a normally maintained intake and a diminished output due to thyroid failure, comes from the faulty information about energy output in the obese, especially in the basal state. In most laboratories, the determination of basal metabolism is expressed in terms of B.M.R. and not in terms of calories. Actually, in the vast majority of patients with mild to moderate obesity, the reported rates of minus 10 to minus 20 per cent really measure the degree of obesity rather than the basal metabolism. In the obese there is no lowering of the basal metabolism and no evidence of thyroid failure. In the occasional patient who has a significant depression of metabolism, there is rarely a marked degree of obesity, and, when it is present, other forms of malnutrition are also present. The thyroid gland is not involved in the obese, and thyroid therapy is ineffectual.

DISORDERS OF THE CENTRAL NERVOUS SYSTEM. The nervous system has much to do with nutrition. Forsythe[3] observed that "improper diet affects the mind as well as the body." Williams[6] speaks of "the serious impairment of the intellectual facilities" in obesity. Many obese persons fit the statement that "fat and stupidity were inseparable companions."[6] Such sweeping generalizations are not tenable. Abundant examples of normal and even superior intelligence in obese persons exist.

The frequency of headache, vertigo, tinnitus and general weakness has been noted, and cerebral arteriosclerosis and cerebral hemorrhage are more common as later developments in obese patients. Impairments in the nervous system thus produced are common, especially in older obese persons.

Interest in recent years has centered around the frequency of neuropsychiatric disorders in the obese. The concept of the jovial, happy fat man is not a true one.[30,54] Hamburger[54] described a series of 18 patients, 16 of whom had genuine neuropsychiatric problems. Nicholson[44] found some emotional disturbance in all of his 93 patients. Others[15,55–59] emphasize the frequency of psychiatric factors in association with obesity. Obesity has been compared[6,30] with the addiction problem in chronic alcoholism. In fact, Hamburger[54] noted chronic alcoholism as an additional factor in some of his obese patients. Suicidal tendencies in the obese are noteworthy,[54] and the suicide rate was 75 per cent greater than normal in a group over 25 per cent above normal weight.[26] Obese patients are subjected to additional psychic trauma in daily life. Ridicule, inability to play games, necessary dress restrictions, lack of social acceptance, conspicuousness in public places, etc., add to the unhappiness of the patient and aggravate other emotional problems.

Just as obesity varies in degree from an ill-defined normal standard, so do emotional disturbances vary around a vague definition of normal limits. Although it may be true that excessive obesity is highly correlated with serious nervous disorders, it is not true that the vast majority of persons who have more modest but real problems of overweight have emotional problems or mood swings which are more acute than those of the great majority of persons who are of normal or below normal weight.

OBSERVATIONS ON THE OBESE STATE: PHYSIOLOGIC

The Physiology of Adipose Tissue. Adipose tissue is a specialized tissue which has for its basic function the storage of fat. It is of mesenchymal origin and is closely related to the reticuloendothelial system.[144] It is a multipotential tissue with an unusual capacity for the storage of fat. Connective tissue may store fat under certain conditions but, when the fat is removed, the properties of connective tissue return, which is in contrast to true adipose tissue. Wells[144] noted that physiologic activities of lipid tissue were relatively independent of the amount of fat present in the cells, and the abundant innervation and blood supply to the parenchyma of this tissue was emphasized.

This subject was reviewed by Wertheimer and Shapiro.[60] Food fat is stored in adipose tissue, and excessive fat feeding affects the composition of the fat deposits. The idea that fat tissue can synthesize fat and the relation of this synthesis to the appearance of glycogen in the fat tissue are new developments. Although glycogen formation in fat tissue has not been shown in normal nutrition, special conditions which involve the flooding of a resting or starved body with carbohydrate may cause glycogen to be formed directly in adipose tissue and thus may be a stage in rapid fat formation. This step perhaps explains some of the peculiar relationships which exist between fat formation and the availability of insulin. It has been noted that alloxan diabetic rats cannot convert glucose into fat in either the liver or adipose tissue but that insulin restores lipogenesis in both. On the other hand, a lack of insulin may precipitate an excessive fat breakdown because of the failure of normal carbohydrate metabolism to supply the energy needed for lipogenesis.[61] Regardless of the mechanisms involved, there is evidently a direct formation of fat from carbohydrate in adipose tissue in which insulin and glycogen play a role. Thus, although fat may be deposited in adipose tissue from the circulating media, it likewise may be synthesized in situ as a direct result of the specific metabolic activities of the adipose cells.

That fat deposits are not static was noted long ago,[5] but the details of the phenomena of incessant formation and breakdown of fat have required modern techniques of study. Factors which regulate the rates of fat exchange are of special interest. Wertheimer[60] reviewed the evidence for the nervous regulation of fat tissue and concluded that "the nervous influence on adipose tissue may be of high importance in the etiology of obesity and leanness, as well as in the localized occurrence of fattening." This influence may be mediated through the hypothalamus, and if so, it serves to emphasize the role of the hypothalamus in problems of nutrition. The endocrine glands also participate in the regulation of fat deposits. The anterior pituitary and the adrenal cortex exert effects which are evident experimentally and clinically, as does insulin, with notable effect on glycogenesis and lipogenesis. The influence of the thyroid gland on fat exchange is by the more obvious route of its effect on total metabolism.

The physiology of adipose tissue has been summarized by Wertheimer:[60] "Adipose tissue is a tissue with special structure and a special type of cell. It is supplied by a comparatively dense capillary network and innervated by sympathetic nerve fibers. Deposition and mobilization of fat in adipose tissue is an active process involving the metabolism of the tissue. Under conditions favoring fat deposition, adipose tissue accumulates glycogen, which is presumably built in the tissue cells themselves. Synthesis of new fatty acids from carbohydrates as well as transformation of one fatty acid into another, proceed continuously in this tissue. All of these metabolic activities are regulated by nervous and endocrine factors."

Morbid Anatomy. In 1896, Duckworth[5] described the normal distribution of fat deposits. "It is naturally found in the face, in the palms of hands, soles of the feet, flexures of joints, around the kidneys (suet), in the mesentery and omentum, in the appendices epiploicae, the subcutaneous areolar tissue; in certain situations, such as the abdominal wall, mammary region, and in the cancellous and canalicular tissue of bones, especially in yellow marrow. No fat is met with in the scrotum or penis, or in the nymphae; nor is there any between the rectum and the bladder. None is found within the cranium." Stengel[110] observed: "The favorite seats of fatty infiltration are the subcutaneous and subserous tissues, the mesentery and omentum, along the fasciae, between the muscles, about the kidneys, and in the liver and heart. The lungs and the central nervous system are rarely and only slightly affected." A large fraction of the total fat is in the subcutaneous deposits.[13]

"Neutral fats are, as everyone knows, lodged, sometimes in enormous quantities, in what are roughly known as fat depots, among which the subcutaneous and intermuscular tissues, the bone-marrow, the mesentery, omentum and retroperitoneal tissues, the epicardium, the tissue about the kidneys, and the tissues of the orbit furnish examples. In very obese persons the fat, after filling these places to their utmost, seems to overflow into the most unexpected localities—adipose tissue extends through the wall of the heart and appears under the endocardium; it pushes apart the lobules of the pancreas, and even spreads round to the free surface of the intestines. In every case the fat is inclosed in cells. In the infant one may readily observe that the adipose tissue falls into lobules which are easily separated. These are seen to be sharply outlined, gland-like structures, provided with an extremely rich capillary circulation, and composed of polygonal cells with very granular protoplasm which contains only the beginnings of the accumulation of oil globules which will ultimately distend them. Such lobules are quite distinct from the surrounding loose connective tissue, which contains no fat, and are very conspicuous in any section which passes through adrenal or thyroid since a comparison with those glands is at once suggested. . . . It would be interesting to be able to show that all adipose tissue is of this nature, but probably in obesity fat accumulates in other connective-tissue cells which have no specific relation to its metabolism."[181]

In obesity, the location of the increased deposits varies somewhat with age and with sex. Young persons tend to have a more uniform deposition with relatively little distortion of the normal outlines of the body, although disfigurement is inevitable as weight becomes excessive. Many young people store enormous quantities of fat in the buttocks. The sex distribution is quite marked up to the age of fifty to sixty. Women notoriously increase the fat pads behind the breasts, the subcutaneous layer of the shoulders, upper arms, legs, and thighs, and especially the deposits in the buttocks. In men the fat is most readily deposited in the abdominal region. As fat men age, deposits occur in the breast areas and buttocks as in the female.

Single or multiple lipomata may occur in persons of normal or even minimal fat content and in a great variety of locations. Occasionally the number of tumors becomes unusually large and may be associated with tenderness or even pain (Dercum's disease). The reason for the localizations of these fat deposits is not clear but, if the hypothesis of the specific nature of fat cells is accepted, it is conceivable that localized alterations in the growth characteristics of these fat cells might occur which are comparable to those found in other cell types of the connective tissue series. When these localized tumors occur in persons who are obese they are usually overlooked but are often noted when excessive weight is removed.

Unusual distribution of fat often occurs in the presence of abnormal endocrine function. Even in the absence of a high degree of obesity, the aggregation of the ordinary fat deposits in unusual areas may be striking. The Fröhlich type of fat distribution is characteristic of the adipose-genital dystrophy often attributed to hypopituitarism. In both sexes the deposition of fat is about the thigh, buttocks, breasts and face in a feminine manner. Adrenal disorders are associated with the "buffalo hump" in the lower cervical and upper thoracic region. The deposition of fat in the face, neck, shoulders and upper chest produces the striking appearance caused by a cortical tumor with Cushing's syndrome. Abnormalities, especially tumors, of the sex organs tend to reverse primary male or female fat distribution. Extraordinary and unexplained localized accumulations of fat, apparently of racial origin, have been described.[144]

Changes in the various organs of the body in association with obesity are not always clearly defined. Williams[6] stated, "That gross obesity is essentially an invasion of normal tissue by adipose tissue is just as true as it is that myxedema is an invasion by what is called mucin." This concept is perhaps not literally true. The deposition of fat between the muscular fasciculi in the voluntary and cardiac muscles is common and not inconsistent with vigorous function of these muscles. Large deposits of fat on the epicardium have given rise to the term "fatty heart." In addition to the superficial deposits on the heart surface, there may be a thin layer of fatty infiltration in the connective tissue directly below the epicardium.[1] The epicardial fat may extend irregularly into the myocardium separating the myocardial fibers and, in severe cases, deep infiltration may lead to atrophy of the muscle fibers. The distinction between infiltration of the muscle and the degeneration of the muscle from associated heart disease is difficult.[62] Anders,[63] in his report on "Fatty Infiltration of the Heart," made a distinction between "sub-pericardial overfatness" which is a common condition associated with obesity and "fatty infiltration." The latter condition may follow "sub-pericardial fatness" but is found only in association with "anemic obesity" of extreme degree and carries a serious prognosis.

The liver in obese subjects has been the subject of recent detailed studies. Colwell[64] noted that patients who were gaining weight rapidly during convalescence from illness showed increased fat in the liver cells obtained by biopsy. The direct relation of the fat deposition to the weight gain was noteworthy. Zelman[28] made an extensive study of the liver in 20 obese females who were 50 to 100 per cent overweight. All showed laboratory and histologic evidence of hepatic disease. The bromsulphonphthalein test was abnormal in all. Glucose tolerance was impaired in 50 per cent. Needle biopsies of the liver showed fatty and pigment changes and periportal fibrosis. None showed normal tissue. The duration of the obesity correlated well with the anatomic changes found. Zelman also noted that experimental hypothalamic obesity and the hereditary obesity of mice were uniformly accompanied by hepatic disease.

Mass Exchange. A body is considered to be in a state of flux, with a constant flow of intake and output. A mass balance may be approximated by quantitative studies of the intake and output factors.

INTAKE	OUTPUT
Food Water	Urine Feces
Oxygen	Carbon Dioxide Water Vapor
Weight Loss	Weight Gain

Unless the intake equals the output, a change in weight will occur. Such balance experiments have been done on many subjects of all weight classifications.

The conduct of balance experiments necessitates a well organized metabolic ward with enthusiastic and well trained personnel. These studies require that conditions for a patient be comparable to the cage studies for animals. The meticulous handling of all food, water, urine and feces day after day for weeks at a time is a formidable task. The intake, food and water, and the output, urine and feces, can be determined directly and with precision. Body weight can also be determined directly.

The insensible loss of weight is the sum of the weight losses due to the weight of CO_2 and water vapor minus the weight of O_2 taken in. The direct measurement of the gas exchange for long periods is not practicable. The weight changes in this exchange are quite large, ranging from one and a half to two ounces per hour under basal conditions for persons of normal size. The determination of this factor is best made by a fine beam balance whereby the weight change per minute can be recorded. However, for long-term studies this method is not feasible. Fortunately, a method has been developed for the determination of the insensible weight loss from the level of heat production. Benedict and Root[65] showed that a constant relationship exists between the basal metabolism and the insensible weight loss in the basal state. If the fundamental relation which exists between basal metabolism and basal insensible weight change holds true for total metabolism to total insensible weight change, a relatively simple method of approximating the insensible weight loss clinically over long periods is available. The total heat exchange can be estimated from the caloric intake and the caloric equivalent of the weight change. By extrapolation from the data of Benedict and Root, an approximation can be made of the insensible weight loss.

In most of the studies of the relationship between total heat production and insensible weight loss, the heat production has been estimated from the observed insensible weight loss. Johnston and Newburgh[66] critically examined the available data and found a close agreement between caloric outputs measured directly and outputs calculated from the insensible weight loss. For persons of normal weight, insensible weight losses varied from 30.5 to 68.4 grams per hour, which corresponded to caloric levels of 1770 to 3570 calories per day. Since the relationship between total caloric output and insensible weight loss appears to be established, the estimation of the insensible weight loss from the total caloric output is justified.

That the results obtained by the estimation of insensible weight loss from the total caloric output are of the same order of magnitude as those obtained from the corrected difference between intake and output is shown by observations made with a normal young girl as the subject, doing sedentary work over a period of 37 days. Her nonwork activities were restricted and no unusual physical activities were noted. The mass factors which were directly measurable are summarized in Table 10. The intake factors totaled 118.0 and the output 69.0 kilograms, giving a difference of 49.0 kilograms. The total caloric output was then estimated from the caloric intake and the caloric equivalent of the weight loss. By extrapolation from the table of Benedict and Root, the insensible weight loss was estimated from the total caloric output to be 44.6 kilograms for 37 days. This value when compared with the weight difference, 49.0 kilograms, indicates a high degree of reliability of the method for determining insensible weight loss.

TABLE 10. INSENSIBLE WEIGHT LOSS OF NORMAL GIRL IN 37 DAYS

INTAKE		OUTPUT	
	Kilo		*Kilo*
Food and Water	117.2	Urine	65.9
Weight Loss	.8	Feces	3.1
	118.0		69.0
Insensible Weight Loss by Difference			49.0
Insensible Weight Loss by Calculation			44.6

Whether estimated by differences in weight or calculated from the total caloric output, the insensible weight loss for this subject was of the order of 20 grams per kilogram per day, two and a half pounds per day, or one and two thirds ounces per hour. Nearly 40 per cent of her total daily mass output was in this form.

The results of a study of mass factors on three patients of normal weight and three who were obese are depicted in Table 11. Only data relative to food, water and urine are recorded.[19] The normal patients averaged a daily intake of food and water of 3.05 kilograms, which represented 5.1 per cent of the average body mass. The urine output averaged 1.75 kilograms per day, or 2.9 per cent of the average body mass.

It is difficult to get reliable data concerning the maintenance requirements of obese patients. The best approximation can be obtained by fixing diets of 2500 to 3000 calories and noting the loss in weight. The three obese women averaged 81 per cent overweight and they lost 160 grams per day on diets of 2500, 2500 and 2900 calories respectively. The intakes were large, averaging 4400 gm. per day, which is nearly 50 per cent above that of the normal group. The urine outputs averaged 2600 gm. which is 48 per cent greater than for the nor-

TABLE 11

METABOLIC DATA IN 3 PATIENTS OF NORMAL WEIGHT*[19]

PT.	AGE	TOTAL WKS.	BODY WEIGHT Ideal	Initial	% Deviation	Final	Total change	WKS. ANAL.	RATE BODY WT. CHANGE GM.	INTAKE Wt.	Per cent	URINE Wt.	Per cent	CALORIES Total	Per kilo
B	23	5	58.5	62.6	+7	61.8	−.8	5	−20	3.17	5.1	1.78	2.9	2390	39
C	33	14	60.8	54.9	−10	56.1	+1.3	6	+60	2.90	4.8	1.64	2.6	2230	39
J	31	9	60.9	57.8	−5	57.2	−.6	4	−20	3.09	5.3	1.84	3.2	1710	29
AVE.					−3			5	0	3.05	5.1	1.75	2.9	2110	36

* Values are in kg. unless specified.

METABOLIC DATA IN 3 OBESE PATIENTS*

PT.	AGE	TOTAL WKS.	BODY WEIGHT Ideal	Initial	% Deviation	Final	Total change	WKS. ANAL.	RATE BODY WT. CHANGE GM./DAY	INTAKE Wt.	Per cent	Per cent ideal	URINE Wt.	Per cent	Per cent ideal	CALORIES Total	Per kilo	Per kilo ideal
Cz	42	2	69.5	149.9	+110	148.4	−1.4	2	−110	4.62	3.1	6.6	2.68	1.8	3.8	2920	19	42
W	38	2	61.4	107.0	+74	104.4	−2.6	2	−250	4.08	3.8	6.7	2.49	2.3	4.1	2500	24	41
N	44	2	61.6	94.7	+54	93.4	−1.3	2	−110	4.53	4.8	7.3	2.60	2.7	4.2	2450	26	40
AVE.					+81			2	−160	4.41	3.9	6.9	2.59	2.3	4.0	2620	23	41

* Values are in kg. unless specified.
(*By permission of The American Journal of the Medical Sciences.*)

mal persons. These patients averaged 23 calories energy intake per kilogram of observed weight and 39 grams of mass intake per kilogram of observed weight. The calorie: gram ratio for these intakes is 0.60 as contrasted to 0.71 for the normal persons, indicating comparatively a greater increased water intake in the obese subjects.

The mass ratios show considerably more individual variation than in the normal groups, but they average 3.9 per cent for intake and 2.3 per cent for urine when calculated on the observed body weight. The mass ratio for intake and, to a less extent, for urine output being slightly lower in the obese than in the normal group is probably related to the fact that in spite of the high mass and high caloric intake, body weight was lost. In other words, even intakes which were 50 per cent greater in weight than for the normal subjects did not maintain the body weights of the obese.

There is evidence that under the conditions of life on a metabolic ward, obese patients exist at a metabolic level of basal metabolism plus 40 per cent. One of our patients who weighed 370 pounds had an average daily insensible weight loss of approximately four and one half pounds, or two and one half ounces per hour. This value, for an inactive person, is more than 50 per cent greater than for a normal person carrying on moderate activities. Similar estimations have been made for many patients of varying degrees of obesity. They all show elevated levels of insensible weight loss which roughly parallel the degree of obesity.

The masses of intake, urine output and insensible weight loss are much higher in the obese than for normal persons. When the observed values are compared with the observed weights of the obese, it is found that the ratios are not widely different from those of normal persons. However the physiologic load of these mass transfers is more clearly indicated by comparing the mass movement with the mass of active tissues of the body as reflected in the ideal weights. The intake mass of the obese was 69 grams per kilogram of ideal weight, or roughly 30 per cent greater than normal. The urine output was nearly 40 per cent greater, whereas the insensible weight loss was over 50 per cent greater than the values for normal persons. These data indicate the enormity of the total daily mass exchange and the metabolic burden that this represents in obese subjects.

Protein Metabolism. The protein metabolism of obese persons is not abnormal. Richter[67] found a normal nitrogen balance in such persons. These observations were confirmed in a study of four patients[68] who were maintained on freely selected diets for an average of five days. Nitrogen equilibrium was at levels averaging 11.0 grams per day, which represented .064 gram per kg. of actual weight. However, when the fat deposits were discounted by recalculating on the basis of ideal weight, the ratio became 0.16 gram per kilogram. The level of nitrogen metabolism observed in these patients falls well within the normal limits. Denis and Borgstrom[69] found a total protein metabolism of approximately 1.1 grams per kg. of body weight, or 0.17 gram of nitrogen per kg., in 233 normal young males. Beard[70] obtained almost identical figures from 400 analyses. *There is no fundamental depression of protein metabolism which is characteristic of obesity.*

The excretion of creatinine in the urine by a person on a meat-free diet was shown by Folin[71] to be constant for the individual and totally independent of the other elements of nitrogen metabolism. Variations among individuals are dependent largely, but not wholly, on variations in body weight. Folin calculated the number of milligrams of creatinine eliminated per kilogram of body weight. Shaffer[72] called this expression the "creatinine coefficient" and substituted, in the expression, the number of milligrams of creatinine nitrogen for the number of milligrams of creatinine. Diet (especially a high meat intake), age, sex and muscle mass and efficiency produce the chief effects on creatinine excretion. In general, the excretion in women is lower than that in men. The lower figure for women was considered by Shaffer to be not an effect of sex itself, but rather of the greater proportion of adipose tissue and of a lower muscular development in the female. The creatinine coefficients of women trained in physical education correspond to those of men.[73,74] Further studies[75,76] showed the relationship of creatinine excretion to muscle mass, thereby supplying a measure of the muscle mass as related to body weight.

McClugage et al.[77] found no appreciable difference in creatinine excretion between five normal and five obese people. However, when the coefficients

TABLE 12. CREATININE NITROGEN EXCRETION OF OBESE AND NORMAL[77]

	CREATININE NITROGEN	OBSERVED WEIGHT
	Grams per Day	Kilo
Obese	0.42	137.0
Normal	0.49	64.6
Variation	0.07	72.4

TABLE 13. CREATININE COEFFICIENTS OF OBESE AND NORMAL[77]

	OBESE	NORMAL
Average Observed Weight (Kg.)	137.0	64.6
Average Ideal Weight (Kg.)	65.4	62.2
Av. Creatinine Coefficient, Observed Weight	3.4	7.7
Av. Creatinine Coefficient, Ideal Weight	6.7	7.9

were calculated, there appeared to be a marked drop in the figure for the obese group: 3.4 as compared to 7.7 for the normal group. If the ideal weight is substituted in the calculation of the obese group, the average coefficient is normal: 6.7. If the relationship between creatinine excretion and muscle mass described above is valid, the hypothesis that the excess weight of the obese is adipose tissue is supported. The demonstration of an essentially normal creatinine coefficient, when calculated on the ideal weight, indicates that the obese have an essentially normal muscle mass.

Carbohydrate Metabolism. The frequent association of diabetes with obesity makes the study of carbohydrate metabolism in obesity of unusual importance. Beeler and Fitz[52] found abnormal glucose tolerance curves in obese persons. Newburgh and Conn[51] observed that obese middle-aged patients with glycosuria, if given a standard diet before testing, oxidized sugar adequately, had diabetic type glucose tolerance curves, and had normal type curves when weight was returned to normal.

The limits of the normal body for handling glucose are not known. Many healthy persons can take in 500 to 600 grams of carbohydrate daily in divided doses without evidence of stress. Experience with diabetic patients shows that 200 to 250 grams per day in divided doses can be handled by most of them. With increasing severity of diabetes, gradually, or abruptly in association with an illness, the carbohydrate-handling capacity can drop rapidly to 100 or even 70 grams per day. On the other hand, with treatment, intrinsic capacity can improve. Normally, about 5 grams of sugar are circulating in the blood in the fasting state. An average carbohydrate meal will be digested and absorbed in about two hours. If the meal contains 60 grams of carbohydrate, the blood must take up and dispose of this load at a rate averaging 0.5 gram per minute as the blood sugar normally returns to approximately 100 mg. within a few minutes. The rate of change of blood sugar in this instance is 10 per cent per minute. A 120-gram carbohydrate meal would require an average of 1 gram per minute to be taken up and then disposed of—a rate of 20 per cent per minute. When the sugar is not removed from the blood as rapidly as it is picked up from the intestine, hyperglycemia and its sequelae develop. Normally, the removal rate parallels the loading rate. Rates of three or more grams per minute are well within the capacity of normal persons, as shown by glucose tolerance tests and by the almost daily experience with the use of 20 to 50 per cent glucose solutions intravenously. Mild diabetics can handle approximately 1.0 to 1.5 grams of carbohydrate per minute, whereas severe cases may be able to deal with only fractional minute loads. This minute-load picture provides a more accurate concept of the dynamic mechanisms and the stresses involved than does the twenty-four hour-load. We may imagine the stream of carbohydrate particles entering and leaving the blood at rates of 1, 2 or even 3 grams per minute for shorter or longer periods of the twenty-four hours. From either the twenty-four hour-load or the minute-load point of view, the carbohydrate-handling capacity of a body is not fixed. It can improve or deteriorate in response to the stresses thrown upon it.

The removal of the sugar from the blood is by a mechanism which produces glycogen and fat in the liver and possibly glycogen and certainly fat in the adipose tissue. Fat is formed directly from carbohydrate not only in the liver but in adipose tissue.[60] Under conditions of very rapid fat formation in adipose tissue, glycogen may be found in the adipose tissue for short periods.[60] The removal of glucose from the blood may be by glycogen production in liver and in adipose tissue, by direct fat production or by fat formation through an intermediate glycogen stage. This fat formation requires a considerable energy transformation which may be provided by the cells by way of two carbon fragments formed by glycolysis of glucose in the cells.[78] Thus, an additional factor of proper intermediary metabolism of glucose molecules comes into play in the formation of fat.

Insulin is an important agent in carbohydrate metabolism—in glycogen and in fat formation from carbohydrate. Wertheimer[60] noted that insulin affects the direct formation of glycogen in fat tissue, and he pointed to the definite loss of fat formation in diabetic animals. Thirty per cent of the daily glucose supplements of the diet of a well nourished animal is converted into fatty acids but, when poisoned with alloxan, producing insulin insufficiency, the rate dropped to 5 per cent of the normal value. No such depression occurred in phlorizinized animals with intact islets.[20] Alloxan diabetic rats cannot convert glucose into fat in either liver or adipose tissue, but insulin restores lipogenesis in both tissues.[61] Factors which favor lipogenesis are those which favor the entry of glucose into cells, and those which exclude glucose from cells increase mobilization of fat.[61] Insulin favors the penetration of glucose into cells. Brobeck[95] found that partially depancreatized rats which were being overfed to produce obesity became diabetic, whereas the others did not. Extra insulin was needed for fat formation with high carbohydrate feeding. Mayer[99] found a strain of mice which readily developed obesity and then diabetes and in which the islands of Langerhans were abnormal. Also, he noted that the factor which limited the food intake of an animal was its capacity to dispose of carbohydrate. Insulin therefore plays an important role in the synthesis of fat from carbohydrate.

The capacity of the body to adapt itself to its environment, nutritional as well as external, is tremendous. The evidence of this adaptive mechanism with reference to carbohydrate handling is to be seen in the "training" of patients for a glucose tolerance test. Patients who have been maintained on low carbohydrate intakes for several days are unusually sensitive to the abrupt load of a glucose tolerance test, but if given diets containing 250 to 300 grams of carbohydrate for several days these same patients show normal tolerance curves. The latent glucose handling capacities are not utilized on low carbohydrate diets but may be mobilized within a day or so by an increased carbohydrate load. There is, however, a limit beyond which the body can no longer adapt itself to an increasing carbohydrate load. When by prolonged excessive carbohydrate intake the carbohydrate-handling capacity is overtaxed, diabetes results.

Relative failure of insulin, from inadequate production or excessive flooding with carbohydrate, results in a failure of the carbohydrate storage as well as the carbohydrate oxidation mechanisms. In developing obesity, the normal carbohydrate-handling mechanism is subjected to a gradually increasing intake load which at first is readily directed into carbohydrate and, especially, into fat stores. As the load continues or increases, the strain on the carbohydrate-removal mechanisms is accentuated by the load of increased metabolism associated with the larger body. Ultimately, the body overtaxes its ability to handle glucose, the "sprain" occurs, and the carbohydrate-handling capacity drops rapidly to below normal levels. Clinical diabetes then develops.

Any factor, congenital, accidental, surgical or infectious which reduces the production of insulin by injuring the pancreas would materially influence this picture. An increased amount of insulin, exogenous or endogenous, would increase the formation of fat only insofar as it is accompanied by an increase in carbohydrate intake.

Not all obese persons have abnormal carbohydrate tolerance.[100] Ogilvie[53] observed that in the early phases of obesity the glucose tolerance was improved and that only after several years was impaired tolerance found. In fact, he believed that the duration of the obesity rather than its intensity was the determining factor in the development of diabetes. It seems probable that these observations may be correlated with the type of diet which produced the obesity. It is our experience that a large number of patients, especially middle-aged women, become obese from the ingestion of a high carbohydrate, low protein diet, in contrast to the many obese who are "gross overfeeders." These persons would have a period of adaption to high carbohydrate diet. As the diet was increased and continued, the adaptation would cause improved tolerance up to a limit where rapid loss of carbohydrate-handling capacity would develop. Clinically, the strain resulting from carbohydrate overload which produced and maintained the obese state can be relieved by giving insulin, by reducing the carbohydrate load to a level which the natural insulin production can handle, and by reducing the body weight, which by reducing the total metabolic as well as the carbohydrate load, may permit a return to normal glucose-handling capacity.

Obesity, therefore, may be related to carbohydrate metabolism and to diabetes. The formation of fat is an active part of the carbohydrate storage mechanism and is increased by excessive carbohydrate and reduced by lowered carbohydrate intake. Insulin is a vital part of this mechanism, and the insulin requirements for fat formation are as important, if not more so, than for carbohydrate oxidation. Clinical diabetes represents a failure of carbohydrate handling both in oxidation and in storage factors, the former being the more serious to life. The nutritional environment which favors the development of obesity also favors the development of diabetes.

Fat Metabolism. A review of the literature on fat metabolism will not be attempted. For detailed information regarding the intermediate metabolism of fat, the reader is referred to the reviews of Gurin,[78] Stadie,[79] and Buchanan and Hastings.[20] Burr and Barnes[80] considered at length the "Non-caloric Functions of Dietary Fats."

In obesity, the observer is always impressed with the masses of apparently inert, semipermanent fat deposits. However, there is vital activity in these fat stores. Buchanan and Hastings,[20] in their discussion of the relation which exists between the structural and storage elements of a body and the metabolic pool, noted that, in time, these apparently stable storage materials reflect the composition of the metabolic pool. Peters and Van Slyke[81] observed that even when the energy requirements are being met by fat, the dietary fat is to a considerable extent laid down in the tissues. What factors determine which fat molecules will be oxidized are unknown. Such a concept of fat metabolism is important for the understanding of the over-all picture of fat formation, transport and mobilization. It restores optimism regarding the efficacy of therapeutic efforts in obesity.

Fat is formed from two carbon chains which may be contributed to the metabolic pool from any source. In practice, carbohydrate is the chief source of fat, although protein and fat, both exogenous and endogenous, can be broken down to usable fragments. The species-characteristic fat is usually synthesized, but under conditions of heavy fat ingestion, unusual fats may be stored temporarily. The possibility that the obese have some unusual facility for the formation of fat has been a source of argument. Lyon[82] described experiments on special strains of mice in which those of one strain became fat more rapidly than those of another. However, it was found that more calories were eaten by the first strain. He found also that there was apparently a higher "efficiency of utilization" in both strains on a high fat (50 per cent fat) diet. Likewise, one strain appeared to possess a mechanism for the oxidation of the extra calories consumed by the high fat diet. Such experiments, if confirmed, would suggest that factors other than the total energy exchange had an influence on obesity. However, it is possible that some of the apparent disappearance of oxygen was related to the more complete desaturation of ingested fats in the slower strain and the direct, temporary storage of food fats by the faster strain. The possibility of a neural regulation of total fat storage, as contrasted to fat distribution, was discussed by Bruch.[59] Gurin[78] reviewed the influence of the extracts of the several endocrine glands on lipogenesis and the facility with which the formation of fat may be influenced by the balance of certain hormones. There is no evidence, however, to show that the balance of these endocrine secretions, as it exists in living persons, has any influence on lipogenesis, which supersedes the basic influence of excessive caloric supply.

The mobilization of fat from fat stores has been studied in the search for evidence that obese people will not give up stored fat on demand as do normal by Von Bergmann,[83] who considered that adiposity was caused by a hereditary constitutional trait of adipose cells which caused them to retain their fat content. Hetenyi[84] postulated that fat, once deposited, could not be released. Bloch,[86] repeating the work of Hetenyi, found no significant differences in the blood fat levels of obese and normal controls at a variety of diet levels and that obese subjects did lose weight when underfed, the weight loss corresponding very closely to the weight loss predicted from an estimation of the caloric deficit. These studies are in harmony with clinical observations that obese persons release fat on demand just as do normal persons.

More recent attempts to explain obesity on the basis of an impairment in the mobilization of fat[87,88] postulate in part a failure of the tissues to break down carbohydrate beyond pyruvic acid and an inhibition by pyruvic acid of the utilization of fat, with a resultant reduction in the rate of mobilization of fat from adipose deposits. This theory provided the basis for a reduction diet high in fat and protein but low in carbohydrate. The theory was reviewed but was not supported by Werner[89] and Hegsted.[90] Werner compared the effects of isocaloric diets with abundant carbohydrate and found the reducing effect of both diets to be the same and to be related to the caloric value of the diet and the energy output of the subjects.

It is believed that a large part of all fat is transported to and from its depots in the body in combination with other substances, notably cholesterol and protein. Much of the work dealing with total blood lipids, cholesterol and lipoproteins has been done on problems of blood fat in its relation to arteriosclerosis. An unusual transportation of fat should be manifest by changes in the cholesterol or lipoprotein concentrations in the blood. The total blood lipids vary but little in obesity with high or with low fat diets. The blood lipids appear to be influenced considerably by the level of caloric intake, regardless of its fat content. It seems possible that the energy requirements of the body are met by the fuel source available at the moment and that the fat transport system is altered continuously according to need. This would account for the blood lipid levels observed in obese persons in view of their known high energy exchange with its inevitable high rate of fat metabolism.

Turner[91] postulates that lipoprotein serves as a carrier for fat in a manner comparable to the transportation of oxygen by hemoglobin. He has evidence that "loaded" and "unloaded" lipoproteins have different characteristics. Likewise, the lipoproteins found after a fat meal differ from those found in starvation, where the fat source is the body reserves. The potentialities for the study of problems of obesity by these methods are great.

Reference has been made to the influence of the endocrine glands upon the location of fat deposits and on fat synthesis. Best and Campbell[92] found that anterior pituitary extract promotes the transportation of fat from body stores to the liver. The adrenal cortex apparently influences fat mobilization. It is said that adrenalectomy inhibits both fat formation and fat mobilization and that these functions are restored by cortisone therapy.[61] The adrenal cortex likewise may have an indirect effect on the intestinal absorption of long-chain fat particles through its control of the normal electrolyte balance.[93] Epinephrine and an intact sympathetic nervous system may also be concerned in the mobilization of fat stores.[61] There is no evidence that the extreme conditions encountered in animal experiments have a parallel in obesity as it occurs in man.

Many concepts of a metabolic abnormality in obesity would indicate that obese persons cannot burn fat for energy on demand. Evidence for such an abnormality has been sought in the intermediary metabolism of fat. The R-Q has been regarded as providing evidence of the fuel source of the energy produced, and it is usually considered that the combustion of glucose gives an R-Q of 1, protein .80, and fat .71 (see Chapter 1). The fasting respiratory quotients in obese persons are lower than they are in normal controls.[85] Table 14, column 1, shows the results observed in one series of normal and obese persons.[94] Although there is considerable

TABLE 14. RESPIRATORY QUOTIENTS OBSERVED BEFORE AND AFTER TEST MEAL[94]

TESTS	BASAL	FIRST HOUR	SECOND HOUR	THIRD HOUR	FOURTH HOUR	SIXTH HOUR	EIGHTH HOUR
Normal							
2	0.790	0.834	0.760	0.767	0.757		
17	0.825	0.860	0.861	0.839	0.871	0.815	0.811
14	0.780	0.830	0.832	0.828	0.864	0.810	0.820
20	0.848	0.870	0.833	0.825	0.860	0.840	0.839
21	0.770	0.796	0.765	0.762	0.765	0.785	0.808
Ave	0.783	0.838	0.810	0.804	0.823	0.812	0.819
Obese							
1	0.788	0.765	0.802*	0.758	0.713		
7	0.758	0.752	0.738	0.775	0.780*	0.842	0.910
24	0.773	0.756	0.852*	0.768	0.708	0.790	0.823
6	0.698	0.700*	0.689	0.700	0.718	0.678	0.692
12	0.830	0.791	0.807*	0.779	0.773	0.806	0.830
14	0.730	0.723	0.794*	0.780	0.758	0.746	
25	0.720	0.733*	0.721	0.705	0.727	0.705	0.719
Ave	0.757	0.746	0.772	0.752	0.740	0.761	0.795

* Peak of heat curve.

(By permission of The American Journal of the Medical Sciences)

variation in the R-Q in both groups, the tendency to lower values in the obese is unmistakable. According to the usual interpretation, that means that the obese are burning more fat than the normals.

Further information is derived by noting the source of the energy being produced after a meal, thus indicating the fuel burned selectively in the presence of supplies of other food types. The remaining columns of Table 14 show the R-Q's observed at the indicated intervals after the ingestion of a standard meal containing 40 grams of protein, 26 grams of fat, and 52 grams of carbohydrate. Here again, the R-Q's suggest that the obese are readily burning fat, and since the quotients obtained, during fasting and after a test meal, are lower in the obese and higher in the normals, the evidence is conclusive that the obese are burning more fat than the normal persons.

Ketone bodies are produced as an intermediary stage of fat oxidation.[20,78,79] If fat is being oxidized incompletely ketone bodies appear rapidly in the urine as is seen in diabetes, severe exercise, starvation and comparable conditions. "Beyond a level of fat metabolism of 2.5 grams per kilogram per day all fat catabolized is not completely oxidized, hence part of the fat catabolized is excreted unburned in the form of ketone bodies."[79] Any inability of the obese to oxidize fat completely should be reflected in ketonuria, but McKay and Sherrell[96] found less ketosis in some obese persons during fasting than in normal controls. Folin and Denis[97] observed no increased ketosis in the obese during starvation. The periods of fasting to which their cases submitted were 5 and 6 days, long enough to eliminate the influence of any greater storage of nonfat fuel substances which the obese may have had. Deuel and Gulich[98] found no increased ketosis in the obese during fasting. Yet the obese during a fast, because of their higher level of oxygen exchange, burn more fuel—which after the exhaustion of stored nonfat fuel substances, comes primarily from fat—than do normal persons. These studies show that, as measured by the degree of ketonuria, obese persons oxidize fat completely and, when under load, more readily than do normal persons. Further evidence regarding the source of the fuel burned in the obese while fasting comes from a study of nitrogen metabolism. In starvation, protein is lost, some of it for fuel. Folin and Denis[97] found no greater loss of body protein in the obese than in people of normal weight. Thus, with a higher level of metabolism, the obese meet the need with greater oxidation of fat instead of exerting greater demands on available protein.

The evidence provided by these studies indicates that obese persons have no barrier to the oxidation of fat as a source of energy. In fact, it seems likely that obese persons oxidize fat more readily than do normal persons, since they usually remain in nitrogen balance when underfed, whereas persons of normal weight do not.[85] It is understandable that the obese should metabolize fat better than normal persons if we consider again the great capacity of a living body to adapt to its nutritional environment. The obese, over years of high energy and high fat metabolism, develop the requisite enzyme systems in an abundance adequate to handle the large fat loads.

Water Metabolism. Large daily variations occur in the weights of the obese. These changes are associated with little or no alteration in the appearance of the subject. It has been assumed that most of this weight shifting is due to changes in water balance. In the obese, the pitting edema of cardiac failure may not be manifest until 10 to 12 pounds of water are stored.[6]

Fluctuations of water balance occur in persons of all states of nutrition, as would be expected from the dynamic concept of a body. The stream of water intake and that formed from food can never exactly balance the output. There must always be an increase or a decrease in retained water.

One method of estimating the amount of the daily water swing is to study subjects under strict metabolic technique. The diet should be as close to maintenance as possible to minimize the effects of tissue changes. The activities should be as uniform from day to day as possible. Under these conditions, observations of changes in weight can be made and the differences noted between the daily fluctuations of weight and the average daily weight change calculated from the total weight change for the period of observation. Data in Table 15 have been selected to show the changes in weight noted in two normal and two obese subjects who were closely maintaining their average weight balances. Included are observations on two thin subjects, who were being rapidly fattened, to show that this same daily fluctuation in weight occurs under these conditions.

0.7 kilograms occurred. The two obese subjects, also on approximately maintenance programs, showed average daily weight shifts and maximum single weight changes of about the same order as the normal subjects. In the thin subjects, the true weight gains were very large, yet the observed daily weights fluctuated above and below the expected weight changes to about the same degree as in the first two groups. These data suggest that daily swings of water balance of a pound are to be expected and that three pound swings are not abnormal.

Proof that these weight swings in normal persons are due to water swings was provided by Newburgh.[85] A normal subject had an absolutely uniform energy output. Utilizing his method of calculating total metabolism, Newburgh

TABLE 15. OBSERVED FLUCTUATIONS OF DAILY WEIGHT DUE TO WATER SHIFTS

	SEX	AGE	TOTAL DAYS	WEIGHT		TOTAL WEIGHT CHANGE		OBSERVED DAILY WEIGHT CHANGE		MAXIMUM WATER SWING					
												Swing Away		Swing Back	
				Initial (Kg.)	Final (Kg.)	Total (Kg.)	Ave. per Day (Kg.)	Ave. of Daily wt. Change (Kg.)	Maximum Daily wt. Change (Kg.)	Day Started	Duration (Days)	Days	Total Weight Change (Kg.)	Days	Total Weight Change (Kg.)
Normal	F	23	37	62.6	61.9	.7	.02	.31	1.3	28	7	3	1.4	4	1.4
	F	38	36	66.7	63.8	2.9	.08	.26	.7	21	7	3	.4	4	.0
Obese	F	53	5	145.3	145.0	.3	.06	.50	.9						
	F	39	7	170.9	170.7	.2	.03	.43	1.5	4	4	1	1.5	3	1.2
Thin	M	35	46	39.0	59.1	20.1	.44	.48	1.4						
	F	25	118	45.6	59.6	14.0	.12	.31	1.8						

The average daily change in weight for the normal women, as determined by dividing the total weight change by the number of days, was 20 and 80 grams. However, the observed daily weight changes averaged 310 and 260 grams, respectively, which is many times the calculated value. Even under the stable environment of these subjects, maximum daily changes of 1.3 and

determined the weight of body tissue destroyed daily and compared this with the weight changes observed on a very accurate beam balance. The daily weight fluctuations of one half pound or more are apparent (Table 16). At the end of the five-day period, the subject actually weighed 115 grams more than he did at the start in spite of the fact that he had destroyed 475 grams of body tissue. On that day he was storing 570 grams of water more than at the beginning of the study.

TABLE 16. CONCEALMENT OF DESTRUCTION OF TISSUE BY RETENTION OF WATER

DAY OF EXPERIMENT	CHANGE IN WEIGHT OF SUBJECT	WEIGHT OF BODY TISSUE DESTROYED	WATER BALANCE
	grams	*grams*	*grams*
1	+285	95	+369
2	−225	95	−105
3	+65	95	+149
4	−125	95	−41
5	+115	95	+198
Totals...	+115	475	+570

(*By permission of The American Physiological Society.*)

Another disturbance of water balance is usually referred to as a "water swing," in which water in appreciable amounts may be retained or excluded from the body for several days before rectification occurs. This phenomenon is quite remarkable in the obese on reduction programs; the same type of reaction, although less extreme, may be noted in normal persons or in the obese on a maintenance program.

The right-hand portion of Table 15 indicates the significant swings noted in three patients. In these three instances, the weight increased on the first part of the swing and later decreased. The reverse is just as frequently observed. In the first patient, on the twenty-eighth day of her study, the weight curve started an upward swing which lasted three days and totaled 1.4 kilograms. In the following four days the curve came back to the base line. The second patient showed a small swing which gradually merged with the base line about the fourth day. The obese patient showed a sharp upward swing in one day and a gradual return to nearly the base line in three days. The large and disturbing water swings seen in reduction programs are quantitatively, but not qualitatively, distinctive.

The effect of the pituitary gland or neighboring hypothalamic structures on water storage is seen in diabetes insipidus. Mayer[100] commented upon the disturbance of water regulation in hypothalamic lesions. Whether mechanisms of these types are operative in the type of water balance fluctuation described above is not known.

Energy Metabolism. The popular prejudice that fat people are frequently "small eaters" and, therefore, have some mystic power of handling food more economically than normal people persists in spite of many reports demonstrating that the metabolism of the obese is within normal limits. "Obesity may not be accounted for on a purely caloric basis."[17] The fact that the fat person actually consumes more energy than he would if he were not obese has been emphasized by many.[11,101,102] Observations have been made repeatedly that the basal calories per day lie between 2000 and 2200 instead of the normal 1400 to 1600. In experimental obesity, fat mice have increased heat production, increased oxygen consumption and increased temperature.[95] Such studies lend no support to the conception of a mysterious economy practiced by the tissue infiltrated with fat.

As in the discussion of mass exchange, energy exchange is best considered by an analysis of its components. On the intake side are the food and the caloric equivalent of the weight loss. On the output side, the total energy loss includes the basal metabolism, the specific dynamic action of food, the work fraction and the nonwork fraction. The caloric equivalent of any weight gain would appear in the output column.

ENERGY EXCHANGE

INTAKE	OUTPUT
Food	Basal metabolism Specific dynamic action of food Work fraction Non-work fraction
Weight loss	Weight gain

ENERGY INTAKE. The food intake is excessive in periods of rapid weight gain.

In periods of so-called "static" obesity, the food intake may be somewhat lower than in the gaining period. This is true particularly in those persons, only moderately obese, who have little or no activity. However, when the total intake of all foods is determined and estimated, the intake even in "static" obesity is higher than it would be for the same person if he were of normal weight. In the grossly obese, even when inactive, the food intake must remain high.

The supposition that obese persons may increase the true food intake, as contrasted to the apparent food intake provided by the diet, by a superiority of digestion efficiency is not supported by facts. Studies of the efficiency of digestion in relation to levels of caloric intake varying from 2000 to 5000 calories have been made.[103] The efficiency of digestion is shown by the ratio of the solid material in the feces to the solid matter in the food. The ratio of fecal solids to food solids varies but little with diets ranging from 2000 to 5000 calories per day (see Table 17). These data indicate that the variation in efficiency of digestion in persons with normal gastrointestinal tracts is relatively small. The efficiency is high at all levels of intake, and the slight variations noted reflect the type of food used rather than any real change in efficiency. The persons studied were underweight or of normal

TABLE 17. RELATION OF FECAL SOLIDS TO FOOD INTAKE

	PATIENT	NUMBER OF WEEKS	INTAKE OF FOOD, CALORIES	FOOD SOLIDS, GM.	FECAL SOLIDS, GM.	RATIO OF FECAL SOLIDS TO FOOD SOLIDS PERCENTAGE
2,000 Calorie Diets						
	1	2	2,150	358	27	
	Average			358	27	7.5
2,500 Calorie Diets						
	15	1	2,410	384	30	
	17	1	2,570	434	19	
	Average		2,490	409	25	6.1
3,000 Calorie Diets						
	1	4	2,920	490	18	
	5	6	2,980	382	57	
	10	3	3,090	485	21	
	14	3	3,060	506	28	
	16	2	3,030	482	20	
	Average		3,020	469	29	6.2
3,500 Calorie Diets						
	10	1	3,510	545	23	
	15	3	3,520	566	33	
	16	2	3,600	560	24	
	18	1	3,710	603	27	
	Average		3,580	568	27	4.8
4,500 Calorie Diets						
	18	2	4,400	707	40	
	Average		4,400	707	40	5.7
5,000 Calorie Diets						
	6	6	5,090	841	37	
	18	4	5,250	854	44	
	Average		5,170	848	40	4.7

(By permission of The American Medical Association.)

weight. They show that digestion efficiency is very good under normal and heavy overload of the gastrointestinal tract. Thus, the possibility of significant improvement in food absorption by obese persons is not great.

The fat content of the stools of obese patients is normal.[89] Nenenschwander-Lemmer[104] determined the caloric value of the feces and their content of nitrogen and fat for three obese and three normal controls. The subjects were confined to bed and the diet fed was below the estimated requirements to maintain weight. The normal and the obese showed the same absorption efficiency of about ninety percent.

Obesity is not the result of an ability of fat people to extract more food from ingested material.

ENERGY OUTPUT. *Basal Metabolism.* Basal heat production is customarily referred to the surface area of the body. Early work on metabolism showed that, pound for pound, obese people in a basal state produce less heat than normals. If height were used as a basis of comparison, the obese would produce much more heat than normal. The value of the surface area as a standard of reference has long been established, particularly for persons of normal body proportions. However, it is important to note the difference between the basal metabolism, which is the estimated heat production per unit of time, and the basal metabolic rate, which is the expression of the deviation of the basal metabolism per unit of body surface from the accepted "standard" values.

In obese persons, the basal metabolic rates are usually within normal limits.[16,105–109] A pudgy woman of 49 years, five feet tall, weighing 294 pounds may have only 6 per cent less energy exchange in the resting state than a man of the same age, six feet three inches tall, weighing ideally 205 pounds. The surface is the same in the two cases, namely, 2.22 square meters. It is apparent, however, that there is a fundamental difference in the two cases. The measure of the physiologic handicap in the obese might better be stated by comparing the metabolism of this obese woman, not with that of a normal person having the same surface—a veritable giant—but with that of a person comparable to her in all respects other than weight and surface. The oxygen consumption of obese persons is high, but the large surface area produces the normal level of basal metabolic rate.[105] That the level of basal metabolism is actually increased is well demonstrated by comparing the heat production with that of a person comparable in age, sex and height but of *normal* weight. This focuses attention upon the metabolic load which the relatively normal amount of active body tissues is carrying.

The data for several series of obese patients have been recalculated[11] to show actual heat production as contrasted with the conventional expression of BMR calculated for both actual and ideal body weights (see Table 18). The

TABLE 18. EXCESS OF WEIGHT, SURFACE AND ENERGY IN THE OBESE[11]

	NUMBER OF CASES	AGE	WEIGHT			SURFACE			TOTAL BASAL CALORIES PER HOUR		
			Ideal	Observed	Excess	Ideal	Observed	Excess	Ideal	Observed	Excess
					per cent			*per cent*			*per cent*
Means	10	37	140	253	80	1.69	2.17	28	62	81	30
Strouse and Wang	10	27	125	207	66	1.57	1.95	24	59	74	25
Strang and Evans	7	37	129	238	83	1.59	2.06	29	58	73	26

average BMR's, as calculated in the usual manner, for these three series of patients were 0 per cent, +1 per cent and —3 per cent, respectively. It is obvious (Table 18, last two columns), however, that the obese persons metabolize in a basal state 25 to 30 per cent more than they themselves would if of normal weight. Ninety-five to 100 calories per hour basal are not unusual in the grossly obese.

A person of normal weight with a level of basal oxygen exchange shown by the obese, representing rates of +20 to +25 per cent, would have symptoms of thyrotoxicity. The obese do not have these symptoms. The marked elevation in rate of heat production, in excess of that which would be normal for them if they were of ideal weight, can be considered as a measure of the physiologic strain involved in dealing with their fat deposits. They can not escape from this extra labor even in their quietest moments. Keys[13] noted that the metabolism per unit of nonfat tissue of the body is not reduced with increasing obesity, but rather that increase in basal metabolism is related to the increased metabolism of the increased obesity tissue. *Obesity is not caused by any diminution of the energy expenditure in the basal state. Actually, the basal heat production is greater than normal.*

Specific Dynamic Action. The specific dynamic action may be defined as the extra heat which is produced in the body as the cost of handling the food. It has been suggested that obesity may result from a reduction in the heat lost following food intake in certain people as compared with normal persons.

Von Noorden[111] showed that a daily excess consumption of 200 calories would lead in the course of a year to a deposition of 17 pounds of fat, or 20 pounds of fat tissue. DuBois[109] calculated that an excess of 89 calories per day would add 8 pounds of weight per year. The excessively obese patient may gain weight at the rate of 20 pounds a year or faster, while the milder degrees approach the lower rate. The caloric excesses, therefore, vary from 90 to 200 calories per day during the period of gain in weight. On the average in normal people, 6 per cent of a mixed meal is used for its specific dynamic effect.[112] Therefore, on an average caloric intake of 2500 calories per day, 6 per cent, or 150 calories, would approximate the extra specific dynamic heat. The development of obesity, as a result of abnormal specific dynamic action, within ten to fifteen years would require a real drop in this 150 calorie factor, to 100 or even 75 calories, a 33 to 50 per cent diminution of the total heat effect in mild and a total absence in the severe grades. A depression of the specific dynamic action of these magnitudes should be readily demonstrable.

Many observers[113–116] suggest that a definite relationship exists between obesity and an abnormality in the specific dynamic action of food. Mason[117] reported that thin states are also associated with an abnormal action. Although Aub and DuBois[118] showed many years ago that the specific dynamic action in persons of unusual shape was normal, Gibbons[119] found a difference between two dogs of the same weight but of different shapes. Some investigators[115,120,121] appear to find large variations in specific dynamic action in pathologic conditions which are frequently associated with abnormal nutritional states, whereas essentially normal results have been found by other authors[122–124] in comparable nutritional disturbances.

The form of expression of the observations which have been made has a great bearing upon their apparent significance. Throughout medical literature, the heat influence of food is expressed in terms of percentage. An attempt to compare the results of different observers shows at once that the meaning to be attached to this percentage factor varies considerably. Mason[114] and Wang et al.[116] reduced their data for successive periods to terms of calories per square meter per hour and determined the percentage variation of the latter values from the basal value. Aub and Means[122] dealt with the total calories per hour and noted the percentage deviation from the basal total calories. In spite of the variations in point of reference, the percentages so obtained are essentially comparable. In some cases the maximum value obtained is used, in others the value obtained after a definite interval of time. However, these forms of expression deal directly or indirectly with rate of heat production. A statement to the effect that Patient A has a specific dynamic action of X per cent, therefore, means that at a certain period of observation the rate of heat production was X per cent above the rate in the basal state. The time factor is ignored.

Two factors exert an important artificial influence upon the numerical values of heat effects when expressed as percentage: the numerical value of the base line and the variations in body surface. The magnitude of the basal value seriously influences the percentage value for a given caloric increment; e.g., a 10-calorie increase at a 60 calories per hour base line is equivalent to 16 per cent, but at 90 calories per hour the same increment is only 11 per cent of the base line. If it is recalled that grossly obese persons characteristically metabolize at levels 40 to 50 per cent higher than normal persons and thin persons considerably less, the significance of this fact in the calculation of the percentage specific dynamic action data after the manner of Aub and Means for obese, thin and normal persons becomes apparent. The second factor of importance appears in the calculations which use calories per square meter per hour as a basis. This expression requires the division of the total calories per hour by the body surface. Aub and DuBois[118] pointed out that subjects with smaller surfaces have distinctly higher percentage increase after food. A 10-calorie increment in a person with a surface of 1.67 square meters would introduce a variation of 6 calories in terms of calories per square meter per hour and proportionate change in basal metabolic rate expressed as percentage. If, however, the surface is 2.2, as in many obese patients, the apparent variation is 4.5 calories per square meter per hour. Although the caloric increase is constant, an apparent variation is produced if the data are reduced to the described forms. Here again an identical change in rate of heat production produces an apparent depression of percentage of specific dynamic action in the obese and an apparent elevation in the thin. This factor may be minimized by the calculation of the basal metabolic rate and its changes on the basis of ideal weight and surface.

The basal metabolic rates calculated on ideal weight are higher than those calculated upon actual weight. Of more immediate importance, it will be seen that the average specific dynamic rate is apparently increased. This increase is due solely to the use of ideal surface as a divisor instead of observed surface in dividing the heat increment. Since the numerical value for the ideal surface is quite comparable to that for normal groups, the percentages for specific dynamic action thus obtained are more essentially comparable to the figures for the percentage specific dynamic action of normals than are the figures based upon actual surface. Many of the alleged depressions in specific dynamic action which have been reported are due to a mathematical expression rather than to an observation of heat effect.

A true appreciation of the thermal effects of a meal is obtained by focusing the attention upon the total caloric increment which may be observed.[112,125,126] "The computation of the percentage of the increment is . . . open to serious criticism, and it is difficult to see how such percentages can have real significance."[112] Attention must be given not only to the intensity but also to the duration of heat reaction. Given repeated observations of time and intensity, the estimation of the total heat effect is mathematically approximated by the determination of the area beneath a smooth curve drawn through the plotted caloric increments and their respective time factors. The value of such a curve is dependent upon the accuracy and

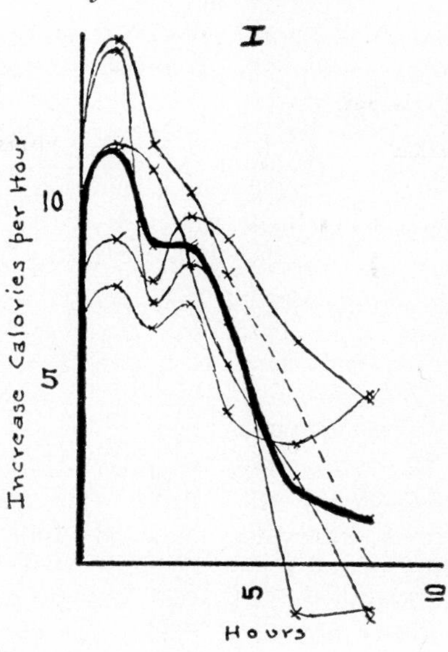

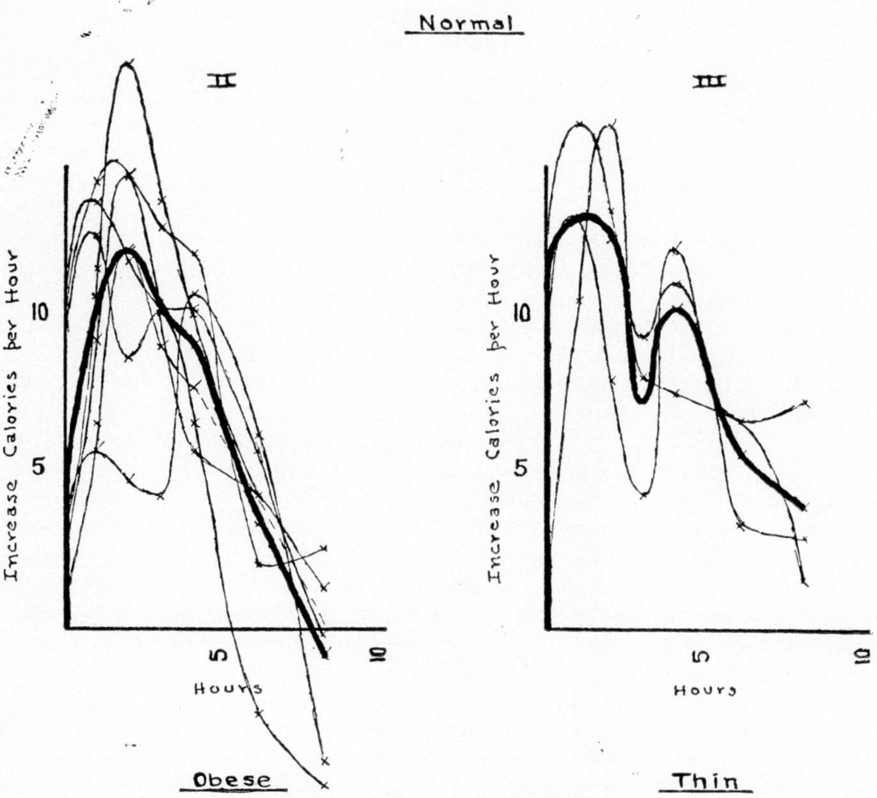

CHART 1. Heat Effect of Test Meal.[94]

TABLE 19. EXTRA CALORIES PRODUCED BY INGESTION OF A TEST MEAL.[94]

TEST	CALORIES PRODUCED						TOTAL CALORIES	FIRST FOUR HOURS	SECOND FOUR HOURS	BASAL CALORIES FOR EIGHT HOURS	INCREASE IN BASAL CALORIES, PER CENT
	First Hour	Second Hour	Third Hour	Fourth Hour	Sixth Hour	Eighth Hour					
Normal....	10	11	9	8	8	5	51	37	14	466	11
Obese.....	8	12	12	10	13	4	58	42	17	571	10
Thin......	11	14	10	9	16	7	67	43	23	449	15

number of observations. Theoretically, points at 15- to 30-minute intervals are desirable. Practically, 1-hour intervals were feasible. The possibility of the failure of the peak of the production to coincide with an observation time undoubtedly tends to diminish the curve area. However, an appreciable deviation from any observed maximum point would result in a very sharp curve peak which in consequence, would have only a minimal influence on the total curve area. In spite of the admitted inaccuracies, the area so described gives the best idea of the true effect of the meal on metabolism.

The curves made from a series of observations of the heat effect of a fixed meal on five normal persons, eight obese and three thin subjects are shown in Chart 1.[94] An analysis of these curves was made by determining the areas beneath them. The averages appear in Table 19.

The data in Table 19 show a heat production of 51 calories and 58 calories for the normal and obese groups, respectively. The average deviations of the individual subjects from these means is 7 and 11 in the two groups, or 14 and 19 per cent from the mean. The thin group averages 67 calories with a 9-calorie deviation, or 14 per cent from the mean. The entire 15 observations average 57 calories ± 17 per cent. As a deviation of but 1 calorie in the base line determination produces an 8-calorie, or 14 per cent, deviation in the 8-hour curve, it may be assumed that the error in the determination of total heat effect is on the average no greater than that of the Tissot apparatus alone. The apparently large percentage error is due to the small numerical value of the total heat effect rather than to the technique.

The curves (Chart 1) show a considerable individual variation in each of the three groups. In each group curves of the high type of short duration and the low type of longer duration are represented. The factors producing these individual variations in heat production may in part be related to the natural variations in stomach emptying time as well as to the less demonstrable factors in the digestion and absorption cycles. The close resemblance in the three groups of not only the total area but also the contour of the composite curve is striking. There is no relation whatsoever between the height of the curve peak and the total area, thus emphasizing the fallacy of confusing maximum rate of heat production with the true specific dynamic action of a meal.

The total heat effect of the test meal does not vary significantly in the different groups of subjects. The observed deviations are small and for the most part explicable as resultants of secondary factors. The individual members of each group show a considerable variation in rate of maximum heat production and in time of occurrence of the maximum rate. However, the total heat production is remarkably constant not only in the three groups but in the entire series. Furthermore, it is not possible to identify special forms of obesity on the basis of variations in the specific dynamic action. Our observations show that, regardless of their varying characteristics all obese persons react in the same manner to a test meal. This is in accord with the findings of Lauter,[126] who failed to differentiate "exogenous," "hypopituitary" and "hypothyroid" types on the basis of specific dynamic action.

The hypothesis of "luxus consumption" was advanced by Grafe.[128] According to this concept, there is a production of heat, apart from specific dynamic action, which is influenced by the amount of food eaten. Wiley and Newburgh[129] undertook to prove or disprove the hypothesis. By a carefully designed experiment they showed that their subject gained weight as expected when given a diet increase of 1800 calories, and that the changes in his heat production which were observed could be well explained on the ordinary basis. They concluded that the phenomenon of "luxus consumption" did not exist.

It may be concluded that the obese differ in no way from normal persons in their response to food. The heat effect of a meal is the same regardless of the nutritional status of the person who eats it. However, the specific dynamic action is not the same for all foods. For protein food the specific dynamic action effect is about 30 per cent of its caloric value, whereas carbohydrate and fat produce about 5 per cent. Hence, obese persons, especially young females, who prefer diets high in carbohydrate and low in protein actually do get a much lower heat loss from specific dynamic action than do normal persons eating normal diets. A simple calculation shows that if a girl takes in 2500 calories as an average mixed diet for which the specific dynamic action effect is probably around 10 per cent, her heat loss will be 250 calories. However, if she selects 2500 calories almost exclusively from carbohydrate food, the specific dynamic action effect will be less than 125 calories—a saving of 100 or more calories a day which can have an important influence on fat production in the course of a year.

There is nothing about obesity per se which influences the specific dynamic action of food. However, an obese person, just as a person of any other nutritional status, can get a high calorie diet with a relatively low specific dynamic action by the improper selection of food.

The Work Fraction. A large portion of the total daily energy output is due to work. Estimates of the amount of energy expended in different occupations were published by Lusk.[22] Passmore[130] recently emphasized that work loads are not uniformly sustained throughout the working period and that the physiologic stress is more accurately evaluated by a consideration of the load per minute. In all of his data the figures given are for total energy output during the periods of observation and include the basal metabolism and any specific dynamic effect of food which may be present. Some of Passmore's data re-

TABLE 20

EXTRA CALORIES PER HOUR ATTRIBUTABLE TO OCCUPATIONS OF MEN[22]

OCCUPATION OF MEN	EXTRA CALORIES OF METABOLISM PER HOUR DUE TO OCCUPATION
Tailor	44
Bookbinder	81
Shoemaker	90
Metal worker, filing and hammering	141
Painter of furniture	145
Carpenter making a table	164
Stonemason chiseling tombstone	300
Man sawing wood	378

EXTRA CALORIES PER HOUR ATTRIBUTABLE TO OCCUPATIONS OF WOMEN[22]

OCCUPATION OF WOMEN	EXTRA CALORIES OF METABOLISM PER HOUR DUE TO OCCUPATION
Seamstress, needle work	6
Typist, 50 words per minute	24
Seamstress, using sewing machine	57
Bookbinder	63
Housemaid (moderate work*)	81
Laundress (moderate work)	124
Housemaid (hard work*)	157
Laundress (hard work)	214

* Cleaning windows and floors, scouring knives, forks and spoons, scouring copper and iron pots.

TABLE 21. ENERGY EXPENDITURE DURING DOMESTIC WORK[130]

REF.	SUBJ.	AGE	SEX	WT., KG.	ACTIVITY	ENERGY COST, CAL/MIN.
84	Av. of 2	22	F	50	Sewing, 30 stitches/min.	1.14
84	Av. of 2	22	F	50	Knitting, 23 stitches/min.	1.17
134	*CN*		F	44	Hand sewing	1.3
134	*CN*		F	44	Sewing with machine	1.6
83	Av. of 4	22	F	50	Sweeping floors	1.7
35	*Al*	43	F	84	Simple work sitting	1.7
20	*C.G.D.*	28	M	58	Brushing boots	2.2
35	*Al*	43	F	84	Washing small clothes	2.3
39	Av. of 5	20	M	71	Polishing	2.4
111	*George*	23	M	69	Peeling potatoes	2.9
130	Av. of 3	31	F	48	Scrubbing standing	2.9
35	*Al*	43	F	84	Stirring	3.0
20	*C.G.D.*	28	M	58	Cleaning windows	3.0
35	*Be*	44	F	65	Washing small clothes	3.0
35	*Al*	43	F	84	Bringing in the wash	3.3
35	*Be*	44	F	65	Kneading dough	3.3
130	Av. of 3	31	F	48	Scrubbing, kneeling	3.4
49	*Bob T.*	28	M	68	Getting in coals	3.5
35	*Ho*	55	F	80	Scrubbing floors	3.6
117	Av. of 10	24	M	61	Cleaning windows	3.7
117	Av. of 10	24	M	61	Tidying beds	3.9
35	*Ho*	55	F	80	Mopping	4.2
39	Av. of 5	19	M	67	Ironing	4.2
35	*Be*	44	F	65	Wringing the wash by hand	4.4
35	*Ho*	55	F	80	Taking out and hanging out the wash	4.5
35	*Al*	43	F	84	Polishing floor	4.8
49	*Bob T.*	28	M	68	Breaking firewood	4.9
49	*Be*	44	F	65	Beating carpets and mats	4.9
49	*Al*	43	F	84	Taking and hanging out the washing	5.0
49	*Ho*	55	F	80	Bed making, bed stripping	5.4
49	*Al*	43	F	84	Clearing floor 'kneeling and bending'	5.9
49	*Be*	44	F	65	Putting washing through mangle	6.0
49	*Al*	43	F	84	Scrubbing	7.0
49	*Ho*	55	F	80	Beating and brushing carpets	7.8
49	*Al*	43	F	84	Putting washing through mangle	8.0

(*By permission of The American Physiological Society.*)

porting the energy output for various occupations are tabulated:

Light industry	1.6 to 2.5	calories per minute
Average industry	2.4	calories per minute
Heavy industry	6.8	calories per minute
Very heavy industry	12.5	calories per minute

Certain very heavy jobs require the expenditure of 14 to 24 calories per minute for short periods. He noted that although the brain has a very high oxygen consumption and uses up about 20 per cent of the total oxygen intake at rest, the increased energy output during mental work is slight when separated from the effects of the associated body movements. The labor involved in modern housework is not comparable to the figures compiled by Lusk for this type of work. Passmore offered a definition of the limit of endurance as a work rate coupled with a rest rate so that the average is not more than 5 calories per minute. Such a level corresponds to 300 calories per hour or 2400 calories per eight-hour day.

These data were compiled for persons of normal weight with normal mechanical efficiency. Lusk[22] showed that big men and big women use up to 25 per cent more energy in a given occupation than small men and women (see Chart 2). However, his subjects were big, not fat, and presumably had normal mechanical efficiency. The efficiency of the obese person as a machine is greatly impaired. He requires more energy to perform a given task than does a normal person.[126] The energy expenditure in the performance of work by an obese person, as for a normal person, is determined by the type of work performed. Although an obese person requires more energy to perform a given task, he sometimes saves work energy by selecting the less strenuous types of work.

Nonwork Fraction. The amount of energy used in the performance of the incidentals of living is hard to estimate. Lusk[22] estimated 200 and 150 calories per day for men and women respectively for such nonmeasurable activities. Passmore[130] found 2.3 to 4.0 calories per minute to be the total rate of heat production during washing, dressing, etc., and that about one hour a day was utilized for these purposes. He further analyzed the energy expenditure in walking, running, and the various recreations. While sitting, writing or card

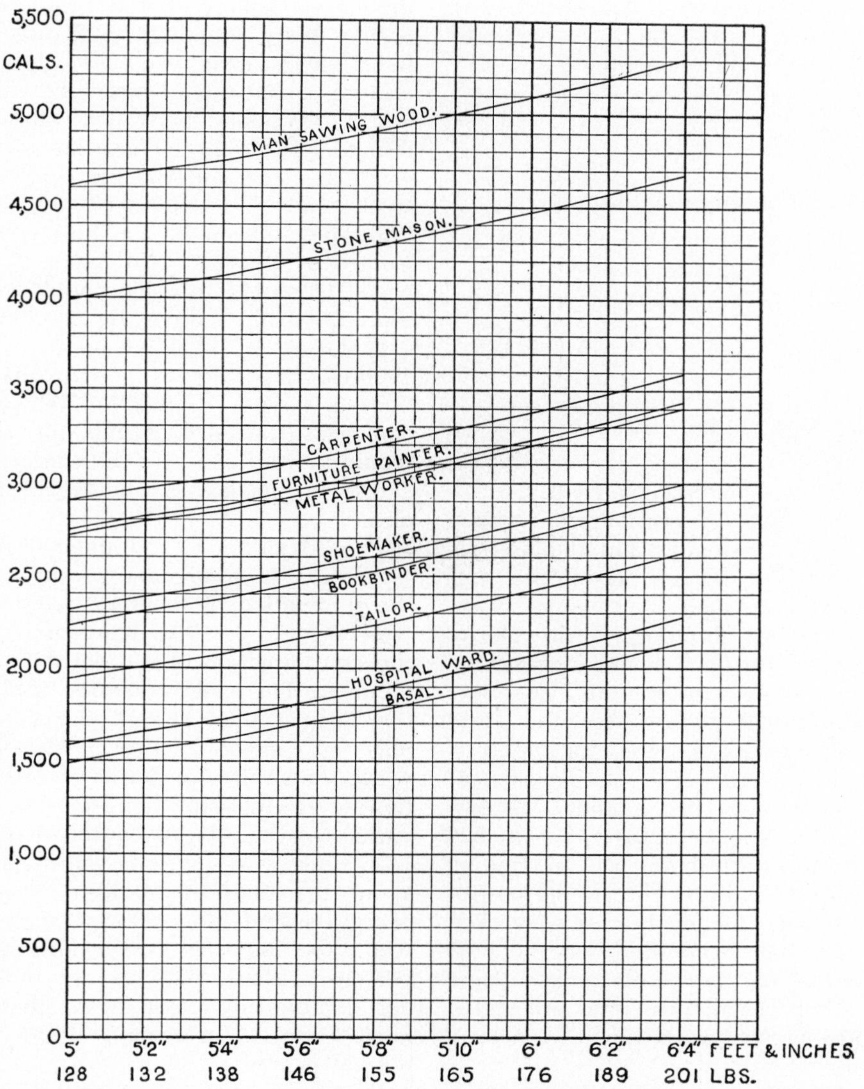

CHART 2. Metabolism in calories per day of men engaged for eight hours in various industrial pursuits.[22]

TABLE 22. ENERGY EXPENDITURE CARRYING OUT PERSONAL NECESSITIES[130]

REF.	SUBJ.	AGE	SEX	WT., KG.	ACTIVITY	CAL/MIN.
125	Av. of 12	8–11	F	34	Dressing and undressing	2.3
125	Av. of 7	9–10	M	35	Dressing and undressing	2.5
20	*C.G.D.*	28	M	58	Washing hands and face, brushing hair	2.5
49	*Bob T.*	28	M	68	Washing and dressing	2.6
35	Av. of 3	43–55	F	70	Washing, dressing and undressing	3.3
111	Av. of 5	21–23	M	73	Dressing, washing and shaving	3.8
39	Av. of 9	18–20	M	69	Dressing	4.0
117	Av. of 4	20–25	M	62	Washing and shaving	2.6
117	Av. of 6	20–25	M	62	Dressing	3.0

(*By permission of The American Physiological Society.*)

TABLE 23. RELATIONSHIP BETWEEN ENERGY EXPENDITURE (Cal/min.) AND SPEED OF WALKING (mph) AND GROSS BODY WEIGHT (LB.)[130]

SPEED MPH	WEIGHT, LB.						
	80	100	120	140	160	180	200
2.0	1.9	2.2	2.6	2.9	3.2	3.5	3.8
2.5	2.3	2.7	3.1	3.5	3.8	4.2	4.5
3.0	2.7	3.1	3.6	4.0	4.4	4.8	5.3
3.5	3.1	3.6	4.2	4.6	5.0	5.4	6.1
4.0	3.5	4.1	4.7	5.2	5.8	6.4	7.0

(*By permission of The American Physiological Society.*)

playing, a person expends 1.4 to 2.5 calories per minute as total output. Driving a car, golf, gardening and dancing require 3.0 to 8.0 calories per minute. Vigorous exercise such as rowing, swimming and hard climbing requires 4.5 to 15 calories per minute with a maximum of 20 calories per minute. Passmore estimated 1500 calories for the eight hours of off-work activities for one average heavy worker (see Table 26). If the basal energy per 8 hours, as estimated from the heat loss at rest, 520 calories, is subtracted, the remaining 1000 calories indicate the energy cost of the activities alone. For this worker, these activities accounted for about 35 per cent of his total daily output. Here again, the over-all principles are stated for persons of approximately normal stature.

The amount of energy utilized by the obese in the performance of these tasks would necessarily be considerably higher. Passmore noted that an 80 pound body walking at 2 miles per hour, on the level, used 1.9 calories per minute, a 100 pound body, 2.2 calories, and a 200 pound body, 3.8 calories per minute (Table 23). These are increases of 15 per cent and 100 per cent respectively, but they include the increased basal metabolism of the larger bodies. For many persons with minor to moderate degrees of obesity, indolence and inertia sharply reduce the potential energy losses. If an active miner expends 1000 calories a day in his nonwork fraction, a saving of 400 to 500 calories could easily result from inactivity which would more than offset the energy wastage from mechanical inefficiency in the obese.

Total Metabolism. Supplementing the estimation of total energy output from the summation of the four components, Newburgh[85] developed a method for the determination of the daily total metabolism. This method can be applied to the 24-hour total energy exchange and may be carried on for long periods while the subject performs his usual activities. His patients represented a wide variety of the alleged causes of obesity. In no case was anything unusual found about the total metabolism. The total energy output was always larger than would be found in comparable normal persons. "These patients certainly did not exhibit any capacity to live at a lesser expenditure of calories than normal persons."[85]

Whether the estimation of the total energy exchange is made by noting the intake or the output factors, the over-all picture is approximately the same. This fact is shown for normal persons in Table 24.[130]

It would appear that the energy exchange picture in an obese patient may be between the extremes of the "plethoric" and the "anemic" types of obesity. The plethoric man is a "gross feeder" whose intake may be 4000 to 5000 calories a day. He has a high basal metabolism and the high specific dynamic action of his 4000 calorie diet. In his early years he is active. His work fraction may be 800 to 1400 calories a day and his nonwork activities may be 1000 to 1500 calories a day. His output equals his intake but both are at a high level. As he slows down with age, the effect on his weight of a drop of 10 to 20 per cent in his work fraction and perhaps a 30 to 40 per cent drop in his nonwork activities on his energy balance is obvious. However, his difficulties as a reduction problem reside almost entirely in his ability to reduce his intake, because his total output of energy, although lessening, is still sufficiently high to obtain a large caloric deficit and a suitable rate of weight loss.

The other extreme is the "anemic type" of woman who has 50 to 100 pounds of flabby fat on a poorly muscled body. She is a "small eater" in that her intake may total 2500 to 3000 calories. Her basal metabolism is high. The specific dynamic action of her food would be 150 to 250 calories less than for her plethoric counterpart not only because of the lower caloric intake but because of the higher percentage of nonprotein foods. However, the big energy difference is in the work and nonwork fraction. These fractions may be reduced to only a few hundred calories each. Her energy output will equal her intake but at levels which, though obviously high for a normal person, are not comparable to those of her plethoric counterpart. These patients tend to gain weight with age more slowly than the high level male. They present much more serious reduction problems because, by tradition and habit, their work and nonwork fractions of energy output are low and the potential caloric deficit by rigid dieting is not great. Furthermore, the poor development of their machines militates against any increased activities which they might be persuaded to undertake.

A review of the several components of an energy balance indicates that the obese obtain their energy from food and body reserves and that they expend their energy in a manner quite comparable with normal persons. *The summation of the four main sources of energy output—basal metabolism, specific dynamic action, work, and nonwork fractions—provides no evidence that the obese person has any unusual mechanisms for the conservation of energy.*

Tables 25 and 26, from Passmore,[130] show the daily expenditure of energy of a 130-pound clerk to be around 2700 calories and of a coal miner weighing 135 pounds to be 3800 calories. The clerk expended 300 calories in work, 870 in nonwork and 1570 in basal energy, a

TABLE 24. SIMULTANEOUS MEASUREMENTS OF DAILY ENERGY EXPENDITURE AND INTAKE[130]

REF.	NO. OF SUBJ.	DAYS OBS.	NATURE OF ACTIVITIES	DAILY CAL. EXPEND.	DAILY CAL. INTAKE	(EXPEND./INTAKE) × 100
111	5	13	Male students, 5 days hard work and 8 days sedentary	3,500	3,610	97
132	77	7	Military cadets, normal training	3,420	3,710	92
39	12	7	Military cadets, normal training	3,430	3,350	102
39	12	7	Military cadets, normal training	3,450	3,410	101
49	10	7	Male clerks in colliery office	2,800	3,040	92
49	19	7	Coal face	3,660	4,030	91

(By permission of The American Physiological Society.)

TABLE 25. ENERGY OUTPUT AND INTAKE OF A CLERK OVER 1 WEEK[130]
Ian C., Age 29, Ht., 66 in., Wt., 66 kg., Occupation, Clerk

ACTIVITY	TOTAL TIME SPENT Hr.	Min.	CAL/MIN.	TOTAL CAL
In bed	54	4	1.13	3,670
Daytime dozing	1	43	1.37	140
Recreational and off work:				
Light sedentary activities	31	14	1.48	2,810
Washing, shaving, dressing	3	18	3.0	590
Playing with child	[illegible]	30	3.2	100
Light domestic work	7	14	3.0	1,300
Walking	8	35	6.6	3,400
Gardening	2	48	4.8	810
Standing activities	6	45	1.56	630
Watching football	2	10	2.0	260
Total recreational and off work	62	32		9,800
Working:				
Sitting activities	22	22	1.65	2,210
Standing activities	25	57	1.90	2,960
Walking	1	22	6.6	540
Total working	49	41		5,710
Grand total	168			19,320
Daily average	24			2,760
Food intake (daily av. determined by diet survey)				2,620

(By permission of The American Physiological Society.)

TABLE 26. ENERGY OUTPUT AND INTAKE OF A COAL MINER OVER 1 WEEK[130]
John H., Age 32, Ht., 69 in., Wt., 67 kg., Occupation, Stripper

ACTIVITY	TOTAL TIME SPENT Hr.	Min.	CAL/MIN.	TOTAL CAL
In bed	58	30	0.94	3,690
Recreational and off work:				
Light sedentary activities	38	37	1.59	3,680
Washing, shaving, dressing	5	3	3.3	1,000
Walking	15		4.9	4,410
Standing	2	16	1.8	250
Cycling	2	25	6.6	960
Gardening	2		5.0	600
Total recreational and off work	65	21		10,900
Working:				
Loading	12	6	6.3	4,570
Hewing	1	14	6.7	500
Timbering	6	51	5.7	2,340
Walking	6	43	6.7	2,700
Standing	2	6	1.3	230
Sitting	15	9	1.63	1,530
Total working	44	9		11,870
Grand total	168			26,460
Daily average	24			3,780
Food intake (daily av. determined by diet survey)				3,990

(By permission of The American Physiological Society.)

specific dynamic action of 260 calories being distributed among these three fractions. These figures break down roughly into 10 per cent specific dynamic action, 10 per cent work fraction, 30 per cent nonwork and 50 per cent basal metabolism. The miner divided his output into approximately 10 per cent specific dynamic action, 30 per cent work, 25 per cent nonwork and 35 per cent basal metabolism, the calories being around 1170 for work, 1030 for nonwork and 1580 for basal, with 400 calories specific dynamic action distributed over the day. These two men had approximately the same basal metabolism. The nonwork fractions differed by 200 calories, but the work fractions differed by 870 calories, which accounted for about 85 per cent of the difference in their total caloric outputs.

These figures are in sharp contrast with those of Newburgh's[85] obese patient who expended 2800 calories a day while at complete rest in bed—100 more calories than did the active clerk. Her basal metabolism, 2100 calories, constituted 75 per cent of her total output. To emphasize the magnitude of this basal output, it may be noted that it was 50 per cent greater than the combined work fractions of the clerk and of the miner. The demonstration that normal persons may expend 800 to 1000 calories per day, roughly one third of their total energy expenditure, in the nonwork fraction and that the combined work and nonwork fractions may equal 40 to 60 per cent of the total output, shows that by indolence and inactivity the obese may retain large portions of their potential outputs.

If the elevations of the basal metabolism due to large mass, of the specific dynamic action due to large food intakes, of the nonwork and work fractions due to the necessity of moving large bodies and the coexistent inefficiency of the muscular system are kept in mind, it is clear that the observed high energy exchanges of the obese are necessary merely for maintenance in the obese state. The great economies in energy output which they may effect in the work and nonwork fractions by selection of occupation and by inactivity should be appreciated. There is no evidence of energy movements in the obese which are not consistent with the law of thermodynamics. "Many novel ways of evading this law [of thermodynamics] have been proposed in the past but we must regard them as emotional and groundless."[131]

These observations point sharply to the problems of the energy relationships which exist in the obese. There is no abnormal sequestration of energy in the basal metabolism or the specific dynamic action of food. Both of these factors may be 10 to 30 per cent greater in the obese than if the patient were of normal weight and eating a normal diet. However, occupation can change the output by 900 to 1000 calories a day. The nonwork fraction can vary 200 to 300 calories in normally active people and can easily drop 400 to 500 calories with inactivity. Just as a careful analysis of the food intake shows the excessive intakes of obese people, an analysis of the output factors reveals the large outputs and where large economies can be effected in anticipated outputs. Thus, the probable effects on weight loss of a properly restricted diet may be predicted by an estimation of the potential caloric deficit.

ETIOLOGY OF OBESITY

It is generally accepted that obesity results from an excess of intake over output of mass and energy. The interest of students has therefore transferred to the related problem: Why do obese people eat too much? The obvious approach is to learn of the mechanisms which regulate the intake-output balance in normal persons and then to note the deviation from the normal pattern which results in obesity.

Etiological Classification. A common classification is:

(1) Exogenous obesity, or alimentary obesity due to obvious overeating

(2) Endogenous obesity, by which metabolic or endocrine causes are indicated.

The endogenous group may be further subdivided according to the endocrine gland dysfunction with which it may be associated:

(1) Pituitary—Fröhlich's syndrome
(2) Hypothalamic — Laurence-Moon-Biedl syndrome.
(3) Simple hypogonadal—eunuchoid obesity
(4) Adrenogenital—usually associated with adrenal tumors
(5) Hypothyroid—usually following thyroidectomy but without myxedema
(6) Pluriglandular obesity.

Bruch[15] divided obese patients into:

(1) "Constitutional type," which is an expression of body build, and
(2) "Symptomatic type," which is an expression of emotional maladjustment and leads to severe degree of obesity.

Another grouping is based upon the possibility of a metabolic abnormality:[61]

(1) Regulatory obesity:
 (a) Psychologic
 (b) Physiologic
(2) Metabolic obesity.

A differentiation between "dynamic" obesity or developing obesity and "static" obesity, a condition of maintenance of the obese state, has been advocated.[87,88]

The meanings of the terms frequently employed have undergone a significant change in recent years. Originally the terms were interpreted literally. Endogenous obesity meant that a person had some alteration in his mechanisms for fat handling which produced obesity regardless of his over-all energy relations. Similarly the other terms—hereditary, endocrine, etc.—indicated specific factors which produced obesity. Such a literal application of the terms is not usually intended at the present time. Rather, the meaning is that a specific factor may have an influence, direct or indirect, upon the caloric intake or output, or both, and thereby may affect the end result of the energy balance. From this approach, the influence of *metabolic, endocrine, hereditary* and *psychic factors* will be considered.

Metabolic Obesity. The possibility that the obese person may have an abnormality of intermediate metabolism which will result in obesity has been postulated. A recent statement of this hypothesis is indicated in the classification of "metabolic obesity." "Such abnormalities of metabolism may involve either excessive fat synthesis or impaired fat degradation. In one instance there is an excess of substrate without an accompanying metabolic disorder; in the other there is an abnormality in the way substrates are handled by cells leading, in turn, to an increased energy intake."[61] According to this concept, the material for this increased fat formation is provided by an increase in food intake.

Primary abnormalities of metabolism in man are known—e.g., the production of alcaptonuria from phenylalanine—but they are rare. The search for an abnormality which might contribute to obesity has involved a great deal of animal experimentation. For man no evidence has been presented[46,85,144] that fat deposits are not synthesized and mobilized directly in relation to the energy demands of the body. The "lipophilia" postulate considers that a primary disorder of the handling of fat exists and that as a result of this disorder an excessive intake of food occurs which results in obesity. The demonstration that fat can be removed from experimental animals as well as from patients by appropriate dietary measures indicates that such metabolic aberrations, if they exist, are not dominant properties of the individuals. Certainly in patients who reduce, the postulated metabolic fault does not operate to divert the food intakes necessary for maintenance into fat tissue at the expense of other tissue requirements. The "anemic" type of obesity might conceivably correspond to a condition in which a normal food intake is diverted for fat formation, but if this were true, there should be evidence of the wastage of protein intake in these patients. All evidence indicates that protein metabolism is normal for the active tissue of the body. Likewise the R-Q, especially after meals, should indicate impaired fat oxidation. No evidence is at hand.

There is no evidence that obesity in man is due to an abnormality of metabolism. The evidence that differences exist in the manner in which certain experimental animals respond to overfeeding is unquestioned.

Hereditary Obesity. Heredity is generally regarded as having a marked influence on the occurrence of obesity. Tanner[4] wrote, "This tendency is seen not only in individuals but in nations: e.g., the Dutch are as stout as the Americans are proverbially thin." Of three series of patients, 50 per cent, 60 per cent and 70 per cent, respectively, of the cases gave a history of obesity in one parent.[1] Fat children seem to have fat parents. Hunt,[17] however, found little or no correlation between the occurrence of obesity in girls and their mothers and only slight correlation between the occurrence of obesity in boys and their mothers. Clinical studies usually describe the immediate parents only. In fact, one report stated that obesity is not transmitted from grandparents.[133] The importance of the hereditary transmission of obesity in association with gout and a tendency to glycosuria has been noted.[1,5]

The clinical evidence of an hereditary factor in obesity has been subjected to much merited criticism. The factors of environmental influence have not been completely evaluated. Duckworth, while discussing heredity, mentioned environment and the effects of customs and practices in different groups in the same region on the production of obesity. Early training influences eating habits. Forsythe[3] wrote, "Adults have many old prejudices to overcome, but the case is different in regard to children. They may be taught to use any kind of food, and what they use when young, they will love when old. If I can introduce a different method of feeding children, my purpose will be answered. This alone will, in time, effect a total change in the general mode of living." Other writers, over one hundred years later, agree that the eating habits of children are greatly influenced by their parents both by precept and by example.[59] Likewise, the social and the economic status of the family play significant roles.[134] Undoubtedly much of the observed relationship between obese parents and obese children is due to environment rather than to heredity.

By definition, hereditary obesity means that the patient has inherited a mechanism which facilitates the development of obesity apart from the ordinary energy balance system. Suggested mechanisms are (1) an abnormal intermediary metabolism, or (2) an alteration of the appetite-satiety mechanism whereby a high intake is secured. In a well studied strain of wild mice, there appears to be a gene which is consistently associated with hyperphagia and obesity.[46] Whether or not there is in man a gene which transmits this trait has not been demonstrated. Evidence is available that metabolic abnormalities may be inherited in man. A disturbance of phenylalanine and tyrosine metabolism, which is related to alcaptonuria, represents such an inherited trait. Other types of inborn errors of metabolism are known, although in many instances the hereditary factor is not clearly established. The potentialities of the hereditary transmission of induced alterations of cellular intermediary metabolism have been described by Bonner.[135]

The existence of an hereditary influence on the development of obesity in man has not been demonstrated either on clinical or statistical grounds. However, the evidence[99] in certain mice of inherited factors which facilitate the development of obesity through hyperphagia, and perhaps through other changes, precludes a positive statement that such an influence does not exist.

Endocrine Obesity. Students of nutrition problems have been aware that some mechanism exists in the body whereby the balance of intake and output is maintained for long periods. Increasing knowledge of the role of endocrine glands as regulators of internal environment of the body made it inevitable that they should be regarded as primary causes of obesity. Classifications of "endogenous," a term used as equivalent to "endocrine," obesity became generally accepted, although McLester[136] described the endocrine subgroup as the "obesity which accompanies" these disorders. Dunlop[137] classified 523 cases and found only 8.2 per cent to fall in the "endogenous" group, 37.2 in the exogenous, and 53.6 per cent were considered mixed types. Likewise, the observation that patients showed stigmata attributable to more than one endocrine gland introduced the idea of a "polyglandular" type.

Endocrine dysfunction is rarely uniglandular. In the case of the predominant disorder of one gland, other glands tend to readjust and adapt the body to the new internal environment. Endocrine glands are regulatory organs. Although they frequently have indirect influences on the intake and output of food, they neither control supply of food nor do they introduce new and more efficient mechanisms of handling food, after absorption, which might result in a positive energy balance and obesity. Endocrine dysfunction is frequently seen in association with obesity, but the same endocrine dysfunctions may be noted in otherwise normal or in thin persons.

In established endocrine disorders it is possible to change the state of nutrition by appropriate control of nutritional factors without altering the endocrine dysfunction. Hyperthyroidism is frequently associated with loss of weight, but a gain can be secured if sufficient food is ingested. One thyrotoxic patient who weighed 102.5 pounds[138] gained, on average intake of 4800 calories per day, 20 pounds in 49 days. Following thyroidectomy he maintained a normal weight with a normal intake. Conn[46] described two patients, with adenomas of the islets of Langerhans, one of whom was obese, the other of normal weight. Removal of the adenoma restored carbohydrate balance to normal in each case, but each returned to preoperative weight as a result of return to the preexisting eating habits. The obese patient then lost 30 pounds by diet regulation, but she regained her lost weight when she resumed her hyperphagia. Examples of weight alteration in other classic forms of endocrine disorder such as "Cushing's syndrome" and "gonadal," "hypothyroid" and "pituitary" obesity by control of nutritional factors have been reported.

Endocrine disorders may contribute to the obesity by influencing, directly or indirectly, the caloric balance. Also, alterations in the caloric balance can significantly influence the function of the endocrine glands, but no useful purpose is served by preserving the classification of obese patients according to apparent gland dysfunction. However, the frequency of the association is such that when obesity is moderate or extreme in degree, a search for endocrine dysfunction, associated with or caused by the obesity, should be made. *The value of the term "endocrine" obesity lies largely in its directing attention to the locations of the fat deposits.*

Neuropsychiatric Obesity. THE RELATION OF NUTRITION TO THE CENTRAL NERVOUS SYSTEM. Why does a person eat as he does? The answer lies in the balance of the two sensations, appetite and satiety; one starts the intake and the other stops it. The sensation of hunger is a primitive sensation[59] which disappears almost immediately after the onset of feeding; hence, it does not determine the size of the meal which may be eaten.[59,139]

Each functioning area of the human body affects other areas and in turn receives influences from the recipient areas. Thus, the processes of nutrition influence the central nervous system and vice versa. The body supplies food for energy and structural elements to the central nervous system, which in turn enables the body to deal with its environment both external, through the higher centers, and internal, through the hypothalamic centers. The nervous system has much to do with the maintenance of the average nutritional level of the body through its influences on energy intake and energy output. The sensations of appetite and satiety occupy key positions in this regulatory process.

With regard to the sensations of appetite and satiety, it may be presumed that the body operates much as it does with other sensations such as pain, sound, sight, etc. Stimuli arise from the environment in the form of odors, tastes and sights, or from the body proper as resultants of changes in the several organs or their internal environments, and are transmitted to the central nervous system where they are integrated and produce sensations which may or may not be perceived. One of the important properties in the production of an effective stimulus is the rate of change of the preexisting physiologic state of the sensitive area in accord with Weber's law. Weber's law probably holds whether the stimuli are transmitted by nerve fibers or by the body fluids. When impulses reach the central nervous system they are received at the lower functioning levels which, anatomically speaking, may include the spinal cord, medulla and hypothalamus. Direct or reflex response to stimuli emanates from these levels. However, reflex responses may be and usually are subjected to conditioning influences which are exerted upon these lower centers from thalamic, subcortical and cortical levels. The end result of these complicated processes of stimulation and integration is a sensation.

Stimulation. The stimuli, related to nutritional problems, may be external or internal in origin. The external stimuli are produced by food and by the environment in which it is served. With regard to food per se, its appearance, manner of serving, temperature, color and other properties produce very important stimuli which influence the physiologic response of the body to its ingestion. Environmental stimuli such as clatter of dishes, cleanliness of equipment or even sunshine and flowers may play important roles in both appetite and satiety.

The internal stimuli which affect nutrition are not so well understood as the external. Many are transmitted to the nervous system by nerves, especially of the autonomic system, but some appear to be carried by less obvious mechanisms through the body fluids. The physiologic state of the body has a great deal to do with the development of the internal stimuli which contribute to the sensations of both appetite and satiety. More important, however, are the physiologic reactions of the body to the loads thrown upon it by the intake of food.

Stimuli arise from the gastrointestinal tract. The early studies on the hunger mechanism by Cannon, Carlson, and others, clearly showed that afferent stimuli from the stomach are transmitted to the reflex centers by the vagi. These studies have thoroughly established the visceral origin of the stimuli, the nerve pathways and the importance of the medulla and hypothalamus in nutritional problems. The stimuli arising from the empty stomach and the factors which modify them are important for hunger sensation, and those from the full stomach and activated intestinal tract following the ingestion of food[139] constitute an important part of the total physiologic response to food and contribute to the sensation of satiety.

Stimuli of metabolic origin have an effect on nutrition. Two possible mechanisms have been described by the study (1) of the mass effect and (2) of the heat effect of ingested food.

The mass effect has to do with the influence which the intake has on the residual mass of material, the body. An attempt was made to visualize the physiologic stresses which are thrown on the body daily by intake and by output.[19] As the first index of the physiologic load, the mass of the intake was compared with the mass of the residual body. Secondly, as one measure of the stresses involved in getting rid of this intake load, the relation of the weight of the urine output to body mass was determined. Included also in the study were data on the caloric intake used (1) to compare the familiar figures for calories per kilo of body weight with data for grams per kilo of body weight and (2) to show the independence of the ratios for mass load and for energy load. The data obtained from three patients of normal weight studied for five to fourteen weeks are summarized in Table 11, p. 551. The average daily intake was 3.05 kilograms—equivalent to 5.1 per cent of the average body mass. It is usually not appreciated that the daily load of intake by mouth approximates one twentieth of the average mass. When it is recalled that the bulk of this load is thrown on the body mechanisms in two or three deposits made within a matter of ten to twelve hours, the physiologic stresses related thereto may be better understood. The rate of change of the body mass at these times is significant. The average energy exchange of these patients was 36 calories per kilo per 24 hours, whereas the average mass exchange was 51 grams per kilo per 24 hours. The average urine output for 24 hours was 1.75 kilo or about 3 per cent of the average mass. The time of the urine output is considerably influenced by the meal schedule, but the rates of change of this output factor would be small because urine formation extends over a much larger portion of the day. Although not considered in this study, the output through insensible weight loss, the other major mass loss, is spread rather uniformly over the twenty-four hours and would have relatively little direct influence on production of stimuli.

What do all these data mean with reference to body maintenance? The figures for normal persons may be interpreted to suggest that an intake load of 5 per cent of the body mass is handled with comfort and that perhaps this loading rate is a component of the sensation of satiety. Certainly these people could have eaten more or less, yet they did what the majority of persons normally do, that is, they maintained their average weights from day to day. The volume of urine was fairly constant. This is also remarkable since additional water was freely available. Perhaps this too is a satiety factor in the sense that a fairly uniform metabolism results in a fairly constant production of waste products requiring excretion and a fairly constant percentage of water retained in the body.

A second type of metabolic stimulus is provided by the specific dynamic action of food. In a preceding section it was shown that the heat effect of a meal was characteristic of the meal, not of the state of nutrition of the recipient. However, the state of nutrition, with its closely related level of basal metabolism, may influence the physiologic response to a fixed increment in heat production. In normal persons, test meals which utilized 40 grams of protein can cause a rise of basal metabolic rate of 20 per cent within an hour after ingestion.[94] Changes in the rate of heat production of such magnitude necessarily produce abrupt alterations in the existing physiologic status.

The physiologic load which is thrown upon the organism by this sudden alteration of the heat production is unique. Many intricate and automatic readjustments are necessitated, especially in the departments of circulation and temperature regulation. Since the reserve capacity of the organism as a whole is usually more than adequate to care for any possible rate of heat production if the alteration is gradual, observations of maximum rate of heat production afford no measure of the physiologic strain. The load lies in the abruptness with which the body is called upon to readjust to new levels of heat production. It is, therefore, measured not by the maximum rate of total heat production but by the rate at which the existing rate of heat production is altered.

An attempt has been made to obtain a relative numerical measure of the physiologic load which was thrown upon normal persons by the test meal. The basic observations are those of total calories per hour for the successive pe-

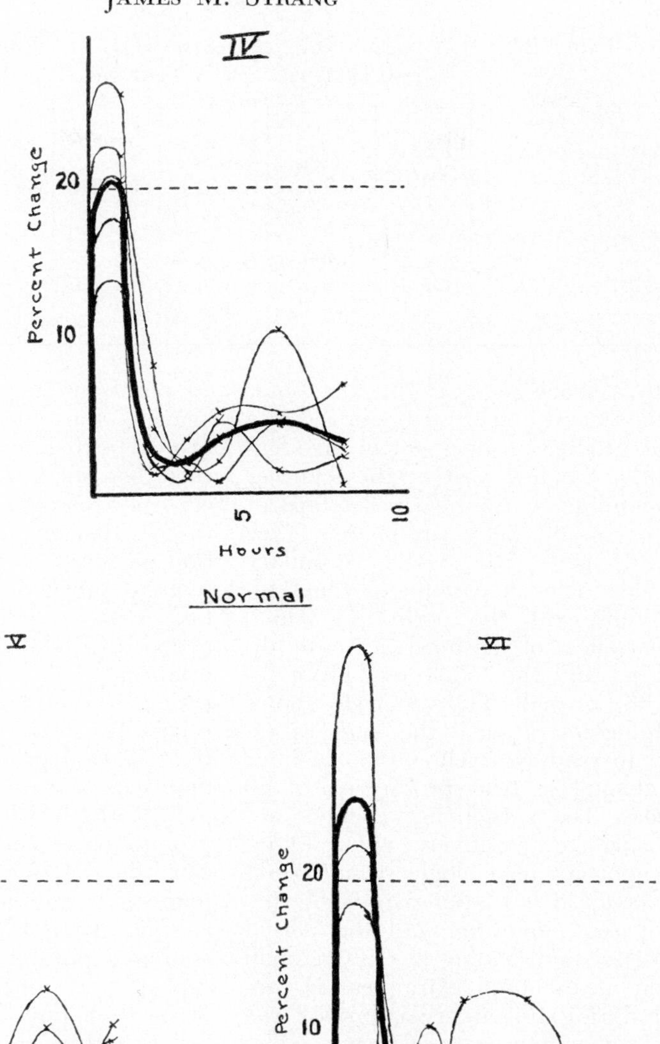

CHART 3. Rate of change of rate of heat production.[94]

riods. However, instead of noting the relationship of each observation to the basal determination, the observation is compared with the rate of heat production for the hour immediately preceding. The numerical difference is then divided by the total heat production of the preceding hour in order to give the percentage change—in other words, the rate of change of the rate of heat production. These data have been plotted in Chart 3 and averaged in Table 27.

It will be seen that, immediately following the ingestion of food, the curve

TABLE 27. RATE OF CHANGE OF RATE OF HEAT PRODUCTION AFTER THE INGESTION OF A TEST MEAL[94]

TEST	BASAL CAL.	FIRST HOUR PER CENT	SECOND HOUR PER CENT	THIRD HOUR PER CENT	FOURTH HOUR PER CENT	SIXTH HOUR PER CENT	EIGHTH HOUR PER CENT
Normal	58.2	20.1	2.4	2.0	3.3	5.5	3.1
Obese	71.4	15.3	4.6	2.9	3.3	7.1	5.7
Thin	56.1	24.7	6.4	7.5	5.1	7.0	3.1

rises to a sharp peak at the first hour. For the second and third hours the rate of heat production does not change significantly, the low part of these curves corresponding to the nearly flat tops of the curves of heat production (see Chart 1, page 565). The secondary short slow rise—maximum in the sixth hour—represents the period in which the heat effect of the meal is rapidly diminishing and the total metabolism returns to normal. This analysis shows that following a meal the body is required to readjust itself within an hour to a change in heat production of 20 per cent. The subsequent changes are small and comparatively unimportant. The important physiologic strain, therefore, occurs in the latter part of the period of food ingestion and the period immediately succeeding it. Only a small fraction of the total extra heat is produced during this interval, but by the time the maximum rate of heat production has developed, the adaptations to this rate will have been complete. It is therefore, important to distinguish sharply between the two phenomena which are depicted, the rate of extra heat production and the physiologic response to this extra heat.

A possible relationship between satiety and the physiologic stress resulting from the specific dynamic action of food is apparent. If this relationship may be assumed, it is probable that when the existing rate of heat production changes at a certain rate, for example, 15 per cent per hour, the body as a whole experiences a feeling of comfort and well-being, but when the rate of change is appreciably increased, for example, to 20 per cent per hour, the body rebels against the load and automatically avoids further insult by preventing further food intake—that is, complete satiety. As a corollary of this hypothesis, it follows that when the total heat production is low, a person on a general diet will be satisfied by a smaller food intake with its smaller specific dynamic action and total calories than when the total metabolism is high. The normal person leading a routine existence has a relatively stereotyped curve of variations of heat production throughout the day, with a resultant constant total output. With the same level of total heat production at corresponding meal times each day, a person on a general diet tends not only to reproduce the same specific dynamic action with its same resultant physiologic load, but also to repeat the same total caloric intake. Some such physiologic mechanism may be related to the well known fixity of individual eating habits, which, in turn, may be related to the equally astonishing relative stability of body weight.

Stimuli arise as a result of alterations in the circulation of blood following the ingestion of food. After a meal appreciable amounts of blood are added to a previously resting splanchnic circulation, and readjustments in the pulse rate and peripheral blood pressure occur. Changes in oxygen requirements for the specific dynamic action of food, as well as the need to remove additional carbon dioxide, introduce additional demands upon the circulation. One of the large loads on the circulation is the need to remove from the body the extra heat produced by the specific dynamic action of the food. Dissipation of heat from the surface of the body occurs and is reflected in the changes in the temperature of the skin. Booth and Strang[140] observed changes in skin temperature following a meal of meat which was designed to produce satiety. In normal subjects, ten minutes after the beginning of the meal there was a rise in the temperature of the skin which amounted to 0.9° C. in 22 minutes when eating stopped. There was further steady increase to 1.8° C. in 40 minutes. The maximum elevation of 2° C. was attained in the third 20-minute period.

The attainment of satiety, as evidenced by the cessation of eating, was also marked by a sensation of warmth in most cases and by the appearance of gross perspiration in some. These phenomena emphasize the importance of the production and dissipation of heat in the response of the body to the ingestion of food. The rapid change in temperature is probably responsible for the sensation of warmth usually experienced, as it has been demonstrated by Bazett[141] that this sensation is the result of the rate of change of the temperature of the tissues surrounding the nerve end-organs in the skin rather than the result of changes in the actual temperature of the tissues. The intensity of the sensation of warmth may be a component of the sensation of satiety. In persons of normal weight the inability to continue eating coincided with a rise of 0.9° C. in only 22 minutes. In any event, it is apparent that stimuli may be produced in the body by the readjustments of the circulation activated by the ingestion of food.

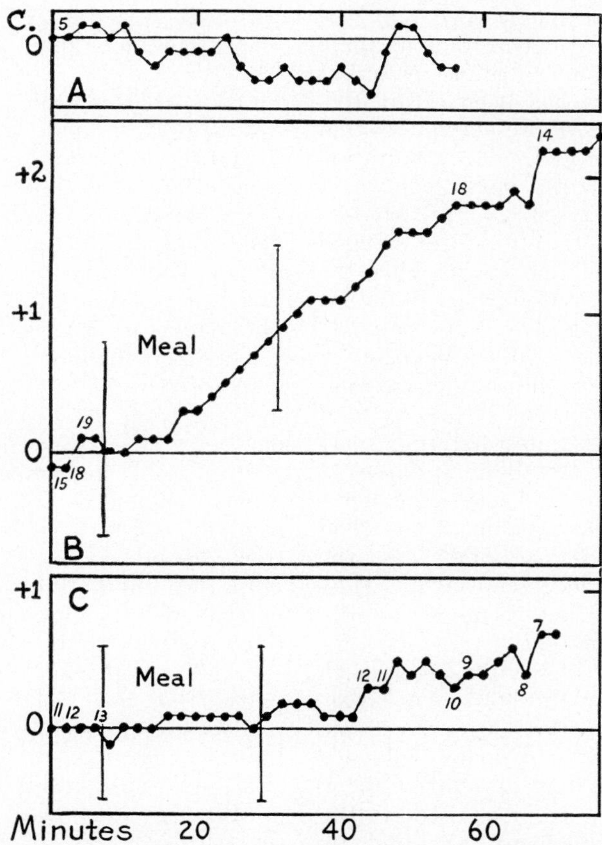

CHART 4. Composite curves of the temperature reactions of the skin during the control period with the meal omitted (*A*) and of persons of normal weight (*B*) and obese persons (*C*) before, during and after a meal of meat to the level of satiety.[140]

Fat tissue has special nerve fibers attached to it (Wertheimer).[60] According to his thesis, one regulatory mechanism of fat deposits is mediated by impulses from fat tissue to the hypothalamus and return. He noted evidence that local deposits of fat can be influenced by stimulation or injury to the nerves in these deposits. "Normal innervation seems requisite for attainment of a dynamic equilibrium in fat tissue. . . . Adipose tissue seems to possess a certain 'tonus' due to constant innervation. . . . The nervous influence on adipose tissue may be of high importance in the etiology of obesity and leanness."[60] Localized alterations in fat storage and mobilization as a result of local nerve injuries have been reported.[59]

Stimulation of the nervous system occurs by changes in the O_2 and CO_2 concentrations of the circulating fluids. A comparable mechanism whereby the effective glucose concentration of these fluids influences the nutrition centers of the hypothalamus has been postulated. Evidence has been presented[61,100] that alteration of this glucose concentration is an important factor in the control of appetite and satiety. Stead[142] reported on the demands of the brain for oxygen which are relatively enormous when the mass of the brain is compared to the remainder of the body. It is possible, therefore, that the relative diversion of O_2 supplies from the autocratic and parasitic central nervous system by food loads in the gastrointestinal tract may be an additional metabolic stimulus to arrest intake of food. There is evidence also that the caloric value of the food intake, per se, has an influence on the total amount of food taken in[139,143] How this metabolic stimulus might be developed is not apparent.

A great variety of stimuli arising both outside and inside the body may be associated with nutrition processes. Some appear to have their major influence upon the sensation of appetite. Others, especially those resulting from the physiologic readjustments required by food loads, affect the sensation of satiety. The limited number of nutritional stimuli described merely outline the pattern showing how factors in the external and internal environment may exert their influence on the intake-output balance by way of the central nervous system.

Integration. The integration of the many stimuli occurs primarily in the reflex areas of the nervous system. The hypothalamus is the location of regulatory centers of many of the homeostatic mechanisms of the body. There is much evidence that it is likewise the location of the feeding centers. Two such centers have been identified in the hypothalamus by experimental methods. Lesions of a center in the region of the ventromedial nuclei result in hyperphagia; lesions of a center in a lateral area result in complete anaphagia. Apparently the lateral area has the dominant influence, since lesions of both areas result in anaphagia even when a previous medial lesion was producing obesity by hyperphagia.[61,95,139,145] Mayer[100] has postulated a glucostatic center in the hypothalamus. This center is sensitive to alterations in the effective concentration of glucose in the blood. Low glucose concentrations would stimulate food intake and high levels restrict intake. The existence of hunger centers and water-regulating centers in the hypothalamus is also probable.

The hypothalamic nutrition centers are subject to important conditioning influences from the higher centers of the nervous system. Emotional tension, both acute and chronic, influences appetite and satiety mechanisms. Intake and cessation of intake can be accelerated or inhibited from influences of this level. Memories, both pleasant and unpleasant, are important factors, and habituation, as distinct from habit, has its effect. This is especially noticeable when an eating pattern has developed as a result of a physiologic stress, and the pattern continues long after the removal of the stress. The sum total of human qualities, personality, will power and the capacity for self-discipline are important conditioning agents for the maintenance of normal nutritional balance.

Sensation. The results of the many stimuli and of their integration by the central nervous system are two sensations, appetite and satiety. Appetite is a sensation which has to do with the initiation of food intake. Observations of human beings and their eating patterns show that this process is much more than a simple reflex. Satiety is a pleasant sensation of comfort and well-being which results when a person has ingested a physiologically satisfactory amount of food. With the attainment of this sensation he stops eating. Undoubtedly many factors, at reflex levels, are important contributors, especially those factors which have to do directly with the disposition of the mass of food load or of its heat effects. It is understandable that sharp rates of change will produce automatic responses which tend to arrest the changes. The initial physiologic state of the body has just as important a role in the reaction as does the food load. The influences of all of the factors of stimulation are more readily demonstrable in the sensation of satiety than of appetite. The influence of conditioning factors is always large. Habit, for example, definitely influences the size of the food load which produces satiety. One has only to consider the satisfaction and comfort resulting from a normal breakfast with its limited physiologic load and the same comfort and satisfaction from a much different dinner. It is not merely a matter of so many grams of protein, carbohydrate and fat, as with animals. Traditional food types for specific meals, times of meals, etc., are equally important factors in determining just how much food is taken in before satiety develops. Skillful cooking and attractive serving are important factors in promoting food intake. The pleasurable environmental influences of a holiday or a banquet alter the normal satiety patterns and permit the ingestion of relatively enormous intakes on these occasions. Conditioning influences likewise make possible the alterations of satiety sensations by training. An undernourished young man maintained an average weight of 115 pounds. By diet, his weight was increased to 160 pounds in several years. He now maintains this weight and its intake-output level with the same comfort as his original level. The reverse picture provides the only hope for the obese patient. He must develop normal satiety reactions at a normal level of intake and output. It is impossible to identify any single stimulus or any single conditioning factor as the sole or even major influence in satiety. The importance of the sensation of satiety for nutrition lies in the number of calories ingested before this sensation is produced.

The Central Nervous System in Relation to Obesity. Much has been written about the neuropsychiatric causation of obesity. It was originally presumed that apart from the intake-output energy relationship some neuropsychiatric factor caused the deposition of fat. At present, however, students prefer to state that a neuropsychiatric disturbance causes a relative hyperphagia and thereby obesity. How neuropsychiatric influences may affect the state of nutrition may be considered by noting the deviations observed in obesity from the normal influences of the central nervous system on nutrition, as described above.

Stimulation. Effective stimulation of the nutrition centers may be diminished in the obese, especially the internal stimuli. In gastrointestinal stimulation, it is obvious that the enlarged stomach of a fat person requires a greater filling than the small stomach of a thin person in order to produce the comparable sense of distention.

With regard to metabolic stimulation we again find evidence of reduced stimulation. The rates of change are diminished because of the greatly increased basic levels of function. The data for the mass exchange of three obese patients were described above in the section on mass exchange (Table 11).[19] These data show that although the obese persons actually took in and put out more than 40 per cent more food than the normals, their rates of mass exchange were appreciably lower and consequently the mass stimulus to the nutrition centers would be reduced. This point is supported somewhat by the observed increase in water intake which might be interpreted as evidence of an attempt on the part of the body to attain a comfortable mass balance. Insofar, therefore, as a rate of mass exchange of around 5 per cent contributes to the development of satiety, it will be apparent that obese people would take in large amounts of material, usually food with real energy content, when available, to supply this mass and thereby maintain or increase their obesity.

The second type of metabolic stimulus described above, the specific dynamic action of food, provides a similar story of ineffective stimulation because the high basal levels of heat production result in lowered rates of change. Five obese patients were studied with regard to their rates of response to a fixed meal in a manner comparable to the normal persons previously described.[94] The data appear in Table 27 and Chart 3 with those of normal and thin persons who were fed identical meals. The general form of the curve of the obese group is quite comparable with that of the normal group. The significant point is that the maximum of the composite curve falls at 15 per cent, which is 25 per cent lower than for the normal group. On the other hand, the thin group as shown in Chart 3 reached its maximum at 25 per cent, which is 25 per cent higher than for the normal group. Hence, although identical meals produce the same total heat reaction in normal, thin and obese persons, the physiologic load of this extra heat production is approximately one fourth less in the obese and one fourth greater in the thin than in the normal—the thin group bears a 66 per cent greater physiologic strain than the obese in the handling of a meal which is identical in protein, fat and carbohydrate and in total calories. The great difference between the various nutritional states lies not in the total extra heat production from food, but in the differences in physiologic load resulting from the same increment of heat.

In the discussion of satiety in normal persons it was assumed that the optimum feeling of well-being paralleled a rate of change of heat production of 15 per cent, and that when this rate increased to 20 per cent a feeling of absolute satiety ensued which prevented further food intake. If these same figures are applied to the curves of the thin and obese groups a striking observation will be made. Whereas in the normal persons satiety, 20 per cent, corresponds to the peak of the heat curve, in the thin the satiety point was passed long before the peak was reached. This may be interpreted to indicate that the test meal was considerably greater in specific dynamic action and, therefore, in total calories than a meal which these persons would voluntarily have selected. On the other hand, the peak of the obese curve fails to reach the satiety level by 25 per cent, and, in fact, coincides with the level of optimum sensation. A comparable interpretation would suggest that the test meal, with its fixed total calories and specific dynamic action, would fail to satisfy these patients. In other words, if we assume that the test meal, with its 40 grams of protein and 610 calories, completely satisfied the normal group, the thin patients, if permitted free selection of food, would have been satisfied with much less food, whereas the obese group would have obtained a far greater intake. The selection of the values, 15 and 20 per cent, for the critical points is quite arbitrary, and more careful investigation may reveal different true levels. However, regardless of the levels selected, the fundamental difference between the three groups will persist. Furthermore, it may later be shown that the peaks of the curves of rate of change of heat production fall earlier in the thin group and later in the obese group than in the normal group. If, for example, the peaks were found to be at 20 minutes, 40 minutes and 60 minutes in the thin, normal and obese groups, the resultant effects upon their respective total food intakes would be accentuations of tendencies described above.

The same factors which operate to produce the fixed eating habits and fixed body weights of normal persons may become perverted in two directions. The resultant extreme in one case is the apparently healthy person who persistently holds a weight 20 to 25 per cent below normal. He functions at a low metabolic level and receives his optimal specific dynamic action stimulus from a small food intake which maintains his weight by a caloric intake equivalent to his output. The other extreme is the likewise apparently healthy person who maintains a weight 50 to 200 per cent above normal and operates at a very high level of metabolism. He holds his weight, or, as usually happens, slightly increases his weight, because of the correspondingly large caloric intake which is required to produce the requisite rate of change of heat production for the optimum sensation of satiety. The persistent small intake of the thin and the large intake of the obese are probably further aggravated by secondary phenomena both psychic and mechanical. In both of these abnormal states vicious habit cycles are firmly established. In neither case does any new abnormal factor in metabolism exist.

The changes produced in the circulatory system by food intake would likewise be less intense in the obese than in normal persons. Obese persons normally have relatively high levels of basal metabolism. As in all conditions of elevated metabolism, an increase in the normal circulatory load results from the need for increased heat dissipation. In the so-called "plethoric" type of obesity, the greatly increased skin circulation with its consequent increased heat loss is usually evident.

The rate of change of skin temperature after eating is much reduced in the obese as compared with normal persons. Not only was the maximum rise in skin temperature in the obese less than one third that of normal, but the onset of the rise occurred after 24 minutes in the obese as contrasted to 10 minutes for the normal subjects.[140] In obese subjects the total production of heat in response to food is probably the same as in persons of normal weight. Although the total production of heat is the same, studies of the specific dynamic action showed a slower rate of change of the rate of production of heat and the maximum point of the rate of change was somewhat delayed. This phenomenon is conceivably reflected in the diminished and delayed elevation of the temperature of the skin in the obese subjects. The resulting decrease in the intensity of the feeling of warmth may be one more factor in the delay of the sensation of satiety.

In the matter of the development of nutritional stimuli the obese show characteristic alterations from the normal patterns. Although only a few facets have been studied, the evidence indicates that effective stimulation, especially of the mechanisms involved in the production of satiety, is absent or delayed. This is particularly true of the stimuli resulting from the physiologic responses of the body to food loads. These minimal stimuli consequently favor the ingestion of larger and larger food intakes in order to promote the development of an adequate sense of satiety.

Integration. The alterations in the integration of nutritional stimuli by the central nervous system of the obese are many. There appears to be no doubt that feeding centers exist in the hypothalamus. They possibly exert an influence on intake and output of food at the reflex level. However, there is no evidence that lesions of these areas are associated with the development of obesity in man.[44,46,100] The possibility of functional alterations in these reflex centers which might be produced in man by training and established habit must be recognized. That such acquired functional alterations may not be permanently dominant properties is shown by the establishment of normal eating patterns by proper reduction programs.

Whether or not alterations in the feeding centers located in the hypothalamus exist in man apart from those resulting from habit, cannot be proved. Conn referred to obese patients being conditioned to a "higher satiety level."[46] Bruch[59] suggested that hypothalamic imbalance can exist either in the form of an increased appetite with normal satiety centers or a normal appetite with hyposensitive satiety centers. Pennington[88] postulated that alterations in the sensitivity of the hypothalamus might produce obesity through an effect on the balance between fat deposition and fat mobilization as well as through a direct effect upon appetite. Although much of the regulation of intake appears to be more or less automatic from reflex levels, it is difficult to separate simple from conditioned reflexes in a sentient animal such as man. The higher centers have the function of selective facilitation or inhibition of the feeding reflexes.[139] In man this higher control is undoubtedly dominantly operative even in what seems to be automatic feeding.

The importance in obesity of alterations in the conditioning areas has been emphasized. Obesity in persons with congenital or acquired brain injury is noted occasionally. Hyperphagia is usually a characteristic of these patients, but apathy and lack of activity contribute to the resultant obesity. Although these problems are not of frequent occurrence in ordinary practice, Mayer[100] described a series of 74 cases of frontal lobotomy of which 70 showed marked increase in appetite associated with laziness and lack of initiative.

Many authors consider obesity to be solely a symptom of emotional instability. Bruch[59] looked upon obesity as the result of a "dissatisfaction of a person accustomed to having his desires met who meets denial." Practically every form of mental disorder has been identified with obesity.[56] Bruch[59,146] emphasized the immaturity of her young patients, noting that many of the children were overprotected and could not dress or bathe themselves until ten years of age. Parson[55] and Kantor[147] described the "intensity of the drive to overeat." The term "addiction to food," mentioned by Evans,[30] was elaborated by Hamburger[54] who grouped his cases into four classes: (1) overeating as a response to nonspecific emotional tensions, (2) overeating as a substitute gratification in intolerable life situations, (3) overeating as a symptom of an underlying emotional illness, especially depression and hysteria, and (4) overeating as an addiction to food.

From the intensity of the neuropsychiatric symptoms, patients may be grouped into mild, moderate and severe. The mild disorders are readily recognized.[54,57] They may be considered as those patients who appreciate the relationship of their overeating to their obesity. Gelvin[8] reported 108 cases of whom 50 per cent stated that they ate too much and one third of the others admitted that they did. Freed[148] reported that 74 per cent of 500 patients were aware that they ate more when they were worried or nervous, 19 per cent ate more when they were "idle, bored, or tired." Darling[57] described his first group: "Although obesity is largely the result of psychological forces, these forces were of no more serious character than those which occur in other 'normal' people whose defences against anxiety take other forms, e.g., overwork, thrift to the point of self-abnegation, fantasy, and so on." The moderately ill persons seem to be unaware of the relationship of the mental disturbance to hyperphagia, although in many other respects they behave in normal patterns.[54,57] Many obese patients have been found to have serious neuropsychiatric disturbances. In addition to the symptomatic hyperphagia, other significant manifestations of personality disorders such as drunkeness, drug addiction, petty thievery and suicidal tendencies have been encountered.[15,54,56]

There can be no question about the frequent association of obesity and neuropsychiatric disturbances. Whether or not the neuropsychiatric disturbance causes the obesity is another matter. Statements such as "psychologic conflicts giving rise to the obese state,"[56] "preponderance of evidence is in form of an emotional cause for the hyperphagia in most patients,"[56] "fact that emotional tension and psychoneurosis will in certain people produce obesity"[44] imply this causal relationship. "The hypothesis is advanced that emotional experiences call into play functional disturbances of the hypothalamus which may be of importance in the large group of obese patients in whom no organic lesion can be detected."[59]

The impression is gained from some reports that all obese patients have neuropsychiatric problems. Perhaps this idea has developed from the fact that a large number of the patients who have been intensively studied represent the more severe forms of obesity or patients who have personality problems and happen to be obese. However, there is not unanimity of opinion on this point. Harvey[149] stated that neuropsychiatric factors may exist in obesity but, if present, they are much less important than heredity, environment or endocrine factors. Kirlander[134] considered that emotional factors may play a role in obesity. Disorganized homes are found no more frequently among obese children than among those of normal weight.[17,100] Mayer[100] called attention to the fact that no adequate statistical study of the incidence of either obesity or psychoneurosis, singly or in association, has been made. The vast majority of mildly to moderately overweight patients seen socially or in office practice present no evidence of variations of behavior patterns greater than those of normal or underweight persons. The careful analytic procedures which have been applied to the more seriously obese have usually elicited neuropsychiatric abnormalities. Hamburger found only one patient in his series with no neuropsychiatric disorder. If these same techniques were applied to normal and thin people, how many would escape comparable neuropsychiatric diagnoses?

No special form of personality change is associated with obesity. The same types of psychic disturbances are noted in all states of nutrition. In fact, phases of overnutrition and undernutrition have been reported in a given patient with a psychiatric disorder.[56] Many of the studies of the interrelationship between obesity and emotional disturbances have developed from the failure of certain obese patients to reduce weight as expected. The frequency of lying, cheating on diets and inability to carry out a regimen was soon detected. Neuropsychiatric studies then demonstrated adequate reasons for this behavior but not necessarily adequate reasons for the obesity.[56,59,147] The fact that these patients are resistant to standard treatment for obesity because of their emotional illness is not evidence that the illness produced the obesity. Likewise, the fact that the neuropsychiatric problem is not necessarily altered when one of these patients does lose weight tends to emphasize the coincidental rather than the causal relationship of these two conditions.

The possibility exists that the emotional disorders associated with the obesity are caused by the obesity. If, in contrast to the practice of describing the emotional factors present in persons already obese, we undertake to note the development of emotional difficulties after obesity has been achieved, such a sequence appears probable. *Obesity is not the result of an impulsive action. It is acquired over long periods of more or less consistent overeating.* The eating habits acquired in childhood tend to carry on in life. Bruch[59] observed that "a person forms his food likes and dislikes early in life" and pointed out the effect of tribal life food habits, of "religion, superstition, climate, industrial progress, advertising." The vast majority of the persons who are mildly or moderately obese have normal personalities. As they continue in the rut of overindulgence, they encounter new social difficulties; they cannot wear stylish clothing nor follow sports as before; they encounter physical difficulties due to overweight; and they are "kidded," then "laughed with," and then "laughed at." They try one or a variety of self-prescribed reduction regimens with limited success and their half-hearted attempts at self-control lead to frustration and introspection. A vicious cycle ensues. "All obese are faced by medical disapproval and severe cultural condemnation."[15] Sooner or later a diagnosable neuropsychiatric situation appears. Rarely does one reach maturity without plenty of psychic trauma. It is not impossible that in these later stages of obesity an unconscious attempt at rationalization might recall to memory real or fancied potentially traumatic childhood experiences which have been dealt with normally for many years. It is probable that much of the psychic trauma observed in the chronic obese subject may be the result of the comment, ridicule and lack of social acceptance which he experiences and which are aggravated by the resultant brooding and introspection. It is more likely that the gradual and unnoticed development of obesity will result in the unfolding of latent personality weaknesses than that personality weaknesses exert some mysterious effect on the energy balance.

In obesity, just as abnormalities of intensity of nutritional stimuli were noted, we also find abnormalities in integration of these stimuli due sometimes perhaps to changes in reflex centers but usually to altered conditioning influences.

Sensation. Aberrations of the sensations of appetite and satiety have much to do with obesity. Abnormalities of stimulation and integration have obvious influences on both sensations, and the consequent delay in the attainment of satiety is a large factor in the production of excessive intakes. However, it is probable that there is also an alteration in the perceptivity of satiety by the obese person. The appreciation of this sensation may be much more acute and the resulting pleasure much more satisfying to him than to another. By training or by intuition musicians and artists are more acutely aware of the sensations of sound and sight than are average persons. There is no reason to assume that obese people are not more responsive than normal to the sensation of satiety. Such a sensitivity is consistent with their "lust for food" and with the difficulties experienced by many otherwise rational persons in the control of their obesity. The intake required for the continuous or even intermittent gratification of this sensualism produces obesity and resists its correction.

In summary, abnormalities of the central nervous system do not cause obesity any more than do endocrine, hereditary or other factors. Obesity is a problem of nutrition, and hence of supply. The central nervous system provides a regulatory mechanism, but if excessive food is not supplied to the body, the regulatory mechanisms are inoperative. Like other regulatory mechanisms, the central nervous system factors may influence the intake-output balance. Abnormalities of the central nervous system are frequently found in association with obesity and, as Conn[46] remarked about endocrine problems, the association is so common that when gross obesity presents, search should be made for a neuropsychiatric disorder. Gross obesity represents a profound weakness in character which may have an hereditary or acquired etiology. This character weakness not only permits the obesity to develop but militates against its correction. When by some circumstance the obesity is corrected, there is not necessarily any alteration in the parents or in childhood experiences of the patient and the neuropsychiatric background has not been altered. Yet those patients with character can maintain their new weight balances. Those without character relapse just as do their equivalent smokers, drinkers and drug addicts. There is no reason to assume that the vast majority of obese persons have any greater personality disorders than that they happen to like the pleasures of satiety more than other pleasures.

Working Classification of Obesity. A discussion of the etiology of obesity must be based on the fact that obesity is a state of nutrition. Nutrition problems are supply problems. They are not problems of regulation, emotion or inheritance. On this basis, a working classification of obesity is offered:

(1) Simple obesity
(2) Obesity associated with
    (a) Metabolic disorders
    (b) Hereditary disorders
    (c) Endocrine disorders
    (d) Psychiatric disorders

This classification emphasizes the fundamental nature of obesity. A positive caloric balance has been maintained for a sufficient length of time to permit the formation of excessive fat deposits. The second group indicates that obesity is encountered in association with certain groups of disorders with sufficient frequency to warrant emphasis of the fact. In many instances, the obesity per se affects the progress and treatment of the disorder. In others, the presence of the disorder promotes or facilitates the development of obesity. The vast majority of the mild to moderately obese people have no discernable associated disorder.

If attention is focussed on the fact of the positive caloric balance in obesity, certain significant contributants may be more clearly appreciated. The standard of living has a great influence on the basic factors of high energy intake and low energy output. The availability of food and the present fortunate economic status markedly influence food intake. Better qualities of meats have higher fat content. Better quality desserts have high carbohydrate and fat content. Prosperity makes more luxuries become necessities. "Soft" living greatly reduces the fuel needs. Warm houses and labor-saving machines eliminate the need for hundreds of calories a day. The automobile, the elevator and similar devices have almost eliminated the energy requirements for the transportation of the body which formerly was one of the important causes of energy output as indicated in Tables 25 and 26, in which it may be noted that walking accounted for over one sixth of the total caloric output of two working men. The economic and social values of these standard-of-living factors are not always paralleled by equivalent physiologic values. The normal standards of daily caloric requirement of a few years ago are far above the present day needs.

Standards of conduct are important if one is to deal with his world in a socially acceptable manner. The key factor in the development of obesity is the failure to control the pleasure of eating. This is a problem of the behavior of man because he alone has such qualities as sensation, choice and values. "Small vices" such as overeating, overdrinking and oversmoking are socially acceptable. However, it is a fine distinction as to when overindulgence in any pleasure becomes habituation.

The prevention and early control of obesity require character. The treatment likewise requires character. It is surprising how frequently an adequate motivation can elicit unsuspected resources of character.

TREATMENT

The treatment of a patient with obesity begins with a complete history, including dietary history, and physical examination. It is rare for an obese patient not to have tried self-treatment many times. Only when trouble develops will a physician be consulted. Therefore, the physician, when an obesity problem presents, should delve beyond the obvious for complicating difficulties. The dietary history directs attention to the malnutrition, especially protein deficiency, so frequently encountered. The usual examinations will disclose associated disorders which may complicate the treatment or even preclude treatment for the obesity. Many secondary factors materially influence the practicability of treatment for a given individual. The economic aspects include the costs of laboratory and professional services, but especially the cost of food. Protein food is, in general, more expensive than carbohydrate food. Home surroundings permit a detailed personal control of food which is not obtainable elsewhere, but social demands which require frequent "party meals" make dieting difficult. If the patient obviously lacks character and power of self-discipline, it is a waste of time and effort to attempt a proper reduction program. The reason the patient presented himself at the particular time very often provides a valuable index as to the indications for treatment as well as the probability of success.

Historical Note. The search for a specific treatment for obesity is of long standing. Tanner[4] quoted from Maccary (1811) a list of curative agents in use at that time. "Thus, we find a tolerable list of remedies in the pages of Maccary, which includes—Bleeding from the arm or jugular vein; Leeches to the anus; Dry Cupping; Prolonged blistering; Vegetable diet with vinegar; Acids—except nitric and phosphoric; Hot baths; Salt-water baths; Baths of Aix, Spa, Foges, Rouen, and Acqui; Occasional starvation; Decoction of guaiacum and sassafras; Scarifications; Salivation; Grief and anxiety to be induced; Purgatives; Issues; Pricking the flesh with needles; Walking with naked feet; and Removal of exuberant fatty tissue with the scalpel." He then added a few of the additional remedies of the first half of the nineteenth century. "Since this ridiculous catalogue was published, Turkish baths, sea-voyages, very little sleep, emetics, digitalis, soap (a relative of Mr. Wadd's ordered a quarter of a hundredweight of Castile soap for his own eating), salt, mercury to salivation, the inhalation of oxygen gas, purgatives, diuretics, the extract of the fucus vesiculosus, and preparations of bromine or of iodine have been freely tried."

The relation which existed between food and obesity was recognized in 1820: "Fat people should not eat freely of oily nourishing diet."[3] By midcentury the importance of dietary regulation in the treatment of obesity was well appreciated. Tanner[4] stated the principles of diet therapy based on the then present knowledge of fat formation and the "influence of respiration in removing carbon from the blood." He noted that foods are nitrogen-containing and non-nitrogen-containing; that the latter are the chief sources of fat formation; that man needs a mixed diet; that while "non-azotized" foods may be reduced, they may not be cut off altogether. These principles have a marked resemblance to our attitudes one hundred years later. The reduction diet, attributed to a William Harvey of that period, was publicized by William Banting about 1863. It is one of the significant milestones in the history of nutrition in its dealing with the basic dietary difficulties of obesity. " . . . He consulted Mr. William Harvey, who cut off the supply of bread, butter, milk, sugar, beer, soup, potatoes, and beans, and ordered the following diet:

Breakfast: Four or five ounces of beef, mutton, kidneys, broiled fish, bacon, or cold meat (except pork); a large cup of tea without milk or sugar, a little biscuit or one ounce of dry toast.

Dinner: Five or six ounces of any fish except salmon (it would have been as well also to have forbidden herrings and eels), any meat except pork, any vegetable except potato, one ounce of dry toast, fruit out of a pudding, any kind of poultry or game, and two or three glasses of good claret, sherry, or Madeira. Champagne, port, and beer forbidden.

Tea: Two or three ounces of fruit, a rusk or two, and a cup of tea without milk or sugar. (Coffee might have been allowed.)

Supper: Three or four ounces of meat or fish, and a glass or two of claret.

For Nightcap, if required, a tumblerful of grog, (gin, whiskey, or brandy without sugar) or a glass or two of claret or sherry."[4]

The diet clearly indicates the principle of adequate protein with lowered carbohydrate and fat intake. This diet was modified repeatedly in the next fifty years. Table 28 shows the analysis of several of these modifications. Other diets of historical interest which still have much merit are the milk and eggs diet of Weir Mitchell (1878) and the milk diet of Moritz (1908). Mitchell[150] prescribed a half pint of milk and an egg every three hours, five or six times a day, for periods of three weeks at a time. Moritz[151] recommended 25 cc. of milk per kilo of normal weight per day. Thus a man who should weigh 80 kilo would receive 2000 grams of milk divided into five parts.

The Dietary History. Medical tradition calls for an organized analysis of the chief complaint, present illness, family history and past history; more recently it has been stylish to inventory the social background and emotional biography. It is not yet a part of the discipline to note routinely the significant details of the patient's diet.

What do you eat? The aim of the dietary history is an estimate of the total ingested foods with respect to both type and amount. There is a considerable difference of opinion among investigators regarding the food intake in obesity. Beaudain[152] found the food intake of obese and normal persons to be about the same and Hunt[17] found that obese children ate as did normal children. On the other hand, Bruch[59] stated that in her children the food intake correlated with the increase in weight, and over 50 per cent of Gelvin's[8] patients admittedly ate too much. "Eating too much" and being a "big eater" are not synonymous terms. "Eating too much" clearly indicates a recognition of the basic principle that the intake is appreciably greater than the output. That some obese persons are not "big eaters," certainly at the time of observation, is understandable when the limitations of their outputs are recognized. However, it should be appreciated that the food intake of most obese persons is not only relatively high but high in absolute terms as well. It is difficult to obtain a true record of the food intake of a patient. Beaudain[152] noted that greater precision in methods of estimation of food intake resulted in much higher caloric values, and Bruch[59] found that a detailed dietary history patiently extracted from an ignorant or reluctant patient showed high values. Trulson[153] never found caloric imbalance when an exact history was obtained.

For hospital patients studied under proper conditions, the matter of amount of intake can be approximated by the weighed diet technique with a "weigh-back" check with a fair degree of accuracy. One such study[154] involved eight obese patients who were instructed to ask for and eat food as they ordinarily ate at home. They ate an average of 2570 calories a day for four days. These patients lost an average of 2 pounds each during the 4 days of this food intake. The patient with the maximum intake of 3690 calories, and who weighed

TABLE 28[1]

AUTHOR	GRAMS PROTEIN	GRAMS CARBOHYDRATE	GRAMS FAT	GRAMS ALCOHOL	APPROXIMATE CALORIES
Banting	172	81	8	(75)*	1,100 (1,600)
Oertel					
Maximum	170	120	45	(60)	1,600 (2,000)
Minimum	156	75	25	....	1,180
Ebstein	102	47	85	(20)	1,300 (1,450)
Hirschfeld					
Maximum	139	67	65	....	1,400
Minimum	100	50	41	....	1,000
Kisch					
Plethoric	160	80	11	....	1,086
Anemic	200	100	12	....	1,116
von Noorden	155	112	28	....	1,366

* The figures in parentheses include the calories from alcohol, if this is administered.
(*By permission of the Oxford University Press, Inc.*)

359 pounds, lost 5 pounds in 4 days, the one on a minimum intake of 1450 calories weighed 207 and lost 4 pounds in 5 days. Another series[155] of six obese women on an average intake of 2510 calories for a total of 70 days showed an average weight loss of .12 Kg. per day, or slightly less than 2 pounds a week. In view of these data one can only speculate on the intakes at home on which these weights were gained and maintained.

The types of food selected by obese patients may greatly affect the problem. Many patients ingest markedly unbalanced diets, with especial disproportions of carbohydrate and protein. Our experience is comparable to that of Duckworth[5] who described the high carbohydrate, low protein, relatively low calorie intake of the anemic type and the high protein, "high everything" diet of the plethoric type of obese patient. *All obese patients have excessive caloric intakes,* and the resulting clinical picture is determined more by the protein intake than by any other factor.

Patients consciously or unconsciously place themselves in the most favorable light during an interview. An adequate history can be obtained only by asking, "What did you eat for breakfast today; for lunch; for supper last night?" and "What did you eat during the morning, the afternoon and the evening?" A review of specific common food items such as bread, potatoes, meat, vegetables, candy bars, crackers, peanuts, pop, beer, etc., helps the patient to recall items which initially were not even considered as food. The use of side dishes of rice, spaghetti, potatoes, etc., is so commonplace with certain races that they are usually forgotten by the patient.

It is not essential that the practicing physician obtain precise information of his patient's food intake. In fact, standards of adequate intake vary for age, sex, occupation, national origin and other features of a patient's life. They also vary with the individual doctor, his information regarding foods and nutrition and more especially with his impressions of how his personal food habits influence his mode of living and his feeling of well-being. It is a great mistake to assume that a reasonably adequate social or economic status of a patient automatically guarantees sensible food patterns. A review of the intake of the common foods in the three main groups is easily obtainable. The amounts of *sugar* and *starch foods* such as bread, potatoes, crackers, candy, pie, cake, etc., and of the *fat foods* such as butter, margarine, gravy, mayonnaise, nuts, fried foods, etc., readily show the main sources of calories. A satisfactory approximation of the protein intake is secured by noting specifically the quantities of *animal protein* ingested and by referring to the rough rule: one egg equals one ounce meat equals one ounce fish equals one ounce cheese equals one glass milk. Each contains about six grams of protein. A normal protein intake should contain at least ten of these protein units. Intelligent, economically stable obese women frequently are found to be bordering on protein insufficiency.

When an obese person states that he does not eat much, he frequently refers to the bulk of his intake rather than the caloric value, and in that sense he is often correct. However, there is a forty-fold spread in the gram-calorie ratio between the lowest and the highest calorie foods. Lettuce has fewer than five grams of carbohydrates—less than twenty calories—per hundred grams, which constitutes a serving. Butter, on the other hand, contains nearly eight hundred calories in one hundred grams, which to the eye would appear to be a much smaller serving than the lettuce. However, the ordinary serving of butter has around one hundred calories; a twenty-calorie serving of butter would be almost unnoticeable. A slice of bread weighs about twenty-five grams and provides about eighty calories or slightly less than the pat of butter. An excess food intake of only one hundred calories a day will, in one year, produce a weight gain of about ten pounds. Thus, a knowledge of a few of the common food equivalents is a help in the approximation of a patient's intake:

1 Glass milk	140 Calories
1 Slice bread	80 Calories
1 Egg	75 Calories
3 Ounces meat	90 Calories
1 Pat butter	90 Calories

There are two important items of information obtained by a dietary history: first, facts about caloric factors; second, and much more vital, data regarding protein intake. A large percentage of obese patients seeking treatment have been previously under treatment by other physicians or by self or fad treatment. The popular forms of self-treatment usually deal exclusively with calories and neglect other food essentials, principally protein. Hence, obesity is frequently complicated by the coexistence of protein starvation. In our experience, the obese patients classed as "anemic" in type, that is, the pale, fat young females, characteristically have an extremely low intake of protein of animal origin. They give an almost stereotyped history of taking coffee and juice for breakfast, a sandwich or salad and coffee for lunch, and a single adequate meal in the evening which may contain only three or even four of the protein units mentioned above. Their intermediate snacks consist of soda, candy, crackers, chocolate bars, etc., none of which have significant protein content.

Alcohol as an accessory food plays two roles: (1) It has significant caloric value and (2) it influences appetite and satiety factors. Williams[6] felt that total abstainers tend to become big eaters by substituting one vice for another, but he pointed out that alcohol "not only increases the desire for food, but enhances the powers of digestion and assimilation." The use and abuse of alcohol contribute to the obese state, especially in the case of the "gross eater." So-called "snack foods" are even more treacherous than alcohol. These readily available foods are usually highly concentrated low protein foods temptingly packaged. A list of commonly encountered snacks[156] which has been widely publicized but patently ignored illustrates this point.

The main purpose of the art of cooking is to induce people to eat more.[6] "It is practically impossible for a person to eat to repletion of such simple unstimulating foods as dairy produce, salads, and raw fruits." Special gravies, sauces, fancy butter-laden cakes and cookies and other triumphs of the culinary art are high in caloric value. "But what was originally intended as an occasional treat . . . has now become the settled daily indulgence of thousands of people."[6] The repetitious daily use of these high calorie luxuries which have become commonplace has contributed heavily to the obesity problem.

When do you eat? Malnutrition is often encountered among patients who have peculiar eating habits. Large numbers of tense jittery people who become exhausted at 10 to 11 A.M. eat little or no breakfast. Late afternoon fatigue and its many associated symptoms frequently reflects a scant or absent lunch. Habitual irregularity in meal timing is a common cause of gastrointestinal irritability. The "snack" and the "coffee break" have become an accepted tradition. For those who eat normal meals the influence of these caloric increments is obvious. For those who neglect their regular meals, these practices, although almost a physiologic necessity, tend further to unbalance the food intake in the direction of high carbohydrate and low protein. The "night-eating syndrome" is an important factor in many obese patients.[58] A careful history discloses the eating habits of a patient, and it is not rare that an attempt to alter this pattern is a major problem of the reduction regimen.

Where do you eat? Where a patient eats may have much to do with the development of his obesity and may influence treatment. If he gets two or more meals at home, a capable cook can purchase and prepare proper food. The serving of the meal, the allowance of a reasonable time for eating and the freedom from turmoil during the meal are

TABLE 29. CALORIC VALUES FOR COMMON "SNACK" FOODS

"JUST A LITTLE SANDWICH"	AMOUNT OR AVERAGE SERVING	CALORIES
Hamburger on bun	3″ patty	500
Peanut butter	2 tablespoonfuls P.B.	370
Cheese	1½ oz. cheese	400
Ham	1½ oz. ham	350
BEVERAGES		
Soft drinks, soda, root beer, etc	6 oz. glass	80
Club soda	8 oz. glass	5
Chocolate malted milk	10 oz. glass (1¾ cups)	430
Ginger ale	6 oz. glass	55
Tea or coffee, straight	1 cup	0
Tea or coffee, with 2 tablespoonfuls cream and 2 teaspoonfuls sugar	1 cup	90
ALCOHOLIC DRINKS		
Ale	8 oz. glass	125
Beer	8 oz. glass	105
Highball (with ginger ale—ladies' style)	8 oz. glass	135
Manhattan	Average	175
Martini	Average	160
Old Fashioned	Average	150
Sherry	2 oz. glass	55
Scotch, bourbon, rye	1 oz. jigger	75
FRUITS		
Apple	1 3-inch	90
Banana	1 6-inch	100
Grapes	30 medium	75
Orange	1 2¾-inch	80
Pear	1 average	100
SALTED SNACKS		
Pecans	10 halves	150
Almonds	10 halves	130
Cashews or peanuts	10	60
Potato chips	10 2″ diameter	110
Buttered popcorn	1 cup	100
Cheese crackers	10 2″ diameter	220

CANDIES	AMOUNT OR AVERAGE SERVING	CALORIES
Chocolate Bars, small size		
Plain	1 bar (1¼ oz.)	190
With nuts	1 bar	275
Chocolate Covered Bar	1 bar	250
Chocolate Cream, Bon Bon, Fudge	1 piece 1″ square	90
Caramels		
Plain	1 piece ¾″ cube	35
Chocolate nut caramels	1 piece	60
DESSERTS		
Pie		
Fruit—Apple, etc	⅙ pie 1 average serving	400
Custard	⅙ pie 1 average serving	300
Lemon Meringue	⅙ pie 1 average serving	350
Pumpkin pie with whipped cream	⅙ pie 1 average serving	460
Cake		
Iced layer—2 layers white cake	1 average serving	345
Fruit—thin slice ¼″	1 average serving	125
SWEETS		
Ice Cream		
Plain vanilla	⅙ qt. serving	190
Chocolate and other flavors	⅙ qt., ⅔ cup	220
Milk sherbet	⅙ qt., ⅔ cup	240
Sundaes, small chocolate nut with whipped cream	Average	400
Ice cream sodas, chocolate	10 oz. glass	255
MIDNIGHT SNACKS FOR ICE-BOX RAIDERS		
Cold potato	½ medium	45
Chicken leg	1 average	90
Milk	7 oz. glass	140
Mouthful of roast	½″ × 2″ × 3″	130
Cheese	¼″ × 2″ × 3″	120
Left-over baked beans	½″ cup	105
Brownie	¾″ × 1¾″ × 2¼″	300
Cream-puff	4″ diameter	450

helpful. Other members of the family should be in sympathy with the patient's efforts to reduce, because nothing undermines the morale more than indifference or ridicule. For those who are dependent upon public restaurants for their meals, the problems multiply. Economic considerations frequently lead to low protein, high carbohydrate meals. Specially ordered meals are more expensive than the standard menus and it is difficult to get many of the simpler low-fat meats cooked without gravies and sauces. The noise and the rush of the restaurant favor bolting of meals, which promotes the ingestion of excess food. It is practically impossible for a person dependent upon public eating places to adhere to an adequate reduction regimen.

Principles of Therapy. The basic principles of treatment provide:

(1) A maximum difference between the intake and output of energy, that is, caloric deficit.
(2) An adequate amount of protein.
(3) The necessary amount of carbohydrate.
(4) An abundant supply of accessory food substances such as minerals and vitamins.
(5) Time.

A maximum difference between the caloric intake and output of energy can be obtained only by a reduction of the intake to minimum safe levels and by maintaining the output at the maximum safe level. Fat is removed from the body directly in proportion to the caloric deficit at the rate of 1 gram for 9.3 calories. The loss in fat tissue is somewhat greater because this includes the weight of associated water and the limited losses of structural materials. In theory, the intake of food can be reduced to the necessary protein and carbohydrate which can readily be obtained in diets of 500 to 600 calories.[11,154,157] The monotony of such diets militates against their use, especially outside a metabolic ward. Diets of 800 to 1000 calories have been shown to contain enough variety in foods to secure the cooperation of patients.

The total energy output of the obese usually exceeds normal. All fractions of output contribute to this over-all result. The big variable in energy output is the nonwork fraction. Indolent, inactive persons conserve large amounts of energy. Obesity tends to minimize spontaneous activities. An increase in output in this fraction of even 500 to 1000 calories per day would be advantageous. Good clinical judgment is necessary to determine how much this factor may be increased by exercise, sports, etc., with proper regard for the total physiologic loads so imposed. The more the activity, the greater is the energy output. Usually it is not the medical contraindication to activity that hampers progress but the difficulty of inducing an adult to change his recreations and habits to forms which utilize significant amounts of energy.

Adequate amounts of protein in the diet are imperative. Zelman[28] noted that liver damage was less with a high fat, low protein diet than with a high carbohydrate, low protein diet. He reasoned that since a reduction diet in itself provided a high fat content of the metabolic mixture, a high protein food intake was indicated. One gram of protein per kilogram of "ideal" body weight is an adequate and safe level provided the protein is of high biologic value. Whether this level is optimum or how much of lower grade protein can be utilized with safety is not known. Nitrogen equilibrium can be established at lower levels of protein intake for short periods but this does not justify the use of low levels of protein in the treatment of obesity, which usually extends over months. The physiologic reactions of the body characteristic of starvation which accompany prolonged protein deficiencies are not seen in obese patients during reduction if adequate protein is eaten.[68]

Carbohydrate is essential in a reduction diet to ensure optimum protein metabolism. How much is required is conjectural. On reduction programs which contained 30 to 40 grams of carbohydrate, certain patients were in negative nitrogen balance persistently, thus suggesting the wastage of protein for its antiketogenic properties.[154] A satisfactory nitrogen balance was maintained with 80 grams of carbohydrate. The effect of the additional 160 calories is probably of less moment than the effect of the low carbohydrate on protein metabolism. In theory, carbohydrate is also necessary to prevent ketosis. How much carbohydrate is necessary for this purpose is influenced by the total energy requirements of the patient and also the facility with which the patient can metabolize fat. The obese have a great ability to utilize fat for energy. Under the metabolic conditions of a reduction program ketonuria was not observed with diets containing over 40 grams of carbohydrate.

Accessory food substances—minerals and vitamins—are required to avoid relative deficiency states. The amounts and nature of these substances contained in food vary greatly. The need of the body for the various minerals and vitamins varies greatly with the type of intake and output of energy. Storage in the body of any of these materials is quite restricted and is regulated to a large extent by the efficiency of the excretory system. In the obese, in view of the large outputs of urine over long periods of time, the possibility exists that the daily mineral exchange exceeds that of normal people. The reduction in mineral intake associated with the reduced food mass of a diet could possibly induce a relative mineral depletion. For reduction programs, oversupply of the foreseeable needs of the body by the use of supplementary polyvalent mineral and vitamin mixtures is justified.

The size of the negative caloric balance determines the rate of weight loss per day. Time determines the total weight loss. The loss of 930 calories is equivalent to 100 grams of fat. Fat tissue differs from fat in its content of protein and water. The maintenance of nitrogen balance indicates that any protein which might be removed from fatty tissue cells goes into the metabolic pool and is reused. It would therefore have no influence on the total caloric exchange. In general, it may be expected that a 930 calorie deficit would correspond to a weight loss of 115 grams, or a one pound weight loss corresponds to about 3700 calories. When reduced to these terms, the possible rate of weight loss for a given caloric deficit may be appreciated. Under very special conditions, weight losses of a pound a day have been secured. The usual caloric deficit obtainable is in the neighborhood of 1000 to 2000 calories per day. The rates of weight loss possible, therefore, range from one and a half to three and one half pounds per week. When appreciable amounts of fat must be removed, it is apparent that time becomes an important factor. If a rate of weight loss of two pounds a week is obtainable and fifty pounds must be removed, twenty-five weeks or roughly one half a year will be necessary.

Diets. The basic principles of a reduction diet as just described must be adapted for practical use. There is a difference between a "safe" diet and a "successful" diet, which must combine the features of biologic adequacy and safety with those of acceptability for a sufficient period of time to secure significant weight loss.

The use of fast periods may produce excellent results and might be satisfactory for the "gross feeder." The omission of one seventh or one sixth of all of his foods each week would entail little risk of specific food deficiencies over a period of months. For the average patient, it should be recalled that total fasting entails the risk of developing serious malnutrition, and the rate of weight loss would be slow.

Many diets based on the use of milk, or milk and eggs, often supplemented with other simple foods, are theoretically adequate, but it is a rare person who can tolerate their monotony for a sufficient time to get significant results.

The weighed diet is most satisfactory for hospital use. Relatively precise information regarding the food intake of sick patients is desirable. Also the educational value of the weighed diet is great. The patient not only has the opportunity of learning food values but also may learn to gauge proper servings of foods. The dietary discipline exhibited by nurses and dietitians helps the patient to appreciate the true importance of diet. For the elderly, the inactive and the sick, who have relatively low energy outputs, a weighed diet offers the only hope of obtaining sufficient caloric deficit to secure a reasonable rate of weight loss. For use in the home, weighed diets are of great advantage when the need for weight loss is urgent.

Five weighed diets are described in detail below. The more liberal diets might be employed for unusually large patients or to obtain patient cooperation. The 500 calorie diet has been used with success when indicated.

NOTES FOR FIVE WEIGHED DIETS. The following five diets were supplied by Miss Mary Borland, Dietitian in charge of Weighed Diet Division, The Western Pennsylvania Hospital.

1. All meats are weighed or measured without bone or visible fat.

2. Roast meats are weighed or measured after they have been cooked.

3. Steak, chops, cutlets, liver and

DIET 1. CALORIES 1000, PROTEIN 60 GM., CARBOHYDRATE 80 GM.

		GRAMS	CARBOHYDRATE	PROTEIN	FAT
Protein	Eggs	100	0	13	11
	Meat, Group I	120	0	24	30
	Milk, skim	360	18	12	3
Carbohydrate	Bread	25	13	2	1
	Cereal	10	7	2	1
	Fruit, Group II	180	23	2	0
	Vegetable, Group I	240	9	3	0
	Vegetable, Group II	120	10	2	0
Fat: Butter		5	0	0	4
			80	60	50

	GRAMS	HOUSEHOLD MEASUREMENT
Breakfast		
Fruit, Group II	60	¼ cup
Cereal	10	¼ cup cooked or ⅓ cup prepared
Milk, skim	120	½ cup
Egg	100	2 eggs
Bread	25	1 slice
Butter	5	1 pat
Dinner		
Meat, Group I	60	2 ounces
Vegetable, Group I	60	green salad or ¼ cup cooked
Vegetable, Group II	120	½ cup
Fruit, Group II	60	⅓ cup
Milk, skim	120	½ cup
Supper		
Meat, Group I	60	2 ounces
Vegetable, Group I	180	1 green salad and ½ cup cooked
Fruit, Group II	60	½ cup
Milk, skim	120	½ cup

Substitutions

(1) 2 ounces Meat, Group I = 2 ounces Meat, Group II and 1 teaspoon butter
(2) 2 ounces Meat, Group I = 2 ounces Meat, Group III and 2 teaspoons butter
(3) 2 ounces Meat, Group I = 2½ ounces haddock and 3 teaspoons butter
(4) 2 ounces Meat, Group I = 1½ ounces American Cheese
(5) ½ cup Fruit, Group II = 1 cup Fruit, Group I
(6) ½ cup Vegetable, Group I = ¼ cup Vegetable, Group II
(7) ½ cup Vegetable, Group II = ¼ cup Vegetable, Group III
(8) ½ cup Vegetable, Group II = 1 cup Vegetable Soup (Heinz)
(9) Sandwich meal may be substituted for either dinner or supper:

Meat, Group II, 2½ ounces	Vegetable, Group I, 1 salad
Bread, 2 slices	Butter, ⅔ teaspoon

DIET 2. CALORIES 1000, PROTEIN 80 GM., CARBOHYDRATE 80 GM.

		GRAMS	CARBOHYDRATE	PROTEIN	FAT
Protein	Eggs	100	0	13	11
	Meat, Group II	110	0	22	17
	Meat, Group III	110	0	22	6
	Milk, skim	360	18	12	3
Carbohydrate	Bread	25	13	2	1
	Cereal	10	7	2	1
	Fruit, Group II	180	23	2	0
	Vegetable, Group I	240	9	3	0
	Vegetable, Group II	120	10	2	—
Fat: Butter		2			1
			80	80	40

	GRAMS	HOUSEHOLD MEASUREMENT
Breakfast		
Cereal	10	¼ cup cooked or ⅓ cup prepared
Milk, skim	120	½ cup
Eggs	100	2 eggs
Bread	25	1 slice
Butter	2	⅓ pat (teaspoon)
Fruit, Group II	60	¼ cup
Dinner		
Meat, Group II	110	4 ounces
Vegetable, Group I	60	1 green salad
Vegetable, Group II	120	½ cup
Fruit, Group II	60	¼ cup
Milk, skim	120	½ cup
Supper		
Meat, Group III	110	4 ounces
Vegetable, Group I	60	green salad and
	120	½ cup cooked
Fruit, Group II	60	¼ cup
Milk, skim	120	½ cup

Substitutions

(1) 4 ounces Meat, Group III = 5 ounces haddock plus 1 teaspoon butter
(2) ½ cup Fruit, Group II = 1 cup Fruit, Group I
(3) ½ cup Vegetable, Group I = ¼ cup Vegetable, Group II
(4) ½ cup Vegetable, Group II = ¼ cup Vegetable, Group III
(5) ½ cup Vegetable, Group II = 1 cup Vegetable Soup (Heinz)
(6) Sandwich meal may be substituted for either dinner or supper:
Meat, Group II, 4 ounces — Vegetable, Group I, green salad
Bread, 2 slices

DIET 3. CALORIES 1200, PROTEIN 60 GM., CARBOHYDRATE 100 GM.

		GRAMS	CARBOHYDRATE	PROTEIN	FAT
Protein	Egg	50	...	7	5
	Meat, Group I	145	...	29	36
	Milk, Whole	360	18	11	14
Carbohydrate	Bread	50	27	5	1
	Cereal	10	7	2	1
	Fruit, Group II	240	31	2	..
	Vegetable, Group I	180	7	2	..
	Vegetable, Group II	120	10	2	..
Fat: Butter		6	...	..	5
			100	60	62

	GRAMS	HOUSEHOLD MEASUREMENT
Breakfast		
Cereal	10	¼ cup cooked or ⅓ cup prepared
Milk	180	¾ cup
Egg	50	1 egg
Bread	25	1 slice
Butter	4	⅔ teaspoon
Fruit, Group II	120	½ cup

DIET 3. CALORIES 1200, PROTEIN 60 GM., CARBOHYDRATE 100 GM. (*Continued*)

Dinner		
Meat, Group I	75	2½ ounces
Vegetable, Group I	60	1 green salad
Vegetable, Group II	120	½ cup cooked
Fruit, Group II	60	¼ cup
Milk	60	¼ cup
Supper		
Meat, Group I	70	2½ ounces
Vegetable, Group I	180	1 green salad and ½ cup cooked
Fruit, Group II	60	¼ cup
Bread	25	1 slice
Milk	120	½ cup
Butter	2	⅓ teaspoon

Substitutions

(1) 2½ ounces Meat, Group I = 3 ounces haddock plus 3½ teaspoons butter
(2) ½ cup Fruit, Group II = 1 cup Fruit, Group I
(3) ½ cup Vegetable, Group I = ¼ cup Vegetable, Group II
(4) ½ cup Vegetable, Group II = ¼ cup Vegetable, Group III
(5) ½ cup Vegetable, Group II = 1 cup Vegetable Soup (Heinz)
(6) Sandwich meal may be substituted for dinner meal:
Bread, 1 slice — Vegetable, Group I, 1 green salad
Meat, Group I, 3 ounces — Fruit, Group II, ¼ cup

DIET 4. CALORIES 1200, PROTEIN 80 GM., CARBOHYDRATE 100 GM.

		GRAMS	CARBOHYDRATE	PROTEIN	FAT
Protein	Eggs	100	...	13	11
	Meat, Group I	100	...	20	25
	Meat, Group III	120	...	24	6
	Milk, skim	360	18	11	4
Carbohydrate	Bread	25	13	2	1
	Cereal	10	7	2	1
	Fruit, Group II	240	31	2	..
	Potato	50	11	2	..
	Vegetable, Group I	240	10	2	..
	Vegetable, Group II	120	10	2	..
Fat: Butter		7	...	..	6
			100	80	54

	GRAMS	HOUSEHOLD MEASUREMENT
Breakfast		
Cereal	10	¼ cup cooked or ⅓ cup prepared
Milk, skim	180	¾ cup
Eggs	100	2 eggs
Bread	25	1 slice
Butter	4	⅔ pat (teaspoon)
Fruit, Group II	120	½ cup
Dinner		
Meat, Group I	100	3½ ounces
Vegetable, Group I	60	1 green salad
Vegetable, Group II	120	½ cup cooked
Potato	50	¼ cup (scant)
Fruit, Group II	60	¼ cup
Milk, skim	60	¼ cup
Supper		
Meat, Group III	120	4 ounces
Vegetable, Group I	180	1 green salad and ½ cup cooked
Fruit, Group II	60	¼ cup
Milk, skim	120	½ cup
Butter	3	½ pat (teaspoon)

Diet 4. Calories 1200, Protein 80 Gm., Carbohydrate 100 Gm. (*Continued*)

Substitutions

(1) 4 ounces Meat, Group III = 5 ounces haddock plus 1 teaspoon butter
(2) ½ cup Fruit, Group II = 1 cup Fruit, Group I
(3) ½ cup Vegetable, Group I = ¼ cup Vegetable, Group II
(4) ½ cup Vegetable, Group II = ¼ cup Vegetable, Group III
(5) ½ cup Vegetable, Group II = 1 cup Vegetable Soup (Heinz)
(6) Sandwich meal may be substituted for dinner meal:

Meat, Group I, 3 ounces	Vegetable, Group I, 1 green salad
Bread, 2 slices	Milk, Skim or Buttermilk, ½ cup

Diet 5. Calories 500, Protein 55 Gm., Carbohydrate 40 Gm.

		Grams	Carbohydrate	Protein	Fat
Protein	Egg	50	..	7	5
	Meat, Group III	100	..	20	5
	Cottage Cheese	80	3	16	1
	Milk, skim	240	12	7	2
Carbohydrate	Cereal	10	7	2	1
	Fruit, Group II	60	8	1	..
	Vegetable, Group I	240	10	2	..
			40	55	14

	Grams	Household Measurement
Breakfast		
Cereal	10	¼ cup cooked or ⅓ cup prepared
Milk, skim	120	½ cup
Egg	50	1 egg
Fruit, Group II	60	¼ cup
Dinner		
Cottage Cheese	80	⅓ cup
Vegetable, Group I	120	½ cup cooked or raw
Milk, skim	60	¼ cup
Supper		
Meat, Group III	100	3½ ounces
Vegetable, Group I	120	½ cup
Milk, skim	60	¼ cup

Substitutions

(1) 3½ ounces Meat, Group III = 4½ ounces haddock plus 1 teaspoon butter
(2) ½ cup Fruit, Group II = 1 cup Fruit, Group I
(3) ½ cup Vegetable, Group I = ¼ cup Vegetable, Group II
(4) ½ cup Vegetable, Group II = ¼ cup Vegetable, Group III
(5) ½ cup Vegetable, Group II = 1 cup Vegetable Soup (Heinz)

fresh fish are weighed or measured before they are cooked.

4. Salad greens and vegetables are weighed or measured raw.

5. Vegetables are weighed or measured after they are cooked.

6. All fruits are either fresh or canned or frozen without sugar.

7. Dinner and supper may be interchanged as whole meals but not in part.

(Vegetable, meat and fruit groups are listed on page 601.)

The measured diet is more generally used in homes and for patients not acutely ill. The household measurements of the first four diets are given in the right hand columns of the tables.

The Four Group Diet. For the large group of relatively healthy office patients for whom speed of weight loss is not vital, the "four group" diet has been developed.[158] This program makes fewer demands on the patient but gets slower results. It is especially useful for those whose home situations preclude strict dieting and for those who must eat in restaurants. It has the advantage that it prepares the patient, mentally and emotionally, for the type of diet regulation he must hereafter maintain. In the four group diet, emphasis is laid chiefly upon safety, and the rate of reduction is made secondary. Adequate protein, which is regarded as the one over-all essential of any reduction plan, comes first and foremost, and sufficient

Vegetable, Meat and Fruit Groups

VEGETABLES:

Group I C-4 P-1 F-0
- Asparagus—fresh
- Asparagus—canned
- Brussels Sprouts
- Broccoli
- Cabbage
- Celery
- Cauliflower
- Cucumber
- Eggplant
- Green Peppers
- Lettuce
- Pumpkin—fresh
- Radishes
- Rhubarb
- Sauerkraut
- Spinach
- Salad Greens
- String Beans
- White Squash
- Tomatoes—fresh
- Tomatoes—canned
- Tomato Juice
- Sauerkraut Juice

Group II C-8 P-2 F-0
- Beets
- Carrots
- Mushrooms
- Onions
- Green Peas—canned
- Rutabagas
- String Beans
- Squash—yellow
- Turnips

Group III C-16 P-4 F-0
- Green Peas—fresh
- Lima Beans—canned
- Corn—fresh
- Parsnips

FRUITS:

Group I C-6 P-1 F-0
- Muskmelon
- Honeydew
- Cantaloupes
- Watermelon
- Strawberries
- *Water Packed*
  - Peaches
  - Pears
  - Fruit Cocktail
  - Apricots

Group II C-13 P-1 F-0
- Apples
- Apricots
- Cherries
- Grapes—as purchased
- Grapefruit
- Loganberries
- Blackberries
- Blueberries
- Lemon
- Oranges
- Peaches
- Pears
- Pineapple
- Plums
- Red Raspberries
- Black Raspberries

Banana-C-20 P-2 F-0

Group III C-76 P-3 F-1
- Dates
- Figs
- Prunes
- Raisins

MEATS:

Group I P-20 F-25
- Roast Beef
- Fillet of Beef
- Beef Tongue
- Ham
- Lamb Chops
- Salt Mackerel
- Turkey
- Tuna Fish

Group II P-20 F-15
- Beef Hearts
- Canned Beef
- Bologna
- Chicken
- Frankfurts
- Roast Lamb
- Roast Pork
- Pork Tenderloins
- Sardines—canned
- Sweetbreads
- Salmon—fresh
- Salmon—canned
- Sirloin Steak
- Veal Chop
- Halibut—smoked

Group III P-20 F-5
- Blue Fish
- Heart—Chicken
  - Veal
- Liver—Veal
  - Beef
  - Calves
  - Chicken
- Herring
- Kidney—beef or veal
- Mackerel—canned or fresh
- Round Steak
- Roast Veal
- Shad
- Smelts
- White Perch
- White Fish
- Veal Tongue
- Halibut—fresh

Group IV P-16 F-1
- Crabmeat—canned
- Clams—hardshelled
- Cod
- Frog Legs
- Flounder
- Sturgeon
- Lobster—fresh or canned
- Haddock

Group V P-25 F-1
- Chicken Gizzard
- Smoked Haddock
- Shrimp—canned

carbohydrate is then provided. The total caloric value, although vital to the rate of weight reduction, is subordinated.

GROUP I. *Food Which Must Be Eaten Every Day:*

1. "X" ounces of lean meat or its equivalent. The number of ounces is determined by the physician as for any reduction diet. It should be remembered that the dictum 1 gram protein per kilogram refers to dry protein. The following foods have approximately 6 grams of protein: 1 ounce of lean meat, 1 egg, 1 ounce of cottage cheese, 1 ounce of fish, 6 ounces of skimmed milk. Those foods with the lowest fat contents are most serviceable but the protein is essential. A 70 gram protein diet would therefore call for approximately 12 ounces of meat or its equivalent. In general the protein should be divided equally between breakfast, lunch and dinner. The patient should develop a working visual image of 3 to 4 ounces of meat.
2. 4 to 6 glasses of water.
3. 1 vitamin capsule per day.

GROUP II. *Eat All You Want of These Foods:*

Since 60 to 80 grams of carbohydrate are desirable and since these foods have about 5% carbohydrate, relatively large quantities may be used with little effect on the calories and considerable benefit in bulk, water, mineral and vitamin factors.

Asparagus, fresh	Sauerkraut
Asparagus, canned	Spinach, fresh
Broccoli	Spinach, canned
Cabbage	String beans, canned
Cauliflower	Summer squash
Celery	Tomato
Chard	Tomato juice
Chicory	Water cress
Cucumber	
Eggplant	
Endive	Cantaloupe
Lettuce	Watermelon
Mushrooms	
Mustard greens	Skimmed milk
Radish	Buttermilk

GROUP III. *Eat In Moderation:*

This group includes a few of the more concentrated foods, such as cereals and whole milk, but chiefly the fruits and vegetables, fresh, frozen or canned unsweetened, which have less than 15% carbohydrate. One portion from this group may be taken with each meal.

Whole milk (180 cc. [6 ounces])
Cereal (15 grams [½ ounce] dry weight)

Oatmeal	Puffed Wheat
Cornflakes	Shredded Wheat
Rice Flakes	

Vegetables, fruits and fruit juices (90 grams [3 ounces])

Artichoke	Apple juice
Beets, fresh or canned	Grapefruit juice
Brussel sprouts	Orange juice
Carrots	Pineapple juice
Chives	
Dandelion greens	Blackberries
Kale	Blueberries
Leek	Raspberries
Okra	Strawberries
Onion	Grapefruit
Peas, canned	Orange
Pumpkin	Tangerine
Rutabaga	
String beans, fresh	Apples
Turnip	Grapes
Winter squash	Peaches, fresh
	Pears
	Pineapple
	Plums

GROUP IV. *Avoid:*

This group includes the concentrated carbohydrate and fat foods which are of importance chiefly for calories.

Corn, sweet	Peas, fresh
Kidney beans	Peas, dry
Lentil	Potato, sweet
Lima beans	Potato, white
Navy beans	Soybeans
Parsnips	Yam
Cream cheese	Margarine
Roquefort cheese	Condensed milk
Swiss cheese	Cream
Butter	Ice cream
Bread, white	Pie
Bread, whole wheat	Pretzels
Bread, rye	Rolls
Cake	Macaroni
Cookies	Spaghetti
Crackers	Noodles
Doughnuts	Rice
Fig bars	Tapioca
Pancakes	Wheat germ
Duck	Bacon
Fat meat	Mayonnaise
Goose	French dressing
Hamburger	Salad dressing
Pork, all kinds	Salad oils
Sweetbreads	Olive oil
Sardines in oil	Nuts
Candy	Apricots, canned
Jams	Apricot, dried
Honey	Avocado
Maple syrup	Banana
Molasses	Cherry
Sugar	Dates
Grape juice	Figs
Apple sauce	Dried fruit
Fruits canned with sugar	Prunes
	Raisins

Certain general instructions apply to all reduction diets:

(1) All of the protein quota must be eaten. This is quite difficult for many women with the so-called "anemic" type of obesity. The daily protein allowance must be divided among three meals.

(2) The food is divided into three approximately equal feedings. The development of uniformly stable eating patterns is important.

(3) The meals are at least four to five hours apart. Breakfast must be eaten around 8 A.M. to enable the patient to eat a proper lunch. This time factor is important for those who have difficulty in eating protein.

(4) Meals should never be omitted.

(5) No food is eaten between meals. If the patient cannot adapt himself to a three-meal schedule, he may use a four- or five-meal schedule. In this event, care must be taken to redistribute the protein.

(6) Lemon juice, vinegar and spices may be used as desired.

(7) Sweeteners are permissible. Psychologically, however, it is better if patients learn, or develop, a taste for the natural flavors of foods.

(8) Water may be taken as desired. Enough fluid, as plain tea, coffee, clear fat-free broth or water, is taken to ensure a urine output of 1000 to 1500 cc. daily.

Adjuvants. ENDOCRINE PREPARATIONS. There is no indication for the use of endocrine preparations in the treatment of obesity. Thyroid has been used for over fifty years to "release the water" because of the erroneous idea that the metabolic status of an obese person corresponds to that of a patient overweight from myxedema. Even in theory, it has no value in the treatment of obesity. Thyroid raises metabolism, especially basal metabolism. As the basal level in obesity is never below normal for the ideal weight and, in gross obesity, the basal heat production may be 40 to 50 per cent above normal values for ideal weight, the need for thyroid stimulation is not apparent. In practice, the use of thyroid has little or no effect on weight reduction[30,44] and when used to excess produces palpitation, precordial distress and nervousness without significant effect on fat loss. Exogenous thyroid inhibits rather than adds to the natural production of thyroid. One vigorous 34-year-old male patient who weighed 406 pounds gave a history of having taken 10 grains of thyroid daily for five years. His basal metabolism was normal. When the thyroid was discontinued, his metabolism remained at the same rate, suggesting that his thyroid gland had resumed normal activity. On the other hand, a relatively inactive woman who weighed 170 pounds following a period of dietary restriction was given 5 grains a day for a few weeks. It was discontinued because of palpitation and nervousness. In the succeeding few weeks she gained twenty pounds and her basal metabolism dropped to low normal levels. She probably ate carelessly in this period, but it is quite possible that the failure of her thyroid gland to resume its normal function contributed much to the picture. Not only is there no indication for thyroid as a reducing agent, but its use may be a real handicap.

No other endocrine product has been shown to affect the treatment of obesity.

SEDATION. Mild sedation is of benefit. Many patients are apprehensive, and the excitement of starting a real diet program aggravates their nervousness. Phenobarbital, 0.25 grain, in the form of the simple elixir taken before meals, helps in establishing desirable eating patterns as well as in reducing tensions. Food addiction is present, to some degree, in obese patients. The withdrawal symptoms of restlessness, tension and emotional instability, common to any other addiction, require sedation. There is more reason for sedatives than for central nervous system excitants, such as coffee, amphetamine, thyroid, etc. In theory, the tranquilizing drugs now widely used should be of great help in reduction programs, but my own experience with them has been disappointing.

AMPHETAMINE. Some years ago amphetamine was found to have anorexic properties, and its use was widely heralded. Its effect upon the appetite is quite transitory, and any weight loss obtained during drug therapy is directly proportional to the reduction in caloric intake. The benefit over any considerable period is negligible.[44] An important objection to the use of amphetamine is that it produces a nonselective reduction in all types of food which can result in serious malnutrition, particularly in protein. Patients suffering from anxiety, restlessness or coronary disease should not be given amphetamine. Amphetamine is frequently given in combination with one of the barbiturates to lessen its effects on the nervous system. It has not been shown that barbiturates do not also remove the effect of the amphetamine on the nervous system, nor has it been shown that the effect of the combination is superior to that of the sedative alone. When amphetamine is used solely as a psychologic prop, its withdrawal may lead to dietary excesses.

VITAMINS. The active body needs vitamins. The relation of certain vitamins, for example thiamine, to the metabolism of a specific food substance is accepted. However, what the vitamin requirements might be under the metabolic conditions of a reduction regimen has not been established. With greatly restricted diet programs, loss of hair may occur after several weeks of strict dieting, but this is corrected by small amounts of viosterol. All reduction diets are in practice supplemented with a polyvitamin capsule to ensure the presence of the known vitamins in adequate amounts.

PSYCHOTHERAPY. Varying degrees of instability of the central nervous system are to be found in association with obesity. What constitutes psychotherapy is a matter of fine definition. Obese patients have bad habits which are firmly established. Most of them derive pleasure from the indulgence of these habits. They must be taught and they must be willing to learn how to eat properly. Insofar as the process of instruction and the supplying of encouragement during a period of personal readjustment constitutes psychotherapy, all patients need it and all get it.

Psychotherapy in its more formal garb is another matter. Most obese patients do not need it any more than does any other segment of society. For those patients who are truly disturbed and happen to be obese, it is apparent that the treatment for the obesity is a secondary matter. Bruch[146] stated, "The fact that they are fat suggests that their life adjustment was poor at the start." The treatment of obesity requires a modest degree of self-control, which these patients lack. The attempts to reduce disturbed patients have uniformly failed.[15,44,54–57,59] The value of psychotherapy prior to reduction procedures is a matter of opinion and experience. Werner[159] called attention to the cost of psychotherapy and to age as limiting factors. Since a large percentage of obese patients are over middle age, it would seem to offer little of value for them. The general therapeutic responses to psychotherapy are not germane to this review. There is no reason to suppose that they would be any better or any worse because of the state of nutrition of the patient.

A diluted, impersonal form of psychotherapy has been advocated. Groups of obese persons have met more or less systematically to discuss their nutritional and other problems.[134,149,160] Modest success, especially at the outset, has been reported by some groups. Apparently the composition, social and educational, of the group is important. The personality of the leader is perhaps the most important factor. The use of such groups for the instruction of patients as a means of saving time and money for hospital clinics has been advocated, but that is somewhat away from the true psychotherapeutic approach. The value of a community approach to a problem which is distinctly personal is questionable.[149]

EXERCISE. Exercise as an adjuvant to a reduction diet is of considerable value when the patient is capable of taking exercise. One of the alleged advantages of the spa treatment is the arrangement of courses of activities of varying intensities which may be prescribed. For obese persons with limited abilities such programs offer a toning-up regimen which may be helpful. The actual increase in energy output would be quite small. Walking is perhaps the safest and most available form of exercise for the ordinary person. An untrained adult can expend 250 to 300 calories in thirty minutes of moderate activity without distress.[161] With more vigorous and more prolonged activities, 500 to 1000 calories can easily be used. One patient who played eighteen or more holes of golf every day while dieting accurately reduced from 224 pounds to his ideal weight of 177 pounds in eleven weeks.[30] When exercise is part of daily labor, the work fraction of total output, values of 3000 to 4000 calories may be secured. It is not common to find obesity associated with this kind of labor. One patient, who had a job which involved lifting one hundred pound sacks several hours daily, weighed 406 pounds; he lost 162 pounds in 9 months while taking a diet of 1200 calories. Most obese patients are totally unable to take such effective exercise because of age, poor muscular development, and particularly, the strain on the already overburdened circulation caused by the necessity of eliminating the heat produced. Exercise, to become a significant factor in weight reduction, must be performed daily and for adequate periods. Rates of heat loss of 500 to 800 calories per hour mean little if maintained for but a few minutes a day. Four to five hours' exercise daily, which has been recommended, can produce a truly important effect on energy output. There is no substitute for good clinical judgment regarding the amount of exercise a patient may take with safety and benefit. Bedroom calisthenics performed casually morning and night have little bearing on the problem. Exercise is a poor substitute for diet. Five hundred to 1000 extra calories may be expended by relatively severe exercise and 1000 to 2000 calories can be avoided by even a moderate diet. In most cases, exercise is sporadic at best. Diet has its uniform effect each day. One of the great drawbacks of exercise on a reduction program is its effect on the appetite. This effect is of little moment for the "anemic" group, but for the "gross-feeders" exercise can be detrimental. It takes little or no effort for these people to offset entirely a 1000 calorie expenditure by an equivalent or greater intake. The appetite factor must be recognized when the form and amount of exercise are prescribed.

Passive exercise, such as hydrotherapy and massage, has no important influence on caloric output. However, it can produce desirable effects in improving sluggish circulations and in increasing muscle tone. A proper course of physiotherapy may do much to get the semi-invalid in condition to take active exercise. One valuable contribution of massage, especially superficial massage, is the improvement which takes place in the skin as a result of increased circulation. Fat may be removed from the skin at a rate faster than the elasticity of the skin can accommodate, with resultant looseness or wrinkling of the skin. This may be conspicuous in the neck, upper arm and thigh areas. If patients are instructed, when they have lost only five to ten pounds, to massage these areas systematically two to three times a day with any simple rubifacient, such as alcohol, much of the worrisome skin problem can be avoided.

WATER AND SALT. Much difference of opinion exists as to the place of water and salt in a reduction program. When circulatory failure exists, the salt and fluids are restricted. Neither salt nor water restriction materially influences the water swings which normally occur from day to day or which are found in women at menstruation. The larger swings noted in the obese have not been related to salt or water intake. Normally functioning kidneys are the most potent regulatory factor in salt and water balance. The relatively high meat intake of a reduction diet makes salt restriction a difficult matter if the meat is to be eaten. The high heat output increases the body needs for water. The reduced water components of the restricted diet tend to reduce the intake of fluid. It seems that restriction of water intake might be irrational. Patients taking unrestricted fluid intakes lose fat without complications.[19] Sufficient salt to enable the patient to eat the necessary food and sufficient fluid to secure a urine output of 1000 to 1500 cc. a day are desirable.

Prevention. The most effective therapy is prevention. If it were possible to prevent a fraction of the fifteen million people who are 10 per cent overweight from joining the five million who are 20 per cent overweight, much would be accomplished. Unfortunately, the insidious development of significant obesity makes it difficult for a person to determine just when he became fat.

It is important to prevent and correct obesity in children. Eating habits with lasting effects are developed in childhood.[3,15,59] Adequate exercise in the young who show early evidence of obesity is important.

Girls 17 to 20 years of age who have already acquired habits of carelessly eating high carbohydrate and low protein foods are setting the stage for difficult reduction problems after the age of 40. These girls show moderate amounts of flabby fat and poor muscular development by the age of 20 to 25. After one or more pregnancies associated with the loss of considerable protein, which is never entirely replaced, we see the classic picture of the "static" obese 40 year old woman. Irregular meals low in protein and high in carbohydrate and fat, nibbling at home, party snacks in the afternoon and evening associated with limited physical activities are so firmly established that reduction is a task. For the men in the 30- to 40-year age group who have acquired habits of heavy eating during their active days, carelessness, indifference, and the "it can't happen to me" attitude are large factors in the development of fat deposits over the ensuing 10 to 15 years. A basic difficulty is the failure to recognize the time when the habits and pleasures of indulgence change into "small vice" and habituation. "It is of utmost importance to check the first propensities to gluttony (and intoxication) as they soon become uncontrollable."[3]

As they grow older, patients tend to change their eating habits. The tendency to reduce the intake of protein food seems to parallel the lessening in physical activities and is often associated with a relative, or absolute, increase in starchy foods. The net result is often a relative obesity in which fat deposits replace the inadequately maintained vital tissues, although the total weight may change but little. As weakness and other stigmata of malnutrition develop, energy output decreases with further increase in fat formation. Much of this type of relative obesity could be prevented by attention to the types of food chosen by people over 50 years of age.

Dangers. The dangers involved in reduction procedures are usually overstated. There is no age group at which overnutrition does not occur nor in which reduction to a proper weight does not improve health. One ten-year-old boy lost 31.5 pounds in 12 weeks with no after-effect but improved general well-being. A 12-year-old girl reduced from 208 to 164 pounds in 20 weeks with marked physical and mental improvement. At the other extreme, a 67-year-old woman had difficulty in walking. She was having 15 to 18 extrasystoles a minute and her blood pressure was 240 mm. Hg systolic and 110 diastolic. She reduced from 278 to 182 pounds in 24 weeks. After only 4 weeks of dieting, her blood pressure was 135 mm. Hg systolic and 80 diastolic, and she was marketing and doing some housework with ease.

Cardiac and renal decompensations, glycosuria and hyperglycemia have been recognized as indications for, rather than contraindications to, a radical reduction diet. Evans and Strang encountered no disasters, nor even minor mishaps, in the patients treated with severely limited diets.

Difficulties sometimes encountered when patients lose weight too rapidly are not caused by the weight reduction per se but by the type of weight which is removed. Rapid losses in weight almost universally mean that large amounts of protein, together with its associated water, are lost. In general, 1 gram of protein tissue is equivalent to 1 calorie. A loss of one pound of protein tissue corresponds roughly to 450 calories, or about one eighth of the value for one pound of fat tissue. On programs in which calories alone are considered, it is easy to see that if the caloric deficit is supplied chiefly from protein tissue the rate of loss in weight will be far greater than when fat alone supplies the calories. Many popular reduction fads utilize diets grossly inadequate in protein. They frequently secure a rapid reduction in weight but at the risk of precipitating serious illness.

Medical writings notwithstanding, no identifiable metabolic aberration resembling thyrotoxicosis occurs as the result of proper reduction programs. There is no contraindication to rapid losses if proper diets are used and if the weight lost is fat tissue.

Reduction Regimen. When a patient starts off on a reduction program he should understand his problem and his objectives. It is human nature to search for a "specific" to dissolve the fat rapidly. Also, it is convenient for the patient to place the responsibility for his obesity everywhere but on himself. He must understand that his obesity is his personal problem, but that it can be corrected. The patient may be overwhelmed by the facts about his problem and its treatment. It takes courage to agree to a dramatic performance such as an operation to relieve the insistent pain of appendicitis. It requires a different kind of courage to face a complete overhauling of one's habits and pleasures. The monotony of a reduction diet is a serious handicap to one who loves the pleasure of eating. There is value in letting the patient know that we appreciate his difficulties.[162]

The patient must be both educated and given a knowledge of general food values, of diets and of the peculiarities of the human body, especially with regard to weight. More particularly, he will learn his own capacity for self-discipline. The training program begins with the establishment of proper habits of eating. His body must learn the normal response to proper meals at proper times.

Many will benefit from an initial period of hospitalization. They can more easily learn about food values, food types and food servings; they can discover lean meats, fat-free vegetables and salads; and they can learn that they will not be hungry on proper diets even with quite low calories and that their weight will come down with dieting. Most important of all, they can see that it can be done and that they can do it. Many a discouraged, unhappy patient has been given a good start by spending two or three weeks in a hospital. Time and expense are the practical deterrents to making this a universal practice.

Spa treatment, which is not as popular in this country as in Europe, likewise provides a protected environment in which the patient may start his reduction program. Under spa conditions the physiotherapy and exercise programs are well organized.

Eventually the patient must carry on his program in his normal surroundings. He is on his own. Encouragement from an understanding family sympathetic with his objectives is to the good. Too often lack of interest in his diet, ridicule or family opposition is too great a handicap to overcome. The selection of a program for a patient must anticipate home problems as far as possible. A complete fast one day a week may be all that one patient can accomplish. Another may require five small feedings a day. Another may have the difficulty of working different "shifts" in weekly cycles. "In practice it will be found that the greatest success in the dietary treatment of obesity lies in the regimen which will least tempt the patient to transgress it."[1]

Postreduction Period. When possible, the problems of the postreduction period should be discussed with a patient prior to discharge. A review of what he has learned about foods, about obesity and about himself is in order. Emphasis is placed upon the physiologic value of protein as contrasted with carbohydrate and fat foods. Food fads, fantastic diets and panaceas must be understood in their true perspectives. The basic relationship of body mass to the balance of intake and output has been established. The relief which the patient has experienced from presenting symptoms and his freedom from the stress and strain of his fat overload should be re-emphasized. An appreciation of his self-mastery is in order. Self-deception about food and weight is no longer permissible.

Most patients wish to know whether the overweight will return. If the weight which was lost was water and protein tissue, it will return, and rapidly, as soon as a normal protein intake is resumed. This is the experience with all of the so-called rapid reduction methods. If the weight lost was fat, the patient may be assured that the fat will not return provided that his caloric balance remains normal. Slowly but inevitably fat will be redeposited directly in proportion to an excessive intake if he returns to his previous habits of eating. It is unfortunately true that the demonstration of sufficient will power to adhere to a restrictive regimen for 6 to 12 months is no guarantee of sufficient character to avert a relapse.

The need for a strict diet disappears with the desired weight reduction. A few guiding principles with reference to follow-up may then suffice:

1. Sufficient protein should be eaten at *each* meal and in any desired quantity, but it should never fall below the level of the reduction diet.

2. In general, fruits and vegetables may be eaten as desired.

3. Fruit should basically replace pastries and other rich foods as dessert. Reserve special desserts for special occasions.

4. Concentrated foods, such as those listed in Group IV, page 602, should be added cautiously. One portion a day may be used at the outset. This may be increased or decreased to hold the weight in balance.

5. Carefully watch "snacks" and "sneaky foods." The extra roll and butter, the extra tablespoonful of mayonnaise, the side dish of potato or spaghetti supply extra calories; the pleasure is insignificant in proportion to the risk.

6. Methods of food preparation can entirely change the basic values of a food. Broiled, roasted and baked foods are always to be preferred to fried foods. Heavy gravies are full of calories. Vegetables covered with melted butter and simple salads decked with rich dressings are in an altogether different class from the plain vegetables. It should be kept in mind that the purpose of special cooking is to induce one to eat more. The habit of plain cooking and simple serving of foods should be cultivated.

7. Alcoholic beverages offer a twofold problem. They have significant caloric value, and they make one less alert to the quantity of food being eaten.

8. Physical activities should be developed. Common sense is indispensable, and the advantages of maintaining a well toned machine are as great as those of a sustained additional energy output.

9. It is not necessary to become pathologically weight-conscious. However, weight should be taken and recorded under uniform conditions once a week.

10. A definite trend toward increasing weight should be arrested at once.

11. As time passes, normal habit patterns, normal physiologic responses and normal sensations become established.

Summary. The removal of the fat from an obese person depends upon the development of an adequate negative caloric balance and a continuance of a suitable regimen for a sufficient period. A properly designed diet will provide a safe, low intake. A carefully regulated program of work and exercise will provide the maximum output consistent with safety. The rate of loss in weight depends upon the regimen, the total loss upon its duration. Certain adjuvants, when indicated, will have beneficial influence on the course. Many object to the consideration of the treatment of obesity as a moral issue. Insofar as the term "moral issue" is related to character and character means capacity to meet the realities of this world, obesity is a moral issue. Regardless of the mechanism of production of weakness in character, it is the fundamental difficulty in the exercise of self-control. No amount of rationalization or explanation increases one's capacity for self-discipline. The successful treatment of obesity, as for alcoholism, smoking and other minor vices, depends upon the will power to deny to oneself certain pleasurable sensations.

"On the part of both physician and patient firmness of purpose and steady perseverance will be needed."[4] "The most ignorant person, however, certainly knows what is meant by excess; and it is in the power of every man, if he chooses, to avoid it."[3]

RESULTS OF TREATMENT

Weight Loss. The demonstration that body weight can be reduced by the application of the principles described above lends support to their validity, but the goal is not weight removal, per se, but fat removal. By proper diet, only fat and its attendant water are removed. Since patients remain in nitrogen equilibrium, there is no evidence that protein is lost from the body. Any protein material which is sacrificed in the breaking down of fat tissue goes into the metabolic pool and is re-utilized, thus having no effect on the over-all balance. Weight losses of this type may be permanent. By improper diet, which usually means one too low in protein, much protein tissue is lost. These weight losses are frequently associated with morbidity and are never permanent. It is commonly stated that a loss of two pounds per week may be expected from a 1000 calorie diet.[1] For many patients this approximation holds. However, the degree of obesity and the amount of physical activity have equally great influence on this factor.

Patients studied under strict hospital conditions lose weight more rapidly than office patients.[1] Five hospital patients[11] had an average weight of 222 pounds, which corresponded to an average excess weight of 72 per cent. After dieting an average period of 17 weeks, these patients weighed an average of 181 pounds, which corresponded to an average excess weight of 40 per cent. These 5 patients lost 47 per cent of their excess weight. The diets employed varied from 600 to 650 calories with 55 to 65 grams of protein. A second series of patients,[154] 13 in number, with an average weight of 259 pounds, dieted for an average of 59 days and lost an average of 35 pounds. The average figures for the diets of this group were 360 calories, 58 grams protein, 14 grams carbohydrate and 8 grams fat.

The series of Evans and Strang include several patients who reduced more than 100 pounds. One unemployed colored woman who remained in the hospital during the total period of dieting reduced from 389 to 169 pounds, 20 pounds of which were accounted for by the removal of an abdominal apron of stretched skin and hypertrophied subcutaneous supporting tissue. She lived in the hospital for two periods of about a year each, with approximately a month's vacation between them during which she gained some 30 pounds. This patient while dieting usually was ingesting less than 5 calories per kg. of actual weight. For the whole period she was well, cheerful and busy about the hospital; she remained in nitrogen equilibrium and maintained a constant index of creatinine excretion, normal as related to her ideal weight.

Short[163] maintained a patient, with an initial weight of 402 pounds, for a period of 18 months on a diet planned to include all the essential foodstuffs but supplying only 700 calories. She lost 239 pounds and during the entire period remained in good health and spirits.

The rate of reduction is related to the caloric deficit, which is reflected usually in the level of intake. Diets containing 500 to 1400 calories are reduction diets.

However, weight loss will occur at any level of intake provided the output is sufficiently high to produce a reasonable caloric deficit. One hospital study[155] involved 6 patients whose intakes averaged 2510 calories per day. In 70 patient days they lost a total of 18.5 pounds. They were all considerably overweight, ranging from 170 to 330 pounds. Four other patients who averaged 2400 calories per day for 23 patient days lost a total of 12 pounds.[68] They also were quite heavy, weighing initially from 320 to 430 pounds. Two of Werner's[89] patients lost weight on diets averaging 2800 calories. His diets were designed to show that the caloric value rather than the types of food employed determined the rate of weight loss. These studies demonstrate that the rate of weight loss corresponds to the caloric deficit. Diets containing 2400 to 2800 calories may be reduction diets for persons who weigh 100 to 180 per cent more than they should, many of whom have basal metabolisms of 2200 to 2400 calories with total energy outputs per day well over 4000 calories. A 1000 to 1500 calorie deficit at these levels produces weight loss just as truly as at the lower levels of total metabolism.

Office-treated patients can also lose weight. Of 111 patients who had dieted for over 4 weeks[157] and averaged 48 per cent overweight, 5 patients were 100 per cent overweight, 11 were 75 to 100 per cent, and 27 were 50 to 15 per cent overweight. Ninety-eight patients were completed cases.

98 patients in 858 weeks lost a total of 2590 pounds:
- Average time on diet, 8.7 weeks
- Average loss per patient, 26.4 pounds
- Average loss per week, 3.0 pounds

111 patients at end of first week:
- 111 patients lost 714 pounds
- Average loss per patient, 6.4 pounds

75 patients at end of four weeks:
- 75 patients lost 1209 pounds in four weeks
- Average loss per patient, 16.1 pounds
- Average loss per week, 4.0 pounds

47 patients at end of eight weeks:
- 47 patients lost 1265 pounds
- Average loss per patient, 26.9 pounds
- Average loss per week, 3.4 pounds

The diets ranged from 550 to 700 calories with the protein level at 1 gram per kilo of ideal weight and carbohydrate from 25 to 50 grams.

Patients will reduce if they follow a proper diet for a sufficient period of time. The above series have included complicating endocrine and metabolic disorders, but none presented psychiatric disturbances of greater intensity than are seen in the usual office practice. Individual cases illustrate more clearly some of the specific problems encountered in office practice.

A 58-year-old man who did sedentary work weighed 248 pounds. His diagnoses included diabetes, cholelithiasis and hypertension. He had lost only 9 pounds in 3 years but paid little attention to his condition prior to an acute attack of angina-like pain. Thoroughly frightened, he reduced to 216 pounds in 4 months and experienced absence of symptoms and a return of his blood pressure to 120/80 from an initial level of 180/110. His gallbladder was removed 3 months later. He grew careless and gained weight to 226 pounds; glycosuria returned and, frightened once more, he resumed his therapeutic diet.

A 16-year-old girl, active and athletic but a lover of candy, weighed 150 instead of 120 pounds. She gained 2.5 pounds in the first 2 weeks of dieting and then, with the same diet, reduced to 136 pounds in the next 10 weeks. This normal girl learned proper eating habits and lost fat consistently, although she probably had a considerable restoration of body protein in the first weeks of dieting.

An 18-year-old college freshman weighed 190 pounds instead of her proper 130 pounds. Although of a socially prominent family, she "sat out" her first two college dances and determined to correct her weight. Between January 1 and April 17 she reduced to 142 pounds. Her weight 5 months later was 143 pounds. After 3½ months of dieting she was able to buy party dresses in a size normal for her age. Pride plus motive can be a potent force.

A 49-year-old executive, hard, self-indulgent and domineering, was offered up-rated life insurance because he weighed 230 pounds instead of 175. He had on two previous occasions lost 10 to 20 pounds by dieting. At this time he reduced to 205 pounds in 5 months. He received his insurance at a normal premium. Eight months later he weighed 226 pounds following a trip to Europe. Having attained his financial objective, he returned to his previous habits of living and regained his lost weight.

A 35-year-old secretary weighed 270 instead of 140 pounds. Both her parents were obese and she had always been heavy. Her menstruation had always been irregular, sometimes lapsing for 6 to 7 months, and she was subject to severe headaches. In 3½ months her weight fell to 228 pounds, but the headaches persisted. Benzedrine was tried for a month with little effect on course or symptoms, and in the fifth month she became careless in her eating. She regularly became very hungry at 4 A.M. She resumed her strict diet, the hunger disappeared and her weight continued to decrease. After 7 months of special diet she felt well and strong and had no headaches. Her weight was 214—a loss of 56 pounds. For the next 6 months her dietary efforts decreased, but she lost another 12 pounds. For several months she had had normal menses. A further loss to 189 pounds was obtained over the subsequent 6 months, and she remained at this general level for 15 years, during which period she married happily. An attempt at further reduction was made by her family doctor, who used 2 to 5 grains of thyroid daily as a supplement. A reduction to 170 pounds was obtained, but thyrotoxic symptoms became so severe that the thyroid was stopped. In the following 8 months, she gained 25 pounds in spite of half-hearted attempts at dieting. After she had resumed a proper diet, her weight dropped 6 pounds in 2 weeks. This woman illustrates the effect of childhood feeding habits, the correction in time of gross obesity by proper diet, the clearing of incapacitating headaches, the return of normal menstrual cycles, the long period of weight maintenance and the results of ill-advised thyroid therapy.

A 34-year-old "small business" man weighed 406 pounds. He performed hard physical labor several hours daily at his work. He had taken 10 grains of thyroid daily for the preceding 5 years. His BMR was −8 per cent, but his calories per hour were 96. His blood pressure was 180 mm. Hg systolic and 110 mm. diastolic, his pulse 96 and his heart "overactive." He lost 19 pounds in 2 weeks in the hospital. He went back to work adhering to a 1200 calorie diet with 90 grams of protein and 80 of carbohydrate. Nine months later he weighed 243 pounds and his pulse and blood pressure were normal. A high energy output with a restricted intake and a large caloric deficit is illustrated.

In contrast to these patients are the large numbers of pathetic moderately obese women like Mrs. X. She is a "modern" mother of three children, active in church, school and social affairs. She knows all about diets and calories and has been on several unsuccessful reduction programs. She weighs 190 pounds and should weigh not over 140. She eagerly anticipates each instruction. In 3 months she lost 27 pounds; in 4 months she regained 7 pounds, and in another 8 months, 14 more. A second reduction trial produced a loss of 9 pounds in a month, but her weight remained around 180 pounds. She has been unable to adjust her social life to the diet restrictions, but above all she is an excellent cook and loves to eat.

These patients were seen in office practice and represent a cross section of those who consult doctors because of obesity. They are ordinary people with likes and dislikes, prejudices and ideas. They differ from patients of normal weight or underweight only in that they like to eat and that their pleasure in eating "got ahead of them." Like any other persons dealing with any other undesirable habits, they can resume control of themselves when they find sufficient reason regardless of ancestors, endocrines or metabolic dyscrasias.

Prognosis. An appreciable percentage of overweight patients can and do succeed in reducing. Dublin[24] reported on one group of 300 overweight employees of whom 81 per cent lost weight. One year later a check of 224 of these patients showed that 32 per cent had lost a few more pounds. Five years later 21 per cent of 193 patients of this series had reduced still further. The principal factor involved in permanent success is the reeducation of the patient's food habits. The long period of self-discipline required of a patient for the removal of significant amounts of weight aids in his self-control, but he must also have learned to like normal types of foods in normal proportions.

The "relapse" rate is high. Howard[1] stated that "invariably, when treatment is discontinued, patients become careless as regards their diet, and a gradual gain in weight results." Others[44,55,59,159] have emphasized the poor long-range results after the cessation of treatment. Even Dublin noted that of his 193 patients seen 5 years after reduction, 79 per cent had regained 18 or more pounds. Our own experience is of the same order. A generalization is that one fourth of the patients never try to reduce, one fourth will carry on for 3 to 4 weeks, one fourth will persist for 2 to 3 months; of the remaining patients who may labor for up to 10 to 12 months, less than half will maintain a truly long-term weight control.

In a large number of cases, the failure to cope with obesity is in reality a failure to deal with a complication rather than with the obesity per se. Neuropsychiatric problems are apparent. However, a fair percentage of the failures in young and middle aged women are failures to deal with the prolonged protein malnutrition with which obesity is associated. These patients exhibit, at the outset, the same physiologic, mental and emotional adaptations to prolonged protein starvation that Benedict and his associates[164] and others later demonstrated in their malnourished subjects. When the protein starvation has been acute, as in many patients who have used improper diets, the restoration of body protein is rapid. A patient who had weighed around 220 pounds lost weight rapidly to 175 pounds by an improper diet. He was practically incapacitated. When placed on a reduction diet adequate in protein although low in calories, he promptly gained 10 pounds and his symptoms were relieved. While continuing on the same diet, he later lost 15 pounds but continued in good health. The gain of several pounds shown by many young girls at the start of a reduction program which is followed by a slow, steady loss in weight may be interpreted as protein replacement followed by fat removal. The problem of the older obese woman who has adapted herself to a low protein intake over many years is difficult. Obese patients will literally force a protein intake which is quite high for them for several weeks and obtain the characteristic weight response. They then enter a plateau phase of slight weight change which is, we believe, due to their failure to keep up their protein intakes because of their habitual dislike of these foods. Studies of the total nitrogen content and daily fluctuations of nitrogen balance for adequate periods have not been made on patients of this type. Hence, information regarding the magnitude of the initial nitrogen deficit and the rate of replacement is not available. Clinically, it seems probable that many of the difficulties in continuing a consistent weight loss in the 30- to 40-year-old obese woman center around the prolonged and very efficient adaptation of her body to a low protein intake and the difficulty of readjusting this mechanism. If a complicating disorder and the adaptations of the body to it remain unrelieved, the chances of an alteration in the state of nutrition of the body are minimized.

"The mental peculiarities and temperament are deeply concerned in every case; the difficulties of treatment are greatly enhanced in persons of indolent and phlegmatic habit, and proportionately diminished in persons of active and energetic disposition."[5] The degree of obesity, per se, is important, for although "the greater the obesity, the greater the rate of weight loss" is true, the bleakness of the immediate future is too much for many really heavy patients. The slow rate of accomplishment seems to them disproportionate to the magnitude of the effort put forth. The complications of the obesity or the conditions which may be associated with it may provide serious obstacles. Organic disease may so reduce energy output that only a very strict program which the patient cannot endure for long will suffice. Mental, emotional and moral difficulties constitute real barriers.

The fundamental determinant of the success or failure of reduction is motive. When a patient has a reason which for him is compelling, he can exert enough self-control to reduce. Whether or not the program continues when the urgent motive is gone is another matter. In our experience, the three chief motives which can sustain a patient are *avarice*, *vanity* and *fear*.

OBSERVATIONS AFTER REDUCTION: CLINICAL

Mortality. "Fat People Who Lose Weight Live Longer" is the title of a paper by Dublin[165] in which he presented statistics to support this thesis. The report was based on a comparison of death rates among 2300 people who had reduced weight sufficiently to obtain improved insurance ratings with the basic data for mortality in the obese. He concluded that as a consequence of reduction there was a substantial lowering of mortality, approximately one fifth in males and one third in females. The study of the causes of death of reduced patients showed that the decline in death rate is greatest in the degenerative diseases. Table 30, which deals with

TABLE 30. PER CENT ACTUAL OF EXPECTED DEATHS AMONG PERSONS 20–64 YEARS OF AGE "RATED" FOR OVERWEIGHT —ALL CASES AND CASES WHICH SUBSEQUENTLY RECEIVED LOWER "RATINGS" AFTER REDUCTION IN WEIGHT[27]

SEX	ALL CASES Moderately Overweight	ALL CASES Severely Overweight	RERATED CASES Moderately Overweight	RERATED CASES Severely Overweight
Males	142	179	113	109
Females	142	161	90	135

Modified from Table 9, *Mortality Among Insured Overweights in Recent Years* by L. I. Dublin and H. H. Marks, Sixtieth Annual Meeting of the Association of Life Insurance Medical Directors of America, October 11–12, 1951. (By permission of the authors and The American Journal of Public Health.)

the same data, provides the "best evidence to date of the value of reduction programs."[27] There is not universal agreement that such statistics actually prove this thesis.[166] It is, however, the prevailing clinical impression that weight reduction definitely prolongs life. Since obesity causes one to age more rapidly, it is understandable that the improvements should be more noticeable in the degenerative disorders.

Symptoms. Relief from symptoms and a generally increased feeling of well-being accompany weight reduction. References are made to weakness and lassitude associated with weight reduction.[167] Burr stated,[80] "The sudden decrease in fat content of the human diet brings complaints from workers that they are unable to do as much work and that their appetites are not satisfied." Such, however, is not the experience of many observers who have followed large numbers of these patients. Perhaps the difference in experience is related to the types of diet employed. Benedict noted such reactions to his semistarvation diets. Brozek[168] found similar symptoms associated with malnutrition. With diets containing proper amounts of protein and carbohydrate, such complaints are rare. Dyspnea on exertion, transient swelling of the feet, sweating and heat intolerance are markedly improved, and digestive disorders such as distention, flatulence, constipation and heartburn are relieved. Headaches and dizziness, common complaints in the obese, may disappear completely. Sleeplessness or restless sleeping, which is often the result of heavy feeding at bed time or of the mechanical handicap of the heavy abdominal wall, is benefited. Joint pains, especially of the feet and knees, are frequently due to chronic sprain alone, but many times degenerative joint changes have developed. Removal of an extra burden promotes the comfort of these joints. Skin disorders (see p. 540) are much more readily controlled.

Lusk[22] described the difficulties of the fat man in hot, humid weather when his metabolism may actually be 50 per cent higher than on a day of moderate temperature because of the thick, ill-conducting layer of adipose tissue. The performance of even light work is penalized in hot, moist weather because of the difficulty experienced in eliminating heat. This inefficiency and waste is relieved by fat removal. In fact, the generally improved physiology which results from the removal of excessive fat is exhibited in every function of the body.

Complications. HYPERTENSION. A striking improvement in hypertension usually follows weight reduction. Preble[16] recorded the blood pressure, by decades of age, of 194 obese patients before treatment and after reducing 10 pounds or more (see Table 31). The average decrease for the entire group was 18 mm. Hg systolic and 10 mm. diastolic.

TABLE 31. BLOOD PRESSURE BEFORE TREATMENT AND AFTER (194 CASES)[16]

AGES, YEARS	0–20	21–30	31–40	41–50	51–60	61–70	71
	BEFORE TREATMENT						
Systolic	130	129	147	157	165	180	179
Diastolic	80	88	101	101	98	113	95
	AFTER REDUCING 10 POUNDS OR MORE						
Systolic	115	127	132	101	143	166	150
Diastolic	70	81	90	89	90	102	86
	Average: Before, 155/96; after, 133/86						

Among the 1000 cases of obesity analyzed by Preble, 62 had a systolic blood pressure of 200 or above. Twenty-two of these were treated by reducing the weight 10 pounds or more, and in them the average systolic dropped from 219 to 176, and the diastolic from 129 to 108.

Evans[30] found the systolic blood pressures of 100 consecutive cases taken without regard to age, sex and degree or duration of obesity to be above 140 in 61 percent. Eleven per cent were above 180, and 10 per cent above 200. The diastolic pressures were above 100 in 36 per cent of these patients. Seven per cent of the total were above 110, and 8 per cent above 120. Treatment reduced the systolic pressure below 135 in 75 per cent of those whose level was from 140 to 180, in 50 per cent of those whose level was 180 to 200, but in only 20 per cent when the pressure was above 200. Many of the patients with the higher pressures, although not attaining normal levels, did show an appreciable reduction. All but one of the patients with diastolic pressures of 100 to 110 and of 110 to 120 attained, with treatment, a diastolic pressure of below 90, but only 20 per cent of those whose diastolic level was above 120 reduced to normal. Wood and Cash[32] found that a drop in blood pressure is commonly associated with reduction and quoted statistics which relate a weight loss of 25 to 30 pounds with a drop of 25 to 30 millimeters systolic and 15 to 20 millimeters diastolic pressure.

However, it is not clear that hypertension is related to obesity rather than to body build. Master and Jaffe[34] found as many of their obese patients to have normal pressure as had high blood pressure but agreed that there is no question of the value of reducing the weight when the blood pressure is elevated.

Clinical and statistical evidence indicates that obese patients with initially high blood pressures who reduce in weight show reductions in systolic and usually in diastolic pressure. An improved application of the cuff on a more normally shaped arm may be a factor in the observed presssure changes.

CARDIAC DISEASE. The improvement which may be observed by the reduction in weight in patients who have diminished cardiac reserve is striking. Persons of normal or slightly increased weight experience the benefits of even small reductions in the basic load which they must transport. In the truly obese, the benefits are markedly increased. It is a common experience that obese patients almost bedfast from their cardiac limitations may become relatively active after the removal of 10 to 50 pounds of fat. Dublin[165] reported on 33 obese patients who reduced weight and who initially had definite physical signs of disease, chiefly hypertension and heart disease. Seventeen, followed 5 years after reduction, had no progression of their conditions and were clinically improved. All but two had maintained a considerably lower weight.

Statistics from Norway dealing with effect of the rigid food restrictions of the war period on mortality from circulatory disease indicate that shortly after the beginning of food deprivation there was a definite reduction in mortality, which reached a minimum in about 3 years.[165,169] After the food restrictions were removed, the mortality rates returned to their previous levels. Although no data regarding weight reduction were quoted, it is probable that this rate change more or less paralleled the weight loss inevitable from a change in diet previously abundant in fat and calories to the meagre war diet. An improvement in mortality from circulatory disease as a result of weight reduction was indicated.

Exceptions to the thesis that normal weight offers a better prognosis than obesity in cardiac disease have been noted by Sprague,[169] who quoted data to indicate that in angina pectoris and in acute myocardial infarction obese patients had a better prognosis than those without obesity. The data indicated the prognosis in relation to the weight observed at the time of acute illness. They gave no indication of the frequency of attacks in the two groups or of the amount of organic change necessary to produce symptoms in the already functionally embarrassed obese as compared with the more adequate normal. Likewise, they have little bearing on the benefits which these patients might have obtained by weight reduction after the onset of the cardiac illness. Walker[170] reported on patients who lost 7 to 40 pounds by dieting over periods up to 8 months with an average weight loss of 1.6 pounds per week. Of 39 patients, 13 of 15 having angina reported significant relief. About half of 25 patients who had ballistocardiograph studies showed improvement with weight reduction.

ARTERIOSCLEROSIS. That weight reduction may arrest the progress of arteriosclerosis or even reverse it has been suggested by Wilens.[38] In his review of arteriosclerosis in autopsy material, he noted the marked difference between the incidence of arteriosclerosis in the obese and in the thin. Also, he observed that a fair number of deaths occur after lingering illnesses in which malnutrition and much weight loss occur. Thus, many patients who were classed as "thin" at autopsy may have been of normal or excess weight for most of their lives. The observed incidence of arteriosclerosis in the "thin" may therefore represent only that of obese patients who have lost weight before death or, if there is a certain basic amount of arteriosclerosis in the normally thin, the failure to increase this number from the numbers of obese known to have lost weight prior to death suggests that the arteriosclerosis previously present in the obese may have disappeared during the period of weight loss. There is no way to settle this question at present.

Investigators who postulate that the development of arteriosclerosis is related to the lipid content of the blood have studied the fluctuations of the several blood lipids with weight reduction. Walker[41,170] found that patients who had lost significant amounts of weight and who had initially elevated lipoproteins, especially in the S_f 12–20 fraction, would probably drop the level with weight reduction and that the permanency of this reduction would be proportional to the initial level. Apparently, variations in cholesterol were not related to weight reduction or cholesterol intake during reduction. Peters and Man[39] found low blood cholesterol values following periods of weight reduction. Young[40,171] observed that phospholipid and cholesterol increased somewhat during weight reduction and in the postreduction periods, although the changes were small. He found a wide fluctuation of blood lipids in women but

TABLE 32. EFFECT OF REDUCTION OF WEIGHT ON DISPOSAL OF DEXTROSE[51]

	WHEN OBESE				AFTER REDUCTION OF WEIGHT			
	Fasting	1 Hr.	2 Hr.	3 Hr.	Fasting	1 Hr.	2 Hr.	3 Hr.
	105	236	256	152	78	126	107	52
	127	303	244	174	93	146	115	59
	168	290	370	302	104	113	90	74
	166	300	344	264	106	153	136	69
	99	212	216	164	82	156	105	70
	162	202	210	240	71	146	129	50
	124	294	125	99	86	154	93	60
	161	300	202	178	91	166	87	51
	148	234	282	176	93	156	136	113
	113	212	200	115	78	178	100	77
	73	188	200	97	93	147	110	94
	115	200	196	196	76	121	109	76
	133	300	236	164	112	149	50	68
	148	314	270	146	89	170	93	57
	113	234	200	164	98	109	88	59
	119	230	185	102	85	135	107	66
	121	172	192	107	89	117	96	96
	141	230	202	156	97	139	84	62
	106	270	252	222	83	154	119	63
	117	238	242	192	92	192	129	58
	300	504	508	428	111	192	76	59
Averages....	136	260	244	183	91	149	104	68
	124*	278	266	111	87	200	188	88

* Only patient showing incomplete recovery after reduction of weight.

observed no constant variation in any factor in relation to pre-diet, rapid or slow weight change. A low fat diet, per se, caused little reduction of serum lipids.[43] The diets, however, had low protein, high carbohydrate and high calories, which caused some patients to gain weight. The great variability in serum lipid pattern may have been influenced by the rapid synthesis of blood lipids from carbohydrate or by the liver damage noted in 20 per cent of patients on these diets. In spite of the many studies of blood lipids, it cannot be definitely stated that blood lipid concentrations are related to the development of arteriosclerosis. Nor can it be shown that weight reduction reduces an already present arteriosclerosis by way of changes in blood lipids or by other mechanisms.

ENDOCRINE DISORDERS. *Menstruation.* Abnormalities of menstruation are frequently noted in association with obesity. Pain and irregularity are the most common complaints. Most of these problems subside as normal weight is secured. Mitchell and Rogers[172] studied 32 women with amenorrhea for 3 to 31 months. Thirteen lost from 13 to 69 pounds and began to menstruate. One woman lost 15 pounds, had two periods, put the weight back on and ceased to menstruate. Fifteen patients lost no weight and had no return of menstruation. Only 2 patients lost weight without a return of menstruation. Mitchell discussed the possible relationship of both obesity and amenorrhea to an underlying emotional disorder. We believe that this form of menstrual disorder is due to the ingestion of a faulty metabolic mixture at a physiologically impressionable period. Exactly the same symptoms are encountered in many grossly undernourished girls. The symptoms seem to be related to long periods of low protein intake. In both the thin and the obese, the symptoms respond to proper protein feeding, whether it is combined with increased calories as in the undernourished or with lowered calories as in the obese. This thesis would tend to explain Mitchell's observation that menstruation appeared after 1 to 4 months of dieting but before the complete correction of the obesity.

A few women have reduced in the hope that loss of weight will cure sterility. Sterility has a great many causes other than obesity, and it is hardly proper to expect diet to control the disorder completely. However, several young women, after years of sterility and obesity, have become pregnant after weight reduction and have carried through to normal deliveries.

Diabetes. The obese diabetic patient improves following weight reduction.[5] Newburgh and Conn[51] reported the glucose tolerance curves of 35 obese, middle-aged patients with glycosuria before and after weight reduction. Twenty-one of the patients dieted sufficiently to obtain normal or nearly normal weight. The data appear in Table 32. In the left columns of the table are shown the characteristic diabetic responses to glucose before reduction in contrast to the quite normal handling of sugar after weight reduction in the right columns. A graphic summary of these data is provided by Chart 4, which shows the composite curves for these patients. It should be noted that these patients after reduction ate any kind of food they desired without glycosuria as long as they did not gain weight. One patient gained weight after her initial reduction and again showed the diabetic type of curve. A normal curve followed a second weight reduction. Thus the permanence of the "cure" of the diabetes was not established.

TABLE 33. EFFECT OF RECURRENT OBESITY ON DEXTROSE TOLERANCE CURVE[51]

OVERWEIGHT, PERCENTAGE	FASTING	1 HR.	2 HR.	3 HR.
45	128	314	322	202
0	91	140	72	61
25	119	230	185	102
0	87	135	107	66

Kinney[173] reported the case of a patient who had weighed over 200 pounds for 8 years prior to the diagnosis of diabetes, and who had gained in 2 years to 300 pounds. His insulin requirements reached 180 units daily. In 5 years he lost 150 pounds and then required no insulin. Comparable but less dramatic experiences occur in daily practice.

In 1942, Newburgh[174] reviewed 62 adult obese diabetics and their response to weight reduction. These patients were not extremely obese. Two thirds of them were less than 40 per cent overweight. Fifty-seven of the 62 patients had normal glucose handling after weight reduction. Attention was called to the fact that the glucose handling difficulty in these adult, obese persons may be different from that of the juvenile diabetic who is rarely obese and, when obese, does not respond to reduction in this manner. It would seem from these and

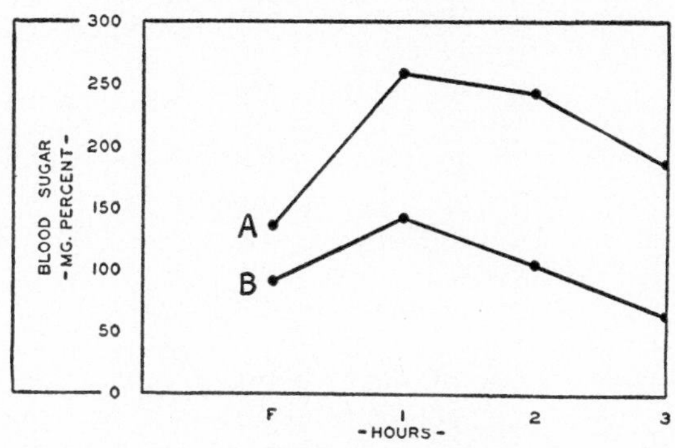

CHART 4. Composite dextrose tolerance curves for twenty-one patients A before and B after reduction of weight.[51]

similar studies that the diabetes found in the adult obese person represents a "sprain" of the sugar handling mechanisms from prolonged excessive carbohydrate feeding rather than a primary disease. With adequate physiologic rest, which is secured in the course of reduction by dieting, the mechanism resumes its normal resiliency. However, as is the case with other forms of "sprain," a lesser trauma a second time will again produce physiologic imbalance. Not only is the diabetes per se much improved, but the frequency and severity of its complications are much reduced following weight reduction.

NEUROPSYCHIATRIC DISORDERS. The mental attitude of the average patient who is reducing or has reduced is usually much improved. Many feel better than they have felt for years and exhibit a vitality in marked contrast to their previous depression and irritability. In some, the discovery that they have a capacity for self-discipline adds to their pleasure and satisfaction.

There are no reports of improvement by reduction in patients who have serious emotional or addiction problems. Rather the reports are almost uniformly to the effect that weight reduction is not possible without psychiatric therapy and quite unsatisfactory with it. Possibly, all grossly obese persons have personality problems. It makes little difference whether the obesity develops with the psychic disturbance or the psychic disturbance progresses as part of the personal adaptation to obesity. Nicholson[44] reported a higher percentage of recoveries with psychotherapy than with any other methods, including diet, but he noted the importance of establishing proper eating habits. Parson[55] had more success with psychotherapy than with diet. There may be lack of success with serious problems even after specific psychotherapy.[15,54,56]

Weight reduction can be accomplished in these patients. It has been done repeatedly. However, they require hospitalization and strict management for long periods. The patient often feels well with his loss in weight and his improved physiology, but he relapses when placed on his own responsibility. It is therefore questionable whether, beyond the demonstration that fat can be removed from any person under proper conditions, it is worth doing. Whether or not appropriate psychotherapy after weight reduction would produce long-term benefits has not been determined.

There are unstable people who are obese and who cannot be reduced by standard methods, and there are as many unstable people who are thin and who cannot be fattened. In many other illnesses, such as cardiac failure or fracture of the femur, the primary illness militates strongly against efficient treatment of an associated obesity. The proper therapy for obesity requires a self-control and character which the unstable person lacks. Significant loss in weight is difficult to attain in these patients. The results of group therapy, as currently practiced, have not been outstanding. The results are "inconclusive but interesting."[175] Kirlander[134] expressed the theory of group therapy as "misery loves company" or "company gives courage." Some people benefit from such therapy, but talking about obesity is not a cure. The fundamental fallacy of group therapy as conducted by nonprofessional people is the neglect of the fact that obesity is a personal problem. It is not known what might be accomplished by a psychiatrist dealing with an appropriately selected group.

OBSERVATIONS AFTER REDUCTION: PHYSIOLOGIC

Mass Exchange. Limited observations on the mass exchange of patients during reduction are available. Data on weight of intake and urine output, comparable to those described above, have been obtained on 4 obese women who were losing weight.[19] They were between 38 and 50 years of age and were initially between 71 per cent and 180 per cent—average 133 per cent—overweight. They were 25 to 119 per cent overweight at the conclusion. The average loss in weight was 32 kilograms. Table 34 shows the rapid reduction obtained by diets of 2 to 9 calories per kilogram. Since the mass balance data for the entire periods of study, from 6 to 26 weeks, were repetitious, only the data from representative portions of the total period are given for each patient, as noted in column 9 of Table 34. The actual weight of the daily intake of these patients averaged 3.56 kilograms—nearly 8 pounds. This value is about 15 per cent greater than for persons of normal weight and only 20 per cent less than for the group of obese patients who were on maintenance intakes. The ratio of weight of intake to body mass was only 2.7 per cent but, when calculated on the ideal weight of these patients, it becomes 5.4 per cent. Thus, the ratio of weight of intake per kilogram of ideal weight, 5.4 per cent, differs but slightly from the value of 5.1 per cent which was observed for normal people. In this series the intake averaged 4 calories per kilogram and 27 grams per kilogram, giving a food concentration of 0.15 calories per gram. This concentration is about one fifth of that of the normal group and one fourth of the concentration of the obese on the maintenance programs. It is obvious from the low caloric intake that the great bulk of this mass intake was water. These obese people ingested enormous quantities of water.

The urine output averaged 2.04 kilograms per day as compared with 1.75 for normal weight persons and 2.3 kilograms for obese persons on maintenance programs. When calculated in relation to body mass, the output was 1.6 per cent of actual weight and 3.1 per cent of ideal weight. The ratio of urine output per kilogram of ideal weight, 3.1 per cent, corresponds to the value of 2.9 per cent found in normal persons. This relatively normal urine output reflects the high rate of weight loss from insensible perspiration which, of course, would be expected from the known high levels of metabolism of these subjects.

What do these data mean with regard to body maintenance? The fat people on reduction diets showed the expected low ratio of intake and urine output to observed body weight. The huge water intakes have been noted. When the data are recalculated on the basis of ideal weight, the masses of intake and of urine output are found to approximate the ratios found for normal people. It is possible that this excessive water intake, which constitutes the principal factor of the intake and urine output, represents a subconscious attempt of the patient to attain at least the mass components of the sensation of satiety with reference to both intake and urine output during the period of sharply restricted food intake.

Protein Metabolism. In any program involving weight reduction, it is important to determine the nature of the material lost. Many studies of undernutrition have been made, among them the classic study of Benedict.[164] General underfeeding is associated with loss of body protein. However, reduction diets in which adequate protein and sufficient

TABLE 34. METABOLIC DATA IN 4 OBESE PATIENTS LOSING WEIGHT*[19]

			BODY WEIGHT						RATE BODY WT.	INTAKE			URINE			CALORIES		
PT.	AGE	TOTAL WKS.	Ideal	Initial	% Deviation	Final	Total change	WKS. ANAL.	CHANGE GM./DAY	Wt.	per cent	per cent ideal	Wt.	per cent	per cent ideal	Total	per kilo	per kilo ideal
Jac 1	39	19	61.2	171.2	+180	134.0	−37.6	6	−310	2.43	1.6	4.0	1.10	.7	1.8	390	3	6.
Jac 2	40	16	61.2	105.1	+71	76.9	−28.2	4	−140	3.10	3.5	5.1	2.05	2.3	3.3	780	9	13.
Re	58	26	70.9	196.4	+177	146.7	−49.7	7	−310	4.25	2.5	5.9	2.39	1.6	3.4	350	2	5.
Wa	38	6	61.4	134.6	+119	123.3	−11.3	5	−320	3.06	2.4	5.0	1.21	.9	1.9	530	4	9.
Cz	42	17	69.5	150.5	+116	117.0	−33.5	4	−360	4.96	3.7	7.1	3.47	2.6	5.0	590	4	9.
AVE.					+133		−32.1	5	−290	3.56	2.7	5.4	2.04	1.6	3.1	530	4	8.

* Values are in kg. unless specified

(By permission of The American Journal of the Medical Sciences.)

carbohydrate are supplied do not result in protein loss. Keeton and Dickson[176] found that most obese persons on a diet yielding 1375 calories and 90 grams of protein maintained nitrogen balance. Newburgh[85] reported three patients in nitrogen equilibrium on reduction diets of 450 calories.

A study on a series of patients being reduced by dietary measures indicates that these patients were in nitrogen balance on protein intakes of 1 gram per kilogram of ideal weight.[68] This level of intake was carried throughout the study. Two diets were employed. The first, taken for an average of 39 days, provided an average of 336 calories, 59 grams of protein, 10 grams of carbohydrate and 7 grams of fat. The second, eaten for an average of 101 days, afforded 444 calories, 61 grams of protein, 29 grams of carbohydrate and 9 grams of fat. The results are shown in Table 35. In the first diet period, the nitrogen intake fell to 0.9 gram per kilogram because of the monotony of the diet, in spite of efforts to maintain the intake at 1.0 gram. The addition of 20 grams of carbohydrate in the second diet produced a more palatable menu. Although less than 450 calories per day were eaten, this diet was followed for 6 to 9 months.

At the outset of the first period a loss of body nitrogen occurred because of the increased output. The average loss was 2.0 grams per patient day, or 78 grams per patient for the period. Since the four patients lost an average of 15.7 kilograms of body weight in the 39 days, 78 grams of total nitrogen lost for the same period indicates a small but appreciable loss of body nitrogen. That this loss is of little practical significance is suggested by a comparison with the nitrogen loss of the undernourished patients of Benedict as analyzed by Lusk.[177] Benedict's men lost 65 grams of nitrogen and 4.5 kilograms of weight in 3 weeks on a 1375 calorie diet. On the basis of Lusk's figure—1 kilogram of body weight contains 30 grams of nitrogen—those subjects lost 2 kilograms of protein tissue. Expressing these facts in another way, Lusk found that they lost 3.2 per cent of the total body nitrogen, but 6.5 per cent of the total body weight.

In the development of a comparable statement for the obese patients, the ideal weight was employed as indicative of the minimal total nitrogen content of the body. On this basis the 78 gram nitrogen loss in five and a half weeks of this first period corresponds to less than 3.9 per cent of the total body nitrogen. Of equal significance, however, is the fact that this nitrogen loss accompanied a loss of body weight equivalent to 10 per cent of the actual weight and to 24 per cent of the ideal weight.

Throughout the second diet period the patients were practically in nitrogen balance. At this time, however, a new phenomenon appeared in the form of successive periods of loss and gain of nitrogen, but such that at the end of six- to eight-week cycles there was no appreciable alteration of the total nitrogen content of the body. The full significance of this phenomenon is not apparent, although it is conceivably related to the temporary protein storage mechanisms. A comparison of the figures for the whole 101 days of this second period of reducing diet with increased carbohydrate with those of Benedict, as above, shows even more striking results (Table 36). The obese patients, on diets of approximately one third of the caloric value of Benedict's, lost but 10 grams of nitrogen in fourteen and a half weeks. This loss is 0.5 per cent of the estimated total body nitrogen, and is to be contrasted with the 21.6 kilograms of total weight loss or its equivalents, 15 per cent of the actual weight and 32 per cent of the ideal weight. Such ratios suggest that relatively little body protein was lost by these patients in the second period.

The fluctuations in nitrogen balance in the successive dietary periods may be in part explained as dependent upon two factors. With the abrupt institution of the low carbohydrate diet at the outset of Period 1, protein was required for its antiketogenic properties. Upon the adaptation of the body to its new en-

Table 35. Nitrogen Exchange of Obese Patients Undergoing Reduction by Dietary Measures[68]

AVERAGE DAILY NITROGEN EXCHANGE. LOW CARBOHYDRATE PERIOD

CASE	DAYS	WEIGHT					INTAKE					NITROGEN OUTPUT			NITROGEN BALANCE, GM.	NITROGEN PER KG. ACTUAL WEIGHT	NITROGEN PER KG. IDEAL WEIGHT
		Initial, kg.	Ideal, kg.	Excess, per cent	Average for period, kg.	Final, kg.	Calories	Protein, gm.	Carbohydrate, gm.	Fat, gm.	Nitrogen, gm.	Urine, gm.	Feces, gm.	Total, gm.			
1	58	170.0	61.2	178	157.3	148.0	330	53	11	8	8.5	9.4	0.4	9.8	−1.3	0.062	0.16
2	43	113.1	65.9	71	109.0	104.0	380	63	11	9	10.0	13.4	0.6	14.0	−4.0	0.120	0.21
3	0	.....	....	...	.....	.....	...	..	..	..	....	....	....	....	.....	.....	....
4	37	193.2	70.9	172	185.2	178.6	325	65	7	4	10.4	10.6	1.0*	11.6	−1.2	0.062	0.16
5	57	160.6	64.5	149	151.7	143.2	308	53	10	6	8.5	9.1	1.0*	10.1	−1.6	0.065	0.16
Average	39	159.2	65.6	142	150.8	143.5	336	59	10	7	9.4	10.6	0.8	11.4	−2.0	0.077	0.17

AVERAGE DAILY NITROGEN EXCHANGE. INCREASED CARBOHYDRATE PERIOD

CASE	DAYS	WEIGHT					INTAKE					NITROGEN OUTPUT			NITROGEN BALANCE, GM.	NITROGEN PER KG. ACTUAL WEIGHT	NITROGEN PER KG. IDEAL WEIGHT
		Initial, kg.	Ideal, kg.	Excess, per cent	Average for period, kg.	Final, kg.	Calories	Protein, gm.	Carbohydrate, gm.	Fat, gm.	Nitrogen, gm.	Urine, gm.	Feces, gm.	Total, gm.			
1	200	148.0	61.2	141	125.1	105.5	586	59	41	20	9.4	8.7	0.6	9.3	0.1	0.078	0.16
2	8	104.0	65.9	58	103.6	103.2	525	65	50	7	10.3	9.7	1.0	10.7	−0.4	0.100	0.16
3	37	145.0	67.1	116	137.5	132.1	383	64	20	5	10.2	10.0	1.4	11.4	−1.2	0.083	0.17
4	139	178.6	70.9	151	161.5	147.3	371	65	16	5	10.4	8.6	1.0*	9.6	0.8	0.060	0.13
5	121	143.2	64.5	122	131.5	122.9	357	53	20	7	8.4	7.0	1.0*	8.0	0.4	0.060	0.12
Average	101	143.8	65.9	118	131.8	122.2	444	61	29	9	9.7	8.8	1.0	9.8	−0.1	0.072	0.15

* Estimated.

TABLE 36. NITROGEN AND WEIGHT LOSS IN UNDERNOURISHED AND IN REDUCTION PATIENTS[68]

	UNDER-NOURISHED *	PERIOD I	PERIOD II
Duration, weeks	3	5½	14½
Diet, calories	1375.	336.	444.
Daily nitrogen output, gm	11.3	11.4	9.8
Daily nitrogen loss, gm	3.1	2.0	0.1
Total nitrogen loss, gm	65.	78.	10.
Estimated initial body nitrogen content, gm	2037.	1970.	1980.
Reduction body nitrogen, per cent	3.2	3.9	0.5
Initial body weight, kilo	67.9	159.2	143.8
Ideal body weight, kilo	......	65.6	65.9
Body weight loss, kilo	4.5	15.7	21.6
Weight loss (initial body weight), per cent	6.5	9.8	15.0
Weight loss (ideal body weight), per cent	......	24.0	32.0

* Lusk.[177]

ergy supplies, this factor diminished rapidly. Subsequently, the maintenance of balance appears to depend upon the ingestion of adequate nitrogen (Period 2). Secondly, the increase of carbohydrate in the diet from a ratio of 1 gram to each 6 of protein to 1 gram for each 2 of protein permits a more palatable menu and, therefore, the desired protein intake while increasing the caloric value roughly only 100 calories.

In view of the marked loss of weight which took place during this period, the maintenance of the initial level of nitrogen metabolism indicates the absence of physiologic starvation with its concomitant depression of nitrogen metabolism. The numerous investigations of starvation[22] characteristically show prompt depressions of nitrogen level amounting to 30 per cent or more in short experiments and to 50 and 80 per cent in those running from three to four weeks. In general, *it seems that a reduction regimen of the type described can be continued for six to nine months without a serious depression of nitrogen exchange below the initial level.*

Further confirmation of the opinion that little protein is lost from the body during dietary reduction is provided by a study of the creatinine excretion.[77] The creatinine coefficient in obese patients is within normal limits. Five patients lost an average of 21 kilograms of weight. The averages of the creatinine coefficients for the first and last weeks of the diet periods were the same, suggesting that no appreciable alteration in the muscle mass had occurred.

Carbohydrate Metabolism. Weight reduction has a marked effect upon the metabolism of carbohydrate (see page 617). Reduction diets usually have carbohydrate contents of 100 grams or less. The period of low carbohydrate feeding has a specific effect in promoting recovery from the prolonged overtaxing of the carbohydrate handling mechanisms which is frequently associated with the production and maintenance of the obese state. Also the removal of fat, per se, takes a great load from the total metabolism and consequently a proportionate load from the carbohydrate metabolism. The need for insulin is reduced, not only that required for the previously increased carbohydrate metabolism, but also that essential for the high level of fat exchange of the obese state. The glucose handling capacity of these reduced patients becomes normal and remains so provided the excessive carbohydrate feeding and its consequent weight gain are not resumed.

Fat Metabolism. The reduction diets which have been described require that a patient obtain a large percentage of his daily energy needs from his fat stores. Concern has been evinced lest an overloading of the fat metabolizing mechanisms which results from the enforced metabolism of 350 to 400 grams of fat might cause a "sprain" of these mechanisms comparable to that found in the obese in their handling of excessive carbohydrate. Excessive ketone production is ordinarily considered evidence of the incomplete metabolism of fat. The frequent occurrence of acidosis has been noted under conditions in which carbohydrate is unavailable because of low supply (as in starvation), prolonged severe exercise or a metabolic defect (as in diabetes). It is therefore of interest to note any evidence of abnormality of fat metabolism in obese patients on reduction programs. Folin and Denis[97] found that obesity itself was not a predisposing cause of acidosis and that repeated fastings habituated the organism to the complete oxidation of fats. The adaptive power of an organism was further shown by the demonstration of Abderhalden and Lampé[178] that fasting progressively increased the power of a dog's blood to split tributyrin.

Much of the earlier work on ketosis centered around diabetes. In 1921, Woodyatt published his concept of the ketogenic and antiketogenic properties of foods. He considered that a fatty acid glucose (FA/G) ratio of 1.5 or less was necessary for the proper oxidation of fat. Newburgh demonstrated improvement in his diabetic patients, the clearing of ketone bodies from the urine and the gradual drop of blood fats to normal levels with diets having ratios of 2.5. Patients remained free of ketonuria for long periods on 2350 calorie diets containing 230 grams of fat and only 25 grams of carbohydrate. The question was raised whether the FA/G ratio of the diet ingested actually expressed the FA/G ratio of the foods as metabolized. The food mixture supplied to these diabetic patients resembles the metabolic mixtures from which obese patients, while on reducing diets, obtain their energy. Mason[107] found no acidosis in a patient who for 70 days obtained 6.9 per cent of her calories from protein, 2.5 per cent from carbohydrate and 90.6 per cent from fat. When diets low in antiketogenic material are fed, the amounts of acetone bodies excreted are the same whether the fat burned is derived from ingested or stored fat.[179]

Every patient taking a reducing diet which is sufficiently limited to attain results is handling a metabolic mixture of a high ketogenic-antiketogenic ratio, yet obese patients burning 3500 to 4000 calories per day, when placed on reduction diets of 400 to 800 calories, will show no ketonuria. The ketogenic-antiketogenic ratios of the metabolic mixture which provides their energy may reach 3.0 to 3.5. A patient weighing 170 kilograms was given, for 58 days, a diet containing 53 grams protein, 11 grams carbohydrate and 7 grams fat. She lost 22 kilograms, and it was calculated that she lost 8 grams of protein per day. Her average daily weight loss of 380 grams corresponded to a loss of 8 grams of protein and 303 grams of fat. The mixture which she was metabolizing therefore approximated 61 grams protein, 11 grams carbohydrate and 311 grams fat. The FA/G ratio of this mixture is 308/77 or 4.0. This patient had no ketonuria after the first few days, and several plasma CO_2 determinations revealed normal values.

The more recent concepts of fat metabolism described by Stadie[79] minimize the interrelationship of carbohydrate and fat metabolism. The total metabolic load apparently is one of the principal factors involved in fat metabolism and the availability of carbohydrate to meet part of this load merely reduces the demand for fat metabolism. When fat is completely metabolized no ketonuria develops. When the requirement for fat is too great, the fat is not completely metabolized and ketonuria is found. Under ordinary conditions 2.5 grams of fat per kilogram of body weight represents the limiting rate of fat metabolism without ketosis.[79] Obese patients, who ordinarily may metabolize over 3000 calories daily, when placed on reduction diets oxidize large amounts of body fat, frequently 200 to 300 grams per day. Many of these patients weigh 100 or more kilograms and hence burn

2 to 3 grams per kilo of observed weight. Since the observed weights are frequently 50 or more per cent greater than the ideal weights, they burn 3 to 4 grams per kilo of ideal weight. If the average weight for the period of study of the patient previously described is used, 157 kilograms, the 311 grams of fat burned daily correspond to 2.0 grams of fat per kilogram. However, if the ideal weight, which is a better measure of the active tissue of the body, is used, the ratio is 311 grams for 61 kilograms, or 5.0 grams per kilogram. It is probable that, given adequate time, the body can sufficiently adapt itself to a metabolic mixture containing a high percentage of fat to avoid ketonuria at minimal levels of activity. The amount of additional exertion in these patients which would produce ketonuria has not been determined.

In theory, the one way to get an increased fat loss without oxidation is by excessive ketone production. In this instance, fatty acid residues which still have high caloric value are excreted from the body. In consequence, the rate of removal of fat would be considerably greater than the heat production as estimated by indirect calorimetry would indicate. This would be a true fat loss. It is conceivable that the encouragement of this outpouring of intermediate fat products might be of value in accelerating the reduction of obese patients. An additional factor which would make the apparent rate of weight loss even greater in the presence of ketosis is the great loss of water which occurs as a result of the relative tissue acidosis. This latter weight loss would be replaced immediately upon the cessation of ketosis and the restoration of normal water balance. However, the physiologic imbalance which results from continued ketosis would more than offset the slight benefit from increased loss of fat.

Hyperlipemia is most frequent when the body is forced to mobilize its fat reserves for fuel because other material is lacking or cannot be utilized, as in fasting, diabetes and malnutrition.[81] As noted above, patients on dietary reduction programs are forced to burn their reserve fat for their energy needs. Newburgh[85] found that the blood fat levels of obese and normal subjects, when subjected to the same types of restricted diets, showed no significant differences. These observations of blood lipids are in accord with the concept that under the conditions of a reduction program, fat is metabolized efficiently.

Obese patients can utilize fat from their body stores as well as normal persons. In fact, certain evidence suggests that they have a superior capacity for completely metabolizing fat. Such an improved fat metabolism is not unexpected in view of the fact that obese people have had to burn extra fat for years.

Water Metabolism. Daily and periodic fluctuations in the water content of the body are greatly exaggerated by the physiologic adjustments which the body makes to a reduction diet. Variations in the water content of the fat tissue are probably responsible for much of this change in weight. The wide variations in the normal capacity of fat tissue to store water are exaggerated during the rapid removal of fat. The rim of cytoplasm of the distended fat cell can swell up with fluids, and the depleted fat cells can become hydropic.[30] Although ordinary fat tissue has a water content of around 15 per cent, this content can vary from 10 to 70 per cent.[102] A person having 100 pounds of excess fat with a water content of 15 per cent would obviously gain or lose 5 pounds in gross weight if he changed this water fraction to 20 per cent or 10 per cent. The conditions which determine these changes are not clear. It might be expected that much tissue water would be removed by the abrupt introduction of a ketogenic diet. The application of this principle for dehydration in disorders of the central nervous system was in vogue a few years ago. The metabolic mixture supplying the body with energy during a reduction program is highly ketogenic. This factor may be responsible in part for the sharp drop in weight sometimes seen in the first three to five days of dieting but would hardly affect the subsequent water swings in view of the evanescence of the ketosis.

Normal water swings are greatly exaggerated under the metabolic conditions of a reduction diet. Gains or losses of water of 10 to 15 pounds in a few days are seen. Abrupt weight losses in the first few days of dieting are sometimes due to excessive water loss. A patient who weighed 194 Kg. showed the following initial response to diet:

	WEIGHT	WEIGHT LOSS	BELOW PRE-DICTED WEIGHT
Initial	193.9 kilo		
3 days later	189.6 kilo	4.3 kilo	3.0 kilo
7 days later	185.5 kilo	8.4 kilo	4.0 kilo

In the course of the next seven to ten days there was but little change in weight, but the removal of fat plus the retention of water restored the weight to the predicted weight line.

Although water swings may occur at any time in the course of reduction, they tend to become more frequent and of longer duration as the diet period continues. The patient referred to above had a "down swing" in her third month of dieting. She had been holding fairly close to her predicted weight curve for three weeks. In one day she gained 1 kilogram, but in the two succeeding days there was no weight change. On the 4th day she lost 1 kilogram, reaching the prediction line. On the fifth she passed 3950 grams of urine, lost 3.6 kilograms and fell 3 kilograms below the expected weight. Eleven days later her weight was again at the prediction value. In contrast, a marked upswing began in the fourth month of her study.

	WEIGHT	WEIGHT LOSS	ABOVE PREDICTED WEIGHT
Initial	162.5 kilo		
17 days later	161.0 kilo	1.5 kilo	3.0 kilo
2 days later	157.4 kilo	3.6 kilo	.0 kilo

In two days this patient, by diuresis and slight diarrhea, removed the excess water which had been accumulating in her tissues over the preceding two and one half weeks. Comparable experiences have been reported by others. Newburgh[85] described graphically the weight curve of a girl who weighed as much on the fifteenth day of dieting as she did at the start. In the next nine days by diuresis, she lost enough water to bring her observed weight close to her predicted weight.

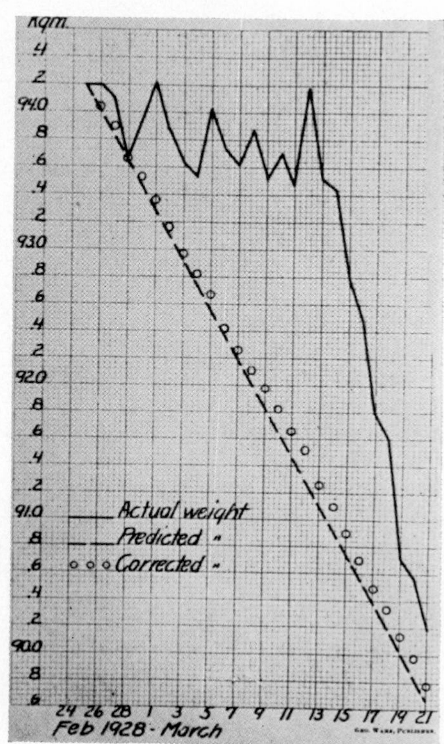

CHART 5. Water retention and loss during reduction diet.[85] (By permission of The American Physiological Society.)

The importance, magnitude and duration of these water swings are frequently unappreciated. A great deal of patient dissatisfaction develops from the discouraging experience of the failure of the scales to show consistent reward for the efforts of dieting. The gain of 3 to 5 pounds which is frequently noted in young girls each month with menstruation is quite upsetting to them. Some patients who are resistant to reduction by dieting are subjects of this water retention problem. If the program is carried on long enough, these water swings correct themselves. It takes a firm control to keep a patient on a diet when

TABLE 37. INFLUENCE OF WEIGHT REDUCTION ON ENERGY EXCHANGE[11]

Case number	BEFORE REDUCTION										AFTER REDUCTION										
		Weight			Surface area			Total basal calories per hour					Weight			Surface area			Total basal calories per hour		
	Age	Ideal	Observed	Excess	Ideal	Observed	Excess	Ideal	Observed	Excess	Duration of reduction	Number of observations	Observed	Excess	Percentile decrease in excess	Observed	Excess	Percentile decrease in excess	Observed	Excess	Percentile decrease in excess
		pounds	*pounds*	*per cent*	*m.*	*m.*	*per cent*	*cal.*	*cal.*	*per cent*	*weeks*	*num-ber*	*pounds*	*per cent*	*per cent*	*m.*	*per cent*	*per cent*	*cal.*	*per cent*	*per cent*
1	50	131	206	57	1.56	1.88	20	55	69	25	20	12	145	10	82	1.63	5	75	53	−3	112
2	29	133	236	77	1.68	2.16	28	62	70	12	17	11	203	52	32	2.01	19	32	61	−1	108
3	32	125	251	100	1.56	2.11	35	57	72	26	20	11	216	72	28	1.95	25	28	69	+21	19
4	41	133	216	62	1.61	1.98	23	58	74	27	19	12	167	25	59	1.79	11	52	62	+7	74
5	28	121	202	66	1.52	1.90	25	56	70	24	9	7	173	43	33	1.77	16	36	60	+6	75
Average 1–5...	36	128	222	72	1.58	2.00	26	58	71	23	17	10	181	40	47	1.83	15	45	61	+6	77

for six weeks the scales show little or no weight change.

Energy Metabolism. BASAL METABOLISM. If an obese patient may have a basal caloric requirement 30 per cent in excess of normal, it becomes important to know what happens to this excess when the weight is reduced. If the basal calories do not change, the reduced person would have a metabolism comparable to that of one with a severe thyrotoxicosis. A study was made of the changes in basal metabolism of five patients who lost from 29 to 61 pounds over periods of nine to twenty weeks.[11] These weight losses correspond to an average reduction of 18 per cent of the initial weight. The true picture of the physiologic status of the patients is shown by restating these data as reductions of excess weight averaging 47 per cent. Five patients, 72 per cent overweight, who had surface areas increased by 26 per cent, used 71 calories per hour, or 23 per cent more than would be normal for them if they had been of normal weight. These patients after prolonged dieting lost 47 per cent of their excess weight, showed a reduction of 45 per cent of their excess surface and a 77 per cent reduction in their excess calories. Before dieting the increase in calories consumed is proportional to surface area increase rather than to weight increase; after dieting, the reduction in excess calories is out of proportion to that of both weight and surface area. The rate of drop in basal calories is more than one and one half times; in one case it was over three times as great as the change in either weight or surface area.

The influence of the diets on the total calories per hour is indicated in Table 38, which shows the average values for all determinations. In general, the drop in basal metabolism was greatest in the first month but continued throughout the reduction period until it approached the normal value for the ideal weight.

In considering these data, one must keep in mind the limits of normal variations in metabolism of an individual. Harris and Benedict[180] showed the extreme variations of metabolism in a given person. Over a period of two years, a 14 per cent variation might be noted. However, in a series of cases studied from one to three months, the coefficients of variation were around 4 per cent of the average metabolism. The variations in metabolism are smaller than the possible errors of the determinations.[109] Variations in the figures for basal metabolic rates in the obese are probably greater than those for normal people because many of the obese probably never attain a truly basal level of metabolism.

The average of these five cases showed a diminution of daily basal energy requirements of 240 calories or 14 per cent of the initial value following weight reduction. Expressed in terms of the physiologic status, these cases, which initially were metabolizing 23 per cent in excess of normal, had reduced to but 6 per cent above ideal metabolism, although they remained some 40 per cent overweight. This was a reduction of 77 per cent of the excess metabolism. These figures, well beyond the limits of normal variations, indicate that weight reduction by dietetic measures does not expose these patients to the danger of thyrotoxicosis. The energy exchange is diminished out of proportion to the reduction in weight. It may be stated that in no instance have the observed calories after reduction been lower than minus 5 per cent of the theoretically normal metabolism. Emphasis is laid upon this point to distinguish between the drop in heat production following reduction of the obese and that of undernutrition.

The physiologic difference between the lowering of basal metabolism of the obese with weight reduction and that associated with starvation is shown by comparing the observations made on the obese with those of Benedict[164] and Lusk[177] in their studies of acute undernutrition, chronic undernutrition and starvation. (In Tables 39 and 40 the data for Squads A and B are taken from Lusk's review of Benedict's work and, in consequence, certain values differ slightly from the original data.)

Comparing the obese with Benedict's subjects, it must be emphasized that his cases were healthy, active males, while our patients were relatively inactive obese females. The men had at the outset normal basal metabolism, but that of the obese was elevated 23 per cent above their normal. In regard to weight loss, none of the undernutrition cases approached the magnitude of loss of the obese. On a percentage basis, the starvation case lost a comparable amount.

Clinically, the response in the two groups differed; the undernourished groups became less ambitious, less energetic and tried to conserve all possible energy. They were depressed, irritable and unstable. In contrast to this, the obese cases showed consistently more initiative, had a desire to do things and felt in all respects better than they had for years.

The physiologic reaction differs in the different groups. The acute undernutrition and the starvation cases dropped 30 per cent of their calories in three weeks. The chronic undernutrition cases dropped 19 per cent in approximately the time in which the obese patients reduced their energy exchange only 14 per cent. This disparity is given more significance when it is recalled that the energy drop in the first three groups represents a lowering of the normal basal metabolic level, whereas the 14 per cent depression in Group IV corresponds rather to a 77 per cent *return of an excessive metabolism toward normal.* This difference is emphasized further by the marked disparity in diets. Group I, on a diet 6 per cent greater than the

TABLE 38. INFLUENCE OF WEIGHT REDUCTION ON CALORIES PER HOUR[11]

CASE NUMBER	OUTSET	FIRST MONTH	SECOND MONTH	THIRD MONTH	FOURTH MONTH	FIFTH MONTH
1	69	65	63	62	53	52
2	70	68	63	64	63	
3	72	75	73	76	72	69
4	74	69	64	65	62	62
5	70	66	58	60		
Average......	71	66	64	65	62	61

TABLE 39. METABOLISM IN VARIOUS FORMS OF UNDERNUTRITION[11]

	TYPE	SUBJECT	BASAL CALORIES BEFORE DIET	BASAL CALORIES IDEAL WEIGHT	DURATION OF DIET	CALORIES OF DIET	WEIGHT LOSS	WEIGHT LOSS	BASAL CALORIES AFTER DIET	PERCENTILE LOSS IN CALORIES
							kgm.	*per cent*	*cal.*	*per cent*
I*	Acute	Squad B	1,745	1,745	3 weeks	1,375 net	4.5	6.5	1,293	32
II*	Starvation	Leveran.	1,432	1,432	3 weeks	0	10.1†	17.0	1,002	30
III*	Chronic	Squad A	1,686	1,686	4 months	1,400 (1,900 net)	5.7 (Held weight)	8.5	1,367	19
IV	Obese		1,700	1,380	17 weeks	620 gross	18.6	18.0	1,460	14

* Essential data from Lusk[177] and DuBois.[109]
† Estimated from graph.

TABLE 40. RATES OF CHANGE OF WEIGHT, SURFACE AND ENERGY[11]

GROUP	TYPE	SUBJECT	I WEIGHT LOSS	II SURFACE LOSS	III BASAL CALORIES LOSS	IV RATIO Calorie loss / Weight loss	V RATIO Calorie loss / Surface loss
			per cent	*per cent*	*per cent*		
I	Acute	Squad B	6.5	<1.0	32.0	4.9	32.0+
II	Starvation	Leveran.	17.0	5.0	30.0	1.7	6.0
III	Chronic	Squad A	8.5	3.3	19.0	2.2	5.9
IV	Obese		18.0	8.5	14.0	0.77	1.6

basal needs, had a depression of 32 per cent in calories and a small loss of weight. Group II, at the time of the lowest metabolism, had a 30 per cent drop in calories, while the weight loss was about one half that of the obese patients. Group III, after the initial weight loss, was holding weight on a diet 42 per cent above the basal needs, while the drop in calories was only 19 per cent of the initial value. In the obese patients, however, on a diet 57 per cent less than the basal needs, the initial metabolism was depressed only 14 per cent, and the patients lost weight consistently.

The reaction in the obese to reduction by diet differs markedly from that in a patient of normal weight to undernutrition. In the latter, there is a severe depression of energy exchange, even though he started at normal levels. In the obese, the depression of energy exchange is very much less in proportion to the limitation of the diet and the weight loss and is only a return toward normal, never beyond, from an initially elevated rate. These observations, and the clinical differences in the two groups of cases, indicate that the obese patients were not physiologically undernourished. When on a limited diet—with sufficient protein—they do not seem to require the protective depression of the energy exchange which Lusk observed in the undernourished. A patient with a lesser degree of obesity, and therefore a smaller initial elevation of the basal metabolism, will have a smaller numerical drop in basal metabolism with reduction of weight in order to attain the level proper for his normal weight.[11,172]

TOTAL METABOLISM. The effect of weight reduction on the total metabolism is the sum of its effects on the four principal components. The excessive basal metabolism reduces to normal levels.

The heat production from the specific dynamic action of food would be somewhat less in view of the reduced food intake. The work fraction would be reduced in proportion to the increase in personal efficiency. The effect on the nonwork fraction would be the balance of many variables. The energy reduction due to increased muscular efficiency might be offset by the greater activities and greater mobility in the reduced state. Since alterations in this fraction can produce great changes in daily energy requirements, it is perhaps correct to state that the maintenance of a good normal level of energy output, which will militate against a recurrence of obesity, will depend to a large extent upon the patient's ability to develop and maintain suitable avocations.

Summary of the Results of Reduction. The results of reducing measures show a loss of weight, the rate of which is determined by the caloric deficit and the total amount by the duration of the program. The benefits of fat loss are reflected in an improved mortality and decreased morbidity. The patient becomes less vulnerable to his environment, with consequent improvement in his outlook on life. The symptoms which are related to obesity, per se, are considerably relieved. Since much of the disability in obesity is due to the associated illnesses, recovery is markedly influenced by their nature and severity. Just as there were physiologic adaptations of the body to meet the demands of the obese state, there are re-adaptations to the altered weight status. The body readjusts to the type of metabolic mixture which supplies its energy by quantitative changes in metabolism, especially in carbohydrate, fat, water and basal metabolism. There are no qualitative changes in metabolism associated with obesity or with weight reduction.

ROLE OF THE PHYSICIAN

In the treatment of obesity, the role of the physician is somewhat different than in most illnesses. Patients have become accustomed in this day of medical miracles to the response to specific vitamins, hormones and antibiotics. The pattern of diagnosis, prescription and recovery is so firmly implanted that it is expected of all adequate physicians for all problems. The corollary, which is most unfortunate for the obese, is that the physician does everything for the patient; the patient does nothing for himself. The obese patient is hardly to be blamed if he searches for a panacea, for a simple way out of his difficulty. When he finally becomes aware of his need for reduction, he tries the hundred easy methods before he admits the need for professional advice. The physician can help his patient to help himself by telling him about his problem, by outlining a program which he can follow and by supplying moral support during the difficult correction period.

Education. Patients must learn that obese people are ordinary everyday persons. They may be tall or short, young, or old, male or female. They may or may not have associated diseases or disorders. The one thing they have in common is that for years they have eaten more food than they have burned up. The facts are that this extra weight is largely fat which represents about 4000 calories per pound and that this fat disappears only in relation to a caloric deficit.

The environmental factors which helped to produce the obesity should be appreciated. Patients need to know the menace of obesity. The "It can't happen to me" philosophy is quite human. The absence of acutely distressing symptoms makes it hard to impress a patient with possible disabilities ten years hence in contrast to present pleasures. He should be told that obesity promotes physiologic imbalances, that it aggravates disease states and that it accelerates the rate of degeneration of the body and the development of old age.

The patient must learn about foods and food values. Many obese people sincerely believe that they are not large eaters. They confuse bulk with caloric value. They do not appreciate that the omission of breakfast or lunch does not necessarily insure that the total daily intake is not excessive, although it sometimes does reduce the amount which otherwise might have been eaten. Hunger is a physiologic guide to start eating. It has little to do with the total daily food intake. It is easily relieved by comparatively small quantities of food and is controlled by the establishment of habit patterns of three or four well spaced meals. Unfortunately, the foods often preferred by the obese are those of high caloric but low satiety value.

The "fun of eating" must be curtailed, and sharply. There is no use in denying the asceticism necessary during the dietary correction of obesity. The aim of therapy is the re-establishment of normal pleasure values. The patient is not to be denied forever the pleasures of eating. He is to re-educate himself with regard to the relationship of the pleasures of eating to the total of pleasures available to a person in this world.

Program Planning. The physician has the important responsibility of planning with the individual patient a reduction program which is possible and practicable. One of the best protections against food fads is a sympathetic analysis of the total problem confronting the patient. Factors such as where he gets his food, the cost of meat, eggs and milk, the social requirements of his business with regard to entertainment, the type of personality, the type of work, the family cooperation and many comparable factors must be considered as well as items of total weight to be lost, water shifts, protein shifts and complicating or coexisting medical problems. The alterations of eating habits, the proper amount of exercise and the possible changes in work and social activities should be discussed. Fundamentally, the most important feature is a proper diet.

For many patients who live normal lives or who have relatively mild obesity a few simple rules suffice. Persons with careless eating habits are taught to become calorie- and protein-conscious, to eat regular meals, to eat protein at every meal, to use fruit for desserts. If they can avoid or minimize the "sneaky foods," the extra hard roll with butter, the side dish of spaghetti, the hors d'oeuvres, the rich desserts, the cocktails and the wine, the problem is solved for many. The majority of patients need a formal diet. It may be a liberal four-group type or a strictly weighed diet.

It should be recognized that some people are not suitable candidates for reduction programs, just as some people are not suitable candidates for thyroidectomy or some other therapeutic procedure. Those patients should not be treated.

Moral Support. Patient and physician alike appreciate that a major alteration in the habit patterns of years requires an unpleasant period of readjustment. Patients have many excuses and explanations as to why it is difficult for them to reduce. After the usual protestations that obesity in his case was the result of a conspiracy against an innocent bystander, the patient is afraid of hunger, of weakness, of ridicule, etc. How to give moral support to these well-intentioned, vacillating persons is a serious matter. If the physician recognizes the motive of the patient in seeking help at this particular time—greed, vanity, fear, etc.—he can often employ this knowledge advantageously. However, it should be recognized by both physician and patient that the responsibility for the success of a reduction program rests with the patient. In much of modern medicine the physician is the actor, the patient the spectator. This passive role is not possible for the obese patient. The physician, no matter how sympathetic, cannot remove one pound of fat from his patient. Nor can he adopt the role of the policeman.

Ultimately, the success of a reduction program depends upon character. It makes little difference whether a weak character is the result of a poor inheritance or poor environment. As with a man who has lost a leg, if it is not there, it is not there. Much ingenuity may be exerted to support and assist an unfortunate disability, but nothing is gained by denying its existence. Such recognition does not at all imply a censorious attitude toward the unfortunate victim. Failures in reduction will occur, but successes are common. A great many pounds of fat have been removed from a great many cooperative patients, and large numbers of these persons have re-established self-mastery with incalculable benefits to their health and happiness.

Obesity should be recognized as a disorder of the state of nutrition of human beings because they are human beings. Successful treatment depends upon education, motivation and character. What will the patient do to help himself? "If people decline to be privy to their own salvation, it is not for us to lure them thither by trickster methods."[6]

References

1. Howard, C. P. and Mills, E. S.: In The Oxford Medicine. New York, Oxford University Press, 1941, vol. 4.
2. Cullen: Quoted by Tanner (Ref. 4).
3. Forsythe, J. S.: Domestic Medicine, London, 1826.
4. Tanner, T. H.: Practice of Medicine. 4th American Ed. Philadelphia, Lindsay and Blakiston, 1867.
5. Duckworth, D.: In Allbutt, T. C.: System of Medicine. New York, The Macmillan Company, 1897, vol. 5.
6. Williams, L.: Obesity. London, Oxford University Press, 1926.
7. Jolliffe, N.: J.A.M.A., *161:*1633, 1956.
8. Gelvin, E. P., McGavach, T. H. and Kenigsberg, S.: Am. J. Digest. Dis., *20:*200, 1953.
9. Robinson, S. C. and Brucer, M.: Am. J. M. Sc., *199:*819, 1940.
10. Mayer, J. and Stare, F. J.: J. Am. Dietet. A., *29:*340, 1953.
11. Strang, J. M. and Evans, F. A.: J. Clin. Invest., *6:*277, 1928.
12. Armstrong, D. B., Dublin, L. I., Wheatley, G. M. and Marks, H. H.: J.A.M.A., *147:*1007, 1951.
13. Keys, A. and Brozek, J.: Physiol. Rev., *33:*245, 1953.
14. Keys, A.: In Overeating, Overweight and Obesity. New York, National Vitamin Foundation, 1953, p. 13.
15. Bruch, H.: Psychosom. Med., *14:*337, 1952.
16. Preble, W. E.: Boston Med. & Surg. J., *188:*617, 1923.
17. Hunt, E. E., Pechos, P. S. and Fry, P. C.: Ref. 14, 73.
18. Dublin, L. I. and Lotka, A. J.: Length of Life, New York, Ronald Press, 1936.
19. Strang, J. M.: Am. J. M. Sc., *221:*537, 1951.
20. Buchanan, J. M. and Hastings, A. B.: Physiol. Rev., *26:*120, 1946.
21. Clarke, H. T.: quoted by Buchanan and Hastings (Ref. 20).
22. Lusk, G.: Science of Nutrition, 4th ed. Philadelphia, W. B. Saunders Company, 1928.
23. Levitt, M. F. and Gaudino, M.: Am. J. Med., *9:*208, 1950.
24. Dublin, L. I.: Am. J. Pub. Health, *43:*993, 1953.
25. Barr, D. P.: Ref. 14, 90.
26. Dublin, L. I. and Marks, H. H.: Mortality of Women According to Build. Proceedings of the Association of Life Insurance Directors of America, *25:*203, 1939.
27. Breslaw, L.: Am. J. Pub. Health, *42:*1116, 1952.
28. Zelman, S.: Arch. Int. Med., *90:*141, 1952.
29. Hartman, H. R. and Ghrist, D. A.: Quoted by Wood and Cash (Ref. 32).
30. Evans, F. A.: In Duncan, G. G. (editor): Diseases of Metabolism. 3rd ed. Philadelphia, W. B. Saunders Company, 1952.
31. Palmer, R. S.: Quoted by Wood and Cash (Ref. 32).
32. Wood, J. E. and Cash, J. R.: Ann. Int. Med., *13:*81, 1939.
33. Robinson, S. C., Brucer, M. and Mass, J.: J. Lab. & Clin. Med., *25:*807, 1940.
34. Master, A. M. and Jaffe, H. L.: J.A.M.A., *153:*1499, 1953.
35. Strang, J. M.: New England J. Med., *200:*167, 1929.
36. Martin, L.: Lancet, *263:*1050, 1952.
37. Short, J. J.: Quoted by Armstrong (Ref. 12).
38. Wilens, S. L.: Arch. Int. Med., *79:*129, 1947.
39. Peters, J. P. and Man, E. B.: J. Clin. Invest., *22:*707, 1943.
40. Moore, N. S., Young, C. M. and Maynard, L. A.: Am. J. Med., *17:*348, 1954.
41. Walker, W. J., Lowry, E. Y., Love, D. E., Mann, G. V., Levine, S. A. and Stare, F. J.: Am. J. Med., *14:*654, 1953.
42. Turner, K. B. and Sterner, A.: J. Clin. Invest., *18:*45, 1939.
43. Hatch, F. T., Abell, L. L. and Kendall, F. E.: Am. J. Med., *19:*48, 1955.
44. Nicholson, W. M.: Am. J. Med. Sc., *211:*443, 1946.
45. Greene, J. A.: Quoted by Nicholson (Ref. 44).
46. Conn, J. W.: Physiol. Rev., *24:*31, 1944.
47. Rogers, J. and Mitchell, G. W.: New England J. Med., *247:*53, 1952.
48. Given, W. P., Gause, R. W. and Douglas, R. G.: New England J. Med., *243:*357, 1950.
49. Joslin, E. P.: Quoted by Howard and Mills (Ref. 1).

50. John, H. J.: Am. J. Med. Sc., *173:*184, 1927.
51. Newburgh, L. H. and Conn, J. W.: J.A.M.A., *112:*7, 1939.
52. Beeler, C. and Fitz, R.: Arch. Int. Med., *28:*804, 1921.
53. Ogilvie, R. F.: Quart. J. Med., *28:*345, 1935.
54. Hamburger, W. W.: M. Clin. North America, *35:*483, 1951.
55. Parson, W. and Crispell, K. R.: M. Clin. North America, *36:*385, 1952.
56. Brozin, H. W.: Ref. 14, 52.
57. Darling, C. D. and Summerskill, J.: J. Am. Dietet. A., *29:*1204, 1953.
58. Stunkard, A. J., Grace, W. J. and Wolff, H. G.: Am. J. Med., *19:*78, 1955.
59. Bruch, H.: Am. J. Dis. Child., *59:*739, 1940.
60. Wertheimer, E. and Shapiro, B.: Physiol. Rev., *28:*451, 1948.
61. Van Itallie, T. B.: Am. J. Med., *19:* 110, 1955.
62. Anderson, W. A. D.: Pathology. 2nd Ed. St. Louis, C. V. Mosby Company, 1953.
63. Anders, J. M.: Am. J. M. Sc., *121:*421, 1901.
64. Colwell, A. R.: Ann. Int. Med., *41:*963, 1954.
65. Benedict, F. G. and Root, H. F.: Arch. Int. Med., *38:*1, 1926.
66. Johnston, M. W. and Newburgh, L. H.: J. Clin. Invest., *21:*357, 1942.
67. Richter, P. F.: Quoted by Howard and Mills (Ref. 1).
68. Strang, J. M., McClugage, H. B. and Evans, F. A.: Am. J. M. Sc., *181:* 336, 1931.
69. Denis, W. and Borgstrom, P.: J. Biol. Chem., *61:*109, 1924.
70. Beard, H.: Am. J. Physiol., *82:*577, 1927.
71. Folin, O.: Am. J. Physiol., *13:*66, 1905.
72. Shaffer, P. A.: Am. J. Physiol., *23:*1, 1908.
73. Tracy, M. and Clark, E. E.: J. Biol. Chem., *19:*115, 1914.
74. Hodgson, P. and Lewis, H. B.: Am. J. Physiol., *87:*228, 1928.
75. Myers, V. C. and Fine, M. S.: J. Biol. Chem., *14:*9, 1913.
76. Hunter, A.: Creatinine and Creatine. New York, Longmans, Green & Co., 1928.
77. McClugage, H. B., Booth, G. and Evans, F. A.: Am. J. M. Sc., *181:*349, 1931.
78. Gurin, S.: Ref. 14, 1.
79. Stadie, W. C.: Physiol. Rev., *25:*395, 1945.
80. Burr, G. O. and Barnes, R. H.: Physiol. Rev., *23:*256, 1943.
81. Peters, J. P. and Van Slyke, D. D.: Quantitative Clinical Chemistry. 2nd ed. Baltimore, Williams & Wilkins Company, 1946.
82. Lyon, J. B., Dowling, M. T. and Fenton, P. F.: J. Nutrition, *51:*65, 1953.
83. Von Bergmann: Quoted by Newburgh (Ref. 85).
84. Hetenyi, C. T.: Quoted by Newburgh (Ref. 85).
85. Newburgh, L. H.: Physiol. Rev., *24:*18, 1944.
86. Bloch, M.: Quoted by Newburgh (Ref. 85).
87. Pennington, A. W.: Ref. 14, 123.
88. Pennington, A. W.: J. Clin. Nutrition, *1:*100, 1952.
89. Werner, S. C.: New England J. Med., *252:*661, 1955.
90. Hegsted, D. M.: Ref. 14, 135.
91. Turner, R. H.: Am. J. Med., *12:*379, 1952.
92. Best, C. H. and Campbell, J.: Quoted by Evans (Ref. 30).
93. Frazer, A. C.: Physiol. Rev., *26:*103, 1946.
94. Strang, J. M. and McClugage, H. B.: Am. J. M. Sc., *182:*49, 1931.
95. Brobeck, J. R.: Physiol. Rev., *26:*541, 1946.
96. McKay, E. M. and Sherrell, J. W.: Endocrinology, *21:*677, 1937.
97. Folin, O. and Denis, W.: J. Biol. Chem., *21:*183, 1915.
98. Deuel, H. J., Jr., and Gulich, M.: J. Biol. Chem., *96:*25, 1932.
99. Mayer, J., Russell, R. E., Bates, M. W. and Dickie, M. M.: Metabolism, *2:*9, 1953.
100. Mayer, J.: Physiol. Rev., *33:*472, 1953.
101. Labbé, M. and Stevenin, H.: Compt. rend. Soc. de biol., *88:*9, 1923.
102. Lauter, S.: Klin. Wchnschr., *5:*1696, 1926.
103. Strang, J. M., McClugage, H. B. and Brownlee, M. A.: Arch. Int. Med., *55:* 958, 1935.
104. Nenenschwander-Lemmer, N.: Quoted by Newburgh (Ref. 85).
105. Means, J. H.: Arch. Int. Med., *17:*704, 1916.
106. Strouse, S. and Wang, C. C.: Arch. Int. Med., *34:*275, 1924.
107. Mason, E. H.: J. Clin. Invest., *4:*93, 1927.
108. Hagedorn, J. C., Holten, C. and Johansen, A. H.: Arch. Int. Med., *40:*30, 1927.
109. DuBois, E. F.: Basal Metabolism in Health and Disease. Philadelphia, Lea & Febiger, 1927.
110. Stengel, A.: Textbook of Pathology, 5th ed. Philadelphia, W. B. Saunders Company, 1907.
111. Von Noorden, C.: Quoted by DuBois (Ref. 109).
112. Benedict, F. G. and Carpenter, T. M.: Food Ingestion and Energy Transformation. Carnegie Institute of Washington, Pub. No. 261, 1918.
113. Bauman, L.: J.A.M.A., *90:*22, 1928.
114. Mason, E. H.: Northwest Med., *26:*143, 1927.

115. Plaut, R.: Deutsche Arch. f. klin. Med., *139:*285, 1922.
116. Wang, C. C., Strouse, S. and Saunders, A. D.: Arch. Int. Med., *34:*573, 1924.
117. Mason, E. H., Hill, E. and Charlton, D.: J. Clin. Invest., *4:*353, 1927.
118. Aub, J. C. and DuBois, E. F.: Arch. Int. Med., *19:*840, 1917.
119. Gibbons, R.: Am. J. Physiol., *70:*26, 1924.
120. Appel, K. E. and Farr, C. B.: J. Nerv. & Ment. Dis., *70:*43, 1929.
121. Foster, G. L. and Smith, P. E.: J.A.M.A., *87:*2151, 1926.
122. Aub, J. C. and Means, J. H.: Arch. Int. Med., *28:*173, 1921.
123. DuBois, E. F.: Arch. Int. Med., *17:*915, 1916.
124. Means, J. H.: J. Exper. Med., *32:*120, 1915.
125. Kraus, E. and Rettig, R.: Deutsche Arch. f. klin. Med., *163:*337, 1929.
126. Lauter, S.: Deutsche Arch. f. klin. Med., *150:*315, 1926.
127. Johnston, M. W.: Quoted by Newburgh (Ref. 85).
128. Grafe, E.: Quoted by Newburgh (Ref. 85).
129. Wiley, F. H. and Newburgh, L. H.: Quoted by Newburgh (Ref. 85).
130. Passmore, R. and Durnin, J. V. G. A.: Physiol. Rev., *35:*801, 1955.
131. Taggart, J. V.: Am. J. Med., *19:*110, 1955.
132. Owen, J. A., Falk, L. J., Crispell, K. R. and Parson, W.: Am. J. Med., *14:*521, 1953.
133. Kisch, E. H.: Quoted by Howard and Mills (Ref. 1).
134. Kirlander, A. B.: J. Am. Dietet. A., *29:* 337, 1953.
135. Bonner, D. M.: Am. J. Med., *8:*90, 1950.
136. McLester, J. S.: Nutrition and Diet in Health and Disease. 5th ed. Philadelphia, W. B. Saunders Company, 1949.
137. Dunlop, D. M. and Murray Lyon, R. M.: Quoted by Howard and Mills (Ref. 1).
138. Strang, J. M.: Pennsylvania M. J., *38:* 493, 1935.
139. Brobeck, J. R.: In Wohl, M. G. and Goodhart, R. S. (editors): Modern Nutrition in Health and Disease. Philadelphia, Lea & Febiger, 1955.
140. Booth, G. and Strang, J. M.: Arch. Int. Med., *57:*533, 1936.
141. Bazett, H. C.: Physiol. Rev., *7:*531, 1927.
142. Stead, E. A.: Am. J. Med., *9:*425, 1950.
143. Adolph, E. F.: Quoted by Brobeck (Ref. 139).
144. Wells, H. G.: J.A.M.A., *114:*2177, 2284, 1940.
145. Anaud, B. K. and Brobeck, J. R.: Proc. Soc. Exper. Biol. & Med., *77:*323, 1951.
146. Bruch, H.: Am. J. Med., *19:*110, 1955.
147. Kantor, S.: Ref. 14, 70.
148. Freed, S. C.: Quoted by Brozin (Ref. 56).
149. Harvey, H. I. and Simmons, W. D.: Am. J. M. Sc., *225:*623, 1953.
150. Mitchell, W.: Quoted by Duckworth (Ref. 5).
151. Moritz, F.: Quoted by Lusk (Ref. 22).
152. Beaudain, R. and Mayer, J.: J. Am. Dietet. A., *29:*29, 1953.
153. Trulson, M. F.: Ref. 14, 87.
154. Strang, J. M., McClugage, H. B. and Evans, F. A.: Am. J. M. Sc., *179:* 687, 1930.
155. Strang, J. M. and Evans, F. A.: J.A.M.A., *104:*1957, 1935.
156. Smith, Kline and French Laboratories: Caloric Values of Common "Snack" Foods. Philadelphia, 1957.
157. Evans, F. A. and Strang, J. M.: Am. J. M. Sc., *177:*339, 1929.
158. Strang, J. M.: In Conn, H. F. (editor): Current Therapy. Philadelphia, W. B. Saunders Company, 1953, p. 353.
159. Werner, S. C.: Am. J. Med., *19:*110, 1955.
160. Kotkov, B.: Psychosom. Med., *15:*243, 1953.
161. Mayer, J. and Stare, F. J.: J. Am. Dietet. A., *29:*340, 1953.
162. Loeb, R.: Am. J. Med., *19:*110, 1955.
163. Short, J. J.: Quoted by Evans (Ref. 30).
164. Benedict, F. G., Miles, W. R., Roth, P. and Smith, H. M.: Carnegie Institute of Washington, Pub. No. 280, 1919.
165. Dublin, L. I.: Ref. 14, 106.
166. Rutstein, D. D.: Ref. 14, 119.
167. Pennington, A. W.: Indust. Med., *18:* 259, 1949.
168. Brozek, J.: J. Clin. Nutrition, *12:*118, 1953.
169. Sprague, H. B.: Ref. 14, 117.
170. Walker, W. J.: Ann. Int. Med., *39:*705, 1953.
171. Young, C. M., Ringler, S. and Greer, B. J.: J. Am. Dietet. A., *29:*890, 1953.
172. Mitchell, G. W. and Rogers, J.: New England J. Med., *249:*835, 1953.
173. Kinney, J. R.: Ann. Int. Med., *40:*1024, 1954.
174. Newburgh, L. H.: Ann. Int. Med., *17:* 935, 1942.
175. Ford, M. J.: Am. J. Pub. Health, *43:* 997, 1953.
176. Keeton, R. W. and Dickson, D.: Quoted by Newburgh (Ref. 85).
177. Lusk, G.: Physiol. Rev., *1:*523, 1921.
178. Abderhalden, E. and Lampé, A. E.: Quoted by Lusk (Ref. 22).
179. Hubbard, R. S.: Quoted by Evans (Ref. 30).
180. Harris, J. A. and Benedict, F. G.: J. Biol. Chem., *46:*257, 1921.
181. MacCallum, W. G.: Textbook of Pathology. 2nd ed. Philadelphia, W. B. Saunders Company, 1921.

CHAPTER 9 *By* RICHARD WAGNER, M.D.

Glycogen Storage Disease and Idiopathic Galactosemia

GLYCOGEN STORAGE DISEASE

(Glycogenosis, von Gierke's hepatonephromegalia glycogenica)

Introduction and Definition. Glycogen storage disease is an inborn and probably familial metabolic error, involving some of the enzymes which catalyze glycogen synthesis and degradation. It has been observed in identical twins. In other cases diabetes mellitus occurs in the ascendency. It was first recognized as a disease entity in childhood by Wagner and Parnas[1] in 1921. The low fasting blood sugar and the negative epinephrine effect were interpreted to be the result of a defect in mobilizable glycogen. Numerous similar cases were described afterwards, and in 1929 von Gierke[2] reported the autopsy findings of a typical case and Schönheimer[3] pointed out the possible underlying enzymatic defect. Thannhauser et al.[4] were the first to call attention to a lowered alkaline phosphatase level in the liver, but not until the investigations of Cori, Cori and co-workers[5] was the enzymatic defect and the glycogen structure in the disease fully understood and a classification in four different subgroups attempted. The most common form is the hepatonephromegalic type in which glucose 6-phosphatase, essential for the maintenance of the normal blood sugar level, is deficient. The structure of the liver glycogen in these cases is normal. This has been demonstrated on liver biopsy and autopsy specimens.

The Enzymatic Defect. Glucose enters the liver as a phosphorylated molecule. Depending upon the demand, it may be synthesized into glycogen or broken down to a great number of intermediates and oxidized to carbon dioxide and water. The complete enzymatic synthesis of glycogen from glucose is now well understood. In Figure 1 a scheme of glycogen synthesis and degradation and of the enzymes catalyzing the individual steps can be seen.

The discovery of the enzymes participating in glycogen metabolism has been contributory to the understanding of glycogen structure. Three enzymes are required for glycogen synthesis and degradation:

1. *Phosphorylase,* which is essential for synthesis as well as breakdown. It makes or breaks only the α-1,4 linkages of the molecule. The other two auxiliary enzymes work only in one direction.

2. *Amylo-1,6-glucosidase,* which is active only in glycogen degradation by breaking the glucose residue in the α-1,6 linkages; this occurs only after phosphorylase has exposed this molecule by breaking off the distal molecules in α-1,4 linkage.

3. *Amylo-(1,4 $\rightarrow$ 1,6)-transglucosidase,* which is active only in synthesis and leads to ramification of the molecule.

TABLE 1. THE FOUR TYPES OF GLYCOGEN STORAGE DISEASE

Enzyme, deficient	Organ involved	Glycogen structure
1. Glucose 6-phosphatase	Liver, kidney	Normal
2. Unknown	Generalized	Normal
3. Amylo-1,6-glucosidase	Liver, muscle	Abnormal; very short outer chains
4 Amylo-(1,4 → 1,6)-trans-glucosidase	Liver, probably generalized	Abnormal; long inner and outer chains

(Cf. Cori, G. T.: Oesterr. Ztschr. Kinderh. u. Kinderfürsorge, *10*:38, 1954.)

From the studies of Cori, Cori et al.[5] it can be concluded that glycogen storage disease is not a uniform disease. Four types were distinguished in regard to the enzymatic deficiency, the organ involved and the structure of glycogen (Table 1).

In *type I* the disease is restricted to liver and kidney. The enzyme glucose 6-phosphatase which is essential for the formation of blood glucose from glucose 6-phosphate occurs only in these two organs. It is also indispensable for the formation of glucose from glycerol, lactic acid, pyruvic acid and amino acids. In severe cases of the hepatonephromegalic type, the Coris[5] found that only 2 to 10 per cent of the normal activity of the enzyme glucose 6-phosphatase is present in liver and kidney. This explains the accumulation of glycogen in these two organs and some of the other manifestations of the disease, such as the lack of response of the blood sugar to epinephrine. Although glycogen degradation in the liver is inhibited, synthesis is not impaired. One of the sequelae of this defect is fat infiltration in the liver. The kidney has normally a low glycogen content (approximately 0.1 per cent). Synthesis and degradation are well regulated. Glycogen does not accumulate. In glycogen storage disease 7.5 per cent was found in the cortex of the kidney. Glucose 6-phosphatase is absent in heart and skeletal muscle under normal conditions; these tissues do not directly participate in the formation of blood sugar. Glycogen does not accumulate here in type I. The structure of glycogen is normal in the hepatonephromegalic type. In the milder cases, when the patient survives beyond infancy the activity of glucose 6-phosphatase is reduced to a lesser extent.

Clinical Manifestations. In most instances the patient is first seen by the

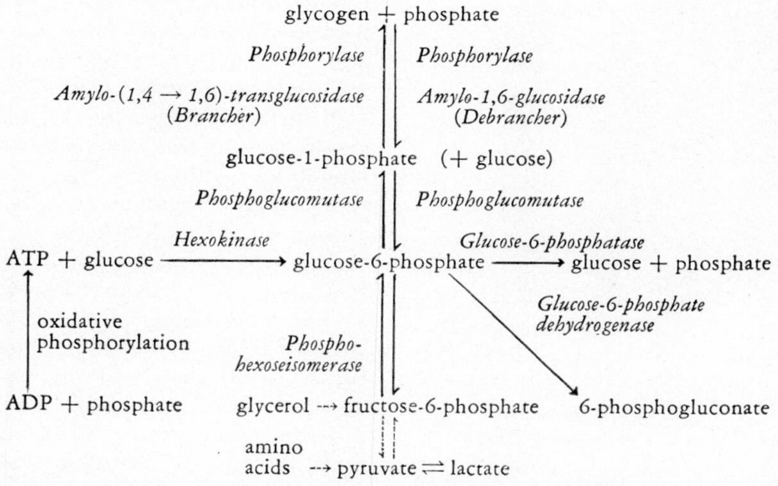

FIG. 1. Enzyme reactions in glycogen synthesis and degradation in the liver. (From Cori, G. T.: The Harvey Lectures, Series *48*:145, 1952–3.)

physician during the neonatal period or in infancy because of an enormously enlarged abdomen and failure to do well. On palpation, hepatomegaly is readily recognized as the cause. The sharp liver edge can be felt below the umbilicus. The organ can be enlarged to such a degree that the right lobe may reach the anterior upper iliac spine. The surface of the liver is smooth and the consistency moderately firm. The left lobe, separated from the right by a deep notch, occupies the entire left hypochondrium and can be mistaken for the spleen. However, the spleen is not enlarged, in contrast to other conditions with hepatomegaly. Jaundice, ascites or other signs of portal hypertension are missing.

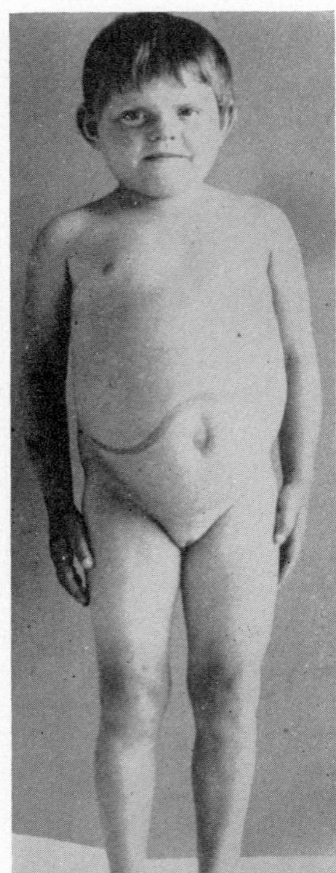

FIG. 2. E. S., 10 years, 40¾ inches, weight 45 lbs. (From Wagner, R., and Parnas, J. K.: Ztschr. f.d. ges. exper. Med., *25*:361, 1921. Julius Springer, Berlin.)

The physical appearance of the patient is characteristic. The face is flabby; there is accumulation of fat on the face, at the nape of the neck, around the shoulders, above the hips and at the mons pubis, in contrast to the rather lean buttocks and extremities. These children are awkward and clumsy. The gait is impaired, resembling that of a pregnant woman. In those who live more than three or four years, a baby-like expression is particularly impressive (Fig. 2). To a certain degree these children resemble cases of adiposogenital dystrophy. The tendency to obesity may be explained by the conversion of unstored sugar into fat. Growth and development in the first year of life is markedly retarded and frequently disturbed by attacks of acidosis. The onset of walking is delayed. The musculature is poorly developed and of diminished tone.

Older children are dwarfish and retarded in skeletal maturation. The body proportions remain at an infantile level. In some cases an eruptive xanthomatosis occurs, with localization of the xanthomatous lesions on the extensor surface of the joints, particularly the elbow and knee joints.

The development of genital and extragenital sexual characteristics is delayed. Pelvis, breasts and external genitalia remain infantile; the gonads do not mature. Pubic and axillary hair is missing. As to the interpretation of the dwarfism and the delayed skeletal differentiation, it is not known whether the increased gluconeogenesis from protein and a negative nitrogen balance are responsible or whether it is a genetic type of dwarfism, comparable to that in other syndromes with multiple congenital anomalies. Although small stature and retarded development are also occasionally observed in cirrhosis of the liver, they are by no means a constant finding, and they differ from the dwarfism in glycogen storage disease in many respects. The anomalous carbohydrate function of the liver in this disease seems to elicit a specific disturbance of growth, ossification and body proportions. A negative nitrogen balance, mentioned before, and an accumulation in the peripheral blood of sugar phosphates which are unable to penetrate the cell membrane might be contributory factors. Although gross mental retardation is not one of the characteristics of glycogen storage disease, the patients usually do not reach higher levels of intelligence.

A rare symptom is a bleeding tendency due to lowered prothrombin activity. The patients are rather susceptible to respiratory infections, which have usually been the immediate cause of death. With the advent of antibiotic therapy, the prognosis has improved, particularly in the age group beyond infancy.

Laboratory Findings. Fasting hypoglycemia represents the most characteristic finding. Although variation of the blood sugar from almost zero to 60 mg. per 100 ml. is encountered, fasting values above 60 mg. per 100 ml. are rarely seen. Ketonuria is common, particularly under fasting conditions and during acute infections. Both acetone and diacetic acid reactions in the urine are positive; even β-oxybutyric acid can be excreted in large amounts. Lipemia may be ten times the normal total blood lipid; hypercholesterolemia with normal partition between free cholesterol and cholesterol esters is frequent, but not a constant finding. An abnormal epinephrine effect, following subcutaneous injection of 0.3 to 0.5 cc. of epinephrine, is characterized by absence of elevation of the blood sugar, a marked increase of ketosis and only a small elevation of blood lactic acid.

Blood glycogen is distinctly higher than in normal children.[6] Values of 30 to 40 mg. per 100 ml. of blood are not unusual. Most of the blood glycogen accumulates in the leukocytes, as shown by Wagner.[7] Values up to 30 to 40 μg. per 1×10^6 leukocytes were observed (normal 3 to 4 μg.). But even the plasma carries considerable amounts of glycogen. The blood sugar curve following ingestion of glucose resembles that of diabetics, with an unusually high rise and a delayed return to the fasting level. At the peak of the curve glycosuria may occur. Following fructose or galactose ingestion there is no rise in the blood sugar level; each of these sugars is rapidly removed from the blood by the liver, converted into glycogen and not released as glucose.

Blood lactic acid levels considerably exceed the normal level of 10 to 20 mg. per 100 ml. When the concentration of glucose in the blood falls below the normal level, blood lactic acid may rise to values between 100 and 150 mg. per 100 ml. Acidosis in glycogen storage disease seems to be partially due to increased lactic acid concentration in the blood.

The protein partition in the blood plasma is normal. There is no increase of the globulin fractions, as in some other liver diseases. Liver function tests other than those related to impaired glycogenolysis are negative. Jaundice is absent, and bilirubin levels in the serum are normal. Leukopenia and relative lymphocytosis are characteristic findings; hypoprothrombinemia is occasionally encountered.

Type II is a generalized glycogenosis, erroneously named the cardiomegalic form of glycogen storage disease. The children die from cardiac failure early in life. The accumulation of glycogen occurs mainly in heart and skeletal muscle. However, the glycogen content of liver, kidney and brain is also above the normal value. On x-ray the heart reveals a large globular shape; the electrocardiogram shows left axis deviation, widening of the QRS complex and inversion of the T wave. Fasting blood sugar, glucose tolerance and epinephrine tests are normal. Acidosis is absent. Deficiency of a specific enzyme is not demonstrable. Glucose 6-phosphatase activity in liver and kidney is normal. Postmortem glycogenolysis in liver and muscle occurs normally, and the structure of the glycogen is normal. It is possible that glycogen degradation is slower than synthesis with gradual accumulation of glycogen in the organs involved.

In *type III* an abnormal structure of liver and muscle glycogen was found by Illingworth and Cori.[5] The liver glycogen has very short outer branches and the muscle glycogen has almost none, resembling a phosphorylase limit dextrin. It seems to be justifiable to conclude that the amylo-1,6-glucosidase activity is low; only the outer branches are broken off, while the inner nuclei of the glycogen molecules remain unbroken and may accumulate in excessive amounts.

In *type IV* the liver glycogen is less branched and has longer inner and outer chains than normal glycogen. The polysaccharide resembles amylopectin in these properties, and also in solubility, x-ray diffraction pattern and absorption spectrum of the iodine complex. The authors assume that transglucosidase activity is reduced in this type. A polysaccharide is synthesized which is less ramified than normal glycogen. Andersen's[8] case of familial cirrhosis of the liver with storage of abnormal glycogen in the reticuloendothelial cells throughout the body as well as in the liver is a representative example of this type.

A genetic etiology of the disease in types I, II and IV is probable, since in many instances, more than one sibling in the same family has been affected. There is little doubt that the disease is genetically transmitted from one generation to another as a recessive trait.

In recent studies, Wagner and co-workers[9] reported a considerable increase of glucose-6- and fructose 6-phosphate in the peripheral blood for the hepatonephromegalic type. The Seliwanoff reaction was found to be positive in deproteinized serum filtrates. The inability of phosphorylated intermediates to penetrate the cell membrane may be one of the factors responsible for the retarded development. The low fasting blood sugar seems to be due not only to the reduced concentration of glucose, but also to the presence of sugar phosphates of a reducing power lower than that of glucose.

So far only type I, the hepatonephromegalic type, is easily accessible to clinical diagnosis and routine laboratory procedures. It is debatable whether or not the other types should be classified under the heading of glycogen storage disease. More cases need to be studied with regard to the structure of glycogen deposits.

Pathology of the Hepatorenal Type (von Gierke). The two most outstanding findings are hepato- and nephromegaly. Increase of the weight of the liver to three times or more the normal weight and that of the kidney to twice the normal weight is not unusual. The spleen is normal in size and weight. The liver and kidney are slightly yellowish in color. The liver glycogen may range from eight to sixteen grams per 100 gm. of wet weight of liver or even more.

On microscopic examination, the liver reveals a rather uniform picture. The regular pattern of a normal liver is replaced by a plantlike appearance of the swollen cells. The individual cell is many times the normal size and is distinctly outlined. The cytoplasm shows double refractive droplets, particularly in the livers of young infants. Stained with Sudan, they appear to be red. With Best's carmine staining, the sections are uniformly red; the cytoplasm is stuffed with small droplets of glycogen. The nucleus is round and located in the center of the cell. It does not contain glycogen. The periportal connective tissue is not increased.

Postmortem glycogenolysis does not occur; however, the glycogen can be readily hydrolyzed by a homogenate of normal liver. On the other hand, a homogenate made from a patient's liver is unable to hydrolyze glycogen obtained from normal liver or other sources.

The kidney is of conspicuously light color. The epithelial cells of the tubules of the cortex are swollen and protrude into the lumen. On Best's carmine staining, glycogen is detected in the tubular system and in Henle's loops, but not in the glomeruli. The medullary portion does not contain glycogen.

In the spleen, lipid and glycogen reactions are negative. In the striated muscles, the medulla and other parts of the central nervous system, deposits of glycogen have been detected.

Differential Diagnosis. There are not many other conditions which can be mistaken for glycogen storage disease. A patient with hepatomegaly without splenomegaly or ascites, with low fasting blood sugar, fasting ketosis and hyperlipemia makes one suspect glycogen storage disease. A liver biopsy and the other laboratory findings will clarify the diagnosis. In Gaucher's and Niemann-Pick's diseases the spleen is always considerably enlarged. Neuroblastoma with metastases to the liver must be ruled out; in this ailment, the liver can reach the size of a glycogenosis liver. Congenital syphilis, amyloidosis, cirrhosis, passive congestion and steatosis (steatose massive du foie[10]) are other conditions to be considered in the differential diagnosis.

Treatment. The treatment should be directed toward compensating for the inability to break down glycogen to form sugar. A normal blood sugar level is essential for the nutrition of all tissues. Since glucose phosphates which are unable to penetrate the cell membrane accumulate in the peripheral blood, glucose should be administered from external sources, either by frequent feedings of glucose or starches, including one or two night feedings, or from a high protein diet taking advantage of gluconeogenesis. Parnas and Wagner[11] were able to demonstrate a considerable rise of the fasting blood sugar following the ingestion of various pure amino acids.

Treatment of acidosis secondary to hypoglycemia is just as important, particularly during infancy. Sodium lactate administration is occasionally hazardous because of an already high lactate level. Bicarbonate is more effective in making base immediately available.[12]

In view of the increased susceptibility to intercurrent infections, antibiotics are indicated during such episodes. Some patients, properly treated, seem to develop satisfactorily. There is a definite improvement with age. Although children beyond the first year of life have better chances to survive, the prognosis is still guarded. Linear growth never approaches a normal level. Mason and Andersen[12] reported the case of a girl who was under observation from the age of 6 months and died at the age of 10½ years. At autopsy multiple hepatomata and congestive right heart failure were found. Other cases reported in the literature reached even the age of 18 years. In these patients the liver has a tendency to shrink, and the fasting blood sugar level has a rising tendency. We have to assume that the excess glycogen is disposed of by oxidation of glucose 6-phosphate to 6-phosphogluconate, a reaction catalyzed by glucose 6-phosphate dehydrogenase. The patient reported by Wagner and Parnas[1] developed diabetes mellitus after several years of observation.

References

1. Wagner, R., and Parnas, J. K.: Ztschr. f. d. ges. exper. Med., *25:*261, 1921.
2. von Gierke, E.: Beitr. z. path. Anat. u. z. allg. Path., *82:*497, 1929.
3. Schönheimer, R.: Ztschr. f. physiol. Chem., *182:*148, 1929.
4. Thannhauser, S. J., Sorkin, S. Z. and Boncoddo, N. F.: J. Clin. Invest., *19:*681, 1940.
5. Cori, G. T. and Cori, C. F.: J. Biol. Chem., *199:*661, 1952; Illingworth, B., and Cori, G. T.: J. Biol. Chem., *199:* 653, 1952; Cori, G. T.: The Harvey Lectures, *48:*145, 1952–53.
6. Van Creveld, S.: Medicine, *18:*1, 1939.
7. Wagner, R.: Am. J. Dis. Child., *73:*559, 1947.
8. Andersen, D. H.: Lab. Invest., *5:*11, 1956.
9. Wagner, R., Meyerriecks, N. and Sparaco, R.: Read before the 67th Annual Meeting of the American Pediatric Society, Carmel, California, June 1957.
10. Debré, R., Polycories. Paris, Gaston Doin & Cie., 1947.
11. Parnas, J. K. and Wagner, R.: Biochem. Ztschr., *127:*55, 1922.
12. Mason, H. H. and Andersen, D. H.: Pediatrics, *16:*785, 1955.

IDIOPATHIC GALACTOSEMIA

Definition. This disorder is a congenital condition transmitted as a homozygous recessive gene.[1] The intermediate between galactose and glucose acts as a toxic agent, affecting liver, lens, brain and kidney. The presence of this metabolite leads to the development of hepatomegaly, jaundice, cataracts, mental retardation, proteinuria, amino aciduria and severe malnutrition. The presence of a reducing sugar in the urine of a child with jaundice from the third day of life on should suggest the possibility that this reducing substance is galactose.

Pathology.[2] The livers of the fatal cases reveal varying degrees of cellular degeneration. In the more severe cases there is complete disruption of lobular architecture and extensive loss of parenchymal cells with collapse and condensation of the reticulin framework. The cells may be arranged in short columns or they may form distinct tubular structures. The cholangioles are usually plugged with bile. The final picture is one of diffuse hepatic fibrosis which is often pericellular and not unlike diffuse syphilitic cirrhosis. The histologic findings are not specific, but a presumptive diagnosis of galactosemia can be made from a microscopic examination of the liver.

Chemical Pathology. Normally, galactose is metabolized in the body by first being phosphorylated to galactose 1-phosphate (Gal 1-P) by galactokinase at the expense of adenosine triphosphate (ATP). Gal 1-P is then converted to glucose 1-phosphate (G 1-P) by two reactions which involve a nucleotide, uridine diphosphate glucose (UDPG) and two specific enzymes:

$$\text{(I) Gal 1-P} + \text{UDPG} \rightleftarrows \text{UDP gal} + \text{G 1-P (P gal transferase)}$$
$$\text{(II) UDP gal} \rightleftarrows \text{UDPG (galacto-waldenase)}$$

The mammalian erythrocyte is known to metabolize galactose. For this reason Schwarz, Golberg, Komrower and Holzel[3] compared the metabolism of galactosemic red cells with that of normal cells under the same conditions, assuming that the presence of a biochemical defect in hepatic parenchymal cells might be shared by the erythrocytes. These authors found that galactosemic erythrocytes, in contrast to normal red cells, do not respire on galactose substrates. Oxygen uptake on glucose substrates is partially inhibited by the presence of galactose. Galactosemic erythrocytes, on exposure to galactose, *in vivo* or *in vitro,* accumulate galactose 1-phosphate. Values up to 20 mg. of galactose 1-phosphate per 100 ml. of blood have been observed. Much smaller amounts accumulate in normal red cells exposed to high galactose concentrations *in vitro,* and very little galactose 1-phosphate is found in normal infants on a milk diet. After exposure to galactose, the O_2 uptake of galactosemic erythrocytes is considerably reduced, while that of normal cells is slightly enhanced. This effect is reflected in the level of phosphorylated intermediates: galactose lowers the ester phosphorus (other than galactose 1-phosphate) of galactosemic cells and raises that of normal cells.

The observations of Schwartz et al.[3] were confirmed and extended by Isselbacher, Anderson and Kalckar,[4] who found that the defect in galactosemia is due to a block in step (I). Hemolysates of normal and galactosemic erythrocytes were incubated with Gal 1-P and UDPG or UDP gal and the reactions measured by specific enzymatic techniques. P gal transferase activity was present in normal cells to the extent of 0.75 μM per hour, but this enzyme was completely lacking in the erythrocytes of ten galactosemic subjects. In contrast, galacto-waldenase was present in equal amounts in normal and galactosemic cells. No inhibitors or absent cofactors were found to account for the block in reaction (I). Furthermore, the absence of P-gal transferase could not simply be explained by the lack of galactose intake by galactosemic subjects, since the enzyme does not disappear from the red blood cells of normal infants on a galactose-free diet up to 18 months.

Another peculiarity of metabolism is amino aciduria, first described by Holzel, Komrower and Wilson[5] and confirmed by several other investigators.[6] The urine α-amino nitrogen excretion is within normal limits while the patients are on a galactose-free diet. There is a two- to threefold increase after d-galactose is added to the diet for 10 days and return to normal after withdrawal of galactose. By paper partition chromatography the amino aciduria is found to be generalized in nature and includes a number of amino acids. These findings suggest that galactose has some direct effect, possibly toxic in nature, upon the renal tubules which permits the α-amino nitrogen to be excreted in excess and prevents its resorption in the normal manner. Amino aciduria does not appear to be related to the liver damage which is characteristic of galactosemia.

According to Komrower, Schwartz, Holzel and Golberg[7] the amino acid pattern is essentially similar in all cases, with a predominance of the neutral simple aliphatic chain type, i.e., serine, glycine, alanine, threonine, glutamine and valine; in addition phenylalanine, lysine, cystine, glutamic acid, methylhistidine, tyrosine and amino-iso-butyric acid have been detected in the urine. The urine amino acid pattern can be restored to normal by feeding the infant a lactose or galactose-free diet. The excretion of amino acids begins on the fifth or sixth day of milk or galactose feeding. The daily urine total nitrogen value as well as the urine urea-nitrogen remains fairly constant. Plasma and blood α-amino-nitrogen levels are either normal or only slightly raised.

Sidbury[8] has recently shown in *in vitro* studies that accumulation of galactose-1-phosphate of the order demonstrated in the cells of galactosemia patients with galactose in their diet is commensurate with marked inhibition of phosphoglucomutase in the cells of these patients. Phosphoglucomutase is essential in various metabolic reactions. Their inhibition would explain the symptoms of patients with galactosemia through inhibition of phosphoglucomutase.

Clinical Manifestations. Idiopathic galactosemia can be detected in the neonatal period and occurs occasionally in siblings. Vomiting, marked weight loss and jaundice of increasing intensity are the most prominent symptoms. The liver and spleen are only moderately enlarged at the onset of the ailment, but the liver increases considerably in size if the disease is not recognized. If not properly treated, it is usually fatal in early childhood. The children are drowsy and inactive. The urine is found to contain protein and a nonfermentable reducing substance, which can be identified as galactose by filter paper chromatography. Amino aciduria is another important finding. In untreated cases bilateral cataracts develop soon after birth. Cases have been reported in which the symptoms did not appear until 3 or 4 months of age or in which the child was not seen until the second year of life and revealed mental retardation, hepatomegaly and cataracts.

Laboratory Findings. Glucose tolerance tests on a milk-free diet are flat. Galactose tolerance tests are abnormal, with a considerable rise of the galactose level in the blood to 200 to 300 mg. per cent between one and two hours, and a slow return to the fasting level. A depression of the blood glucose level at the peak of the galactose tolerance test has been reported by several investigators; even slight signs of a hypoglycemic reaction, characterized by pallor and sweating, may occur. When milk is discontinued in the diet, the blood galactose level drops rapidly and galactose can no longer be detected in the urine. The proteinuria, like the other anomalies of metabolism, diminishes rapidly following the cessation of milk feeding and disappears entirely after a few days.

Urinary excretion of sodium and potassium during a period of milk intake is within normal limits. Acidosis, observed by several investigators, is considered a renal acidosis similar to that found in hyperchloremic renal acidosis. Komrower et al.[7] showed a definite reduction in the amounts of inorganic and ester phosphorus in the erythrocytes after a regimen of galactose feeding. Galactose 1-phosphate was estimated at the same time and showed a considerable increase.

The most satisfactory concept of the pathogenesis of galactosemia has been developed by Komrower and co-workers.[7] The classic symptoms of the disease seem to result from a disturbed cell metabolism due to the accumulation of galactose 1-phosphate in the tissues.

The presence of amino aciduria, proteinuria and metabolic acidosis indicates a disturbance of the renal tubule which is corrected when milk or galactose is withdrawn from the diet. It has been suggested that the metabolic block is not always complete. The severity of the defect varies from patient to patient. There is also a considerable variation in the time of onset of symptoms and also in their severity. If the child survives into the second year of life, hepatomegaly, cataracts and mental retardation are usually the presenting symptoms.

The etiology of the hypoglycemia associated with galactosemia is not yet well understood. Komrower and coworkers[7] assume that galactose 1-phosphate accumulated in the liver may inhibit glycogenolysis and may lower the blood glucose level. From *in vitro* experiments on erythrocytes one may conclude that galactose itself has no toxic effect on normal cells. It seems to be the accumulation of galactose 1-phosphate which is responsible for the partial inhibition of glucose metabolism. The rate of accumulation and disappearance of galactose 1-phosphate is determined by the relative amounts of galactokinase and of the uridyl transferase and galacto-waldenase system in a particular tissue.

Treatment. Successful treatment depends on recognition of the defect as soon as possible after birth. It consists of replacement of the milk in the diet by a milk substitute. In this way the infant is enabled to develop normally. Intravenous fluid therapy is required in situations where vomiting, dehydration and critical loss of weight are encountered.

References

1. Holzel, A., and Komrower, G. M.: Arch. Dis. Childhood, *30:*155, 1955.
2. Bowden, D. H., and Donahue, W. L.: Am. J. M. Sc., *230:*305, 1955.
3. Schwartz, V., Golberg, L., Komrower, G. M., and Holzel, A.: Biochem. J., *62:*34, 1956.
4. Kalckar, H. M., Anderson, E. A., and Isselbacher, K. J.: Biochim. et biophys. acta., *20:*262, 1956.
5. Holzel, A., Komrower, G. M., and Wilson, V. K.: Brit. M. J. *1:*194, 1952.
6. Hsia, D. Y., Hsia, H., Green, S., Kay, M., and Gellis, S. S.: A.M.A. J. Dis. Child., *88:*458, 1954.
7. Komrower, G. M., Schwartz, V., Holzel, A., and Golberg, L.: Arch. Dis. Childhood, *31:*254, 1956.
8. Sidbury, J. B., Jr.: Report of the 27th Annual Meeting of the Society for Pediatric Research, Carmel, California, May 29, 1957.

CHAPTER 10

By WALTER BAUER, M.D.,
AND EVAN CALKINS, M.D.

Gout

Gout is a metabolic disease the most obvious biochemical manifestation of which is an increase in the serum uric acid concentration. When clinically overt, it is manifested by recurrent attacks of acute arthritis, which follow a characteristic pattern, and, in many cases, by urate deposits, chiefly in and about the joints of the extremities.

Gouty arthritis was known as a clinical entity long before its relationship to uric acid metabolism was suspected. To the historians of medicine, the disease has had an unusual appeal. Recordings of its ancestry are found in the earliest medical literature. Its pedigree is a most distinguished one, and no disease has enjoyed a more royal patronage. Descriptions of its dramatic appearance, the ensuing pathos and the whimsical aspects of the disease have been documented by the ablest authors in fiction and biography. The excellent clinical accounts of gout ascribed to Aretaeus of Cappadocia, Caelius Aurelianus, Hippocrates and others testify to the intimate knowledge of its varied features possessed by the Greek and Roman physicians.[1]

The term gout, introduced in the 13th century, is derived from the Latin *gutta*, a drop, and refers to the belief that the disease is due to a poison of some sort falling, drop by drop, into the joint. It is an admirable name in that it connotes no theory, has little nosologic significance and implies no specific pathogenesis. The earlier writers often failed to differentiate gouty arthritis clearly from other joint disorders until Sydenham, the modern Hippocrates, emphasized this distinction.[2] His masterly clinical portrayal of the disease, based in part on his thirty-four years of personal affliction, remains unsurpassed.

The relation of uric acid to gout was not established until the development of chemistry made available the necessary analytic methods. Shortly after Scheele (1776)[3] had discovered uric acid as one of the constituents of a kidney stone, Wollaston (1797)[4] and Pearson (1798)[5] succeeded in demonstrating the same substance in the "chalkstones" (tophi) of patients suffering from gout. Garrod's discovery (1848) by the "Thread Test"[6] of increased amounts of uric acid in the blood of gouty patients finally established a relationship between this substance and gout. Evidence that uric acid is the end-product of human purine metabolism was provided by a series of independent investigations.[7,8] It remained for Emil Fischer[9] to prove the chemical constitution of uric acid and to establish its structural relationship to purines. Since then, the role of purine metabolism in the pathophysiology of gout has been accepted. The introduction by Folin[10] of a reliable method of determining the uric acid content of the blood, and its improvement by Folin[11] and Benedict,[12] have aided greatly in the subsequent metabolic and clinical studies of this disease.

Gout may be primary or secondary.

Primary gout is one of the diseases which are characterized by specific heritable metabolic defects, the chemical analogues of structural malformations. Secondary gout may occur in patients with myeloid metaplasia, polycythemia vera, chronic leukemia, chronic hemolytic anemias and certain other hematologic conditions in which there is accelerated nucleoprotein turnover; no inherited predisposition is required.

The relationship of hyperuricemia and clinical gout is not as clear as is frequently stated. The fact that all patients with gout at some time have elevated serum uric acid concentrations has fostered the belief that the hyperuricemia and the clinical manifestations have a cause and effect relationship. There is abundant evidence that, in patients with primary gout, prolonged elevation of serum uric acid concentration may be accompanied by the deposition of urate crystals in many portions of the body, and, in many instances, by the formation of kidney stones. On the other hand, prolonged elevation of serum uric acid due to conditions other than primary gout, such as chronic renal disease or leukemia, is not usually accompanied by the deposition of urates in the tissue parenchyma. In a given patient, acute attacks of arthritis do not necessarily occur at times of highest serum uric acid concentrations. The experimental introduction of uric acid into the blood stream or joints of gouty patients has not precipitated acute attacks of arthritis.[13] Furthermore, the most effective agent in the treatment of acute gouty arthritis, colchicine, has not yet, to our knowledge, been demonstrated to have any effect on uric acid metabolism.

For these reasons, it has been suggested that "tissue factors" may play a role in gout. The nature of these, if present, is totally unknown. An alternative possibility is that the clinical manifestations of the disease, especially acute gouty arthritis, may be due to some other as yet undetected defect in the metabolism of purines or other substances, which is related only indirectly to that of uric acid metabolism.

Whatever the relationship may be between uric acid metabolism and the clinical manifestations of gout, alterations in uric acid concentrations constitute the biochemical label by which these patients are most easily identified. It is not surprising therefore, that studies of the abnormal metabolism of this substance have occupied the forefront of research on the pathogenesis of this disease.

URIC ACID METABOLISM*

Sources of Uric Acid in the Body. Uric acid excreted in the urine of man may be derived from three sources (Fig. 1):

A. It is the chief end-product of the catabolism of endogenous purines.
B. It can result from conversion of ingested purines.
C. Uric acid may be synthesized directly from glycine and other simple precursors without prior incorporation into tissue purine nucleotides.

These three sources will be considered separately.

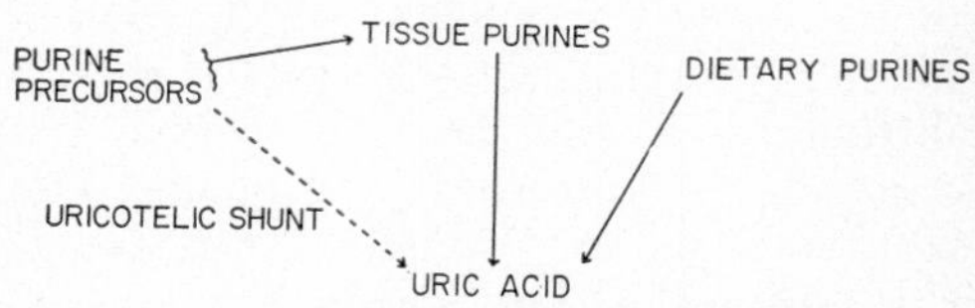

FIG. 1. Origin of uric acid in man.

A. CATABOLISM OF PURINES. Nucleoproteins are contained in the nuclei and cytoplasm of all living tissues and by suitable techniques can be separated into a protein moiety and a large complex polymer called nucleic acid. The basic unit of the nucleic acid is the nucleotide, a complex of one molecule of a base (either a purine or pyrimidine), one molecule of a pentose (ribose or desoxyribose) and one molecule of phosphoric acid. The chemical formula of a typical nucleotide, adenylic acid, is shown

* The reader is urged to consult published reviews for further details concerning uric acid metabolism[14–19] and the chemistry of purines.[20, 22]

in Figure 2. Larger aggregates of nucleotides form nucleic acids, which, together with specific proteins, make up nucleoproteins. The many nucleotides which comprise a nucleic acid molecule are thought to be linked by ester bonds between phosphoric acid and hydroxyl groups of the pentose.

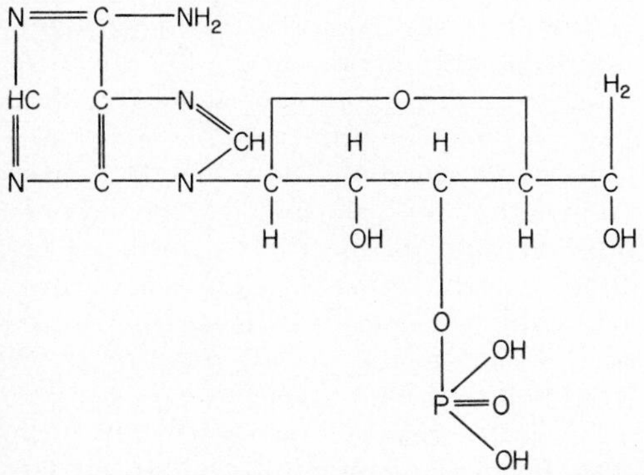

FIG. 2. Chemical formula of adenylic acid, a typical nucleotide.

The nucleoproteins which predominate in cellular nuclei and cytoplasm have certain basic differences, which permit their separation into two large classes, the desoxyribonucleic acids (DNA) and ribonucleic acids (RNA), as shown in Figure 3. The increasing awareness that the nucleotides are essential components of coenzymes[23] suggests that the nucleoproteins may serve as a reservoir of readily available material for use as coenzymes.

	RNA	DNA
Purines	Adenine Guanine	Adenine Guanine
Pyrimidines	Uracil Cytosine	Thymine Cytosine (Methyl-Cytosine)
Carbohydrate	Ribose	Desoxyribose

FIG. 3. Some differences in the chemical components of two classes of nucleoproteins: ribonucleic acids (RNA) and desoxyribonucleic acids (DNA).

Of the bases which comprise the nucleotides, the pyrimidines[22] are not related to uric acid synthesis or, so far as we know, to gout. The purine nucleotides, adenylic acid and quanylic acid, however, are broken down sequentially to uric acid.[24,25]

Although the mechanism by which the compounds are transformed through the various steps is not completely understood, a large number of intermediates have been identified chemically. The present concept concerning their metabolic interrelationship is shown in Figure 4.

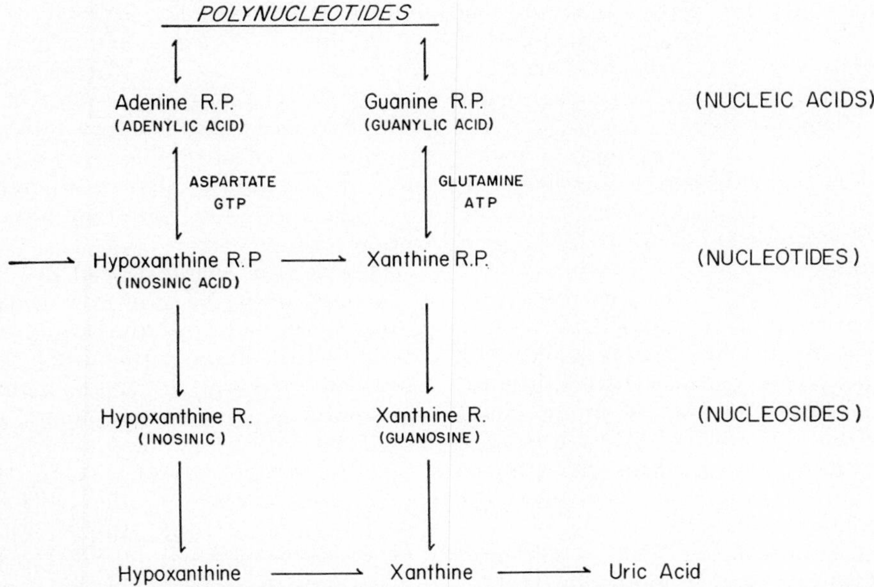

FIG. 4. Probable metabolic interrelationship of some biologically important purines.

The metabolic precursors of the purine molecule, and therefore of the derived uric acid molecule, have been determined by administering a variety of isotopically labelled compounds in vivo and by enzymatic studies in vitro.[26–33] As shown in Figure 5, the source of the

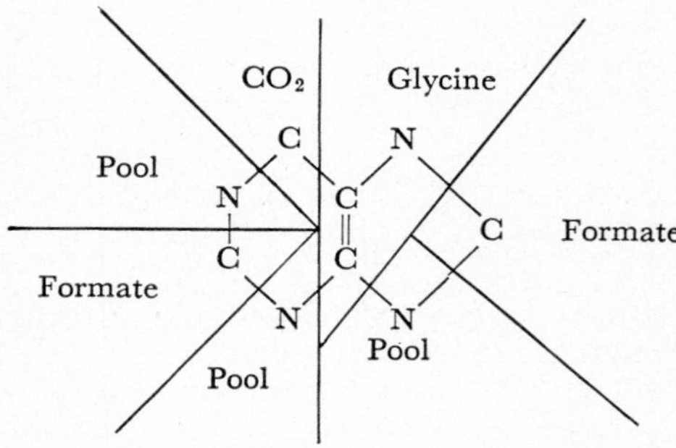

FIG. 5. Source of atoms comprising the purine ring.

various atoms can be traced ultimately to glycine, formate, CO_2 and the common metabolic pool of amino groups. Although the numerous individual steps in this process are still being investigated, the elucidation of purine biosynthesis is one of the major accomplishments of recent biochemical research.[34–45] The present concept of this pathway is shown in Figure 6.

Stetten[19] has suggested that the composition of a polynucleotide or nucleic acid may depend on the composition of the mixture of available mononucleotides. The fact that adenosine triphosphate (ATP) is required to make guanine nucleotides while guanosine triphosphate (GTP) is required to make adenine nucleotides may constitute a self-regulatory mechanism for preserving the proper ratio of available mononucleotides.

Nucleotides exist, in free form, in plants as well as in animals. For example, caffeine and theobromine are both methylated purines. In contrast to the nucleotides of animal origin, however, these compounds are not transformed into uric acid in the human body, but are excreted unchanged or partly demethylated.[46–49]

B. RELATIONSHIP OF DIET AND URIC ACID METABOLISM. It is a remarkable fact that carnivorous animals synthesize the purines which are present in their cells from small molecular fragments, rather than by conversion of dietary purines. The ingested nucleic acids, which are liberated by pepsin and trypsin hydrolysis, are further broken down by duodenal enzymes to nucleotides and nucleosides. The manner in which these compounds are absorbed and incorporated into the metabolic pool is not fully understood. It is known, however, that they are not incorporated as such into the purine pool of the body. It is also known that both normal and gouty persons on high purine diets exhibit an increase in the rate of excretion of uric acid and transiently, at least, in the serum concentration of this substance.[50,51] It is believed that ingested purines are to a large degree converted into uric acid. Even on a moderately high purine diet, however, the amount of urinary urate attributable to this source does not equal the amount which derives from catabolism of endogenous purines.

Alterations of dietary components other than the purines may be followed by changes in uric acid excretion. Thus, the uric acid excretion has been shown to be increased by a high protein diet[52,53] or by a diet high in glycine and other amino acids[54,55] and may also be influenced by changes in total caloric or fat intake.[56,57] These alterations are best understood by considering the effect of the changes on the size of the pool of amino acids:[18] factors increasing the amount of available amino acids and nitrogen tend to increase the rate of uric acid formation and, therefore, excretion.

There is some evidence that uric acid is excreted into the digestive tract in gastric juice, bile and duodenal secretions.[58–62] Utilization of this uric acid by intestinal organisms, to yield ammonia, may constitute a minor site of uric acid breakdown.

C. "URIC ACID SHUNT." As a third source, uric acid may be derived by direct biosynthesis from simple precursors, along the pathway outlined in Figure 6, without prior nucleotide formation and without incorporation into nucleic acids or functional nucleotides such as adenosinetriphosphate. Although such a "shunt" is probably quantitatively of little importance in normal persons, there is increasing evidence that it may underly the hyperuricemia of gout. This evidence will be considered in greater detail later.

Distribution and Excretion of Uric Acid. Although it is rare to see concentrations of uric acid higher than 15 mg. per cent in the serum of gouty patients, one may achieve a concentration as high as 27 mg. per cent following the adddition of this substance to the serum of gouty patients *in vitro*.[63] Uric acid is distributed between red blood cells and serum according to the Gibbs-Donnan equilibrium.[63] The maximal serum concentration for normals, cited by various authors, depends to a great extent upon the method used. According to the method currently in widest use (Folin), the maximal concentration for normal males is considered to be 6 mg. per 100 ml. and for premenopausal females 5 mg. per 100 ml.[64] This sex differential, which has been amply established by several different chemical methods,[65] is not present in preadolescent children. The plasma uric acid concentration in normal boys is the same as that in normal girls.[66] The serum uric acid concentration in young relatives of gouty patients is not significantly elevated prior to puberty.[64] In female relatives of gouty patients there is a significant tendency for the serum uric acid concentration to rise following menopause.[68] One is tempted to postulate that these differences in serum uric acid concentrations might reflect the increase in 17-ketosteroid secretion in adult males and, to a lesser extent, in postmenopausal females. Determination of the 17-ketosteroid excretion in gouty patients, however, indicates that it is either normal[70] or reduced.[67]

The serum uric acid concentration may be elevated above normal in several states which are not associated with gouty arthritis. The commonest of these conditions is renal insufficiency, with inability of the kidney to excrete nitrogenous end-products. Serum uric acid is one of the components of "nonprotein nitrogen" and is never elevated in renal disease without corresponding elevation of other nitrogenous substances, particu-

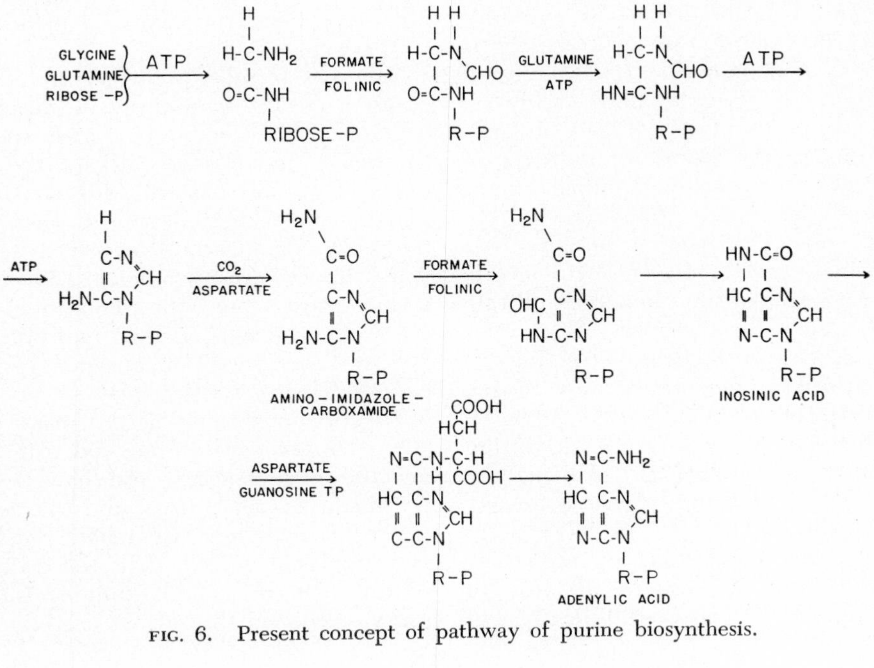

FIG. 6. Present concept of pathway of purine biosynthesis.

larly blood urea. Serum uric acid concentration may also be increased in a variety of conditions associated with rapid breakdown of tissue, and hence of nucleoproteins. Acute myocardial infarction,[71] starvation,[72] carcinoma of the stomach,[73] eclampsia and severe infections are examples which are not associated with clinical gout. Other conditions, in which the increased purine breakdown is more sustained, such as myeloid metaplasia,[74] polycythemia vera,[75,76] pernicious anemia in remission[77] and chronic leukemia, may also be associated with elevated serum uric acid levels. These patients exhibit typical attacks of acute gouty arthritis with greater frequency than one would expect in the general population.[65]

In both normal and gouty persons, the serum uric acid level may vary with time. In females it is apt to reach a peak just prior to the onset of menstruation. In males it may follow a cycle of approximately two to three weeks' duration.[78] For this reason, it is usually wise to obtain a series of serum uric acid determinations approximately twice weekly in a given individual, before concluding that he does or does not have gout on the basis of this determination.

Although in some animals, such as the frog[79] and chicken,[80] there is evidence for tubular excretion of uric acid, it is agreed that in man uric acid is filtered through the glomerulus and largely reabsorbed by the tubules in a manner analogous to the excretory patterns of many other substances. Comparison of uric acid and inulin clearance of both normal and gouty persons suggests that approximately 90 per cent of the uric acid appearing in the glomerular filtrate is subsequently reabsorbed.[13,81–83]

The total uric acid excreted per 24 hours by normal persons on a low purine diet varies between 300 and 600 mg.,[84] the rate being somewhat greater during the day than at night.[50,85,86] An increase in the rate of excretion of uric acid may theoretically be due to an increase in the rate of degradation of the body purines, to an increase in the rate of glomerulus filtration, or to a decrease in the rate of tubular reabsorption. Although the former of these mechanisms underlies the uricosuria in many disease states (see below), alterations in the renal factors, especially tubular reabsorption, is the usual mechanism of the uricosuria seen with various uricosuric agents. Although the uricosuria due to ACTH and corticosteroids was initially thought to be due to increased purine breakdown,[87,88] subsequent evidence implicates decreased tubular reabsorption of uric acid.[89–91]

The increased uric acid excretion in Dalmatian coach hounds as compared with other dogs has long been known.[92] At first this peculiarity was believed to be due to a defect in the breakdown of uric acid to allantoin, an hypothesis which was weakened somewhat by the demonstration of normal uricase activity in these dogs.[93] Recently, by the use of renal clearance studies, it has been demonstrated[94,95] that the uricosuria of the Dalmatian coach hound can be attributed to a defect in the reabsorption of uric acid in the renal tubule with the result that essentially all uric acid filtered by the glomerulus appears in the urine. This provides an interesting explanation for the previously observed fact that tubular blocking agents, such as salicylate, have been shown to be ineffective in these dogs.[95,96]

Whereas in most animals, uric acid is catabolized almost entirely by means of uricase to allantoin, and in many species to urea (Fig. 7), the bulk of the evidence suggests that this does not take place to any large degree in man. Attempts to demonstrate uricolytic activity by human tissues *in vitro* have been unsuccessful, but the conditions of study may have been less than optimal. Despite the apparent absence of uricase in man, some workers[97,98] have been able to recover in the urine only 60 to 80 per cent of labelled uric acid injected intravenously and have found N^{15} in the excreted urea, and to a lesser extent in ammonia. Benedict, Forsham and Stetten[99] found that the rate of synthesis of uric acid, estimated isotopically, exceeded the rate of excretion by

20 to 40 per cent. The most likely explanation for this discrepancy is that the small amounts of uric acid excreted into the intestines may be transformed by intestinal bacteria into ammonia and reabsorbed. Wyngaarden and Stetten[100] repeated their study following administration of large doses of oral sulfonamides, however, with essentially the same results. This does not exclude the possibility of destruction of uric acid by bacteria. The hypothesis that uric acid is catabolized by the human body remains to be proved.[101] If this theory were true, a decrease in this rate of destruction would represent a possible cause of at least some cases of hyperuremia.

Uric Acid Metabolism in Patients with Gout. Numerous studies have been carried out in human beings, by means of N^{15} or C^{14} labelling of uric acid and potential precursors, in an attempt to establish the nature of the metabolic defect in this disease. Most of these studies fall into one or two categories: (*a*) After the administration of isotopically labelled uric acid (usually by vein), the specific activity of uric acid in the urine is followed in terms of time. This is the so-called "isotope dilution technique." (*b*) After the administration of N^{15} labelled glycine, the rate of incorporation of N^{15} into urinary uric acid is determined.

When a known amount of isotopic uric acid is injected, the degree of its dilution with endogenous nonisotopic uric acid will depend on the quantity with which it has been mixed, the so-called miscible pool. The concentration of the isotopic uric acid in the body falls rapidly as it is diluted by newly formed uric acid and is excreted in the urine. From an analysis of the rate of this isotopic dilution and the absolute value of the initial "miscible pool" it is possible to calculate the rate at which uric acid is being synthesized in the body. In order to make these calculations one has to make several assumptions: (*a*) that uric acid is freely diffusible in the body

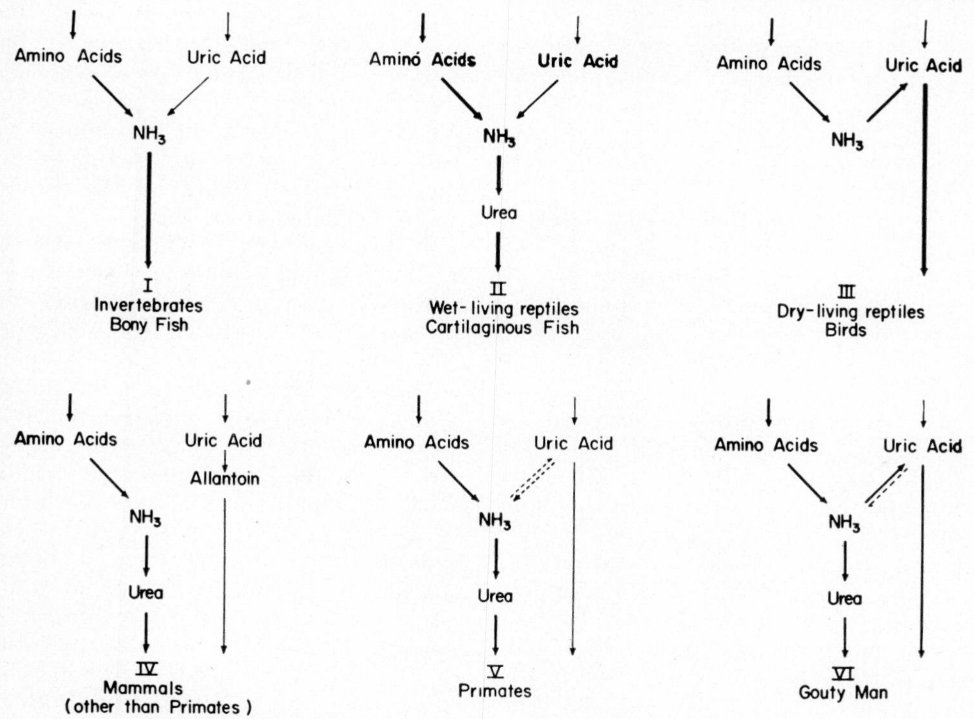

FIG. 7. A comparison of the modes of excretion of nitrogen and uric acid in various species, emphasizing that the postulated defect in gouty man represents a minor variation and follows a well established biologic pattern.

and that the labelled material mixes readily with the miscible pool; (*b*) that labelled uric acid acts, metabolically, the same as the unlabelled material; (*c*) that there is no new labelling of uric acid as a result of resynthesis from breakdown products of the labelled material; (*d*) that the specific activity of the urine is a true index of the specific activity of the uric acid of the body. Recent examination of some of these assumptions has indicated that they may not be entirely valid.[102] Nevertheless, certain conclusions from these studies seem fairly well established.

The miscible pool in normal persons is approximately 1 gram.[101–103] In gouty patients without clinically evident tophi the pool is moderately increased to approximately 2 to 4 grams.[103] In patients with clinically evident tophi the pool is markedly increased, values as high as 30 grams being reported.[90] Successive extracts of a tophus excised on the ninth day following injection of N^{15} labelled uric acid revealed decreasing specific activity of the extracted nitrogen,[90,99] indicating that the superficial layers contained more labelled material than the deeper layers. This indicates that in such patients the miscible pool does not approximate the total body uric acid.

The isotope dilution studies referred to above have indicated that the normal person synthesizes approximately 700 mg. of uric acid a day, which represents a daily turnover rate of about 50 to 75 per cent of the body's miscible pool of uric acid.[99,103]

The rate of synthesis estimated by this means exceeds the daily excretion rate by approximately 100 to 250 milligrams per day and provides further support for the belief that some destruction of uric acid may be taking place in normal man. This method is more difficult to interpret in gouty patients because of the unknown exchange rate of the isotope with the uric acid in tophi, but the evidence available suggests that there is an increased rate of uric acid synthesis. The total body uric acid is generally increased to such a degree, however, that the percentage of the miscible pool which turns over each day is reduced.[99,103]

Somewhat better measurements of the relative rates of uric acid synthesis are provided by the N^{15} glycine experiments. Following the oral administration of N^{15} labelled glycine to a patient on a very low purine diet, the percentage of the ingested dose of N^{15} appearing in the urine as uric acid each day was plotted in a cumulative fashion for a nine-day period. The amount of labelled glycine appearing in the uric acid provides an index of the amount of uric acid synthesized during this time. By this means it was shown that gouty patients who excrete normal amounts of urate usually have a normal rate of urate synthesis.[104–106] On the other hand, in gouty patients with increased uric acid excretion rates the uric acid synthesis was also increased.[106,107] One recent study, using C^{14} labelled glycine,[108] indicated an increased rate of uric acid synthesis in all gouty patients studied, but further investigation, using this technique, has demonstrated a normal rate of uric acid synthesis in other gouty persons.[109,110] Whether this apparent difference reflects different underlying metabolic defects or different phases of the disease cannot be stated at present.

In those patients in whom studies using N^{15} labelled glycine indicated an increased rate of uric acid synthesis, the N^{15} appeared in urinary uric acid very promptly—too rapidly to be accounted for by prior incorporation of the purine molecules into tissue nucleotides. Additional evidence has come from studies with 4-amino-5-imidazole-carboxamide —which, though not a normal purine intermediate, can be converted by the body to its natural riboside. Labelled samples of this material given to gouty subjects resulted in the appearance of isotopic material in the urine in 12 to 18 hours.[111] The speed of isotopic incorporation into uric acid from both of these precursors suggests that in gouty patients there may be a more direct pathway between glycine and uric acid than via functional purines in tissue, this being the third possible source of uric acid mentioned earlier.

Parenthetical support of this concept of a direct synthesis of uric acid in man comes from a review of the manner with which other animal species excrete their primary nitrogenous end products (Fig. 7). Baldwin[112] has advanced the intriguing hypothesis that the major controlling variable in the development of this mechanism is the amount of water which is available to the animal to wash away the highly toxic ammonia. According to this hypothesis, the invertebrates and bony fish living in a highly aquatic environment are able to excrete ammonia directly. The amphibia and the elasmobranchs excrete primarily urea. In birds, lizards and most insects living under relatively dehydrated circumstances, an accumulation of urea, with its high osmotic properties, would drastically upset their water balance. Instead, they transform the ammonia into uric acid, which is osmotically less active. In most mammals, including the primates, this is not necessary, inasmuch as the flow of material in the blood placenta provides a moderately hydrated environment. They have continued to excrete primarily urea. The recent evidence reported above suggests that the patient with primary gout may have developed, to some extent, a biochemical process analagous to that seen in the birds, snakes and lizards.

The few metabolic studies performed in secondary gout indicate that quite a different mechanism is at work in these cases.[113–115] Although the total cumulative incorporation of administered N^{15} labelled glycine in urinary uric acid was found to be increased in secondary, as in primary gout, the rate of incorporation of N^{15} was far more gradual in the former condition. It would appear that in secondary gout direct formation of uric acid is not increased, but rather the increased rate of uric acid formation is the secondary result of a more rapid over-all synthesis and degradation of nucleic acids. This excessive uric acid is derived indirectly from tissue nucleotides rather than directly from simple precursors.

One cannot leave the subject of the metabolic abnormalities in gout without reminding the reader that the precise manner in which uric acid metabolism is related to acute gouty arthritis is by no means understood. There is much evidence to indicate that the relationship is an indirect one at best. In the future there may be more fruitful areas for investigation in this disease than uric acid metabolism per se. The recent demonstration that there is an increased excretion of 8-hydroxy-7-methyl guanine in gouty patients during acute attacks[116] may represent the first observation in such an area.

CLINICAL MANIFESTATIONS OF GOUT

Incidence. The incidence of gout is unknown. The statistics reported for various sections of the United States of America and other countries are difficult to evaluate.[117–120] They range from a small fraction of 1 per cent among meat-eating people[117] to 7 per cent in natives of India, who are largely vegetarians and teetotalers.[119] These astonishing variations are due partly to the differences in populations studied and the diagnostic standards applied and to the variable degree in which physicians are familiar with and aware of this disease. Undoubtedly many more cases are seen in private practice than in hospitals because acute gouty arthritis is, as a rule, self-limited and of short duration. Nevertheless, disagreement concerning the incidence of gout is also present in pathologic studies. Beitzke,[121] who examined 200 unselected cadavers over twenty years of age, found histologic proof of gouty arthritis in ten cases. Heine,[122] in postmortem studies on 1002 patients ranging from fifteen to ninety-five years of age, noted an incidence of 1.1 per cent. Considering such marked discrepancies and the lack of definite clinical data, the authors do not accept as established views that gout is a rare or even declining disease.[123,124] In our opinion, the diagnosis frequently is not made because the patient does not exhibit the classic features of chronic gout. Alertness to its early manifestations and application of modern diagnostic means will enable us to gain more reliable knowledge concerning the incidence of the disease.

HEREDITY. From the time the first clinical observations on gout were made, medical writers have stressed its hereditary nature. More recent specific reports vary greatly, some[125–127] showing a low, others[128–130] a significantly high familial incidence. There can be little doubt that the frequency with which one obtains affirmative information on this point depends upon the thoroughness with which the inquiry is pursued. Circumspect questioning on repeated visits and interviews with the patient's relatives have often procured a positive family history where it had been denied previously. The propensity of the disease to pass over one or more generations has long been a hindrance to the investigation of the genetics of gout. The discovery, however, that asymptomatic hyperuricemia is quite common among relatives of gouty patients[131–133] has paved the way for genealogic studies of this disease.[134–139]

These studies have shown that hyperuricemia is a single dominant gene, but only a fraction of those affected by hyperuricemia ever develop clinically recognizable gout. The inheritance of hyperuricemia is not sex-linked. This becomes apparent if allowance is made for the fact that the statistical upper limit of normal serum urate concentration in woman is about 1 mg. lower than in man. "Hyperuricemia" of 5 to 6 mg. per cent is not uncommon in female relatives of gouty patients. This level, although apparently abnormal and an indication of the inherited characteristic, is not usually sufficient to permit precipitation of urate in tissues and the development of clinical symptoms of gout. Although genetic studies indicate that familial hyperuricemia is an essential prerequisite for gouty arthritis, they offer no explanation of the mechanism by means of which the carrier state of hyperuricemia is transformed into that of the manifest disease. Slightly over 95 per cent of all patients afflicted with gouty arthritis are males. Symptomatic gout is very rare in infancy. Acute gouty arthritis is seen occasionally in the teens. Acute arthritis occurs with increasing frequency from the second to the sixth decade, being most common in the forties. However, the first evidence of the disease may not appear until late in life. Cases are on record demonstrating the initiation of symptoms in the sixties, seventies and eighties. In such instances, the attacks as well as the subsequent course tend to be mild. The converse is likewise true: onset at an early age frequently portends severe seizures, often polyarticular in distribution, and may lead to extensive crippling and severe vascular nephritis before middle life.

There is at present no accurate information concerning the relevance to gout of either race or climate. Allegedly a disease of the temperate zones, it is known to occur in the tropics, and does affect Negroes, Chinese and East Indians. Those who believe that gout is the nemesis of high living quote a higher incidence among people whose occupations are conducive to overindulgence in food and drink. However, until we have more comprehensive analyses, further discussion will be baseless.

Clinical Manifestations and Course. The symptomatic or articular manifestations of gout have been designated by various terms. The acute attacks which are followed by complete remissions are best referred to as acute gouty arthritis, in distinction to chronic gout, signifying chronic gouty arthritis, with or without tophi.

The onset of the first attack of acute gouty arthritis is, as a rule, dramatic. The person, usually a healthy-appearing middle aged man, is suddenly seized with severe, sometimes excruciating pain, often in one of the metatarsophalangeal joints. Although such attacks frequently begin at night, they may occur at any time. Within a few hours of the onset, the afflicted joint is swollen, red, hot and exquisitely tender. The swelling may appear so rapidly that within a few hours the patient may be unable to remove his shoe without cutting it. The inflammatory edema is much more marked than in other acute arthritides and often extends some distance beyond the joint margins. Effusions into the larger joints are not uncommon. At the peak of the attack, the intense swelling of the foot, accompanied by redness and increased heat, resembles septic inflammation or an extensive cellulitis. There may be an associated lymphangitis. The skin is red, tense and shiny. The superficial veins are distended. The pain, often described as "crushing," usually worse at night, generally confines the patient to his bed or room because weight-bearing is intolerable.

As tenderness and redness subside, pitting edema is demonstrable. With the disappearance of the swelling, the overlying skin appears loose and thin, and desquamation of the cutis and itching may follow. The combination of these findings is rarely encountered in other types of acute arthritis, and therefore is of singular diagnostic significance. The attack usually subsides spontaneously, within a few days to a few weeks, with complete restoration of normal joint function.

Approximately 50 per cent of the initial attacks are confined to the first metatarsophalangeal joint, but the neighboring metatarsal and tarsal joints or those of the opposite foot may be involved simultaneously or in rapid succession. A bursa, more commonly that over the olecranon or patella, may be the site of an attack. The younger the person, the more likely is the attack to be polyarticular and migratory. Fever, again more prominent in young patients, usually is mild, rarely lasts for more than a few days, and may be absent. The severity of the initial attack varies greatly. In some persons the acute illness is extremely mild and lasts only a few days. Occasionally one sees abortive attacks.

Physical examination at the time of the first attack of gouty arthritis is usually negative except for the articular findings. Maximal joint tenderness is usually present on the medial aspects of the involved joint. A tophus, unknown to the patient, may be found in the helix of the ear, indicating the presence of the disease.

The clinical course subsequent to the initial attack usually conforms to a distinct pattern. Recurrent attacks of acute arthritis are followed by remissions during which the patient experiences no articular symptoms. These periods become progressively shorter until acute episodes occur once or twice yearly, often with a certain regularity. Some patients, for unexplained reasons, are taken ill each spring or fall. At this stage of the disease the patient frequently passes through episodes during which attacks involving multiple joints recur at extremely short intervals. Effusions in the large joints are apt to develop and often last weeks or even months. Complete remissions are less likely to occur when the disease is approaching or has entered upon the phase of chronic gouty arthritis or chronic gout. Such periods of rapidly recurring attacks, however, do not always represent the beginning of the chronic stage and may occasionally be followed by complete remissions, as in a patient of ours who was bedridden for three months and then remained entirely free from symptoms for the ensuing three years.

Although usually the disease follows a gradually progressive course, its clinical picture is one of extreme variability. Very rarely the patient remains symptom-free for many years, as exemplified by one instance in which the initial seizure at twenty-seven years of age was succeeded by the second one sixty-two years later.[140] In the benign form two to six attacks may be scattered over a period of thirty to fifty years, or they may be concentrated in one of the middle decades of life. In very few instances, most of which belong to the juvenile form, the disease is chronic from the onset. More frequently a period of five to forty years separates the initial attack from the chronic phase.

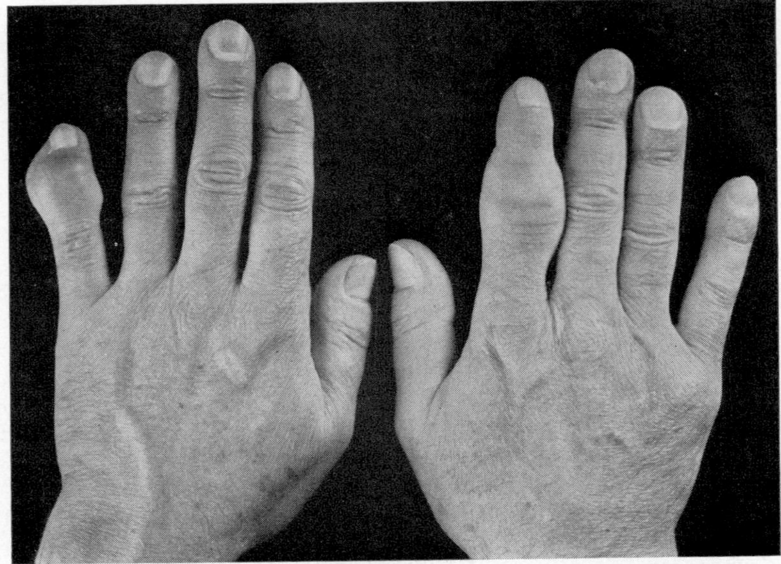

FIG. 8. Knob-like deformities of a terminal and a midphalangeal joint due to tophaceous deposits.

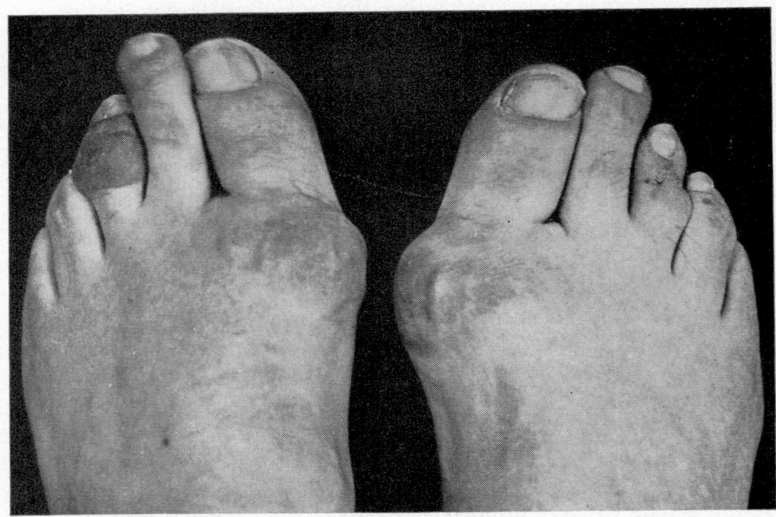

FIG. 9. Deformities of the first metatarsophalangeal joints caused by bony and soft tissue urate deposits. Tophi are present in both third toes. On the right, the tophaceous deposit is considerably reduced in size because of previous extrusion of the chalk-like material.

In the advanced stages of the disease, an increasing number of joints are affected, particularly those of the feet, hands, ankles, wrists, knees and elbows. Subcutaneous tophi, representing deposition of urates in periarticular and bursal tissues, are then frequently found and are responsible for the knobby deformities of the knuckles and the interphalangeal joints (Figs. 8 and 9). They may also be seen about the knee and elbows and along the tendons of the fingers, toes, ankles and wrists. Tophaceous deposits occur in nonarticular cartilage; indeed, their most common site in chronic gout is the helix of the ear (Fig. 10). They vary in size from a barely palpable nodule to deposits measuring as much as 5 cm. in diameter. Their presence in cartilage may be unattended by any symptoms, but in subcutaneous tissue visible inflammatory reaction usually results. Here, the deposits appear first as slightly reddened elevations, which gradually develop into white, cream-colored or yellow nodules of varying size (Fig. 11). The skin overlying a tophus may ulcerate (Fig. 11*B*) and discharge a white, chalky material which on microscopic examination shows the characteristic acidular crystals of sodium urate (Fig. 12). Such ulcerating lesions may occur anywhere on the body surface but are more common

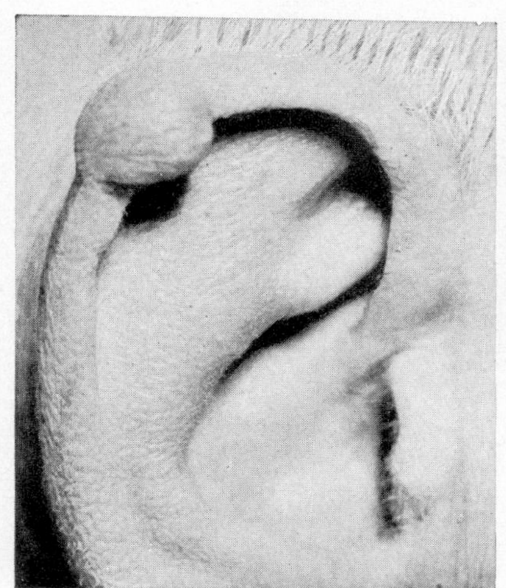

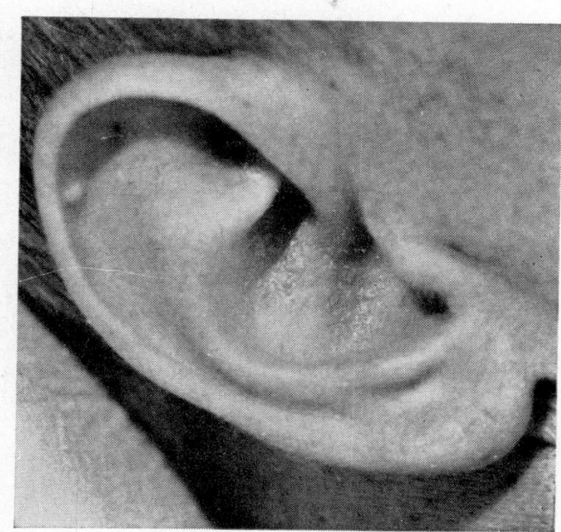

FIG. 10. Tophi on the helix of the ear.

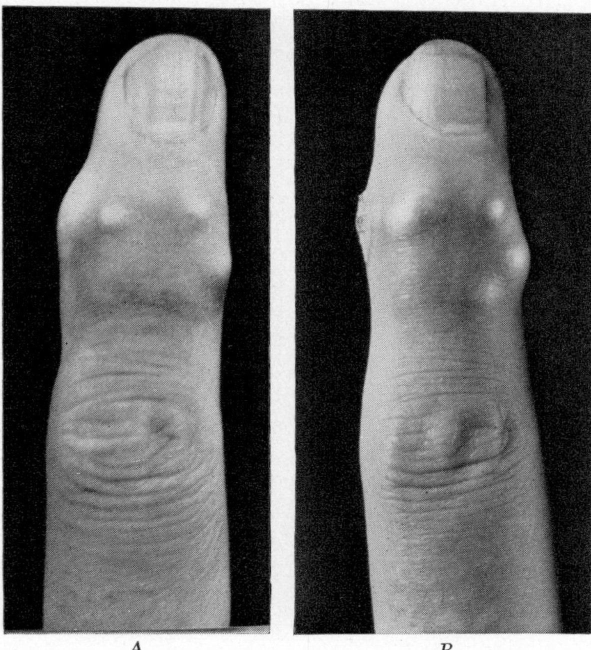

A *B*

FIG. 11. Tophaceous deposits about the terminal phalangeal joint of an index finger (*A*), which subsequently increased in size causing breakdown of the overlying skin and discharge of urates (*B*).

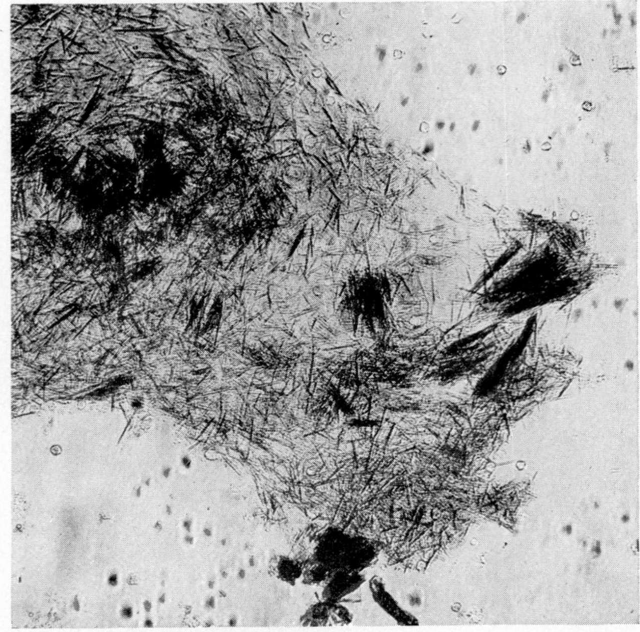

FIG. 12. Sodium urate crystals removed from a tophus. Unstained preparation.

in hands and feet. They rarely become infected.

Tophi are found in about 50 per cent of all cases of gout. In some they antedate the acute joint disease; in others they are not found until ten to thirty years after the initial attack. They should not be confused with the subcutaneous nodules of rheumatic fever and rheumatoid arthritis. Because they constitute the one pathognomonic lesion of gout, they should always be searched for. Regardless of whether a nodule has the characteristic clinical appearance of a tophus, it is unwise to accept it as such until it has been needled, the monosodium urate crystals (Fig. 12) have been demonstrated and a positive murexide test* has been obtained.

The term *irregular gout,* still used by some writers, designates a group of nondescript symptoms which do not resemble the characteristic findings of symptomatic gout. The patients, usually women, suffer from an arthritis which is insidious in onset and is slowly progressive, without remissions. As a rule, these persons show only a slightly higher than normal blood uric acid value. Tophi are not seen. A family history of gout is rarely obtained. If such a syndrome is indeed due to gout, it must be rigidly proved to be so by histologic examination, by demonstration of uric acid crystals in the tissues and by a favorable response to colchicine.

PREMONITORY SYMPTOMS. The specific changes which presumably take place in the gouty subject between birth and the onset of the clinical illness have not been studied. Whether hyperuricemia is ever present at birth, we do not know, but hyperuricemia has been demonstrated in adults prior to the appearance of articular symptoms.[131–133,135,136] We do not understand the bodily alterations immediately preceding the gouty seizure—the so-called larval state. Many patients experience no premonition of the impending attack; some even claim to feel their best at that time. Others, however, complain of anorexia, nausea, indigestion, melancholia, stiffness, aching, polyuria and nocturia. These prodromata remain unexplained.

* A few crystals are evaporated with a drop of concentrated nitric acid, and the residue moistened with ammonia. The formation of a purple color indicates uric acid. This test is best performed in a porcelain dish.

Precipitating Factors. Considerable importance is generally attached to a number of factors said to precipitate attacks of arthritis in a patient with latent gout. Their true significance in relation to the disease has not been determined, and it is difficult to evaluate how often they are chance associations.

TRAUMA. Minor or major trauma has long been considered the most common precipitating factor. Ebstein[141] postulated that urate deposition secondary to trauma was dependent on the presence of tissue necrosis. The prevalent involvement of the joints of the large toes has been attributed to chronic strain on these articulations sustained in walking or from pressure of ill-fitting shoes. Many similar examples of injury as an antecedent to gouty arthritis can be cited. The precise role of trauma in gouty arthritis should be determined by exact experimental studies.

FOOD. The belief that certain foods are promotive of gouty arthritis is one of the oldest medical traditions and is still accepted by many competent clinicians. The proponents of this theory contend that the ingestion of purine-rich foods by the gouty subject results in an accumulation of uric acid in the blood, thus inducing an acute attack of gout. Habitual dietary excesses are considered predisposing factors, whereas periodic indulgence supposedly serves as a precipitating factor.[120] It has been found, however, that most gouty subjects do not show an adverse response to occasional excess purine feedings and that in well controlled studies covering an extended period, the frequency of seizures does not vary in alternating intervals of high and low purine intake.[142] The incidence of gout among vegetarians is much higher than is generally assumed.[119]

The natural course of the disease is characterized by very sudden changes in an erratic, unpredictable pattern. The temptation to both patient and physician to fasten the responsibility for these to some tangible factor is great, but the evidence quoted here should caution us against accepting as verified the influence of dietary habits on the development and progress of gout.

It has also been stated that certain foods, regardless of their purine content, are capable of producing attacks regularly in some gouty patients, supposedly as an allergic manifestation. A specific brand of cheese or wine or a particular kind of fruit or vegetable has been held responsible. We have not made similar observations. Attacks have been observed subsequent to the institution of a ketogenic or high fat diet. Lockie[143] proposed that the latter be used as a provocative test. Others[144,145] have not found it successful as such.

ALCOHOL. Some clinicians consider ingestion of alcohol the most important of all precipitating factors. Fermented beverages are thought to be much more provocative than distilled liquors. Attempts have even been made to relate the incidence of gout in a given community to the type of alcoholic beverage prevalently consumed. Others hold the mode of use a significant circumstance, considering that people who overindulge in meat habitually partake of red wine and malt liquors, and therefore sustain the combined effect of two inciting agents. All are agreed that certain gouty individuals fare sumptuously with some regularity and that some of their attacks follow dietary and alcoholic indiscretions. However, this sequence more often does not exist, even in the same patient. One subject experienced but two attacks in twenty years, although his debaucheries continued throughout the symptom-free interval. Another suffered ten attacks in ten years during middle life and none during the subsequent fifteen years, while his habits of eating and drinking remained unchanged. Instances like these are by no means exceptional and serve to emphasize that the instrumentality of alcohol in precipitating gouty arthritis is unproved. Actually, chronic alcoholics[140] have been said to show no higher and teetotalers no lower than the average incidence. Only the collection of accurate data from a significant number of cases will give us the final answer.

MEDICINAL PREPARATIONS. The sudden withdrawal of ACTH or cortisone may precipitate an attack of gouty arthritis.[146] Attacks are said to have followed the administration of liver extract intramuscularly, of Salyrgan, ergotamine tartrate, insulin, decholin, thiamine chloride and other medicinal agents. The case reports are too sparse to allow a conclusion as to cause and effect.

OPERATIONS. Hench[147] has repeatedly stressed that gouty arthritis should be suspected when arthritis occurs during the first seven days following a surgical procedure. Talbott[148] has reviewed the records of eighteen untreated gouty patients on whom thirty-four surgical operations had been performed. He reports an incidence of postoperative gouty arthritis in 86 per cent of the operations.

MISCELLANEOUS FACTORS. Coincidental diseases such as leukemia, polycythemia and chronic glomerular nephritis, as well as marked blood loss and transfusions, are said to have activated latent gout. Severe purgation, foreign protein therapy, exposure to cold and dampness and emotional upsets have been accused of producing attacks.

Diagnosis. CLINICAL DIAGNOSIS. The diagnosis of joint disease is relatively easy, in most instances, when based upon a detailed medical history and a complete physical examination. A few well chosen laboratory tests or a therapeutic trial with specific medication are often valuable adjuncts. Biopsy may be necessary. The passage of time and further observation are indispensable.

A history of recurrent attacks of acute arthritis spaced by completely asymptomatic intervals should always suggest a diagnosis of gout, particularly in a middle-aged male. Provided the presence of the disease is suspected, confirmation in most instances is relatively simple. The abrupt onset of severe articular pain, usually without known cause, followed rapidly by a red, hot swelling of the joint, extending beyond the articular margins, is of great diagnostic significance, especially in a first attack. Additional aids are a positive family history, positive identification of tophi and the occurrence of cuticular desquamation as the edema subsides, a finding highly characteristic of gouty arthritis. The dramatic response to full doses of colchicine, rarely, if ever, observed in any other types of arthritis, is of real diagnostic significance. However, failure to improve following adequate treatment with colchicine has been observed in a few cases of proved gout and does not therefore rule out the diagnosis of gout.

LABORATORY FINDINGS. Our experience with gout has led us to conclude that hyperuricemia is an almost invariable if not constant feature of the disease. Its presence, therefore, if not attributable to other causes, constitutes evidence of prime importance. We have rarely found serum uric acid values lower than 6 mg. per cent. In the few exceptions (less than 2 per cent) they varied between 5.2 and 5.8 mg. per cent. Normal or low serum uric acid values are of no diagnostic significance if the patient has received recent treatment with salicylates, ACTH, adrenal corticoids or Benemid, since these drugs are capable of reducing hyperuricemia to normal levels.

For the determination of uric acid, we use either one of the two most commonly employed methods, that of Folin[11] or that of Benedict.[12] Some workers prefer more recent modifications of these procedures.[149,150] All these methods depend upon reduction of complex tungstate reagents to colored compounds. This reaction is not strictly specific for uric acid and may be enhanced or inhibited by unrelated substances present in the blood. While neither test offers undue technical difficulties, only the use of carefully prepared and fresh reagents and frequent control of determinations assure reliable results. The use of serum is preferable to that of whole blood. Since the distribution of urates between plasma and red cells is a function of the bicarbonate, it has been suggested[132] that specimens should be collected and centrifuged under oil. In our experience this precaution has proved unnecessary since the variations that occur because of loss of carbon dioxide are insignificant compared with the unavoidable errors involved in the determination of uric acid. Folin's[151] method for unlaked whole blood is free from the objections to other whole blood methods, but since it is doubtful whether diffusion of urates from the cells is ever complete, the method should not be used if sufficient blood can be obtained for a determination on serum. Blauch and Koch[152] determined the uric acid content of normal whole blood with the aid of the specific enzyme, uricase, and found values ranging from 1.04 to 3.83 mg. per cent. Others[153,154] have modified this procedure and adapted it to the use of serum. These methods correct for the error due to non-uric acid reducing substances. However, they give low values since they do not eliminate the loss of uric acid which invariably occurs during the precipitation of proteins. Because they depend on a colorimetric procedure, they are, like other methods, affected by various substances which inhibit or enhance the formation of color. We see little reason for the routine use of uricase methods on serum, since in this case the nonspecific color formation is insignificant, usually corresponding to less than 0.5 mg. per cent of uric acid. Recently a procedure has been devised based on the change of the absorption of ultraviolet light in a sample that is acted upon by uricase.[155] In principle this procedure is free from the inherent errors of the usual colorimetric procedures but, unfortunately, it is limited essentially to the research laboratory. From these considerations it will be immediately apparent that one cannot interpret serum uric acid values correctly unless the standard for each method used has been established by a sufficient number of determinations on normals. Comparison of the values obtained in different laboratories has shown wide discrepancies which may partially be accounted for in this manner.

We have had an opportunity to analyze the synovial fluid from numerous effusions in gouty arthritis. The detailed findings in twenty-three cases, compared to normal values[156] are given in Table 1. Urate crystals are occasionally observed in synovial fluids of patients with gout, but the infrequency of this observation is such that it seldom provides diagnostic assistance.

Patients with acute gouty arthritis generally have a mild to moderate leukocytosis. The mononuclear count is frequently increased. The sedimentation rate may be elevated and frequently remains high in the intervals between attacks. In several cases, we have seen rates as high as 2 mm. per minute (the upper limit of normal for the method we employ being 0.4 mm. per minute).[157] Evidence of mild renal impairment is commonly met. Achlorhydria occurs no more frequently in gouty patients than in other persons. An abnormal sugar tolerance curve, occasionally present, is of no diagnostic significance, but may indicate coincidental diabetes mellitus.

ROENTGENOLOGIC FINDINGS. The roentgenographic findings most suggestive of gout are well defined, punched-out areas, usually 5 mm. or more in diame-

TABLE 1. SYNOVIAL FLUID IN GOUTY ARTHRITIS

	NORMAL			GOUT		
	Average	Low	High	Average	Low	High
Leukocytes, per cu. mm.	63	13	180	13,317	1000	70,600
Polymorphonuclears, per cent	7	0	25	71	0	99
Relative viscosity	235	5.7	1160	17	2	68
Protein, gm./100 cc.	1.72	1.07	2.13	4.18	2.82	5.02
Globulin, gm./100 cc.	.05	......	....	1.54	.92	2.13
Mucin nitrogen, gm./100 cc.	.104	.068	.135	.058	.002	.099
Mucin glucosamine, gm./100 cc.	.087	.050	.132	.040	.006	.070
Sugar, mg./100 cc.	Essentially same as in serum			86	15	113
Uric acid	Essentially same as in serum			Essentially same as in serum		

Number of effusions 23
Number of patients 18

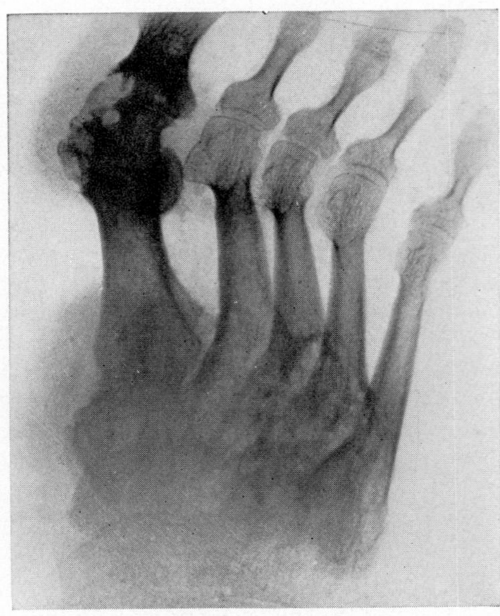

FIG. 13. Characteristic punched-out areas seen in the bones of the first metatarsophalangeal joint.

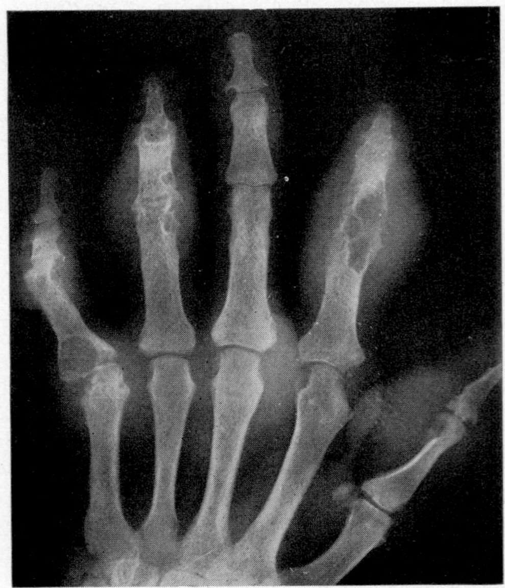

FIG. 14. Extensive destruction of the phalangeal and metacarpophalangeal joints of a patient suffering from chronic gouty arthritis.

ter; they are commonly observed in the subchondral bone at the bases or head of the phalanges. In contrast to rheumatoid arthritis, the bones surrounding these areas are usually of normal density (Figs. 13 and 14). Lesions similar to those seen in gout may be produced by gummata of syphilis, by leprosy and yaws, as well as by tuberculosis and Boeck's sarcoid. The occurrence of these lesions in gout is more directly related to the severity of the disease than to its duration. Thus, in 19 per cent of one series,[158] patients with gout for twenty-eight years or longer exhibiting tophi and hyperuricemia failed to show subchondral lesions radiographically. The lesions are often seen in joints which have never been involved clinically. This is especially apt to be true in the feet, but it may also be true in other joints, such as the sacroiliacs (Fig. 15). Occasionally tophaceous deposits result in bone expansion (Fig. 16) or bone expansion and destruction (Fig. 17), thus simulating, roentgenographically, a bone tumor. In addition to such abnormalities, one may find soft tissue

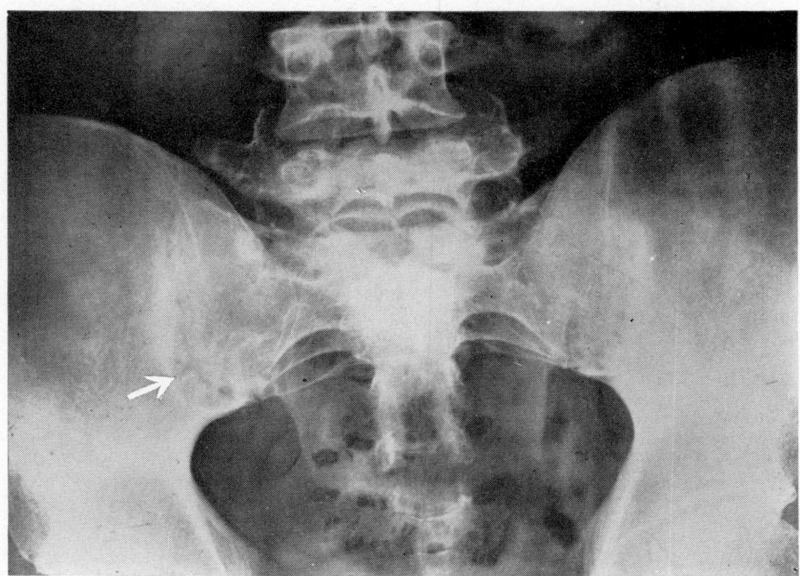

FIG. 15. The punched-out areas in the region of the sacro-iliac joints of this roentgenogram, indicated by the arrow, are due to urate deposition.

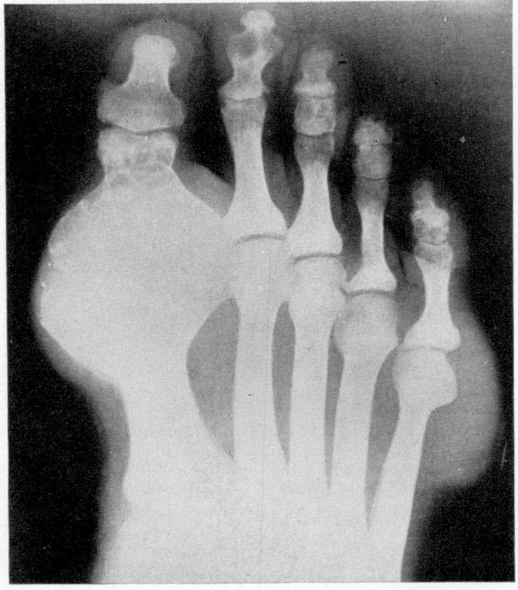

FIG. 16. In this instance urate deposits caused expansion of the bones of the first metatarsophalangeal joint, thus giving the appearance of a bone tumor.

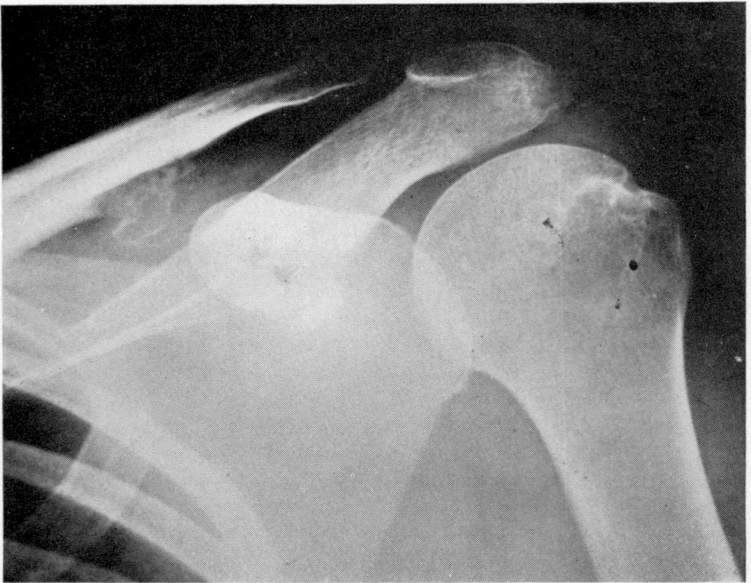

FIG. 17. Destruction of the cortex of the clavicle due to urate deposition. The mass of extruded material is clearly illustrated.

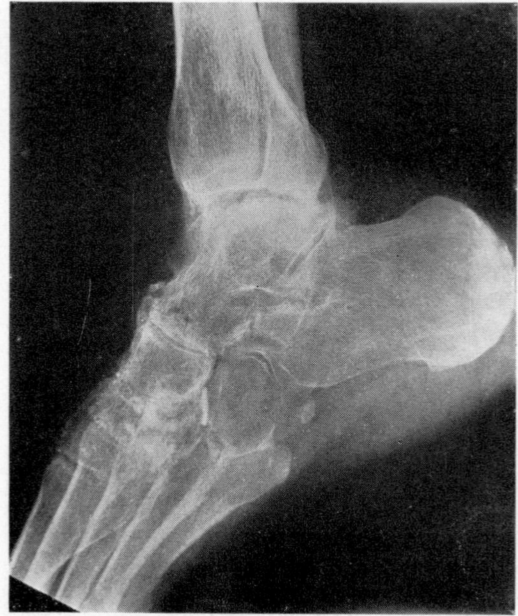

FIG. 18. Lateral view of a foot, showing marked decalcification, destruction of the joint spaces and ankylosis. This patient had widespread ankylosis at the age of twenty-eight years.

thickening often extending far beyond the affected joint, joint narrowing, conspicuous marginal overgrowth of bone and marked destruction of the articulating surfaces.

Decalcification is rarely seen except in patients who have suffered prolonged severe attacks involving the small joints of the feet and wrists. In these exceptional instances, the marked decalcification, joint destruction and obvious ankylosis closely approximate the changes seen in specific infections or rheumatoid arthritis (Figs. 18 and 19). Premature arteriosclerosis is frequently demonstrable in the vessels of the legs and feet.

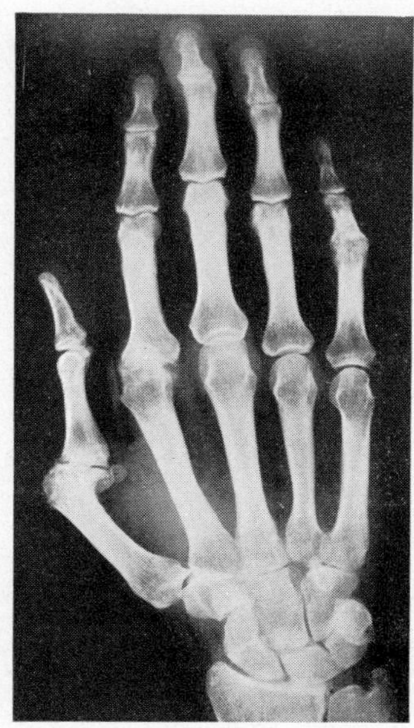

FIG. 19. Hand of the patient referred to in the legend of Fig. 18. The phalangeal joints are narrowed. The midphalangeal joint of the little finger is fused. There is obvious destruction of the metacarpophalangeal joints of the first and second fingers.

Although the x-ray findings in gouty arthritis are characteristic and consistent, they cannot be considered specific. The roentgenologist's impression should therefore be taken only as corroboration of a clinical diagnosis.

DIFFERENTIAL DIAGNOSIS. Occasionally gouty arthritis may be confused with traumatic joint disease, cellulitis, rheumatic fever, one of the specific infectious arthritides, rheumatoid arthritis, Heberden's nodes and acute bursitis, particularly when the latter is associated with a hallux valgus deformity.

Traumatic arthritis is as a rule readily diagnosed. Articular pain and swelling follow almost immediately upon a known injury. Marked inflammatory reaction of the periarticular tissue is not discernible and the symptoms always remain confined to the affected joint. The patient exhibits none of the characteristics of the gouty person, and his arthritis never responds to colchicine therapy. However, it should be remembered that trauma may mark the onset of acute gouty arthritis as well as of infectious arthritis. In such cases differentiation is greatly aided by aspiration and analysis of the joint fluid. An acute traumatic effusion contains rarely more than 1000 leukocytes per cubic millimeter with polymorphonuclears ranging from 0 to 20 per cent, in contrast to the higher values usually found in the other acute arthritides.[159]

Cellulitis or septic inflammation is frequently suspected; in fact, sometimes it is diagnosed before it becomes evident that one is actually dealing with acute gouty arthritis. Occasionally, the affected joints have been incised and drained. One can readily appreciate the diagnostic difficulties offered by a patient who presents himself with a painful, red, hot swelling of the dorsum of the hand or foot with or without lymphangitis and fever. Failure to find a skin abrasion or other portal of entry for an invading organism and careful elucidation of the past history will generally lead to the correct diagnosis.

Rheumatic fever, especially in younger individuals, can be simulated by recurrent attacks of gouty arthritis as in the following case history. A young man of nineteen years entered the hospital with a provisional diagnosis of rheumatic fever. At the age of nine he suffered from a hip affliction which was considered tuberculous in origin and was treated by immobilization in plaster casts. Between the ages of fourteen and nineteen he experienced numerous attacks of polyarthritis, migratory in nature, accompanied by fever. They were always followed by complete recovery and diagnosed rheumatic fever, although he did not develop endocarditis. When first seen by us, he had a blood uric acid level of 9.2 mg. per 100 cc. Since then the fasting serum values have varied between 12.3 and 14.8 mg. per 100 cc. and he has developed tophi. Undoubtedly a good many similar cases of juvenile gout are mislabeled rheumatic

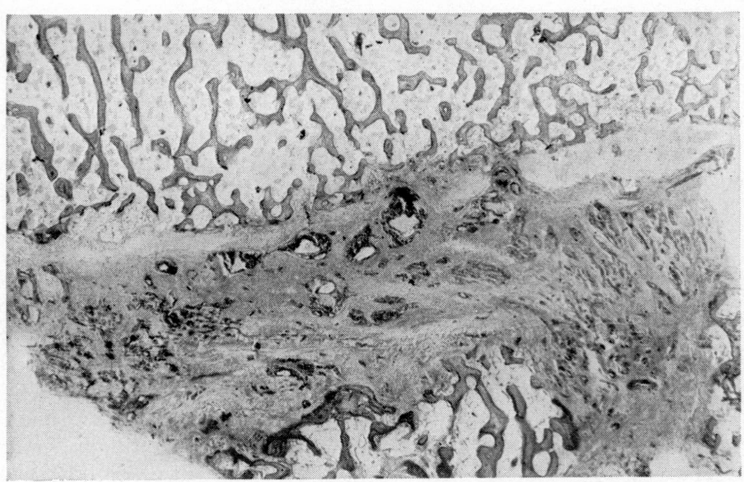

FIG. 20. Fibrous ankylosis of the astragalotibial joint (low magnification, × 10). A few small strips of eroded articular cartilage adjacent to the astragalus remain. The numerous light areas in the connective tissue are deposits of monosodium urate, surrounded by zones of marked chronic inflammation.

fever. The clinical differentiation, however, should not be difficult. The arthritis or rheumatic fever usually follows an upper respiratory infection or other precipitating factor by seven to fourteen days. Patients frequently exhibit weight loss, nosebleeds, skin eruptions, subcutaneous nodules, tachycardia and precordial pain. The electrocardiogram often shows a prolonged P-R interval and other alterations. The ultimate development of valvular heart disease is of the utmost diagnostic importance.

Specific infectious arthritis, due to a pyogenic organism, in the acute phase more nearly resembles acute gouty arthritis than does any other type of joint disease, particularly since it may occasionally be recurrent. In such instances, usually caused by the gonococcus, the clinical picture may show some similarity to that of gout, as in the case of a patient who entered the hospital suffering from his eighth attack of arthritis. He stated that recovery from the previous seven seizures had been complete. Differentiation was facilitated by a history of genitourinary infection and such constitutional symptoms as chills and fever preceding in close parallelism every exacerbation of arthritis. It was confirmed by the finding of the organism in prostatic smear. Although the inflammatory swelling of specific infectious arthritis may be severe, it rarely is as marked or occurs as precipitously as in gouty arthritis. The duration of the gouty attack is usually much shorter than that of infectious arthritis of equal severity, and it is almost never accompanied by chills. Fever, if present, does not usually last longer than two or three days. Particularly with the aid of synovial fluid findings, one should not encounter serious diagnostic difficulties.

Typical *rheumatoid arthritis,* ushered in by constitutional, vasomotor and neurologic symptoms of insidious onset and characterized by symmetrical joint involvement, should rarely if ever be mistaken for gouty arthritis. However, in 18 per cent of all cases, rheumatoid arthritis is marked by an atypical onset and in 7 per cent it may remain atypical for a long time. In this form, an apparently healthy person experiences an acute attack of arthritis without prodromata, preceding acute illness or obvious focus of infection. The joint involvement may be polyarticular, migratory or occasionally monarticular. Recovery from the first attack is often complete and the remission may last for a few months or even years. The patient may have a number of attacks before the disease becomes chronic. Careful clinical observations and determination of the blood uric acid concentration will facilitate the distinction between the two diseases.

The clinical features of chronic gouty arthritis with ankylosis may resemble those of rheumatoid arthritis even more closely. We have seen two such cases, in a relatively early stage of the disease, and others have been reported.[160,161] In one[162] the onset of gout at twenty-one years of age was followed by chronic arthritis within five years. Widespread ankylosis was demonstrable at the age of twenty-eight. The diagnosis of gout was confirmed by the identification of sodium urate crystals in tophi of the ear, in the finger, the olecranon bursa and the tissues of four joints examined. Of particular interest were the findings in the astragalotibial joint. Extensive pannus formation, responsible for complete fibrous ankylosis, simulated strikingly the gross pathologic changes of rheumatoid arthritis. Even the microscopic appearance of the synovial tissues might have been difficult to distinguish from that of rheumatoid arthritis except for innumerable small urate foci (Figs. 20 and 21). Such unusual forms of gouty arthritis are admittedly rare. They should not be confused with rheumatoid arthritis. Clinical differentiation is greatly aided by painstaking inquiry into the past and family histories. Biopsies of nodules, tophi and synovial tissue will often ascertain the correct diagnosis. Synovial fluid analysis may or may not help to distinguish one from the other. Association of the two diseases is ex-

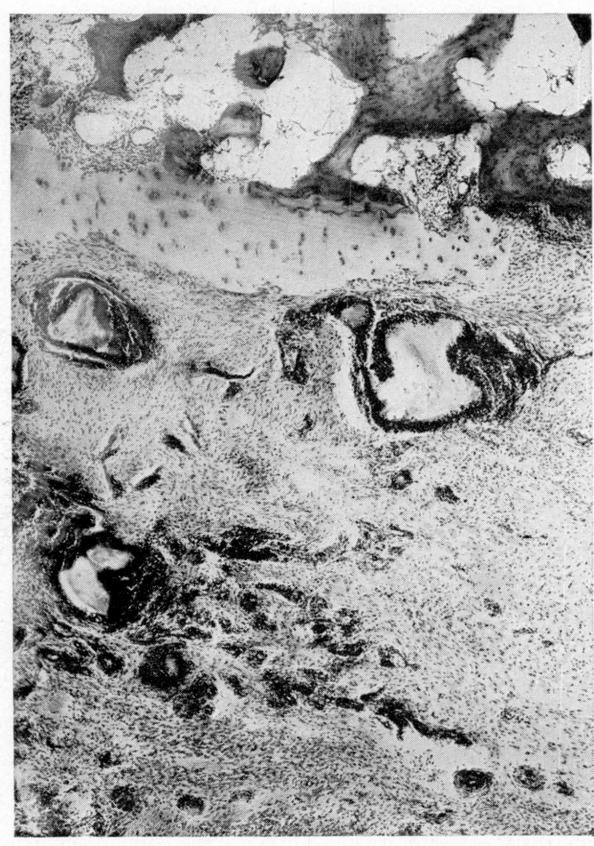

FIG. 21. High power photomicrograph of an area of the section illustrated in Fig. 20, showing invasion and destruction of articular cartilage of urate-containing fibrous tissue which has extended into subchondral bone spaces.

tremely rare. A few cases have been reported, but we know of no authenticated instance.

Bursitis, particularly as a manifestation of a hallux vulgus deformity, has probably been mislabeled gouty arthritis on innumerable occasions. This diagnostic error can be avoided if the affected part is carefully examined. In bursitis, the swelling is limited to the bursa and the immediately adjacent tissue, and the distended sac may be easily palpated. The metatarsophalangeal joint motions are painless within a limited range.

Heberden's nodes, classic stigmata of degenerative joint disease, consist of hypertrophic osseous changes at the articular margins of the terminal interphalangeal joints. They are insidious in development, not usually productive of severe symptoms, and may readily be differentiated from tophaceous deposits in the skin and deeper tissues surrounding these joints. Occasionally, however, Heberden's nodes are acute in onset and have then frequently been confused with gouty arthritis. The distal finger joints may be painful, reddened, bulbous, fluctuant and extremely tender. Numbness and tingling of the involved fingers may also occur. Heberden's nodes occur predominantly in women and affect the index and middle fingers more often than the other phalanges. Tophi are much more common in males and are discernible by their yellowish color. It is well known, of course, that the two disorders may be associated coincidentally or casually.

Complications. CARDIOVASCULAR LESIONS. Premature vascular disease and the anatomic and physiologic alterations resulting therefrom constitute the important complications of gout. Some authors contend that "the gout is to the arteries as the rheumatism is to the heart."[163] Others opine that "gout has nothing to do with arteriosclerosis,"[164] and that hypertension is a chance finding. Actually, the incidence of arteriosclerosis and hypertension is higher in gouty subjects than in a control group of comparable age.[165–168] Hypertension is usually a late manifestation. The triad of arteriosclerosis, nephrosclerosis and increased arterial tension frequently leads to hypertrophy of the left ventricle. Extensive coronary and cerebral vascular disease may be the immediate cause of death. Terminal pericarditis has been reported. Some of the older writers[140,169] have stressed the high incidence of venous thrombosis, a finding which has been rare in our observation.

RENAL DISEASE. The majority of gouty patients die from uremia. There are a number of ways in which gout may lead to renal disease.[170] The incidence of urinary calculi in gouty subjects is relatively high, amounting to 12 per cent in Hench's series.[158] An occasional patient may experience one or more bouts of renal colic prior to the first gouty seizure. More frequently, this complication develops in patients with long-standing disease. Deposition of urates in the walls of the collecting tubules and the renal pelvis is frequently seen. Urinary obstruction by these deposits or by stones predisposes to pyelonephritis, which in turn may increase the tendency to renal lithiasis. Diffuse infiltration of the renal parenchyma with urates is often observed; this is discussed more fully in the section on pathology. Finally, the patients with gout exhibit an increased tendency to vascular sclerosis (see above). Involvement of the renal vasculature is one of the most important causes of renal impairment in these patients.

Some writers have suggested that secondary gout may be caused by chronic renal disease. From our experiences we have concluded that such instances represent latent gout complicated by renal disease. In establishing the presence of a causal relationship between clinical gout and an underlying disease which may be manifested by hyperuricemia, it is important to obtain a detailed family history and if possible blood uric acid determination on the patient's relatives.

It was assumed at one time that gout was prevalent among lead workers; hence the term, saturnine gout. It, too, was considered an example of gout secondary to renal disease due, in this instance, to the vascular nephritis of plumbism. Although gout is more rarely a complication of lead poisoning than was previously assumed,[171] it may of course be associated by chance with the vascular nephritis of plumbism. Other types of arthritis occurring in a patient with hyperuricemia due to renal damage from lead poisoning may in the past also have been erroneously diagnosed as gout.

PATHOLOGY

Although our knowledge of the pathogenesis of gout is incomplete, it appears well established that the pathologic manifestations of the disease are dependent upon the deposition of sodium urate in various tissues and the inflammatory and degenerative changes resulting therefrom. The urate deposits surrounded by tissue exhibiting inflammatory and foreign body reactions constitute the one pathognomonic lesion of the disease and are readily demonstrated, provided that the tissues to be examined are properly fixed and stained.[*172] For a long time this may be the only discernible lesion. Many of the anatomic alterations observed in the late stages of gout are the result of the ill-understood arterial and arteriolar sclerosis which frequently manifest themselves as the disease advances.

The local tissue changes which make possible the precipitation of uric acid in the form of sodium urate are unknown. Deposition of urates is much more prone to occur in relatively avascular structures. Ebstein[141] insisted that, irrespective of the tissues affected, a previous injury or tissue necrosis was a prerequisite. This theory has a certain appeal, but since no histologic studies are available demonstrating the earliest changes in an acute attack, it can be neither proved nor disproved. There is equally good reason for assuming that uric acid is deposited in normal tissues and that the necrosis seen is a secondary phenomenon. The reaction of the tissues to urate deposition is extremely variable. When it occurs in the soft tissues, an acute inflammatory reaction of the severest grade usually results, yet marked precipitation in the cartilaginous structures of joints, ears and nose may take place unknown to the patient. Such a reaction is sometimes followed by the appearance of a visible tophus; in other cases the offending urates may be completely absorbed. Again, we are without a satisfactory explanation for these differences, although they are probably accounted for by the amount of uric acid set free in the tissue and the vascularity of the part affected.

The Gouty Joint. Urate deposits in the articular structures are the cause of the most frequent disability resulting from gout. Postmortem studies have demonstrated that the articular cartilages are the most common and at times the exclusive sites of urate deposition. The accumulations are always much more pronounced in the central avascular part than in the more vascular joint margins. An affected joint surface appears as though it has been imperfectly coated with white lacquer or a mortar-like material (Fig. 22). The extent of the articular surface deposit varies greatly from joint to joint. In some it is confined to irregularly placed, small white specks and streaks; in others, a considerable portion of the articular cartilage is covered by large white plaques.

No joint is exempt, although certain ones are more frequently involved,[160,173,174] for instance, the joints of the lower extremities, as compared to those of the arms. The metatarsophalangeal joints of the great toes are more regularly involved and may be the only site. Next in order of frequency are the small joints of the feet, the ankles, hands and wrists. The knees, elbows, shoulders and hips are less commonly involved; occasionally urate deposits may be found in the sacroiliac and the sternoclavicular joints, and in the articulations of the spine, jaw and larynx. Massive deposits of urates are not infrequently encountered in joints which have never been the site of acute gouty arthritis.

* The fresh tissue should be fixed immediately in absolute alcohol and later stained according to the method of de Galantha.

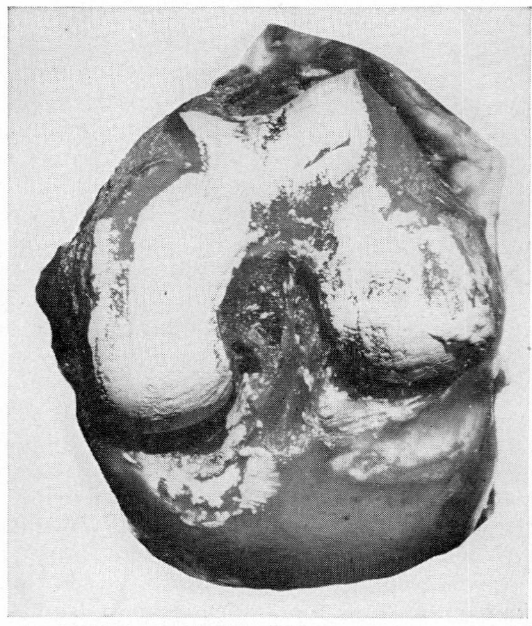

FIG. 22. Extensive urate deposition in the articular cartilage of the femur and the synovial membrane of the knee joint. One further notes degenerative changes of the cartilage and secondary marginal overgrowth at the perichondrial margins. (This specimen was prepared by Dr. S. B. Wolbach for the Warren Museum, Harvard Medical School.)

Conversely, deposits may not be found in the tissues of a joint which has been subjected to recurrent attacks of acute gouty arthritis.

GROSS EXAMINATION of a joint which is the site of urate deposition may reveal no changes other than the presence of the urates. Often, however, in chronic gout the affected joints are enlarged and grossly deformed because of extensive tophaceous deposits and bony destruction (Figs. 8 and 9). In such instances urates may be demonstrable in the articular cartilage, perichondrium, ligaments, synovialis and such periarticular structures as tendons, bursae, bone marrow, subcutaneous tissues or even the overlying skin. Practically all specimens in this phase show the gross characteristics of degenerative joint disease, including marginal overgrowths or exostoses to a more marked degree than is ordinarily seen at a corresponding age.[162] The synovial membrane usually presents only minimal changes, although urate deposition may be sufficiently marked to cause extensive proliferation and fibrous tissue ankylosis. Even bony union may ensue, but such severe changes are rare and generally confined to the smaller articulations.

MICROSCOPIC EXAMINATION. Microscopic examination discloses that the urate deposits in cartilage, although superficial, are actually embedded in the intercellular matrix. They are almost always confined to the upper layers of cartilage, although they occasionally extend into bone. On the articular surface, the urate deposits appear as a coating of amorphous material (Fig. 23). This is most dense near the joint cavity and grows progressively thinner as it penetrates into the middle or lower portion of the cartilage. Where the deposit is most sparse, the characteristic acidular crystals are seen most often (Fig. 24). The reaction of cartilage to the infiltration is directly proportional to the amount of urate present. Microscopic examination of cartilage strips from which the urates have been dissolved shows profound alterations in those portions of the matrix where urate deposition had been heaviest. Little or no reaction is discernible in the areas which contain only minute foci. When urates are present in large amounts, one finds cartilage changes such as pits, depressions, fissures, crevices and thinning of a more severe grade than is compatible with the age of the subject.[162] In addition, one notes diminution in number, scattering and clumping of the cartilage cells.

The striking predilection of urate deposits for articular cartilage rather than other body tissues remains unexplained. They occur most often in the avascular central area, which derives a portion if not all of its nourishment from synovial fluid. The latter normally, as well as in gout, contains the same amount of urate as the blood plasma. Urates, being freely diffusible, undoubtedly gain access to normal cartilages as do other freely diffusable constituents of synovial fluid. In the gouty subject an excess of urates is thus made available to cartilage. The prevalence of urate crystals in some joints and their complete absence in others cannot be explained adequately and indicate that factors other than an increased urate concentration must be operative.

Urate deposits in the synovial mem-

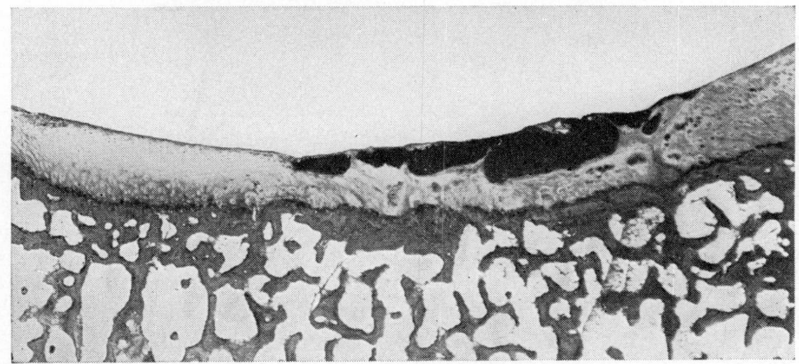

FIG. 23. A photomicrograph (×60) of the phalangeal side of a first metatarsophalangeal joint. One observes a heavy deposit of urates in the upper half of the articular cartilage associated with marked degenerative changes.

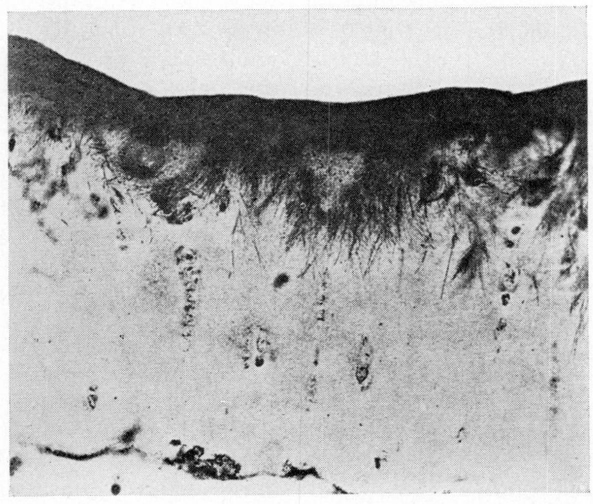

FIG. 24. Heavy precipitation of urates in the upper third of the articular cartilage. In the deepest portion the characteristic sheaths of urate crystals are clearly shown. (A. M. Brogsitter's monograph, Histopathologie der Gelenk-Gicht, 1927, F. C. W. Vogel, Leipzig.)

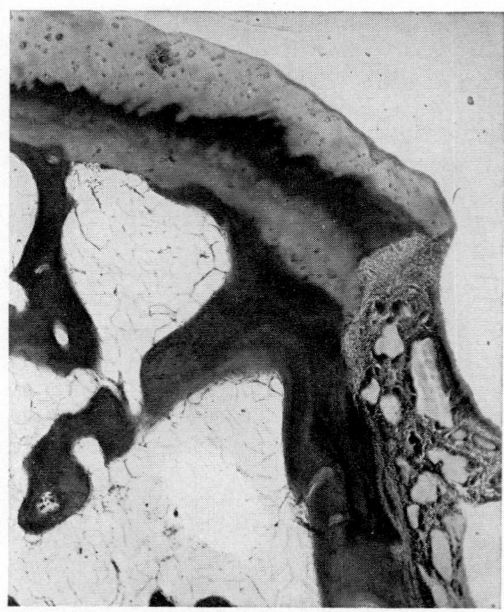

FIG. 25. Characteristic foreign body reaction accompanying urate deposition in the synovial tissue at the perichondrial margin of a finger joint. It has resulted in pannus formation which has extended onto the articular cartilage surface. (× 60.)

brane and capsular tissue are presumed to cause the nonspecific, inflammatory reaction which characterizes the acute stage of gouty arthritis. Failures, reported in the past, to demonstrate the foreign substance in the soft articular tissues may have been due to improper fixation and staining. In appropriately prepared material, obtained from a joint which has been subjected to repeated attacks, the crystals are easily recognized microscopically. The lesion consists of a central mass of urates, often amorphous in appearance, embedded in vascular granulation tissue. Crystals, enmeshed in interstitium, are more readily seen in the smaller foci. Older urate deposits may be surrounded by a relatively avascular fibrous tissue capsule. In their immediate neighborhood, one finds mononuclear phagocytes, giant cells, polymorphonuclear leukocytes, eosinophils and plasma cells. Focal areas of lymphocytes are numerous, and vascular sclerosis is frequently seen.[160,162] Heavy precipitates in the synovial lining and subsynovial tissues result in marked proliferative activity, and occasionally in the formation of a pannus which spreads onto the articular surfaces and may envelop them completely. In consequence, there result invasion and destruction of cartilage (Fig. 25) which in some instances lead to fibrous and/or bony ankylosis (Figs. 20, 21).

Extra-articular Pathology. The term tophus (chalk stone or concretion) has through general usage come to denote urate deposits in tissues other than joints. They are most commonly seen in the helix or antihelix of the ears, the olecranon and patellar bursae, the tendons of fingers, hands, wrists, toes, feet, ankles and heels (Figs. 26, 27). Less frequently they are met in the skin of the palms and soles, the tarsal plates of the eyelids, the nasal cartilages, the finger tips, the tendinous expansion of muscles and in the cornea and sclerotic coats of the eye.[175] The kidneys may also be the seat of urate precipitates. Very rarely deposits have been found in the corpus cavernosum and prepuce of the penis,[169] the aorta, myocardium and aortic valves, the tongue,[176] epiglottis, vocal cords and the arytenoid cartilages. Occasionally the crystals have been recovered from the sputum of gouty sub-

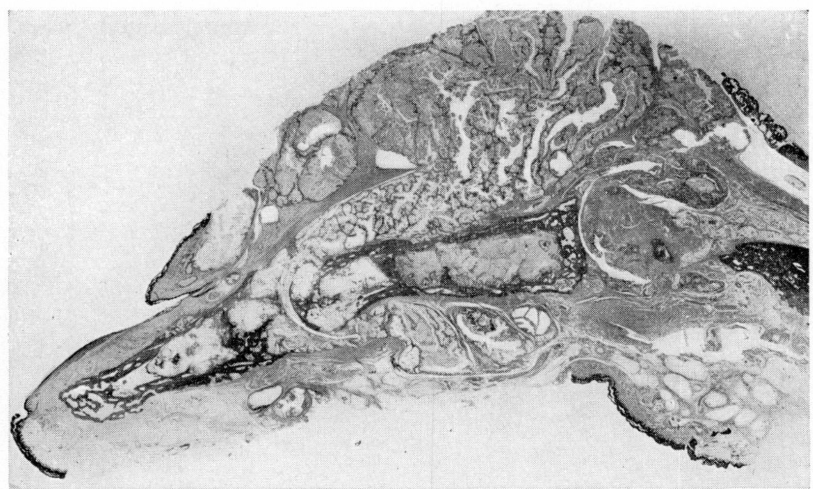

FIG. 26. Microscopic section through an index finger, showing extensive tophaceous deposits which have largely replaced the bony structures and the adjacent subcutaneous tissue. In this instance protrusion of the chalky urate material had taken place.

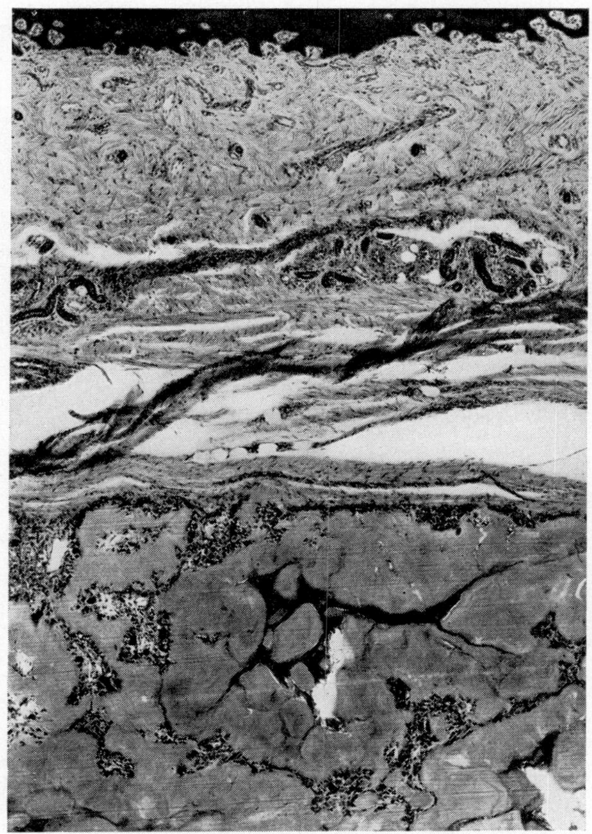

FIG. 27. Section through the tophaceous deposit in the subcutaneous tissues of the finger illustrated in Fig. 26. The large masses of urates are surrounded by small connective tissue septa which contain foreign body giant cells and chronic inflammatory cells. ($\times 60$.)

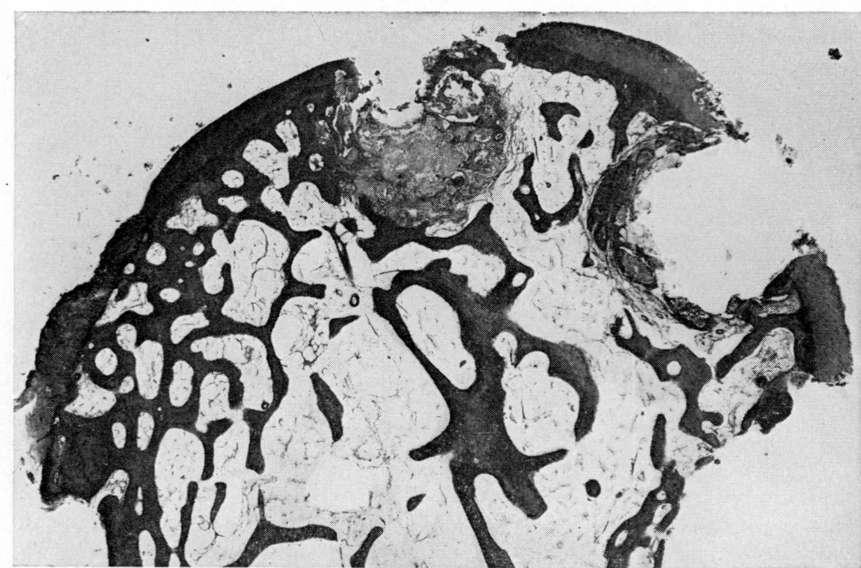

FIG. 28. Proximal phalanx of a finger. The surface of the articular cartilage is frayed and uneven. There is cartilaginous and bony overgrowth (lipping) at the articular margins. The two large circular defects (punched-out areas) in the articular cartilage and subchondral bone were lined with fibrous tissue infiltrated with large numbers of inflammatory cells and studded with numerous masses of sodium urate crystals. Isolated urate deposits were seen in the bone marrow of this phalanx. (× 20.)

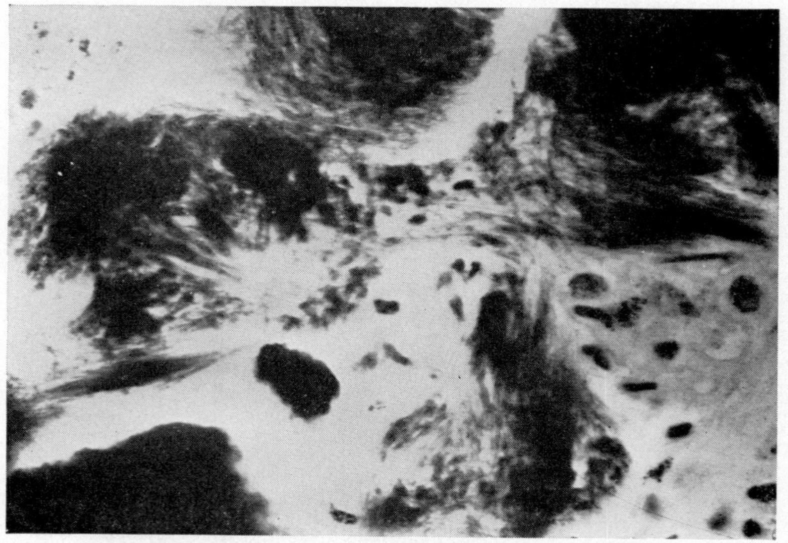

FIG. 29. Showing acicular urate crystals in tophaceous deposits. This section was taken from a subcutaneous nodule and stained by the de Galantha method. (× 900.)

jects.[169] Isolated reports of urates in the central nervous system and its coverings have not been verified. Such extra-articular deposits are followed by the foreign body inflammatory reaction previously described and varying in extent and degree with the vascularity of the affected tissue. When present in the bone marrow, they may represent a direct extension of articular pannus containing uric acid foci or a primary deposition of urate.[160] In either instance they result in lacunar absorption of adjacent trabeculae and replacement of the marrow by fibrous tissue (Fig. 28). These tophaceous deposits consist of sodium urate, the crystals of which are readily demonstrable (Fig. 29).

KIDNEY LESIONS. The renal lesions observed in gout have been called gouty nephritis, gouty form of Bright's disease, interstitial or arteriosclerotic nephritis and renal impairment of gout. This varied terminology indicates that no unanimity of opinion has existed concerning the nature of these changes, but all authors are agreed that the incidence of kidney disease is higher in gout than in other chronic disorders (rheumatoid arthritis, diabetes mellitus and pernicious anemia). However, few, if any, would argue that anatomic alterations of the kidney can be demonstrated as the primary cause of gout.

Grossly, the kidneys are reduced in size, their capsules being moderately adherent to an irregular surface.[177,178] The cortex is diminished in thickness. The extent of such changes is proportional to the severity and duration of gout. Urate deposits may be seen on the cut surface of the kidney. They appear most commonly as punctate foci in the cortex or as long white streaks in the medulla, where they call forth the same type of inflammatory reaction as in other vascular tissue. Because of these inflammatory changes it is difficult to decide whether such urate deposits have originated in the interstitial tissue or in the collecting tubules.[178] Tubular blockage by small urate concretions may occur and, in turn, lead to both abscess formation and pyelonephritis. The glomeruli show varying degrees of fibrosis. Although glomerular nephritis may be present, it is probably unrelated to gout.[179] We agree with others[179,180] that the renal lesion incident to gout is primarily a vascular sclerosis similar to that seen in other portions of the vascular system. Indeed, generalized arterial and arteriolar sclerosis can readily be seen in many gouty patients at postmortem examinations.[181]

COMPARATIVE PATHOLOGY. A condition resembling chronic tophaceous gout is known to occur spontaneously in birds[182–185] and may be produced experimentally by prolonged and abundant feeding of protein,[182,186] by ligation of the ureters or by removing or poisoning the kidneys.[141,187,188] These procedures may result in blood uric acid levels as high as 400 mg. per cent. Under these conditions, urate deposition in the joint cartilages takes place and large tophi appear in the extremities. Urate precipitates may appear in practically all tissues. Acute attacks simulating those in human gout have not been described.

A disorder occurring in hogs is of particular interest because it constitutes the only known disturbance in intermediary purine catabolism. Virchow[189] and later Mendelson[190] described crystalline deposits resembling guanine in muscle and joints of pigs. This finding was confirmed by chemical analysis.[191] Pecile[192] discovered guanine in the urine of a "gouty" pig. Since this substance is not normally present,[193] it appears that inability to deaminize guanine accounts for this rare disorder. Nothing is known about the clinical appearance of these animals, since the various observations were made postmortem in the course of inspection for *Trichinella spiralis.*

TREATMENT OF ACUTE GOUTY ARTHRITIS

Although newer agents, singly or in conjunction with colchicine, have been used successfully in refractory cases, *colchicine* remains the most effective drug for the relief of acute attacks of gout in the majority of patients.[194] The probable chemical structure of this drug is shown in Figure 30.

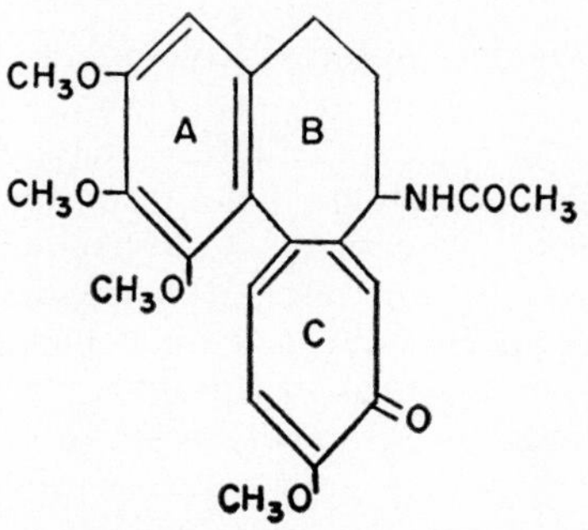

FIG. 30. Probable chemical structure of colchicine.

The mechanism of action of colchicine remains unknown. It is clearly not a uricosuric agent, since it influences neither the renal excretion of urate nor its serum concentration,[195] nor does it alter the magnitude of the miscible pool of uric acid.[196,197] It is not an analgesic. Its most striking pharmacologic property is that of altering nuclear mitosis at the metaphase. Although this usually requires large doses, it is notable that the dose of colcemid, a close derivative of colchicine which has been reported to be effective in the treatment of acute gouty arthritis, is approximately equal to the dose which, when given daily, has been shown to display a marked leukopenic effect in chronic leukemia. In view of the probable relationship of gout to nucleoprotein metabolism, at least by way of its end product, uric acid, it is tempting to speculate whether colchicine may not exert its benefit by way of an elusive effect on purine metabolism.

The chief use of colchicine is in the treatment of acute gouty arthritis. In most cases we recommend 0.5 mg. every hour for 5 doses, followed by 0.5 mg. every 2 hours until the patient experiences relief or until watery diarrhea, nausea or vomiting commences. For the diarrhea we then prescribe paregoric 5 cc. after each movement. The total required dose of colchicine rarely exceeds 12 mg. The patient usually begins to experience relief within 12 hours and the symptoms are largely gone in 24 to 72 hours. Once the optimal nontoxic dose has been established in a given patient, it can usually be repeated in slightly smaller doses for subsequent acute attacks without causing the above mentioned symptoms. Colchicine should always be used in pure (tablet) form, since the wine or tincture may deteriorate on standing. Tolerance does not develop to the drug. A course may be repeated in 48 hours, if necessary, but this is rarely indicated once proper interval treatment is instituted.

Colchicine has several uses in the less acute stages of gout. A dose of 0.5 or 1.0 mg. every 2 hours for 3 or 4 doses, taken upon the appearance of prodromal symptoms or the first twinges or articular pain, will frequently abort an attack. When acute attacks recur with considerable frequency, ingestion of 0.5 or 1.0 mg. nightly, or 0.5 or 1.0 mg. every 12 hours will often keep the patient symptom-free.[198] Toxic manifestations from long term use of this sort are seldom if ever encountered. A dose of 0.5 mg. t.i.d. for several days before and after surgery will greatly reduce the high postoperative incidence of acute attacks of gouty arthritis.

Colchicine, administered intravenously, has been reported to provide a safe, rapid and effective method of treatment of acute attacks of arthritis, without unpleasant gastrointestinal manifestations. A dose of 0.25 to 3 mg. in 1 to 3 cc. of normal saline is administered in a single injection followed by 0.5 mg. every 6 hours until pain subsides. The total should not exceed 4 mg. in 24 hours.

Colcemid (desacetylmethyl colchicine) is presently undergoing clinical trial. This alkaloid from the willow saffron (*Colchicum autumnale*) differs from colchicine structurally in the replacement of the acetyl by a methyl radical. Most extensively used in the treatment of chronic leukemias, it has been stated that this drug displays the clinical effects of colchicine in some patients with gout, without the undesirable side effects.[199,200] More recently, serious side effects have been encountered—notably suppression of blood elements—and the suitability of this drug for wide usage in the treatment of gout is subject to considerable question.

Phenylbutazone (3,5-dioxo-1,2-diphenyl-4-n-butyl-pyrazolidine, [Butazolidin]) is a cogener of aminopyrine and antipyrine. It is a potent analgesic and anti-inflammatory agent which, though nonspecific for gout, is very effective in the treatment of acute attacks.[201] An initial dose of 200 mg. every 4 to 6 hours for 1 day is recommended, followed by decreasing dosage, such as 200 mg. every 8 hours for 2 days, 200 mg. every 12 hours for 2 days, and 100 mg. every 12 hours for 2 days. Phenylbutazone has proved to be a highly effective therapeutic agent in many patients with severe acute gouty arthritis unresponsive to colchicine. Although, in contrast to colchicine, it is a potent uricosuric agent,[202,203,204] its mode of action in acute gouty arthritis is probably unrelated to this property. Because of the severe toxic effects of this drug[205] it should be employed only in those cases which cannot be managed by other means. Its use is contraindicated in patients with peptic ulcer and other gastrointestinal diseases, varicose ulcers, liver, kidney and heart disease and severe hypertension, and it should be discontinued at once if a skin rash appears. It should never be used as a uricosuric agent for months on end.

ACTH and corticoid therapy. In patients with acute gouty arthritis who fail to respond to colchicine or Butazolidin, it may prove helpful to give ACTH, in an initial dose of 50 mg. intramuscularly every 6 hours, followed by decreasing doses over a 5-day period.[198] Comparable intravenous therapy can also be employed. It is usually advisable to give, in addition, colchicine 0.5 mg. two to four times daily to lessen the chance of a flare-up following cessation of ACTH. Cortisone is thought to be less effective than ACTH, perhaps because inadequate doses have been used. With the introduction of prednisone and other of the newer corticoids, which can be given in large doses if necessary, it is probable that ACTH therapy will seldom be indicated in gouty patients.

TREATMENT OF CHRONIC GOUT

Experience of recent years has confirmed the fact that adequate therapy with uricosuric agents will prevent the most distressing ravages of chronic gouty arthritis. The most effective uricosuric agent is probenecid (Benemid). This agent was introduced in the treatment of gout by Gutman[206] following the observation of Wolfson that caronamide exerted a uricosuric effect[207] (Figs. 31 and 32). It acts by inhibiting the reabsorption of uric acid by the renal

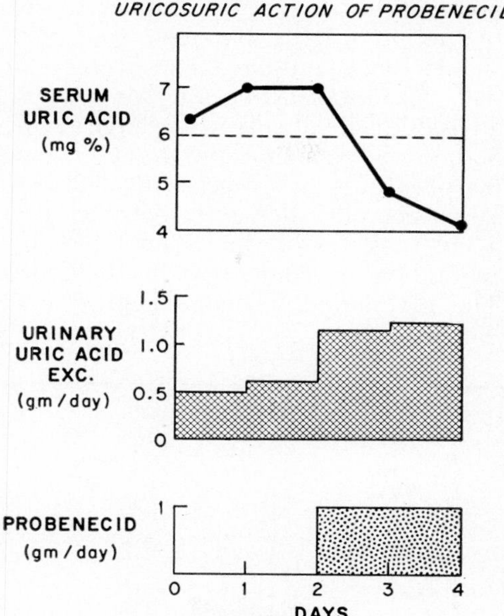

FIG. 31. The uricosuric action of probenecid in a 46-year-old man (Q.N.) with excellent renal function. Note the rapid fall in serum uric acid concentration and the sharp increase in daily urinary excretion of uric acid.

tubules.[208,209] The required daily dose varies from one patient to another, ranging between 0.5 gm. per day, which is effective in approximately 10 per cent of patients,[210] to 3.0 gm. per day. In 50 per cent of patients 0.5 gm. twice a day is sufficient. Efficacy of the drug is indicated by the response (see Fig. 33). The serum uric acid concentration usually falls to normal or nearly normal levels within a few days of initiation of therapy. This is accompanied by a marked increase in urinary urate excretion which, in patients on a low purine diet, lasts as long as mobilizable stores remain in the body. In normal subjects this is a matter of only a day or two, but in advanced tophaceous gout the increased uricosuria may persist for years. Since the only way to be certain that one is accomplishing one's objective depends on the chemical findings, we make it a practice to obtain at least three determinations of serum uric acid concentration and two 24-hour urinary urate excretion determinations prior to starting therapy. Because of the possibility of forming kidney stones during the period of hyperuricemia, the patient should force fluids to 2.5 to 3 liters per day. Alkalinization of the urine is also advisable in patients with large tophi. Sodium or potassium citrate, 1 heaping teaspoonful 4 to 5 times daily will usually accomplish this objective; the latter agent is preferable in patients with hypertension or congestive heart failure. The *p*H should be maintained at 6 or higher.

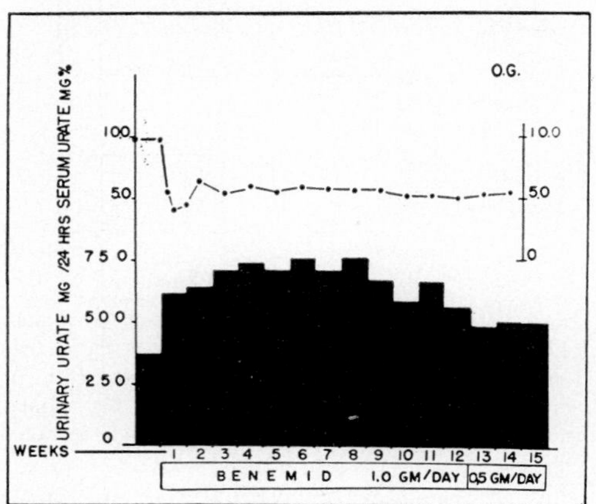

FIG. 32. Note that the initial sharp increase in rate of uric acid excretion disappeared after three months, presumably as the pool of available urate reached normal. Thereafter, despite a more nearly normal rate of uric acid excretion, the serum uric acid level remained at a low level. This figure is reproduced, by permission of the authors, from A. B. Gutman and T. F. Yu's initial description of the uricosuric action of probenecid (Tr. A. Am. Physicians, *64:*281, 1951).

Since acute attacks of gouty arthritis do not decrease in frequency in the early weeks of therapy with probenecid, and, indeed, may increase in frequency and severity during this time,[198,209] the objectives of treatment should be explained to the patient and the occurrence of acute attacks should not be interpreted as reason for discontinuing treatment.

Follow-up studies over the course of years have confirmed initial optimism concerning the benefit of treatment with probenecid. Tophi often gradually decrease in size,[210] and estimates of the miscible uric acid pool have shown a significant decrease.[211] Ulcerated tophi with persistently discharging sinuses heal. Areas of rarefaction by x-ray may decrease in size. Surprisingly, there is usually a concomitant decrease in the symptoms of chronic arthritis. Chronic joint stiffness and pain are lessened, and acute attacks become less frequent and severe. Whether the changes in the kidneys in relatively early stages of gouty nephritis will be reversed has yet to be proved.

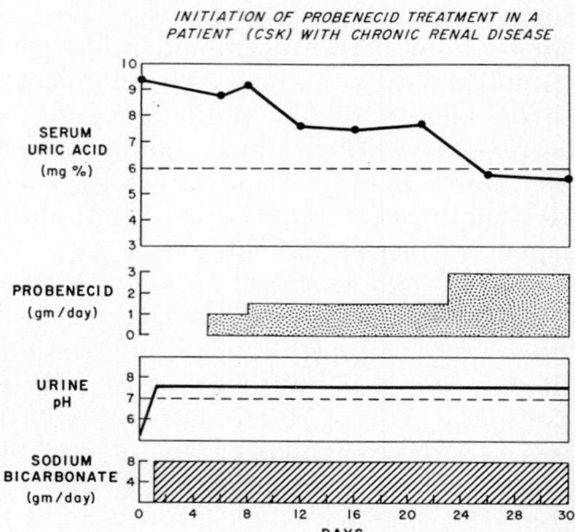

FIG. 33. The initiation of uricosuric therapy in a 59-year-old man (C.S.K.) with chronic tophaceous gout and chronic renal disease. (NPN was 47 mg. %, creatinine clearance 74 liters per 24 hours.) The patient was placed on a low purine diet and was required to force fluids to 3000 to 4000 cc. per day in order to decrease the likelihood of kidney stones. He measured the *p*H of his own freshly voided urine. The data emphasized the fact that the dose of sodium bicarbonate and probenecid in a given patient must be adjusted to achieve the desired physiologic result, and not in accordance with any preconceived schedule.

Toxic reactions to probenecid are rare. Morning nausea is the most common one; hypersensitivity reactions are very rarely seen. Probenecid may be ineffective in patients with severely impaired renal function. The earlier observation that salicylates given concomitantly with probenecid nullify the uricosuric effect of the latter[198,213] has not been borne out by more prolonged clinical trial.[212]

Salicylates. The uricosuric effect of large doses of salicylates has been recognized for eighty years,[215,216] but most investigators have found that maintenance of the necessary dosage has been impractical because of toxic effect.[198,217,218,219] Recently Marson has advocated the use of sodium salicylate as a uricosuric agent in daily doses of 5 to 6 grams.[214,219,220] In his hands this program has been both tolerable and effective, duplicating in most respects the results reported above with probenecid. These results require further confirmation before this mode of therapy can be considered an alternative to probenecid. The reader is reminded that doses of salicylates in the range of 1 to 2 grams a day usually have no uricosuric effect; indeed, they may cause retention of uric acid.[221,222] Maintenance salicylate therapy, in doses of approximately 3.6 to 5.4 gm. per day, may be of value in lessening smoldering articular symptoms often occurring between acute attacks.

Diet. The value of diet in the control of chronic tophaceous gout, already under considerable suspicion, has been further de-emphasized by two recent observations. The demonstration that uric acid is derived from simple metabolites, which are constantly available from dietary ingredients as well as from endogenous purine breakdown, has made it appear unlikely that avoidance of foods with high purine content will significantly decrease the uric acid pool. The advent of probenecid has provided an agent whose effectiveness would seem to far outweigh whatever contribution dietary purines might make. For this reason, it is recommended that patients with gout, who are maintained on probenecid, eat a normal well balanced diet, avoiding only those foods of extraordinarily high purine content, such as sweetbreads, liver, kidney, brain, anchovies, sardines and leguminous vegetables.

During the last five years the combined efforts of chemists, physiologists and clinicians have led to tremendous strides in the treatment of this old disease. The management of acute gouty arthritis has been improved to the extent that few, if any, patients need suffer the severe manifestations of an acute attack. The use of uricosuric agents has demonstrated that the accumulation of excessive amounts of uric acid in patients with gout can be prevented. One is encouraged to hope that many and perhaps all of the chronic manifestations of the disease can also be prevented. The extent to which this is true, however, only time can tell.

References

1. Garrod, A. B.: The Nature and Treatment of Gout and Rheumatic Gout. London, Walton and Maberly, 1859.
2. Sydenham, T.: Tractatus de Podagra et Hydrope. London, G. Kettilby, 1683.
3. Scheele, K. W.: Examen Chemicum Calculi Urinarii, Opuscula II, p. 73, 1776. Cited from Levene, P. A. and Bass, L. W., Nucleic Acids Chemical Catalog Company, New York, 1931.
4. Wollaston: Phil. Tr. London, *87:*386, 1797.
5. Pearson, G.: Phil. Tr. London, *88:*15, 1798.
6. Garrod, A. B.: Medico-Chir. Tr. London, *31:*83, 1848.
7. Miescher, F.: Hoppe Seyler; Medizinisch-Chemische Untersuchungen, p. 441, 1871.
8. Kossel, A.: Ztschr. f. physiol. Chem., *3:*284, 1879; *4:*290, 1880; *5:*152, 1881; *10:*248, 1886; *12:*241, 1888.
9. Fischer, E.: Untersuchungen in der Puringruppe. Berlin, Julius Springer, 1907.
10. Folin, O. and Denis, W.: J. Biol. Chem., *13:*469, 1912–1913.
11. Folin, O.: J. Biol. Chem., *106:*311, 1934.
12. Benedict, S. R. and Behre, J. A.: J. Biol. Chem., *92:*161, 1931.
13. Berliner, Robert W., Hilton, James G., Yü, T. F. and Kennedy, T. J., Jr.: J. Clin. Invest., *29:*396, 1950.
14. Brochner-Mortensen, K.: Medicine, *19:* 161–229, 1940.
15. Peters, J. P. and Van Slyke, D. D.: Quantitative Clinical Chemistry Methods. Baltimore, Williams & Wilkins, 1931, Vol. 1.
16. Christman, A. A.: Physiol. Rev., *32:*303–348, 1952.
17. Umbreit, W. E.: Metabolic Maps, Minneapolis, Burgers Publishing Co., 1952.
18. Bishop, C. and Talbott, J. H.: Pharmacol. Rev., *5:*231, 1953.
19. Stetten, DeW., Jr.: Ann. Rheumat. Dis., *15:*404, 1956.
20. Cold Spring Harbor Symposium, 1947.
21. J. Cell. & Comp. Physiol., *38:* Supp. 1, 1951.
22. Carter, C. E.: Ann. Rev. Biochem., *25:* 123, 1956.

23. Soodak, M.: In Methods of Enzymology. New York, Academic Press, 1955, Vol. 1, p. 612.
24. Horbaczewski, J.: Monatschr. d. Chem., *10:*624, 1889.
25. Spitzer, W.: Arch. f. d. ges. Physiol., *76:*192, 1899.
26. Sonne, J. C., Buchanan, J. M. and Delluva, A. M.: J. Biol. Chem., *166:*395, 1946; *173:*69, 1948.
27. Buchanan, J. M., Sonne, J. C. and Delluva, A. M.: J. Biol. Chem., *173:*81, 1948.
28. Shemin, D. and Rittenberg, D.: J. Biol. Chem., *167:*875, 1947.
29. Abrams, R., Hammarsten, E. and Shemin, D.: J. Biol. Chem., *173:*429, 1948.
30. Karlsson, J. L. and Barker, H. A.: J. Biol. Chem., *177:*597, 1949.
31. Heinrich, M. R. and Wilson, D. W.: J. Biol. Chem., *186:*447, 1950.
32. Sutton, W. B., Schlenk, F. and Werkman, C. H.: Arch. Biochem., *32:*85, 1951.
33. Marsh, W. H.: J. Biol. Chem., *190:*633, 1951.
34. Abrams, R. and Bentley, M.: J. Am. Chem. Soc., *77:*4179, 1955.
35. Goldthwait, D. A.: Fed. Proc., *15:*263, 1956.
36. Goldthwait, D. A., Greenberg, O. R. and Peabody, R. A.: Biochim. et biophys. acta, *18:*148, 1955.
37. Greenberg-Manago, M., Ortiz, P. J. and Ochoa, S.: Science, *122:*907, 1955.
38. Kornberg, A., Lieberman, I. and Simms, E. S.: J. Am. Chem. Soc., *76:*2027, 1954.
39. Levenberg, B. and Melnick, I.: Fed. Proc., *15:*117, 1956.
40. Lieberman, I.: J. Am. Chem. Soc., *78:* 215, 1956.
41. Lukens, L. N. and Buchanan, J. M.: Fed. Proc., *15:*305, 1956.
42. Shive, W., Ackermann, W. W., Gordon, M., Getzendaner, M. E. and Eaken, R. E.: J. Am. Chem. Soc., *69:*725, 1947.
43. Stetten, M. R. and Fox, C. L., Jr.: J. Biol. Chem., *161:*333, 1945.
44. Warren, U. and Flaks, J. G.: Fed. Proc., *15:*379, 1956.
45. Wyngaarden, J. B. and Stetten, DeW., Jr.: J. Biol. Chem., *203:*9, 1953.
46. Krüger, M.: Ber., *32:*2818, 3336, 1899.
Krüger, M. and Schmid, J.: Arch. f. exper. Path. u. Pharmakol., *45:*259, 1901.
Krüger, M. and Schmid, J.: Ber., *32:*2677, 1899.
Krüger, M. and Schmid, J.: Ztschr, f. physiol. Chem., *32:*104, 1901; *36:*1, 1902.
47. Minkowski, O.: Arch. f. exper. Path. u. Pharmakol., *41:*375, 1898.
48. Buchanan, O. H., Christman, A. A. and Block, W. D.: J. Biol. Chem., *157:*189, 1945.
49. Myers, V. C. and Hanzal, R. F.: J. Biol. Chem., *162:*309, 1946.
50. Galinowski, Z.: Arch. f. Verdauungskr., *60:*165, 178, 1936.
51. Wilson, D. W., Bishop, C. and Talbott, J. H.: J. Appl. Physiol., *4:*560–565, 1952.
52. Folin, O.: Am. J. Physiol., *13:*66, 1905.
53. Raiziss, G. W., Dubin, H. and Ringer, A. L.: J. Biol. Chem., *19:*473, 1914.
54. Lewis, H. B., Dunn, M. S. and Dorsy, E. A.: J. Biol. Chem., *36:*9, 1918.
55. Christman, A. A. and Mosier, E. C.: J. Biol. Chem., *83:*11–19, 1929.
56. Harding, V. J., Allen, K. D., Eagles, B. A. and Van Wyck, H. B.: J. Biol. Chem., *63:*37, 1925.
57. Aldersberg, D. and Ellenberg, M.: J. Biol. Chem., *128:*379, 1939.
58. Harpuder, K.: Klin. Wchnschr., *ii:*436, 1923.
59. Brugsch, T. and Rother, J.: Ztschr. f. physiol. Chem., *143:*48, 1925.
60. Williams, J. L. and Dick, G. F.: J.A.M.A., *100:*484, 1933.
61. Lucke, H.: Ztschr. f. d. ges. exper. Med., *74:*329, 1930.
62. Ferrannini, A. and Conese, G.: Arch. per le sc. med., *87:*187, 1949.
63. Talbott, J. H. and Sherman, J. M.: J. Biol. Chem., *115:*361, 1936.
64. Smyth, C. J., Cotterman, C. W. and Freyberg, R. H.: J. Clin. Invest. *27:* 749, 1948.
65. Gutman, A. B.: Ann. Int. Med., *39:*1062, 1953.
66. Wolfson, W. Q., Hunt, H. D., Levine, R., Guterman, H. S., Cohn, C., Rosenberg, E. F., Huddleston, B. and Kadata, K.: J. Clin. Endocrinol., *9:*749, 1949.
67. Wolfson, W. Q., Guterman, H. S., Levine, R., Cohn, C., Hunt, H. D. and Rosenberg, E. F.: J. Clin. Endocrinol., *9:*497, 1949.
68. Stecher, R. M., Hersh, A. H. and Solomon, W. M.: Ann. Int. Med., *31:*595, 1949.
69. Marson, F. G. W.: Quart. J. Med., *22:* 331, 1952.
70. Butt, W. R. and Marson, F. G. W.: Brit. M. J., *2:*1023, 1952.
71. Sarkady, L.: Klin. Wchnschr., *21:*884, 1942.
72. Lennox, W. G.: J.A.M.A., *82:*602, 1924.
73. Ficarra, B. J.: Surgery, *19:*223, 1946.
74. Hickling, R. A.: Lancet, *1:*57, 1953.
75. Tinney, W. S., Polley, H. F., Hall, B. E. and Giffin, H. Z.: Proc. Staff. Meet., Mayo Clin., *20:*49, 1945.
76. Videbaek, A.: Acta. med. scandinav., *138:*179, 1950.
77. Riddle, M. C.: J. Clin. Invest., *8:*69, 1929.

78. Mason, R. M.: Proc. Roy. Soc. Med., *44:*289, 1951.
79. Lueken, B.: Pflueger's Arch. f. d. ges. Physiol., *229:*557, 1932.
80. Shannon, J. A.: J. Cell. & Comp. Physiol., *11:*135, 1938.
81. Coombs, F. S., Pecora, L. J., Thorogood, E., Consolazio, W. V. and Talbott, J. H.: J. Clin. Invest., *19:*525, 1940.
82. Smith, H. W.: The Kidney: Structure and Function in Health and Disease. New York, Oxford University Press, 1951.
83. Friedman, M. and Byers, S. D.: Am. J. Med., *9:*31, 1950.
84. Hanzlik, P. J. and Hawk, P. B.: Proc. Soc. Exper. Biol. & Med., *6:*18, 1908.
85. Leathes, J. B.: J. Physiol., *35:*125, 1906.
86. Simpson, G. E.: J. Biol. Chem., *59:*107, 1924.
87. Forsham, P. H., Thorn, G. W., Bergner, G. E. and Emerson, K.: Am. J. Med., *1:*105, 1946.
88. Fajans, S. S., Conn, J. W., Johnson, D. V. and Christman, A. A.: Endocrinology, *49:*225, 1951.
89. Ingbar, S. H., Kass, E. H., Burnett, C. H., Relman, A. S., Burrows, B. A. and Sisson, J. H.: J. Lab. & Clin. Med.,
90. Benedict, J. D., Forsham, P. H., Roche, M., Soloman, S. and Stetten, DeW., Jr.: J. Clin. Invest., *29:*1104, 1950.
91. Gutman, A. B. and Yü, T. F.: Am. J. Med., *9:*24, 1950.
92. Benedict, S. T.: Harvey Lect., *11:*346, 1915.
93. Klemperer, F. W., Trumble, H. C. and Hastings, A. B.: J. Biol. Chem., *125:* 445, 1938.
94. Friedman, M. and Byers, S. O.: J. Biol. Chem., *175:*727, 1948.
95. Miller, G. E., Danzig, L. S. and Talbott, J. H.: Am. J. Physiol., *164:*155, 1951.
96. Friedman, M. and Byers, S. O.: Am. J. Physiol., *154:*167, 1948.
97. Stetten, DeW., Jr., Geriatrics, *9:*163, 1954.
98. Buzard, J., Bishop, C. and Talbott, J. H.: J. Biol. Chem., *196:*179, 1952.
99. Benedict, J. D., Forsham, P. H. and Stetten, DeW., Jr.: J. Biol. Chem., *181:*183, 1949.
100. Wyngaarden, J. B. and Stetten, DeW., Jr.: J. Biol. Chem., *203:*9, 1953.
101. Geren, W., Bendich, A., Bodansky, O. and Brown, G. B., J. Biol. Chem., *183:*21, 1950.
102. Bishop, C., Garner, W. and Talbott, J. H.: J. Clin. Invest., *30:*879, 1951.
103. Talbott, J. H., Bishop, C. and Garner, W.: Tr. A. Am. Physicians, *63:*201, 1950.
104. Muller, A. F. and Bauer, W.: Proc. Soc. Exper. Biol. & Med., *82:*47, 1953.
105. Bishop, C., Rand, R. and Talbott, J. H., Metabolism *4:*174, 1955.
106. Benedict, J. D., Yü, T. F., Bien, E. J., Gutman, A. B. and Stetten, DeW., Jr.: J. Clin. Invest., *32:*775, 1953.
107. Benedict, J. D., Roche, M., Yü, T. F., Bien, E. J., Gutman, A. B. and Stetten, DeW., Jr.: Metabolism, *1:*3, 1952.
108. Wyngaarden, J. B.: J. Clin. Invest., *36:* 1508, 1957.
109. Wyngaarden, J. B.: Metabolism, *1:*374, 1958.
110. Seegmiller, J. E., Laster, L. and Liddle, L.: Metabolism, *7:*376, 1958.
111. Seegmiller, J. E.: Combined Staff Clinic, Am. J. Med., *22:*816, 1957.
112. Baldwin, E.: Dynamic Aspects of Biochemistry. 2nd ed. Cambridge, The University Press, 1952.
113. Yü, T. F., Wasserman, L. L., Benedict, J. D., Bien, E. J., Gutman, A. B. and Stetten, DeW., Jr.: Am. J. Med., *15:* 845, 1953.
114. Laster, L. and Muller, A. F.: Am. J. Med., *15:*857, 1953.
115. Yü, T. F., Weissinann, B., Sharney, L., Kupper, S. and Guterman, A.: Am. J. Med., *21:*901, 1956.
116. Gutman, A. B., Yü, T. F. and Weissinann, B.: Tr. A. Am. Physicians, in press.
117. Van Breeman, J.: Proceedings of the International Congress on Rheumatism and Hydrology and the Bicentenary Congress on Chronic Rheumatism. London, Headly Brothers, 1938, p. 302.
118. Kahlmeter, G.: Proceedings of the International Congress on Rheumatism and Hydrology and the Bicentenary Congress on Chronic Rheumatism. London, Headly Brothers, 1938, p. 298.
119. Das Gupta, S. C.: Indian M. Rec., *55:*97, 1935.
120. Hench, P. S.: In Barr, D. P., ed.: Modern Medical Therapy in General Practice. Baltimore, Williams and Wilkins Company, 1940, vol. III, p. 3395.
121. Beitzke, H.: Ztschr. f. klin. Med., *74:*215, 1912.
122. Heine, J.: Virchow's Arch. f. path. Anat., *260:*521, 1926.
123. Thomson, F. G.: Brit. J. Rheumat., *1:*25, 1938.
124. Aldred-Brown, G. R. P.: J. Roy. Inst. Pub. Health & Hyg., *1:*298, 1938.
125. Cohen, A.: Am. J. M. Sc., *192:*488, 1936.
126. Monroe, R. T.: M. Clin. North America, *18:*999, 1935.
127. Futcher, T. B.: J.A.M.A., *39:*1046, 1902.
128. Scudamore, C.: A Treatise on the Nature and Cure of Gout. 4th ed. London, Longman, Hurst, Rees, Orme and Brown, 1823.
129. Hutchinson, J.: M. Times and Gaz., *1:*543, 1876.
130. Luff, A. P.: Gout: Its Pathology, Forms, Diagnosis and Treatment. London, Cassell and Company, 1907.

131. Folin, O. and Denis, W.: Arch. Int. Med., *16:*33, 1915.
132. Jacobson, B. M.: Ann. Int. Med., *11:*1277, 1938.
133. Talbott, J. H.: J. Clin. Invest., *19:*645, 1940.
134. Smyth, C. J., Stecher, R. M. and Wolfson, W. Q.: Science, *108:*514, 1948.
135. Smyth, C. J., Cotterman, C. W. and Freyberg, R. H.: J. Clin. Invest., *27:* 749, 1948.
136. Stecher, R. M., Hersh, A. H. and Solomon, W. M.: Ann. Int. Med., *31:*595, 1949.
137. Smyth, C. J.: Practitioner, *166:*62, 1951.
138. Smyth, C. J.: Bull. Rheumat. Dis., *2:*7, 1951.
139. Wilson, D., Collins, D. H. and Mason, R. M.: Proc. Roy. Soc. Med., *44:*285, 1951.
140. Roberts, W.: Albutt's System of Medicine. New York, The Macmillan Company, 1900, Vol. 3, p. 155.
141. Ebstein, W.: Die Natur und Behandlung der Gicht. Wiesbaden, J. F. Bergmann, 1882.
142. Talbott, J. H.: Gout and Gouty Arthritis. Modern Medical Monographs. New York, Grune and Stratton, 1953, p. 78.
143. Lockie, L. M. and Hubbard, R. S.: J.A.M.A., *104:*2072, 1935.
144. Hench, P. S.: J.A.M.A., *113:*1064, 1939.
145. Bauer, W.: J.A.M.A., *113:*1065, 1939.
146. Hellman, L.: Science, *109:*280, 1949.
147. Hench, P. S.: M. Clin. North America, *19:*551, 1935.
148. Linton, Robert R. and Talbott, J. H.: Ann. Surg., *117:*161, 1943.
149. Brown, H.: J. Biol. Chem., *158:*601, 1945.
150. Forsham, P. H., Thorn, G. W., Prunty, F. T. G. and Hills, A. G.: J. Clin. Endocrinol., *8:*15, 1948.
151. Folin, O.: J. Biol. Chem., *101:*111, 1933.
152. Blauch, M. B. and Koch, F. C.: J. Biol. Chem., *130:*443, 1939.
153. Buchanan, O. H., Block, W. D. and Christman, A. A.: J. Biol. Chem., *157:* 181, 1945.
154. Block, W. D. and Geib, N. C.: J. Biol. Chem., *168:*747, 1947.
155. Praetorius, E.: Scandinav. J. Clin. & Lab Invest., *1:*222, 1949.
156. Ropes, M. W., Rossmeisl, E. C. and Bauer, W.: J. Clin. Invest., *19:*795, 1940.
157. Rourke, M. D. and Ernstene, A. C.: J. Clin. Invest., *8:*545, 1930.
158. Hench, P. S., Vanzant, F. R. and Nomland, R.: Tr. A. Am. Physicians, *43:* 217, 1928.
159. Ropes, M. and Bauer, W.: Synovial Fluid Changes in Joint Disease. The Commonwealth Fund, Cambridge, Harvard University Press, 1953.
160. Brogsitter, M.: Histopathologie der Gelenk-Gicht. Leipzig, F. C. W. Vogel, 1927.
161. Pommer, G.: Mikroskopische Untersuchung über Gelenkgicht. Jena, Gustav Fischer, 1929.
162. Ludwig, A. O., Bennett, G. A. and Bauer, W.: Ann. Int. Med., *11:*1248, 1938.
163. Huchard, H.: Traite clinique des maladies du coeur et de l'aorte. Paris, O. Doin, 1899, p. 174.
164. Aschoff, L.: In E. V. Cowdry, ed.: Arteriosclerosis. New York, The Macmillan Company, 1933, p. 10.
165. Schnitker, M. A. and Richter, A. B.: Am. J. M. Sc., *192:*241, 1936.
166. Mathieu, L., Collesson, L. and Choltus, R.: Ann. de méd., *35:*124, 1934.
167. Sydenstrucker, E.: In E. V. Cowdry, ed.: Arteriosclerosis. New York, The Macmillan Company, 1933, p. 131.
168. Alvarez, W. C. and Stanley, L. L.: Arch. Int. Med., *46:*17, 1930.
169. Futcher, T. B.: In Osler, W. and McCrae, T.: Modern Medicine, Volume I. Philadelphia, Lea Brothers, 1907.
170. Fineberg, S. K. and Altschul, A.: Ann. Int. Med., *44:*1182, 1956.
171. Aub, J. C., Fairhall, L. T., Minot, A. S. and Reznikoff, P.: Lead Poisoning. Baltimore, Williams and Wilkins Company, 1926.
172. de Galantha, E.: Am. J. Clin. Path., *5:*165, 1935.
173. Scudamore, C.: A Treatise on the Nature and Cure of Gout. 4th ed. London, Longman, Hurst, Rees, Orme, and Brown, 1823.
174. Moore, H.: Tr. Path. Soc. London, *33:* 271, 1881–1882.
175. Weve, H. J. M.: Aver Keratitis Urica en andere Vormen van Jichtig Ooglijden. Rotterdam, W. J. Van Hengel, 1924.
176. Schlesinger, M. J.: Unpublished data. Beth Israel Hospital, Boston, Mass.
177. Levinson, F.: Ztschr. f. klin. Med., *26:* 293, 1894.
178. Brown, J. and Mallory, K. C.: New England J. Med., *243:*325, 1950.
179. Schnitker, M. A. and Richter, A. B.: Am. J. M. Sc., *192:*241, 1936.
180. Brogsitter, A. M. and Wodarz, H.: Deutsch. Arch. f. klin. Med., *139:*129, 1922.
181. Trout, E. F., Knight, A. A., Santo, P. B. and Passerelli, E. W.: J.A.M.A. *156:*591, 1954.
182. Kionka, H.: Arch. f. exper. Path. u. Pharmakol., *44:*186, 1900.
183. Fox, H.: Diseases in Captive Wild Mammals and Birds: Incidence, Description, Comparison. Philadelphia, J. B. Lippincott Company, 1923.
184. Kaupp, B. F.: Poultry Diseases, Including Diseases of Other Domesticated Birds. Chicago, Alexander Eger, 1923.

185. Schlottenhauer, C. F. and Bollman, J. L.: J. Am. Vet. M. A., *85:*98, 1934.
186. Schlottenhauer, C. F. and Bollman, J. L.: Am. J. Digest. Dis., *3:*483, 1936.
187. Galvani, 1766. Cited from Ebstein, W.: Die Natur und Behandlung der Gicht. Wiesbaden, J. F. Bergmann, 1882.
188. Schröder, W.: Arch. f. Physiol., Supp., p. 113, 1880.
189. Virchow, R.: Virchow's Arch. f. path. Anat. u. Physiol., *35:*358, 1866; *36:* 147, 1866.
190. Mendelson, W.: Am. J. M. Sc., *95:*109, 1888.
191. Salomon, G.: Virchow's Arch. f. path. Anat. u. Physiol., *97:*360, 1884.
192. Pecile, D.: Ann. der Chem., *183:*141, 1876.
193. Schittenhelm, A. and Bendix, E.: Ztschr. f. physiol. Chem., *48:*140, 1906. Schittenhelm, A.: Ztschr. f. physiol. Chem., *66:*53, 1910.
194. Bauer, W. and Singh, M. M.: New England J. Med., *256:*171, 214, 1957.
195. Talbott, J. H.: Gout and Gouty Arthritis. Modern Medical Monographs. New York, Grune and Stratton, 1953, pp. 79–134.
196. Benedict, J. D., Forsham, P. H., Roche, M., Soloway, S., and Stetten, DeW., Jr.: J. Clin. Invest., *29:*1104, 1950.
197. Bishop, C., Garner, W. and Talbott, J. H.: J. Clin. Invest. *30:*879, 1951.
198. Gutman, A. B. and Yü, T. F.: Am. J. Med., *13:*744, 1952.
199. Kuzell, W. C., Schaffarzick, R. W. and Naugler, W. E.: Arch. Int. Med., *96:* 153, 1955.
200. Colsky, J., Wallace, S. and Banowitch, M. M.: New England J. Med., *253:* 730, 1955.
201. Kuzell, W. C.: Am. J. Med., *16:*212, 1954.
202. Kuzell, W. C., Schaffarzick, R. W., Brown, B. J. and Mankle, E. A.: J.A.M.A., *149:*729, 1952.
203. Wyngaarden, J. B.: J. Clin. Invest., *34:* 256, 1955.
204. Yü, T. F., Sirota, J. H. and Gutman, A. B.: J. Clin. Invest., *32:*1121, 1953.
205. Mauer, E. F.: New England J. Med., *253:*404, 1955.
206. Gutman, A. B. and Yü, T. F.: Tr. A. Am. Physicians, *64:*279, 1951.
207. Wolfson, W. Q., Cohn, C., Levine, R. and Huddleston, B.: Am. J. Med., *4:* 744, 1948.
208. Sirota, J. H., Yü, T. F. and Gutman, A. B.: J. Clin. Invest., *31:*692, 1951.
209. Talbott, J. H.: Bull. Rheumat. Dis., *2:* 1, 1951.
210. Gutman, A. B. and Yü, T. F.: J.A.M.A., *157:*1096, 1955.
211. Bishop, C., Rand, R. and Talbott, J. H.: J. Clin. Invest., *30:*889, 1951.
212. Boger, W. P. and Smith, R. T.: Nord. med., *51:*2021, 1954.
213. Pascale, L. R., Dubin, A. and Hoffman, W. S.: J.A.M.A., *149:*1188, 1952.
214. Marson, F. G. W.: Ann. Rheumat. Dis., *13:*233, 1954.
215. Byasson, H.: J. de therap., *4:*721, 1877.
216. See, G.: Bull. Acad. de méd., Ser. 2, *6:*689, 717, 759, 803, 926, 937, 1008, and 1024, 1877.
217. Bauer, W. and Klemperer, F.: New England J. Med., *231:*681, 1944.
218. Combined Staff Clinic: Am. J. Med., *9:* 799, 1950.
219. Marson, F. G. W.: Quart. J. Med., *22:* 331, 1953.
220. Marson, F. G. W.: Lancet, *2:*360, 1955.
221. Klemperer, F. and Bauer, W.: J. Clin. Invest., *23:*950, 1944.
222. Yü, T. F. and Gutman, A. B.: Proc. Soc. Exper. Biol. & Med., *90:*542, 1955.

CHAPTER 11

By C. J. WATSON, M.D.

Porphyrin Metabolism

INTRODUCTION

The porphyrins exist in nature in both a free and a combined state. The iron porphyrin protein compounds such as hemoglobin, myohemoglobin, cytochrome and catalase are outstanding representatives of the latter type. Other metal complexes occur which differ from the heme-proteins; in the human being these are limited with but rare exception to the zinc complex of either copro- or uroporphyrin, both of which also exist in the body, in part, in the free state. These are the principal endogenous porphyrins of the excreta, whereas the respiratory pigments such as cytochrome and catalase contain protoporphyrin complexly bound with iron and protein. It should be noted, however, that very small amounts of free proto- and coproporphyrin are found in the circulating erythrocytes, bone marrow and liver. The white matter of the central nervous system contains minute quantities of free coproporphyrin. The present chapter will deal mainly with the problem of the free porphyrins, including metal complexes which are not heme-protein in character.

The basic structure of the porphyrins is a porphin skeleton composed of four pyrrol nuclei joined by four methene or CH bridges. As seen in Figure 1, there are eight carbons at which substitutions may occur; protoporphyrin is a divinyl dipropionic tetramethyl porphin; coproporphyrin is a tetramethyl tetrapropionic porphin; uroporphyrin is a tetraacetic tetrapropionic porphin. Metal complexes are formed by attachment to the nitrogens in the interior of the ring. H. Fischer's choice of prefixes for the naturally occurring porphyrins was based principally on the major site of occurrence or source of initial isolation.[1] Thus proto- is related to the widespread representation in various parts of the body, copro- and uro- to isolation from the feces and urine, respectively. The latter terms have become relatively unsatisfactory, as neither porphyrin is limited in occurrence to feces or urine, and it has become increasingly evident, as will be apparent in the following, that both have intrinsic metabolic significance, being concerned at least indirectly with heme synthesis. It may be emphasized that the porphyrins have mainly or perhaps wholly *anabolic* significance, in contrast to the bile pigments, which are mainly *catabolic*.

ORIGIN AND SIGNIFICANCE OF THE FREE PORPHYRINS

Great advances have been made in recent years in our knowledge of the biosynthesis of the porphyrins. Shemin and co-workers[2–7] discovered that glycine and acetate are the main primary building blocks on the pathway to porphyrin. Later studies in Shemin's laboratory revealed that glycine and a succinyl derivative form an intermediate known as delta-amino-levulinic acid.[8,9] Two molecules of this substance condense to yield porphobilinogen, the primary pyrrolic precursor of the porphyrins.[9–13] Westall[14] crystallized this compound from acute porphyria urine, and its constitution was established by Cookson and Rimington.[15] It is evident that four molecules of porphobilinogen may combine to yield a uroporphyrin. The heating of porphobilinogen in vitro gives rise mainly to the asymmetric uroporphyrin III.[16,17] Since the protoporphyrin of the hemoglobin molecule has the same configuration, corresponding to aetioporphyrin III, it was logical to consider that the pathway of porphyrin biosynthesis on the way to heme was via uroporphyrin III and coproporphyrin III. Subsequent studies have failed, in the main, to provide evidence that these porphyrins are intermediaries between porphobilinogen and protoporphyrin.[22,23] Very recently, however, strong evidence has been described indicating that the reduced form, or porphyrinogen, is the actual intermediary and that the porphyrins themselves are side products. Thus Neve, Labbe and Aldrich[24] found that if reduced uroporphyrin III was incubated with chicken red cell hemolysate the synthesis of heme as measured by the uptake of Fe^{59} was greatly enhanced, whereas this was not true with uroporphyrin. More direct evidence on this point has recently been obtained in a study with Bashour and Schwartz* in which N^{15} uroporphyrin I and C^{14} uroporphyrin III were incubated, either with liver homogenate or chicken red cell hemolysate. In both instances there was clear evidence of formation of the corresponding coproporphyrinogen, and when C^{14} uroporphyrinogen III was used, protoporphyrin formation was also observed. It was evident early in the study of porphyrin chemistry that various isomers of the porphyrins may occur and that some form of standard nomenclature was necessary. H. Fischer, whose work clarified the structure of many of the porphyrins, based his classification on the four relatively simple aetioporphyrin isomers[1] which do not occur in nature. These have four methyl and four ethyl groups in varying positions on the porphin ring (Fig. 1). Fischer first recognized that

* Unpublished.

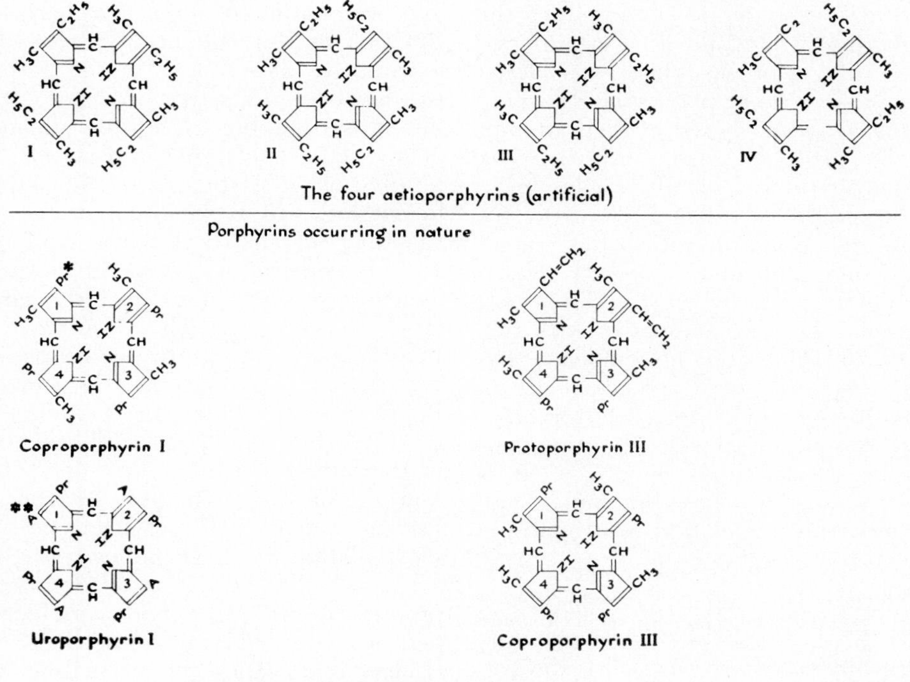

FIG. 1. Important naturally occurring porphyrins and classification of isomers based on the four artificial aetioporphyrins, according to H. Fischer.[1]

at least two of the four isomer types (see Fig. 1) are represented in nature, i.e., I and III. He spoke of this as the "dualism" of the porphyrins. The protoporphyrin of the heme-proteins has a configuration corresponding to aetioporphyrin III;* some of the copro- and uroporphyrins, however, have the same configuration as that of aetio-I. Under certain pathologic conditions, notably in porphyria, a marked overproduction of the symmetric type I porphyrins is observed. In Figure 1 it may be seen that these differ from type III only by virtue of the opposite position of the substituents of methyl and ethyl groups on pyrrol nucleus 4. Derivation of one series from the other would obviously require a disruption of the porphin ring, 180° rotation of nucleus 4 and resynthesis of the porphyrin without any other change in configuration. There is no evidence that this occurs.

In comparison with the heme-proteins, little is known about the free porphyrins or their zinc complexes. Whether the latter are fundamentally related to the site and mode of origin of the porphyrins is unknown. Certain evidence in favor of this will be considered in the discussion of porphyria elsewhere in this chapter; however, no attempt will be made to distinguish between free porphyrin and metal complex; most of the available quantitative data for copro- and uroporphyrins in the excreta and tissues depend on methods which split out any zinc which is present and determine the total amount of each free porphyrin. Thus far no evidence has been described for the occurrence in human excreta of copper, iron or other metal complexes, which might not be split by the methods employed. It is true that zinc has been identified with certainty only in relation to uroporphyrin; the belief that it is also attached to a portion of the coproporphyrin, at least in the urine, rests upon absorption spectrum and chemical behavior, especially the concentration of hydrochloric acid required for splitting.

The urinary coproporphyrin is excreted in considerable part as a colorless and nonfluorescing porphyrinogen or precursor.[25] This is probably identical with the reduced form of coproporphyrin obtained by treatment with sodium amalgam. It was this compound which was used in the above mentioned experiments of Neve and Aldrich,[24] also by Bashour and Schwartz in porphyrin biosynthesis, in which it was shown that the pathway of biosynthesis proceeds over the porphyrinogen rather than the free porphyrin itself. Conversion of porphyrinogen to porphyrin is readily achieved by exposure to iodine or ultraviolet light. The latter is more efficient in the conversion of uroporphyrinogen to uroporphyrin; the former is superior in the case of coproporphyrinogen.

A. Formation of Free Porphyrins in Relation to Hemoglobin Synthesis. The pathway of biosynthesis of the porphyrins has been discussed in the foregoing, but it is desirable to consider in more detail some metabolic aspects of the porphyrins in particular relationship to hematology. In seeking the origin and functions of the free porphyrins, primary consideration must be given to the developing normoblasts and the circulating erythrocytes. The occurrence of small amounts of free protoporphyrin in the erythrocytes was noted by van den Bergh in 1928.[26] Subsequent studies[27,28] revealed that it was especially plentiful in the reticulocytes but that under certain circumstances, notably in iron deficiency anemia and pernicious anemia shortly after the liver-induced reticulocyte peak, the correlation of erythrocyte protoporphyrin (EP) with reticulocyte percentage was greatly diminished.[28] It is clear that among the circulating "fluorescytes,"[29] there are porphyrin-containing red blood cells which do not take up supravital stain and which rep-

* Actually, there are 15 possible protoporphyrins, corresponding to the 15 more readily prepared mesoporphyrins.[1] The latter are tetramethyl, diethyl, dipropionic acid porphins. The protoporphyrin of the hemoglobin molecule corresponds in configuration to mesoporphyrin 9; hence it is properly designated as protoporphyrin 9, type III.

resent forms intermediate in maturity between reticulocytes and ordinary erythrocytes. Schwartz and Wikoff[30] and Watson[20] have shown that the circulating red cells also contain very small amounts of coproporphyrin which was crystallized[30] and shown to consist mainly of coproporphyrin III, although isomer analyses in experimental phenylhydrazine anemia reveal a 60:40 ratio for III to I.[30] These studies as well as observations in various anemias seen in man[20,31] have revealed a close correlation of erythrocyte coproporphyrin (ECP) with reticulocyte percentage, under most circumstances, lead poisoning and porphyria being somewhat exceptional, as will be noted presently. The concentration of erythrocyte coproporphyrin follows the reticulocytes faithfully in cases of pernicious anemia after liver or B_{12} therapy.[20a] The peak value lags very slightly behind that of the reticulocytes, while that of the erythrocyte protoporphyrin is considerably later (Fig. 2). It may be emphasized that in pernicious anemia in relapse, the erythrocyte coproporphyrin values are zero, at least with the amounts of blood used in the determination.[20b] Normal values for erythrocyte protoporphyrin and erythrocyte coproporphyrin and values more often observed in other anemias are seen in Table I in relation to the urinary coproporphyrin (UCP), to be discussed later. The contrast between

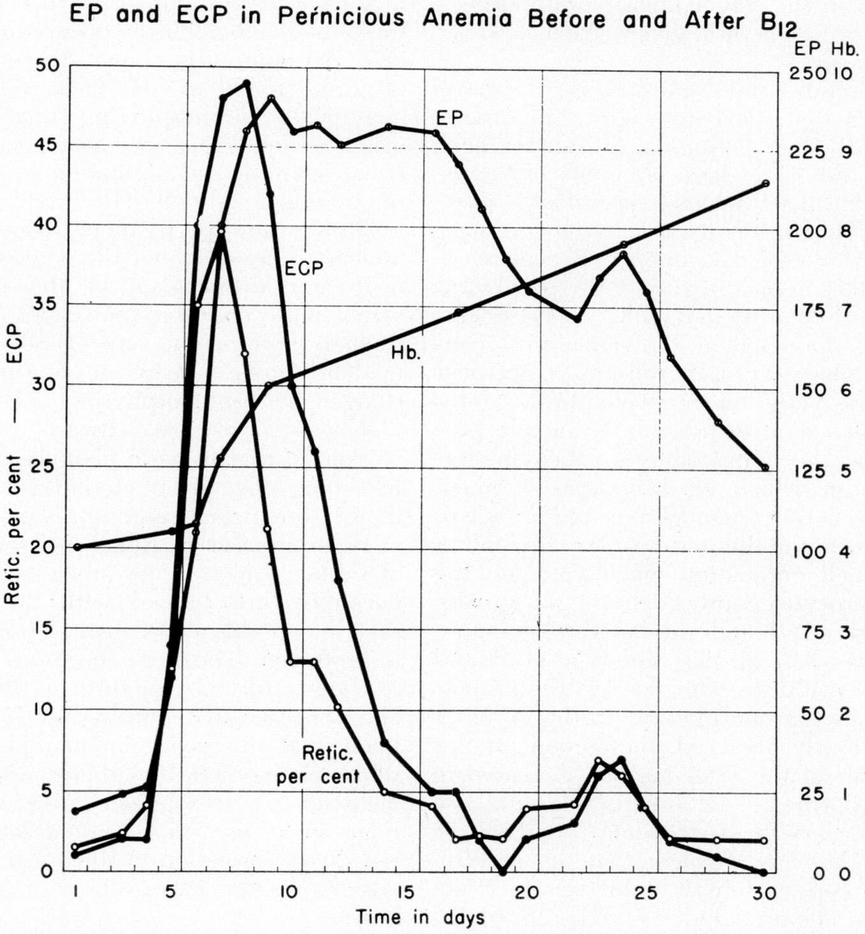

FIG. 2. The erythrocyte porphyrins in relation to the reticulocyte response to vitamin B_{12} in pernicious anemia administered on day 1. (From A.M.A. Arch. Int. Med., 86:797, 1950.)

the values observed in the iron deficiency and hemolytic anemias is noteworthy. The available evidence indicates that the coproporphyrin III of the reticulocytes is derived by oxidation of its porphyrinogen, the latter being directly involved in the biosynthesis of the hemoglobin protoporphyrin, as discussed above. It seems likely that whatever proportion of coproporphyrin I may be found in different conditions is similarly derived from its porphyrinogen, but no conclusive evidence has thus far been reported in support of the view that some fraction of the type I porphyrinogen is converted to a type I protoporphyrin and heme.

Additional observations supporting the belief that coproporphyrinogen type III is in the direct line of protoporphyrin formation are given briefly in the following.

Schmid and co-workers[32,33] have shown that the bone marrow in experimental lead poisoning in rabbits contains relatively large amounts of coproporphyrin III, which is presumably present primarily as its porphyrinogen, converted during the extraction process or possibly in part in vivo to the porphyrin. The circulating red cells in these animals, examined at the same time, contain chiefly protoporphyrin in marked excess, with but relatively little coproporphyrin. In experimental anemia produced by administering phenylhydrazine, in which erythropoiesis is much more active, hemoglobin synthesis apparently uninhibited and the circulating red cell population much younger, the erythrocyte coproporphyrin is greatly increased though under these circumstances it is 60 per cent type III,[30] and there is a distinct increase in the proportion of coproporphyrin I in the urine; as previously observed, the amount of this isomer in the feces may be increased in cases of hemolytic anemia[31,34,35] and also in dogs with experimental hemorrhagic anemia.[36,37] It is clear that the erythrocyte coproporphyrin value serves as another chemical index of the rate of hemoglobin synthesis, or attempted synthesis. It is usually, but not always, parallel with the percentage of reticulocytes. In the presence of a hindrance to hemoglobin synthesis, as occurs in lead poisoning, the erythrocyte coproporphyrin may be elevated without corresponding increase in reticulocytes; this may well reflect an attempted synthesis which is partially blocked or inhibited by the lead, with a resultant accumulation of coproporphyrin III in the developing and, to a lesser extent, in the circulating red blood cells. Porphyria erythropoietica, as discussed in the following pages, also constitutes an exception to the usual correlation existing between the erythrocyte coproporphyrin and reticulocyte percentage.

In conditions associated with a marked stimulus to erythropoiesis and in which there is also a disturbed synthesis of hemoglobin as occurs in acute lead poisoning, the bone marrow and urine are found to contain considerable amounts of uroporphyrin. Indeed, the urine under these circumstances generally contains small amounts of porphobilinogen as well. The uroporphyrin is mainly the type I isomer. This would appear to indicate that the lead induces a greater disturbance in the type I series between uro- and coproporphyrinogen while in the type III series it is evidently greater between coproporphyrinogen and protoporphyrin.

It was shown by Schwartz and coworkers[38a] that if acute phenylhydrazine poisoning plus the photodynamic activity of rose bengal and ultraviolet light is superimposed on the lead poisoning of rabbits, much larger amounts of uroporphyrin are formed with the result that a veritable experimental porphyria is produced. The urine becomes brown or even dark red because of the presence of excessive porphyrins. It seems likely that this condition in rabbits has some analogy for the photosensitive or congenital erythropoietic porphyria in man, since, as will be noted later, the porphyrin formation in this form is likewise associated intimately with erythropoiesis.

Normally, very small amounts of uroporphyrin are excreted in the urine and feces. We can fully confirm Lockwood's identification[39] of the normal urine uroporphyrin as the type I isomer. Whether this is a side product of normal erythropoiesis or of heme synthesis in other locations such as the liver is unknown. It may be the source of the uroporphyrin which has been observed in embryonic bone and in the epiphyses of growing animals. It is interesting that if uroporphyrin is injected in young animals it deposits where calcium is being laid down.[40] Since uroporphyrin in vitro is readily adsorbed on calcium phosphate, it seems likely that this is a physical chemical coincidence rather than representing any fundamental relation to bone formation.

B. Formation of Free Porphyrins Apart from the Synthesis of Hemoglobin. There can be little doubt that small amounts of free porphyrins are formed in sites other than bone marrow, and unrelated to hemoglobin synthesis. Klüver[41,42] discovered that the white matter of the central nervous system of warm-blooded animals regularly contains small amounts of free coproporphyrin. The concentration is in the neighborhood of 2 to 3 μg/100 gm. of nervous tissue.[43] The coproporphyrin of normal beef brain has been crystallized and identified as the type III isomer by Blanchard.[44] It is of interest that it was accompanied by a much smaller amount of a uroporphyrin, isomer type unidentified.

Various studies have made reasonably clear that the central nervous system porphyrin is formed in situ rather than being transported to the nervous system from some other point of formation. Its function is unknown; the fact that its occurrence is almost limited to the white matter, while cytochrome is chiefly in the gray, appears to make a relationship unlikely. It is possible that it may serve to govern the rate of utilization of oxygen, this concept being based on Granick and Gilder's observations[45] on the metabolism of certain bacteria, in which coproporphyrin is a competitive inhibitor of protoporphyrin, thus reducing the respiratory activity of heme. The complete failure to detect coproporphyrin in the nervous system of cold-blooded animals[42] is also not explained, but it is perhaps not incompatible with the concept just referred to.

There is no reason to doubt that porphyrin biosynthesis in the liver in relation to cytochrome, catalase or other heme enzymes proceeds along the same pathway as that for hemoglobin in the bone marrow. Thus it is probable that small amounts of uro-, copro- and protoporphyrin are provided as side products of this synthesis. Our information thus far is quite inadequate as to the amounts or isomer types of these porphyrins.

Nothing is known about formation and liberation of free porphyrins in still other tissues, but it is reasonable to believe that this may occur in trace amounts in relation to the synthesis of protoporphyrin for the various hemes of cellular metabolism.

NORMAL AND PATHOLOGIC EXCRETION OF THE PORPHYRINS

The Coproporphyrins

The quantitative determination of the porphyrins is best carried out by means of their intense red fluorescence in ultraviolet light. Light of the wave length of the porphyrin Soret band (in the region of 400 mμ) is most efficient in exciting fluorescence. Colorless solutions lacking discernible absorption bands, still exhibit strong fluorescence (Fig. 6 E, p. 703).

The normal range of urinary coproporphyrin (UCP) for adult humans of both sexes using very little alcohol is from 60 to 280 μg./24 hour urine sample.[46,53] The values for males are distinctly higher than those for females. A consistent increase is noted with increasing alcoholism[53] (see Fig. 3). This is considerably higher than the values obtained with previous methods[47,48] partly because they neglected the colorless, nonfluorescing porphyrinogen, partly because of improved collection of samples and fluorimetry. Most of the data obtained with the earlier techniques are comparable to a normal

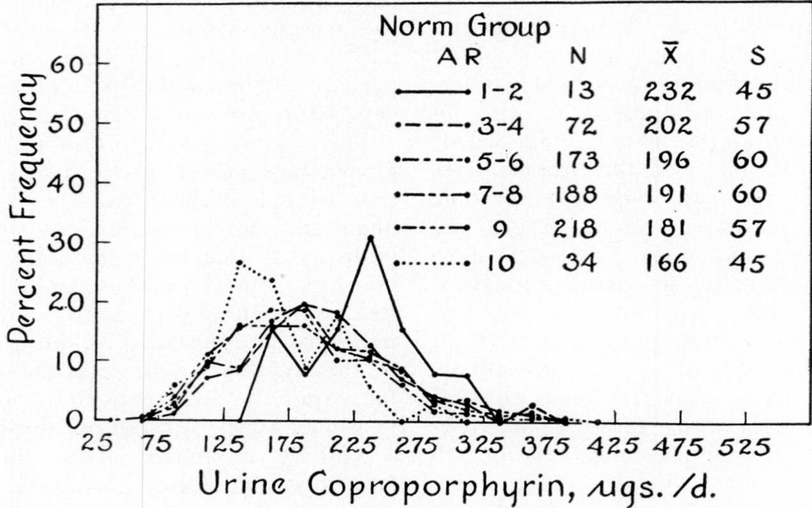

FIG. 3. The range of urinary coproporphyrin excretion in normal persons and the effect of alcohol. AR = Alcohol rating; 1–2 greatest intake, 10 none. (From Zieve, Hill, Schwartz and Watson, J. Lab. & Clin. Med., *41*:663, 1953. Reproduced by permission of the publishers, C. V. Mosby Co., St. Louis.)

range of 20 to 100 μg.[48] The first isolations of coproporphyrin from human urine indicated a distinct preponderance of the type I over the type III isomer.[49,50] Grotepass[51] isolated 200 mg. of crystalline coproporphyrin from 10,000 liters of pooled urine presumably from normal persons; this consisted of about equal parts of types I and III. Nevertheless, in a later study[48] of fifty-four normal persons in this laboratory, a preponderance of type I was found, the percentage of type III ranging from 8 to 54, usually from 20 to 40. While the basis for the difference from Grotepass' results is not certain, the possibility was considered that the higher proportion of type III in his crystalline material was due to a contribution to the pool by one or more persons with asymptomatic chemical or heavy metal toxicity or idiopathic coproporphyrinuria (*vide infra*). It is well established that alcoholic excess often causes significant increases of type III isomer in the urine.[52,53] There is also a distinct possibility that this can be due to a chronic mild toxicity related to contamination of drinking water or atmosphere.[48] This latter question merits further study, particularly in view of the recent report of Comfort and coworkers[118] that in a normal group studied in London, type III was preponderant.

The total urinary coproporphyrin (UCP) is increased under a great variety of circumstances.[31,37,47,54,55] The idea has been advanced in the past that the urinary coproporphyrin was derived in part from blood or bacteria in the colon. More recent studies,[56] however, have failed to offer support for this belief. The ingestion of hemoglobin, blood or coproporphyrin itself was not followed by increases in the urinary coproporphyrin. Insofar as bacterial metabolism is concerned, it has now been observed repeatedly that tetracyclines do not affect the excretion of urinary coproporphyrin, although they generally abolish that of stercobilinogen[57] formation, which is due to bacterial activity in the colon.

In chemical and heavy metal toxicity, of which lead poisoning is the prototype, the increases are often large and are due in the main to the type III isomer. Values of 1000 to 4000 μg. are often found in the 24 hour sample, although in asymptomatic cases the increases are generally not so marked. It is now clear that an increased urinary coproporphyrin is a very sensitive indicator of undue lead exposure,[58] one which can be used to much advantage in industry. It is likely that this is also true for other heavy metals and chemicals. Considerable increases have been observed in relation to gold, arsenic, benzene, carbon tetrachloride, methyl chloride and others. Distinct increases of type III are also observed in many cases of refractory or aplastic anemia,[31,37] in which chemical toxicity often appears to be implicated, while in pernicious anemia, hemolytic anemias, iron deficiency anemias and most cases of leukemia, the urinary coproporphyrin either is not increased or a moderate increase is more often due to the type I isomer.[31] In exceptional cases of leukemia, for reasons that are not clear, a preponderance of type III isomer has been noted.[31] In Hodgkin's disease it is interesting that the type III isomer is often increased in the urine, especially in febrile and cachectic cases; this may represent an endogenous chemical toxicity, although there has been no definite correlation with the presence or absence of necrosis.[31] Excessive type III coproporphyrin excretion in the urine has been observed in certain cases of miliary tuberculosis. Whether this is due to "toxemia" or to production of coproporphyrin III by tubercle bacilli is unknown. It may be noted that many bacteria are capable of elaborating coproporphyrin III and that the diphtheria bacillus in culture does this in rough proportion to toxin production. The crude precipitate discarded in the course of diphtheria toxin production is a rich source of coproporphyrin III.*

In the study of anemias and diseases of the blood-forming organs it is of some interest and even practical value to compare the data for the erythrocyte porphyrins and the urinary coproporphyrin in different conditions. The values shown in Table 1 are the ranges commonly encountered in the majority of the cases of the diseases listed. As already mentioned, there are exceptional instances of leukemia in which the values observed are not in agreement with the ranges in Table 1.

In cases of hepatic disease there is often an increase of the urinary coproporphyrin, usually from 200 to 800 μg./24 hours, at times exceeding 1000.[54,55] In viral hepatitis and infectious mononucleosis this has been due almost entirely to the type I isomer.[54] It appears quite likely that this represents simply a diversion to the general circulation and thence to the urine of coproporphyrin normally excreted by the liver into the bile and then lost with the feces. This is probably due in part to hepatocellular failure and in part to a

* With Schwartz and Keprios, unpublished.

TABLE 1. USUAL RANGES OF URINARY AND ERYTHROCYTE PORPHYRINS IN SOME OF THE PRINCIPAL ANEMIAS

	URINARY COPROPORPHYRIN μg./24 hr.	ISOMER % I	III	ERYTHROCYTE PROTOPORPHYRIN μg./100 cc.	ERYTHROCYTE COPROPORPHYRIN μg./100 cc.
Normal	60–280	60–80	20–40	15–60	0–2.0
Iron deficiency	40–200	60–80		200–1200	1–6
Pernicious anemia (relapse)	100–400	60–80		15–40	0
Hemolytic	100–300	60–80		60–150	5–40
Hypoplastic	150–1000		50–90	20–100	0–4
Leukemia	100–400	60–80		20–100	0–10
Hodgkin's	200–2000		variable*	40–200	0–10
Azotemia	0–30	60–80		50–500	0–10
Heavy metal	600–7000		80–99	300–3000	1–20
Chemical	200–800		60–80	100–400	1–10

* Ratios over a wide range, from 10–90% III.

regurgitation of bile into the blood, the two factors undoubtedly varying in importance from one case to another, depending on stage and type of involvement. In the late stage, after icterus has long disappeared, excessive urinary coproporphyrin is often encountered and probably is due to residual hepatocellular functional impairment; and in the stage of jaundice the factor of biliary regurgitation may be of at least equal significance. The blood serum usually contains demonstrable although very small amounts of coproporphyrin in cases of regurgitation jaundice, whether hepatic or extrahepatic obstructive in origin. (It has not been possible to demonstrate any under normal circumstances.) The urinary coproporphyrin is likewise regularly increased in cases of the latter type, and again the increase is due to type I rather than III. Thus the coproporphyrin excretion has proved of little value in the diagnosis of jaundice, although marked increases point more toward a parenchymal than a mechanical type.[54]

In hepatic cirrhosis significant increases of the urinary coproporphyrin are usual, but not uniform.[55] In many instances, especially when jaundice is present, values from 500 to 1000 μg. are noted. If serial determinations are made, considerable variation from day to day is often observed. The reason for this fluctuation, which is also observed in other diseases, is unknown.

The urinary coproporphyrin isomer ratio in cases of cirrhosis is generally quite different with respect to type.[55] Thus in the chronic alcoholics with Laennec's, or primarily fatty cirrhosis, a preponderance of type III isomer is usually found, although in certain instances in which hemolytic anemia has supervened or where there has been abstinence from alcohol for long periods prior to the determination, the majority of the porphyrin has been type I. Acute alcoholism, without cirrhosis, is usually accompanied by at least transitory increases of type III coproporphyrin in the urine,[52] but in chronic alcoholics with cirrhosis the preponderance of type III commonly persists for months or years after cessation of drinking.[55] In milder cases of fatty liver with early or slight fibrosis, rest, abstinence and a good diet may be followed fairly soon by a return of the total urinary coproporphyrin to within the normal range, but the percentage of type III often remains high. This appears to indicate an actual reduction in the formation of type I, but it may be that this isomer is now being excreted more efficiently by the liver. Serial studies of the urine and fecal porphyrins in such instances have not been reported. As noted in the following, a distinct difference may exist between isomer ratios in urine and feces at the same time, under some circumstances.

In the group of cirrhoses which are primarily nonfatty (nonalcoholic-dietary), whether posthepatitic, pigmentary (hemochromatosis), or idiopathic, the excessive urinary coproporphyrin is nearly always represented by the type I isomer, in contrast to the alcoholic group.[55]

The fundamental significance of the above findings in the cirrhosis material thus far studied is not clear. The excessive type III coproporphyrin excretion in the urine in the alcoholic group, and its frequent persistence long after alcohol was stopped, may well be related to a disturbance of cellular metabolism in the liver. Thus far, no data on porphyrins of bone marrow and liver in these cases are available, so that the exact origin of the urinary type III isomer is unknown. It may be noted, however, that in several cases of acute alcoholism, at a time when such excesses were present in the urine, the erythrocyte coproporphyrin (*vide supra*) was not increased.

In cases of cirrhosis in which the excessive urinary coproporphyrin is composed of type I it is not yet clear whether this represents simply diversion, as already discussed, or actual overproduction. Much more information about fecal and urinary porphyrin, acquired simultaneously, is needed to determine this point.

The question of origin and amount of the fecal coproporphyrin (FCP) may now be considered briefly. Under normal circumstances this is chiefly type I isomer. Significant increases have been observed by various investigators in relation to heightened erythropoiesis, whether induced by hemorrhage or hemolytic agents, or in cases of hemolytic jaundice.[31,34,35,36,37,47] It has been postulated that these increases represent a formation in definite ratio to protoporphyrin, as a side product of hemoglobin synthesis.[37] However, there are many cases of outspoken hemolytic anemia in which no increase of fecal coproporphyrin can be demonstrated.[31] Furthermore, in many cases of hyporegenerative or aplastic anemia the fecal coproporphyrin is well within the normal range and not decreased, as one might anticipate if there were a definite quantitative relationship with erythropoiesis.[31] To what extent contributions of porphyrin from the fecal flora may affect these variations is not certain.

The range of normal values for total fecal coproporphyrin is from 300 to 1400 μg./24 hours of which 70 to 90 per cent is type I.*[31] The preponderance of type I may be maintained even when most of the urinary coproporphyrin is type III; for example, this has been observed in lead poisoning.[50] On the other hand, there are probably many circumstances under which the fecal coproporphyrin is mainly type III. In acute poliomyelitis, the feces as well as the urine in some cases has been found to contain an excess of type III, though many more observations are necessary to determine just how uniform a finding this may be. In some situations, at least, the amount of type III (by actual isolation) in the feces greatly exceeds that in the urine. In a case of so-called "chronic poliomyelitis anterior" studied recently, which could not be classified with accuracy either during life or at necropsy, the feces contained from 2500 to 4000 μg. of coproporphyrin per 100 gm., of which 72 per cent was type III, a greatly increased amount, readily permitting crystallization. The urine in this case was examined many times during the several months of illness, the urinary coproporphyrin and isomer ratio always being in the normal range. The serum coproporphyrin, however, was regularly increased, ranging from 5 to 10 μg. per 100 cc. While these findings are not readily explained, they reveal the need of a systematic study of porphyrin metabolism in various diseases of the nervous system.

An unusual condition has been described in which remarkable increases of coproporphyrin III are observed in both urine and feces, in otherwise normal persons.[60a] There have been no associated symptoms, the abnormality having been detected accidentally. Because of the lack of increase of uroporphyrin or of any appearance of porphobilinogen it has seemed best not to designate these cases as examples of porphyria (*vide infra*), but rather as idiopathic coproporphyrinuria. However, Berger and Goldberg[60b] have recently called it "coproporphyria." In this category must also be placed certain cases of abdominal pain in which, curiously enough, the amounts excreted are of much smaller magnitude than in the asymptomatic group just referred to.

Uroporphyrin

Uroporphyrin is regularly demonstrable in extremely small amounts in normal urine. Lockwood[39a] mentions a range of 15 to 30 micrograms per 24 hours (6 subjects). Bashour* in this laboratory has found from 1 to 37 μg. (47 subjects). The studies of Schwartz[38b] and Lockwood[39b] have shown that this is mainly type I isomer. Uroporphyrin excretion has been studied in a variety of diseases other than porphyria. With[61] has found distinct increases in certain cases of hepatic disease. Bashour† has observed very significant increases in some cases of cirrhosis and also in lead poisoning. It is evident, however, that there need not be any increase of the urinary uroporphyrin despite a considerable increase

* With P. Lowry.

† Unpublished.

of the urinary coproporphyrin. The ratio has not, thus far at least, proved to be of value in diagnosis except in relation to porphyria (*vide infra*). A urotype porphyrin is also demonstrable in small amounts in the normal feces. Bashour* has noted a range of 20 to 60 μg. per day (12 subjects). The possibility exists that this is partly derived from the fecal flora. Bashour* found that the fecal uroporphyrin in cases of complete biliary obstruction was usually less than 5 μg., but in two cases 14 and 38 μg. were observed. At the present time at least, the value of determination of the fecal uroporphyrin appears to be limited mainly to the porphyria problem (*vide infra.*)

Protoporphyrin and Closely Related Porphyrins

Protoporphyrin is regularly found in the feces, and very small amounts are often demonstrable in the bile.[35] It is probable that the majority of the fecal protoporphyrin under ordinary circumstances is exogenous, derived principally from the hemoglobin of meat in the diet. Increases are often observed with gastrointestinal bleeding. In hemolytic anemias and in certain cases of porphyria (*vide infra*) larger amounts have been encountered, believed to be endogenous, although of unknown source.

Blood in the intestinal tract is generally productive of some deutero- in addition to protoporphyrin. This is derived, however, by a primary bacterial reduction of hematin to deuterohematin (the vinyl groups being removed by reduction), after which splitting out of iron results in formation of free deuteroporphyrin.[1] So far as can be determined, this is not of metabolic significance but is derived only from hemoglobin altered by the bacterial flora of the colon. It should be mentioned, however, that deuteroporphyrin seldom represents more than a minor fraction of the total hemoglobin in the feces, the majority being excreted as hematin or deuterohematin. Certain additional porphyrins probably derived from protoporphyrin are at times demonstrable in the feces, especially in association with hemolytic anemias. These are very similar in physical behavior to deuteroporphyrin, and hence have been designated as "pseudodeuteroporphyrins."[35] They may be identical with what Schumm[62] earlier referred to as "saproporphrins."

In the author's experience, protoporphyrin has been encountered but very rarely in the urine, so seldom as to be of negligible significance. This is not in accord with the reports of Boas[63] or Brugsch.[64] Since the appearance of Brugsch's paper a renewed search has failed to confirm the concept that protoporphyrin is a regular urinary constituent.

* Unpublished.

PORPHYRIA

This term has been generally used to connote a peculiar constitutional fault or "inborn error"[65] of porphyrin metabolism characterized by marked overproduction of uroporphyrin and related substances. As will be seen, however, there is some uncertainty as to whether such overproduction always represents a constitutional disturbance or whether in rare instances it may appear as a sequel to some other disease, such as an infectious or toxic state. The relatively frequent occurrence of latent forms of porphyria make it extremely difficult to determine in such questionable cases whether the infection or toxic effect of any given disease has served simply as a precipitating factor in making a porphyria manifest. This problem will become more apparent in the following discussion.

The classification of porphyria proposed many years ago by Günther[66,67] has been widely used in the past. He clearly recognized the three main clinical forms of the disease, but his nomenclature is conflicting. He described porphyria congenita, porphyria acuta (idiopathic and toxic) and porphyria chronica. In the first of these, photosensitivity is the outstanding feature, appearing early in life. Although in some instances the red urine is evident at birth, the disease usually does not become manifest until months or years after birth. In these the term congenital can be applied only as it relates to the latent trait, and there can be no doubt that it is just as applicable, in this sense, to many of the cases designated as acute or chronic porphyria in Günther's classification. The latter are frequently familial and congenital, though symptoms rarely appear before adult life. The term chronic is also unfortunate, as the photosensitive (congenital) form is usually chronic in the extreme, and the acute type is either intermittent or the attacks are so frequent and prolonged or the residues so enduring that a degree of chronicity is often achieved. Information gained in recent years has permitted a new and much more basic classification, as follows:

1. *Porphyria erythropoietica*—early photosensitivity, increased hemolysis and erythropoiesis, splenomegaly. Excessive and abnormal porphyrin formation in the developing red blood cells of the bone marrow.
2. *Porphyria hepatica*—excessive and abnormal formation of porphyrin precursors and porphyrins in the liver.
   a. intermittent acute type—abdominal and/or nervous manifestations
   b. "Cutanea tarda" type—photosensitivity and frequent hepatic dysfunction.
   c. Mixed or combined type—photosensitivity with abdominal and/or nervous symptoms and frequent evidence of liver affection.

Porphyria Erythropoietica (*Porphyria Congenita, Günther*)

The fundamental basis for this disease appears to be a constitutional fault in porphyrin synthesis in relation to hemoglobin formation in developing normoblasts of the bone marrow.[68,69] Occurrence in siblings is often noted, and there is little doubt that the disease is due to transmission of a non sex-linked, recessive gene. Contrary to previous belief, both sexes are equally affected. Borst and Königsdörffer,[70] studying the famous case Petry at necropsy, first observed the porphyrin fluorescence in nucleated erythrocytes in the bone marrow. They believed these were megaloblasts and considered that the patient had pernicious anemia. In retrospect, however, it appears more likely that he was suffering from a chronic hemolytic anemia. As will be seen, this is a frequent complication in this form of porphyria. In the case Petry (Fig. 4) death occurred at age 32; by this time the great overproduction of porphyrin since early in life had been responsible for a rich deposit in various organs and tissues, including the liver and spleen, bones, kidneys, intestines and skin. This was so extensive that conclusions could not be drawn as to an individual site of origin.

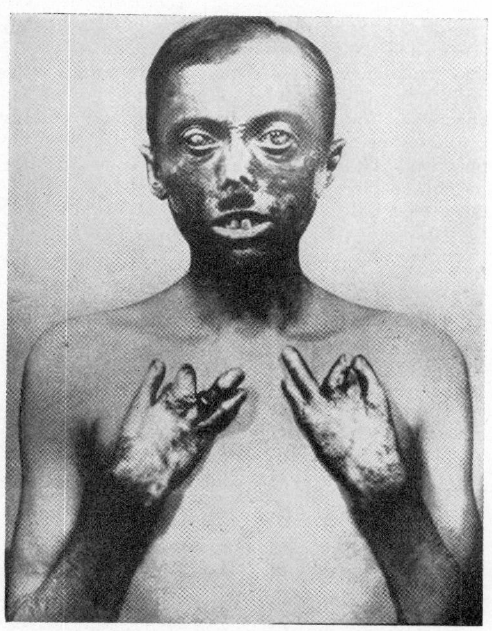

FIG. 4. Porphyria congenita (Günther) (porphyria erythropoietica): the famous case Petry.[67,70] (From chapter by Günther "Hämatoporphyrie" in Schittenhelm's "Die Krankheiten des Blutes und blutbildenden Organe." Bd. II, Enzyklopaedie der Klinische Medizin. Berlin, J. Springer, 1925. Reproduced by permission of the publishers.)

TABLE 2. DISTRIBUTION OF PORPHYRINS IN A CASE OF PORPHYRIA ERYTHROPOIETICA (M.H., ♀, 7)

DATE		ERYTHROCYTES µg./100 cc.	SERUM µg./100 cc.	BONE MARROW µg./100 cc.	SPLEEN µg./100 gm.	LIVER µg./100 gm.	URINE µg./24 hr.
3-8-51	Uroporphyrin	11.0	0	2635.0			3000
	Coproporphyrin	5.6	10.0	302.0			4500
	Protoporphyrin	55.0	0	124.0			0
6-18-51	Uroporphyrin	440.0	5.0		3415.2	869.1	52,300
to	Coproporphyrin	150.0	26.0		735.5	429.6	2800
6-21-51	Protoporphyrin	105.0	0		104.6	45.4	0

(*From Schmid, Schwartz, and Watson.*[68])

Note: The bone marrow values relate to the entire sample obtained by puncture. Because of dilution it is clear that the actual porphyrin concentration in the marrow was considerably higher. It is probable that the concentration in the second period was considerably higher than in the first, but the amount of marrow was too small for actual determination. The appearance of the normoblasts in the fluorescence microscope indicated the presence of large amounts of porphyrin.

Values for the fecal porphyrins for 4-2 to 4-6-51 were as follows: Uroporphyrin 136 µg./24-hr; coproporphyrin 43,400 µg./24 hr. The latter was 98 per cent type I. While these values are not directly comparable in point of time, they nevertheless permit an interesting comparison with the urinary and blood data, especially the much higher values noted for the serum coproporphyrin.

Recently, however, studies of cases in early childhood have permitted a better perspective, at least with respect to the relative importance of bone marrow and liver.[68] In these it was clear that the amount of porphyrin in the developing normoblasts greatly exceeded that in the liver (Fig. 6 b). It was of special interest too that the formation of porphyrin appeared to be initiated in the normoblast nuclei. It was also evident that only certain normoblasts were involved in the excessive formation of porphyrin.[68,69] Otherwise morphologically indistinguishable cells exhibited no increase under the fluorescence microscope. The nuclei of the fluorescing normoblasts were noted in addition to contain benzidine positive inclusions, either hemoglobin or a closely related substance.[69] In these cases there were splenic enlargement and increased hemolytic activity. In the first case of this type which was studied, the hemolytic anemia was outspoken and threatening to life. Splenectomy resulted in dramatic improvement. The patient at once lost her hemolytic anemia, the porphyrin excretion declined to a very small fraction of what it had previously been and the photosensitivity disappeared. Nine years have now elapsed and there has been no recurrence of either anemia or photosensitivity. The patient has developed normally and has been able to have normal activities in the sun. In other cases, however splenectomy has not had such a beneficial result. In one case, despite significant reduction in porphyrin formation and excretion, the photosensitivity has persisted and there has been a variable although mild anemia. The spleens in these cases contain great excesses of uro- and coproporphyrin I which may be ascribed to storage of porphyrins derived from the excessive destruction of porphyrin-laden erythrocytes. In the first case mentioned above the conclusions as to relative amounts in the bone marrow, liver and spleen rested mainly on observations of the intensity of fluorescence in ultraviolet light, rather than actual assay. In subsequent cases an improved microtechnique has been used. Data from such an instance are given in Table 2.

Of special fundamental interest in Table 2 is the contrast in values for bone marrow, circulating red blood cells and urine. This suggests that the relatively large amounts of urinary porphyrin are actually derived in considerable part by release from intact, developing erythrocytes in the bone marrow. Any other explanation would appear to require so rapid a rate of destruction of normoblasts as to appear quite unreasonable.

The prompt and marked decline in porphyrin formation which may follow splenectomy in these cases[68,71] can perhaps best be explained on the basis of reduced need for new red cells incident to reduced hemolysis, hence a diminished erythropoiesis and with this a reduction of hemoglobin and porphyrin formation.

The clinical features of the erythropoietic form are primarily cutaneous. Photosensitivity appears early in life, in some cases being manifest even within a few days after birth. Often it is postponed to the second or third year of life or later. The first manifestation of light sensitivity, the so-called "hydroa aestivale seu vacciniforme," is characterized by vesicles or bullae on the light exposed surfaces of the skin (Fig. 6 a). As the name implies, these are much more common and troublesome in the spring and summer months, when light is more intense and exposure greater. Certain isolated observations suggest that porphyrin formation and excretion may be greater in relation to increased light exposure. In Anderson's case,[74] the first in which the relationship of porphyrinuria and photosensitivity was clearly established, the patient's urine became much more colored with increasing sun exposure prior to the appearance of vesicles. We have observed a similar sequence.[68] Experimental studies have shown that ultraviolet light in the presence of certain stimuli, such as lead, enhances porphyrin formation.[72] This is much more marked if photodynamic action is promoted by a substance such as rose bengal.[73]

As time goes on, the vesicles of hydroa give rise to scarring, which is promoted by secondary infection. With continued exposure to sunlight there is progressive destruction of more and more areas, with mutilation of hands and face (Fig. 4). The nose and ears are often deformed, and there may be considerable scarring of the eyelids and even of the conjunctivae. Parts of digits are lost, and the hands and fingers may become severely deformed.[67] Increased pigmentation is often noted, especially between the areas of scar. The condition may superficially resemble xeroderma pigmentosum, in which photosensitivity is prominent, but without disturbance of porphyrin metabolism.

Hypertrichosis is not infrequent in these cases. It does not appear to be related to photosensitivity. It is usually most marked on the arms and legs.

The spleen is often enlarged, even in earlier childhood. The enlargement is usually progressive as time goes on.[75] Hemolytic anemia may appear at any age. It is probable that a compensated, mild hemolytic activity is frequently present in the absence of a manifest anemia. The reticulocytes and fecal urobilinogen are often increased. The bone marrow is hyperplastic—normoblastic. As already mentioned, certain of the normoblasts contain relatively large amounts of uro- and coproporphyrin of type I, while others do not evidence any increase in porphyrin content (Fig. 6 b). Considerable increases are found in the circulating erythrocytes and plasma.[68] It is probable that the plasma uroporphyrin is responsible for the photosensitivity, perhaps only after actual deposition in the skin, although information on this point is lacking. It should be noted that it has not been possible thus far to reproduce vesicles with artificial light,[71,76] although sunlight is clearly effective. Uroporphyrin I is very light-sensitizing in mice, but so far as can be determined it has not been shown experimentally to have photodynamic activity in man. The experiments thus far described have probably not reduplicated the type and duration of the exposure to light in the disease in man, and it seems most likely that uroporphyrin is responsible for the skin lesions of porphyria.

The urine contains large amounts of uro- and smaller amounts of copro-porphyrin I, while the reverse is found in the feces.[71] The porphyrin in the urine is present at least mainly as the free porphyrin, not as a metal (zinc) complex, as in the other forms of the disease (*vide infra*). The porphyrins are readily separated and isolated in crystalline form. Uroporphyrin is insoluble in ether and is commonly present in such high concentration in this type of the disease that it precipitates when the urine is acidified with acetic acid. The precipitate may then be collected, dissolved and esterified according to well established methods.[1,77,78] The coproporphyrin is readily extracted by ether from the acidified urine. It may be concentrated by extraction from the ether by hydrochloric acid, then esterified and crystallized. The methyl esters of the porphyrins generally crystallize very well from hot chloroform-methyl alcohol;[1] as the chloroform boils off, the esters separate from the methyl alcohol. Pure uroporphyrin I methyl ester melts at 290 to 293° C. with marked shrinking from 284°; copro- I methyl ester melts at 250° C.

The Ehrlich reacting chromogen, porphobilinogen, has not been demonstrable in the urine in the erythropoietic form of the disease, and this is perhaps one of the most important fundamental differences from the other forms, especially in relation to the basis for their differing clinical manifestations.

Treatment has been limited until recently to supportive and protective measures, the latter with particular relation to sunlight exposure. Climate, occupation, clothing, hats, gloves, parasols, ointments and lotions all deserve consideration. Further investigation is needed as to protective ointments or innocuous substances to be given internally to impregnate the skin, which absorb light in the region of the Soret band, i.e., 400 to 410 mμ.

The information thus far available about splenectomy is too meager to permit definite conclusions as to the regularity or permanence of its effect. In the two cases observed by the author, outspoken reductions of porphyrin excretion have been noted; in the first of these, there has been essentially no recurrence of light sensitivity and no anemia for eight years. In the second case there was again a distinct though not as marked diminution in porphyrin excretion, but vesicles have continued to appear and there has been no definite improvement in any respect. In an earlier case reported by de Marval and Pons,[79] splenectomy was followed by a significant reduction in hemolytic activity and some improvement of photosensitivity. Quantitative data were not given, but it was indicated that the porphyria itself was unaffected. Gray and Neuberger[80a] and Rosenthal and co-workers[80b] have reported cases in which benefit was only mild or transitory.

As mentioned earlier, it seems not unlikely that the deposition of uroporphyrin in developing bone is related to its physical affinity for calcium phosphate. This probably explains the red bones and red teeth (erythrodontia) in the erythropoietic type of porphyria. Red teeth are not a constant feature. Mackey and Garrod[75] regarded erythrodontia as evidence that the porphyria had already existed in utero. This applies, of course, to the deciduous teeth. In two cases studied in this laboratory in which the porphyria first became manifest at ages 2 and 4 respectively, there was not any definite erythrodontia in ordinary light, but in both patients the teeth exhibited marked red fluorescence in ultraviolet light.

Porphyria Hepatica

As already indicated, this term is used on the basis of recent evidence that in the forms comprising this group, the liver, rather than the bone marrow, is principally responsible for the formation and release of abnormal porphyrins or porphyrin precursors. The clinical subdivision into the two main forms (intermittent acute and "cutanea tarda") is based chiefly on the presence or absence of photosensitivity versus abdominal and/or nervous manifestations. The latter symptoms characterize the intermittent acute type in which photosensitivity is lacking. Conversely, in the pure cutanea tarda form abdominal and nervous symptoms are not a feature. There are cases which are best classified as mixed or combined in that they exhibit in varying degree combinations of photosensitivity with abdominal and/or nervous phenomena. Rimington[81,82] believes that the acute and cutanea tarda types are quite independent diseases of distinct etiology. He regards cases of the mixed type as representatives of the cutanea tarda group in which abdominal or nervous symptoms have been added to the photosensitivity. He has stressed a markedly increased fecal porphyrin excretion in relatively asymptomatic cutanea tarda cases as indicating a fundamental difference from the acute type, in which it is true that the fecal porphyrin excretion is usually less marked. Nevertheless, acute cases have been observed repeatedly in which the fecal porphyrin excretion during remission was as high as that noted in some cutanea tarda cases.[83] It should be emphasized that in the acute form the main abnormality is an excretion of colorless, non-fluorescing precursors including δ-amino-levulinic acid, porphobilinogen and porphyrinogen. Porphobilinogen is excreted only in the urine. δ-Amino-levulinic acid has thus far been demonstrated only in the urine,[84] and studies of its presence in the feces have not yet been reported. The excretion of uroporphyrinogen is mainly in the urine. Thus it is evident that in the acute form of the disease, even in remission, the representatives of abnormal porphyrin metabolism are excreted largely in the urine and to a much lesser extent in the feces. In the pure cutanea tarda type, in which porphobilinogen is not seen, much larger amounts of porphyrin, especially coproporphyrin, are found in the feces, and during asymptomatic periods it is true that these amounts may be considerably greater than in the urine. During relapse, especially that characterized by outspoken hepatic functional impairment, there is a considerable shift of porphyrin to the urine. In this connection it should be noted that in both forms there is a general tendency toward an increase in the uroporphyrin-coproporphyrin ratio with relapse, and under all circumstances much larger proportions of the uroporphyrin are excreted in the urine. The shift of porphyrin to the urine in relapse is regarded simply as an evidence of diminished hepatic function. This has been well documented with respect to coproporphyrin in other conditions, both human[47] and experimental.[119]

Certain cases of the mixed or combined type are of fundamental interest in that at one time at which abdominal or nervous manifestations are most prominent the liver porphyrin content is relatively low and that of precursor and of the amount of porphobilinogen in the urine relatively high, whereas at another time at which photosensitivity alone is the symptom in evidence the liver contains much larger amounts of preformed porphyrin, and relatively little precursor.[68] This variation in itself points toward a fundamental relationship between the two forms and suggests that the difference is due simply to a shifting location of the disturbance in the pathway of porphyrin biosynthesis. Another important fact in favor of a fundamental relationship is the repeated observation of families in which both types of the disease as well as examples of the mixed form are represented. The most striking families of this type have been reported in detail by G. Dean[85,86] in South Africa. Here the disease is relatively common, because, as Dean has shown, of the pure family strains which have now come down through 12 generations from the time of the first colonists. Dean's observations clearly confirm the belief that the hepatic porphyriac trait is dominant and not sex-linked. It is of interest that of his numerous families, all are descendants of the same mating three centuries ago. Within the hepatic group of cases, the cutanea tarda type is more common in the male and the intermittent acute type in the female.

It is quite possible that there are differing genetic forms of the acute type. Waldenström's experience in Sweden and Lapland fails to reveal cases of acute and cutanea tarda porphyria in the same family, although as already mentioned, this concurrence is quite common in South Africa, the United States and elsewhere. This may well be due to a fundamental genetic difference, but it is also possible that climatic or environmental factors are of importance. In the author's experience, both types of families have been encountered, some having only representatives of the acute form, others of the cutanea tarda disease, and still others of both varieties or the mixed type in the same individual. Again it is not yet clear whether these differences are purely genetic—in other words, fundamentally different but clinically similar disorders—or whether constitutional or environmental factors impinge in such a way on a single disease as to produce these various forms of hepatic porphyria. Further study of this question is needed.

As implied by the name, the *intermittent* acute type is characterized by individual attacks of longer or shorter duration, with varying periods of remission during which the patient is symptom-free. In some cases the attacks are of such long duration as to be subacute or even chronic, but as a rule they are rather abrupt in onset and sufficiently short to be designated as acute. In this connection, however, it should be emphasized that the acute attacks are seldom less than 48 hours in duration and that very brief attacks of pain lasting but for a few minutes or even a few hours with complete remission are not at all suggestive of acute porphyria.

The manifestations of the disease are abdominal or nervous, or both. There is evidence that various chemicals, especially barbiturates, are at times active in precipitating attacks, although the fundamental mechanism is not understood. Waldenström[87] gave barbiturate to a person who had never had previous attacks but whose latent porphyria was discovered when a sister's manifest disease led to study of the other members of the family. Following the barbiturate an attack occurred, with heightened porphyrin excretion. A similar experiment and result were reported by Jorgenson and With.[88] Attacks have followed the ingestion or administration of many other chemicals including Sulfonal, Trional, Phanodorm, Sedormid, ergot preparations and chloroquine. Interestingly enough, BAL (British anti-lewisite) has been reported to alleviate attacks,[89] but cases have also been observed in which acute relapse followed its use. Alcoholic beverages are at times of apparent significance, and the author is aware of several instances in which an acute attack has followed a period of acute alcoholism. Studies with alcohol in this laboratory[52] resulted in heightened porphyrin excretion in several instances and a distinct, although mild attack in one.

There is strong reason to believe that psychic and emotional disturbances may precipitate acute attacks. A clear history of a single severe stressful situation or an outspoken emotional disturbance preceding an attack has often been obtained. These patients commonly have a "nervous" constitution or background, as emphasized by Günther,[67] who referred to this as "porphyrismus." This, however, has never been objectively defined.

The manifestations during relapse are extremely varied, so much so that Waldenström[90] has termed the disease "the little simulator." Abdominal pain is often very severe, frequently colicky in type, either generalized or localized. Pain in the back or loins is also common. Various conditions have been simulated, including appendicitis, bowel obstruction, renal or biliary colic, perforated ulcer and pancreatitis. The importance of porphyria in surgical diagnosis has repeatedly been stressed, more recently by Calvy.[91] The severe constipation which is usually present increases the likelihood of confusion with bowel obstruction. The abdomen is usually soft, and tenderness is not marked; rebound tenderness is generally lacking. Fever and leukocytosis are unusual but may occur. X-ray of the abdomen often reveals areas of distention in the colon, caused by trapped gas, proximal to an area of spasm.[92] Very rarely, volvulus and gangrene may supervene.[93] There is often lack of any bowel movement, with empty rectum, for many days. In exceptional cases, however, diarrhea is noted.

The nervous manifestations are perhaps best divided into (1) peripheral neuropathy, (2) bulbar, (3) psychic and (4) autonomic. The first category is characterized by pain in the extremities, especially the legs, weakness or outspoken flaccid paralysis and often quadriplegia. This is not an ascending symmetric paralysis of the Landry type; it develops rather, in an unpredictable fashion, the involvement at times being widespread simultaneously and at others first in one then another muscle group or extremity without any fixed sequence.[90] Paralysis of abdominal or other trunk muscles and respiratory paralysis occur less frequently. The latter is one of the chief causes of death. Upper motor neuron signs are usually lacking. A curious contrast is at times observed in that ankle clonus may occur in the absence of patellar reflexes. Sensory phenomena, other than the pain in the extremities, are seldom observed.[94] Bulbar signs are not infrequent in the more severe cases, and are often associated with respiratory paralysis. Difficulty in swallowing, regurgitation and aspiration point to bulbar involvement. Vocal cord paresis with a weak, hoarse, high pitched voice is noted in some cases. Tachycardia may be marked; quite possibly it may be due to vagal nuclear involvement or to peripheral vagal neuropathy. This may also be the basis for electrocardiographic changes of nonspecific type that are at times noted.[95]

Among the psychic changes a pseudohysteria is quite common. Many cases have been wrongly classified, at least for a time, as neurasthenia or hysteria. Patients subject to intermittent acute porphyria have often been excessively "nervous" for long periods, even many years before the attack. Günther's "nervous" constitution or "porphyrismus," has already been referred to.

In some cases the porphyria masks under the appearance of schizophrenia or of a manic or depressive state.

It is difficult to assign manifestations to autonomic involvement, although a relationship appears reasonable. Pigment deposition in autonomic ganglia has been observed,[92] although the character of the pigment has not been defined. It is not unlikely that abdominal pain is a result of autonomic disturbance rather than a direct effect of porphyrin or porphobilinogen on the intestinal wall, as has been supposed.[96] This is supported by the relative frequency with which temporary relief is obtained from ganglion blocking agents such as tetraethylammonium (*vide infra*) and the considerable benefit often obtained from chlorpromazine. In one of the author's cases bilateral splanchnicectomy has been followed for a prolonged period by complete relief of abdominal pain, although the underlying porphyria was unaffected. In some cases the symptoms are solely abdominal, in others nervous, but in the majority both are represented at least in some degree.

Hypertension, quite likely neurogenic, is relatively common and may be marked.[97] The author has repeatedly observed cases in which outspoken hypertension and irregular attenuation of retinal arterioles occurred during relapse but disappeared completely during remission. Convulsions may occur in association with the hypertension, but without headache or choked disk, so that it is doubtful that they may be ascribed solely to hypertensive encephalopathy. Oliguria is also noted at times, but albuminuria and hematuria are lacking, thus serving to differentiate the condition from acute glomerulonephritis or eclampsia.

Pregnancy has been observed in association with porphyria; in some cases fatal relapses have occurred at the time of delivery, although there is no definite evidence that relapse is due to the pregnancy or the delivery itself. Nevertheless, this is suggested at least in certain instances. In a remarkable case recently studied by the author, the symptoms of porphyria, chiefly pain in the extremities, came on at a considerable interval after the first pregnancy, which was uneventful. For several years the pain has been remarkably cyclic in character, starting shortly after the middle of the menstrual period, at a time corresponding roughly with ovulation and continuing just to the onset of the menses, then disappearing until the next mid-menstrual period. This patient's second pregnancy was attended by rather severe symptoms attributable to the porphyria. In a subsequent pregnancy the symptoms were so severe that interference with the pregnancy was deemed essential.

In one of the author's cases a severe relapse followed the use of an ergot preparation taken in an unsuccessful attempt to induce abortion during the early months of pregnancy. The relapse itself probably later resulted in a spontaneous miscarriage and in this instance remission occurred soon after the uterus had emptied. The same patient had a later pregnancy and spontaneous (?) abortion without evidence of relapse of the porphyria. In one case[98] in which the mother died in relapse eight days after delivering a healthy baby, it was found that for the first twelve hours of life the infant's urine was port wine colored and contained uroporphyrin and excessive coproporphyrin, after which it rapidly became quite normal. This suggested a considerable transfer of these substances across the placenta, although the possibility is not wholly excluded that there was transitory formation in the infant's tissues.

Pigmentation of the skin is noted in some cases. In one of the author's cases pigmentation and weakness of the extremities had led to prolonged but unsuccessful treatment for supposed Addison's disease; prior to this the patient had had an appendectomy for abdominal pain and a thyroidectomy for nervousness and weakness, both procedures also to no avail. Exceptional cases have been recorded in which a very striking generalized pigmentation of the skin has been present.[99] The nature of the pigment is unknown; porphobilin, as described in the following, deserves consideration in this respect.

Treatment during relapse has been limited until recently to attempts to relieve pain and limit nervous activity, and at the same time to administer chemicals sparingly. Barbiturates are to be avoided entirely. Such sedatives as paraldehyde or chloral hydrate have not been shown to precipitate or aggravate attacks. Nor have opiates been indicted in this respect, and they may be required for severe pain not relieved by other medication. Demerol is of much value, though seldom effective for more than three or four hours even with 100 mg. subcutaneously. The value of chlorpromazine was first realized when it was used in a case of porphyria in an attempt to reduce the Demerol requirement.[100] It was at once beneficial and the patient soon went into remission. This has been the experience in a number of subsequent cases, as reported by Melby[100a] and Monaco et al.[100b] In this study it was evident that, although chlorpromazine did not cause any immediate decline of porphyrin or porphobilinogen excretion, a remission of symptoms rather regularly supervened. This experience led to the concept that the chlorpromazine may interrupt a vicious cycle of nervous disturbance, permitting the onset of remission. There is some evidence that chlorpromazine ameliorates autonomic nervous injury of various types, and it is quite possible that this is the mode of action in acute porphyria. In any event, it has proved to be superior to any other remedy thus far used in the treatment of pain and nervousness. There has been no effect on established paralyses. In the majority of instances thus far studied, 25 mg. four times daily has been adequate to provide relief. In certain cases, however, as much as 100 mg. intramuscularly three or four times daily has been required at the outset of treatment.

ACTH or cortisone has been used in many cases of acute porphyria with some apparent success.[83] This is, however, unpredictable and many cases have been reported in which there has been complete failure to obtain any benefit.

The *urine* in the *intermittent acute form* is characterized by a mixture of porphyrin precursors which is quite different from and more complex than that in porphyria erythropoietica. In this disease colorless precursors are largely represented both in the urine and in the liver and preformed porphyrins are present only in minor degree. The freshly passed urine is often normal in color, darkening greatly on standing (Fig. 6 g). The Ehrlich aldehyde reacting chromogen, porphobilinogen, is present in large amount during relapse, often, but not always diminishing and at times disappearing entirely with remission.

Dean emphasizes that in the South African cases of acute porphyria, the porphobilinogen regularly disappears during remission, only rarely being demonstrable and then in minor degree, whereas it is characteristic of the cases in Sweden that the porphobilinogen persists during remission. Nevertheless, Waldenström has noted certain instances in which there has been complete disappearance. In the United States there are all manner of variations in this respect. At times very large amounts persist indefinitely despite long continued complete remission. The values may diminish remarkably, and at times there is complete disappearance. The author's experience in this regard would not permit a separation of two distinct forms of acute porphyria, although this is certainly suggested by the experience in Sweden and in South Africa.

The porphobilinogen aldehyde compound is insoluble in chloroform in striking contrast to that of urobilinogen.[101] (Fig. 6 h). The simple test depending on this characteristic is of considerable aid in diagnosis, though not entirely pathognomonic. This test consists simply in mixing 3 ml. of urine and 3 ml. of Ehrlich's reagent* and shaking together briefly. Six ml. of saturated aqueous solution of sodium acetate are then added and thoroughly mixed. Five ml. of chloroform are next shaken with the aqueous solution and allowed to separate. The urobilinogen aldehyde compound is extracted by the chloroform to which it imparts a pink or deep red color, depending on amount. The porphobilinogen aldehyde is not extracted by the chloroform, its red color remaining in the aqueous. Viewed with a spectroscope this compound exhibits a strong α absorption band with maximum intensity at 560 mμ. This is indistinguishable from the band of urobilinogen aldehyde, but the latter does not exhibit the fainter β absorption band (max., 520 mμ) which is characteristic of the porphobilinogen aldehyde in more concentrated solutions. In carrying out the above test smaller or larger amounts of urine and reagents may be employed, in the same proportions. It is essential that all of the hydrochloric acid in the Ehrlich's reagent be converted by sodium acetate to acetic acid. The final aqueous solution should be negative to Congo red paper. Weak or borderline (pink) reactions are at times encountered in instances in which the presence of porphyria cannot be proved, and in which it is conceivable that a similar or identical compound is excreted in small amount as an expression of some other abnormality. It is possible that other unrelated pyrrols of indole type are at times responsible for weak color reactions of this type. Weak or questionable reactions should not be the basis for the diagnosis of porphyria. It is safe to say that if the patient is having active symptoms due to intermittent acute porphyria, the porphobilinogen reaction is outspoken and unmistakable and the above mentioned absorption bands are readily seen. It should be mentioned that certain indicators in hydrochloric acid alone and hence in the presence of Ehrlich's reagent exhibit a red color similar to that of the porphobilinogen aldehyde and also insoluble in chloroform. A supposed porphobilinogen reaction was recently found to be due, in several instances, to the presence of methyl red in the urine. In these a Zephiran solution containing methyl red had gained access to the sample. If there is any question of admixture with an indicator, the simple addition of hydrochloric acid alone will resolve the matter. Ingested pyridium may give rise to a confusing orange-pink color.

The well defined porphobilinogen, as isolated by Westall,[14] exhibits an Ehrlich aldehyde reaction in major degree as soon as the Ehrlich reagent is added; urobilinogen develops its color to any considerable extent only after the sodium acetate solution is added.[17]

* 0.7 gm. p-dimethylaminobenzaldehyde, 150 cc. concentrated HCl, 100 cc. H_2O.

Schwartz, in this laboratory, first observed atypical porphobilinogen-like substances in acute porphyria urine which behave more like urobilinogen in this respect, and also in being extracted from the urine by ethyl acetate, unlike porphobilinogen. Schwartz also found that the aldehyde compound of the Westall porphobilinogen is not extracted by butyl alcohol, unlike that of the atypical porphobilinogen(s). These observations have been confirmed repeatedly;[17,93] attempts to purify the latter compound by either the Westall method or other techniques have thus far been unsuccessful. No definite evidence of conversion to porphyrin by heat has yet been obtained. Schwartz has also found that crystalline porphobilinogen is readily converted to the atypical compound by heating under pressure in a sealed tube in dilute hydrochloric acid, exactly as is done in decarboxylating uroporphyrin.[102] The nature of the alteration which occurs has not yet been determined. The aldehyde compound of the atypical or altered porphobilinogen obtained in this fashion or encountered in the urine does not exhibit the β absorption band at 520 mμ.

Rarely, porphobilinogen and excessive uroporphyrin are encountered in cases of well defined disease entities not exhibiting the manifestations of porphyria. The author has now observed this peculiarity in certain cases of Hodgkin's disease, carcinomatosis, hepatic cirrhosis and nervous system affection.[17] It is unknown whether the appearance of these substances in such cases is related to a latent porphyria or a constitutional tendency to it. The latter is perhaps suggested by the fact that such an association has been lacking in most cases of Hodgkin's disease and cirrhosis.

Distinct increases of δ-amino-levulinic acid, porphobilinogen and uroporphyrin are observed in the urine in lead poisoning. The first of these substances may be found in great excess.

Although the acute porphyria urine is characterized mainly by the presence of colorless precursors, it is usually possible even in freshly passed urine to observe the absorption spectrum of a preformed uroporphyrin metal complex (Fig. 5). Although it is true, as Waldenström[103] observed, that if an alkaline urine is passed this spectrum may no longer be visible, the urine nevertheless contains the immediate precursor of the

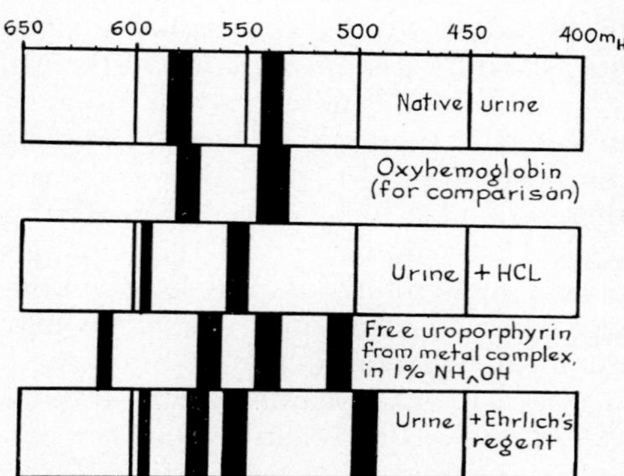

FIG. 5. Absorption bands of zinc complex of uroporphyrin in acute porphyria urine, and from top downward, oxyhemoglobin, porphyrin hydrochloride spectrum formed by adding HCl to native urine (with the same treatment hemoglobin yields hematin with absorption in the red, thus easily distinguishing it from the porphyrin metal complex), the free porphyrin spectrum in dilute ammonia, and last, the spectrum produced by adding Ehrlich's aldehyde reagent to the urine. In the last the hydrochloride spectrum of the preformed porphyrin is again seen; the strong band at 560 mμ between the two bands of the hydrochloride is that of the porphobilinogen aldehyde; the strong band at the right is that of the dark brown porphobilin.

FIG. 6. (*Continued*)

D. Section of liver biopsy from case of hepatic cutanea tarda porphyria; unstained photograph in fluorescence microscope under ultraviolet light to show large amounts of porphyrin. The normal liver exhibits only bluish green fluorescence.

E. Red fluorescence of coproporphyrin solutions in ultraviolet light. That on the left was weakly colored, that on the right almost colorless.

F. Porphyria hepatica, cutanea tarda. E. G., male, 72. The patient also had bullous, ulcerating and scarring lesions on the face and hands.

G. Urine in acute porphyria. The sample on the left was freshly passed; that in the middle is the same urine after exposure to the air and light for several days. The sample on the right, from another patient, had stood for some time.

H. Chloroform solubility of the urobilinogen aldehyde compound (left) vs. porphobilinogen aldehyde (right), the latter a sample of urine from a patient with acute porphyria.

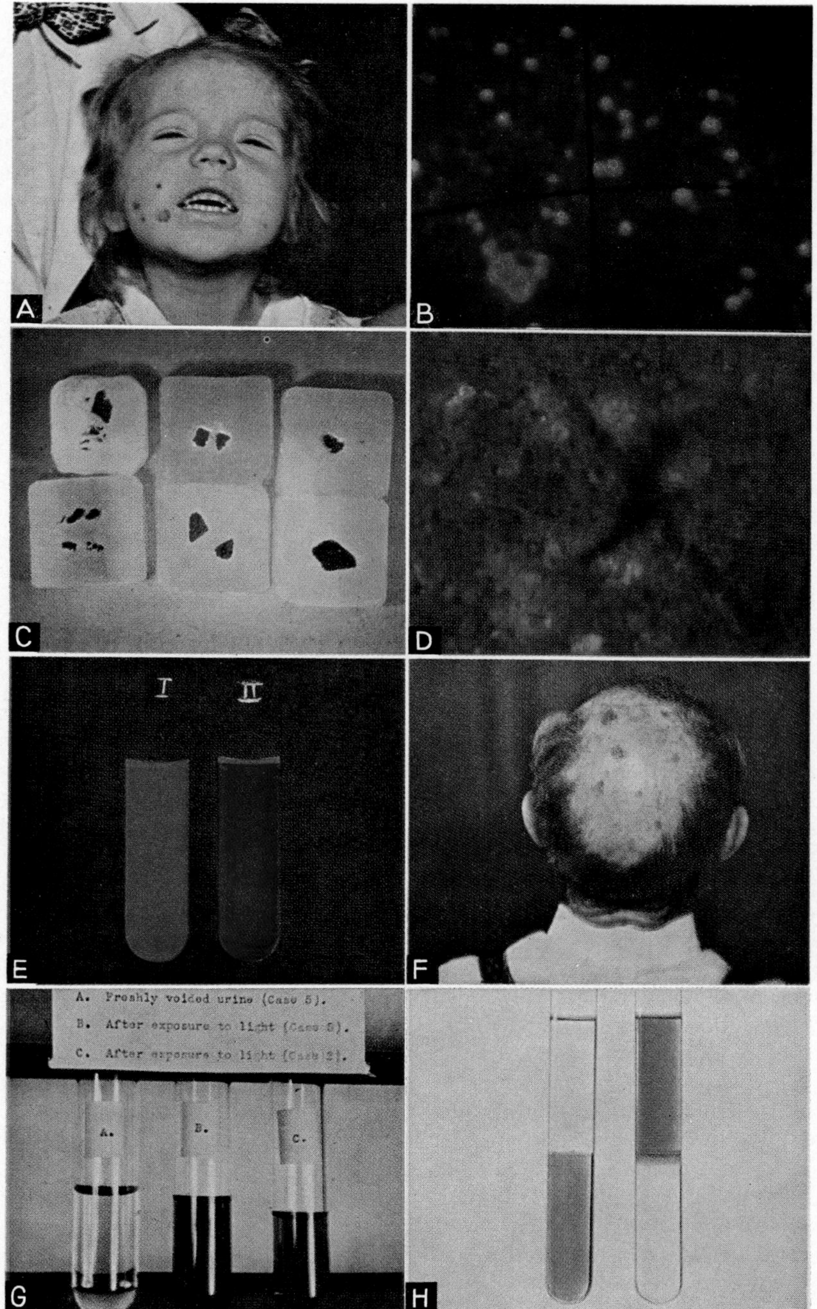

FIG. 6. Various aspects of porphyria.

A. D. H., female, 4. Porphyria erythropoietica; hydroa aestivale; early erythrodontia. This patient had hemolytic anemia and splenomegaly.

B. Porphyrin-laden normoblasts from bone marrow of same case. Unstained preparation photographed in fluorescence microscope, with ultraviolet light. (From Schmid, Schwartz, and Watson: A.M.A. Arch. Int. Med., *93:*167, 1954. Reproduced by permission of A.M.A.)

C. Paraffin blocks of liver biopsies photographed under ultraviolet light: (1) porphyria erythropoietica, (2) porphyria hepatica, cutanea tarda, (3) porphyria hepatica, intermittent acute. It is evident that the amount of porphyrin is large in 2, small in 1 and 3. (From Schmid, Schwartz, and Watson: A.M.A. Arch. Int. Med., *93:*167, 1954. Reproduced by permission of A.M.A.)

(*Legend continues on facing page.*)

porphyrin, i.e., its reduced form or porphyrinogen. As already mentioned, it is likely that this is in any event of greater significance from a metabolic viewpoint. If the acid urine is heated at 80° for one half hour, a very great increase of porphyrin is commonly observed. In certain samples, however, the urine on heating may become dark without any significant increase of porphyrin, but with disappearance of porphobilinogen and formation of the brown pigment porphobilin (Fig. 6 G).

It may be emphasized that the appearance of porphobilinogen is at times quite transitory, in relation to the acute attack. In one of the author's cases,[17] a woman of 29 had had ten laparotomies in eight years for recurrent abdominal pain, without relief from attacks. On the last admission a diagnosis of neurosis had been made, but a porphobilinogen test, as the attack was subsiding, was found to be positive. At this time the blood serum contained 9 μg./100 ml. of coproporphyrin. Twenty-four hours later the porphobilinogen reaction was much weaker and after 48 hours it was quite negative; at this time the serum no longer contained demonstrable coproporphyrin. The urine uro- and coproporphyrin concentrations were normal throughout these observations.

As mentioned earlier, the urine in cases of acute porphyria, at least in relapse, also contains relatively large amounts of the immediate precursor of porphobilinogen, δ-amino-levulinic acid.[10,13,84,105] Goldberg[106] has shown that porphobilinogen is harmless in small animals in acute experiments. The possibility has not been excluded that it or some derivative may be implicated in the human disease, and the same is true for δ-amino levulinic acid.

Earlier studies in this laboratory had shown that the Waldenström uroporphyrin complex as crystallized from acute porphyria urine, without preliminary heating, usually contains a preponderance of type I isomer.[77,78] This complex is often separable on a calcium carbonate column into a major component of uroporphyrin I and a minor component of a 7-carboxyl type III porphyrin. This form of complex was designated as the type A Waldenström porphyrin (Waldenström[107,108] having been the first to crystallize such a complex from acute porphyria urine). In other instances the Waldenström porphyrin ester behaves as an entity on the calcium carbonate column, but on decarboxylation the coproporphyrin mixture may be shown to consist mainly of type I isomer.[78,83,109] Rimington and his coworkers[111,112] in a series of more recent papers have stated that the Waldenström complex is mainly composed of uroporphyrin III and only to a minor extent of the type I isomer. This problem has now been studied extensively* in the author's laboratory, and the main fact to emerge is that with heating and disappearance of the porphobilinogen there is a very great increase of a Waldenström type porphyrin, which is now composed mainly of type III, as might be expected from the observation that heating of crystalline porphobilinogen alone produces mainly uroporphyrin III. The *unheated* urine samples from a number of cases of acute porphyria, subjected to various methods of isolation, have yielded a uroporphyrin complex which in most instances contains more type I than type III. It is of special interest that the *porphyrinogen* in fresh acute porphyria urine, separated from any preformed porphyrin and then converted to porphyrin by atmospheric O_2 and ultraviolet radiation, has been found to be mainly type I.* A few exceptions have been noted in which the only porphyrinogen in the urine was that of the 208 or 7-carboxyl type III porphyrin. Chu and Chu[110] have recently reported that in certain instances of acute porphyria the Waldenström ester was found to consist of approximately equal parts of uroporphyrins I and III and smaller amounts of a 7-carboxyl type III porphyrin. They found the latter in larger amount in cutanea tarda cases. In our own experience, the 7-COOH type III porphyrin has been present in varying amounts in all of the forms of hepatic porphyria,

* With Berg, Schwartz, Hawkinson and Bossenmaier, to be published.

often excreted in large part as colorless porphyrinogen.

In acute porphyria the preformed coproporphyrin is mainly type III. This simply indicates that there is relatively little transition from uroporphyrinogen to coproporphyrinogen in the type I series, while in the III series this appears to be more efficient.

During prolonged remissions of acute porphyria a marked reduction may be noted in the amount of porphobilinogen, uro- and coproporphyrin in the urine. In some cases there is complete disappearance of the porphobilinogen aldehyde reaction and the uroporphyrin may decline into the normal range. Opportunity has recently been afforded to re-examine a patient who had a severe acute attack of porphyria with quadriparesis 14 years ago. A number of the members of this patient's family were also found to have latent porphyria. The patient, at the time of the acute attack a young woman of 25, has had no further symptoms of the disease, has been married and had a normal pregnancy several years ago (the child is well and the urine exhibits no evidence of porphyria). The urine at the present time is quite negative for porphobilinogen and the uro- and coproporphyrin values are 14 and 234 μg. per day, respectively. Also, the fecal uro- and coproporphyrin values were normal.

As already mentioned, the broad category of porphyria hepatica also includes the "*cutanea tarda*" type of Waldenström and a mixed or combined form with features both of the acute disease and of cutaneous photosensitivity. In Günther's classification these forms were undoubtedly embraced by the term "chronic" porphyria. The designation "cutanea tarda" is apt in expressing the late appearance of skin lesions which are related at least in part to photosensitivity (Fig. 6 F). The onset is commonly postponed until the fourth to sixth decades. The skin lesions are often not as severe as in the most advanced stages of porphyria erythropoietica (congenita), possibly simply because of the late onset and the relatively short duration of photosensitivity. Bullous lesions are also common in this form, and the factors of trauma and heat appear to be of greater significance in their production than is true in porphyria erythropoietica. In some cases it has seemed that one or the other of these factors alone, without light exposure, was responsible for the development of bullae. Nevertheless, the lesions are almost entirely limited to the light exposed surfaces of the skin. Considerable scarring and at times some ulceration are observed (Fig. 6 F). Pigmentation of the skin and in some cases a curious purplish facies have been emphasized, especially by Brunsting,[113] for this form of the disease.

In the *combined* form of *hepatica porphyria* the abdominal and nervous manifestations are quite similar to those already described for the intermittent acute cases. The prognosis is somewhat better and the term "chronic" is more applicable, in accord with Günther's early observations.

It should be noted, however, that long and complete remissions occur in some cases. In these the urine porphyrin excretion may diminish markedly and porphobilinogen may disappear.

Hepatic manifestations appear to be somewhat more prominent in the "cutanea tarda" or combined forms. Jaundice has been observed repeatedly, ascites rarely. Spider nevi are seen in some cases. Alcoholism has been unduly frequent in patients with this disease,[113] in one of our cases the administration of alcohol under controlled circumstances clearly resulted in an increased excretion of porphyrins (both uro-type and copro-) and porphobilinogen in the urine. An association with diabetes mellitus appears to be more than casual.[114] To what extent the tendency to fatty liver manifested by these conditions is related to the porphyria, either as a causal or a precipitating factor, is unknown. The latter appears more reasonable. Cirrhosis is not infrequent, although exact figures as to its incidence are lacking. Laboratory evidences of liver functional impairment, such as reduced serum albumin, reversal of A/G ratio, positive cephalin cholesterol flocculation, thymol turbidity and bromsulphthalein retention, are often noted. It is interesting that any marked degree of urobilinogenuria is quite infrequent, either in the mixed or in the intermittent acute forms of porphyria. The reason for this is not clear.

Porphobilinogen is usually not found in the urine of the "cutanea tarda" cases, except when abdominal or nervous manifestations are also present, as in the "mixed" form; then it is often noted in large amount.[68] The uro- type porphyrin which is present behaves similarly to the Waldenström porphyrin isolated from the intermittent acute cases. On the average, however, the melting point of the methyl ester is significantly higher,[115] commonly from 265 to 275° C. because of a somewhat larger proportion of uroporphyrin I. The observations thus far available indicate that, as in the intermittent acute cases, the porphyrin is excreted as the zinc complex. The meager data available on the coproporphyrins indicate that a mixture is usual, with a preponderance of type III which is not as marked as in the intermittent acute form. In one case of combined type studied in considerable detail in this laboratory,[116] the feces contained coproporphyrin III and protoporphyrin 9 (type III), in addition to small amounts of a Waldenström uro-type porphyrin. The porphyrin formation in this case was studied with the aid of N^{15} glycine, as shown in Figure 5. The purely anabolic aspect of the porphyrins is noted, in contrast with stercobilin.

With respect to treatment of the cutanea tarda or combined types of the disease, little can be added to what has already been said in the foregoing about the treatment of abdominal and nervous manifestations or photosensitivity. Thus far there has been insufficient experience with the use of chlorpromazine in the management of nervous symptoms or pain, but it is to be anticipated that it will have the same usefulness in these cases as in the ordinary intermittent acute type. Insofar as the cutaneous lesions are concerned, protection against sunlight exposure is required just as in the erythropoietic group. There is perhaps greater need for the avoidance of trauma, as it appears that minor trauma, including heat, plays a greater role in the formation of vesicles in this form than in the porphyria erythropoietica. Further studies on this point are needed. There is evidence that avoidance of alcohol is of considerable moment in ameliorating the symptoms of the hepatic cutanea tarda or combined types of the disease. A number of our patients have become completely asymptomatic and have remained so for long periods after complete abstinence was begun. This factor, however, also requires further critical study before any final judgment of its basic significance can be determined.

Fluoromicroscopic examination of hepatic biopsy material in the "cutanea tarda" type has regularly revealed large amounts of native porphyrin[68] (Fig. 6 C, D); extraction and fractionation have shown that this is mainly a uro-type porphyrin, with smaller but definitely increased amounts of coproporphyrin. The amount of porphobilinogen (as determined by boiling aqueous suspensions of the fresh liver) has been small or nil, in marked contrast with the intermittent acute type. This is in accord with the finding earlier alluded to, that in acute porphyria the disturbance of porphyrin metabolism is represented in the urine by colorless precursors including δ-amino-levulinic acid, porphobilinogen and tetrapyrrolic porphyrinogens. The bone marrow in the two forms of porphyria hepatica shows essentially no increase of porphyrin over the normal either before or after heating, in striking contrast to the large amounts found in porphyria erythropoietica.

The possibility that this differing site of origin is also responsible for the consistent excretion as the zinc complex in the hepatic types and as free porphyrin in the erythropoietic form deserves further exploration. Photosensitivity has been observed in cases in which most of the urinary porphyrin was excreted as the zinc complex. Although the fluorescence of the zinc complex is less intense than that of the free porphyrin, it may be sufficient, nevertheless, to accord with a possible photodynamic activity. The finding that the porphyrin is excreted as the zinc complex does not, of course, give adequate insight as to the internal status of the porphyrin, and it is possible that free porphyrin is present in the blood or skin in amounts sufficient to cause photosensitivity. In a "mixed" type of case studied a number of years ago,[117] in which death was due to hepatic cirrhosis and coma, the liver contained large amounts of a uro-type porphyrin, obviously a much greater concentration than in any of the other tissues or organs studied. As first extracted by dilute ammonia, the porphyrin appeared to be mainly or entirely zinc complex, quite in accord with that in the urine, but it is possible that free porphyrin had become combined with (hepatic) zinc during the process of extraction.

The finding that abnormal porphyrin metabolism in acute porphyria is represented mainly by porphobilinogen or porphyrinogen, as previously discussed, probably explains the lack of photosensitivity in this group. It is clear that large amounts of porphobilinogen may be present in the urine, and that it may be demonstrable in the liver and blood, in the absence of photosensitivity, but regularly associated with abdominal or nervous manifestations. At the same time, it should not be assumed that these latter symptoms are due to porphobilinogen. As mentioned above, Goldberg[106] failed to find any damaging effect of porphobilinogen in small animals. Yet it is true that the administration in these experiments was over a relatively short period of time and perhaps not comparable to the human cases of porphyria, nor have species differences in response been excluded. Nevertheless, the presently available evidence fails to support the concept that porphobilinogen itself is the injurious agent in the acute disease. It has recently been reported that δ-amino-levulinic acid is photosensitizing in the rat.[106b] In this study it was suggested that this precursor is converted to uroporphyrin in the cells of the skin. This observation is difficult to reconcile with the lack of photosensitivity in acute porphyria, in which the largest amounts of urinary δ-amino-levulinic acid are found, while in the cutanea tarda cases the increase is slight or lacking. In cases of porphyria having photosensitivity, whether porphyria erythropoietica or the hepatic cutanea tarda cases, the highest concentrations of uro- and coproporphyrin are found in the blood, but in these abdominal and nervous symptoms are lacking. Thus the concept advanced by Carrie[96] that the abdominal and nervous features of acute porphyria and of lead poisoning are "porphyrinopathic" appears unlikely. In this connection a study* in this laboratory may be mentioned in which increasing amounts of coproporphyrin III were given intravenously in a normal volunteer. There was no adverse effect after rapid injection of as much as 5 mg. of the free porphyrin.

EXPERIMENTAL PORPHYRIA

A section on porphyrin metabolism would be incomplete without at least brief discussion of the experimental production of porphyria. Methods are now available by which experimental erythropoietic and hepatic types can be produced. In respect to these conditions, the term porphyria is used arbitrarily and does not connote any constitutional or inborn error, as has been discussed in the foregoing in relation to the human disease.

A very great elaboration of porphyrin and precursors related to a disturbed hemoglobin synthesis in the developing normoblasts is produced by the combined administration of lead, phenylhydrazine and a photodynamic insult such as that which can be administered with rose Bengal and ultraviolet light.[73,38a] The lead and phenylhy-

* With W. Terry, unpublished.

drazine alone cause a marked increase in excretion of porphyrins, but this is further augmented by the photodynamic effect. Under these circumstances many of the normoblasts in the bone marrow exhibit intense red fluorescence under ultraviolet light, most of the porphyrin being in the nucleus. In this respect the condition is quite similar to that seen in human erythropoietic porphyria. In the acute experimental disease, however, the urine of the afflicted rabbits also contains porphobilinogen in considerable amounts.[38a] As noted in the foregoing, this is not true in erythropoietic porphyria.

An hepatic type of experimental porphyria may be produced by means of Sedormid (allylisopropylacetylcarbamide),[120] and also by isopropyl acetamid.[106a] The effects of the former have been studied in more detail. It has been shown that the excessive porphyrin and porphobilinogen excretion in the urine and bile is associated with a progressive decline of the concentration of catalase in the liver.[121] In this form the liver porphyrin and porphobilinogen concentration is very high and that in the bone marrow is entirely normal.[120,122] The concentration of the colorless precursor, including porphobilinogen in the liver, is much higher than that of preformed porphyrin. Nevertheless, some excess of the latter is regularly observed under ultraviolet light, and the amount in the biliary tract is often so large that the gallbladder and bile ducts fluoresce intensely red. The porphobilinogen excretion and most of the uroporphyrin excretion are limited to the urine, the bile containing large amounts of proto- and coproporphyrin. The latter is also moderately excessive in the urine.

Rabbits with porphyria produced by Sedormid exhibit apparent weakness of the extremities.[120] Whether this is actually a result of peripheral neuropathy or simply of the marked sedation which the Sedormid induces is not entirely clear. Goldberg[106a,123] has found that allylisopropylacetamide also causes porphyria in rabbits but no evidence of paresis of the legs and no evidence of sedation. This suggests that it is the sedation alone which is responsible for the weakness in the rabbits with Sedormid toxicity. However, in our experience the acetamide does not cause the outspoken degree of porphyria which is seen with Sedormid, so that the question of difference in degree must also be given consideration. In the rabbits receiving Sedormid the actual cause of death is usually a very marked distention of the stomach, often with perforation.[120] This appears to be due to profound pylorospasm. Spasm is also noted in the intestine. These changes are reminiscent of the smooth muscle spasm which occurs in human acute porphyria.

The pattern of porphyrin isomer excretion in experimental porphyria differs somewhat from that seen in porphyria of the human. Thus, in the above mentioned lead-phenylhydrazine erythropoietic type the coproporphyrin excreted is mainly type III, as in ordinary lead poisoning but unlike human erythropoietic porphyria.[38a] The uroporphyrin, however, is much the same, being mainly type I. In the hepatic porphyria due to Sedormid most of the uroporphyrin in the urine appears to be type III,[120] unlike the preformed Waldenström porphyrin, which is found in the unheated urine of human acute porphyria (see above).

References

1. Fischer, H. and Orth, H.: Die Chemie des Pyrrols, Bd. II. Leipzig, Akad. Verlagsgesellsch., 1937.
2. Shemin, D. and Rittenberg, D.: J. Biol. Chem., *159:*567, 1945.
3. Shemin, D. and Rittenberg, D.: J. Biol. Chem., *166:*621, 1946.
4. London, I. M.: J. Clin. Invest., *28:*1255, 1949.
5. London, I. M. and West, R.: J. Biol. Chem., *184:*359, 1950.
6. London, I. M., Shemin, D. and Rittenberg, D.: J. Biol. Chem., *173:*797, 1948 and *183:*749, 1950.
7. Shemin, D., London, I. M. and Rittenberg, D.: J. Biol. Chem., *183:*757, 1950.
8. Shemin, D. and Kumin, S.: J. Biol. Chem., *198:*827, 1952.
9. Shemin, D. and Russell, C. S.: J. Am. Chem. Soc., *75:*4873, 1953.
10. (a) Neuberger, A. and Scott, J. J.: Nature, London, *172:*1093, 1953.

(b) Gibson, K. D., Neuberger, A. and Scott, J. J.: Biochem. J., *58:*xli, 1954.
(c) Gibson, K. D.: Ciba Foundation Symposium, Porphyrin Biosynthesis and Metabolism. London, J. and A. Churchill, 1955, p. 24.
11. Schmid, R. and Shemin, D.: J. Am. Chem. Soc., *77:*506, 1955.
12. Granick, S.: Science, *120:*1105, 1954.
13. (a) Neuberger, A., Scott, J. J. and Gray, C. H.: Biochem. J., *58:*xli, 1954.
(b) Berlin, N. J., Neuberger, A. and Scott, J. J.: Biochem. J., *64:*80 and 90, 1956.
14. Westall, R. G.: Nature, *170:*614, 1952.
15. Cookson, G. H. and Rimington, C.: Nature, London, *171:*875, 1953.
16. Cookson, G. H. and Rimington, C.: Biochem. J., *57:*476, 1954.
17. Watson, C. J.: Arch. Int. Med., *93:*643, 1954.
18. Neuberger, A., Muir, H. M. and Gray, C. H.: Nature, *165:*948, 1950.
19. Grinstein, M., Kamen, M. D., Wikoff, H. M. and Moore, C. V.: J. Biol. Chem., *182:*715, 1950.
20. (a) Watson, C. J.: J. Clin. Invest., *23:* 69, 1944.
(b) Watson, C. J.: Arch. Int. Med., *86:*797, 1950.
21. Salomon, K., Richmond, J. E., and Altman, K. L.: J. Biol. Chem., *196:*463, 1952.
22. Dresel, E. I.: Ciba Foundation Symposium, Porphyrin Biosynthesis and Metabolism. London, J. and A. Churchill, 1955, p. 72.
23. Schwartz, S. and Ikeda, K.: *Ibid.*, p. 209.
24. Neve, R., Labbé, R. and Aldrich, R. A.: J. Am. Chem. Soc., *78:*691, 1956.
25. Watson, C. J., Pimenta de Mello, R., Schwartz, S., Hawkinson, V. E. and Bossenmaier, I.: J. Lab. and Clin. Med., *37:*831, 1951.
26. Hijmans van den Bergh, A. A. and Hyman, A. J.: Deutsch. med. Wchnschr., *54:*1492, 1928.
27. Watson, C. J. and Clarke, W.: Proc. Soc. Exper. Biol. & Med., *36:*65, 1937.
28. Watson, C. J., Grinstein, M. and Hawkinson, V.: J. Clin. Invest., *23:*69, 1954.
29. Seggel, K. A.: Ergebn. d. inn. Med. u. Kinderheilk., *38:*382, 1940.
30. Schwartz, S. and Wikoff, H. M.: J. Biol. Chem., *194:*563, 1952.
31. Watson, C. J.: A.M.A. Arch. Int. Med., *99:*323, 1957.
32. Schmid, R., Schwartz, S. and Watson, C. J.: Proc. Soc. Exper. Biol. & Med., *75:*705, 1950.
33. Schmid, R., Hanson, B. and Schwartz, S.: Proc. Soc. Exper. Biol. & Med., *79:*459, 1952.
34. Watson, C. J.: J. Clin. Invest., *14:*110, 1935.
35. Watson, C. J.: J. Clin. Invest., *16:*383, 1937.
36. Dobriner, K. and Rhoads, C. P.: J. Clin. Invest., *17:*105, 1938.
37. Dobriner, K. and Rhoads, C. P.: Physiol. Rev., *20:*416, 1940.
38. (a) Schwartz, S., Keprios, M. and Schmid, R.: Proc. Soc. Exper. Biol. & Med., *79:*463, 1952.
(b) Schwartz, S.: Veterans Admin. Tech. Bull. 10–94, Dec. 1, 1953.
39. (a) Lockwood, W. H.: Australian J. Exper. Biol. & M. Sc., *31:*457, 1953.
(b) Lockwood, W. H. and Bloomfield, B.: Australian J. Exper. Biol. & M. Sc., *32:*733, 1954.
40. Fränkel, E.: Arch. path. Anat., 248:125, 1924.
41. Klüver, H.: Science, *99:*483, 1944.
42. Klüver, H.: J. Psychol., *17:*209, 1944.
43. Chu, E. J. H. and Watson, C. J.: Proc. Soc. Exper. Biol. & Med., *66:*569 1947.
44. Blanchard, T. P.: Proc. Soc. Exper. Biol. & Med., *82:*512, 1953.
45. Granick, S. and Gilder, H.: Science, *101:* 540, 1945.
46. Schwartz, S., Zieve, L. and Watson, C. J.: J. Lab. & Clin. Med., *37:*843, 1951.
47. Watson, C. J. and Larson, E. A.: Physiol. Rev., *27:*478, 1947.
48. Watson, C. J., Hawkinson, V., Schwartz, S. and Sutherland, D.: J. Clin. Invest., *28:*447, 1949.
49. Fink, H. and Hoerburger, W.: Die Naturwissenschaften, *18:*292, 1934.
50. Watson, C. J.: J. Clin. Invest., *15:*327, 1936.
51. Grotepass, W.: Ztschr. f. physiol. Chem., *253:*276, 1938.
52. Sutherland, D. and Watson, C. J.: J. Lab. & Clin. Med., *37:*29, 1951.
53. Zieve, L., Hill, E., Schwartz, S. and Watson, C. J.: J. Lab. & Clin. Med., *41:*663, 1953.
54. Watson, C. J., Capps, R. C., Rappaport, E. M. and Hawkinson, V.: J. Clin. Invest., *28:*621, 1949.
55. Watson, C. J., Sutherland, D. and Hawkinson, V.: J. Lab. & Clin. Med., *37:*8, 1951.
56. Larson, E. A. and Watson, C. J.: J. Clin. Invest., *28:*452, 1949.
57. Sborov, V., Jay, A. R. and Watson, C. J.: J. Lab. & Clin. Med., *37:*52, 1951.
58. Maloof, C. C.: Arch. Ind. Hyg., *1:*296, 1950.
59. Rimington, C.: Compt. rend. trav. lab. Carlsberg, serie chim., *22:*454, 1938.
60. (a) Watson, C. J., Schwartz, S., Schulze, W., Jacobson, L. O. and Zagaria, R.: J. Clin. Invest., *28:* 465, 1949.
(b) Berger, H. and Goldberg, A.: Brit. M. J., *2:*85, 1955.

61. With, T. and Peterson, H. C. A.: Lancet, *2:*1148, 1954.
62. Schumm, O.: Ztschr. f. physiol. Chem., *169:*62, 1927.
63. Boas, I.: Klin. Wchnschr., *12:*589, 1933.
64. Brugsch, J.: Porphyrine. Leipzig, J. A. Barth, 1952.
65. Garrod, A. E.: Inborn Errors of Metabolism. London, Henry Froude, 1923.
66. Günther, H.: Deutsch. Arch. f. klin. Med., *105:*89, 1911.
67. Günther, H.: Hämatoporphyrie. In Schittenhelm's Die Krankheiten des Blutes u. der blutbildenden Organe. Berlin, H. J. Springer, 1925.
68. Schmid, R., Schwartz, S. and Watson, C. J.: A.M.A. Arch. Int. Med., *93:*167, 1954.
69. Schmid, R., Schwartz, S. and Sundberg, R. D.: Blood, *10:*416, 1955.
70. Borst, M. and Königsdörffer, H.: Untersuchungen über Porphyrie. Leipzig, S. Hirzel, 1929.
71. Aldrich, R. A., Hawkinson, V., Grinstein, M. and Watson, C. J.: Blood, *6:*685, 1951.
72. Pimenta de Mello, R.: Proc. Soc. Exper. Biol. & Med., *76:*823, 1951.
73. Pimenta de Mello, R.: Proc. Soc. Exper. Biol. & Med., *72:*292, 1949.
74. Anderson, T. M.: Brit. J. Dermat., *10:*1, 1898.
75. Mackey, L. and Garrod, A. E.: Quart. J. Med., *19:*357, 1926.
76. Blum, H. F. and Pace, N.: Brit. J. Dermat., *49:*465, 1937.
77. Grinstein, M., Schwartz, S. and Watson, C. J.: J. Biol. Chem., *137:*323, 1945.
78. Watson, C. J., Schwartz, S. and Hawkinson, V.: J. Biol., Chem., *137:*345, 1945.
79. de Marval, L. and Pons, R.: Arch. argent. pediat., *5:*220, 1934.
80. (a) Gray, C. H. and Neuberger, A.: Lancet, *1:*851, 1952.
    (b) Rosenthal, I. M., Lipton, E. L. and Asrow, G.: Pediatrics, *15:*663, 1955.
81. Rimington, C.: Acta med. scandinav., *143:*161 and 177, 1952.
82. Macgregor, A. G., Nicholas, R. E. H. and Rimington, C.: A.M.A. Arch. Int. Med., *90:*505, 1952.
83. Watson, C. J.: Advances Int. Med., *6:*235, 1954.
84. Granick, S. and Vanden Schrieck, N. G.: Proc. Soc. Exper. Biol. & Med., *188:* 270, 1955.
85. Dean, G.: Brit. M. J., *2:*1291, 1953.
86. Dean, G. and Barnes, H. H.: Brit. M. J., *2:*89, 1955.
87. Waldenström, J.: Acta med. scandinav., Suppl. 82, 1937.
88. Jorgensen, J. and With, T. K.: Nord. med., *27:*1341, 1945.
89. Peters, H. A.: Dis. Nerv. System, *17:*2, 1956.
90. Waldenström, J.: Acta psychiat. et neurol., *14:*375, 1939.
91. Calvy, G. L.: Surg., Gynec. & Obst., *90:* 716, 1950.
92. Mason, V. R., Courville, C. and Ziskind, E.: Medicine, *12:*355, 1933.
93. Watson, C. J., Schmid, R. and Varco, R. L.: Am. J. Med., *22:*980, 1957.
94. Denny-Brown, D. E. and Sciarra, D.: Brain, *68:*1, 1945.
95. Eliaser, M. and Kondon, B.: Am. Heart J., *24:*696, 1942.
96. Carrié, C.: Die Porphyrine ihr Nachweis, ihre Physiologie und Klinik, Leipzig, G. Thieme, 1936.
97. Watson, C. D. and Larson, E. A.: Oxford Med., Chap. IV-A, 228 (1), 1951.
98. Woody, N. C.: Pediatrics, *4:*47, 1949.
99. Pohl, A. W. and Roberts, J. R.: Ann. Int. Med., *27:*1028, 1947.
100. (a) Melby, J. D., Street, J. P. and Watson, C. J.: J.A.M.A., *162:*174, 1956.
     (b) Monaco, R. N., Teeper, R. D., Robbins, J. J. and Calvy, G. L.: New England J. Med., *256:*309, 1957.
101. Watson, C. J. and Schwartz, S.: Proc. Soc. Exper. Biol. & Med., *47:*393, 1941.
102. Edmondson, P. and Schwartz, S.: J. Biol. Chem., *205:*605, 1953.
103. Waldenström, J. and Vahlquist, B.: Ztschr. f. physiol. Chem., *260:*189, 1939.
104. Waldenström, J. and Vahlquist, B.: Acta med. scandinav., *117:*2, 1944.
105. Shuster, L.: Biochem. J., *64:*101, 1956.
106. (a) Goldberg, A., Paton, W. and Thompson, J.: Brit. J. Pharmacol., *9:*91, 1954.
     (b) Jarrett, A., Rimington, C. and Willoughby, D. A.: Lancet, *270:*125, 1956.
107. Waldenström, J.: Deutsches Arch. klin. Med., *178:*38, 1935.
108. Waldenström, J., Fink, H. and Hoerburger, W.: Ztschr. physiol. Chem., *233:*1, 1935.
109. (a) Watson, C. J. and Berg, M.: J. Biol. Chem., *214:*537, 1955.
     (b) Watson, C. J., Berg, M., and Hawkinson, V.: J. Biol. Chem., *214:* 547, 1955.
110. Chu, T. C. and Chu, E. J.: J. Biol. Chem., *227:*505, 1957.
111. Rimington, C.: Acta med. scandinav., *143:*161 and 177, 1952.
112. Nicholas, R. E. H. and Rimington, C.: Biochem. J., *55:*109, 1953.
113. Brunsting, L. C., Mason, H. L. and Aldrich, R. A.: J.A.M.A., *146:*1207, 1951.
114. Sterling, K., Silver, M. and Ricketts, H. T.: Arch. Int. Med., *84:*965, 1949.
115. Watson, C. J., Lowry, P. T., Schmid, R., Hawkinson, V. E. and Schwartz, S.: Tr. A. Am. Physicians, *64:*345, 1951.

116. Lowry, P. T., Hawkinson, V. E. and Watson, C. J.: Metabolism, 1149, 1952.
117. Watson, C. J. and Schwartz, S.: J. Clin. Invest., *20:*440, 1941.
118. Comfort, A., Moore, H. and Weatherall, M.: Biochem. J. *58:*177, 1954.
119. Hoffbauer, F. W., Watson, C. J. and Schwartz, S.: Proc. Soc. Exper. Biol. & Med., *83:*232, 1953.
120. Schmid, R. and Schwartz, S.: Proc. Soc. Exper. Biol. & Med., *81:*685, 1952.
121. Schmid, R., Figen, J. F. and Schwartz, S.: J. Biol. Chem., *217:*263, 1955.
122. Schmid, R., Schwartz, S. and Watson, C. J.: Acta. haematol., *10:*150, 1953.
123. Goldberg, A. and Rimington, C.: Proc. Roy. Soc. London, s.B, *143:*257, 1955.

CHAPTER 12 *By* GARFIELD G. DUNCAN, M.D.

Spontaneous Hypoglycemia

INTRODUCTION

Spontaneous hypoglycemia, occurring in episodes regular or irregular in pattern depending upon the underlying cause, is common to multiple clinical disorders which disturb the blood sugar regulatory mechanism in one or more ways, as a result of which withdrawals of sugar from the blood exceed its replacement. Effective over a sufficient period, these disturbances lead to a lowering of the concentration of sugar in the blood to abnormally low levels—60 mg. per cent by the Folin-Wu method[1] and true glucose values below 45 mg. per cent by the Somogyi-Nelson method.[2] The clinical effects of these changes vary with the nature of the underlying disorder as well as with the rate, intensity and duration of its effect. The hypoglycemia may occur as a complication or manifestation of a disease in its mildest form or it may occur later and may be of grave import. When one considers the variety of possibilities and modes of action involving disturbances in glycogenesis, glycogenolysis and gluconeogenesis and the influences which disturbances in the adenohypophysis, adrenal gland, pancreas, liver, and a variety of functional stresses may exert, it is not surprising that varied and bizzare symptoms are associated with spontaneous hypoglycemia.

Symptoms caused by the relative degrees of hypoglycemia in a variety of disorders are similar. It appears best to consider this common feature—hypoglycemia per se—in its different aspects separately rather than jointly with each of the hypoglycemia-producing disorders.

Epinephrine response symptoms and cerebral manifestations, psychiatric and neurologic (see Table 1), occur at one time or another according to the degree, the speed of development and the duration of the hypoglycemia. These manifestations may overlap or phase one into the other, but in general the epinephrine response and the psychiatric and neurologic manifestations represent respectively mild, moderate and severe prolonged hypoglycemic states. The degree or severity of symptoms varies with the level of the blood sugar, the rate at which the concentration of sugar in the blood has been reduced and the period of time over which the sympathetic nerve impulses are stimulated to increase the production of epinephrine. The early symptoms of hypoglycemia, when the decrease in the blood sugar is rapid, are attributed to this *epinephrine response* and are identical, in several respects, with those produced by the administration of epinephrine. They are fainting, tremulousness, "inward trembling," emotional disturbances, excessive perspiration, chilliness, circumoral numbness, mild degrees of mental cloudiness, hunger, apprehension and paresthesias, and cardiac palpitation. Objectively, there are pallor, dilated pupils, tachycardia with a bounding pulse, excessive perspiration and moderate elevation of the blood pressure. A rapid reversal to normal shortly after the ingestion of a carbohydrate-containing food is characteristic.

TABLE 1. SYMPTOMATOLOGY AND SIGNS ASSOCIATED WITH HYPOGLYCEMIA

PROMINENT FEATURES	PHYSICAL SIGNS
Epinephrine Response	
Nervousness	Emotionally upset
General weakness	Skin pale and wet with perspiration
Weakness and trembling of extremities	Pupils dilated
Emotional instability	Tachycardia*
Hunger and faintness	Blood pressure* moderately elevated
Apprehension	Fixed facial expression
Circumoral numbness	
Psychiatric Manifestations	
Restlessness	Above findings may be present with:
Emotional instability	Failure to obey commands
Mental confusion	Restlessness
Personality changes	Maniacal behavior
Negativism	Delirium
Resistance to treatment	
Difficulty in concentration	
Amnesia (retrograde)	
Neurologic Manifestations	
Thick speech	May be unconscious
Aphasia	Muscle tone increased with twitching of muscles
Visual disturbances	Inarticulate speech
Cloudy vision	Aphasia
Diplopia	Tendon reflexes hyperactive*
Tonic and Clonic contractions of muscles	Babinski reflexes positive in all severe cases
Convulsions	Monoplegia
Unconsciousness	Hemiplegia
Headache	Paraplegia

* When a patient is *in extremis*, the blood pressure is below normal and there are marked tachycardia and hypoactive or absent reflexes.

The epinephrine response is most prominent when the decrease in the blood sugar occurs rapidly, but it may not be detectable when the hypoglycemia develops slowly, in which case, and after prolonged hypoglycemia, symptoms involving the nervous system tend to overshadow all others—hence the term cerebral type of hypoglycemia. When the hypoglycemia develops slowly, adaptive mechanisms protect the patient from symptoms until the concentration of sugar is much lower than in the case when a decline in the blood sugar is rapid. This, it would appear, accounts for the fact that a patient may have severe symptoms with a blood sugar level of 45 or 50 mg. per cent on one occasion and yet exhibit no clinical manifestations of hypoglycemia on another when the concentration of sugar in the blood is as low or lower. This feature is seen in the clinical management of diabetes in which a hypoglycemia from a rapidly acting insulin causes symptoms typical of an epinephrine response, whereas, there may be no symptoms when the same degree of hypoglycemia occurs as the result of an overdosage of a long acting insulin. Fasting alone, or with exercise added, intensifies the rate at which the concentration of sugar in the blood decreases.

Cerebral manifestations may be the only clinical evidences of hypoglycemia when the blood sugar decreases very gradually. Headache, visual disturbances, thick speech, twitching of muscles, awkward locomotion, transitory hemiplegia, paraplegia, catatonia, tonic and clonic muscular spasms, urinary incontinence, convulsions and unconsciousness may appear in various combinations. They are, in the more advanced states, indicative of hypoglycemia of severe degree and of considerable duration. Lacking correction, a severe attack may prove fatal. *Psychi-*

atric manifestations, especially restlessness, negativism, personality changes, emotional instability, maniacal behavior and even physical resistance to treatment may be prominent.

In prolonged attacks, *neurologic manifestations,* with sensory and motor disturbances, predominate. Prolonged hypoglycemias of severe degrees may cause irreparable cerebral damage with mental deterioration to the degree of permanent idiocy.

Bizarre *neurologic and psychiatric manifestations* of a repetitive nature and with a definite relation to fasting from food and to increased physical activities should suggest the possibility of a hypoglycemia in otherwise ill defined cases. It is not surprising that, more often than not, the first specialist seen by these patients is the neurologist or the psychiatrist.

As the hypoglycemia feature of the disorder progresses, a variety of combinations of symptoms appear. Headache, difficulty in concentration, emotional disturbances, difficult speech, disorientation and mental confusion appear and increase in severity. Dizziness, faintness, diplopia, cardiac palpitation and coldness of the extremities occur. The patient has a staring or blank facial expression during attacks. He may be unable to walk, or, if he can, he may appear to be inebriated. He may be melancholic or restless and maniacal. Unless recognized and treated, the condition causes, in the severe cases, loss of consciousness, muscle twitching, generalized convulsions, following which there is a retrograde amnesia. Patients may be amnesic as a result of mild attacks of hypoglycemia. During severe attacks the normal color of the mucous membranes is maintained, but there is pallor of the skin; the blood pressure is elevated and the pulse is full and bounding; tendon reflexes are usually exaggerated, and a Babinski reflex is almost invariably present when a severe attack is at its worst. A subnormal blood pressure and a weak pulse occur in patients who are *in extremis;* hence, these are ominous signs.

In bona fide cases of hyperinsulinism (organic) the blood sugar levels during attacks are invariably below 50 mg. per 100 cc. and usually below 35 mg. (Folin-Wu).[1] Blood sugar values by the Somogyi-Nelson method[2] are, in general, 18 to 26 mg. lower than those obtained by the Folin-Wu method.

Complete, sudden and dramatic relief from these symptoms and signs is the rule upon the administration of dextrose by vein. However, residual disturbances of the nervous system may remain in isolated cases.

GENERAL CONSIDERATIONS AND CLASSIFICATION

Spontaneous hypoglycemia may be classified according to whether the underlying disorder is the result of *organic structural changes* or whether it is secondary to *functional derangements.*

The respective groups are presented in Table 2. In general, the disturbances are more profound and progressive when the cause is organic than when they are due to functional disorders. The urgency for an early diagnosis is greater when the cause is organic, since few of the organic disorders causing hypoglycemia can be overlooked without grave risks. This is not so when the disorder is of a purely functional nature. The hypoglycemia of functional nature is the response to (1) *excessive stimulative demands* or to (2) *excessive response* to *normal stimulation* of normal pancreatic islets or (3) to *retarded glycogenolysis* when the threshold of glycemia which initiates release of glucose from hepatic glycogen is lower than normal. In the first instance the nature of the demand on the islets is normal but the degree of demand is such that the physiologic responses of the insulin-producing mechanism, under these circumstances, are extended, and as a result the concentration of sugar in the blood is reduced to subnormal values. Rarely are extreme degrees of hypoglycemia found when the cause is functional. Furthermore, in these cases, the disorder tends to remain static over long periods. In contrast, the hypogly-

TABLE 2. CAUSES OF SPONTANEOUS HYPOGLYCEMIA*

I. Organic Structural Changes
   A. Hyperinsulinism due to tumors, benign or malignant, of the islets of Langerhans.
   B. Adrenal cortical insufficiency due to:
      (1) Idiopathic adrenal cortical atrophy
      (2) Destructive lesions, e.g., meningococcemia, acute hemorrhagic fever and invasive neoplasm
      (3) Adrenalectomy
      (4) Congenital adrenal hyperplasia—inability to produce hydrocortisone in normal amounts
   C. Adenohypophysis—impaired or absent function due to:
      (1) Tumors—notably chromophobe adenoma, craniopharyngioma and cystic disease
      (2) Destructive processes—postpartum hemorrhage with thrombosis and necrosis (Sheehan's disease) and abscess
      (3) Irradiation
      (4) Atrophy (pituitary cachexia, Simmond's disease)
      (5) Hypophysectomy
   D. Diseases of, or affecting, the liver
      (1) Hepatitis
         (a) Viral
         (b) Poisoning, e.g., phosphorous, arsphenamine, carbon tetrachloride
      (2) Cholangiolitis—ascending infectious
      (3) Neoplasm—primary or carcinomatosis
      (4) Fatty degeneration or fatty metamorphosis
      (5) Cirrhosis
      (6) Chronic passive congestion due to myocardial insufficiency
      (7) Glycogen storage disease (glycogenosis, von Gierke's hepato-nephromegalia glycogenica)
   E. Miscellaneous—certain fibromas and sarcomas, progressive muscular dystrophy, status thymico lymphaticus and hypothyroidism (cretin)

II. Functional Disorders
   A. Hypoglycemia due to:
      (1) Functional hypertrophy of the islets of Langerhans—functional hyperinsulinism
      (2) Altered gastrointestinal function following gastrectomy, gastroenterostomy, rapid administration of glucose into duodenum via tubes and (rarely) thyrotoxicosis
      (3) Relative hyperinsulinism with neurogenic disturbances
      (4) Ganglion blocking agents, notably hexamethonium, pentolium bitartrate and mecamylamine
   B. Adrenal cortical insufficiency—possible causes
      (1) Abrupt withdrawal of prolonged corticoid therapy
      (2) Spontaneous adrenal failure and stress associated with fulminating infections
   C. Idiopathic spontaneous hypoglycemia of infancy
   D. Miscellaneous causes—prolonged physical exercise, lactation, renal glycosuria, severe and continuous cachexia and diarrheal states.

* Modified after Conn and Seltzer.

cemic states of organic origin tend to progress unfavorably until eventually they exceed the capacity of the usual physiologic adaptive or homeostatic mechanisms to correct them. The only apparent control exerted over the production of insulin by an islet cell adenoma is the extent to which it can produce, and as the tumor enlarges or multiplies by metastasizing, its capacity to produce insulin becomes enormous. The production of insulin by the tumor has no apparent physiologic deterrent—normal physiologic controls are bypassed or overwhelmed. The forces at work may be compared to a revolution in which the normal garrison is completely overrun by an overwhelming rebel force which is not bound by the usual modifying restraints of a well disciplined community. Functional hypoglycemias may be likened to disturbances in the community, but by going to unusual lengths the garrison continues, in general, to exercise effective, if not entirely perfect, control.

SPONTANEOUS HYPOGLYCEMIA CAUSED BY ORGANIC STRUCTURAL CHANGES

Hyperinsulinism (Organic)

History. The background for the identification of organic hyperinsulinism was established by several pioneer workers. Langerhans (1869), while a medical student, described the islets in the pancreas in "Beiträge zur mikroskopischen Anatomie der Bauchspeicheldrüse. Von Mering and Minkowski (1890), by removing the pancreas of a dog, produced a fatal diabetes. Laguesse (1893) supported Langerhans' conclusion in "*Sur la Formation des Ilots de Langerhans*" and indicated, on the basis of the work of Von Mering and Minkowski, the possible endocrine nature of these islets. Ssobolew (1900), by causing atrophy of the acinar portion of the pancreas, leaving the islets intact, did not produce diabetes; the possibility that the islets contain a substance that might be of value to diabetic patients was suggested. Opie (1901) postulated that diabetes, the antithesis of hyperinsulinism, is due to alterations in the islets of Langerhans. Nicholls[3] recorded the findings in the case of the first tumor to be identified as an islet cell tumor. Allen and his associates, Copp and Barclay,[4] focused further attention on the function of the islet cells in their work with experimental diabetes. Banting and Best[5] recovered a hypoglycemic agent from isolated islets of Langerhans. (Insulin was the name given to this agent by McLeod, in whose laboratory it was discovered.) Campbell and Fletcher[6] observed the symptoms of hypoglycemia following an overdose of insulin. Gibson and Larimer[7] concluded that clinical conditions existed in which hypoglycemic states occurred without the administration of exogenous insulin. Harris[8] introduced the term *hyperinsulinism* to explain the clinical condition which simulated that produced from overdosage of insulin. Finally, Wilder and his co-workers[9] established the anatomic concept of organic hyperinsulinism when they reported the first islet cell tumor to be removed from a patient. Large amounts of insulin were recovered, both from the parent tumor and from metastatic growths in the liver. From Wilder's observations and subsequent experience, it is clear that islet cell tumors elaborate insulin, the export and action of which overwhelm the capacity of normal processes which ordinarily maintain blood sugar values within a circumscribed range.

Howland[10] reported the first cure of a case of hyperinsulinism following the removal of an adenoma of the islets of Langerhans. Whipple,[11] prior to 1938, collected 74 cases of tumors of the islets of Langerhans; 56 were found at operation and 18 at autopsy.

The insulin content of the serum in 9 of Willebrand's[12] 11 cases of organic hyperinsulinism was found to be greatly increased. The technique of determining the insulin content of the serum was the glucose uptake by the rat diaphragm. That this tenuous progress has borne fruit is indicated in the recent reviews of this subject—notably in those of Crain and Thorn,[13] Howard and coworkers,[14] and Conn and Seltzer.[15]

Clinical Considerations. Organic hyperinsulinism is a clinical entity in which there is an excessive production of insulin by a functioning tumor—an insulinoma, also referred to as a nesidioblastoma[16]—or tumors, benign or malignant, arising from the islets of Langerhans of the pancreas. Metastatic lesions, in cases of malignant islet cell tumors, also produce insulin in large amounts. The enormity of the excess of insulin which gains access to the blood is such that at certain times—after exercise and during fasting hours—the usual control and adaptive mechanisms are overwhelmed, sugar is taken from the blood more rapidly than it is replaced and varying degrees of hypoglycemia occur.

Clinical attacks caused by the hypoglycemia are periodic, irregular, and they vary in degree in relation to the intake of food and to exercise. Attacks or spells are prone to occur before breakfast—at the end of the longest period in the 24 hours without food. There may be difficulty in arousing the patient. Attacks may be precipitated by delaying a meal and especially if vigorous exercise is used as an added provocative measure. Attacks are more severe if undernutrition and low carbohydrate regimens are adopted and if a loss in weight occurs. Other factors may exert an unfavorable influence in precipitating attacks. In two of my patients, attacks were more likely to occur and to be more severe during menstruation than they were at other times.

Attacks tend to be fewer and less severe if a liberal diet is allowed and especially if nourishments are taken between regular meals and at bed time, if a gain in weight occurs; during the course of an acute infection, and in the absence of the usual amount of physical exercise as observed when these patients are subjected to the inactivity associated with hospitalization. Any feature which tends to increase the need for insulin in the diabetic patient is likely to have some ameliorative effect on attacks of hypoglycemia.

Adenomas of the islets may be devoid of apparent function. Actually, over 80 per cent of these tumors—based on findings at autopsy—were considered to be nonfunctioning.[17,18] *Of 274 functioning adenomas the tumors were almost equally distributed in the head, body and tail of the pancreas.*[14] Tumors in the head may not be visible. Indeed, they may be so imbedded as to be difficult to detect by careful palpation of the gland at operation. Usually the tumor is firmer than normal pancreas tissue and is not likely to be missed if the pancreas is mobilized sufficiently to permit appropriate palpation.

It is no longer believed that benign islet cell tumors undergo malignant changes, but nearly 10 per cent of functioning islet cell tumors are malignant and show evidence of metastases.[17] Malignant tumor of the islets is a disorder of the adult; none has been reported in persons under 18 years of age.[14] Adenomas of the islets, however, do occur in children. Two such diagnoses were confirmed in children under five years of age in Howard's[14] 264 hypoglycemic patients who were subjected to surgery, and normal islet tissue was found in 3 other children, also under five, who were hypoglycemic subjects.

Spontaneous hypoglycemia occurs in adenomatosis involving, in the same individual, not only the islet cells of the pancreas but the adenohypophysis and the parathyroid gland. It is probable that this syndrome is of genetic origin. Gastric and duodenal ulcers frequently occur in patients with adenomatosis of the endocrine glands.

Diagnosis. The recognition of clear-cut cases of organic hyperinsulinism is a simple matter. A history of "weak spells" before breakfast or before other meals, especially if delayed; attacks being more frequent and more severe after strenuous exercise; the repeated finding of low fasting blood sugar values—below 60 mg. per cent (Folin-Wu Method) as well as the still lower values, usually below 45 mg. per cent, during an attack; and the prompt relief from glucose administered intravenously combine to make the diagnosis rather certain in the otherwise healthy person. The diagnosis is not always as simple as it would appear, however. In mild cases, fasting blood sugar values may be normal, and the patient unknowingly may obscure the clinical picture by taking food frequently—a practice, he has learned, which makes him feel better. Also, we have witnessed the complete cessation of attacks when the patient was at relative rest in the hospital. Provocative tests may be conducted in doubtful cases, or for completeness of objective proof of the diagnosis. Circumstances which increase the likelihood of a hypoglycemia are created by (a) restricting the carbohydrate and caloric content of the diet for 3 days. The diet recommended by Conn[15] fulfills these requirements. It contains protein 50 gm., carbohydrate 50 gm. and fat 88 gm. (1200 calories). Daily fasting blood sugar values are obtained for 3 days and if hypoglycemic levels of diagnostic value—below 50 mg. per cent (Folin-Wu Method)—do not develop, it is unlikely that a functioning islet cell tumor (insulinoma) is present. However, this is not always the case and as an early diagnosis and cure are of importance, the provocative testing is intensified (b) by withholding all food on the fourth day and, failing to provoke a hypoglycemia by this means, (c) the fast is extended to the fifth day of the test and 2 hours of vigorous exercise on a stationary rowing machine or bicycle is included during the forenoon. Failure to precipitate a diagnostic hypoglycemia before midday rules out insulinoma with reasonable certainty. Women are especially sensitive to provocative tests during the early part of the menstrual period.

It is significant that patients subject to attacks of functional hypoglycemia

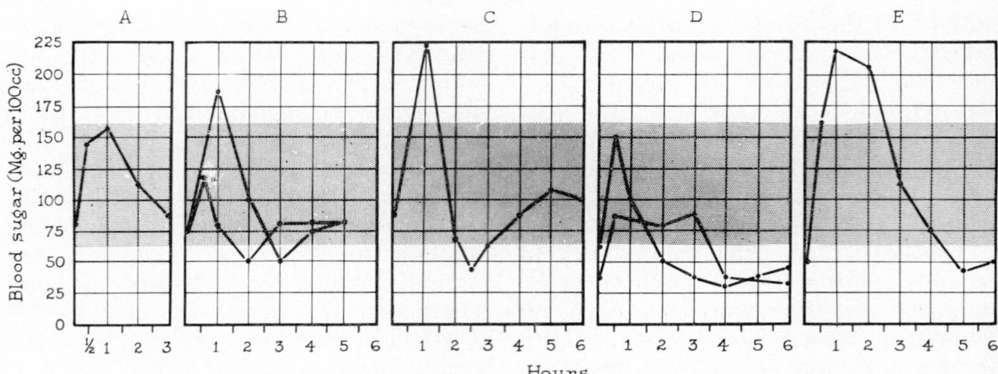

FIG. 1. Responses to glucose tolerance tests (100 gm. glucose given orally to adult patients). The shaded zone indicates the extent of normal fluctuations of the blood sugar levels during the tests.

A. The normal response. The peak of the curve does not exceed 160 mg. and the 2 hour value is below 120 mg. per 100 cc.

B. Functional hypoglycemia with relative hyperinsulinism. The initial elevation of the blood sugar, but usually not in excess of normal, followed by mild degrees of hypoglycemia at the second and third hours is characteristic.

C. Curve obtained in a case of functional hyperinsulinism subsequent to gastrectomy. The prompt hyperglycemia is rapidly followed by hypoglycemic values at 2, 2½, and 3 hours with normal levels prevailing at, and after, the fourth hour.

D. Organic hyperinsulinism. Two illustrative curves show an initial but relatively slight rise in the blood sugar and the relatively flat subnormal values at the fourth, fifth and sixth hours —the outstanding characteristic of this test in this disorder.

E. Hepatogenic hypoglycemia. The low fasting value, the prompt development of hyperglycemia and the return to subnormal levels between the fourth and sixth hours are illustrative.

will tolerate the foregoing tests without developing episodes of hypoglycemia. In practice these are the cases in which the full diagnostic study outlined above is necessary. The diagnosis of organic hyperinsulinism can be made short of such extensive investigation as a rule.

The glucose tolerance test is widely used in the attempts to identify the various causes of hypoglycemic states (Fig. 1). As a single study it is likely to mislead unless the patient is prepared for the test with a diet including 450 to 500 gm. of carbohydrate daily for three to five days. This preparation is based on the probability that the function of the normal islets is depressed by the prolonged production of great amounts of insulin by the insulinoma, and that their productivity is restored after several days of stimulation with a diet high in carbohydrate content. While islet function is suppressed, a diabetic type of glucose tolerance curve is not uncommon, but when sensitivity and normal responsiveness of islet cell function is restored, a low, relatively flat type of curve is the rule. Such curves are illustrated in the case of Miss J. G. and are shown in Figure 2.

This patient (J. G.) illustrates several common features in this condition. Repeatedly the fasting blood sugar values were normal but following the omission of breakfast and lunch and with 20 minutes of cycling in each hour, the values fell to 41 mg. per cent (Folin-Wu) after the third hour; without further exercise at the eighth hour, the blood sugar level was 39 mg. per cent. There were no subjective symptoms whatever and no neurologic nor mental symptoms during the eight hour test.

The most characteristic feature of the glucose tolerance curve is, in the appropriately prepared patient, *the flat hypoglycemic values at 4, 5 and 6 hours after the glucose is taken* (see D, Fig. 1). The three-hour value may be equally low, but this is not regularly the case. The early part of the curve is quite variable in bona fide cases. The values in the first two, or even the first three hours, may be indistinguishable from a normal response or they may be low normal values.

Responses to the glucose tolerance test in cases of organic hyperinsulinism —insulinoma—are contrasted in Figure 1 with those obtained in cases of functional hypoglycemia and hepatic disease and with a normal response.

Treatment. Islet cell tumors should be removed surgically. To delay, once the diagnosis is established, is to invite preventable complications. Early removal promises a prompt and complete cure, unless the tumor is malignant,* safeguards against irreversible complications, notably damage to the central nervous system, and guards against the development of extreme degrees of obesity, which hampers subsequent surgery.

ACTH or *hydrocortisone* is given preoperatively to elevate the blood sugar level by inducing resistance to the activity of excessive quantities of insulin and on the likelihood that the steroids might prevent the highly fatal and mysterious "idiopathic hyperthermia" that sometimes follows within four days of the removal of a functioning islet cell tumor. Conn[15] gave three patients 120 units of aqueous ACTH intramuscularly daily preoperatively and postoperatively, and uneventful recovery followed. A fourth patient, who received no steroids, suddenly developed a hyperpyrexia of 107° F. 36 hours after the operation and expired within two hours. No cause for the febrile episode was found at autopsy.

Glucose administration for one or two hours prior to and during operation will guard against a hypoglycemia, though there is no evidence that manipulation of the tumor at operation increases its output of insulin. If the glucose is administered at a constant rate, a prompt rise in the level of the blood sugar, as observed by McMillan,[19] within one half hour of removal of the tumor is presumptive evidence that no functioning islet cell tumor remains. A transitory hyperglycemia appearing promptly after operation and persisting a few hours to a few days is of greater significance as the possible complicating factor of glucose administration will not need to be discounted.

Multiple tumors occurred in 18.6 per cent of Porter's[20] series. Tumors may escape detection unless the pancreas is mobilized sufficiently to permit thorough palpation of the gland between the thumb and fingers. The peritoneum is divided around the duodenal curve and along the superior or inferior border of the body and tail of the gland to accomplish this essential detail.[20]

It may be tempting to remove a prominently visible tumor and retire from the abdomen without methodical exploration of the entire pancreas. This is a trap into which only the inexperienced will fall. The vicinity of the pancreas should be explored for the ectopic tumors which rarely occur.

When preliminary and reliable studies have excluded other causes of the hypoglycemia and on methodical exploration of the pancreas no tumor is detected, the course to pursue varies. Porter's practice is, in adult patients, to remove that portion of the pancreas to the left of the superior mesenteric vessels and to do a splenectomy. If an experienced surgical pathologist can find no tumor in the segment of pancreas, most of the head of the pancreas is then removed. If no tumor is found in this specimen, it is warranted to complete the radical pancreaticoduodenectomy at this first procedure. The remainder of the gland is removed by the usual techniques for duodenal and bile duct resections.[20] In one such radical procedure an undetectable islet cell tumor at the ampulla of Vater was identified on section. In support of the foregoing comprehensive procedure, it is noted that of available patients each adult in whom no tumor or other cause of hypoglycemia was found originally had to be re-explored.

In the rare cases of adenomatosis, because of the multiplicity of functioning

* In view of the long survival in many cases in which malignant changes are suspected in the islet cell tumors, metastases are considered by some to be necessary criterion for the diagnosis of a malignant islet cell tumor.

foci, the more extensive removal of the pancreas would be determined when the nature of the lesion is identified.

Functioning islet cell tumors are rare in the first decade of life, more so than idiopathic spontaneous hypoglycemia. On the better than an even chance that the attacks of spontaneous hypoglycemia will cease without benefit of surgery, the administration of ACTH is given a trial in this age group. If appreciable benefit does not accrue, surgical exploration is indicated (Porter). The therapy recommended by McQuarrie[21] should be given a thorough trial before resorting to surgery, and the extent to which the surgery should be carried if no tumor is found is problematical. This author's inclination is that if no tumor is found after a methodical search further surgery should be abandoned. There is a real likelihood that the attacks will subside spontaneously; failing this a tumor may be detectable on a second exploration after a liberal lapse of time. If no tumor is then found, resection of the tail of the pancreas may be justified. The removal of a portion of the pancreas containing hyperplastic islets, however, should be looked upon as an artificial correction of a disorder which possibly still holds the potential of returning to normal spontaneously.

Alloxan therapy for the control of hyperinsulinism due to functioning islet tumors, benign or malignant, has been unsuccessful. Indeed, its failure to destroy these sources of insulin and the risk that normal islets will be sacrificed, causing diabetes, prohibits the therapeutic use of alloxan. An extract of the adenohypophysis, because of its known diabetogenic effect, experimentally failed to benefit two patients with organic hyperinsulinism.[15] The intensification of the hypoglycemia which resulted from this treatment could hardly have been expected.

Case Report.

Patient J. G. (77094), female, aged 26 years, a secretary, experienced on one occasion in December 1945 an attack of "light headedness" before a delayed dinner. At the same time she appeared to others as though she were intoxicated. After dinner she was quite well but was unable to recall what she had eaten. On December 14, 1946, on the first day of her menstruation and after a physically active day, she had a second attack in the mid-afternoon. She became talkative, appeared confused and when queried could not recall her name. She had a "vacant expression" and her speech became slow. Her pupils were dilated and there was a mild degree of tachycardia and a blood pressure of 126 mm.Hg systolic and 74 mm. diastolic. Subsequent pressures were appreciably lower, e.g., 108/60. Her tendon reflexes were hyperactive.

A history of recent headaches, numbness and tingling of lips, tongue and chin, and episodes of blurred vision was obtained.

Before forced carbohydrate feeding, a glucose tolerance test resulted in a curve which in the first three hours was typical of that seen in the presence of mild diabetes (Fig. 2). After 5 days of a diet containing 400 to 500 gm. of carbohydrate, the first 2-hour portion of the curve was indistinguishable from a normal response, but the succeeding four hypoglycemic values, third, fourth, fifth and sixth hours, revealed what it the most consistent feature of this test in a case of hyperinsulinism due to an islet cell tumor.

The exercise test was positive in that the blood sugar fell to 39 mg. per cent by the fourth hour, the patient having exercised on a stationary rowing machine twenty minutes in each hour.

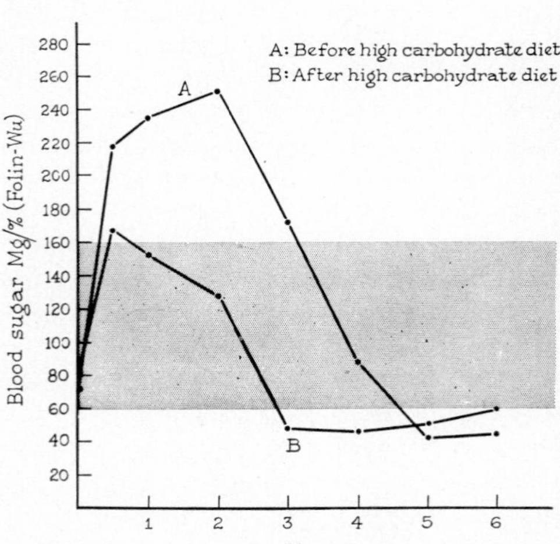

FIG. 2. Two responses in a case (Patient J. G.) of organic hyperinsulinism—islet cell tumor—to glucose tolerance tests.

A. Without preparation with a high carbohydrate diet, a diabetic type of curve was obtained.

B. After 5 days of a diet high in carbohydrate (400 to 500 gm.), the test reveals the characteristic third, fourth, fifth and sixth hour values which vary but little, and each is in the hypoglycemic zone.

At operation on November 25, 1946, a small purplish nodule, 1 cm. in diameter and slightly raised was found in the body of the pancreas. Small blood vessels were observed on the surface of the growth. The nodule was easily outlined by palpation. The entire pancreas was mobilized to permit careful palpation between finger and thumb throughout the organ. No other masses nor abnormalities of other viscera were detected. The tumor was enucleated with the removal of only a small fragment of pancreatic tissue. Free bleeding, indicative of the high degree of vascularity of the tumor, was encountered.

Following operation a febrile response, with temperature reaching 102° F., occurred but subsided by lysis over the three succeeding days.

Small amounts of glycosuria for two days and a mild degree of hyperglycemia (fasting value 148 mg. per cent—Folin-Wu) were looked upon as substantial evidence that no functioning islet cell tumor had escaped detection. There has been no recurrence of the hypoglycemia.

Microscopically, fibrous tissue containing nests of epithelial cells, the proportions being 1 to 3, were seen. There were minor variations in the morphology of the cells but all had abundant, faintly acidophilic cytoplasm with central vascular nuclei. The cytoplasm of many of the cells was finely granular, suggesting specific granules, but with the Gomori stain only a rare cell was observed to contain beta granules. The individual cells were twice as large as those in the islets of the accompanying fragment of normal pancreatic tissue. Though there was scattering of the cells in the tumor, there was a definite ductlike pattern. Small buds were observed to project from discrete isolated ducts. Where the lesion joined the pancreatic tissue there was no sharp capsule of small islands of tumor cells blending with neighboring acinar elements.

An assay showed that the insulin content of the extract was 4.60 units per cc.; this corresponded to 60.9 units per gram of tissue in contrast to the normal of 1.7 units.

Adrenal Cortical Insufficiency (Addison's Disease)

Deficiency of the adrenal cortex may cause a hypoglycemia which may be mistaken for hyperinsulinism. Welty[22] reports two such cases. One patient was seen in coma at which time the blood sugar level was 40 mg. per 100 cc. Consciousness was promptly regained following glucose (dextrose) therapy. A six-hour glucose tolerance test revealed progressively lower blood sugar levels, below 60 mg. per 100 cc., at the fifth and sixth hours. A later attack was fatal, there being no apparent response to glucose and the administration of adrenal cortical hormone. Fibrocaseous tuberculosis of the adrenal glands and a healed primary pulmonary tuberculosis were found at autopsy.

The foregoing notwithstanding, it is extraordinarily rare to find hypoglycemia as the only evidence of adrenal cortical insufficiency.

The underlying causes of adrenal cortical insufficiency as enumerated in Table 2 include (1) idiopathic adrenal cortical atrophy, (2) destructive lesions such as occur in certain infectious processes, notably tuberculosis, a meningococcemia (Friderichsen-Waterhouse syndrome), acute hemorrhagic fever and invasive neoplastic processes, (3) adrenalectomy, a cause which is assuming increasing importance with the upward trend in adrenalectomies for the alleviation of other diseases, and (4) congenital adrenal hyperplasia, due, it would appear, to an inability to produce hydrocortisone in normal amounts.[23]

The clinical features of Addison's disease should obviate the danger of confusing this disease with hyperinsulinism in most cases. In Addison's disease, there are muscle weakness, languor, hypotension, bradycardia, anorexia, hypochlorhydria and vomiting. The pigmentation of the skin and mucous membranes is characteristic of Addison's disease. There is an intensification of the dark color in normally pigmented areas, especially about the nipples. Black "freckles," cutaneous and in the mucous membranes of the mouth and vagina, and bronzing, tanning or dirty brown coloring of the skin are classic signs of this disease. There are increased loss of sodium, a rise in the serum potassium, general dehydration and depression of sexual functions. Hypoglycemia, though uncommon in these cases, may occur and may be the immediate cause of death.

Symptoms of hypoglycemia, when present, tend to occur at higher blood sugar levels than in organic hyperinsulinism.

More significant than the hypoglycemic feature are the clinical and chemical findings already alluded to. The normal decrease of 50 per cent or more in the circulating eosinophils found four hours after the intramuscular administration of 25 mg. of ACTH to the fasting patient does not occur in the presence of adrenal cortical insufficiency.

To detect whether the hypoglycemia encountered in such a case is the result of an insufficiency of the adrenal cortex or of the adenohypophysis, a 48 hour ACTH (adrenocorticotrophic hormone) test is helpful. This test is as follows: The urine voided for 24 consecutive hours is collected for a control quantitative determination of 17-ketosteroids and 11-oxysteroids. ACTH, 10 mg., is thereafter given at 6 hour intervals for 7 doses, and eosinophil counts are done at the end of 24 and 48 hours. The urine voided in the 24–48 hour period is collected also for quantitative determinations of the 17-ketosteroids and 11-oxysteroids. An eosinopenic response of less than 50 per cent or no appreciable increase in the amounts of steroids excreted in the second 24 hour collection of urine in contrast with the first indicates a primary adrenal cortical insufficiency. False positive eosinopenic responses may occur rarely in allergic persons; hence, the value of the combined studies—the eosinopenic response plus the testing of the capacity to increase the steroid excretion when stimulated with ACTH.

The control of the hypoglycemic component in adrenal cortical insufficiency by small doses of cortisone acetate (17-hydroxy-11-dehydrocorticosterone), formerly known as compound E (Kendall), is of diagnostic as well as therapeutic value.

Congenital Adrenal Hyperplasia. Clinical attacks of hypoglycemia, precipitated by stress, have been observed in a girl aged 4 years who had congenital virilism, in a twenty-six month old male with macrogenitosomia praecox and in a girl aged 2 years with congenital adrenal hyperplasia.[23] In the last mentioned the attacks were precipitated by infection. Depletion of sodium occurs in some cases and not in others.

It is believed that in congenital adrenal hyperplasia the normal requirement for hydrocortisone exceeds the productive capacity of the adrenal glands. This deficiency serves as an excessive stimulus to produce adrenocorticotrophic hormone (ACTH), and hyperplasia of the adrenal cortex ensues. Large amounts of steroids, other than hydrocortisone, are produced, much of which are excreted as 17-ketosteroids.

Under these circumstances stress conditions fail to bring about a normal increase in hydrocortisone in the blood, and sugar values significantly below normal are encountered in some of these patients.

ACTH intensifies the pathologic processes and hence is contraindicated as a form of therapy. Replacement therapy by administering hydrocortisone is the treatment of choice.

Anterior Pituitary (Adenohypophysis) Insufficiency—Panhypopituitarism

Spontaneous hypoglycemia is one of many but not a consistent manifestation of panhypopituitarism. When it occurs it follows the destruction of the adenohypophysis and is attributed to a lack of trophic hormones and the secondary atrophy of the adrenal cortex, to malnutrition of severe degree (Simmonds' cachexia) and to a lesser extent to hypothyroidism (pituitary myxedema).

Fisher et al.[24] found that in hypophysectomized animals the oxidation of glucose is greatly accelerated. Clinically, this may be a factor in increasing the likelihood of the hypoglycemia states in patients with insufficiency of the adenohypophysis.

The patient may be deprived of a functioning adenohypophysis as the result of tumors (notably chromophobe tumors), craniopharyngiomas and metastatic lesions (rarely), infrapituitary cyst, occlusion of the blood supply to the adenohypophysis by thromboses or embolism, abscess, atrophy of the adenohypophysis of undetermined cause and certain therapies such as irradiation and hypophysectomy.

Cushing in 1912 reported a case of

chromophobe tumor in which the blood sugar value was 30 mg. per cent. Similar reports have appeared since. Howard[25] mentions the case of a middle-aged truck driver who was subject to recurrent episodes of unconsciousness due to hypoglycemic attacks which were promptly corrected by administering glucose. The patient died in an attack and an autopsy revealed a large chromophobe adenoma which had expanded the sella turcica but had failed to involve the optic chiasm.

Postpartum necrosis of the adenohypophysis (Sheehan's disease) on an occlusive vascular basis is being recognized with increasing frequency. While hypoglycemia may occur and may be the cause of alarming episodes complicating this as well as other causes of panhypopituitarism, a careful clinical appraisal will readily detect the broader spectrum of abnormalities secondary to the lack of trophic hormones.

Not all of these patients are subject to attacks of hypoglycemia, but all appear to lack the normal steroid response to a hypoglycemia provoked by administering a small dose of insulin. It follows that for those patients who are prone to develop spontaneous hypoglycemia, there is no steroid of the "sugar hormone" type to come to the rescue. Fatalities from hypoglycemia under these circumstances are not surprising.

Clinical manifestations and laboratory evidences of hypothyroidism, hypoadrenocorticalism and hypogonadism, as they occur in patients with panhypopituitarism, simplify the differentiation between the spontaneous hypoglycemia of this disorder and that of organic hyperinsulinism.

Diseases of, or Affecting, the Liver

Spontaneous hypoglycemia occurs in a wide variety of hepatic disorders, which, for the most part, are due to toxins of chemical or infectious nature, to replacement of functioning with nonfunctioning tissue in the liver, or to disturbances in function resulting from vascular changes (see Table 2).

Hypoglycemia is not, however, to be considered a characteristic of these states. Even though hypoglycemia is suspected as a complication of hepatic disease, its occurrence is unusual but not rare. This infrequency might give a false indication of its seriousness. Inasmuch as it is an outcome of a reduced capacity of the glycogenetic, gluconeogenetic and glycogenolytic functions of the liver, it is usually an indication of grave and diffuse parenchymal disease. Hence, its detection and control may be life-saving.

Mann (1927) produced profound hypoglycemia in dogs by hepatectomy and mild hypoglycemia by partial hepatectomy. Hypoglycemia was first identified with acute and profound parenchymal disease of the liver resulting from phosphorus (1927) and arsenical poisonings (1930), and it was observed to occur in primary neoplasms of the liver (1929).

The list of disorders of the liver, primary and secondary, in which hypoglycemia may be encountered has grown into a broad spectrum of possibilities (see Table 2).

Any disease causing extensive damage to the liver may cause a hypoglycemia, especially after fasting, and as these patients have no appetite and often must depend on nourishment by vein, they are, at best, on an undernourishing regimen.

Patients acutely ill from hepatic disease and presumed to be bordering on, or already in, hepatic coma have been restored to consciousness by correcting a hypoglycemia. Disturbed mental behavior, associated cirrhosis of the liver and disturbed hepatic function in some cases of chronic myocardial failure are due to hypoglycemia, though this feature may readily escape consideration in the presence of the more obvious clinical manifestations.

Conn and his associates[26] have reported chronic hypoglycemia due to an ascending cholangiolitis. In one patient attacks of unconsciousness occurred from nine to twelve hours after the evening meal, and the blood sugar values, while the patient was fasting, ranged from 14 to 18 mg. per 100 cc. Symptoms typical of a severe hypoglycemia were promptly corrected by giving glucose (dextrose) intravenously. A gallbladder containing a calculus and 2 or 3 ounces (60 to 90 cc.) of pus was removed. A biopsy of the liver revealed an active chronic cholangiolitis, biliary cirrhosis, cloudy swelling and fatty infiltration. After operation the level of the blood sugar became normal as the evidence of hepatic damage gradually disappeared, and there were no recurrences of the spontaneous attacks of hypoglycemia.

Hepatocellular damage of severe degree and predisposing to the production of abnormally low blood sugar levels is detected by an increased thymol turbidity and cephalin cholesterol flocculation, decreased cholesterol esters in contrast to the total cholesterol and a decreased prothrombin. If these tests are normal, a hypoglycemia of hepatic origin will not occur—with one rare exception, Von Gierke's disease (see Chapter 9).

The 24-hour fast or restricted carbohydrate intake is not necessary, nor indeed are they advisable in cases of severe hepatic disease. The glucose tolerance test (for standard tests, see p. 798) in patients with hepatogenic hypoglycemia gives a characteristic result as depicted in curve E, Figure 1.

The fasting value is subnormal, usually below 50 mg. per cent (Folin-Wu). A marked hyperglycemia develops within one hour and is sustained through the second hour, after which the hyperglycemia subsides and hypoglycemic levels tend to ensue after 5 to 7 hours.

Hypoglycemic tendencies not otherwise obvious may be revealed by this prolonged test. In such cases the fasting value is usually a low normal, but the remainder of the curve is as described above.

Patients with hypoglycemic tendencies of hepatic origin cannot tolerate fasting without causing a hypoglycemia, and as fasting is inadvisable for these patients, unusual fasting should not be used as a test. They will have evidences of extensive hepatocellular disease, and they will give a characteristic response to a glucose tolerance test.

Hypoglycemic episodes as an outcome of altered hepatic function in congestive heart failure are probably overlooked because of unawareness that they occur and because of the overshadowing effects of the primary disease.

The ups and downs of myocardial failure may confuse the issue; a transient attack of failure may be responsible for temporary disruption of hepatic function sufficient to produce a hypoglycemia without the usual manifestations of hepatic damage being clinically apparent. An awareness that hypoglycemic attacks may occur in these cases will indicate objective studies for their recognition and measures for their prompt correction. It has been intimated that hypoglycemia as a feature of chronic myocardial insufficiency has been largely unrecognized.[27]

It is beyond my objective here to consider fully the treatments for the variety of disorders responsible for hepatogenic hypoglycemia. Therapy should be directed at controlling the primary disorder. To control and prevent hypoglycemia, multiple (6 to 8) nourishments per day are desirable. In the acute phase of the hepatic disorder a diet low in protein, 20 to 40 gm. per day, may be advisable, but when this restriction is no longer needed the amounts of protein are increased until 2 gm. per kilogram of the ideal body weight is reached. Liberal allowances of carbohydrate, up to 400 grams per day, are incorporated in the multiple feedings.

Nourishment via vein may be imperative. If it is given very slowly, the risk of hypoglycemia "between administrations" will be reduced. There is evidence that the mild degree of hyperglycemia attending the infusion of glucose has a sparing action on the liver.[28]

In Von Gierke's disease (glycogenosis) hypoglycemic values are found, but curiously enough the symptoms usually associated with such values are absent. This disorder is presented in Chapter 9.

Certain Fibromas and Sarcomas

Large sarcomatous or fibromatous tumors are rare causes of hypoglycemia.

Less than a score of cases have been reported. The tumors have no apparent connection with the pancreas. One, a massive fibroma, was located superior to the left lobe of the liver. Another, a spindle cell sarcoma weighing 2700 grams, arose from the diaphragm. Others were adherent to one or the other kidney and several arose in the retroperitoneal space. In each of the 14 cases available for review the tumor was large and enlarged rapidly until massive in size.

It has been postulated that the tumors produce a hypoglycemic agent, that they consume selectively very large amounts of glucose,[15] that they are actually atypical functioning islet cell neoplasms,[29] and that they produce a less well defined disruptive effect, by pressure or stretching, on unknown receptors in the abdomen and a blocking of sympathetic impulses to the liver. A potent insulin, or insulin-like agent, has been recovered from one of these tumors[29a] and an apparent cure followed its removal.

Hypoglycemic episodes disappear with removal of the tumors, but in 5 of 8 cases the tumor eventually recurred and hypoglycemic attacks were again a prominent feature.

Skillern and co-authors[29] support the hypothesis that these neoplasms are atypical functioning islet cell tumors of low grade malignancy. In favor of this concept, they noted that they grow rapidly to a large size and that they are composed predominantly of spindle-shaped cells—usually a malignant feature but not always; metastasis to the liver occurs; and protracted delay of recurrence after removal of the tumor—7 years in one instance and 2 years in another—is a characteristic of this disorder. This concept has not been verified by others.

Case Report.

Patient P. S. (79933), aged 48 years, was admitted to the Pennsylvania Hospital in July, 1947. He had had a nephrectomy at another hospital in 1944 because of a tumor involving the left kidney. Sections revealed a diagnosis of "leiomyosarcoma—probably of the kidney." In 1947 he complained of progressive abdominal enlargement, increasing fatigue and episodes of weakness and dizziness, which were proved to be due to hypoglycemia and which were promptly relieved by the taking of food. A second operation was done, and a retroperitoneal cystic mass the size of a football was found. Serosanguinous fluid and friable tissue were aspirated and a frozen section disclosed the characteristics of a sarcoma. The symptoms became progressively worse, and when the patient was seen by us in 1947 food was necessary every hour to prevent attacks of sweating, lethargy, confusion and deepening stupor. The blood sugar, postprandial, was 48 mg. per cent (Folin-Wu). If food and glucose were withheld, hypoglycemic attacks followed without fail.

Rapid enlargement of the abdominal mass occurred while the patient was under observation, and his clinical course declined until he died suddenly after 114 days of observation.

Autopsy revealed an embolus occluding the left pulmonary artery, which was considered to be the immediate cause of death. There was a huge retroperitoneal tumor arising in the left but also filling the right half of the abdomen. The neoplasm weighed 20 kg. and microscopically proved to be a fibrosarcoma. There was a generalized splanchnomegaly involving the lungs, heart, spleen, pancreas, liver, right kidney, adrenal and thyroid glands.

There was no evidence of an islet cell tumor. The islets in the pancreas appeared normal, as did the other organs except for their increase in size. The hypophysis was enlarged, weighing 1 gm. A diagnosis of acromegaly was made based on acidophilic hyperplasia of the adenohypophysis, generalized splanchnomegaly and somatic giantism.

Mild degrees of hypoglycemia have been reported to occur in progressive muscular atrophy and status thymicolymphaticus and in cretins. The hypoglycemic feature is incidental in contrast to the other significant findings in these patients.

SPONTANEOUS HYPOGLYCEMIA CAUSED BY FUNCTIONAL DISORDERS

Hyperinsulinism Due to Functional Hypertrophy and Hyperplasia of the Islets of Langerhans

Increased islet cell function in newborn infants of mothers whose diabetes was out of control during the latter months of pregnancy has been supported by the finding of hypertrophy and hyperplasia of the islets of Langerhans in these infants. The otherwise unexplained death of an apparently normal infant answering the foregoing qualifications occurred at the Pennsylvania Hospital and was attributed to a hypoglycemia. At autopsy, hypertrophy and hyperplasia of the islets were outstanding.[30]

The widespread custom of depriving infants of diabetic mothers of nourishment in the first 24 hours of life suggests that there is not widespread acceptance of the theory that functional hyperinsulinism occurs in the infant. Nevertheless, as the result of a well controlled study, Helwig[31] states, "I am forced to conclude that some infants of diabetic mothers have definitely larger amounts of insular tissue than infants of nondiabetic mothers." It should be added that these changes occurred in large infants, possibly influenced by increased growth hormones, and that some of the pancreases of infants of diabetic mothers were considered to be normal.

The hypoglycemia in the newborn is a potential, though admittedly uncommon danger that should not be overlooked. As a cause of death, it is rare. We[32] consider that an otherwise unexplained and significant reduction in the mother's need for insulin in the last trimester of pregnancy is due to hyperinsulinism in the fetus. Nourishment is given to such infants every 2 hours for the first 3 days following delivery.

Ideal control of the diabetes during pregnancy is not always achieved, but it would appear that the likelihood of the infant's developing hyperinsulinism is in direct relation to the degree of poor control of the diabetes (see section on pregnancy).

Hyperinsulinism Due to Altered Gastrointestinal Function

Circumstances which permit excessively rapid absorption of carbohydrate from the small intestine provide the stage for postprandial hypoglycemia. A gastrectomy or a gastroenterostomy permits an uninterrupted flow from the stomach to the duodenum. The carbohydrate is exposed to a larger absorptive surface of the duodenum more quickly than is the case when a normal pylorus is controlling the rate at which food leaves the stomach. As a result, a greater amount of carbohydrate is absorbed per unit of time than occurs normally. The rapid elevation of the blood sugar to hyperglycemic levels (Fig. 1) which follows has an abnormally great stimulative effect on normally functioning islets of Langerhans.

An overcorrection of the hyperglycemia follows with the production of a hypoglycemia. The same effect can be provoked in the normal person by instilling carbohydrate directly into the duodenum via tube, in this manner bypassing the pyloric control of egress of the carbohydrate from the stomach.

Postprandial hypoglycemia is occasionally encountered in thyrotoxicosis. This, also, is attributed to excessively rapid absorption—a characteristic of thyrotoxic persons. In these patients, however, the nature of the disorder tends to neutralize insulin activity. Hence, it is not surprising that hypoglycemia following the stimulative effect of rapid absorption of carbohydrate in thyrotoxic patients is unusual.

Gastric surgery is the forerunner of practically all cases of postprandial stimulative hyperinsulinism. Many reports of the postgastrectomy hypoglycemic syndrome indicate that this is not an uncommon condition, and the increasing incidence with which gastrectomy is being performed will add further to its frequency.

There should be no difficulty in differentiating postprandial or stimulative hypoglycemia from fasting hypoglycemia. In the former the stimulative effect on the insulin-producing mechanism is greatest within one half to one hour after the ingestion of a meal, i.e., during the hyperglycemic phase. A precipitous decline to subnormal blood sugar values occurs in the second hour, but increases to normal are usual by the fourth or, at the most, by the fifth hour (see curve C, Fig. 1).

The fasting blood sugar is always normal in these patients, and there is no evidence whatever of the hypoglycemic syndrome before breakfast.

Symptoms of hypoglycemia occur, as a rule, between one and one half and three hours postprandially. They may be troublesome for only a short time following surgery in some cases; others require control therapy for long periods.

The hypoglycemic syndrome should not be confused with the "dumping syndrome." There is no hypoglycemic syndrome associated with the latter, which begins within ten to fifteen minutes after eating and which has been attributed to distention of the jejunum with fluid.· There is, however, rather good evidence that jejunal hypermotility may actually be the cause of the symptoms which result.[32a] These are weakness, nausea, abdominal cramps, sweating and a sensation of bloating in the epigastrium. Cardiac palpitation may be a complaint. These symptoms subside before sufficient time has elapsed for the hypoglycemic syndrome to become manifest. Furthermore, they may be controlled by antispasmodic agents; Dactil is particularly effective.

Treatment. Retarded absorption of carbohydrate from the intestine is the aim of therapy. In this manner the hyperglycemic phase may be averted so that the excessive stimulative effect on the pancreatic islets and hypoglycemia are avoided.

Diets low in carbohydrate value (75 to 100 gm.) are employed with a liberal allowance of protein (from 100 to 140 gm. as tolerated by the individual patient) with a quota of fat sufficient to maintain the total calories within the desired range.

Patients who have some residua of the hypoglycemia when the total diet is divided into three meals benefit from a small portion of the day's allowance in the midforenoon, midafternoon and at bedtime. A small dose of unmodified or crystalline (rapidly acting) insulin one half hour before each meal—the aim being to prevent the hyperglycemic or stimulative phase[33] has been suggested. This measure is neither welcomed by the patient nor is it necessary. It is an alternative, however, when the foregoing measures are not completely satisfactory.

Resection of a portion of the pancreas is contraindicated. A satisfactory result can be obtained without this radical procedure. It should not be overlooked that there is a gradual adaptation of the altered physiologic state which may permit relinquishing, considerably or indeed entirely, the restriction of the carbohydrate intake.

Relative Hyperinsulinism with Functional Neurologic Disturbances

Spontaneous hypoglycemia occurring in persons with disturbances in the vegetative nervous system is a mild and relatively innocent condition. It is important chiefly because it is a common malady affecting the great majority of patients subject to hypoglycemic tendencies and because, if mistaken for organic hyperinsulinism, it may lead to needless surgery involving the pancreas. The understanding of this cause of hypoglycemia is not as precise as that due to functioning islet tumors. Unfortunately, the term functional hyperinsulinism implies that the disorder is pancreatic in origin.

Unlike the functional hyperinsulinism following gastrectomy, in which the prompt hyperglycemia following the taking of carbohydrate is succeeded by a period of hypoglycemia attributable to overstimulation of the islet cells, rarely indeed, in my experience, is there any hyperglycemia (see Fig. 1, curve B) to cause undue stimulation of the islet cells, and there is no proof that insulin is produced in excess of normal. It seems more likely, in view of the absence of a stimulative hyperglycemia and the mildness of the degrees of hypoglycemia, that a mild variant from normal in the homeostatic control of the blood sugar level is at fault and, as these patients usually exhibit other evidences of disturbances in the vegetative nervous system, notably anxiety states and neurocirculatory asthenia, suspicion is cast on the sympathico-adrenal component of the regulatory mechanism.

The maintenance of a precise equilibrium between withdrawals and additions of sugar to the blood is subject to a variety of influences, among the most significant of which are the automatically controlled discharge of insulin, the release of sugar from the liver through the process of glycogenolysis and the influence which the sympathico-adrenal system exerts on this mechanism. The feature we are concerned with is the combination of regulatory influences which come into play in preventing the development of hypoglycemia and those at fault when, on a purely functional basis, a hypoglycemia is permitted to occur. Abnormally great amounts of insulin would account for the latter, but as hyperglycemia, after the ingestion of food, is not a feature in these cases, the evidence that this is the cause of the hypoglycemia is conjectural. Soskin et al.[34] have shown that as the degree of glycemia decreases it reaches a threshold at which the liver begins to discharge glucose. If this threshold is lower than normal, a corresponding hypoglycemia occurs before the glycogenolytic process is set in motion. They believe that it is the level of the blood sugar which retards glycogenolysis after the ingestion of carbohydrate and which stimulates glycogenolysis to prevent hypoglycemia when the immediate effects of the ingested carbohydrate have subsided. The sympathico-adrenal nervous system also affects glycogenolysis. Much is known about the hyperglycemic effect resulting from the stimulation of this system, but little is known of its influence on retarding glycogenolysis.

Clinically, in view of the multiple indications of disturbances in the vegetative nervous system in these patients, it is not unreasonable to suspect that they play a part in producing the hypoglycemia or a retarding effect on glycogenolysis via the sympathico-adrenal system.

It is not entirely clear what exact and entire part each of these three influences—insulin, lowered threshold of glycogenolysis and the sympathico-adrenal system—plays in the production of functional hypoglycemia or whether the aberration from normal is really a combination of two or of all three.

This type of hypoglycemia is regularly and spontaneously corrected if allowed to remain untreated, and this is in keeping with the hypothesis that a relatively mild deviation from normal physiologic processes is at fault. If the sympathico-adrenal system is capable of retarding glycogenolysis, or if the threshold at which hepatic glycogenolysis is initiated is lower than normal, a normal production of insulin would appear to be excessive; for this reason it is not surprising that the condition has been labeled by some as functional hyperinsulinism. That there is an apparent hyperinsulinism effect is probably agreed to by all. Indeed, as long as the possible chain of events is understood and the threat of needless pancreatectomy is clearly avoided the term *relative hyperinsulinism* is acceptable.

Relative hyperinsulinism, as observed in emotionally unstable persons is the most common form of spontaneous hypoglycemia. It accounts for more cases of spontaneous hypoglycemia than all other causes combined. The neurologic demeanor of these patients is out of proportion to the apparent disturbance in the blood sugar controlling mechanisms. They exhibit anxiety states, vasomotor instability, cardiac palpitation and excessive perspiration of hands and feet and in the axillae. The "irritable colon syndrome" with irritability and fatigue may be outstanding. Neurocirculatory asthenia and excessive generalized perspiration are common. These patients do not, however, have a preference for cool temperatures. They never lose consciousness as the result of the hypoglycemia,* and the blood sugar for the most part is in the low normal zone, rarely below 50 mg. per cent (Folin-Wu) during attacks which characteristically occur 2 hours after meals.

* One of my patients lost consciousness on several occasions, but these attacks were due to hysteria and were not related to hypoglycemia.

Diagnosis. 1. Clinical attacks of hypoglycemia of this functional type are postprandial; they never occur before breakfast, nor are hypoglycemic values caused by a diet low in carbohydrates nor by fasting alone or with exercise added.

2. The subjective manifestations are out of proportion to the degree of hypoglycemia, which is of a mild degree. The symptoms are indistinguishable from those caused by a small overdose of rapidly acting insulin (see p. 713) with a distinct neurotic overlay. Improvement usually follows the taking of food, but it is not as dramatic as in cases of severe degrees of hypoglycemia. Indeed, recovery occurs spontaneously if no treatment is given.

The hypoglycemic feature is not progressive. Over long periods the clinical features tend to follow a constant pattern with subjective symptoms, but not the hypoglycemic features, worse at times of challenge—such as a change of occupation, a promotion to greater responsibilities and increased anxieties.

3. GLUCOSE TOLERANCE TEST. The results of this test are distinctive. The fasting blood sugar is normal; the increase in the blood sugar response at one hour is usually normal but may be slightly elevated; a hypoglycemic phase, to 50 mg. per cent (Folin-Wu) or lower, follows between two and three hours with return to pretest levels in three to four hours. Illustrative results of glucose tolerance tests are presented in Figure 1 (curve B).

It is common to obtain a low or flat type of curve without a significant degree of hypoglycemia at any time, though symptoms identical with those associated with previous attacks are usual when the blood sugar is at its lowest—between two and one half to three and one half hours after the glucose is taken.

A low carbohydrate, low caloric diet (protein 55 gm., carbohydrate 55 gm. and fat 88 gm. = 1200 calories) for 3 days does not provoke a hypoglycemia, as it does in cases of functioning islet cell tumors. A fourth day of complete fasting with exercise (see page 717) can be added without producing significant hypoglycemia values.

Treatment. Therapy consists of special diet and psychiatric guidance, preferably by an internist.

The "staying effect" of a liberal protein intake, 100 to 130 gm., is advantageous when well tolerated. The stimulative effect on insulin production is reduced by curtailing the carbohydrate. The quota of fat makes up the remaining calories. An illustrative diet is: protein 120 gm., carbohydrate 150 gm. and fat 146 gm. (2400 calories). This diet, given in three meals, may be adequate to control symptoms, but not infrequently better control is obtained if the diet is divided into three main meals and midforenoon, midafternoon and bedtime snacks (see illustrative diet, Table 3).

Due consideration to the neuroses—a part of this phenomenon—is important. Excessive stimulants, notably caffeine, are reduced or eliminated. This applies to tobacco also. A suitable tranquilizing drug may be remarkably effective. Reduction or removal of causes of anxiety is helpful, and reassurance is of value.

*Spontaneous Hypoglycemia and Ganglion Blocking Agents (Methonium Compounds, Pyrrolidinium Bitartrate and Mecamylamine)**

Patients may be deprived of the emergency neurovegetative (sympathico-adrenal) effect in combating hypoglycemia when taking ganglion blocking agents—a common therapy for severe grades of hypertension (Fig. 3). Quite different from the normal response, there is no apparent inhibition to the development of hypoglycemia when an overdose of insulin is given to such a patient. We have observed this phenomenon in diabetes and consider it probable that some spells of weakness in nondiabetic patients receiving these drugs are due to the blocking of the neurogenic impulses and the mild de-

* These observations were made by Dr. William K. Jenson while a Research Fellow in Medicine at the Pennsylvania Hospital, Philadelphia.

TABLE 3. ILLUSTRATIVE DIET FOR THE TREATMENT OF FUNCTIONAL HYPOGLYCEMIA
120 gm. Protein, 146 gm. Fat, 150 gm. Carbohydrate
2400 Calories—Six Feedings

NO. EXCHANGES	FOOD* EXCHANGE	LIST NO.	SAMPLE MENU	HOUSEHOLD MEASURE	WT. GM.	P	F	C
Breakfast								
1	Fruit	3	Orange juice	½ cup	100	...	...	10
2	Meat	5	Eggs	2		14	10	
1	Bread	4	Bread	1 slice	25	2	...	15
4	Fat	6	20% cream	2 oz.	60			
			Butter	2 tsp.	10	...	20	
1	Milk	1	Milk, whole	1 cup	240	8	10	12
						24	40	37
Mid-morning								
1	Milk	1	Milk, whole	1 cup	240	8	10	12
½	Bread	4	Graham Crackers	1	10	1	...	8
						9	10	20
Lunch or supper								
4	Meat	5	{Cold cuts	2 sl.	90			
			{Cottage cheese	½ cup	90	28	20	
1	Vegetable	2A	Tomato & Lettuce	1	100			
1	Bread	4	Bread	1 slice	25	2	...	15
1	Fruit	3	Applesauce	½ cup	100	...	...	10
3	Fat	6	Butter	2 tsp.	10			
			Mayonnaise	1 tsp.	5	...	15	
1	Milk	1	Milk, whole	1 cup	240	8	10	12
						38	45	37
Mid-afternoon								
1	Milk	1	Milk, whole	1 cup	240	8	10	12
½	Bread	4	Saltines	2–3	10	1	...	8
						9	10	20
Dinner								
4	Meat	5	Roast Beef	4 oz.	120	28	20	
1	Vegetable	2A	Cucumber Salad	1	100			
1	Vegetable	2B	Carrots	½ cup	100	2	...	7
1	Bread	4	Potato	1 small	100	2	...	15
3	Fat	6	Salad oil	1 tsp.	5			
			Butter	2 tsp.	10	...	15	
1	Fruit	3	Peaches	1 medium	100	...	...	10
						32	35	32
Bedtime								
1	Meat	5	Cheese	1 oz.	30	7	5	
½	Bread	4	Saltines	2–3	10	1	...	8
						8	5	8
					Total	120	145	154

* For Food Exchange System see Chapter 15.

grees of hypoglycemia which may ensue.

Adrenal Cortical Insufficiency

Functional hypoglycemia is a potential possibility when adrenal cortical function is temporarily impaired. Prolonged treatment with cortisone (17-hydroxy-11-dehydrocorticosterone, compound E [Kendall]) deprives normal adrenal cortices of their usual stimulation. They become relatively quiescent and incapable of abrupt response to the stimulative effects of physiologic need if the corticoid therapy is suddenly withdrawn without the dosage being gradually decreased. Under these circumstances, there is danger of adrenal cortical failure but especially if there is added stress, notably that caused by acute infections, surgical procedures and trauma. The gradual withdrawal of cortisone therapy—over a period of 7 to 10 days—with or without the adrenal cortical stimulation of ACTH, will prevent functional adrenal insufficiency and avoid the potential risk of a hypoglycemia.

Adrenal failure may be precipitated spontaneously by the severe stress of fulminating infection, less frequently in surgical and traumatic cases and now rarely in thyroid storm. Being mindful of the possibility of this dangerous complication is the first requisite to its detection and control. The treatment is identical with that employed in cases of adrenal crises.

Idiopathic Spontaneous Hypoglycemia of Infancy

This entity, well known to pediatricians, may exhibit a spectrum from minor symptoms to convulsive seizures in the absence of a detectable organic lesion. Favorable response to the ingestion of sugar may be the first clue to the diagnosis. Mental retardation and neurologic abnormalities may result from long episodes of unrecognized hypoglycemia which may be erroneously attributed to epilepsy.

Tumors of the islets of Langerhans are rare in infants. Other causes of hypoglycemia presented by McQuarrie[21] in their relative frequency in 40 cases of hypoglycemia of infancy are as follows: adrenal insufficiency, 6; panhypopituitarism (pituitary dwarf), 1; glycogen storage disease of hepatic type (Von Gierke), 3; hypothyroidism (cretin), 1; solitary pancreatic beta cell tumor, 1; congenital galactosemia, 1; infants of diabetic mothers, 2; and persistent spontaneous hypoglycemia, cause undetermined, 25.

The cause of idiopathic spontaneous hypoglycemia of infancy and childhood is not known. Conn[35] suggests that a pituitary insulotropic principle or a hypothalamic abnormality may be the offender rather than a congenital deficiency of the alpha cells of the islets of Langerhans. Eleven of the 25 cases (44

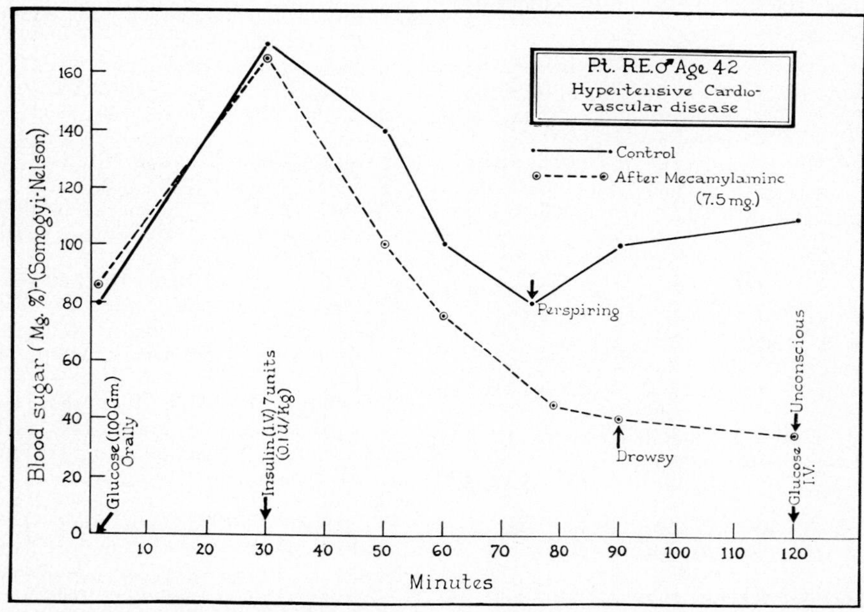

FIG. 3. Interruption, by a ganglion blocking agent, of normal mechanisms of preventing and spontaneously correcting a hypoglycemia. The control blood sugar values (solid line) after the administration of glucose and insulin are contrasted with those (broken line) obtained under identical circumstances except that, in the latter study, the patient had received mecamylamine (Inversine) 7.5 mg.

per cent) exhibited a familial or genetic trait of spontaneous hypoglycemia.

The fact that idiopathic hypoglycemia of infancy subsides spontaneously emphasizes the need for a correct diagnosis, adequate control of the condition to prevent damage to the brain and the avoidance, or at least the deferring, of surgical intervention. It may be impossible to differentiate between this condition and that of a functioning islet cell tumor, but as malignant tumors of the islets do not occur in infancy or childhood, watchful waiting is justified until the true nature of the disorder becomes reasonably apparent.

Treatment is begun with corticotropin (ACTH) given intramuscularly in doses of 4 mg. per kilogram of body weight per day, at 6 hour intervals for 4 days. For the succeeding week one quarter of this amount is given night and morning in the form of H.P. ACTHAR gel (Armour). The dosage is then adjusted as needed. As little as 2 mg. ACTHAR gel on alternate days may suffice. Reduction of the dosage to the point of complete withdrawal within a few months has been accomplished without a return of the hypoglycemia (McQuarrie).[21]

Miscellaneous Causes of Hypoglycemia

The hypoglycemia is a relatively unimportant and innocent feature in prolonged physical exercise, lactation, severe cachexia and some diarrheal states.

References

1. Folin, O. and Wu, H.: J. Biol. Chem., *41:*367, 1920.
2. Nelson, N.: J. Biol. Chem., *153:*375, 1944.
3. Nicholls, A. G.: J. Med. Research, *8:*835, 1902.
4. Copp, E. F. F. and Barclay, A. J.: J. Metab. Research, *4:*445, 1923.
5. Banting, F. G. and Best, C. H.: J. Lab. & Clin. Med., *7:*251, 1922.
6. Campbell, W. R. and Fletcher, A. A.: J.A.M.A., *80:*1641, 1923.
7. Gibson, R. B. and Larimer, R. N.: J.A.M.A., *82:*468, 1924.
8. Harris, S.: J.A.M.A., *83:*729, 1924.
9. Wilder, R. M., Allan, F. N., Power, M. H. and Robertson, H. E.: J.A.M.A., *89:*348, 1927.
10. Howland, G., Campbell, W. R., Maltby, E. J. and Robinson, W. L.: J.A.M.A., *93:*674, 1929.
11. Whipple, A. O.: J. Internat. chir., *3:*237, 1938.
12. Willebrands, A. F. and Groen, J.: Diabetes, *5:*378, 1956.
13. Crain, E. L., Jr. and Thorn, G. W.: Medicine, *28:*427, 1949.
14. Howard, J. M., Moss, N. H. and Rhoads, J. E.: Surg. Gynec. & Obst., *90:*417, 1950.
15. Conn, J. W. and Seltzer, H. S.: Am. J. Med., *19:*460, 1955.
16. Laidlaw, G. F.: Am. J. Path., *14:*125, 1938.
17. Lopez-Kruger, R. and Dockerty, M. B.: Surg. Gynec. & Obst., *85:*495, 1947.
18. Bockus, H. L.: Gastro-Enterology. Vol. 3. Philadelphia, W. B. Saunders Company, 1946.
19. McMillan, F. L. and Scheib, J. R.: Am. J. Surg., *82:*759, 1951.
20. Porter, M. R. and Frantz, V. K.: Am. J. Med., *21:*944, 1956.
21. McQuarrie, I.: Am. J. Dis. Child., *87:*399, 1954.
22. Welty, J. W. and Robertson, H. F.: Am. J. M. Sc., *192:*760, 1936.
23. White, F. P. and Sutton, L. E.: J. Clin. Endocrinol., *11:*1395, 1951.
24. Fisher, R. E., Russell, J. A. and Cori, C. F.: J. Biol. Chem., *115:*627, 1936.
25. Howard, J. E.: Veterans Admin. Tech. Bull. 10-108, 1955, p. 5.
26. Conn, J. W., Newburgh, L. H., Johnston, M. W. and Sheldon, J. M.: Arch. Int. Med., *62:*765, 1938.
27. Mellinkoff, S. M. and Tumulty, P. A.: New England J. Med., *247:*745, 1952.
28. Soskin, S. and Levine, R.: Carbohydrate Metabolism. Chicago, University of Chicago Press, 1946, p. 250.
29. Skillern, P. G., McCormack, L. J., Hewlett, J. S. and Crile, G., Jr.: Diabetes, *3:*133, 1954.

29a. August, J. T. and Hiatt, H. H.: New England J. Med., *258*(No. 1):17, 1958.

30. Bauer, J. T. and Royster, H. A., Jr.: Bull. Ayer Clin. Lab. Penna. Hosp., *3:*109, 1937.
31. Helwig, E. B.: Arch. Int. Med., *65:*221, 1940.
32. Duncan, G. G. and Fetter, F.: Am. J. M. Sc., *187:*347, 1934.

32a. Jordan, G. L., Jr., Overton, R. C. and DeBakey, M. E.: Ann. Surg., *145:*471, 1957.

33. John, H. J.: Endocrinology, *17:*583, 1933.
34. Soskin, S., Essex, H. E., Herrick, J. F. and Mann, F. C.: Am. J. Physiol., *124:*558, 1939.
35. Conn, J. W. and Louis, L.: J. Clin. Endocrinol., *5:*247, 1945.

CHAPTER 13 *By* GARFIELD G. DUNCAN, M.D.

Diabetes Insipidus

Definition. Diabetes insipidus is an uncommon chronic disease resulting from a deficiency of an antidiuretic hormone (ADH) believed to be identical with vasopressin (Pitressin) which, under normal conditions, is produced, stored in and released from an integral unit, the hypothalamoneurohypophyseal system. Polyuria occurs as a result of relative or absolute deficiency of this hormone, which, under the influences of changes in the osmolarity of the blood plasma and other probable factors, normally regulates the facultative reabsorption of water by the distal segments of the renal tubules. Disturbances in water economy which ensue are indicated by the frequent passing of excess quantities of pale urine free from sugar and having a low specific gravity (varying between 1.001 and 1.005), by dehydration of the tissues and by an intense thirst which becomes intolerable if the intake of fluid is reduced to normal amounts. Alterations in electrolyte metabolism, plasma protein concentration and hematocrit values, as well as in water balance, occur in this disease.

Willis (1682) differentiated the nonsaccharine characteristic of the urine in diabetes insipidus from the sweet urine of diabetes mellitus, and Frank (1794) observed that the aglycosuric polyuria of diabetes insipidus was a permanent disorder of extrarenal origin. Schafer (1906) revealed a relationship between the action of the posterior lobe of the pituitary gland and urinary excretion. It was Cushing (1912)[1] and Biedl,[2] one year later, who associated the onset of polyuria with the removal of the neurohypophysis and von den Velden[3] and Farini[4] (1913) who independently observed that preparations of the posterior lobe of the pituitary gland alleviated the polyuria and thirst of diabetes insipidus. Aschner (1912)[5] found that if the hypothalamic centers and the tuber cinereum were not disturbed, hypophysectomy did not precipitate diabetes insipidus but that destruction of the hypothalamic centers produced the typical manifestations of this disorder.

Any pathologic condition, whether infection, tumor, infiltrative process, trauma or congenital disorder, may cause diabetes insipidus by disturbing

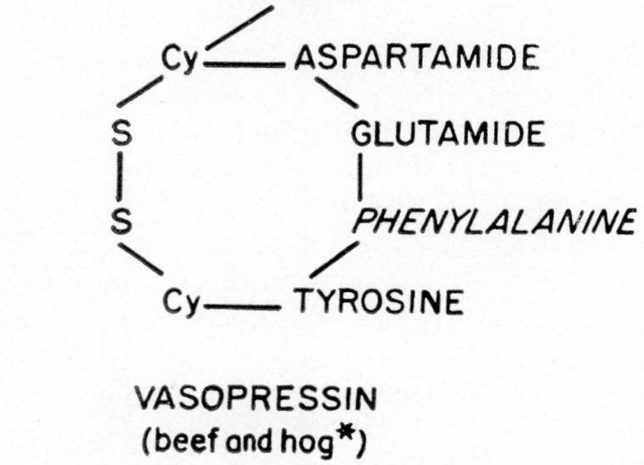

FIG. 1. Structure of vasopressin as synthesized by du Vigneaud and associates.[6]

the function of the hypothalamoneurohypophyseal system in varying degrees, according to the intensity and site of the abnormality. The recent synthesis of the hormone (Fig. 1) from the posterior pituitary gland, customarily referred to as the neurohypophysis, by du Vigneaud and his co-workers[6] has added to our understanding of this disorder.

PATHOGENESIS

The hypothalamoneurohypophysis must be intact, physiologically and anatomically, for the normal elaboration of the antidiuretic hormone. A bilateral injury to the supraopticohypophyseal tract is known to disturb the function of an intact adenohypophysis (anterior lobe of the pituitary gland) and cause diabetes insipidus.

Continued function of the adenohypophysis plays a part in producing polyuria in diabetes insipidus.[7] A complete hypophysectomy does not cause diabetes insipidus. Whether the adenohypophysis produces a diuretic agent or whether its effect is a secondary one exerted through the thyroid and adrenals is not known. It is known that thyroidectomy reduces the polyuria of diabetes insipidus and that there is a failure of the normal response to the ingestion of water in adrenal cortical insufficiency.

Fisher and his associates[8] induced diabetes insipidus at will in cats and monkeys by interrupting the supraopticoneurohypophyseal tract. Furthermore, they found that atrophic changes took place in the supraoptic and paraventricular nuclei and in the posterior or neural lobe of the pituitary gland as a result of these injuries. Destruction of these hypothalamic nuclei is followed by atrophy of the posterior lobe, with disappearance of the parenchymal cells —large glial cells found throughout the neurohypophysis and known as pituicytes. Furthermore, destruction or enucleation of the posterior lobe leads to atrophy of these nuclei. A sharply defined lesion, transection of the hypophyseal stalk without trauma to the base of the brain or to the hypophysis, produced diabetes insipidus in man (Dandy).[9] Diabetes insipidus ensued when the hypothalamic centers were injured, but without division of the pituitary stalk, in the removal of a craniopharyngioma.[10] The functional capacity of this supraopticoneurohypophyseal unit is dependent upon the integrity of each part and the unit as a whole.

Formerly it was generally accepted that the hormone now identified as vasopressin (Pitressin) was a product of the posterior or neural lobe of the hypophysis, but recent advances in neurophysiology indicate that this hormone may originate in the hypothalamic nuclei and may be stored in the posterior lobe of the hypophysis.[11,12,13] If the neurohypophysis serves as a reservoir and not as the source of vasopressin, this may account for the fact that isolated removal of this lobe, without otherwise injuring the hypothalamoneurohypophyseal unit, does not always cause diabetes insipidus.

This unit, having hormonal and nerve capacity, is integrally dependent on the normal functioning of each part. Each part contains specifically staining "neurosecretory granules." This unit is comprised of (a) supraoptic and paraventricular nuclei and nuclei tuberes in the hypothalamus, (b) a tract of unmyelinated nerve fibers arising in these nuclei, pursuing a course down through the hypothalamus near the tuber cinereum via the median eminence, comprising much of the floor of the third ventricle and the infundibular stalk, and terminating in (c) the neurohypophysis, which consists of the median eminence of the tuber cinereum, the infundibular stem and the infundibular process (Fig. 2). The connecting nerve fibers, designated as the hypothalamoneurohypophyseal tract, were discovered independently by Pines[14] and Greving.[15] Experimentally, interruption of more than one half of the tract of nerve fibers produces diabetes insipidus.[16] This results also from division of the infundibulum, with detachment of most of the median eminence or complete removal of the neurohypophysis including the median eminence, or from the destruction of more than 95 per cent of the supraoptic nuclei.[8]

It has been suggested that adrenal cortical dysfunction plays a part in the pathologic physiology of diabetes insipidus.[16a] There is a failure of a normal response to the ingestion of water in adrenal insufficiency, but the association, if any, of disorders of the adrenal cortex with diabetes insipidus is not established.

FUNCTIONAL UNIT RELATED TO PRODUCTION, STORAGE AND RELEASE OF ANTIDIURETIC HORMONE

Fisher and his co-workers[8] established that the hypothalamoneurohypophyseal system is an anatomic and functional unit. They believed, though this belief is questioned by some, that impulses arising in the supraoptic and paraventricular nuclei regulate the secretion and release of the antidiuretic hormone from the neurohypophysis and that diabetes insipidus develops when the production of the hormone by the neurohypophysis is less than the amount required for physiologic purposes.

The concept, on the other hand, that the antidiuretic hormone is produced in the hypothalamus and migrates to and is stored in the neurohypophysis is receiving increasing acceptance. This change of concept is based on Scharrers'[11] observation that in fish evidences of both nerve and glandular properties were demonstrable in the hypothalamic nuclei. This was the first identified indication that specialized cells of the nervous system secrete physiologically active substances. Changes in the staining qualities of cells in the supraopticohypophyseal system suggest that a substance related to the antidiuretic hormone is produced by cells in the supraoptic nuclei and is transported to the neurohypophysis along the axons of the communicating neural tract.[12,13] Experimental stimulation in the supraoptic region causing antidiuresis[17] is interpreted as indicating that there is a release of antidiuretic hormone stored in the neurohypophysis through the medium of stimuli traversing this supraopticohypophyseal tract. The site of production of the antidiuretic hormone, whether in the neurohypophysis or in specialized cells in the supraoptic nuclei, is unsettled, but evidence is accumulating in favor of the latter.

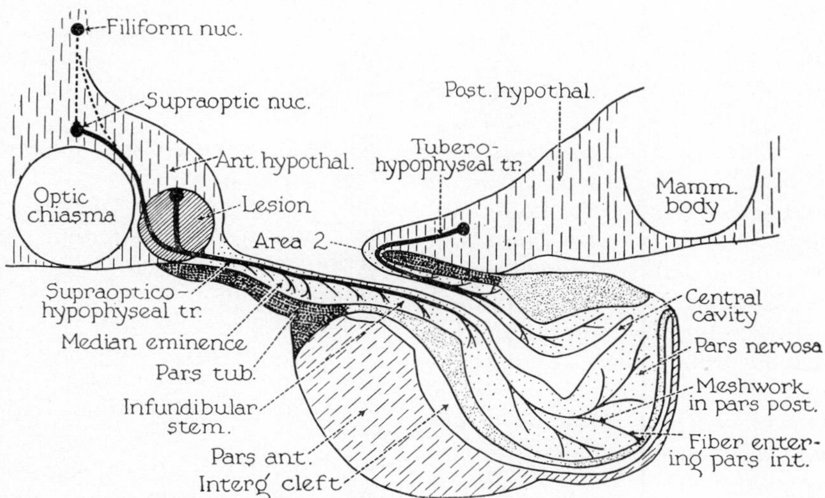

FIG. 2. Diagram of a midsagittal section through the hypothalamus and hypophysis of the cat, showing the two divisions of the hypothalamicohypophyseal tract, the supraopticohypophyseal and the tuberohypophyseal tracts. The broken lines indicate proposed filiformsupraoptic connections and the tractus paraventricularis-cinereus of Greving. The obliquely striped circle indicates the position of a typical lesion designed to produce diabetes insipidus. (Fisher, Ingram and Ranson, "Diabetes Insipidus," Edwards Bros., 1938.)

Polyuria and Polydipsia of Diabetes Insipidus. Fisher and co-workers[8] concluded that the polyuria of diabetes insipidus is primary and that the polydipsia is secondary to it. It has been observed,[18,19] however, that thirst associated with diabetes insipidus may occur in animal and man out of proportion to the degree of the actual deficit of fluid. Even in the presence of adequate hydration, thirst occurs in the patient with diabetes insipidus and to a degree that is seen normally only in the presence of dehydration. Excessive thirst and the taking of abnormally great quantities of water have been observed to precede the polyuria,[20] and a primary polydipsia was demonstrated in dogs with experimental diabetes insipidus. Also, excessive thirst has been produced by stimulation of the hypothalamus[21] without a preceding diuresis. These observations are not in accord with Fisher's conclusions and they challenge the usually accepted belief that polyuria is primary and that polydipsia is secondary to the great quantities of water lost as urine. It has been suggested that the antidiuretic hormone may influence centers regulating thirst and the sensitivity of osmotic receptor centers in the hypothalamus and that it may regulate the reabsorption of fluid by the distal portions of the renal tubules.

Diabetes insipidus in the absence of the adenohypophysis (anterior pituitary gland) is relatively mild, probably because of secondary atrophic changes in the thyroid and adrenal gland hormones which normally may promote diuresis.[22]

The pattern of diabetes insipidus depends on the degree and site of the lesion which disrupts the integrity of the hypothalamoneurohypophyseal unit or system.

The part played by the thyroid gland in causing and preventing diabetes insipidus is controversial. Keller[23] believes that the presence of the thyroid gland is essential to the production of diabetes insipidus. Fisher and his co-workers refute this with convincing evidence that thyroidectomy decreases the severity of but does not abolish diabetes insipidus.

Diabetes insipidus occurring as a result of disturbances in the areas already referred to is revealed clinically by a reduced ability on the part of the kidneys to retain water; as a result, polyuria ensues. Thyroidectomy abruptly halts the transitory diuresis provoked by destruction of the infundibular process and it depresses somewhat the diuresis following a total neurohypophysectomy.[21]

Factors Regulating the Release of the Antidiuretic Hormone. By exerting its antipolyuric effect, the antidiuretic hormone makes it possible for the body to conserve water and for the kidneys to excrete concentrated urine which is hypertonic to blood.[24] The latter condition is attributable to the influence of the hormone on the reabsorptive activity of the distal portions of the renal tubules.

Rare instances occur in which renal tubules are refractory, on the basis of a congenital disturbance, to antidiuretic hormone.[22,56] Under normal conditions production and release of the antidiuretic hormone are enhanced by stimulating (a) the hypothalamic nuclei by noxious agents and psychic stress[25,26] and by certain drugs, notably nicotine,[27] and (b) osmoreceptors when the osmolarity of the blood is increased by administering hypertonic saline solution intravenously.

Nicotine was used as a hypothalamic stimulant by Dingman et al.[28] in their study of the secretory activity of the neurohypophysis. Evaluation of this function was based on the presence or absence of antidiuresis following the administration of nicotine. Two diabetes insipidus subjects showed no antidiuretic response with nicotine or hypertonic saline administration. This is interpreted as signifying complete loss of neurohypophyseal function. In three other patients there was a significant antidiuresis following nicotine but none after the administration of hypertonic saline solution. These findings were interpreted as indicating the presence of functioning neurosecretory activity in the hypothalamus containing antidiuretic hormone in an amount sufficient to prevent a diuresis, and it was suggested that the absence of antidiuresis following the administration of 3 per cent saline solution was due, in these subjects, to a selective failure of osmoreceptor function. This type of response has been observed by Lewis and Chalmers.[29]

Dingman and his associates[28] indicate that other disease processes specifically involving the osmoreceptors accounted for the failure to produce an antidiuretic effect when hypertonic saline solution, 3 per cent, was given intravenously. Calcified internal carotid arteries (bilateral) with possible involvement of the osmoreceptors, infarct of the adenohypophysis and metastatic carcinoma were identified as probable causes in the three respective cases.

In one instance there was infiltration and destruction of the neurohypophysis and stalk by tumor cells but without involvement of the hypothalamus. These findings suggest that the osmoreceptors are located in the neurohypophysis or in the stalk. These investigators intimate that other hypotheses may explain their findings, that an intact neurohypophysis may be necessary for the transmission of secretory impulses, or that no such structures as osmoreceptors exist and "that hypertonic saline entering the hypophyseal circulation may merely promote the secretion into the blood stream of antidiuretic hormone which has accumulated about blood vessels in the posterior pituitary region."

It is apparent that the function of the osmoreceptors may be abolished by organic disease processes and yet the ability to produce antidiuretic hormones may be preserved. If only the hypertonic saline test is employed, the results would not distinguish nonfunctioning osmoreceptors from a primary neurohypophyseal failure. In the three cases observed,[28] about the same degree of antidiuresis resulted from small doses of Pitressin as from nicotine, indicating that the antidiuretic hormone released as the result of stimulation of the hypothalamic nuclei by nicotine was probably adequate to maintain a satisfactory fluid balance.

Under normal conditions, adjustments in the release or suppression of antidiuretic hormone through the regulatory influence of sensitive osmoreceptors increase or decrease the renal output of water as needed.[30] If water is taken in excess, extracellular solutes are diluted, the osmotic pressure decreases, the release of antidiuretic hormone is suppressed and the excess water is excreted as dilute urine. A deficit in the intake of water has the opposite effect: an increase in the output of antidiuretic hormone occurs and water is conserved. The urine under these circumstances becomes concentrated and its volume is greatly reduced.

The mechanism which regulates the release of the antidiuretic hormone involves osmoreceptors within the hypothalamus which are sensitive to changes in the concentrations in the blood. Minute decreases in the concentration of solutes are reflected in the response of the osmoreceptors, which is that of retarding the release of the antidiuretic hormone. Contrariwise, minute increases in the concentration of solutes cause, also through the medium of the function of the osmoreceptors, an increase in the release of antidiuretic hormone.

This hypothesis, put forth by Verney,[30] provides a logical explanation of the control of water conservation as influenced by the antidiuretic hormone, the release of which is controlled by osmoreceptors, which in turn are sensitive to changes in the solute content of extracellular fluids. In diabetes insipidus this mechanism fails because of insufficient amounts, or complete absence, of antidiuretic hormone.

Substances having an antidiuretic effect, though much less than normal, are known to exist in the plasma or serum even though a complete hypophysectomy has been performed. The hypothalamus is one source of these materials.[31]

Results in assaying the antidiuretic hormone content of the blood have been contradictory. Croxatto et al.[31] found no difference between the antidiuretic hormone content of the serum of patients with diabetes insipidus and that of normal subjects. They also found that the antidiuretic agent of the blood is present in free, dializable and in bound forms, and they assume that in diabetes insipidus there is an imbalance of the mechanism by which the transformation of an inactive prehormone of neurohypophyseal origin into the active antidiuretic hormone is effected.

The antidiuretic hormone is inactivated by the liver and to a lesser degree it is excreted in the urine.[32] In hepatic disease retarded destruction of this hormone may lead to the retention of water.[33]

The effect of changes in the volume of extracellular fluids has been stressed by Smith[34] as a regulating influence on the rate of release of antidiuretic hormone. It has been suggested that the osmoreceptors may be sensitized to varying concentrations of individual electrolytes.[35]

Whether the osmoreceptors are stimulated by changes in the osmotic pressure of the blood, by composition and volume of the extracellular fluid or by psychic and chemical stimuli, or by combinations of these factors, it remains that *the central control of water metabolism is dependent on an intact hypothalamoneurohypophyseal unit.*

Experimental and Clinical Diabetes Insipidus with a "Normal Interphase." The acute onset of diabetes insipidus, caused experimentally by dividing the infundibular stalk and clinically as the result of damage to the hypothalamoneurohypophyseal unit, follows a definite pattern as observed by Fisher et al.[18] and by Mudd and his co-workers.[36] The immediate result is a transient phase during which manifestations of diabetes insipidus appear and persist for four or five days. During this period there is excessive thirst and the passing of large quantities of urine, 10 to 12 liters or more, having a low specific gravity (1.001 to 1.005). Following this initial phase there is a so-called "normal interphase" of several days during which the thirst and polyuria subside and the specific gravity of the urine increases to normal. This transitory phase of normalcy has been attributed to a temporary resumption of the secretion and escape of vasopressin (Pitressin) from cells of the median eminence and the neurohypophysis.[37,38] It is probably due to the release of stored antidiuretic hormone from the neurohypophysis while this portion of the hypothalamoneurohypophyseal system is undergoing degeneration, as suggested by O'Connor.[39] This interphase does not appear if a total hypophysectomy is performed.[40]

This trend of events does not prove that the antidiuretic hormone is secreted by the posterior pituitary gland. It is still possible that the hormone is produced in the hypothalamus and stored in the neurohypophysis. Permanent diabetes insipidus becomes apparent after this transitory interphase. Experimentally and clinically, diuresis is a prominent feature during the initial transient and during the permanent phase of diabetes insipidus, but the diuresis is corrected and prevented during the "normal interphase." Also, the intravenous administration of hypertonic saline, known to increase the amount of antidiuretic hormone in the urine under normal conditions, does not accelerate the depletion of the reservoir of antidiuretic hormone during the interphase.[36] Release of the antidiuretic factor, which accounts for the normal interphase, could not be suppressed by the administration of excessive amounts of water, making it appear that an antidiuretic effect, not sensitive to normal regulatory influences, occurred during this phase. This effect was analagous to that which follows a large depot dose of vasopressin which is not subjected to the mechanisms normally regulating the release of the antidiuretic hormone. These features—the failure to influence the duration of the interphase by administration of hypertonic saline (3 per cent solution) and the failure to suppress a pathologic antidiuretic activity by overhydration—led to the conclusion that "the normal interphase of experimental diabetes insipidus is a period of excessive and pathologic antidiuretic activity which is not affected by factors that regulate antidiuretic activity in normal animals."[38]

An illustrative experiment reported by Mudd and his co-workers[36] reveals the initial transient diuretic phase which followed section of the infundibular stalk at the median eminence without removing any portion of the neurohypophysis. The "normal interphase" with the decreased output of urine with a normal specific gravity is also indicated, as is the permanent phase which was controlled by administering vasopressin (Pitressin). A similar course of events is noted in the case of a boy, aged 17 years, who was subjected to a prefrontal lobectomy for the removal of a craniopharyngioma. In this case, reported by Randall and his co-workers,[10] the initial transient phase developed abruptly a few hours after the operation (Fig. 3). The oral intake of fluid increased to 12,625 cc. and the volume of urine to 11,720 cc. This phase was succeeded on the fourth postoperative day by the "normal interphase," which after two days gave way to the permanent phase of diabetes insipidus. The antipolyuric effect and the influence on the specific gravity of the urine which posterior pituitary powder exerts in this phase are demonstrated. It is believed[10] that this sequence of events was precipitated by injury to the hypothalamus without division of the pituitary stalk.

Disturbances in Water and Electrolyte Balances. Of approximately 125 cc. of fluid normally filtered through the renal glomeruli per minute, only 1 cc. is excreted as urine in contrast to the 7 cc. or more excreted by patients with diabetes insipidus. In diabetes insipidus the flow of plasma through the kidney is actually decreased; there is a slight increase in the glomerular filtration fraction. Nevertheless, the glomerular filtration is not significantly altered. In transit through the proximal portion of renal tubules, 85 to 87 per cent of the water and 97 per cent of the solutes—glucose

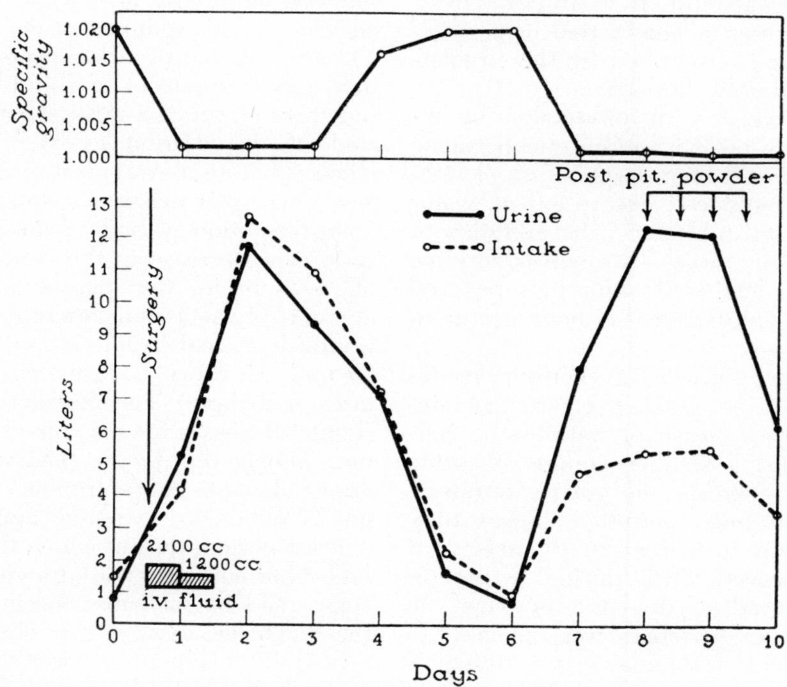

FIG. 3. The initial transitory diuretic phase, the "normal interphase," the onset of permanent diabetes insipidus and its response to antidiuretic hormone following a prefrontal lobectomy are indicated respectively by the changes in the intake of fluid and the volume and specific gravity of the urine. (After Randall et al.[10])

TABLE 1. CONTRASTING VALUES IN ELECTROLYTES, HEMOGLOBIN AND PROTEIN CONTENTS OF THE BLOOD AND IN BODY WEIGHT ASSOCIATED WITH CONTROL AND LACK OF CONTROL OF DIABETES INSIPIDUS*

	NORMAL HYDRATION (Diabetes insipidus under control)	DEHYDRATION (Diabetes insipidus not controlled)	NORMAL HYDRATION (Diabetes insipidus under control)
Cl (mEq./L.)	100.2	106.8	99
HCO_3 (mEq./L.)	30.3	31.7	30.3
Na (mEq./L.)	148	162	148
Hgb (gm. %)	17.6	21	17.5
Protein (gm. %) (total)	6.6	8.0	7.5
Body weight (kg.)	67.6	64.3	57.1

* After Blomhert.[40]

and electrolytes—are reabsorbed into the circulation. This process going on in the proximal portion of the tubules, designed as the *obligatory phase* of reabsorption, is purely passive and accounts for reabsorption of 85 to 87 per cent of filtered water. The second phase of reabsorption, believed to occur in the distal portion of the tubule, accounts for, at most, 13 to 15 per cent of filtered water.[24] This active or *facultative phase* is controlled by the circulating antidiuretic hormone.

Interference with production or effectiveness of the antidiuretic hormone leads, through reabsorption of electrolytes and reduced absorption of water in the distal tubules, to the excretion of a hypotonic urine. Normal hypertonic urine of decreased volume is restored when an antidiuretic hormone is administered.

Nicotine given intravenously[41] or inhaled, as in smoking cigarettes,[42] increases the release of antidiuretic hormone, and a smaller volume of urine having higher specific gravity results.

In a carefully controlled clinical study of diabetes insipidus, by Blomhert,[40] it was observed that, during a preliminary period of dehydration when no antidiuretic hormone was given, (1) the patient was unable to excrete a concentrated urine; (2) that the protein and hemoglobin concentrations of the plasma increased; (3) the concentrations of sodium and chloride in the plasma were increased; and (4) the sodium balance was at first strongly positive but an increase in the output to equal the intake in the presence of excessively high plasma sodium concentrations followed. When normal hydration and the antidiuretic hormone were restored, the body weight promptly increased and appreciable reductions in the concentrations of plasma proteins, chlorides, and sodium ensued (Table 1). The volume of urine decreased remarkably; the output of chloride varied but little (from 61.2 mEq./L. in the period of dehydration to 64.8 mEq./L. when hydration was restored); there was a markedly negative sodium balance —the excretion of sodium increased in spite of a decrease in the concentration of sodium in the plasma; and the amount of potassium excreted in the urine decreased from 71 to between 35 and 41 mEq./L. This positive potassium balance accompanied only a slight decrease in the blood potassium. When the blood potassium was at its lowest concentration, the output of potassium increased appreciably. A third period, during which the antidiuretic hormone was withdrawn, was accompanied by an enormous increase in the intake of water. Other changes observed in this doubly controlled study are included in Table 1.

Changes similar to these, though much less pronounced, observed in a normal subject in negative water balance imply that all of the changes noted are not the result of direct action on the renal tubules but are partially, at least, attributable to the improved hydration established by supplying the lacking hormone.

Dreifus et al.[43] have shown, by making simultaneous determinations of osmotic pressures of the blood and of the urine, that the urines of four patients with uncontrolled diabetes insipidus were hypotonic to the blood; i.e., the ratio of concentration in the urine to that in the blood was less than 1 in uncontrolled diabetes insipidus. Also, there was an increased excretion of sodium, potassium, chloride and total solute when a 2.5 per cent solution of sodium chloride was infused intravenously in the patient with uncontrolled diabetes insipidus. No such increase was observed when vasopressin (Pitressin) was administered simultaneously. It was also shown that the ratio of concentration in the urine to that in the blood exceeded 1 after vasopressin was given.

DIAGNOSIS

General Considerations. Diagnostic studies may be few and readily interpreted, or they may be complex and, though they will clearly indicate the characteristics and the variations of diabetes insipidus, the exact identity of the underlying cause may remain obscure. Newer methods of evaluating these disorders have greatly reduced the number of those which can not be identified with certainty.

Criteria used in evaluating a case of diabetes insipidus are those which establish (1) the diagnosis of diabetes insipidus: (a) a clinical appraisal, (b) the degree of polyuria, (c) the specific gravity of the urine, and (d) special tests—not all of which are necessary in every case—which ascertain the effects of the administration of vasopressin (Pitressin), depriving the patient of water and the administration of hypertonic saline intravenously; and (2) the etiologic diagnosis, which may involve extensive and repeated evaluations before clear definition of the primary disorder is reached. Especially valuable are the neurologic resurveys and comparative studies of the visual fields.

The more common approaches to establishing the etiologic diagnosis, besides the clinical appraisal of the patient, are roentgen ray studies of the cranium and of the sella turcica, and when indicated, an air encephalography and examination of the spinal fluid and its hydrodynamics. Also, a search for evidences of *syphilis, tuberculosis, leukemia, pellagra, sarcoidosis, lymphoma, disease of the upper respiratory tract, acute infectious processes including abscesses of the brain* and *hormonal disturbances* as possible primary causes is warranted.

Diagnosis of Diabetes Insipidus. Several disorders with which polyuria may be associated may be mistaken for diabetes insipidus. A careful clinical appraisal of the patient by means of special tests will, however, detect the true characteristics of diabetes insipidus when they are present.

1. EFFECT OF VASOPRESSIN ON POLYURIA AND SPECIFIC GRAVITY OF URINE. The prompt and complete relief from polyuria, elevation of the specific gravity to or above 1.015 and the clearing of evidences of dehydration following the administration of a therapeutic dose of vasopressin (Pitressin) are significant indications of diabetes insipidus. The recurrence of the manifestations of uncontrolled diabetes insipidus after the effect of the injection of vasopressin is exhausted is positive evidence.

2. DIFFERENTIATING ANTIDIURETIC HORMONE RESPONSE TEST. This test is of special value in differentiating diabetes insipidus of neurohypophyseal origin from the nephrogenic diabetes insipidus of Williams.[44] It is performed while the symptoms are unabated and involves the withdrawal of therapy temporarily from the patient in whose case a precise diagnosis has not been made but treatment has been started.

Technique. (a) Collect the total urine for 2 hours immediately prior to the administration of vasopressin for measurement of the volume and the specific

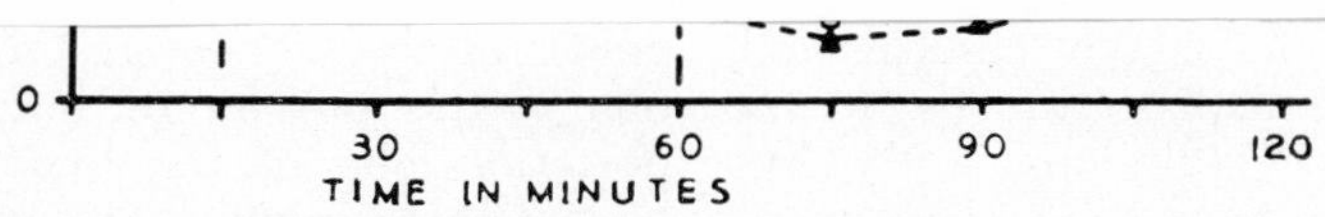

FIG. 4. Results of the hypertonic saline infusion test. The lack of antidiuretic response to hyperosmosis of the plasma in a case of diabetes insipidus is contrasted with the response in a normal subject and one with psychogenic polydipsia. (After Carter and Robbins.[46])

gravity. (b) Vasopressin (U.S.P.), 20 units, is then given subcutaneously and the urine for the succeeding 2 hours is collected.

A great decrease in the volume of urine and an increase in the specific

increase in the specific gravity of the urine occurs, (b) the volume of urine decreases, and (c) there is little or no change in body weight or hematocrit values. In the face of these data, bitter complaints of thirst do not preclude the

instances of selective blocking of osmoreceptor function with the hypothalamic nuclei remaining intact (p. 736). This test, as recommended by Cates and Garrod[47] with minor modifications, involves the administration of 1 to 3 mg. of nicotine base (given as nicotine salicylate) at a time when polyuria is pronounced. The injection should be given slowly. The response in normal and polydipsic subjects is indicated by reduction of the urinary output by approximately 80 per cent. Diabetes insipidus subjects show little or no response to this test. Collection of the urine via an indwelling catheter and recording the volumes at 15 minute intervals just prior to and during the acute observation period make the results more precise.

Etiologic Diagnosis

It has been customary to classify diabetes insipidus of hypothalamoneurohypophyseal origin into the *primary* or *idiopathic* form, in which no organic cause is demonstrable, and the *secondary* form, the cause of which is discernible. This classification is still valid, but cognizance must be taken of the great increase in the percentage of cases that are accounted for on an organic basis and the proportionate decrease in those of the presumably primary or idiopathic type.

Fink[48] reported autopsy evidence in 107 cases of diabetes insipidus that all were secondary to other disease processes of trauma: 63 per cent were due to tumors at the base of the brain or in the posterior cranial fossa; 13 per cent were due to syphilis—a basal meningitis or a gumma in, or near, the hypophysis; 6 per cent were due to tuberculous meningitis; 8 per cent were due to other infectious agents and 10 per cent to trauma.

Zanchi,[49] in collecting 92 cases of diabetes insipidus in which clinical and anatomic studies had been made, found that in 98 per cent lesions in the hypothalamic-hypophyseal system were demonstrated.

There are differences in the features of the primary and the secondary forms of diabetes insipidus. The cases having an hereditary basis are characteristic of the former. In one family of 220 members reported by Weil[50] there were, in five generations, 35 who had diabetes insipidus. Males were more frequently afflicted than females. Blotner[51] and Williams[52] have reported families in which diabetes insipidus had an hereditary basis. The primary, or idiopathic, diabetes insipidus usually appears in infancy and persists throughout life without affecting the patient's general health or longevity. In some cases the disorder appears and disappears, and in others it subsides entirely. It may be associated with congenital, physical and mental defects, among which is the Lawrence-Moon-Biedl syndrome.

Highly selective and primary degenerative changes, of unknown cause, involving the supraopticohypophyseal system in cases of diabetes insipidus, have been observed by Blotner.[52a] There was a marked loss of nerve cells in the supraoptic nuclei and a similar but less extensive decrease in the cells of the paraventricular nuclei. Sections of the neurohypophysis, stained by Gomori's method, revealed no neurosecretory granules.

Injury by a preexisting infection no longer present doubtless accounts for some cases of diabetes insipidus which persist throughout life without affecting the patient's general health.

Diabetes insipidus may be the first clinical evidence of malignant growths elsewhere in the body. For example, metastases from bronchogenic carcinoma may injure the supraopticohypophyseal unit for varying periods and may cause diabetes insipidus before the appearance of any other clinical evidence, subjective or objective, of the primary growth.

In some cases of diabetes insipidus the polydipsia and polyuria, which are readily corrected and the concentrating power of the kidneys restored by injection of the antidiuretic hormone of the posterior lobe of the hypophysis, may be the only symptoms. In another group the polyuria is accompanied by the permanent loss of renal ability to concentrate chlorides, bicarbonate and basic elements, though the normal urine volume is restored by hormonal therapy. In some cases the diuresis is largely overcome, being reduced to 2 liters or thereabouts in 24 hours, but without restoration of the ability of the kidneys to concentrate the urine.

Clinical evidence of the secondary nature of diabetes insipidus is exemplified in the following cases. Frank[53] in 1912 reported an injury in which a bullet lodged in the sella turcica and precipitated diabetes insipidus. The disease has been attributed to developmental abnormalities and it has followed both trauma due to a fracture at the base of the skull and acute infections, notably measles, diphtheria, pertussis, scarlet fever, chicken pox, mumps, erysipelas, influenza, meningitis and encephalitis. It has been seen as a sequel to a post-vaccinal encephalitis and chronic infections, notably syphilis (congenital or acquired), tuberculosis and actinomycosis. Neoplasms, either primary or metastatic, or benign cysts in the base of the brain may be the cause. Warkany and Mitchell[54] recorded as causes of diabetes insipidus different types of tumors occurring at the base of the pons, in the pineal body and in the regions of the sella turcica, optic chiasm, third ventricle, infundibulum and in the interpeduncular region. In short, tumors of the diencephalopituitary region are apt to cause diabetes insipidus. Infiltrations such as occur in syphilis (notably gummata), leukemia, sarcoidosis, lymphoblastoma or lymphadenoma (Hodgkin's disease), and in xanthomatoses, and which are part of the Hand-Schüller-Christian syndrome and involve the hypothalamic area, are known causes of diabetes insipidus.

Xanthomatosis is among the more frequent causes of diabetes insipidus in early childhood. Of 103 cases of xanthomatosis in children reported by Atkinson,[55] symptoms of diabetes insipidus were observed in sixty-one. Pellagra, infarcts of the pituitary gland and subarachnoid hemorrhage have been reported as causes of this disease. The foregoing agents produce diabetes insipidus either by direct destruction of the tissues in the hypothalamohypophyseal area, by pressure exercised directly or by an internal hydrocephalus.

The morbid anatomy seen in non-idiopathic or secondary diabetes insipidus comprises the evidences of trauma, infection, new growths or abnormal infiltrations in the hypothalamic and hypophyseal areas. There is a scarcity of records of studies of anatomic changes in the hypothalamus and in the pituitary gland in cases of idiopathic diabetes insipidus. In both the secondary and idiopathic types of this disease it is common to find enlarged hyperemic kidneys and a dilated bladder with hypertrophied walls. The ureters and the pelves of the kidneys may be dilated.

A "nephrogenic diabetes insipidus" has been described by Williams.[56] This rare disorder closely simulates the diabetes insipidus associated with disorders of the hypothalamoneurohypophyseal system. Presumably, it occurs only in males who are born with the disease, which is transmitted only by females. The specific gravity of the urine is low and is not increased following the administration of vasopressin or by the deprivation of liquids. Neither is the volume of urine reduced by these measures. A congenital defect in the distal portion of the renal tubules, rendering them insensitive to vasopressin (Pitressin), is believed to be the cause of nephrogenic diabetes insipidus.

SYMPTOMATOLOGY

The untreated patient suffers from polyuria and an intense thirst. Five to 15 liters of colorless urine are excreted daily. Amounts up to 43 liters have been recorded (Trousseau). The polyuria may be reduced during febrile disturbances and is less while the patient is at rest than while he is active. An excessive appetite for food is not infrequent. The caloric intake is considerably in excess of that ordinarily estimated as necessary to maintain a constant body weight. It seems likely that this is a compensatory response to neutralize a heat debt incurred by drinking large quantities of water the temperature of which is below that of the body. Fatigue and mental depression, resulting from disturbed rest necessitated by the frequent need for urinating, are common. There is a dryness of the mouth with the formation of thick tenacious mucus in the mouth and pharynx. Dryness of the skin is a manifestation of a general dehydration, and there is an abnormal sensitiveness to cold. The body temperature tends to be subnormal unless some complication intervenes. Obstinate constipation is common. The disorder usually develops abruptly, and it may be transitory or, as is often the case, it may remain stationary without serious impairment of health throughout life with thirst and polyuria the only symptoms. Bed wetting may be the first symptom of the disease in children. The symptoms may be alleviated or intensified during pregnancy. The outcome of the disorder secondary to other processes is dictated by the behavior of the underlying abnormality.

The symptoms may change from those of an apparent functional derangement to those of increased intracranial pressure. This is especially prone to occur in cases of neoplasm in the diencephalo-pituitary area. In some cases the field and acuity of vision are gradually reduced. Edema of the optic disks, ocular palsies (especially of the sixth nerve, with one-sided, bitemporal or homonymous hemianopsia), strabismus with inequality of pupils, tremor and convulsions also develop as a result of tumor growth. Intense frontal headache, nausea, vomiting, dizziness, pains in back and legs, transitory hemiplegias, mental deterioration and infantilism also occur. These are the general symptoms of increased intracranial pressure and localizing signs, depending on the site of the lesion. Precocious sexual development is an unusual complication in these cases, occurring when the tumor involves the pineal body. Loss of weight to the degree of extreme cachexia may occur, though obesity associated with endocrine disorders is not an unusual complication. Edema of the extremities may follow if the disturbances in nutrition are marked. The profound emaciation and exhaustion with disturbed function of the anterior lobe of the hypophysis predispose to impotence, cessation of menses and, rarely, to acromegaly. Dystrophia adiposogenitalis also occurs as a result of involvement of the anterior lobe of the pituitary gland. Intractable diarrhea and a terminal pneumonia with drowsiness progressing to coma and death are not uncommon in cachectic patients with increased intracranial pressure.

Diabetes insipidus is easily recognized as a symptomatic entity, but it may be difficult to ascertain the underlying etiologic process.

PROGNOSIS

Depending upon the cause, the course of diabetes insipidus may be relatively benign. It may cause little, if any, emaciation. Indeed, the patient may experience no ill effect except the thirst and polyuria. In these cases life is not shortened by the disease. The prognosis is not related to the degree of polyuria but rather to the nature of the etiologic abnormality, be it infection, trauma, new growth, abnormal infiltrations or congenital defect. Cachexia is common, and there is predisposition to terminal intercurrent infections.

TREATMENT

The treatment for diabetes insipidus comprises correction of the primary cause, if this is practicable, and substitution therapy with antidiuretic hormone as needed.

Removal of a tumor or tumors which interfere with the functioning of the hypothalamoneurohypophyseal tract may relieve pressure and is desirable when feasible. Irradiation may be helpful when advantages of surgery are denied. Suitable antibiotic therapy, when infection is the cause, may be helpful as in cases of tuberculous, syphilitic and other infections for which specific remedial agents are at hand. The response to one or other of the foregoing measures may

Suggestive Signs of Pathologic Conditions Associated with Diabetes Insipidus (After Warkany and Mitchell)[54]

Symptoms and Signs Which Aid in Differential Diagnosis	Associated Pathologic Conditions	Comment
Familial occurrence	Idiopathic-hereditary form	More frequent in males; general health and development usually normal
Polydactylism, syndactylism, retinitis pigmentosa, obesity, hypogenitalism, retarded mentality	Laurence-Moon-Biedl syndrome or other defect or lesion of diencephalon	
History of abortion or miscarriage	Syphilitic involvement of pituitary gland or diencephalon	
Trauma of head (usually basal skull fracture)	Injury (hemorrhage or scar formation) of pituitary gland or diencephalon	Diabetes insipidus may follow quickly or after interval of several months; in some cases obesity, failure of sexual development, involvement of cranial nerves
Age period	Congenital (hereditary type); early childhood (xanthomatosis); later childhood (tumors, postencephalitic conditions)	
General health	With hereditary type, unaffected; with other types, dependent on underlying condition	
Body temperature	With inflammatory lesions, elevated; with involvement of hypothalamus, elevated or subnormal	
Sexual precocity	Pineal tumor	
Retardation of growth	Tumor of brain; xanthomatosis; postencephalitic lesions of diencephalon	
Generalized lymphadenitis	Leukemia; xanthomatosis; syphilis; lymphogranulomatosis	
Harelip or cleft palate	Developmental defect of diencephalon	
Beefy red tongue	Pellagra	
Gingivitis, loss of teeth	Xanthomatosis	
Necrotic exudate on tonsils	Leukemia	
Roentgenograms of lungs	May show characteristic changes in case of tuberculosis, xanthomatosis, sarcoids, leukemia	
Cardiac enlargement	Chronic nephritis	Absent with idiopathic-hereditary form
Bradycardia	Tumor of brain; hydrocephalus; pellagra	
Hepatosplenomegaly	Xanthomatosis; leukemia; chronic nephritis (from cardiorenal disease)	
Anemia and hemorrhagic manifestations	Leukemia; xanthomatosis	
Roentgenogram of bones	With pineal tumor, advanced epiphysial closure; with Laurence-Moon-Biedl syndrome or other defect or lesion of diencephalon, delayed epiphysial closure; with syphilis or xanthomatosis, characteristic changes	
Pseudo spina ventosa	Schaumann-Besnier-Boeck disease (sarcoids)	Other sarcoids in skin, lungs or bones
Increased intracranial pressure (nausea, vomiting, headache)	Tumor of brain, xanthomatosis, etc.	Nausea, vomiting and headache occur also in cases of water intoxication

SUGGESTIVE SIGNS OF PATHOLOGIC CONDITIONS ASSOCIATED WITH DIABETES INSIPIDUS (*Continued*)

SYMPTOMS AND SIGNS WHICH AID IN DIFFERENTIAL DIAGNOSIS	ASSOCIATED PATHOLOGIC CONDITIONS	COMMENT
Enlargement of head	Tumor of brain, xanthomatosis, etc.	
Mental deficiency	Laurence-Moon-Biedl syndrome; encephalitis and other lesions of brain	Intelligence usually normal with idiopathic-hereditary type, but behavior may be capricious or "neurasthenic"
Exophthalmos	Xanthomatosis; also perhaps with tumors and hydrocephalus	
Loss of vision (atrophy of optic nerves, choked disk)	Tumor of brain, xanthomatosis, etc.	Retinitis pigmentosa with Laurence-Moon-Biedl syndrome
Deafness	Trauma (basal fracture); xanthomatosis	
Cutaneous lesions	With all forms, dry skin and acrocyanosis; with xanthomatosis, bronzing, xanthomas; with pellagra, typically distributed pigmentation, etc.; with leukemia, infiltrative skin lesions and later purpura; with Schaumann-Besnier-Boeck disease, sarcoids	
Basal metabolism	Decreased in many forms	Has been reported as normal with idiopathic-hereditary type
Hypercholesterolemia	Xanthomatosis	Not always present
Roentgenograms of skull	With trauma, fracture; with hydrocephalus, increased convolutional markings, separation of sutures, enlargement of ventricles (encephalograms); with xanthomatosis, typical changes; with tumor, distortion of sella turcica, etc.	

be gratifying, but this is the exception rather than the rule.

Prompt institution of substitution therapy is indicated when the diagnosis of diabetes insipidus is established. Withdrawal of the antidiuretic hormone is subject to the successful correction of the etiologic abnormality and its effect on the production of antidiuretic hormone.

Because of its relative uniformity of action and retarded effect, *Pitressin tannate in oil*, 5 pressor units per cc., is the therapeutic agent of choice. Depot injections given intramuscularly control the manifestations of the disorder for one to five days. The usual dose, 1 cc. of Pitressin tannate in oil, is repeated as often as necessary to control the clinical manifestations of the disorder. A great reduction in the polyuria from 10 liters or more to a normal or nearly normal output with a higher specific gravity and with an attendant alleviation of the thirst and dehydration occurs as a result of this treatment in nearly all patients with this disease. Overdosage does not cause oliguria. Patients receiving this substitution therapy are instructed to take only enough water to satisfy their thirst. Should this counsel be ignored, symptoms of "water intoxication" as described by Snell and Rowntree[57] may be precipitated. Patients with postencephalitic mental changes must be carefully supervised in this respect. Water intoxication should be suspected if otherwise unexplained restlessness, mental confusion, poor muscle coordination, hypothermia, headache, nausea and vomiting are encountered at such times. Convulsions, coma and death may ensue.

A few patients derive no benefit from the pituitary extract; others, although relieved of the thirst and polyuria, become pale and experience nausea, intestinal cramps, diarrhea and cardiac palpitation shortly after the injection. In this event smaller doses may be given at more frequent intervals. Latent anaphylactoid reactions to the pituitary preparations have been reported. Atrophy of the subcutaneous fat at the site of the injection sometimes follows repeated injections in the same area.

Pitressin in aqueous solution, by intranasal spray or by subcutaneous injection, has a prompt controlling effect on the disorder when administered in the amount of 0.5 to 3.0 cc. daily. This effect, lasting ordinarily four to eight but occasionally as long as 48 hours, depends on the amount given and upon the response of the individual patient. This agent may be used for short term observations, but for prolonged therapy Pitressin in oil is substituted for it. Patients who have an unfavorable sensitivity to the oil vehicle may be obliged to rely on the aqueous solution or on nasal insufflations of powdered posterior lobe of the pituitary gland.

If circumstances dictate the use of the aqueous solution and a single daily injection suffices, it is best given in the evening in order to have greatest freedom from symptoms during the night. In this manner one of the most distressing features of the disease, nocturia, is overcome. In the milder cases 0.5 cc. of the aqueous solution, once daily, may suffice, but usually two injections, one in the morning and one in the evening, are needed.

Obstetric pituitrin, as well as surgical pituitrin, has the same effect as Pitressin, but the side effects, particularly abdominal cramps and looseness of the bowels, render them undesirable.

Nasal insufflations of powdered posterior lobe of the pituitary gland, in doses of 40 to 50 mg., alleviate the symptoms of this disease. The powder, now generally available, is snuffed or is blown into the upper portion of the nasal chamber at three- or four-hour intervals during the day and once during the night. The powder may be mixed with a bland nasal jelly and applied to the nasal mucous membrane.

This form of therapy is gaining in popularity and may be recommended because it is effective; it can be conducted without hypodermic injections; the technique of administration is simple, convenient, without danger, and it is relatively inexpensive. Furthermore, no untoward symptoms are produced by it with the exception of the mild stinging sensation when the powder comes in contact with the nasal mucous membrane. Intranasal administration of the hormone is less effective during attacks of coryza.

Preparations from the posterior pituitary gland are ineffective when given orally or by rectum.

Except for the rare case in which spontaneous remission occurs or in those cases in which relief from the manifestations of diabetes insipidus follows successful correction of a precipitating cause, hormone therapy is necessary for the remainder of the patient's life. Alleviation of polyuria with increasing specific gravity of the urine occurs within a few minutes after the administration of Pitressin; excessive thirst subsides more slowly—usually in several hours. Objectively, the indications of dehydration gradually disappear within a matter of hours. The body weight and blood volume increase, and the hematocrit, serum protein, sodium and chloride decrease to normal values.

No response to the antidiuretic hormone occurs in less than 10 per cent of cases of diabetes insipidus. The cause of this refractoriness is not known. A specific defect in the renal tubules rendering them insensitive to functional regulation by the antidiuretic hormone may be responsible. Patients having "nephrogenic diabetes insipidus" are refractory to the antidiuretic action of pitressin.[52]

For infants, sufficient water is allowed to promote a normal weight curve. The quantities of water ingested can be regulated somewhat on the basis of studies of the osmotic pressure of the plasma. Regular determinations of this component and of the different electrolytes in the plasma is recommended by Mathé[58] in a review of the subject of diabetes insipidus.

Benemid has been proposed[59] as a therapy for diabetes insipidus because of a modifying effect which it exerts on the reabsorption of fluid by the renal tubules. Thyroidectomy[60] has been suggested, especially when the Parkinson syndrome is associated with diabetes insipidus.

Irradiation of the hypophyseal area in case of idiopathic diabetes insipidus has been recommended.[61]

Diet. Curtailed salt intake is of little value in most cases, but in some this restriction seems to increase the effectiveness of the hormone therapy. Restriction of protein seems inadvisable as its effect is minor and malnutrition is common in these patients. Diets low in fat are indicated if hypercholesterolemia is present, and if pellagra is suspected, a diet high in caloric and vitamin B content and fortified by large doses of niacin is of value, though no effect on the diabetes insipidus *per se* need be expected.

References

1. Cushing, H.: The Pituitary Body and Its Disorders. Philadelphia, J. B. Lippincott Company, 1912.
2. Biedl, A.: Innere Sekretion. 2nd ed., Berlin, Urban, 1913, Vol. 1.
3. von den Velden, R.: Berlin klin. Wchnschr., *50:*2083, 1913.
4. Farini, A. and Ceccaroni, B.: Gazz. d. osp. Milano, *34:*879, 1913; Clin. med. ital., Milano, *52:*479, 1913.
5. Aschner, B. Referred to by Mathé, G., ref. 58.
6. du Vigneaud, V. et al.: J. Am. Chem. Soc., *75:*4880, 1953.
7. von Hann, F.: Frankfurt. Ztschr. Path., *21:*337, 1918.
8. Fisher, C., Ingram, W. R. and Ranson, S. W.: Diabetes Insipidus and the Neurohormonal Control of Water Balance, Ann Arbor, Edwards Bros., 1938.
9. Dandy, W. E.: J.A.M.A., *114:*312, 1940.
10. Randall, R. U., Clark, E. C. and Dodge, H. W.: Proc. Staff. Meet., Mayo Clin., *32:*109, 1957.
11. Scharrer, E. and Scharrer, B.: Neurosekretion. In Handbuch der Mikroskopischen Anatomic des Menschen. Berlin, Springer, 1954, pp. 953–1066; Recent Prog. Hormone Research, *10:*183, 1954.
12. Bargmann, W. and Scharrer, E.: Am. Scientist, *39:*255, 1951.
13. Drager, G. A.: Proc. Soc. Exper. Biol. & Med., *75:*712, 1950.
14. Pines, I. L.: Ztschr. f. d. ges. Neurol. u. Psychiat., *100:*123, 1925.
15. Greving, R.: Deutsche Ztschr. Nervenh., *89:*179, 1926.
16. Fisher, C.: Proc. Inst. Med. Chicago, *13:*117, 1940.
16a. Lichtwitz, D., Hioco, D. and Delaville, M.: Ann. endocrinol., *16:*819, 1955.
17. Harris, G. W.: Neural Control of the Pituitary Gland. London, Edward Arnold, 1955.
18. Veil, W. H.: Ergebn. d. inn. Med. u. Kinderh., *23:*648, 1923.
19. Bellows, R. T. and Van Wagenen, W. P.: J. Nerv. & Ment. Dis., *88:*417, 1938.
20. Barker, J. P., Adolph, E. F. and Keller, A. D.: Am. J. Physiol., *173:*233, 1953.
21. Greer, M. A.: Proc. Soc. Exper. Biol. & Med., *89:*59, 1955.
22. Williams, R.: Textbook of Endocrinology, 2nd ed., Philadelphia, W. B. Saunders Company, 1955, p. 88.
23. Keller, A. D.: Proc. Soc. Exper. Biol. & Med., *36:*787, 1937.
24. Smith, H. W.: The Kidney: Structure and Function in Health and Disease. New York, Oxford University Press, 1951.
25. Verney, E. B.: Lancet, *2:*739, 1946.
26. Mirsky, I. A., Stein, M. and Paulisch, G.: Endocrinology, *55:*28, 1954.
27. Burn, J. H., Truelove, L. H. and Burn, I.: Brit. M. J., *1:*403, 1945.
28. Dingman, J. F., Benirsche, K. and Thorn, G. W.: Am. J. Med., *23:*226, 1957.
29. Lewis, A. A. G. and Chalmers, T. M.: Clin. Sc., *10:*137, 1951.
30. Verney, E. B.: Proc. Roy. Soc., London, *135:*25, 1947.
31. Croxatto, H. et al.: Metabolism, *3:*32, 1954.
32. Grollman, A. and Woods, B.: Endocrinology, *44:*409, 1949.
33. Ralli, E. P., Robson, J. S., Clark, D. and Hoagland, C. L.: J. Clin. Invest., *24:*316, 1945.
34. Smith, H. W.: Fed. Proc., *11:*701, 1952.
35. Groethuysen, U. S. et al.: Proc. Staff Meet., Mayo Clin., *33:*99, 1957.
36. Mudd, R. H. et al.: Proc. Staff Meet., Mayo Clin., *32:*99, 1957.
37. Heinbecker, P. and White, H. L.: Am. J. Physiol., *133:*582, 1941.
38. Heinbecker, P., White, H. L. and Rolf, D.: Endocrinology, *40:*104, 1947.
39. O'Connor, W. J.: Quart. J. Exper. Physiol., *37:*21, 1950.
40. Blomhert, G.: Acta med. scandinav., *155:*101, 1956.
41. Burn, J. H., Truelove, L. H. and Burn, I.: Brit. M. J., *1:*403, 1945.
42. Walker, J. M.: Quart. J. Med., *18:*51, 1949.

43. Dreifus, L. S., Frank, M. N. and Bellet, S.: New England J. Med., *251:*1091, 1954.
44. Williams, R. H. and Henry, C.: Ann. Int. Med., *27:*84, 1947.
45. Hickey, R. C. and Hare, K.: J. Clin. Invest., *23:*768, 1944.
46. Carter, A. C. and Robbins, J.: J. Clin. Endocrinol., *7:*753, 1947.
47. Cates, J. C. and Garrod, O.: Clin. Sc., *10:*145, 1957.
48. Fink, E. B.: Arch. Path., *6:*102, 1928.
49. Zanchi, M.: Folia endocrinol., *8:*15, 1955.
50. Weil, A.: Arch. f. klin. Med., *93:*180, 1908.
51. Blotner, H.: Am. J. M. Sc., *204:*261, 1942.
52. Williams, R. H.: J. Clin. Invest., *25:*937, 1946.
52a. Blotner, H.: Metabolism, *7* (No. 3): 191 1958.
53. Franke, E.: Berl. klin. Wchnschr., *49:*393, 1912.
54. Warkany, J. and Mitchell, A. G.: Am. J. Dis. Child., *57:*603, 1939.
55. Atkinson, F. R. B.: Brit. J. Child. Dis., *34:*28, 1937.
56. Williams, R. H.: J. Clin. Invest., *25:*937, 1946.
57. Snell, A. M. and Rowntree, L. G.: Endocrinology, *11:*209, 1927.
58. Mathé, G.: Revue du Practicien, *6:*580, 1956.
59. Bachman, H.: Klin. Wchnschr., *32:*783, 1954.
60. Blotner, H. and Cutler, E. C.: J.A.M.A., *116:*2739, 1941.
61. Bernstein, M., Moore, M. T. and Fishbach, D. B.: Arch. Int. Med., *62:*604, 1938.

CHAPTER 14 *By* ABRAHAM CANTAROW

Melituria

NORMAL URINE SUGAR

In the normal person, glucose is excreted by the renal glomeruli but, constituting one of the so-called "threshold bodies," it is practically completely reabsorbed into the blood stream through the tubular epithelium. A very small amount, however, which escapes this conservation process, is eliminated in the urine. The amount of copper-reducing substance or substances in the normal urine varies considerably (0.5 to 1.5 gm. daily), and only a small portion is glucose.[1] Hassan[2] found glucose to be present (osazone test) in 20 to 30 per cent of cases one to two hours after a carbohydrate meal, in 12 to 15 per cent after four to five hours, and in 7 per cent after twelve hours. On the other hand, the output of glucose is less after the ingestion of 50 gm. of pure glucose than following an ordinary mixed meal, and the administration of even as much as 200 gm. of glucose is not followed by glycosuria. After meals of bread, and particularly in concentrated urine specimens, the ordinary reduction tests may yield positive results. According to Sumner,[3] the urine of normal subjects contains reducing substances in concentrations varying from 0.05 to 0.15 per cent in terms of glucose; about 60 per cent of the reduction is due to sugar. Values of 0.25 per cent are to be considered with suspicion and 0.3 per cent as definitely pathologic, especially if the urine is not concentrated.

RENAL THRESHOLD

The concept of a threshold limit of renal "impermeability" to glucose has served as a convenient basis for the classification of various forms of glycosuria. The renal threshold may be defined as that concentration of sugar in the blood which must be reached before an excessive quantity of glucose is eliminated in the urine. This "threshold value" is generally assumed to be about 140 to 160 mg. per 100 cc. of whole blood and 170 mg. per 100 cc. of plasma.

The concept of renal threshold as a barrier or dam is inconsistent with established facts. Glucose passes freely into the glomerular filtrate from the blood, its concentration in the former being approximately the same as in the plasma. Under normal conditions it undergoes practically complete reabsorption in the tubules, probably in the proximal convoluted tubules. A process of phosphorylation appears to be involved in the reabsorptive mechanism. When its concentration in the glomerular filtrate, and in the blood about the tubules, is unusually high, the tubular absorptive mechanism becomes inadequate, and some glucose escapes in the urine. The total quantity of glucose which passes the glomerular filter is of greater significance in determining the occurrence of glycosuria than is the concentration of glucose in the blood. The normal kidney is capable of reabsorbing 300 to 450 mg. of glucose per minute under optimal test conditions; similar values have been obtained in patients with diabetes.[4] When the quantity of glucose that passes through the glomerular filter per minute exceeds these values, its reabsorption in the tubules is incomplete, regardless of the blood sugar level. The concept of a renal threshold for sugar is acceptable clinically if it is applied to this entire phenomenon of filtration and reabsorption, inasmuch as the quantity of glucose entering the tubules per minute is dependent upon the concentration of glucose in the blood plasma under normal conditions of glomerular filtration. From a practical standpoint, therefore, it is satisfactory to assume that tubular reabsorption of glucose becomes incomplete and glycosuria occurs when the blood sugar concentration rises to an excessively high level.

Excretion of glucose in the urine is dependent upon three factors:[5] (a) the concentration of glucose in the arterial blood reaching the glomeruli, (b) the rate at which the glomeruli filter it out of the blood and (c) the rate of reabsorption of the filtered glucose by the tubular epithelium. Inasmuch as the concentration of glucose in the glomerular filtrate is the same as in the blood plasma, the quantity of glucose entering the tubules per minute is represented by the product of the glomerular filtration rate (i.e., the inulin clearance) and the concentration of glucose in the blood plasma. When the former is 125 cc. and the latter 100 mg. per 100 cc., 125 mg. of glucose will enter the tubules per minute. Since, under normal conditions, the tubules can reabsorb up to 250 to 350 mg. per minute, there will be no glycosuria. If the blood sugar is 300 mg. per 100 cc., 375 mg. will enter the tubules per minute, 25 to 125 mg. of which may escape reabsorption and pass into the urine. This is the condition in diabetes mellitus. However, if the glomerular filtration rate is simultaneously reduced to 80 cc. per minute, only 240 mg. of glucose will enter the tubules per minute and glycosuria may not occur despite a blood sugar level of 300 mg. per 100 cc. This might occur in diabetes mellitus complicated by nephrosclerosis or nephritis, unless there was at the same time sufficient tubular damage to diminish tubular reabsorption to the same extent as glomerular filtration.

If these physiologic considerations are borne in mind, the clinical use of the term "renal threshold" for sugar may be of practical value. It must be recognized, however, that the "threshold value" is variable, differing not only among individuals but also in the same individual at different times. In addition to the factors indicated above, the following facts are of importance in this connection:

1. The "permeability" of the kidney for sugar is dependent not only on the level of blood sugar at that moment but also upon the duration of an existing hyperglycemia.

2. Blood and urine (bladder) removed at the same time do not represent simultaneous specimens, for the rate of urine formation varies as does the blood sugar concentration during and prior to the period of urine formation.

3. The concentration of sugar in venous blood may not always be a true index of its concentration in the arterial blood supplying the kidney.

4. The relationship between the level of sugar in the blood and its excretion in the urine varies with both rising and falling blood sugar values. It has been found that following the administration of glucose, its elimination in the urine began when the blood sugar concentration was 150 mg. per 100 cc. and continued until it had dropped to 60 mg. This may be due to the fact that, prior to the excretion of the sugar, the holding capacity of the tissues, including the kidneys, is exceeded, thus producing a local functional strain with the consequence that the glycosuria, once begun, does not stop when the blood sugar has fallen to the threshold value or even lower.

If one admits the practical value of the concept of a renal threshold for glucose, it must be realized that the threshold level possesses a wide individual variation and is capable of extreme variation in normal persons under certain circumstances. Glycosuria has been observed in normal persons with a blood sugar concentration of 60 mg. per 100 cc. and, as in a patient with ether anesthesia reported by Mackay,[6] glycosuria may not occur in the presence of a blood sugar level of over 350 mg. per 100 cc. The renal threshold is believed to be lowered during pregnancy. It is frequently elevated in nephritis and arteriosclerosis, and in patients with diabetes after long periods of insulin therapy. In such cases of diabetes, blood sugar values as high as 425 mg. per 100 cc. have been reported without concomitant glycosuria. With these facts in mind, the statement may be made that glucose is excreted in the urine when the level of blood sugar has risen above the normal "threshold level" for that individual. If the commonly accepted threshold values of 140 to 160 mg. per 100 cc. are considered as normal, persons with glycosuria may be classed in two divisions: (1) with normal renal threshold and excessive hyperglycemia, and (2) with low renal threshold and normal blood sugar (renal glycosuria).

MELITURIA[7*]

The term "melituria" is properly employed to designate the presence, in the urine, of an abnormal amount of sugar. When the sugar is glucose the condition is termed "glycosuria"; when fructose, it is called "fructosuria"; when pentose, "pentosuria"; when lactose or galactose, "lactosuria" and "galactosuria." Since all meliturias are not glycosuria, the identification of the sugar becomes a matter of considerable moment.

Tests for the Detection of Sugars

Metallic Oxide Reduction Tests. The most widely used routine method for the detection of sugar in the urine is one of the copper reduction tests of which the Benedict test is perhaps the most satisfactory. It yields positive results when glucose is present in as low a concentration as 0.1 per cent, and the Benedict reagent is less susceptible to reduction by nonsugar substances than is the Fehling reagent. These substances include uric acid, nucleoprotein, conjugate glycuronates and chloroform, when present in sufficient concentration. Creatinine may, by dissolving cupric oxide, mask slight degrees of reduction caused by small amounts of sugar.

The following sugars are capable of reducing metallic oxides in alkaline solution: glucose, fructose, galactose, pentose, lactose and maltose.

Fermentation Test. The fact that certain sugars are fermentable by yeast has been the basis for the widespread use of the fermentation test in the identification of urinary sugars. The statement is ordinarily made that glucose, fructose and galactose are fermentable by yeast and that maltose and sucrose are fermentable only after hydrolysis by the enzymes maltase and invertase present in the yeast. Lactose is said to be nonfermentable by ordinary bakers' yeast. One possible source of error has been indicated by Neuberg,[8] who demonstrated that yeast possesses the property of splitting off carbon dioxide from the carboxyl group of amino acids normally present in the urine. Another important observation has been made by Castellani and Taylor,[9] who found that ordinary bakers' yeast is not pure and usually consists of one or two species of saccharomyces with a contaminating gram-positive bacillus. They showed that most cultures of so-called "pure-yeast" ferment glucose, fructose, galactose, sucrose, maltose and, in many instances (15 per cent), lactose. Obviously, positive differentiation of urinary sugars on the basis of this test is impossible.

Castellani[10] has elaborated a method of differentiating various sugars on the basis of fermentation by specific fungi and gas production by specific bacteria. For example, glucose alone is fermented by *Monilia balcanica;* glucose and fructose are fermented by *Monilia krusei; B. coli* forms gas with lactose, whereas *B. paratyphosus* does not. The combined use of reduction tests and gas production by specific fungi and bacteria is of great

* This section is taken largely from "Clinical Biochemistry," by Cantarow and Trumper, Fifth Edition. Philadelphia, W. B. Saunders Company, 1955.

value in the positive identification of urinary sugars.

Phenylhydrazine Reaction. This reaction depends upon the formation of a crystalline osazone, the structure of which is typical, to a certain degree, for various sugars. Glucose and fructose form osazone crystals of identical structure. The identification of lactose by this test is not practicable, for the lactosazone crystals, although typical, are formed with difficulty in urine. At times the determination of the melting point of these crystals is utilized as a means of differentiating the sugars, but it is not a procedure of practical clinical value.

Specific Rotation. The degree of rotation of polarized light, determined by means of a polariscope or polarizing saccharimeter, may be employed as an aid in the identification of urinary sugars. This procedure is not frequently resorted to clinically. Furthermore, glucose and lactose cannot be differentiated by this method.

Glucose Oxidase. This enzyme, which is available commercially, catalyzes the oxidation of glucose to gluconic acid and hydrogen peroxide. The latter may be detected by its oxidizing action on certain indicator dyes, e.g., orthotolidine, in the presence of peroxidase. This test is quite specific for glucose,[11] and is therefore particularly useful clinically in rapid identification of a reducing substance in the urine.

Other tests which are of value in the positive identification of urinary sugars will be dealt with in discussing the various types of melituria.

GLYCOSURIA

The term "glycosuria" signifies the excretion in the urine of abnormal amounts of glucose. Glucose may be identified in the urine on the basis of the following tests:

1. Positive reduction test.
2. Fermentation with bakers' yeast.
3. Typical glucosazone crystals with phenylhydrazine.
4. Gas production with *Monilia balcanica*.[10]
5. Specific rotation of polarized light.
6. Oxidation by glucose oxidase.

As has been indicated, the properties of reducing power and fermentation by yeast are shared by many sugars and are therefore not specific for glucose. The following criteria may be established for the positive *identification of glucose:*

1. Typical osazone crystals with phenylhydrazine in the presence of a negative Seliwanoff reaction (resorcinol-hydrochloric acid) to exclude fructose, or
2. Gas production with *Monilia balcanica,* or
3. Specific rotation of polarized light (—52.5°) in the absence of a positive mucic acid test to exclude lactose, or
4. Oxidation by glucose oxidase.

The several forms of glycosuria may be conveniently classified clinically under two headings:

1. Glycosuria unassociated with hyperglycemia, or "nonhyperglycemic glycosuria."
2. Glycosuria associated with hyperglycemia, or "hyperglycemic glycosuria."

Nonhyperglycemic Glycosuria. Glucose may appear in the urine in the presence of a normal concentration of sugar in the blood. This condition may be produced experimentally by the administration of phlorizin. It is observed clinically in so-called "renal glycosuria" (renal diabetes), during pregnancy and, as some believe, in the condition commonly termed "alimentary glycosuria."

PHLORIZIN GLYCOSURIA. The administration of phlorizin is followed by glycosuria associated with a normal and, indeed, in many instances a subnormal blood sugar concentration. There appears to be little doubt that phlorizin glycosuria is in the true sense of the term a renal glycosuria. There is rather convincing experimental evidence that this substance produces its glycosuric effect by inhibiting reabsorption of glucose from the renal tubules, probably by interfering with the process of phosphorylation, which is apparently involved in the reabsorptive mechanism.

RENAL GLYCOSURIA. The frequency of

incidence of this condition, also known as "renal diabetes," "benign" glycosuria and "diabetes innocens," is perhaps not so great as is commonly supposed. When rigid diagnostic criteria are applied, the reported incidence is usually less than 1 per cent of cases of glycosuria, although this condition has been reported as comprising 9 to 26 per cent of all cases of glycosuria in army recruits. The following standards have been set for the diagnosis of true renal glycosuria:[12]

(1) Fasting blood sugar within normal limits and a normal (or supernormal) glucose tolerance curve. (2) Glucose should be present in every specimen of urine, whether voided in the fasting state or after a meal. The quantity of sugar in the urine should be largely independent of the diet, although it may vary somewhat depending on the amount of carbohydrate ingested. (3) Carbohydrate utilization should be normal, as evidenced by determinations of respiratory quotient and serum inorganic phosphorus after glucose ingestion. (4) There should be no disturbance of fat metabolism, ketosis being more likely to develop when the patient fasts than when he overeats. (5) Moderate doses of insulin should have little or no effect on the glycosuria.

The condition is believed by many to be hereditary and familial, and it seems likely that, once developed, it persists throughout the life of the person. The importance of its recognition depends upon its apparent harmlessness; so far as can be determined, it never results in diabetes mellitus nor in any metabolic derangement whatsoever. Practical danger in making the diagnosis of renal glycosuria lies in the confusion of this condition with potential or mild diabetes mellitus. The patient must be watched carefully over a prolonged period before the diagnosis of renal glycosuria can be established definitely.

Inadequacy of the mechanism for tubular reabsorption of glucose is the fundamental defect that determines the occurrence of glycosuria in this condition, as in phlorizin glycosuria. There is presumably congenital deficiency in one of the enzyme systems involved in glucose transport across the renal tubular cells. No metabolic disturbance occurs in subjects with renal glycosuria as long as the carbohydrate intake is adequate to compensate for the amount lost in the urine. Deprivation of carbohydrate may cause hypoglycemia, increased sensitivity to insulin and ketosis more readily than in normal subjects.

GLYCOSURIA OF PREGNANCY. Glycosuria may occur in 15 to 25 per cent of apparently normal pregnant women, particularly in the later months and more frequently in primigravidae than multigravidae. Some reports place the incidence as high as 35 to 60 per cent, but such figures must be accepted with caution. Many have regarded this as a form of renal glycosuria, since the fasting blood sugar is not elevated. However, more extensive use of tolerance tests suggests that decreased glucose tolerance, perhaps physiologic, may form the basis for the glycosuria of normal pregnancy. Great care must always be exercised to exclude the possibility of latent diabetes. It must also be borne in mind that lactose, which gives a positive reduction test, may be present in the urine in late pregnancy and should not be mistaken for glucose.

"ALIMENTARY" GLYCOSURIA. Opinion is divided regarding the metabolic status of this condition. The term is employed to designate the urinary excretion of glucose by certain apparently normal subjects after ingestion of excessive amounts of cane sugar, glucose or, at times, starch. The occurrence of glycosuria under such circumstances must be due either to a "lowering of the renal threshold" for glucose or to absorption of glucose from the intestine at a rate too rapid to allow of its adequate removal from the circulation by the liver, e.g., in hyperthyroidism.

It has been shown that the *normal* person can utilize glucose injected intravenously in amounts up to 0.8 gm. per kg. of body weight per hour; when this rate is exceeded glycosuria occurs.[13] It has also been demonstrated that the absorption of glucose from the intestine proceeds normally at a maximum rate of 1.8 gm. per kg. of body weight per hour, regardless, within wide limits, of the quantity of sugar ingested. Consequently, if the liver removes a minimum of 1 gm. per kg. per hour, allowing 0.8 gm. to pass into the general circulation, glycosuria should not be expected to occur in normal persons. In the absence of any abnormality of hepatic or tissue glycogenic function, alimentary glycosuria might be explained on the basis of increased permeability in the intestinal mucosa for glucose resulting in its absorption at a rate more rapid than can be adequately handled by the liver; it therefore reaches the tissues, including the kidneys, in excessive amount, with the result that a portion is eliminated in the urine. This hypothesis does not necessarily imply the existence of venous hyperglycemia for, tissue utilization being unimpaired, slight grades of arterial hyperglycemia may possibly be corrected and the concentration of glucose in the blood leaving the tissues may be within normal limits. This possibility has been supported by studies of capillary and venous blood sugar tolerance curves in benign glycosuria.[14] Some authorities believe that alimentary glycosuria, in most instances, is in reality renal glycosuria. Others maintain that many such cases are dependent upon some disturbances of intermediary carbohydrate metabolism originating in the liver, endocrine glands or tissues (muscle). No such disturbance can be demonstrated unequivocally in most instances.

The capacity of the normal organism for metabolizing sugar may be influenced by diet. In a person whose habitual carbohydrate intake is low, or who has been subjected to carbohydrate restriction, ingestion of an excessive quantity may result in glycosuria. This is due to an excessive rise in blood sugar concentration (Staub-Traugott effect).

GLYCOSURIA IN NEPHRITIS AND NEPHROSIS. Glycosuria occurs at times in a considerable number of patients with glomerulonephritis, nephrosclerosis and nephrosis.[15] In a great majority of such persons glucose is excreted in the urine in larger quantities than in normal subjects, gross glycosuria occurring in many (30 to 50 per cent in some reported series). In some cases of nephritis and nephrosclerosis this glycosuria is associated with fasting hyperglycemia or diminished glucose tolerance or both. However, in many such cases and in patients with nephrosis, the glycosuria appears to be dependent upon failure of the renal tubules to reabsorb glucose completely from the glomerular filtrate as a result of the degenerative changes in the tubular epithelium. In such cases the urine may contain more than 1 per cent of glucose after a carbohydrate-rich meal. The probable reason for the inconstant occurrence of glycosuria in glomerulonephritis is the fact that the glucose load delivered to the tubules, i.e., the amount filtered through the glomeruli per minute is decreased as a result of glomerular damage and may therefore remain within the resorptive capacity of the damaged tubule cells.

FANCONI SYNDROME.[16,17,18] This condition, originally described in children, is characterized by: rickets, impaired growth, glycosuria, increased urinary excretion of calcium, phosphorus, ammonia and organic acids (including amino acids), a hyperchloremic type of acidosis, and hypophosphatemia. The glycosuria in such cases is unaccompanied by hyperglycemia. These metabolic aberrations are attributed to a common fundamental defect, i.e., an anomaly of the function and, perhaps, structure of the renal tubule, rendering it incapable of reabsorbing certain constituents of the glomerular filtrate in a normal manner. This is, therefore, a type of renal glycosuria, similar to that which occurs occasionally in acquired renal lesions. A perhaps related type of renal glycosuria occurs occasionally in hepatolenticular degeneration (Wilson's disease), which is also characterized by aminoaciduria.

Hyperglycemic Glycosuria. The occurrence of glycosuria in association with hyperglycemia is readily understood. If one accepts the normal "renal threshold" value as 140 to 160 mg. per 100 cc., the elimination of glucose in the urine may be expected in the presence of higher blood sugar levels. The fact must be kept in mind, however, that the renal threshold may exhibit rather wide variations in different individuals and under different conditions. Obviously, the causes of hyperglycemia are potential causes of glycosuria. These include the following: (1) diabetes mellitus, (2) hyperthyroidism, (3) hyperpituitarism (acromegaly, basophilic adenoma), (4) hyperadrenalism (adrenal cortical hyperplasia or tumor; pheochromocytoma; excessive mental strain, emotional excitement, severe exercise, etc.), (5) increased intracranial pressure (brain tumor, cerebral hemorrhage, fractured skull, etc.) (6) arterial hypertension, (7) hepatic disease, (8) ether anesthesia and (9) asphyxia. These conditions are discussed elsewhere (p. 803).

FRUCTOSURIA

Fructose (levulose) reduces metallic oxides in alkaline solution, is fermentable by bakers' yeast and yields an osazone with phenylhydrazine which is morphologically identical with glucosazone. Fructose may be identified in the urine by the following methods:

1. Gas production with *Monilia krusei* but not with *Monilia balcanica* to exclude glucose.

2. Characteristic osazone crystals and positive Seliwanoff (resorcinol-hydrochloric acid) or Borchardt reactions, to exclude glucose. The presence of nitrites or indican in excess interferes with the development of the characteristic yellow color of Borchardt's reaction. Glucose, in large amount (2 per cent) may yield a positive Seliwanoff reaction.

3. Rotation of polarized light to the left in the absence of other levorotatory substances, such as conjugate glycuronates and betahydroxybutyric acid.

Fructose may appear in the urine under the following circumstances:

1. In severe cases of diabetes mellitus, always in association with glucose.

2. Alimentary fructosuria, following the ingestion of large quantities of fructose, particularly in patients with hepatic functional impairment. This has been used as a test of hepatic function, but is unsatisfactory for this purpose. Approximately 10 per cent of normal individuals eliminate fructose in the urine following the ingestion of 100 gm. of fructose.

3. Essential fructosuria, implying the occurrence of fructosuria in the absence of the factors just mentioned, is a rare condition. Silver[19] regards it as a specific, probably inborn error of metabolism, localized primarily in the liver where, he believes, a specific enzyme deficiency exists, resulting in impaired ability to fix fructose as glycogen. The metabolism of other carbohydrates is undisturbed. A few cases have been reported in which there was a total absence of tolerance for fructose, the sugar being eliminated if any whatsoever was ingested. Heeres and Vos[20] state that regardless of the amount ingested, about 14 per cent is eliminated. Insulin has no influence on this condition; no rise in the respiratory quotient follows the administration of fructose to such individuals, indicating failure of utilization of this sugar. It is said that rectal administration produces more severe fructosuria than does oral administration.

PENTOSURIA

Pentoses reduce metallic oxides in alkaline solution and are not fermentable by bakers' yeast. They may be identified in the urine by the following methods:

1. Positive Bial reaction (orcinol-hydrochloric acid).

2. Positive Benedict reaction and negative fermentation test with bakers' yeast in the absence of lactose and nonsugar reducing substances.

3. Characteristic pentosazone crystals with phenylhydrazine.

4. Positive Benedict reaction, gas production with *Bacillus coli communis* and *B. paratyphosus B* (to exclude lactose) and no fermentation with *Monilia tropicalis* (to exclude galactose).

Pentose may appear in the urine under the following circumstances:

1. **Alimentary Pentosuria.** This is a temporary condition, occurring in normal individuals after the ingestion of large quantities of fruits which have a high pentose content (prunes, cherries, grapes, plums). It is of no clinical significance apart from the fact that it may be mistaken for glycosuria because of a positive copper-reduction test. The urinary pentose in this condition is L-arabinose.

2. **Diabetes Mellitus** (some cases).

3. **Essential Pentosuria (Chronic Pentosuria).** This is a relatively rare and extremely interesting condition which is analogous to essential fructosuria. L-Ketoxylose is more or less constantly present in the urine, the quantity excreted bearing no relation to the amount ingested. It is of no known clinical significance, since the utilization of other carbohydrates is unimpaired. It appears to be familial and hereditary in nature, occurring practically exclusively in Jewish subjects, predominantly in males. As in the case of alimentary pentosuria, its chief importance lies in the possibility of mistaking it for glycosuria.

LACTOSURIA

Lactose reduces metallic oxides in alkaline solution (Benedict, Fehling solutions, etc.) and, in about 15 per cent of cases, is fermented by bakers' yeast. It may be identified in the urine by the following methods:

1. Positive Benedict test, gas production with *B. coli communis* and no gas production with *B. paratyphosus B* (to exclude pentose).
2. Positive mucic acid test and negative phloroglucinol reaction (Tollens) to exclude galactose.
3. Characteristic lactosazone crystals with phenylhydrazine. This test is usually unsatisfactory.
4. If positive Benedict test and no fermentation with bakers' yeast, negative Bial test to exclude pentose.

Lactosuria occurs in a considerable proportion of women during the period of lactation. Although this condition has generally been regarded as being confined to the puerperium, recent studies indicate that small amounts of lactose may be found in the urine in about 50 per cent of all pregnant women, the incidence increasing as the pregnancy advances. It appears more frequently in the afternoon, and in primigravidae.

GALACTOSURIA

Galactose reduces metallic oxides in alkaline solution and is fermented by most samples of bakers' yeast, although usually not so actively as are glucose and fructose. It may be identified in the urine by the following methods:

1. Positive mucic acid test to exclude all other reducing substances except lactose, and positive phloroglucinol-hydrochloric acid reaction (Tollens) to exclude lactose.
2. Positive Tollens reaction and no absorption bands upon spectroscopic examination (to exclude pentose and glycuronic acid).

Galactosuria is not frequently observed except following the ingestion of supertolerance doses of galactose. It has been found to occur in nursing infants in association with derangements of gastrointestinal function (from lactose). The excessive excretion of galactose in the urine following ingestion of this sugar has been utilized as indication of hepatic functional impairment. A similar phenomenon occurs in hyperthyroidism, due apparently to acceleration of the rate of absorption of sugar from the intestine.[21]

A condition of "congenital galactosemia" has been described in infants exhibiting the following characteristics: (a) athrepsia, with insatiable hunger; (b) hepatomegaly; (c) lamellar cataract; (d) galactosuria and occasionally (e) mental retardation.[22] It has been found to be due to congenital absence or deficiency in the enzyme, galactose-1-phosphate uridyl transferase, which catalyzes the transformation of galactose-1-phosphate to glucose-1-phosphate. This is an essential step in the normal metabolism of galactose, by which it enters the general pathway of glucose utilization. The enzymatic defect has been demonstrated in the erythrocytes and liver of galactosemic infants.[23] Excessive aminoaciduria may also be present, apparently of renal origin.

There have been reports of rapid improvement in the physical condition and, apparently, prevention of or delayed development of mental deterioration and liver damage when the infant is maintained on a galactose-free diet (i.e., lactose-free).

References

1. Neuwirth, I.: J. Biol. Chem., *51:*11, 1922.
2. Hassan, A.: Biochem. J., *22:*1332, 1928.
3. Sumner, J. B.: J. Biol. Chem., *62:*287, 1924–1925.
4. Goldring, W. et al.: J. Clin. Invest., *19:*739, 1940.
5. Mirsky, T. A. and Nelson, N.: Arch. Int. Med., *71:*827, 1943.
6. Mackay, R. D.: Brit. M. J., *1:*892, 1928.
7. Cantarow, A. and Trumper, M.: Clinical Biochemistry. 5th ed. Philadelphia, W. B. Saunders Company, 1955.
8. Neuberg, C. et al.: Biochem. Ztschr., *31:* 170, 1911; *32:*323, 1911; *37:*60, 68, 76, 1911.
9. Castellani, A. and Taylor, F. E.: J.A.M.A., *78:*651, 1926.
10. Castellani, A.: J. State Med., *39:*621, 1931.
11. Adams, E. C. et al.: Science, *125:*1082, 1957.
12. Marble, A.: Am. J. M. Sc., *183:*811, 1932.
13. Sansum, W. D. and Woodyatt, R. T.: J. Biol. Chem., *30:*155, 1917.
14. Friedenson, M., Rosenbaum, M. K., Thalheimer, E. J. and Peters, J. P.: Arch. Int. Med., *43:*633, 1929.
15. Hawkins, J. A.: J. Clin. Invest., *8:*107, 1929.
16. Fanconi, G.: Jahrb. f. Kinderh., *147:*299, 1936.
17. McCune, D. J. et al.: Am. J. Dis. Child., *65:*81, 1943.
18. Cooke, W. T. et al.: Arch. Int. Med., *80:* 147, 1947.
19. Silver, S. and Reiner, M.: Arch. Int. Med., *54:*412, 1934.
20. Heeres, P. A. and Vos, H.: Arch. Int. Med., *44:*47, 1929.
21. Althausen, T. L.: Am. J. M. Sc., *199:*342, 1940.
22. Goldbloom, A. and Brickman, H. F.: J. Pediat., *28:*674, 1946.
23. Anderson, E. P., Kalckar, H. M. and Isselbacher, K. J.: Science, *125:*113, 1957.

CHAPTER 15

By GARFIELD G. DUNCAN, M.D.

Diabetes Mellitus

Definition. Diabetes mellitus is a chronic disease which, in the uncontrolled state, is manifested by multiple disturbances in the metabolic processes of the body, which are directly attributable to an insufficient supply of insulin. Furthermore, they are controlled by the appropriate administration of insulin or by the reduction of the obese diabetic patient's weight by decreasing the caloric intake. Primary essential (or idiopathic) diabetes, as ordinarily seen, is rarely, if ever, cured. On the other hand, cures are not uncommon in cases of the relatively rare secondary diabetic state caused by excessive steroids, either in therapy or in association with steroid-producing tumors. The greatest apparent disturbance caused by this disease is in the utilization of carbohydrate, though the metabolism of fat and protein and, indeed, the total food and mineral metabolism is affected. An insufficient secretion of insulin by the pancreatic islets of Langerhans, no matter what the cause, will precipitate the clinical syndrome of diabetes mellitus. Diabetes is not, however, as simple as this would make it appear. Primary failure of the *beta* cells of the islets of Langerhans may be the cause of diabetes in those patients who develop the disease on the basis of an hereditary defect and overstimulation of the islets. In others, and much less commonly, the primary fault may be quite remote from the pancreas. Diabetogenic influences of the adenohypophysis, the adrenal cortices and, to an insignificant extent, the thyroid, may be involved singly or in combination, but what relation these glands have in the production of clinical diabetes, as generally seen, is not known. In some instances, it seems that the insulin insufficiency is relative and not absolute and that there may be a normal amount of insulin produced but that its effect is neutralized to a greater or lesser degree by some antagonist.

Practically, whether the insulin inadequacy is relative or absolute, the immediate result is the same. Disturbances in physiologic processes occur in proportion to the degree of insufficiency of insulin; the rate of utilization of sugar and the respiratory quotient decrease; hyperglycemia and glycosuria ensue. Nourishment is thus lost. As the loss of sugar increases, *protein* is drawn upon in an attempt to replace sugar to supply energy and, as a result, a negative nitrogen balance ensues and wasting of muscle becomes prominent. There is an increased output of sugar from the liver. Synthesis of fat from carbohydrate is reduced or even stopped. Also, the catabolism or breaking down of *fat* is speeded up in direct proportion to the reduction of carbohydrate utilization. As the metabolism of fat is accelerated, a point is reached when ketones are produced in quantities beyond the capacity of the tissues to utilize them, and the excretion of ketones in the urine follows.

Unless these processes are favorably influenced by treatment, they tend to progress until the capacity of the kidneys to excrete ketone bodies is reached.

It is at this stage that the retention of ketone bodies in the blood becomes detectable in increasing amounts. Unchecked, these processes, with great latitude in the ranges of progressiveness, will lead to a fatal outcome.

Stetten,[1] in investigating biologic processes by the isotope technique, has shown that under normal conditions a considerable portion of the body fat is broken down and resynthesized daily and that insulin is quantitatively more involved in the synthesis of fat from carbohydrate than it is in the synthesis of glycogen. Indeed, about ten times as much sugar goes into the formation of fat as into the formation of glycogen. In the diabetic, both of these processes—fat and glycogen production—are interfered with to a great degree, and sugar, normally used in fat and glycogen production, is not utilized in normal amounts but accumulates in the blood and is excreted. It is clear why untreated diabetic patients lose weight so rapidly and why they gain so readily when insulin is supplied.

The disturbances in metabolism in diabetes are remarkably accelerated and increased in degree by *acute infections* and *toxemias*. Facilities now at hand have reduced almost to the disappearing point the risks which these complications formerly held. Fifty years ago, Joslin[2] reports, 63.8 per cent of the patients died of diabetic coma, whereas now a death due to this complication is unusual—1.3 per cent of the total deaths in 1950–1955.[3]

Formerly, attention was focused on the changes recorded above and their immediate ramifications. The picture has changed. Diabetes, by lending itself well to control with diet and insulin, has been subdued and life has been remarkably prolonged. As the acute difficulties yielded to therapy and longevity was improved, chronic changes became increasingly evident until now degenerative diseases have replaced acute complications as the most common causes of death in the diabetic population. I refer especially to premature arteriosclerosis and the hazards it presents. Prominent among these is insufficiency of the coronary circulation. Occlusive processes involving one of the coronary arteries have become the most common causes of death of adult diabetic patients. Diabetic retinopathy, intercapillary glomerulosclerosis and the diabetic neuropathies have assumed positions of increasing importance. The great reduction of the mortality from diabetic gangrene does not mean that the underlying cause has been conquered. Peripheral vascular disease continues to be a great hazard and is more prevalent than ever. This is not surprising with the average age at death now being sixty-four instead of forty-four years (1898–1941).[2] Methods of treating the complications which immediately threaten life have improved to such a degree that a false sense of security is understandable, but nothing should detract attention from the underlying menace of arteriosclerosis and from attempts to solve the problems it poses.

The understanding of *uncomplicated diabetes* and the individualized considerations necessary, the early recognition of and treatment for *acute complications* —ketosis, infections, thyrotoxicosis, etc. —and the acceptance of the challenge which the *degenerative diseases* present are essential if maximum benefit is to accrue for these patients.

CLASSIFICATION OF DIABETES

There is no entirely satisfactory classification of diabetes owing to the failure to identify the primary defect or deviation from normal in the type of diabetes (primary or essential) ordinarily encountered. However, as components of the puzzle have fallen into place, a reasonable classification has evolved. Grades of severity of diabetes may alter as the variety of influences to which these patients are subject assert themselves. The diabetes may recede so far into the background that it is not detectable in some obese patients who reduce adequately their caloric intake; others may be neglectful and experience unfavorable progression of the disorder. The diabetes in one patient may be classified differently at different times: for example, the obese patient with primary or essential diabetes may, because of neglect or ignorance, lose weight because of the degree of glycosuria. When he becomes underweight under these influences he has increased his sensitivity to insulin, he has become more prone to ketosis than he formerly was and his diabetes is less stable than it had been. This transition from one phase of the disorder into another does not alter the practicability of the classification (Table 1) if it is used in the light of good clinical judgment.

TABLE 1. CLINICAL CLASSIFICATION OF DIABETES MELLITUS*

I. Primary, or essential, diabetes with an inherited predisposition
  A. Relatively stable
    Onset in adult life
    Overweight is usual (80%+)
    Relatively insensitive to insulin
    Not prone to develop ketosis, in the absence of acute complications
  B. Unstable—juvenile type
    Onset usually in childhood or youth
    Very sensitive to insulin
    Very susceptible to ketosis
II. Secondary diabetes
  A. Endocrinologic causes
    1. Hyperadrenalism
      a. Cortical
        (1) Cushing's syndrome
        (2) Aldosteronism (primary)
        (3) Corticoid therapy
      b. Medullary—Pheochromocytoma
    2. Hyperpituitarism
      a. Acromegaly
      b. Pituitary basophilism
      c. Therapy—adrenicotrophic (ACTH) and growth hormone
    3. Hyperthyroidism (rarely, if ever, a cause of clinical diabetes)
      a. Thyrotoxicosis
      b. Thyroid and tri-iodothyronine therapies
  B. Destruction or excision of pancreatic islet tissue
    1. Hemochromatosis
    2. Pancreatitis
    3. Cystic disease or neoplasm of pancreas
    4. Removal of pancreas
    5. Trauma to pancreas (?)

* After G. G. Duncan, courtesy of New York Academy of Medicine.[4]

Primary, or essential, diabetes, because of its great frequency, our inability, not knowing its cause, to do more than reduce predisposing influences, and its predilection to cause or accentuate the progression of degenerative disorders, presents a major clinical problem.

It is significant that ketosis, the progressive degenerative disorders and an hereditary influence, as occurs characteristically in primary diabetes, are not *characteristic* features of secondary diabetes. Furthermore, secondary diabetes is curable if the cause is identified and if it is practicable to remove it: for example, removal of a corticoid tumor, discontinuance of corticoid therapy, or the removal of a pheochromocytoma.

Two potentially possible causes of diabetes have not been included. First, glucagon, the hyperglycemic factor found in the pancreas, has not been shown to produce diabetes when administered in physiologic amounts. Second, an hepatic origin of diabetes has not been proved. The high incidence of fatty infiltration in the liver in uncontrolled diabetes and particularly in obese subjects makes it likely that the hepatic disorder may be the result, and not the cause, of diabetes.

Of the patients with primary diabetes, those who are overweight and have not received insulin have a *mild diabetes.* This is true irrespective of the degree of hyperglycemia which is present. Restriction of the caloric intake, as illustrated on page 810 shows that the diabetes is readily controlled by reducing the patient's total metabolism through the combined effects of a decreased caloric intake and a reduction in body weight. Insulin, or other hypoglycemic agent, is not necessary or advisable in the treatment of such patients, except during acute complications which aggravate the diabetes temporarily. During such episodes, insulin therapy is not only desirable but is imperative if needless risk is to be avoided.

The juvenile or relatively unstable type of diabetes is characteristic of the young but occurs also in some adults. The *underweight adult* with a fasting hyperglycemia characteristically has a *severe diabetes,* as has the *child diabetic.* These patients are so labeled because to restore good health or, in the case of the child, to maintain normal growth, an increase in body weight, and hence in total metabolism, is necessary, and to accomplish this end insulin therapy is imperative. There is little prospect of these patients being able to discontinue insulin. The amount of insulin a patient can tolerate is not always an accurate measure of the severity of the diabetes. The fat patients with mild diabetes may, and indeed frequently do, tolerate much larger amounts of insulin than their thin brethren. This, in our estimation, is wasted insulin—insulin that is given when the diabetes can be controlled and a good nutritional state can be maintained without it. In fact, insulin given under such circumstances makes reduction in body weight difficult to achieve and by virtue of this influence may expose overweight patients to the natural penalty observed in the longevity records of the obese. There is no escaping the facts that the fat diabetic would not need insulin nor tolbutamide if the body weight were reduced to normal by restricting the caloric intake and that the underweight adult and the child diabetic, in practically all instances, could not achieve a normal weight without insulin or, in cases of some thin adults, tolbutamide.

Between these two extremes fall other grades of severity of diabetes. All are subject to undulations concomitant with complications, changes in endocrine and physical activities, as well as changes in diet.

HISTORY OF DIABETES

A better understanding of the modern conception of diabetes mellitus may be aided by a historical summary.

Allen,[5] following Cantani, has divided the history of diabetes into four periods as follows:

Ancient Period (to 1675) A.D.). The passing of frequent and large quantities of urine was recorded in the papyrus Ebers, a copy of an Egyptian medical journal already old in the time of Moses (Saundby). Celsus (30 B.C.–50 A.D.) wrote concerning, "polyuria without pain but with emaciation and danger." Aretaeus (30–90 A.D.) described diabetes and gave to it the Ionic Greek name meaning "to run through a siphon." He wrote of its progressiveness and of the fatal prognosis.

A Chinese physician, Tchang Tchong-king (200 A.D.), described diabetes as "the disease of thirst." He observed that a diabetic patient might drink ten liters of liquids per day, with an equal amount excreted as urine. Further Chinese medical writings of about 600 A.D. mention polyphagia, polydipsia and polyuria. Later furunculosis and (in the fifteenth century) tuberculosis were recognized complications of diabetes. The sweetness of the diabetic urine was first mentioned in the Ayur Veda of Susruta (Chunder Rose). It was noted also that ants flocked to the patient's urine. Weakness, emaciation, polyuria and carbuncles were recorded as being associated with diabetes. Avicenna (980–1037 A.D.) gave the first description of diabetic gangrene, and Paracelsus (1493–1541) was the first to evaporate the urine and recover "salt." Lipemia in the diabetic patient was first recorded by Helmont (1578–1644).

Second, or Diagnostic, Period (1675–1796). Willis (died 1675) observed that the urine of the diabetic patient was "wonderfully sweet as if imbued with honey or sugar." Willis became the author of the first carbohydrate or undernutrition "cure." Morton (died 1698) was the first to make clear the hereditary characteristics of diabetes, though they were noted as early as the seventh century. Dobson in 1775 grasped the fact for the first time that the sweetness of the urine was due to sugar.

In 1788 Cawley gave the first description of a fatal case of diabetes with abnormal changes in the pancreas. There were multiple calculi and much destruction of pancreatic tissue. Cullen (1709–1890) added the adjective "mellitus" to the disease in order that it might be distinguished from diabetes insipidus.

Francis Home isolated sugar from the urine and observed that on the addition of yeast the urine lost its sweetness, thus proving the fermentability of the sugar.

Third Period, or Period of Empiric Treatment (1796–1850). This period saw Rollo's (1796) restriction of the diet to animal food and a few green vegetables of low food value, occasionally permitting some milk and a little bread. Drugs were given to decrease the appetite. Rollo (1796) was the first to record the significance of diabetic cataracts.

The odor of decaying apples—doubtless acetone—was noted on the breath of a young diabetic patient by Marshal (1798). Chevreul (1815) found that the sugar present in the urine of diabetic patients was identical with glucose. Prout, according to Naunyn (1820), was the first to advocate restriction of protein in the treatment of diabetes. He also introduced washed bran in the treatment of this disease. Furthermore, he was the first to mention coma as a typical termination of diabetes.

Modern, or Experimental, Period. (1850 to present). At the outset of this period M. Gregor demonstrated a fermentable sugar in the blood of diabetic patients. Trommer reported his qualitative test for sugar in the urine in 1841, and Fehling a quantitative test in 1850. Claude Bernard (1885) founded the theory of sugar formation from glycogen. He discovered glycogen and the glycogenic function of the liver and he postulated that the increased blood sugar concentration was an overproduction of sugar by the liver. Mialhe in 1845 recommended large doses of alkali in the treatment of diabetes. Bouchardat (1806–1886) revived the Rollo treatment but modified it by substituting fat and alcohol for carbohydrate; he individualized his patients' needs, advocated small diets and instituted occasional days of fasting; he devised the practice of cooking vegetables and discarding the water, in this manner reducing the starch content. This practice has been abandoned only since 1922. Bouchardat introduced gluten bread and hence originated the idea of substitutes for bread; he noted the advantage of exercise in the treatment of diabetes and he advocated daily testing of the urine for sugar.

Petters (1857) obtained from the urine of a patient in diabetic coma positive reactions for acetone, but it was Kussmaul in 1874 who gave the first detailed clinical description of diabetic coma. The characteristic breathing of "air hunger" bears his name. Cantani (1837–1893) isolated his diabetic patients and allowed only lean meat and various fats. "Fast days" and exercise were employed and after two months without glycosuria, green vegetables and later a greater variety of foods were resumed. Cantani insisted on complete freedom from glycosuria.

Baumel was the first to set up the hypothesis that all diabetes is pancreatic in origin. Ehrlich called attention to the so-called glycogenic degeneration of the renal tubules in diabetes. Kutz (1845–1895) discovered oxybutyric acid in the urine of diabetic patients and recognized the advantage of exercise for the patients having mild diabetes and the absence of benefit if the diabetes was severe. He tested, individually, the carbohydrate tolerance of each patient.

Langerhans, in 1869, discovered islet-cell formations in the pancreas which bear his name. Von Mering and Minkowski in 1889 discovered diabetes in a dog following pancreatectomy. They established the doctrine of the *internal secretion of the pancreas.* Minkowski also discovered the low CO_2 content of the blood in diabetic coma. Naunyn introduced the term acidosis and recognized clinical renal glycosuria. He believed that diabetes was a uniglandular (pancreatic) disease, and that underlying everything in most cases was the diabetic "anlage" or inherited constitutional predisposition. His treatment consisted of a low carbohydrate and, if necessary, a low protein intake with adequate fat to prevent undernutrition.

A number of carbohydrate "cures" for diabetes were advocated. Among these were Smart's "milk cure," von During's "rice cure," Dujardin-Beaumetz's "potato cure," and von Noorden's "oat cure." Blum in 1911 established the fact that patients who did well on carbohydrate "cures" had essentially mild diabetes. It is now obvious that the benefit secured was from the undernutrition which was invariably associated with the "cures."

The swelling of the beta cells of the islets of Langerhans, formerly designated hydropic degeneration and now recognized as being due to engorgement of these cells with glycogen, was observed by Weichselbaum and Stangle, but it was Opie (1901) who put forward the hypothesis that diabetes is due to alterations in the islets of Langerhans.

Guelpa introduced a treatment of fasting, purging and undernutrition until the patients could tolerate a diet rich in carbohydrate. Patients having mild diabetes could tolerate this treatment, but for those having severe diabetes it was inevitably disastrous. A new era was introduced by Allen (1914), who demonstrated the advantages of undernutrition in the treatment of diabetes. Foster (1915) supported Naunyn's treatment but employed stricter undernutrition with better results. Roulston and Woodyatt used "high fat" diets. Through the influence and example of Joslin the undernutrition treatment advocated by Allen received general adoption. Joslin found that by decreasing the fat content of the diet the patient's health was improved. The undernutrition regimen of Allen was suggested when (1) diabetes apparently disappeared in various forms of cachexia, (2) fasting alleviated the diabetes of depancreatized dogs and (3) Joslin observed that, accompanying the rapid emaciation of tuberculosis, there was in one carefully studied patient a diminution of both glycosuria and acidosis.

Allen investigated diabetic therapy by experiments on partially depancreatized dogs on the premise that diabetes is a disorder of the total metabolism and not of carbohydrate utilization alone and that the maintenance of the entire body mass constituted a load upon the internal secretion of the pancreas. Experimental and clinical proof that the diabetic patient's carbohydrate tolerance was affected by the total caloric value of the diet and that greater benefits could be obtained by restricting the total diet than could be obtained when carbohydrate alone was restricted promptly followed.[6] This new doctrine, which introduced the *Allen era* (1914–1921), was rapidly accepted. These principles are still employed by Allen, Joslin and their pupils in the treatment of diabetes. Because of insulin the extremes of undernutrition, formerly essential, are no longer necessary.

The *Banting era* (1922–1936) was introduced with the discovery of insulin.[7] Enthusiasts for each dietetic regimen found this new remedy of inestimable value in the treatment of diabetic patients and in the management of diabetes during complications. A trend to diets with higher carbohydrate and lower fat contents ensued.

A period of enlightening experimental work which has revolutionized our ideas concerning the cause of diabetes was begun when Houssay and Magenta (1924) found that the removal of the pituitary gland from a dog increased the animal's sensitivity to insulin. In 1929 Houssay and Potick discovered that the insulin hypersensitiveness of the hypophysectomized toad was diminished by treatment with preparations from the *pars glandularis* of the hypophysis. Then Houssay and Biasotti (1930) found that in toads and dogs hypophysectomy diminished the severity of diabetes produced by pancreatectomy. A transitory diabetes was provoked by giving a normal animal an injection of anterior pituitary extract (Houssay, Biasotti and Rietti; Evans, et al.; Bauman and Marini, 1932), and diabetes was made more severe by treatment with anterior pituitary extracts (Houssay and Biasotti; Houssay, 1936). These brilliant observations were brought to a climax in 1937 when Young[8] produced permanent diabetes in dogs by injecting intraperitoneally increasing amounts of crude extract of the anterior lobe of the hypophysis. Long and Lukens (1936) attenuated the diabetes by removing the adrenal cortex from depancreatized cats. Lukens and Dohan (1938), by giving large doses of cortin, aggravated the diabetic state in depancreatized and adrenalectomized dogs.

Clinically, insulin hydrochloride (unmodified), although of great value, had the distinct disadvantage that because of its short period of action, four to eight hours, multiple doses were usually necessary to secure a continuous effect. Hagedorn[9] succeeded in reducing the immediate effect and prolonging the action of insulin by adding protamine and thus began the *Hagedorn era* (1937–1943).

The resulting product, *protamine insulin,* was relatively unstable, but Scott and Fisher,[10] by adding small amounts of zinc, prolonged its activity and made the product more stable. Abel[11] obtained insulin in crystalline form in 1927. Zinc insulin crystals in solution were made commercially available in 1938 following the demonstration of its clinical value by Sahyun and Altschuler. This product is purer than unmodified insulin, contains less protein and is less likely to give rise to allergic reactions. The clinical effect is indistinguishable from that of regular (unmodified) insulin (Marble, Ricketts and Wilder, and Duncan [1939]).

Globin insulin, the first commercial insulin with an intermediate action, was made available in 1942 (Reiner, Searle, and Lang).[12] A modification of protamine zinc insulin, in Hagedorn's laboratory, led to the production of isophane (NPH) insulin[13] (N = neutral, P = protamine, H = Hagedorn), which also has an effect intermediate between that of protamine zinc insulin and regular insulin.

Lukens and Dohan[14] have shown experimentally that insulin therapy in the partially depancreatectomized animal may restore to normal hydropically degenerated islets of Langerhans (the degenerative changes having been brought about by injecting an extract of the anterior hypophysis), provided the treatment was conducted before these changes reached an irreversible state. This work confirms the observations of Allen, and of Copp and Barclay, who produced hydropic degeneration of the islets by functional overstrain of the remnant of pancreas remaining after partial pancreatectomy. Furthermore, Haist, Campbell and Best[15] have found that the production of diabetes by injection of the anterior pituitary extract is prevented if large doses of insulin are given at the same time as the pituitary extract. They also found it impossible to provoke diabetes by injection of the pituitary extract if the animal was on a starvation regimen or a high carbohydrate diet.

The *Charles H. Best era*—a research era—dates from 1944 to the present and was so named to do honor to Dr. Best on account of his pre-eminence in research and notably research in diabetes. Many advances recorded in this book have their foundation in Best's laboratory.

The selective destruction of the *beta* or insulin-producing cells of the islets of Langerhans by the intravenous injection of alloxan (Jacobs, 1937; Dunn, et al., 1943; Bailey and Bailey, 1943; Goldner and Gomori, 1943) presented a new approach to the study of diabetes. Also, the administration of glutathione, a normal component of the body, protects against the diabetogenic effects of alloxan. Alloxan can be derived from uric acid. The development of hyperglycemia and glycosuria following injections of ACTH is reversed by administering glutathione (Conn, 1949).

Hyperglycemia in cats, maintained by intraperitoneal injections of glucose, has been shown to produce diabetes, and it has been demonstrated that control of the diabetes in the early stages reverses the pathologic processes and produces a cure (Dohan and Lukens, 1947).

Tagging nutritional components of a diet with radioactive labels and observing their behavior and fate is affording a means of making an infinitely more profound chemical analysis of disturbed values in diabetics than has been possible heretofore (Stetten, 1947–1957).[16,17]

Hyperglycemia and glycosuria have been produced in rabbits by intraperitoneal injections of uric acid after reducing blood glutathione concentrations to a low level by means of a diet deficient in cystine and methionine (Lazarow, 1946, and Griffiths, 1948). The two principles of this process—glutathione and uric acid—are normal constituents of the human body.

Hormonal imbalance and its management in pregnant diabetic patients (Smith, Smith and Hurwitz, 1944; White, 1948) and the importance of hypopotassemia immediately following therapy for diabetic coma (Guest, 1942; Holler, 1946; Nadler et al., 1948) are among the significant advances in reducing the mortality rate from these complications. The elaboration of the value of electrocardiography in detecting hypopotassemia during therapy for diabetic coma by Bellet et al. (1950) also is of great clinical significance. The far-reaching benefits derived from sulfonamide and antibiotic therapies should be included in a listing of historical landmarks dealing with progress for the diabetic patient.

The "lente insulins"—semi-lente, lente and ultra-lente—developed by Hallas-Møller and his associates[18] contain no added protein and yet possess a spectrum of activities—rapid, intermediate and long acting effects (see page 837).

The hypoglycemic effect of certain sulfonamides when taken orally was observed by Janbon and his colleagues[19] and further explored and developed by Loubatieres.[20] Several symposia dealing with two aryl-sulfonyl-urea compounds indicate the interest they have aroused.[21–25] It is not entirely clear how they reduce the blood sugar, but there is evidence that they stimulate the production of endogenous insulin. Other possible modes of action include the inhibition of certain hepatic enzymes in such a manner that the transformation of nonglucose precursors to glucose is inhibited. However, Houssay and his associates[26] have shown that the effect of administered insulin is enhanced in depancreatized eviscerated animals. In some patients, tolbutamide—the sulfonyl urea in common use—replaces insulin therapy for indefinite periods. In others, its effect wears off after a few months.[27] It has been claimed to render labile diabetes less labile on prolonged therapy,[28] and in the exceptional patient the diabetes appears to be made worse.

INCIDENCE OF DIABETES

Total Number of Cases. The incidence of diabetes, though not accurately known, is steadily increasing. There were more than a million known diabetics in the United States in 1951, and newly identified cases are currently amounting to 55,000 annually.[29] On the basis of surveys made by the United States Public Health Service in Oxford, Massachusetts,[30] it was estimated that known and newly detected diabetics total 1.7 per cent (nearly 5000) of the population. If this incidence is applied to the country as a whole, the total diabetics—known and unknown—would reach approximately 2,900,000. Of these, 5 per cent, or 145,000, are children under fifteen years of age. It is estimated that diabetes will ultimately develop in 4 per cent of the women and 2 per cent of the men now living in the United States.[31] Combined, these totals exceed 5,000,000. The increasing incidence of recognized cases is due, in part, to a newly awakened public interest and action arising from the educational activities of the American Diabetes Association and its subsidiary branches, and partly to the broadening scope of regular check-up and insurance examinations. Absolute increases in the incidence of diabetes are attributable to the greater numbers of our population in the older age groups, to the improvement in treatment which permits diabetics a span of life closely approaching that of the normal, and to the increasing number of young diabetics who marry and have children who are more likely to develop diabetes than are children of normal parents. The total number of diabetics has been underestimated. The high incidence of diabetes found in the course of Selective Service examinations indicates a higher frequency of this disease among the younger age group than was formerly considered.[32]

Age and Sex. The National Health Survey (1935–36) revealed that the incidence of diabetes increased steadily until the seventh decade of life in both sexes. There is little difference in the sex incidence in childhood (Fig. 1). This fact has been confirmed by Danowski[33] in an unselected series of 595 juvenile diabetics of whom 309 were males and 286 females. There has been no significant change so far in the twentieth century in the age at onset of the diabetes in any of the decades of life. The peak incidence for the onset of diabetes for both sexes occurs between fifty and seventy years of life, as indicated in Figure 1.

The constantly increasing life expectancy of diabetic patients, on the one hand, with no significant change in the age at onset of the diabetes, on the other hand, is a prominent factor in the increasing incidence of diabetes in the older age groups.

Diabetes occurs more frequently in the female than in the male. Spiegelman and Marks[31] estimated that 2 per cent of the male population and 4 per cent of the female population will become diabetic. In the National Health Survey,[34] 9182 diabetics were encountered and 64.2 per cent of these were female. Women live longer and are less active physically than men and are more prone to become obese between forty and seventy years of age than are the men.

The chances of eventually becoming diabetic, by age and sex, are presented in Table 2.

The incidence of diabetes is higher in married than in single women over forty-five years of age[35] and especially higher in women who have borne children. Married women who have had children weigh more than single women. This increased body weight undoubtedly influences the incidence of diabetes unfavorably. The security enjoyed by the average married woman over forty-five years of age influences the likelihood of gaining in body weight and hence a greater likelihood of devel-

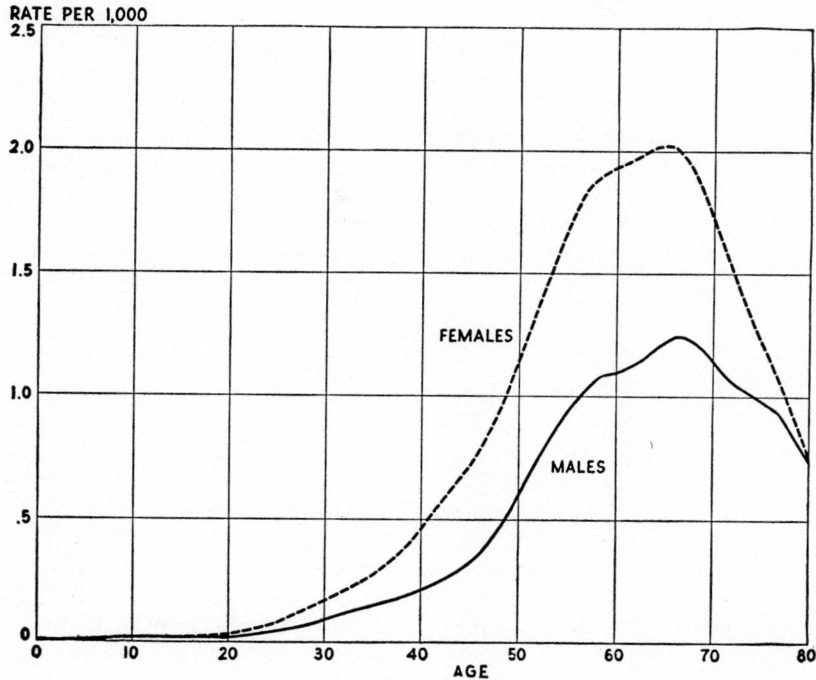

FIG. 1. The respective ages at onset of diabetes per 1000 males and females in the United States.[34]

TABLE 2. CHANCES PER 1000 OF EVENTUALLY BECOMING DIABETIC, BY SEX AND AGE, UNITED STATES (MARKS)[29]

AGE	MALES	FEMALES
Under 15	22.1	41.5
15–19	22.4	42.0
20–24	22.6	42.3
25–29	22.8	42.6
30–34	22.8	42.6
35–39	22.7	42.2
40–44	22.4	41.3
45–49	21.9	39.4
50–54	20.7	36.2
55–59	18.1	30.7
60–64	14.8	23.8
65–69	11.3	16.6
70–74	7.7	10.0
75–79	4.6	5.2
80–84	2.0	2.0
85–89	0.4	0.4

oping diabetes. There is an increasing incidence of diabetes in women over forty-five years of age out of all proportion to that observed in the male population (Fig. 1). The increase in the mortality rate of this group over male diabetics of the same age is striking (Fig. 3).

Occupation. Diabetes is more prevalent in urban than in rural communities. This is true also of the mortality from diabetes, which is between 60 and 70 per cent higher in urban areas. The disease occurs more frequently among the employing and professional groups and among those engaged in selling and serving food and drinks.

The mortality rates as applied to the various occupations illustrate well the beneficial effects of occupations calling for ample physical activity and at the same time highlight the hazards of ownership and other occupations in which there is relatively little need for much physical activity. Hired help on farms do more physical work than the farm owner and are less likely to develop diabetes than their employers. Mechanization of labor will tend to increase rather than decrease the incidence of this disease and the complications which arise as a result of it.

Race. Members of the Jewish race, particularly women, and especially those over forty years of age, are more prone to develop diabetes than the population as a whole. Jews comprise approximately 3.5 per cent of the population of the United States and yet among 5000 new diabetic patients Joslin found 810, or 16.2 per cent, to be Jews. It is conservatively estimated that diabetes is one and one-half times as common among the older Jews as it is in the average population.

Probably the most important cause is the in-breeding of this race, with occupation and obesity as precipitating rather than essential causes. The effects of occupation, prosperity and well-being in predisposing to diabetes are exemplified in the higher incidence of diabetes in the Irish in the United States than occurs in the same race living in Ireland. Diabetes is common among the Teutonic races and uncommon among the Slavs and Latins. The Negro race was formerly, and erroneously, believed to be relatively free from diabetes. With the improvement of social standing and prosperity with larger numbers of Negroes doing less physical work, obesity and diabetes have increased with greater frequency in the colored than in the white race. Approximately 35 per cent of the patients attending the Out-Patient Diabetic Clinic at the Pennsylvania Hospital are of the Negro race.

Diabetes is relatively infrequent among the Chinese and Japanese and severe forms of the disease are unusual in these races.

Diabetes rates at best are inaccurate. In some countries the incidence is calculated most reliably by using the mortality rates. The lack of uniformity in recording the causes (actual and contributory) of death makes most figures speculative.

Mortality. Lack of uniformity in reporting causes of death detracts from the value of these vital statistics. Often, the diabetes has not been recorded on the death certificate if the patient also had cancer. Mortality rates from 1949, when the Sixth Revision of the International List came into use, through 1955 are comparable and show a moderate decline in the death rate attributable to diabetes from 16.9 in 1949 to 15.5 per 100,000 in 1955 (Table 3). Because of the method of recording, the level of mortality (crude death rates) ascribed to diabetes since 1949 is sharply reduced below that prior to the adoption of the Sixth Revision—26.4 per 100,000 for 1944, 26.6 for 1945, 24.8 for 1946, 26.2 for 1947 and 26.4 for 1948, as compared with 16.9 for 1949, 16.2 for 1950, 16.3 for 1951, 16.4 for 1952, 16.3 for 1953, 15.4 for 1954, and 15.5 for 1955.

TABLE 3. TOTAL DEATHS AND CRUDE DEATH RATES PER 100,000 DIABETICS

	TOTAL DEATHS FROM DIABETES	CRUDE DEATH RATES
1949	25,089	16.9
1950	24,419	16.2
1951	25,047	16.3
1952	25,474	16.4
1953	25,796	16.3
1954	24,820	15.4
1955	25,488*	15.5*

* Provisional figures based on a 10 per cent sample (United States). (Current Mortality Analysis of the National Office of Vital Statistics of the U. S. Public Health Service.)

The estimated death rates from diabetes by age in the United States in 1954 and 1953 (Table 4) indicate that the highest mortality is in the higher age groups and the lowest rate is in children. Diabetes is the eighth of the major causes of death in the United States (Table 5). It accounted for 2

TABLE 4. ESTIMATED DEATHS AND DEATH RATES FROM DIABETES BY AGE
United States, 1954 and 1953
(Based upon the returns from a 10 per cent sample of death certificates)

	DEATH RATES PER 100,000*		NUMBER OF DEATHS	
Age groups	1954	1953	1954	1953
All ages	15.4	16.0	24,830	25,390
Under 1	0.8	0.6	30	20
1–14	0.4	0.5	190	220
15–24	1.3	1.4	270	300
25–34	2.2	2.5	520	610
35–44	4.2	4.4	940	980
45–54	11.0	12.1	2,040	2,200
55–64	38.5	41.9	5,510	5,880
65–74	91.5	93.6	8,450	8,540
75–84	152.7	158.8	5,680	5,740
85 & over	154.9	120.5	1,180	880
Not stated			20	20

* Excludes Armed Forces overseas.
Source: Monthly Vital Statistics Reports—Annual Summaries for 1954 and 1953, Part 2. National Office of Vital Statistics of U. S. Public Health Service.

TABLE 5. ESTIMATED DEATH RATES FOR THE TEN LEADING CAUSES OF DEATH: UNITED STATES, 1956

RANK	CAUSE OF DEATH		DEATH RATE	PER CENT OF TOTAL DEATHS
	ALL CAUSES		936.1	100.0
1	Diseases of heart	410–443	361.8	38.7
2	Malignant neoplasms, including neoplasms of lymphatic and hematopoietic tissues	140–205	146.6	15.7
3	Vascular lesions affecting central nervous system	330–334	107.1	11.4
4	Accidents	E800–E962	56.4	6.0
5	Certain diseases of early infancy	760–776	38.7	4.1
6	Influenza and pneumonia, except pneumonia of newborn	480–493	28.3	3.0
7	General arteriosclerosis	450	19.4	2.1
8	Diabetes mellitus	260	15.8	1.7
9	Congenital malformations	750–759	12.7	1.4
10	Cirrhosis of liver	581	10.7	1.1
...	All other causes	Residual	138.6	14.8

Source: Monthly Vital Statistics Report, U. S. Department of Health, Education, and Welfare, U. S. Public Health Service *5* (No. 13): 8, 1957.

per cent of deaths in 1956. The death rates from this cause for 1954 and 1955 were lower than for the preceding five years, and the rate for 1956 was increased to 15.8 from 15.5 in 1955 and 15.4 in 1954.

The total deaths due to diabetes in 1955 were 25,488, of which 9242 and 13,714 were white males and females, respectively, and 840 and 1692 were nonwhite males and females, respectively. The total death rate (per 100,000) was 15.5, of which 12.8 and 18.5 were white males and females, respectively, and 9.7 and 18.6 were nonwhite males and females respectively.

Three fourths of 3543 deaths at the New England Deaconess Hospital in Boston were attributable to cardiovascular and renal complications of the diabetes (Table 6). These and the relative frequencies of other causes of death are shown in Figure 2. In 188 consecutive deaths of diabetic public ward patients at the Pennsylvania Hospital prior to July 1957, the causes of death were as follows: coronary occlusion 41, cerebrovascular accidents 38, arteriosclerotic or hypertensive cardiovascular disease 19, cancer 13, uremia 7, diabetic coma 7, pulmonary embolus 6, cirrhosis of the liver 4, staphylococcal septicemia 3, mesenteric thrombosis 2, pulmonary tuberculosis 1, and miscellaneous causes 47.

The mortality rate of diabetic patients increases steadily until the eighth decade of life. The older age groups have absorbed the increased mortality rates. This result naturally follows the reduced rates in groups under fifty years of age, the aging of the population—diabetic and general—and the more frequent diagnosis of diabetes in elderly persons.

Sex exerts influences on the mortality rates as well as on the incidence of diabetes. In persons over thirty-four years of age, the death rate in females exceeds increasingly that of males (Fig. 3), until in the later decades it exceeds twice that recorded for the males. This is, in more or less degree, the experience of other countries as well as in the United States and Canada.

TABLE 6. THE CAUSES OF DEATH OF DIABETIC PATIENTS, 1950–1955*
(Experience of the Joslin Clinic, Boston, Mass.)

CAUSE OF DEATH	NUMBER OF DEATHS	PER CENT OF ALL CAUSES
All causes	3,543	100.0
Diabetic coma (primary)	47	1.3
Cardio-renal vascular	2,690	75.9
Arteriosclerotic	2,666	75.2
Cardiac	1,714	48.4
Coronary and angina	1,176	33.2
Renal, total	350	9.9
Diabetic nephropathy	211	6.0
Typical or unqualified	189	5.3
Probable	22	0.6
Cerebral	470	13.3
Gangrene	66	1.9
Site unassigned	66	1.9
Other circulatory and rheumatic heart disease	24	0.7
Infections, total	193	5.4
Pneumonia and respiratory	122	3.4
Gall bladder	10	0.3
Appendicitis	4	0.1
Kidney, acute	16	0.5
Abscesses	6	0.2
Other infections	35	1.0
Cancer	367	10.4
Tuberculosis	28	0.8
Diabetes—(i.e., unknown)	22	0.6
Accidents	75	2.1
Suicides	16	0.5
Insulin reactions	7	0.2
Other diseases	98	2.8

* Deaths reported through Dec. 1, 1955.

Diabetes in overweight patients shows relatively the greatest excess mortality among the major causes of death—approximately 4 times the expected rate.[36]

ETIOLOGY

Introduction. The exact cause of clinical diabetes appearing spontaneously is unknown. The circumstances which sur-

union developing diabetes are less than 50 per cent if the nondiabetic parent, who may or may not be a carrier, has a diabetic brother or sister. If the nondiabetic parent has a distant relative with diabetes it is unlikely, but possible, that the children will develop diabetes. (3) If neither parent has diabetes but each had a parent who had diabetes the chances are 1 in 4 for the development of diabetes in their children; if a child of carrier parents develops diabetes the chances are 1 in 4 that the brothers and sisters will develop diabetes also; if a diabetic or diabetic carrier marries a nondiabetic from a nondiabetic family none of the immediate offspring will develop diabetes. The "breeding out" of diabetes falls within the realm of possiblity. To achieve this a consistent union of descendants of diabetic patients with those of nondiabetic families for several generations would be essential.

Granted an hereditary basis for diabetes exists, the onset of the disease is modified by body weight, age, pregnancy, endocrine disturbances, occupation, infections and, possibly, by race.

Obesity. It is known as a result of Allen's observations, which have been amply confirmed, that diabetes is ameliorated when the body weight is reduced by decreasing the caloric intake. Also, the need for insulin increases remarkably with increasing body weight. The *obese diabetic is relatively resistant to insulin.* Nevertheless, the obese diabetics, excepting those who have become obese by virtue of insulin plus a diet high in calories, have mild diabetes. Yet, if insulin is administered to such patients relatively large amounts may be necessary to make much impression on the hyperglycemia. Hence, judging from the amount of insulin needed to control the diabetes, one might erroneously assume that the diabetes is severe. This is not so. An obese diabetic may be given insulin in excess of 100 units daily to correct a moderate hyperglycemia, and yet when this large dosage of insulin is suddenly and completely withdrawn no acute manifestations result and, indeed, the blood sugar concentrations increase but little. This is in contrast to the underweight diabetic patient who may be taking less than one half this amount of insulin daily and who is sensitive to insulin, the sudden withdrawal of which would expose him to the risk of prompt and serious consequences. From these clinical observations it is logical to conclude that pre-diabetic obese persons maintain a normal blood sugar and delay or prevent the onset of diabetes by producing enormous amounts of endogenous insulin and that this increased demand leads eventually to an exhaustion of the islet cells and the onset of clinical diabetes in persons also predisposed by heredity to this disease. It appears unlikely that the explanation for these changes at this stage is to be found in a hormonal imbalance, although the initial onset of the metabolic abnormality may be so related. Alterations in the total metabolism by a combination of reducing weight and a low caloric intake on one hand and an increasing total body mass and increasing weight on the other, offer a working clinical hypothesis which is merely a continued application of the principles laid down by Allen and which are applicable to the majority of adult diabetic patients when first seen by a physician for treatment.

Approximately 80 per cent of diabetic patients are, or give a history of having been, overweight, and yet in the reception room of a physician specializing in the treatment for diabetes there is no such predominance of the obese. Many have lost weight, prior to seeking help, from the progressiveness of the diabetes. This results from loss of sugar and, at times, ketone bodies with no concomitant reduction in caloric intake. Under these circumstances the insulin-producing islet cells are subjected to a sustained stimulation to produce maximum amounts of insulin and the diabetes becomes intensified in direct proportion to the ensuing islet cell exhaustion.

Race. All comprehensive studies of

the racial incidence of diabetes show a higher frequency of this disease among Jewish males and females. White and Pincus[38] contrast a positive family history of diabetes in 30.3 per cent of Jewish males with 23 per cent in all males, and 29.1 per cent in Jewish females with 26.5 per cent in all females. Inbreeding tends by virtue of the predisposition by heredity to intensify this increased incidence of diabetes among Jews.

Endocrine Factors. Clinically, the coexistence of diabetes with other endocrine disorders is not frequent. However, its occurrence in patients with hyperfunctioning of the anterior pituitary and adrenal glands, as seen in Cushing's syndrome, and experimental studies leave no doubt concerning endocrine antagonisms. Over 25 per cent of acromegalic patients develop diabetes.

THE PANCREAS AND DIABETES. It is in the experimental field that most of our knowledge concerning disturbed harmony between the endocrine glands in diabetes has been gained. Permanent diabetes has been produced (1) by removal of the pancreas (von Mering and Minkowski),[39] (2) by partial pancreatectomy—removing nine tenths of the gland—with subsequent overfeeding (Allen),[40] (3) by the injection of saline extracts of the anterior pituitary gland (Young),[8] (4) by the injection of alloxan,[41] and (5) by intraperitoneal injection of glucose in the cat (Dohan and Lukens).[42] Transient diabetes has been produced by injecting uric acid into glutathione-deficient rabbits.[43]

Allen proved the necessity of removing nine tenths of the pancreas before diabetes could be produced by overfeeding, and his co-workers, Copp and Barclay,[44] found that control of the diabetes prevented progressive degeneration of the islets of Langerhans and that so-called hydropically degenerated cells in the diabetic animal could be rescued by controlling the diabetes with insulin and diet. Lukens and co-workers,[45] who confirmed these observations, believed that it is the hyperglycemia that is responsible for the degenerative changes in the islets. These studies are of great importance to the physician treating diabetes. They provide experimental support to the clinical conclusions of authorities in this field that control of the diabetes is an important force in preventing progression of degenerative changes in diabetic patients.

When Young[8] produced permanent diabetes in dogs by injecting increasing amounts of an extract of the anterior pituitary gland he observed that a reduction in the number of islets resulted. Haist[46] found a great reduction in the insulin content of the pancreas of animals made diabetic by Young's method. Similarly, Scott and Fisher[47] found that the average amount of insulin in the normal human pancreas was 1.7 units per gram in contrast to the average of 0.4 units per gram in the diabetic. A decreased production of insulin by the pancreas of the diabetic could explain the presence of diabetes in some cases. But, in the large number of patients who require much more insulin to control the diabetes than is produced by the normal pancreas, as judged by the insulin need of the depancreatized human, other factors must be at work. There may be profligate waste of insulin in the body in a manner not known. This may be due to neutralization of insulin, blocking of enzymatic processes, destruction or inhibition by insulin antagonists or proteolytic enzymes, any one or any combination of which may conceivably influence the onset of diabetes.

It is surprising that a depancreatized man needs only 20 to 50 units of insulin daily to maintain good control of the diabetes which results. Is this because an anti-insulin mechanism or factor is also removed with the insulin-producing portion of the gland? Although removal of an anti-insulin mechanism is possible, no conclusive proof of this has been presented.

When the pancreas is the only endocrine gland to be affected in causing diabetes, as is the case when a pancreatectomy is performed, a mild diabetes results. When, however, diabetes is precipitated by a primary excess of anterior pituitary or adrenal hormone a more severe form of the disease develops and large amounts of insulin are usually needed to preserve good health. Also, the temporary diabetes resulting from injections of adrenocorticotropic hormone (ACTH) is relatively resistant to insulin.

Following removal of the pancreas from the dog the blood sugar rises above normal, the glycogen stores, particularly those in the liver, become depleted and sugar is lost in the urine in large amounts (Table 7). As the diabetes remains unchecked nitrogen excretion in the urine increases, indicating a sacrifice of protein in an attempt to meet the deficiencies incurred by the reduced metabolism of carbohydrate. The synthesis of fat is reduced drastically and the catabolism of fat is increased. The latter process becomes intensified and eventually to a point at which more acetone bodies are produced in the breakdown of fat than can be oxidized. As a result acetone appears in the urine and, barring relief from treatment, acetone bodies eventually accumulate in the blood, giving rise to ketosis which, in the advanced stages, causes coma and death following a progression of the derangements mentioned above and the dehydration, hemoconcentration, loss of base, and peripheral vascular collapse which are associated with them in the final stages.

TABLE 7. RESULTS OF PANCREATECTOMY

Absence of insulin
Reduced glucose utilization
Increased gluconeogenesis
Decreased glycogenesis
Increased glycogenolysis
Increased protein breakdown with a negative N balance
Increased output of 17-ketosteroids, leading to:
- Hyperglycemia
- Glycosuria
- Polyuria
- Loss of sodium, chlorides, ketones, phosphate, potassium, nitrogen and calcium

Resulting in:
- Ketonuria, increased ketonemia, metabolic acidosis, vomiting, paralytic ileus and air hunger

Culminating in:
- Hemoconcentration
- Anoxia
- Coma
- Shock—and death

THE PITUITARY GLAND AND DIABETES. The anterior pituitary gland exerts a major influence on carbohydrate metabolism. A growth hormone has a diabetogenic potential, as have prolactin or the lactogenic hormone, adrenocorticotropin (ACTH) and to a less degree thyrotropin. One of the uncommon causes of diabetes is an hormonal imbalance associated with basophilic adenomas of the pituitary gland. Houssay[48] (1936) observed that the removal of the pancreas from an animal deprived of its pituitary gland caused a more attenuated diabetes than was the case when a normal dog was subjected to pancreatectomy. Evans and Houssay caused a transitory diabetes in dogs by injecting crude extracts of the anterior pituitary gland. Young[49] by pyramiding the dosage of such extracts, produced, in adult dogs, a permanent diabetes. Destruction of the islets of Langerhans occurred as a result of the administration of pituitary extracts. Haist[50] prevented the development of diabetes in this manner by giving protecting injections of insulin, and diets rich in fat made it difficult to cause diabetes by injecting pituitary preparations. Undernutrition diets served also, but to a lesser degree, in preventing the development of permanent diabetes, and Lukens[51] caused a reversal of the untoward trend when the blood sugar was reduced by phlorizin administration. It would appear from the work of Lukens and his co-workers that the prevention of hyperglycemia protected the islet cells. Temporary diabetes in normal human subjects has followed the injection of preparations of pituitary adrenocorticotropic hormone (ACTH).[53]

The anterior pituitary gland plays an important part in the development of experimental diabetes, and that it is a factor in cases of secondary diabetes in man is certain. The relative importance of disturbed function of the pituitary gland, on one hand, and obesity in per-

TABLE 8. EVIDENCES OF A RELATIONSHIP BETWEEN THE PITUITARY GLAND AND DIABETES

EXPERIMENTAL	CLINICAL
1. Injection of extract of the anterior pituitary gland causes diabetes.	1. Diabetic children were formerly believed to be taller than normal at the onset of their diabetes, but this has been disproved.[52]
2. Amelioration of diabetes and increase in sensitivity to insulin following removal of the pituitary gland.	2. The peak incidence of diabetes in children occurs at puberty, and the secondary sexual characteristics are more advanced at the onset of the diabetes than in normal controls.
3. Reduction of the insulin content of the pancreas following the injection of an extract of the anterior pituitary gland.	3. Diabetes in 25 to 40 per cent of cases of acromegaly.
4. Injection of insulin protects the pancreas from the effect of injections of the extract of the anterior pituitary gland.	4. Pituitary basophilism.
5. Removal of the pituitary gland lowers the blood sugar level 20 to 30 mg. per 100 cc.	5. Compared with the normal increased concentration of the follicle stimulating hormone in the serum and increased excretion of ketosteroids in the urine.

Despite the impressive relationship between experimental diabetes and the pituitary gland *there is no clinical evidence that a similar association exists at the onset of diabetes in the vast throng of middle-aged, overweight diabetic patients.*

sons predisposed to diabetes by heredity, on the other, is not clear. Clinically, the latter outstrips the former, and experimentally the reverse is true (Table 8).

THE ADRENAL GLANDS AND DIABETES. The hormone of the adrenal medulla—epinephrine (Adrenalin)—affects carbohydrate metabolism but is not diabetogenic. When epinephrine is injected subcutaneously an elevation of the blood sugar and even glycosuria occur as a result of a rapid immobilization of sugar from the glycogen stores in the liver. This response is identical with that which follows stimulation of the sympathetic nervous system as occurs in injuries to the head—trauma and certain infections—and shock. The response is rapid, causing an appreciable rise in the blood sugar within a few minutes, but its effect is quite transitory.

Epinephrine does not increase protein breakdown, and its effect on carbohydrate metabolism is apparently limited to its antagonism to insulin through the rapid transformation of glycogen in the liver to glucose. This effect is made use of when a rapid increase in the blood sugar level is desired, such as during hypoglycemic reactions or at times of great emergencies—danger, fear and need for sudden defense. Actually, the spontaneous correction of mild degrees of hypoglycemia is due to increased epinephrine production, and the symptoms associated with mild to moderate hypoglycemic reactions are identical with those which follow the subcutaneous injection of epinephrine. The regulating influence which epinephrine exerts on the blood sugar level gives it a position of some importance in dealing with diabetes, even though it is not diabetogenic. Its hyperglycemic effect is greatest in the well fed, well nourished person who has a big supply of glycogen in the liver. This effect is least when these features are reversed.

The *adrenal cortex* is the effector tissue of the pituitary:adrenocortical axis; viz., adrenocorticotropic hormone → adrenal cortex → 11-oxy-steroids (cortisone). Adrenal cortical activity is involved in the metabolism of protein, of carbohydrate and of fat. Furthermore, the stability of the sodium and potassium electrolyte balance comes under the influence of the adrenal cortex. These features are of importance in diabetes and in its complications. They are summarized as follows: Adrenalectomy obliterates the excessive protein breakdown in the diabetic animal and hence eliminates the excess nitrogen excretion in the urine; it reduces hyperglycemia, glycosuria, and ketonuria in the diabetic animal and causes hypoglycemia after mild degrees of starvation in the nondiabetic because of the interference with the release of glucose from glycogen and protein sources. It causes depletion of carbohydrate stores in muscles, liver and body fluids, and the sensitivity to insulin is increased.

These changes are reversed by the administration of cortisone: protein breakdown is stimulated, the severity of diabetes is increased, the tendency to hypoglycemia is abolished, the sensitivity to insulin is decreased, and the tolerance for glucose is depressed.

The clinical counterparts of decreased adrenal cortical function are seen in patients with Addison's disease and especially in those rare cases of Addison's disease and diabetes. The effects of increased adrenal cortical hormones are illustrated in cases of Cushing's disease.

Experimental studies and the clinical evaluation of cases of disturbed adrenocorticotropic hormone have aided in the understanding of the part played by the adrenal cortex in diabetics and nondiabetics. The adrenal glands influence greatly the availability of glucose and its utilization in the tissues. Both of these features are of importance in clinical diabetes.

THE THYROID GLAND AND DIABETES. Prolonged administration of excessive amounts of thyroid hormone has produced permanent diabetes (metathyroid diabetes) in partially depancreatized or incompletely alloxanized animals *but not in animals with intact pancreases.*[54] Clinically, the thyroid gland affects carbohydrate metabolism in direct proportion to the metabolic rate over which it maintains a most important control. In thyrotoxicosis carbohydrate is absorbed more rapidly than normal—a feature which may lead to faulty interpretation of glucose tolerance curves (see p. 804). Diabetes tends to be intensified by excessive thyroid therapy or thyrotoxicosis and lessened with the development of hypothyroidism. However, the thyroid hormone is not a diabetogenic hormone in the same sense as are the pituitary gland and the adrenocorticosteroids.

Miscellaneous Factors. AGE. The fact that the onset of diabetes is most frequent between the ages of forty-five and sixty-five has been presented as evidence in favor of a pituitary influence at an age when, in women, the concentration of the anterior pituitary hormone in the blood is high. The onset of diabetes at puberty, though with a much lower peak, is considered to be due, in part at least, to the increased production of the same hormone. The onset of diabetes does not occur in direct relation to aging, the frequency of new cases decreasing steadily after the mid sixties.

The tendency to become overweight in the forties and fifties with the resulting increase in total metabolism has a definite bearing on the increased incidence of new cases of diabetes at this age.

INFECTIONS. Infections play little, if any, part in causing diabetes. Most infections, especially pyogenic infections, causing leukocytosis and fever intensify the severity of diabetes while they persist. It is not surprising, therefore, that diabetes, undetected at other times, may be recognized for the first time during the course of such infections. Viral infections and infections which do not cause leukocytosis, notably tuberculosis, have much less effect than pyogenic infections in increasing the severity of the diabetes during the course of the complication. In fact, occasionally the progressive emaciation attending tuberculous infections has been noted to decrease instead of increase the severity of the diabetes. It would appear that the decreasing total metabolism in such cases has a great insulin-sparing effect which more than neutralizes the effect of the infection, and a decreasing insulin need ensues. Infections involving the biliary and pancreatic tracts may conceivably cause secondary islet cell destruction with an ensuing diabetes. The disturbing effects which infections exert on existing diabetes is dealt with in the section on complications.

ARTERIOSCLEROSIS. Arteriosclerosis *per se* is not a cause of diabetes. If it were, the incidence of this disease would not be decreasing during the phase of life in which arteriosclerosis is on the increase.

TRAUMA. Direct and extensive injury to the pancreas could conceivably cause diabetes, although this is extremely unlikely. Injury to other parts of the body will not affect the carbohydrate function except through inactivity, fever, temporary stress reactions and changes in body weight that might result. Injuries to the head causing glucosuria do not cause diabetes.

Summary

Persons most likely to develop diabetes are of diabetic families, are overweight, are between forty-five and sixty-five years of age and lead a sedentary existence.

Heredity is the outstanding predisposing cause of diabetes. It establishes the susceptibility to the disease according to the mendelian pattern, carrying recessive characteristics.

Obesity, from the clinical aspect, is the most important precipitating cause of diabetes, occurring in 75 to 85 per cent of patients whose diabetes first becomes manifest in adult life. Obesity, probably by virtue of the stepped-up turnover of fat and especially of lipogenesis as well as the increased total metabolism producing a starvation effect, tends to make the diabetic patient relatively resistant to insulin. It would appear that these same influences in the pre-diabetic state and in the person made susceptible to diabetes by heredity account for the exhaustion of the inadequate pancreas and the precipitation of clinical diabetes.

SYMPTOMATOLOGY

Symptoms may suggest a diagnosis of diabetes but nothing more. The varied symptomatology in a typical case is indicative of some systemic disorder. General weakness, loss of weight, excessive appetite and thirst, the frequent passing of large quantities of urine without discomfort, rising at night to void, itching of the skin (which in the female occurs particularly about the vulva) and backache are the most common symptoms of uncontrolled and uncomplicated diabetes. Impotence in the male is common.

It has been estimated that as high as 12 per cent of adults with unrecognized and untreated diabetes have no symptoms of the disorder. This observation is based on the finding of glycosuria in applicants for insurance and those undergoing routine health examinations.

General Weakness. The only symptom may be general weakness. This symptom has been the most common complaint of my diabetic patients on the occasion of their first visit. It is common to many debilitating diseases and gives little indication of the nature of the underlying disorder.

Rapid Loss of Body Weight. A rapid loss of body weight in the afebrile patient, especially in the young patient, should suggest the possibility that diabetes may be the cause. This symptom is readily accounted for. Sugar is lost in the urine in amounts varying from mere traces to as much as 15 per cent of sugar. One has but to recall that each gram of sugar lost represents a body deprivation of approximately 4 calories. Sugar in the urine means lost nourishment. It is an odd form of starvation but accounts for the seeming paradox which exists when with increased appetite the food intake greatly exceeds that of the normal and yet loss of weight continues. There is excessive protein breakdown with abnormally large quantities of nitrogen excreted in the urine. Weight loss is due in part to the diuresis resulting from hyperglycemia. Further loss in weight is encountered in the presence of ketosis. In this instance dehydration and loss of nourishment in the form of ketone bodies are additional factors.

Great importance attaches to body weight and its changes in diabetes. A person with untreated and uncontrolled diabetes loses weight on an unrestricted diet. The diabetes at the same time becomes more severe. Loss of weight in this manner is injurious. This is true even in the obese patient because it leaves less weight to be reduced by a method which improves and controls the diabetes. The other method of weight reduction is brought about by reducing the patient's total food intake. This restriction lessens the immediate demand on the islet function of the pancreas and at the same time consolidates this gain, since it reduces the total metabolism by virtue of the reduced body weight which ensues. Risking monotony in repetition concerning one of the most important aspects of clinical diabetes, I will restate: A loss of weight, a decrease in total metabolism by restriction of the total diet, decreases the food loss, gives the pancreas functional rest, and affords the overweight patient with uncontrolled diabetes a remarkable improvement in carbohydrate and total food tolerance. A loss of weight due to the activity of the diabetes, whether due to ignorance or wilful neglect, destroys food tolerance, the diabetes becomes more severe, and the need for insulin increases. A previously obese patient who becomes emaciated because of the activity of the diabetes has lost all of the advantages of a reduction in weight by appropriate treatment, and the necessity of using insulin indefinitely is usually inescapable. I hope this is clear. It is of vital importance. It represents one of the fundamental considerations of diabetes, the understanding of which we owe to Frederick M. Allen.

Excessive Appetite and Thirst. These symptoms are in direct relation to the amount of glycosuria and polyuria until ketosis intervenes. Anorexia then appears. Excessive appetite is a compensatory effort to replace lost nourishment; polydipsia, to replace lost fluids. Thirst and the frequent voiding of large amounts of urine are among the most common symptoms of diabetes occurring in about three-quarters of all cases. It is in this group of patients that backache is common. This symptom can be reproduced in normal persons by the intake of large quantities of water. Distention of the renal capsule by increased activity of the kidneys with greater than usual volumes of fluid passing through them is responsible. Fatigue in the debilitated patient accentuates the backache.

Diabetic patients who are free from symptoms are not immune to complications, nor is the diabetes innocent in such cases. A routine urinalysis for every patient will reward one for the effort put forth. Diabetes will be found by this simple test more often than is supposed. Further, it will be found earlier when the diabetes is mild, when it is easily controlled without exacting treatment, and drug therapy—insulin or tolbutamide—will usually not be needed.

Complications of diabetes often prompt the patient to seek treatment. The discovery of diabetes, the presence of which the patient may be entirely ignorant, is often made on such consultations. Acute infections are the most common causes for hospitalization.

The symptoms of the various complications of diabetes will be dealt with later in this chapter, but for the sake of completeness the more common are recorded here. They are: pain, coldness and gangrene of the extremities, dimness of vision (cataract and retinitis), skin disorders (furuncles, carbuncles, intertrigo, epidermophytosis) and symptoms of diabetic neuropathy. Loss of appetite should make one suspect the development of ketosis, especially if the thirst and polyuria are exaggerated and are accompanied by vomiting, intense fatigue, sleepiness and pain in the abdomen.

PHYSICAL FINDINGS

Many diabetic patients have no physical evidence of the chronic disease from which they suffer. However, the more carefully the examination is made, the more often will the search be rewarded by the discovery of abnormalities which when correlated with the symptoms are found to be more or less characteristic, notably, the appearance of *fatigue,* the *looseness* and *fine wrinkling of the skin* observed in patients who have lost in body weight and *dryness* of the skin in those patients who suffer from excessive thirst and polyuria. A mild degree of *pallor* characterizes the skin of many diabetic patients. This is particularly noticeable in those who are overweight and have advanced disease of the arteries. Vascular disease and not anemia is the cause of the pallor which is especially common in patients suffering from disease of the coronary arteries. In the young patients, particularly females, taking large amounts of insulin, the skin may have a *waxy transparency* with a smoothing out of wrinkles of the face. This has been referred to as an "insulin face." It is noticeable shortly after insulin therapy is begun and is due to water retention in the skin and subcutaneous tissues. This condition tends to disappear when the diabetes is controlled over a period of months.

Other *skin disorders* may occur as a result of the diabetes, namely, *xanthelasma, xanthochromia* and rarely, *xanthoma diabeticorum* and *necrobiosis lipoidica diabetica.*

Though all shades of health from the robust, normal-appearing, diabetic patient to one critically ill with ketosis are observed, it is well to emphasize that most physical abnormalities observed in these patients are due to complications of the diabetes. The untreated diabetic patient is especially susceptible to *staphylococcic infections,* e.g., furuncles, carbuncles and bacteremia. He is unusually prone to develop pulmonary *tuberculosis.* This complication is most common among young patients who have had an attack of diabetic coma. Root and Bloor[55] found that 17.8 per cent of patients admitted in diabetic coma developed active tuberculosis within five years. Observation of a patient presenting himself with any of these disorders may bring to light a coexisting diabetes.

The physical examination frequently reveals *degenerative changes,* especially cataracts, diabetic retinitis and generalized disease of the arteries (particularly the coronary arteries). Coldness of the extremities, cyanosis of feet in the dependent position and gangrene of the toes, heel or foot occur as a result of extensive changes in the arteries. *Irritation of the skin,* either general or about the genitalia as a result of pruritus, is common as are *moniliasis* infections; these infections involve the feet, between the toes most frequently, but may be found elsewhere on the body. The physical signs of diabetic coma are considered in detail later.

PATHOLOGY

Introduction. Few diseases cause more widespread pathologic changes than does diabetes. Most of the characteristic changes are those associated with premature aging; degenerative diseases of the arteries are outstanding. Because of the inconstancy of cellular abnormalities, the occurrence of normal tissues in patients with severe diabetes and the occurrence of the occasional identical changes in the pancreas of the diabetic and of the nondiabetic, diabetes can be diagnosed on morphologic grounds alone in but a small percentage of cases.

The most consistent pathologic changes in diabetes are those of accelerated degenerative processes. These are especially discernible in the circulatory system, the eyes, kidneys and nervous system. Changes in the pancreas are disappointingly inconsistent. Infiltrations of glycogen may be seen in the nuclei of the liver, in the Henle's loops of the kidneys, in myocardial muscle fibers, in the stratum corneum and epithelium of hair follicles and sweat glands in the skin and in the pigmented epithelium of the iris.

Pancreas

Acute Changes. *Acute degenerative changes, notably so-called hydropic degeneration* of the islets of the pancreas, can be produced in experimental diabetes. Normal islets are illustrated in Figure 4, and acute hydropic degeneration of the islets—a reversible state—is depicted in Figure 5. Partial pancreatectomy—nine tenths of the pancreas being removed—followed by overfeeding causes hydropic degeneration and, barring relief by appropriate treatment, exhaustion and death of the islet cells. Also, in producing diabetes by injecting an extract of the anterior pituitary gland this form of degenerative change is noted[49] (see p. 777), and when hyperglycemia is maintained by intraperitoneal injection of glucose, engorgement of the islets with glycogen, formerly recognized as hydropic degeneration of the islets, occurs (see p. 776). Engorgement with glycogen does not occur in alloxan diabetes, in which case there is chemical destruction of the insulin-producing cells—the *beta* cells—in contrast to the overworking, exhaustion and functional death of these cells brought about by overfeeding the partially depancreatized animal and by the administration of an extract of the anterior pituitary gland. On the basis of these changes, observed at will in experimental diabetes, it is highly probable that hydropic degeneration of the islets occurs in nearly all, if not all, diabetic patients at one time or another. The fact that hydropic degeneration, first noted by Weichselbaum (1901), is detected only occasionally on examination of tissue secured at autopsy, or by biopsy, in the human is no evidence that this degenerative change is not an essential feature in the development of clinical diabetes. If one could select the time that would be most propitious for observing hydropic degeneration, it would be in that period shortly after the onset of the clinical manifestations of diabetes and when the intensity of these manifestations were not modified by treatment, or during the progression of a fulminating diabetes. The impracticability of this procedure doubtless deprives us of the positive proof that hydropic degeneration is an indispensable phase in the pancreatic change in diabetic patients. Hydropic degeneration is an acute and transitory process.

Hydropic degeneration is, in some cases, accompanied by attempts at regeneration by the islet cells. Mitotic figures may be seen, particularly at the periphery of the islet clusters. That these new cells may be more readily destroyed than the more mature cells by the functional overstrain that exists is possible, and this phenomenon could explain why they do not save the situation. Furthermore, the stimulus to new cell production may subside with control of diabetes. One might speculate that, if it were possible to stimulate islet cell hyperplasia or regeneration and yet keep the diabetes under control, adequate cells might reach maturity in sufficient numbers to cure the diabetes. There is much experimental evidence that, if there is adequate treatment before irreparable degenerative changes have taken place, hydropically degenerated cells can be redeemed and all manifestations of diabetes can be overcome.

Lymphocytic infiltration of the islets occurs in children with severe diabetes and is considered an acute process. *Acute inflammatory changes* in the pancreas are not characteristic of diabetes, and yet diabetes not infrequently follows repeated attacks of pancreatitis when most of the organ is destroyed.

Chronic Changes. Chronic manifestations of diabetes are detected with greater frequency than are the acute and transient changes. Among the chronic changes there is a *reduced number of islets of Langerhans*—although this is not invariably so—and in keeping with this, significantly less insulin is recovered from the pancreas of the diabetic—0.4 units per gram—than from that of the nondiabetic—1.7 units per gram.[47]

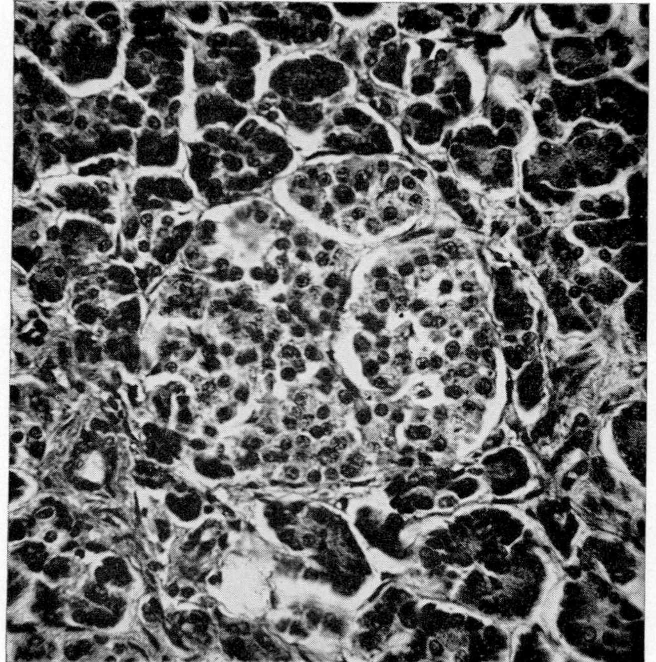

FIG. 4. Normal islet of Langerhans.

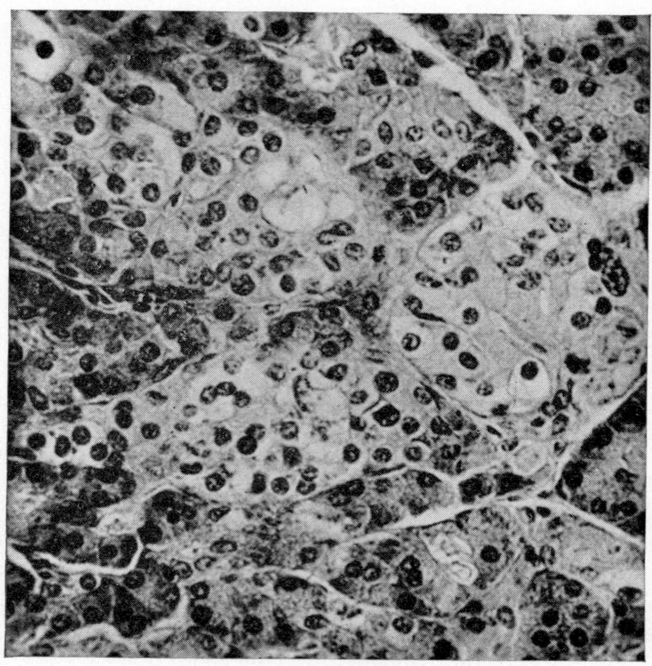

FIG. 5. An advanced stage of "hydropic degeneration" of the cells of the islets of Langerhans. (Courtesy of F. M. Allen.)

Replacement of the islet cells by a hyaline substance is the most common finding in autopsy material of diabetic patients (Fig. 6). This type of degeneration is not limited to the pancreas. The arteries and kidneys are particularly involved by the laying down of hyaline material. Hyalinization of the islets is more common in patients over forty years of age, but it is related more to the duration of the diabetes than it is to the age of the patient or to the degree of severity of the diabetes. The source of the hyaline and the reason for its selective localization in the islets are unknown. Hyalinization is a slow process, but eventually it destroys the function of the islets which it invades, and with progressive involvement of islets the functional capacity of the insulin-producing mechanism is reduced proportionately. It is not known whether hyalinization is a cause of, or the result of, diabetes.

Fibrosis is next in frequency to hyalinization as a chronic change in the pancreas of the diabetic patient. Also, it is primarily a lesion of the islets and there is little extension into the acinar tissue. It is present in slightly over half of these patients; the cause of the fibrosis is not known; extension is along the course of the vessels of the islets, and it is most common in patients over forty years of age.

Pancreatic Lesions with Secondary Diabetes. *Pancreatic calculi* are uncommon. They may be multiple and scattered throughout the pancreas or solitary with the calculus obstructing the duct of Wirsung and, by setting up a retrograde autolysis, they may destroy the pancreas. The acinar portion succumbs first and the islets later. This is an uncommon cause of diabetes.

Infiltration of the pancreas by *neoplastic growths* and by changes with deposits of iron as seen in *hemochromatosis* are uncommon causes of diabetes.

Characteristics of other known causes of diabetes, as listed in Table 1, may be observed.

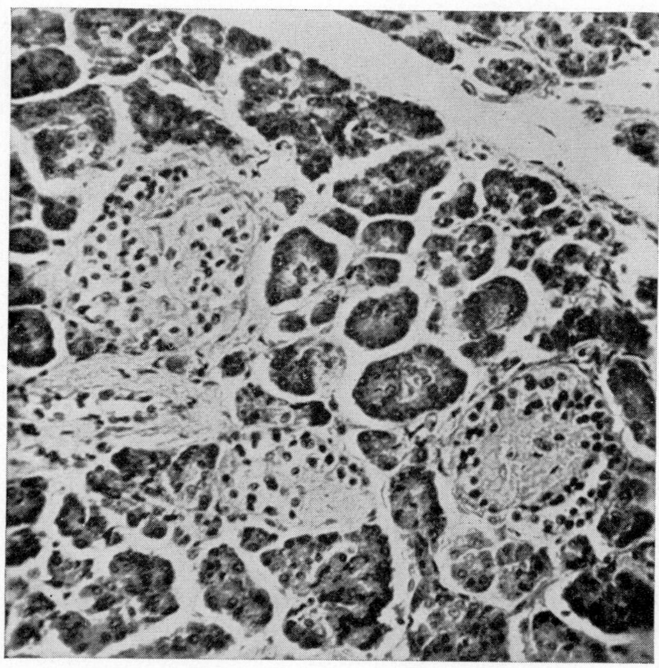

FIG. 6. Bands of interacinar fibrosis and three islets which have undergone extensive hyaline degeneration. (Courtesy of F. M. Allen.)

Extrapancreatic Changes

Liver. Fatty livers develop in diabetic animals maintained on a diet deficient in choline and without insulin.[56] Fatty deposits also occur in the liver of untreated diabetic patients and more especially in the diabetic child. These deposits disappear quickly and the size of the liver rapidly lessens when the diabetes is controlled adequately, especially when choline or one of its precursors is administered freely. In the patient with uncontrolled diabetes and impending coma, hepatic glycogen disappears from the cytoplasm of the liver cells but the nuclei of these cells become engorged with glycogen. These changes are reversible.

Skin. The skin is an organ of considerable importance as a storehouse for glycogen. In uncontrolled diabetes the glycogen stores in the skin become depleted, while the sugar content of the skin may be nearly treble that of the nondiabetic because of the systemic hyperglycemia. Other cutaneous evidences that may be associated with diabetes and characterized by deposits of lipids—chiefly cholesterol—in the skin are xanthelasma palpebrarum, xanthomas and necrobiosis lipoidica diabetica.

Furuncles and carbuncles are common complications of diabetes. Infections of the skin were the second most common complication, accounting for 358 of 3564 consecutive admissions to the public wards of the Pennsylvania Hospital because of acute complications (see p. 892). Xanthochromia, a yellow discoloration of the skin of the palms of the hands, soles of the feet and nasolabial folds, less common since insulin has permitted a more nearly normal diet than previously, is due to a pigment derived from foods rich in carotene, notably the yellow foods, e.g., egg yolk, butter, carrots and sweet potatoes. Diabetic patients who ingest more yellow foods than is normally the case are also more likely to exhibit xanthochromic deposits in the skin.

Eyes. Sclerotic changes in the arteries, hemorrhages and exudates predominate as positive retinal findings in diabetic patients. There are patches of waxy exudates, deposits of lipids, rounded areas of deep hemorrhage and atheromatous changes in the larger and hyaline thickening of the media of the smaller arteries. The source of the waxy exudates is not known but they have been attributed to the leakage of proteins and red blood cells from thin-walled capillary aneurysms. Capillary aneurysms in the inner nuclear layer of the retina may be mistaken for petechial hemorrhages. Superficial flame-shaped hemorrhages are arterial in origin and occur more frequently in the hypertensive diabetic. Increased capillary fragility is a common finding in these cases. Minute discrete saccular aneurysms appearing singly or in clusters in the retinal capillaries are the most distinctive and often the earliest ocular sign of diabetes. The aneurysms are not present in newly formed capillaries and are not dependent on hypertension, arteriosclerosis nor atherosclerosis. The smaller aneurysms, 20 to 30 microns in diameter, are barely visible but larger ones are easily seen. The appearance of diabetic retinopathy during pregnancy and its disappearance after the termination of pregnancy, the increased excretion of oxysteroids in patients with diabetic retinopathy, the production of ophthalmoscopic changes resembling diabetic retinopathy in alloxanized animals by the administration of cortisone and corticotropin, the similarity of the pathologic changes in the retinal vessels with intercapillary glomerulosclerosis and the absence of retinopathy in diabetics with Addison's disease have led to the hypothesis, not entirely accepted, that the cortisone or related substance has an etiologic relationship to the changes seen in the pancreas, kidneys and retinae of diabetes.[57,58,59]

A proliferative retinitis may take the form of a dense white fibrous membrane developing in hemorrhagic areas or the formation of new vessels to be seen most frequently about the optic disk. Both of these abnormalities are common. Hemorrhages into the vitreous, detachment of the retina and glaucoma are more common in diabetics than in the general population.

Advanced grades of diabetic retinopathy are most common in patients with poorly controlled diabetes over long periods. A serious complication, rubeosis iridis diabetica, with new formation of vessels on the iris and often associated with secondary glaucoma, is uncommon. Cataracts, indistinguishable from senile cataracts, are somewhat more common, but not strikingly so, in the older diabetics than in the nondiabetic population. True diabetic cataracts, which may develop with amazing rapidity, are seen in young patients. Fortunately they are rare.

Kidneys. *Intercapillary glomerular nephrosclerosis,* as described by Kimmelstiel and Wilson,[60] is of major importance because of its frequency and because its incidence is increasing. In its advanced stage this disorder is indicative of diabetes. There is a hyaline material laid down between the capillary loops or, as claimed by some, in the walls of the capillaries, progressing until all segments of the glomerular tuft are involved and forming rounded hyaline masses in the glomerulus. Multiple segments of the tufts may be involved with eventual replacement of the entire glomerulus (Fig. 7), leaving it functionless. Hyaline thickening of the efferent as well as the afferent arterioles is common and is distinctive of diabetes. The source of the hyaline is obscure. If it is associated with disturbances in the mucopolysaccharide metabolism, as has been suggested, it is probable that the hyaline changes begin in the capillary walls rather than between them as the basement membrane of the capillary walls is composed of mucopolysaccharides.[61] An advanced degree of arteriosclerosis with its subintimal deposits of hyaline substance is usual in these cases (Figs. 8 and 9). The clinical counterpart is indicated by edema, retinopathy, arterial hypertension and albuminuria. The reduction of renal function ultimately causes uremia. This disease process occurs in a mild form in both diabetic and nondiabetic subjects. It may remain relatively stationary for long periods, but when the edema and albuminuria are of great degree and the serum albumin is reduced the duration of life is measured in months and not in years.

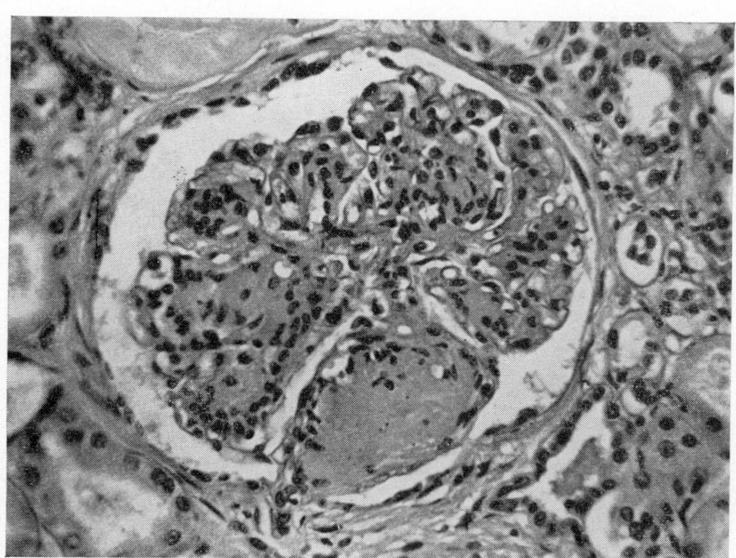

FIG. 7. Intercapillary glomerulosclerosis in diabetes mellitus. Note characteristic nodular hyaline thickening in one segment of the tuft and the diffuse intercapillary sclerosis.

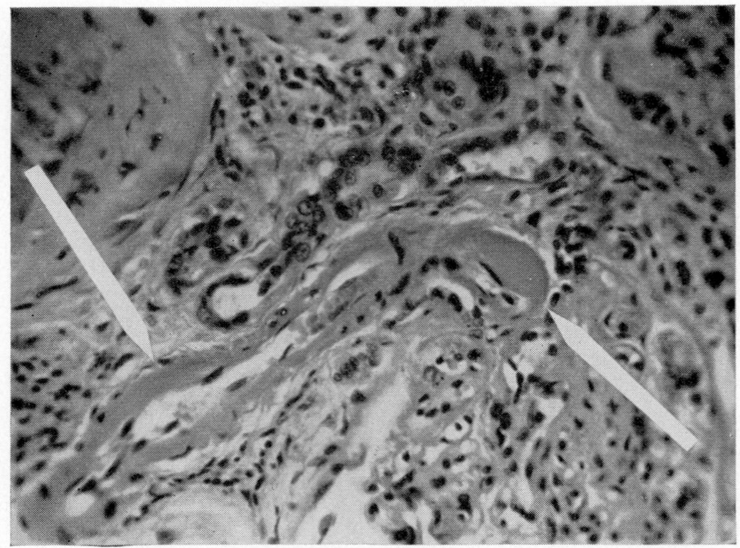

FIG. 8. Arteriosclerosis of an afferent arteriole leading into a glomerulus (lower right) in a kidney of a diabetic patient.

Arteriosclerosis involving the renal arterioles is the most common renal disorder associated with diabetes. It is more frequent in diabetic than in nondiabetic subjects, but the morphologic changes are the same in both. In diabetic patients over fifty years old, it is found in 77.6 per cent, or about five times as frequently as in nondiabetic controls.[62] The characteristic changes, i.e., subintimal deposits of hyaline, are much more intense in diabetic subjects. In fact, thick homogenous deposits of hyaline substance in afferent and efferent renal arterioles present strong presumptive evidence of diabetes. This change, illustrated in Figures 8 and 9, is contrasted with normal renal arterioles as depicted in Figure 10.

The degree of arteriosclerosis appears to have a direct relation to the degree of arterial hypertension in patients under fifty years of age, though arteriosclerosis occurs, even in severe degrees (Fig. 9), in diabetic patients without hypertension. In patients over fifty years of age the degree of involvement is related more to advancing age than it is to the degree of hypertension.

Diabetes, in some manner, intensifies the speed and degree with which the hyaline deposits in the arterioles are made.

Malignant hypertension, a rapidly progressive form of hypertension with uremia secondary to thrombonecrosis, glomerulitis or intimal fibrosis, may be encountered in association with diabetes but there is no specific relationship between the two diseases.

Pyelonephritis is a common complication of diabetes. Of 142 of our diabetic patients coming to autopsy, 41 (28.8 per cent) had evidences of active or healed pyelonephritis. The disease may take an acutely destructive form—necrotizing renal papillitis—with extensive abscess formation and necrosis of the papillae.[63]

Arteries. Lesions of the vascular system are responsible for death in more than 50 per cent of patients who have had diabetes for more than fifteen years. Sclerotic changes in the coronary arteries predominate as do similar changes in the arteries of the pelvis, legs and feet (Fig. 11). Irreversible changes are represented by swelling and hyaline degeneration of the ground substance of the intima and the infiltration of lipids and subsequent calcification. These processes—atheromatous

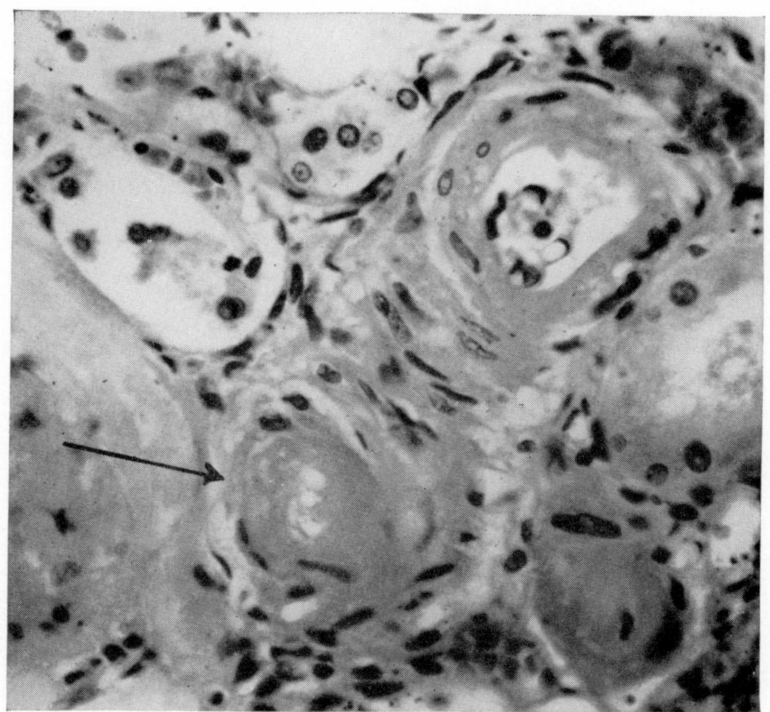

FIG. 9. Severe renal arteriolarsclerosis in a diabetic patient.

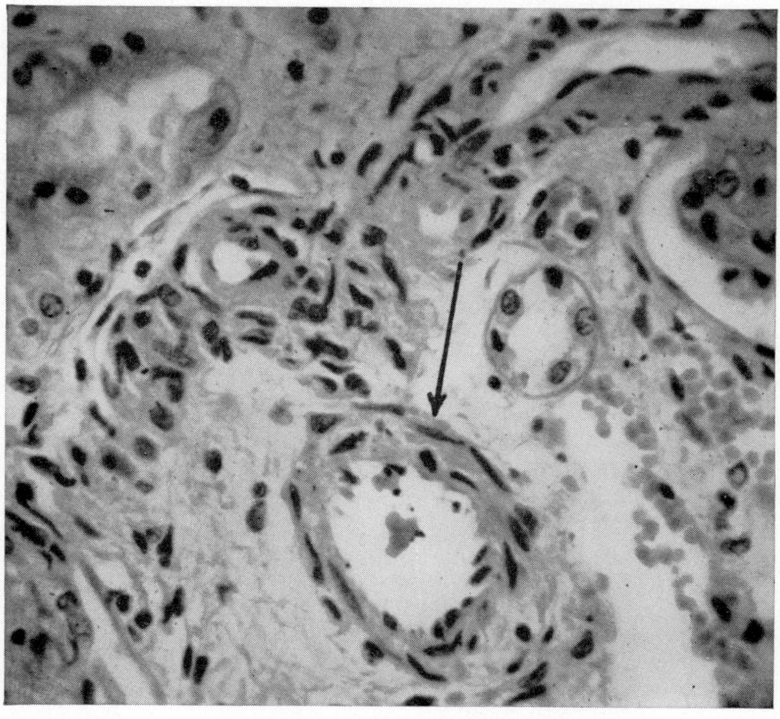

FIG. 10. Normal renal arterioles.

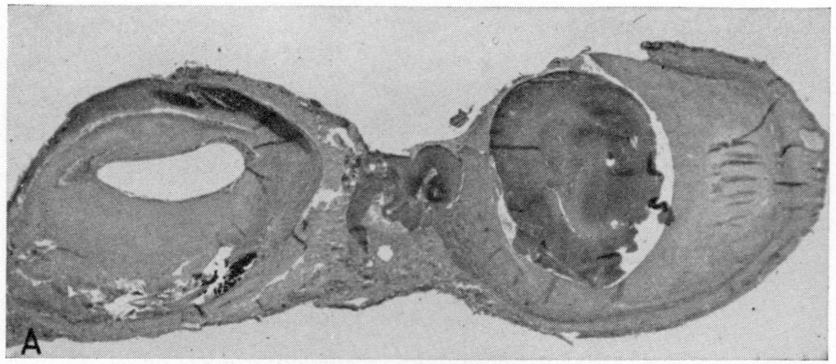

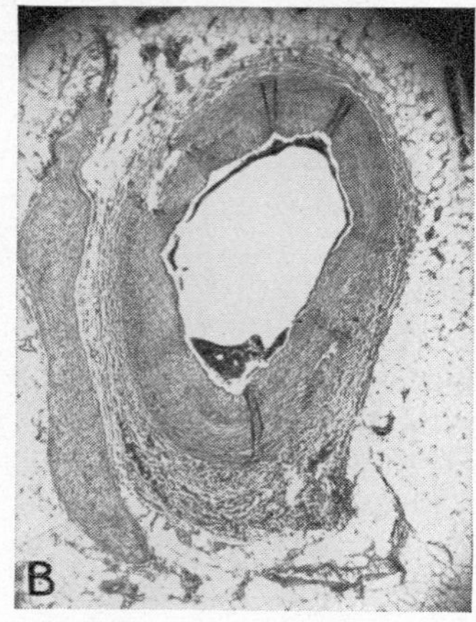

FIG. 11. A. A section of two medium-sized arteries near their junction. Each shows a marked encroachment of the lumen by a hyaline thickening of the intima and one shows, in addition, the occlusion of the lumen by a thrombus. B. A section of a normal artery of approximately the same size is shown for comparison.

and arteriosclerotic—are seen most frequently in the aorta, the coronary arteries, and the vessels of the extremities. Hence, the predisposition to occlusion of the coronary arteries and to occlusive vascular disease of the extremities is not surprising. Primary, or essential, diabetes in some unknown manner accelerates the development of atherosclerosis. This effect is not nearly so apparent in secondary diabetes, i.e., in experimental diabetes produced by alloxan and in diabetes caused by destructive lesions in the pancreas, as in cases of tumor, infection and hemachromatosis. Atherosclerosis is a manifestation of a disturbed lipid metabolism, other manifestations of which are seen in xanthelasmic and xanthomatous eruptions.

In "diabetic atherosclerosis" deposits of lipids occur not only in the large arteries, as is usually seen in the nondiabetic atherosclerotic subject, but in the small arteries and arterioles as well. The coronary arteries are involved in both the male and female to about the same degree. Hence, it is not surprising to find coronary occlusive disease as common in the female as in the male diabetic.

There is increasing evidence of a corelation between atherosclerosis and hyperlipemia. Diets high in fat and inadequate control of the diabetes are probable contributing factors in the production of atherosclerosis. Disturbed integrity of the complex mucopolysaccharides of the ground substance or intercellular material, leading to deposits of lipids in the vessel wall and the production of atherosclerosis, is a promising hypothesis.

A third type of vascular degeneration,

Mönckeberg's sclerosis, involves the medium-sized vessels, causing irregular medial necrosis and calcification without lipid deposition.

Nervous System. Not much is known of the pathologic changes in the neurologic complications of diabetes. Demyelinization of the nerves occurs in cases of *diabetic neuritis,* which is the predominating acute and reversible neurologic complication of diabetes. The degenerative changes of the *diabetic neuropathies*—the characteristically chronic neurologic complications —occur in the peripheral nerves, anywhere in the entire nervous system, and in the spinal cord, particularly in the posterior and lateral columns, and are identical with those seen in pernicious anemia. These changes account for the disturbances in sensation, the so-called diabetic tabes, and in rare cases, changes in the bones and joints of the feet, indistinguishable from Charcot's joints[64] and trophic ulcers of the feet (see p. 872). These neurologic changes have been attributed to arteriosclerosis. This is not the whole answer, however, as they occur in some instances in the absence of significant arteriosclerosis. Infection is the apparent cause in some but not all cases. The degenerative changes of advanced degree, in which not only demyelinization of the distal portions of the nerves but actual destruction of the axis cylinders has occurred, are irreversible. These are distinct from those in which acute inflammatory changes, and possibly, disturbances in "nerve metabolism" predominate.

Alloxan Diabetes. Islet cells of the rabbit's pancreas are selectively destroyed and diabetes is caused by a single intravenous injection of alloxan,[65,66] 150 to 200 mg. per kg. of body weight. Diabetes is produced in dogs when 50 to 75 mg. of alloxan per kg. are given. Larger doses cause uremia plus diabetes. An initial hyperglycemia, lasting fifteen minutes to one hour, follows the injection of the alloxan. This, in turn, is followed by a marked hypoglycemia with convulsions. The hypoglycemia is due, presumably, to insulin released from damaged islet cells. Finally hyperglycemia and permanent diabetes ensue.

The damage to the islets is completed with great rapidity—alloxan is not detectable in the blood for longer than five minutes after its injection intravenously.

Alloxan diabetes is of great interest to investigators because alloxan is chemically related to uric acid—a normal constituent of the body; the glutathione concentration normally present in the blood is greatly reduced after the administration of alloxan; glutathione administered in large doses protects against the islet cell destruction by alloxan, and transient diabetes has been reported to follow the intraperitoneal injections of uric acid in rabbits,[43] but this occurred only when the blood glutathione levels were reduced by means of diets deficient in cystine and methionine. Purified adrenocorticotropic hormone (ACTH) produced in man a transient diabetes associated with loss of tolerance for carbohydrate, increased endogenous purine metabolism and depressed levels of blood glutathione.[67]

The clinical significance of alloxan diabetes is that it permits the exploration of this problem from a new approach. Hopes for clinical usefulness of alloxan in cases of functioning islet cell tumors have not materialized. In fact, it causes chemical destruction of the normal islets without affecting the cells of the tumor.[68]

DIAGNOSIS

General Considerations. Positive features detected in the history and on physical examination may suggest diabetes as the diagnosis. A family history of diabetes is significant, especially if the patient is over forty years of age and is overweight; mothers of infants weighing over ten pounds at birth are prone to have, or to develop, diabetes; a history of glycosuria whether or not it was associated with thyrotoxicosis, pregnancy or acute infection is a common forerunner of diabetes; ophthalmoscopic findings showing the characteristics of diabetic retinopathy and symptoms and signs of a diabetic neuropathy may be the first clue to the diagnosis of diabetes. Symptoms—notably fatigue, polyuria, polydipsia, polyphagia and loss of weight—also are highly suggestive, but the diagnosis cannot be established without finding sugar in the urine and hyperglycemia under usual or special conditions. Special tests may be necessary to detect or to exclude a mild diabetes.

Any evidence of diabetes should instigate an investigation calculated to confirm or disprove the diagnosis. The important considerations, with the diet unrestricted, are:

1. Glycosuria—occurring concomitantly with a hyperglycemia.
2. Hyperglycemia—fasting blood (venous) sugar values above 120 mg. per 100 ml. (Folin-Wu) and postprandial values in excess of 160 mg. per 100 ml., or if capillary blood is used the fasting value for sugar above 120 or a postprandial value above 190 mg. per 100 ml. The diagnosis should not be made on the basis of only one determination of the level of the blood sugar. Transitory hyperglycemia and glycosuria are not uncommon in cases of head injuries, intracranial infection, thyrotoxicosis, hyperpituitarism, conditions affecting the adrenal glands, emotional disturbances, diseases of the liver, during anesthesia, asphyxia and poisoning from chemicals.
3. Special tests for doubtful cases:
   a. Effect of a meal containing 100 gm. of carbohydrate on the level of the blood sugar. Values above 160 mg. per 100 ml. two hours after the meal are indicative of diabetes, provided there is no complication which might alter the carbohydrate tolerance.
   b. Glucose tolerance tests.

The Urine

Glycosuria. In general, the term "glycosuria" is loosely used to mean sugar in the urine and is not restricted to glucose in the urine as occurs in diabetes. A relatively innocent glycosuria occurs in some nondiabetic subjects who have permanently low renal thresholds for glucose and in others whose renal thresholds are temporarily reduced, as occurs during pregnancy and in hyperthyroidism. Other sugars, as discussed in Chapter 14 may be excreted in the urine, but this is an uncommon occurrence and is of little clinical significance.

Glucose, a fermentable, dextrorotatory, copper-reducing sugar appearing in the urine in amounts demonstrable by the Benedict and other tests in common use (see p. 793), should be attributed to diabetes until proved otherwise. It is a simpler matter to establish the diagnosis of diabetes and thereby identify the sugar as glucose indirectly than to identify the sugar by chemical means. A search for hyperglycemia after the strain of a meal usually will give the answer if the patient has diabetes, but if doubt still exists special tests are resorted to (see p. 797). Glycosuria is the most common, though not the most sensitive, indication which leads ultimately to the diagnosis of diabetes mellitus. Ordinarily glycosuria is the result of hyperglycemia, sugar being lost when the venous blood sugar level exceeds the renal threshold, usually between 160 and 180 mg. per 100 ml. Glycosuria is of special importance because it is tested for in a routine urinalysis; hence, the likelihood of its discovery is great and the detection of the diabetes is more likely in contrast with the more delicate, but less frequently performed, test for diabetes, viz., determination of the level of the blood sugar.

There is a copper-reducing substance in normal urine but the quantity is so minute that it escapes detection by the usual tests. Sugar in the urine in concentrations below 0.1 per cent may be considered normal. Glucose when boiled with an alkaline copper solution (Benedict's test, p. 794) reduces the copper to cuprous oxide, thus changing the color of the solution from blue to green, greenish yellow, orange or brick red with increasing concentrations of sugar. Ordinarily, glucose occurring in sufficient quantities in the urine to be detected by the Benedict test indicates a pathologic condition. Glycosuria may occur in some normal persons for short periods after an unusually great carbohydrate intake. This is *alimentary glycosuria* and may be attributed to a lowered renal threshold or to absorption of glucose from the intestine at a rate too rapid for its prompt removal from the circulation. Starving persons may have glycosuria upon the resumption of feeding (*hunger glycosuria*). These are innocent forms of glycosuria.

The glycosuria which occurs as the result of diabetes varies from scarcely detectable traces to large amounts, 10 per cent or more. In the case of a patient having a mild diabetes, glycosuria is least likely to occur in the morning before breakfast—at the end of the longest period without food—and *an evening specimen, not the first one voided in the morning, is the one most likely to contain sugar.* In contrast, the severe grades of diabetes cause continuous glycosuria until corrected by appropriate treatment.

When sugar is found in the urine, and the blood sugar values are normal both before (fasting) and two hours after a liberal meal, and when the patient is subjected to a glucose tolerance test, the diagnosis of a nondiabetic melituria is justified.

False positive reactions to tests for glycosuria are common. The copper used in qualitative tests for glycosuria is slightly reduced and may be mistaken for sugar when large quantities of conjugated glycuronates occur in the urine. They appear in decomposing urine and may be avoided by examining freshly voided specimens. The glycuronates appear in the urine in considerable quantities and give a mildly positive Benedict's test after the ingestion of salicylates, menthol, chloral hydrate and aminopyrine. As a group, the glycuronates reduce the copper in Benedict's and Fehling's solutions but, unlike glucose, are nonfermentable.

The homogentisic acid of alkaptonuria reduces the alkaline copper solutions, thus giving false positive tests for sugar. In this disorder, if the urine is allowed to stand and become alkaline by ammoniacal putrefaction or if alkali is added, it assumes a black or gray color. Alkaptonuria is a rare condition. Sugars, other than glucose, and other reducing substances do not react positively to the specific enzymatic test for glucose.

TESTS FOR GLYCOSURIA. For mass examinations, for office and clinic practice, the following simplified tests for sugar and acetone in the urine are satisfactory. Also they are employed as routine by diabetic patients who test their own specimens.

Enzymatic Tests for Glycosuria. An enzyme—*glucose oxidase*—converts glucose to glyconic acid and is specific for glucose in the routine testing for glycosuria. Two commercial products of this nature* with suitable color charts for the purpose of contrast are available in this country. One of these (Tes-Tape), besides identifying the glucose, gives a crude appraisal of the degree of glycosuria. This qualitative-quantitative reaction is registered on enzyme-impregnated paper, the degree of color obtained depending on the formation of hydrogen peroxide during the reaction.

The commercial test kits permit the removal of sufficient enzyme-impregnated testing material to make one test—usually 1 to 1½ inches. The tape is dipped in the urine, removed and allowed to stand for one minute, at which time the color which has developed is compared with standard colors. The color reactions with Tes-Tape differ from those in tests formerly used and may be confusing at first to the patient familiar with Benedict's or Clinitest. With the enzyme test a blue color is indicative of 4 plus glycosuria (2 per cent or more); greenish blue, 3 plus (approximately 1 per cent); green, 2 plus (approximately 0.5 per cent); greenish yellow, 1 plus (approxi-

* Tes-Tape: Eli Lilly Company, Indianapolis, Indiana; Clinistix: Ames Company, Inc., Elkhart, Indiana.

mately 0.25 per cent); yellowish green, a trace (approximately 0.10 per cent); and a yellow color indicates the absence of glycosuria.

Clinitest for Glycosuria.† This convenient modification of Trommer's test permits a qualitative, and crudely quantitative, test for sugar in the urine. The test is made by placing 5 drops of urine in a test tube; the dropper is rinsed and 10 drops of water are added; then one Clinitest reagent tablet—containing anhydrous copper sulfate, anhydrous sodium hydroxide, citric acid and sodium bicarbonate—is added. Heat is generated by the chemical reaction in the tube, causing the solution to boil. *The test tube is not to be shaken while the solution is boiling.* The result is read after the boiling has ceased for at least fifteen seconds. There is no sugar in the sample tested if the resulting color is blue. Sugar is present if the final color is dark green, yellow, orange, brown or rust red. The amount of sugar present, up to 2 per cent, can be determined with a fair degree of accuracy by contrasting the color obtained with the standard color scale.

Galatest for Glycosuria.‡ This test for sugar in the urine is accurate, simple, requires no boiling and gives a prompt reaction. It is performed by placing on plain white paper an amount of the Galatest reagent—containing a bismuth salt, sodium hydroxide and sodium silicate—sufficient to cover one third of a dime. To this is added one small drop of urine. The result is read after thirty seconds have elapsed. If the powder takes on the amber color of urine the specimen tested contains no sugar. The color changes from a light gray to black with increasing concentrations of sugar. The approximate amount of sugar present is estimated by comparing the color obtained with the standardized color scale.

† The American Diabetes Association has endorsed the distribution to the public through pharmacies of a simple equipment—the Self-tester—with which anyone can test the urine for sugar. This equipment is prepared by the Ames Company, Inc., Elkhart, Indiana.

‡ Galatest equipment is obtainable from the Denver Chemical Mfg. Co., Inc., 163 Varick St., New York 13.

Benedict's Qualitative Test[69] *for Sugar in the Urine (Modified):*

Equipment:

1. Qualitative Benedict's Solution (when purchasing testing solution, specify *Qualitative* Benedict's Solution; Benedict's *Quantitative* Solution does not change color when boiled with glucose).
2. Test tubes marked at 5 cc. and at 2.5 cc. levels.
3. Dropper pipette.
4. Water-bath.

Technique:

1. Put 2½ cc. (approximately ½ teaspoonful) of Benedict's Solution in a test tube.
2. Add 4 drops of the urine to be tested. Hold pipette perpendicularly while adding drops.
3. Shake tube to mix urine and Benedict's solution thoroughly.
4. Put the tube in a water-bath of boiling water and boil for five minutes.
5. Let cool and read reaction.

Interpretation:

Clear blue solution: no sugar. Light greenish-yellow: faint trace of sugar. Yellow to orange: moderate amount of sugar, about 1 per cent. Chocolate-brown or brick-red: large quantities of sugar, over 2 per cent.

Millard Smith's Micro-modification of Benedict's Quantitative Test for Sugar in the Urine.[70]

Equipment:

1. One small ring stand with test tube clamp, a micro Bunsen burner or small alcohol lamp.
2. A Pyrex test tube (18 by 160 mm.).
3. A Millard Smith pipette No. 2 and a 1 cc. Ostwald pipette.

Technique:

1. Transfer 1 cc. of Benedict's quantitative solution to the test tube (held in ring stand clamp) and add 0.2 to 0.7 gm. of anhydrous sodium carbonate. Bumping is prevented by adding a thoroughly dried pebble, a piece of quartz or a pinch of talcum powder.
2. The mixture is raised to and kept at the boiling point.
3. The urine is added slowly from the Smith pipette until all of the blue color disappears. Care should be taken to allow time

for complete reduction before adding more urine. The test is done slowly and care must be taken not to pass the end point. The percentage of sugar present is read directly from the pipette without calculation.

Urine containing less than 1 per cent of sugar is titrated directly. When larger amounts of sugar are present, the urine is diluted, 1 to 10 or 1 to 20 before titration.

Specific Gravity. The specific gravity of the urine usually increases in direct proportion to the amount of sugar present. A specific gravity of 1.030 or above obtained on a pale urine is almost without fail due to sugar. However, a normal specific gravity, 1.008 to 1.025, is common even though glycosuria is present.

Urine Volume. In untreated diabetes the twenty-four-hour urine volume characteristically exceeds the average normal of 1500 cc. In fact the quantities may reach several gallons. The great increase in the volume of urine gives but little index of the severity of the diabetes, but in general the greater the volume the greater is the amount of sugar present. Occasionally the polyuria is so great that amounts totaling more than 50 per cent of the body weight may be voided in twenty-four hours. Control of the diabetes restores the rate of urine excretion to normal.

Ketonuria. Ketonuria is the first recognizable sign of ketosis though it is of little importance in the diagnosis of diabetes. It results when, from insulin lack and insufficient carbohydrate intake, the metabolism of fat is accentuated and ketones are produced in greater than normal quantities. Ketones are also derived from certain amino acids. Ketonuria occurs in a mild form in healthy nondiabetic patients whose food intake, especially the carbohydrate, is greatly curtailed. It is common in the diabetic patient without other evidence of ketosis. This was especially so in the preinsulin era when diets high in fat and low in carbohydrate contents were popular. A considerable quantity of ketones may be excreted in the urine without their accumulation in the blood or without a reduction of the carbon dioxide combining power. Failing appropriate treatment during the course of acute complications, notably acute infections, the rate of production of ketones may exceed the rate at which they can be excreted. It is then that qualitative reactions for ketones in the plasma or serum become positive and it is then that the acetone odor appears on the breath. Stadie[71] has indicated that ketones accumulate because of a coincident breakdown of the fatty acid chains and not because of an interference in the process of fat metabolism at the acetone body stage.

The ketone bodies are *acetone, diacetic acid,* and *β-hydroxybutyric acid.* Acetone and diacetic acid appear under similar conditions and as the latter is, by far, the more injurious of the two it receives chief consideration. Both are identified by a modified Rothera test* or more convenient still, the "Acetest."†

An increasing loss of beta-hydroxybutyric acid in the urine accompanies a deepening ketosis. In severe ketosis it is in this form that most of the ketones are lost, amounting to as much as 200 gm. in twenty-four hours. The tests for acetone and diacetic acid in the urine are strongly positive before appreciable amounts of hydroxybutyric acid are excreted.

Ketonuria is a guide for further investigation. The amount of ketones excreted is of less immediate importance than the amount of these products which has accumulated in the tissues

* Bedside test for plasma acetone and diacetic acid (Rothera-Wishart): Two drops of plasma, or serum, are placed in a Wassermann tube and supersaturated with ammonium sulfate crystals and shaken. Two drops of approximately 5 per cent sodium nitroprusside solution are added and shaken. Two drops of ammonia water are added and shaken. Allow to stand for three minutes.

Interpretation:

Permanganate color
—trace of plasma acetone.
Light blue—moderate
Deep blue or almost black
—heavy reaction for plasma acetone.

† Acetest reagent tablets are manufactured by Ames Co., Inc., Elkhart, Ind.

and in the blood. It has been shown that mild degrees of ketonuria may persist for months and years without apparent harm, whereas, a 4 plus reaction for ketones in the blood from a patient who also has glycosuria is diagnostic of diabetic coma.

QUALITATIVE TESTS FOR ACETONE. *"Acetest" Test.* This test for acetone is simple and reliable. One drop of freshly voided urine or freshly secured sample of plasma or serum is added to a tablet which contains amino-acetic acid, disodium phosphate and sodium nitroprusside. The color of the tablet is noted after thirty seconds have elapsed. Interpretation of the test:

White or cream color	negative test
Purple tint	1 plus reaction
Lavender	2 plus reaction
Moderate purple	3 plus reaction
Deep purple	4 plus reaction

Rothera's Test.‡ To 5 or 10 cc. of urine add about 1 gram of ammonium sulfate and 2 or 3 drops of fresh concentrated sodium nitroprusside solution and overlay with strong ammonia water. A reddish purple ring shows the presence of acetone.

Acetone Test (Denco). This simple and accurate test for acetone is executed by depositing on a dry white paper sufficient of the Acetone Test (Denco) reagent—containing sodium bicarbonate, ammonium sulfate and sodium nitroprusside in anhydrous form —to cover one-third of a dime and by moistening this *entire amount* of powder with 2 or 3 drops of urine, or plasma, to be tested. In the presence of acetone a shade of purple will develop within thirty seconds; a trace of acetone yields a light lavender color and with increasing amounts the color will be darker, a dark blue indicating a 4 plus reaction. In the absence of acetone a grayish yellow color is the result.

‡ Todd, Sanford and Wells: Clinical Diagnosis by Laboratory Methods. 12th Ed. W. B. Saunders Company, Philadelphia, 1953.

Note: Special reagent strips (Ketostix) manufactured by Ames Co., Inc., Elkhart, Ind., provide a simple means of detecting ketones in urine and plasma.

We use this test routinely in examining the urine and the blood plasma, or serum, for acetone.

Clinically, we do not employ the test for diacetic acid but rely on the tests for acetone as indication of the degree of ketonuria.

The Blood

Sugar Content. Hyperglycemia is the most decisive indication of diabetes. Without it the diagnosis cannot be made with certainty. A concentration of sugar in a specimen of venous blood, taken after an eight- to fourteen-hour fast, in excess of 130 mg. per 100 ml., or a value exceeding 160 mg. after a hearty meal is usually due to diabetes. There is practically no difference in the sugar concentration in venous and arterial (capillary) blood in the fasting state. After a meal, however, and in the normal person, the arterial blood sugar level is from 20 to 50 mg. per 100 ml. higher than that in the venous blood. This difference represents utilization of sugar by the tissues and the difference is reduced in untreated diabetes and the normal variation is restored by adequate treatment.

A diagnosis of diabetes should never be made on the basis of a single blood analysis unless the hyperglycemia is accompanied by glycosuria and characteristic symptoms. The most certain criteria of diagnosis are repeatedly elevated fasting blood sugar values and glycosuria. It is significant that in the patient with an untreated but mild diabetes, glycosuria tends to subside toward morning—at the end of the longest period without food. It is then also that the blood sugar level is the lowest in the twenty-four hours.

Sugar is present in the blood of normal persons in concentrations varying from 70 to 110 mg. per 100 ml., fasting (Folin-Wu method). The blood sugar levels in the average untreated diabetic patient without acute complications range betwen 180 and 300 mg. per 100 ml. Most clinical laboratories still employ the Folin-Wu method, but for research purposes Nelson's modification of the Somogyi method* is almost universally used. This latter method measures only glucose, and the values are often referred to as "true glucose" values, which are from 15 to 20 mg. per ml. lower than those obtained by the Folin-Wu method.

The hyperglycemia and glycosuria of diabetes behave in a characteristic manner. Liberal additions to the carbohydrate and total caloric intake tend to increase their severity, while restricted carbohydrate and total food allowance have the opposite effect.

Hyperglycemia may be present for only short periods, one to four hours after each meal, with normal fasting values in patients having mild diabetes. The likelihood of identifying these mild cases is enhanced by taking the blood specimen for determination of the sugar value two hours after the biggest meal of the day. Values in excess of 170 mg. per 100 ml. and an accompanying glycosuria make the diagnosis obvious.

The degree of hyperglycemia alone is not an accurate index of the severity of the diabetes. An untreated obese patient may have a blood sugar level of 500 mg. or more per 100 ml. and yet the mildness of the diabetes is apparent when the hyperglycemia is corrected by merely restricting the total food intake. It is a reliable rule to consider that *every untreated overweight diabetic patient has a mild diabetes, despite the degree of the hyperglycemia that is found.* In contrast, the underweight patient with untreated diabetes has a severe diabetes, though the blood sugar level may not exceed 250 mg. per 100 ml. To restore the underweight patient to good health, a gain in weight is imperative. This end is achieved only by a liberal food intake and insulin therapy. The degree of hyperglycemia, in the light of the relationship of the patient's weight with that of the normal, is a reliable index of the severity of the diabetes. *The fat diabetic patient has a mild diabetes and the lean diabetic patient with a persistent fasting hyperglycemia has a severe or moderately severe diabetes.*

Other departures from the normal composition of the blood (Table 9) are not of special value in arriving at a diagnosis of diabetes. They are, for the most part, observed during complications of this disorder and will be dealt with under the respective complications, i.e., alterations in the hemoglobin, the urea nitrogen, concentration in the blood plasma acetone, carbon dioxide combining power, plasma or serum chlorides, the blood volume as seen in ketosis, and cholesterol and fatty acid values.

Special Tests for Doubtful Cases

Test Meal and Modified Glucose Tolerance Test. The use of a test meal in detecting diabetes has fallen into relative disuse. Variations in the rate of absorption of the various foods make a test dose of glucose preferable to a meal of mixed foods. A simplified glucose tolerance test, which we have used as a screening test for nine years at the Benjamin Franklin Clinic, comprises (1) the giving of 100 grams of glucose in a pint of water flavored with lemon and (2) taking a single specimen of venous blood two hours later. If the blood sugar value (Folin-Wu method) is below 120 mg. per 100 ml., one can safely conclude that there is no detectable evidence of diabetes. If the value exceeds 140 mg., the diagnosis of diabetes is indicated, provided suitable precautions, outlined by Parkhurst and Betsch,[72] are taken. Values between 120 and 140 mg. are inconclusive and the test should be repeated several weeks later. This diagnostic procedure is not so cumbersome as the usual glucose tolerance test, and I do not believe its simplicity sacrifices in the slightest its diagnostic value. Its

* When true venous blood glucose values are employed, as determined by the Somogyi or other method, concentrations in excess of 110 mg. per 100 ml. fasting and 150 mg. after a meal usually established the diagnosis of diabetes.

Capillary blood sugar values above 140 mg. fasting and 210 mg. per 100 ml. after a meal (Folin-Malmros method) indicate diabetes, as do true glucose values of capillary blood above 120 mg. fasting and over 200 mg. per 100 ml. after a meal.

TABLE 9. ALTERATIONS IN THE COMPOSITION OF BLOOD ASSOCIATED WITH DIABETES MELLITUS*

CONSTITUENT	NORMAL RANGE	IN UNTREATED DIABETES
Base—Total (mEq./L)	155	Decreased in ketosis
Chlorides (mEq./L)	103	Decreased in ketosis
as NaCl (mg./100 ml.)	576 –612†	Decreased in ketosis
CO_2 capacity (Volumes %)	55 – 65†	Decreased in ketosis
(mEq./L)	27	Decreased in ketosis
Nonprotein nitrogen (mg./100 ml.)	22 – 29†	Increased in ketosis
Urea nitrogen (mg./100 ml.)	9.6– 17.3†	Increased in ketosis
Potassium—as K (mEq./L)	5	Increased in untreated ketosis
—as mg./100 ml	14.8– 16.8	Decreased after onset of treatment for ketosis
Sodium—as Na (mEq./L)	142	Decreased in ketosis
—as Na (mg./100 ml.)	307.5–316	Decreased in ketosis
Sugar—as total reducing substance arterial whole blood† (mg./100 ml.)	80 –110†	Increased
venous, (mg./100 ml.)	70 –100†	Increased
Sugar (True glucose) mg./100 ml	50 –100	Increased
Cholesterol—Total (mg./100 ml.)	150 –190†	Increased
Fatty acids—Total (mg./100 ml.)	290 –420	Increased
Lipid phosphorus—lecithin (mg./100 ml.)	12 – 14	Increased
Total acetone bodies (as acetone)(mg./100 ml.)	1.3– 2.6	Increased in ketosis
Acetone—qualitative test on plasma	negative	++++ in diabetic coma

* The values are those obtained on plasma or serum taken under fasting conditions unless otherwise indicated.

† Extracted from Sunderman and Boerner's Normal Values in Clinical Medicine, W. B. Saunders Company, Philadelphia, 1950.

simplicity should encourage widespread adoption, particularly in the screening of possible candidates for diabetes, notably overweight relatives of diabetic patients.

Some latitude is permissible in establishing the diagnosis of diabetes in the thyrotoxic patient. We allow a moderate degree of hyperglycemia, 20 mg. per 100 ml. above that of the nonthyrotoxic patient, before considering it diagnostic of diabetes. Even then, this diagnosis should be tentative, in the borderline cases, until the thyrotoxicosis is corrected and the usual methods of evaluating the diabetes are applicable.

Standard Glucose Tolerance Test. It is in diabetes mellitus that gross alterations in carbohydrate tolerance are most frequently observed. It is in the detection of this disease in its mildest states that use is made of the fact that normal persons can ingest considerable quantities of carbohydrate with but trifling changes in the concentration of sugar in the blood. This is in contrast with the diabetic in whom the blood sugar level is profoundly affected by sudden and large demands made on the blood sugar regulating mechanisms.

The standard glucose tolerance test is a reliable test in determining, in doubtful cases, the presence or absence of diabetes. The value of this test is as a diagnostic aid and not as an indicator of the severity of the diabetes. However, if the patient is underweight and has a high fasting blood sugar value, the diabetes is almost certain to be severe. In these cases results similar to those shown in Figure 12, curve C, would be found, i.e., a hyperglycemic fasting blood sugar value with continued increases in the degree of hyperglycemia throughout the three hours subsequent to the oral administration of 100 grams of glucose. I wish to emphasize that in clinical practice a confirmed fasting blood sugar value of 130 mg. per 100 ml. or higher, with glycosuria, would establish the diagnosis and make a glucose tolerance test unnecessary. The curve (C) is presented as an illustration of the values encountered in such a case and not as a recommendation that a glucose tolerance test be done when the diagnosis is obvious without it. Glucose tolerance tests in such cases are needless. In spite of this, the practice of performing these tests on patients obviously diabetic is widespread.

INDICATIONS. In general, the glucose tolerance test is indicated when the diagnosis of diabetes, or its exclusion, cannot be clearly made without it. Persons for whom the test is employed will fall into one, or a combination, of the following categories, namely:

History of glycosuria—applicants for life insurance are the most frequent subjects for a glucose tolerance test under the circumstance of having a history of glycosuria.

Family history of diabetes—for many reasons it is important for one with a family history of diabetes to establish the presence or absence of this disorder. Contemplation of marriage, the selection of occupation and the adoption of preventive or palliative measures are examples of these reasons.

Transitory glycosuria and *hypergly-*

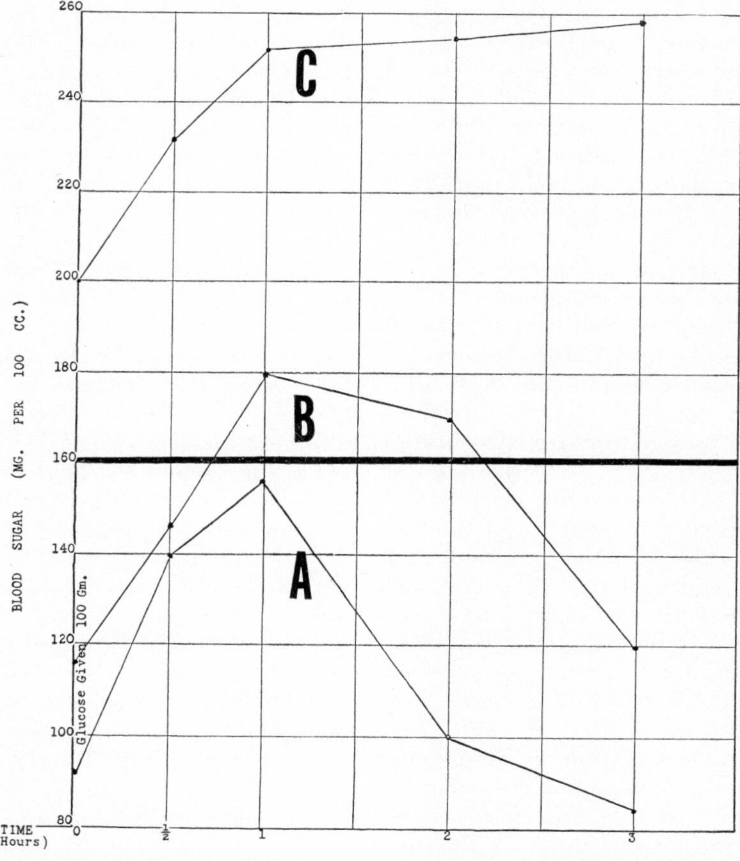

FIG. 12. Three glucose tolerance curves. *A* depicts the normal glycemic response to the oral administration of 100 gm. of glucose. The rise in the blood sugar level is rapid, but a normal value is restored in two hours. In *B* the glycemic response is slower and normal values are not restored until the third hour as is found in mild diabetes. *C* depicts the fasting hyperglycemia and the continued increase in the blood sugar level even at the third hour as seen in severe diabetes. Glycosuria usually occurs when the blood sugar level is maintained for varying periods above 160 mg. per ml. as depicted by the heavy black line.

cemia during other complications, e.g., pregnancy, hyperthyroidism, hepatitis, staphylococcic infections—particularly furuncles and carbuncles—and following a starvation regimen. Follow-up tolerance tests are of special value in this group.

Glycosuria without hyperglycemia as occurs in renal glycosuria, e.g., nephrosis and in some cases of pregnancy and of thyrotoxicosis. The value of such a study is emphasized when one recalls seeing patients who have been needlessly and ineffectively dieting and taking insulin when the disorder was one of renal glycosuria.

Women who give birth to abnormally large babies.

CONTRAINDICATIONS. It is important, when practicable, to perform this test in the absence of conditions other than a possible diabetes, that would influence the tolerance unfavorably. For this reason the glucose tolerance test for the detection of diabetes is contraindicated during the course of *infections, hepatic disturbances* and *dietary restrictions*, especially a starvation regimen, or a low carbohydrate diet or a high fat diet low in carbohydrate content which, though they do not alter the true capacity of pancreatic islet cell function, do exhibit temporary alterations which are adaptations to a reduced demand for insulin (Allen).

The glucose solution occasionally causes nausea. This delays absorption and distorts the blood sugar concentration curve; hence, if the curve does not conform to that for a normal tolerance in the event of nausea, the test should be repeated after a lapse of seven to ten days. Tests done before a week has elapsed may mislead, as in mild diabetes a rapid succession of tests tends to show a progressive improvement in the tolerance for glucose. Also, active exercise during the course of the test will have a similar effect. Contrariwise, prolonged rest in bed tends to reduce the tolerance for glucose and permits slightly higher curves than are obtained when the subjects are ambulatory. Any disorder, but notably a severe degree of visceroptosis, which delays emptying of the stomach, may delay the absorption of the glucose and hence retard the decrease in the blood sugar, simulating the findings in mild diabetes. This difficulty is by-passed in such cases by employing the intravenous glucose tolerance test.

TECHNIQUE OF STANDARD GLUCOSE TOLERANCE TEST. The patient reports in the morning, having had a daily intake of at least 300 grams of carbohydrate for at least three days immediately prior to the test but having had no food since the previous evening. The bladder is emptied, a sample of venous blood (5 ml.) for sugar determination is taken and 100 gm. of glucose, or 1.75 gm. per kg. in children, dissolved in 300 ml. of water and flavored with the juice of a lemon, is given by mouth. Specimens of blood and urine for sugar determinations are secured one half hour later, and at one, two and three hours.

INTERPRETATION. Two values in the curve depicting the various concentrations of sugar in the blood are of outstanding importance, as it is upon them that the real value of the test depends. They are (a) *the fasting blood sugar value* and (b) *the value obtained two hours after the ingestion of 100 gm. of glucose (or 1.75 gm. per kg. of body weight in the case of a child.)*

Fasting Venous Blood Sugar. The normal range of the fasting blood sugar concentration is between 70 and 100 mg. per 100 ml. Values in excess of 130 mg. are indicative of diabetes unless proved otherwise.

Two-hour Blood Sugar Value. The normal person is able to restore the blood sugar level to 120 mg. or lower two hours after the ingestion of the glucose. A more liberal interpretation is permissible in the presence of thyrotoxicosis, which mildly depresses the carbohydrate tolerance. In these instances two-hour values up to 150 mg. are considered nondiabetic if the three-hour value is below 120 mg. per 100 ml. Such curves are common in cases of thyrotoxicosis, the correction of which restores normal responses to glucose tolerance tests and, in so doing, justifies the lenient interpretation in such cases.

Peak Values. The maximum concentration of sugar in the blood normally is found thirty or sixty minutes after the ingestion of glucose. Some authorities believe that if the peak value exceeds 170 mg. per 100 ml. it is indicative of diabetes. We give little heed to the peak of the curve even if it exceeds 200 or 220 mg. per 100 ml., provided the two-hour value is restored to 120 mg. or below. A blood sugar regulating system which, between the one-hour and two-hour intervals, can eradicate such a degree of hyperglycemia is, most probably, not lacking in insulin. Unusually high peaks at one-half and one hour are more likely to be due to an unusually rapid rate of absorption, as is known to occur in cases of a functioning gastroenterostomy and of thyrotoxicosis. Nevertheless, it is a good practice to recheck the test annually in such cases.

Barring conditioning influences already mentioned, a *normal curve* reveals a fasting value below 120 mg. and a two-hour value at or below 120 mg. per 100 ml. *Tolerance curves are indicative of diabetes,* if the clinical evaluation is in keeping with the diagnosis, and if the fasting blood sugar exceeds 120 mg. and if the two-hour value exceeds 130 mg. per 100 ml. It is agreed that the fasting blood sugar may be normal, and indeed it usually is, in cases in which the glucose tolerance test is used properly. This being so, *the value which is of utmost importance is that obtained at the end of two hours.* Indeed, in the majority of cases, the test and interpretation may be simplified and the expense reduced by doing only one blood sugar determination—two hours after the glucose has been taken. This is assuming that previous fasting blood sugar values have been normal. Barring, again, the conditioning influences mentioned below, a two-hour value above 130 mg. is indicative of diabetes. This test detected diabetes in 267 (4.4 per cent) of patients in a survey of 6088 patients visiting the Benjamin Franklin Clinic.

Glycosuria may influence the type of curve. Large quantities of sugar in the urine, occurring concomitantly with blood sugar values on the borderline, would weigh in favor of a diagnosis of diabetes in the belief that had no, or very little, glycosuria resulted the concentration of sugar in the blood would have been higher.

Urine, collected simultaneously with the collection of each blood sample, permits a study of relationship of glycosuria to the degree of glycemia as well as some evaluation of the renal threshold.

The excretion of glucose in the urine depends upon: (a) the concentration of sugar in the arterial blood reaching the glomeruli of the kidneys, (b) the rate at which the glomeruli filter the sugar out of the blood and (c) the rate at which the filtered glucose is reabsorbed by the renal tubules.

The renal threshold is usually considered in terms of the concentration of sugar in venous blood, which is an unreliable index of the concentration of arterial blood reaching the renal glomeruli for at least several hours after the ingestion of food.

Some authorities prefer capillary blood to venous blood for sugar determinations. The former is subject to much greater range of concentration and is likely to be misleading to those inexperienced with the method.

The greater stability of the venous blood sugar values over those of capillary blood would appear to make the former the more reliable for clinical purposes.

Glucose-Cortisone (11-Oxy-Steroid) Tolerance Test. This more exacting test has been suggested by Fajans and Conn[73] for the detection of the potentiality for diabetes in relatives of diabetics who respond normally to the usual glucose tolerance test. They found previously undetected diabetes in 19 per cent of 152 relatives of diabetic patients and in only one of 50 control subjects. Of 75 relatives of diabetics exhibiting normal responses to the standard glucose tolerance test, 57 (76 per cent), in contrast to 97 per cent of control subjects, showed negative responses.

The technique of the test comprises the same preparation and the same number of blood sugar determinations as the standard test (p. 798). Cortisone acetate, 50 mg., was given eight and one-half hours and two hours preceding the ingestion of the glucose to subjects weighing less than 160 pounds. For those in excess of this weight, two doses of 62.5 mg. of cortisone were substituted.

The clinical value of this test will be determined by the ultimate outcome in those subjects in whom it gives the only objective indication of the potentiality for diabetes.

Similar tests, using 10 mg. of prednisone or prednisolone, were shown by West[74] to be much more potent than cortisone in their hyperglycemic effect. It is doubtful that such severe tests are warranted in routine clinical use.

One-Hour, Two-Dose Glucose Tolerance Test (Exton-Rose). This test has not been found, in our experience, to be as reliable an index of disturbed carbohydrate tolerance as the foregoing standard glucose tolerance test. It is convenient in that it is simple to perform, requires fewer venipunctures than the three-hour glucose tolerance test and is completed in one hour—a desirable feature in office practice. The results are dependable if the blood sugar values clearly indicate that diabetes is present. It is noted, however, that there is a broad zone in which the interpretation can indicate only a presumptive diagnosis of diabetes when the blood sugar values are in the upper portion of the zone, or the presumption that diabetes is not present if the values are somewhat lower. The high incidence of inconclusiveness which attends the use of this test in doubtful cases has led us to abandon it in preference to the standard glucose tolerance test. Furthermore, the Exton-Rose test has been based on a misconception concerning the underlying physiologic processes which account for the types of curves obtained.[75] It is agreed that the maximum rate of absorption of glucose from the gastrointestinal tract is 0.85 gm. per kilo of body weight per hour or about 60 gm. per hour for the average-sized man.[76] There is evidence that the maximum absorption is carried on at a slower rate than this, namely, 43 gm. per hour. This being so, a one-hour study cannot possibly give an accurate measure of the patient's ability to dispose of 100 grams of glucose, much of which is still in the intestinal tract at the end of this period.

Furthermore, it is not the second dose of glucose which causes the blood sugar values to fall in the second half hour of the test but rather the accelerated utilization of sugar by the tissues and cessation of the production of sugar from glycogen by the hepatic processes which are set in motion when the blood sugar is initially increased. This mechanism, once in action under normal conditions, continues until the blood sugar is slightly subnormal. The blood sugar concentration begins to fall from its peak when the rate of sugar utilization surpasses the rate of absorption from the gastrointestinal tract and this occurs even while maximum absorption is taking place and is not affected by an additional dose of glucose given one half hour after the initial dose. Minor changes in the rate of absorption, and not necessarily in the rate of utilization, may determine whether the higher concentration of sugar in the blood occurs one half hour or one hour after the administration of the initial dose of glucose. This is also true when the standard three-hour glucose tolerance test is used but, in this case, the longer period permits a greater degree of correction than is possible in one hour.

It is for the foregoing reasons that the Exton-Rose glucose tolerance test is *not* recommended for the detection of diabetes in doubtful cases.

Intravenous Glucose Tolerance Test. This test is not recommended for general clinical use. However, in the unusual case when it is important to circumvent abnormalities of absorption of glucose from the intestine, such as occurs in thyrotoxicosis, hypothyroidism, visceroptosis, gastrectomy, steatorrhea, sprue and gastroenterostomy subjects, this test may be of value.

Techniques. Glucose, 0.5 gm. per kilogram of the normal body weight, is given intravenously as a 20 per cent solution in distilled water at a uniform rate over a period of twenty minutes. Blood (5 cc.) is withdrawn for sugar determination before the infusion is begun, at one half hour, one, two and three hours after the infusion has been completed.

Interpretation. Normal result: The initial blood sugar level is normal; the concentration of sugar in the blood does not exceed 120 mg. per cent two hours after the infusion has been completed. Glycosuria is common even though the curve indicates the absence of diabetes.

Miscellaneous States Affecting Tolerance Test. The degrees to which carbohydrate tolerance is depressed in a multitude of clinical disorders are so slight as to cause no confusion in differentiating the usual case from that of diabetes. These changes are noted in rheumatoid arthritis, senility, neoplastic diseases, cardiac decompensation, arterial hypertension, nephritis, pregnancy, obesity, apoplexy, ulcerative colitis, cirrhosis of the liver, cholecystitis and bronchial asthma. It can be gathered from the foregoing remarks that every diabetic patient when suitably studied will exhibit an elevated and prolonged glucose tolerance curve but that *every high and prolonged curve is not indicative of diabetes.* When the results are inconclusive a subsequent test or tests are indicated. If employed wisely and interpreted in the light of good clinical judgment, glucose tolerance tests will rarely mislead.

In diabetes the blood sugar does not return to normal (below 120 mg. per 100 ml.) within two hours of completing the infusion.

DIFFERENTIAL DIAGNOSIS

Diabetes may be confused with other disorders which cause glycosuria and hyperglycemia. The life of an unconscious patient who has glycosuria and a hyperglycemia as the result of an intracranial hemorrhage may be jeopardized should the condition be mistaken for diabetic ketosis and large amounts of insulin be given. The absence of detectable ketonemia would eliminate diabetic coma (see p. 877).

Glycosuria. The presence in the urine of substances which reduce copper in solution to cuprous oxide may be mistaken for glucose. These are pentose, lactose, levulose, maltose and rarely galactose, conjugated glycuronates, homogentisic acid, vitamin C and creatinine. The recognition of these various factors is dealt with on page 805. Glucose appearing in the urine of a nondiabetic patient is apt to be especially misleading. It occurs in *renal glycosuria* and *following intracranial injuries* and in *shock.*

Renal Glycosuria. Glucose appearing in the urine in the presence of a normal blood sugar concentration is known as renal glycosuria, referred to also as "benign glycosuria" and "diabetes innocens." Renal glycosuria is a symptomless and innocent condition requiring no treatment. It has to do with alterations in the renal threshold for glucose and represents a reduction in the ability of renal tubules to reabsorb sugar which has passed through the glomeruli. The blood sugar level above which glycosuria occurs is the so-called *renal threshold* for glucose. If the venous blood sugar level in the normal person is increased artificially, glycosuria occurs between 160 and 180 mg. per 100 ml. In longstanding diabetes the renal threshold is often higher, even as high as 250 mg. per 100 ml. On the other hand, in renal glycosuria glucose appears in the urine without any elevation of the blood sugar above the normal concentration (70 to 110 mg. per 100 ml.). This innocent disorder occurs in two forms: The one in which there is a constant loss of glucose in the urine, the quantity of which is not altered by changes in the diet and only with difficulty by giving insulin, and the other in which there is a temporary lowering of the renal threshold as observed during pregnancy and hyperthyroidism. Renal glycosuria

TABLE 10. THE RELATIONSHIP OF THE BLOOD SUGAR LEVEL AND THE SUGAR IN THE URINE IN A CASE OF RENAL GLYCOSURIA

1 P.M.	1:30 P.M.	2 P.M.	2:30 P.M.	3 P.M.
Blood Sugar per cent 0.100	Urine Sugar per cent 1.5	Blood Sugar Mg. per cent 0.108	Urine Sugar per cent 1.4	Blood Sugar Mg. per cent 0.098

is not a forerunner of diabetes. Experimentally this condition is produced by giving phloridzin to animals.

Importance is attached to renal glycosuria because of the danger of mistaking it for diabetes. The combination—diabetes and a low renal threshold for glucose—occurs occasionally.

Renal glycosuria is probable if, when the diet is restricted or when insulin is given, there is no decline in the amount of glycosuria. Furthermore, from day to day there is little change in the amount of glycosuria. These inconclusive observations are suggestive, but it is only by parallel examinations of the blood sugar level and the urine that the condition is clearly demonstrated.

A simple method of identifying a renal glycosuria is as follows: The bladder is emptied and the urine is discarded; 8 oz. (240 ml.) of water is given; a sample of venous blood is taken; thirty minutes later a specimen of urine is obtained and at the end of another thirty minutes blood is again obtained. If both blood sugar values are normal (70 to 110 mg. per 100 ml.) and if there is a considerable amount of sugar in the urine collected at the midway period, the diagnosis of a low renal threshold is confirmed. One may carry the test further by securing a second urine specimen and a third blood sugar value as illustrated in Table 10.

Pregnancy and the Renal Threshold. In more than 10 per cent of normal pregnant women there is a lowering of the renal threshold for sugar, allowing glucose to escape in the urine. Lactosuria is common during lactation. Lactosuria and glycosuria may be observed simultaneously in the same patient. The renal threshold for glucose returns to normal after the lactation period has ended.

Hyperthyroidism. In hyperthyroidism it is not unusual to find a lowering of the renal threshold for glucose. The problem is not as simple, however, as that which occurs during pregnancy. These patients are apt to have a hyperglycemia, and it is not rare for the same patient to have diabetes as well as hyperthyroidism. What appears to be a transitory diabetes may be observed. The tolerance for carbohydrate in these patients frequently is restored to normal by appropriate treatment of the hyperthyroidism. Unfortunately this is not always the case.

Nephrosis. The renal threshold for glucose is lowered in nephrosis, in which condition degenerative changes in the tubular epithelium impair the absorption of glucose from the glomerular filtrate. The associated clinical evidences of nephrosis remove any diagnostic difficulties.

Alimentary Glycosuria. It is believed by some that alimentary glycosuria represents a decreased renal threshold for sugar but that the threshold is sufficiently high to prevent continuous glycosuria, and that sugar appears in the urine after extra "loads" of carbohydrate. This interpretation should be accepted with reserve and a careful study of the patient's carbohydrate tolerance should be made in each instance. So-called "alimentary glycosuria" may be due to a reduced renal threshold for sugar or to an increased permeability of the intestinal mucosa for sugar. Both causes are innocent. It should be suspected, however, until proved otherwise, that the glycosuria is due to diabetes.

Diseases of the Hypophysis. Hyperglycemia and glycosuria, indistinguishable from that occurring in uncomplicated diabetes, are common in *acromegaly.*

The diabetes which occurs as the result of changes in the hypophysis in the acromegalic patient doubtless has its origin in the excessive activity of the pituitary gland. The fact that irreparable changes take place in the pancreas as a result of these changes has been conclusively shown experimentally by Young.[49]

The important consideration is that acromegalic patients who have hyperglycemia and glycosuria have two disorders, acromegaly and diabetes, and should be treated accordingly.

PITUITARY BASOPHILISM (Cushing's disease). This disease, due to tumor growth of the basophilic cells of the anterior lobe of the pituitary gland, also causes hyperglycemia and glycosuria. Here also at least two disorders—basophilism and diabetes—coexist. The diabetes is due indirectly to the changes in the hypophysis.

Diseases of the Adrenal Glands. Hyperglycemia and glycosuria may occur as the result of a *tumor of the adrenal cortex.* The diabetes is indistinguishable from the chronic diabetes ordinarily seen except that it is not characteristically associated with the degenerative changes seen in primary or essential diabetes, and it is cured by removal of the adrenal tumor.

The subcutaneous, intramuscular or intravenous injection of epinephrine (Adrenalin), the active principle of the adrenal medulla, provokes hyperglycemia and may cause glycosuria. This is a transitory effect lasting only a matter of minutes. It neither causes nor predisposes to diabetes. The hyperglycemic response is due to a liberation of glucose from the liver. The same mechanism, under control of the sympathetic nervous system, operates in shock, fear and anger, and permits unusual effort to resist threatened danger.

Intracranial Injury. Clinically glycosuria and hyperglycemia are common after intracranial trauma. This may result from violent accidents in which the base of the brain is injured and in event of intracranial hemorrhage as a result of injury or disease of the vascular system, or from injury caused by intracranial tumors and acute infectious processes. Glycosuria of this type is in no way related to diabetes.

Melituria. Melituria is a term employed to include all sugars which may appear in abnormal amounts in the urine. Sugar being detected by the usual tests is likely to be *glucose* but it may be fructose, pentose, lactose—during lactation—or very rarely galactose, maltose, mannoheptulose—following the ingestion of avocados—and sucrose, which does not give a positive reaction for sugar with Benedict's test until hydrolyzed with hydrochloric acid. Sucrosuria is to be suspected when a urine free from albumin has a specific gravity above 1.035.

The clinical significance of the nondiabetic meliturias is, first, the danger that they may be regarded as being due to diabetes with the prospect of a lifetime of treatment; second, that a reducing substance in the urine, especially glucose in hyperthyroidism and during pregnancy and lactose during lactation, may be taken for granted as being due to the current complication and the possibility of a co-existing diabetes be overlooked; and third, *all meliturias are clinically benign and relatively innocent except the glycosuria due to diabetes* and that uncommonly seen in extensive hepatocellular disease, in which case the patient is seriously ill. The problem resolves itself into a question: *Is this sugar in the urine due to diabetes or is it not?* Methods employed in making the diagnosis in problem cases are dealt with on page 797.

From the point of view of the scientist it may be important to identify the sugar, especially if it is not glucose and not due to diabetes. Clinically the melituria is of little importance if it is not diabetic in origin and if it does not lead to an incorrect diagnosis. More details on the subject of melituria are given in Chapter 14.

PROGNOSIS

The outlook for the diabetic patient should be evaluated from: (1) the standpoint of *a possible cure* of the diabetes and the advantages of *good control* of the disorder in its chronic form (2) the prospects of acquiring *complications* with the influences that play for or against their development, and (3) *life expectancy*.

Possibilities of Curing Diabetes. A cure cannot be promised in any case of primary, or essential, diabetes. Yet those who have seen many of these patients have encountered occasionally one whose diabetes apparently disappears following appropriate treatment. At least, the diabetes is no longer detectable using the usual diagnostic measures. This is an unusual occurrence and one that should not be looked upon as a cure until many years pass with normal responses to annual diagnostic tests. I have had a special interest in three children followed for many years after all detectable signs of an acute diabetes had disappeared. In one it was possible to record the onset of symptoms to a certain afternoon. It is highly probable that in such cases acute reversible processes are taking place in the islets of Langerhans and that prompt and adequate treatment rescues a number of "knocked-out" functioning units sufficient to produce insulin in amounts adequate to erase evidences of diabetes.

Allen and his associates[44] have demonstrated that, in animals, islet cells in a state of hydropic degeneration can be redeemed by relieving the functional overstrain on these cells by restoring to and maintaining the blood sugar at normal concentrations by means of diet and insulin. Lukens and Dohan[51] have confirmed these observations.

Illustrative of the transient disappearance of diabetes is a male, aged thirty-eight years, height 6 feet, weight 180 pounds, who, while en route to the United States by air from Okinawa, developed excessive thirst and polyuria. Treated at the Pennsylvania Hospital in November, 1945, he had fasting blood (venous) sugar values as high as 294 mg. per 100 cc. and to control his diabetes 24 units of protamine zinc and 8 units of regular insulin daily were needed. His improvement was progressive and his insulin was discontinued on May 4, 1946. He was subjected to a glucose tolerance test on May 7, 1946 in order to complete the data necessary for him to secure a pension. The fasting blood (venous) sugar value was 119 mg. per 100 cc. and values after taking 100 gm. of glucose were: one-half hour, 137 mg.; one hour, 88 mg.; two hours, 96 mg.; and three hours, 93 mg. Subsequent tests repeated at regular intervals were normal until February, 1950, when two postcibal blood sugar values of 270 mg. and 190 mg. per 100 cc. were found. There had been no increase in weight and no other aggravating causes for this unfavorable change were detected. Such remissions, as illustrated by this case, are rarely observed in adults but they are not rare in children.

A third group—the middle-aged overweight patients—provides, not infrequently, candidates whose diabetes is pushed back and off the stage of detection by a reduction in weight through the agency of a reduced caloric intake. The onset of the diabetes in these patients is not acute; the "disappearance," *but not a cure*, of the diabetes is due to the reduced total body mass and hence the total metabolism by a means which spares islet cell function, and to the reduced need for insulin when the synthesis of fat from carbohydrate is reduced. This is in contrast to the deleterious effect that accompanies the loss of weight due to the activity of the diabetes, features of which are hyperglycemia and the excretion of large quantities of sugar and acetone in the urine.

The benefits of the reduction in weight by virtue of a restricted caloric intake form the basis of Allen's[77] undernutrition treatment. Benefits from undernutrition are obtainable in the insulin era, in properly selected cases (see p. 766), as previously demonstrated.[78,79,80] Newburgh[81] also found support for the undernutrition regimen in the treatment of obese diabetic patients. The diabetes is not cured by the reduction in weight by undernutrition. In spite of normal responses to glucose tolerance tests for varying periods, a return of the former degree of obesity is accompanied by evidences of diabetes. Also, without a gain in weight, diabetes becomes apparent during the course of acute infections, notably pyogenic infections. It would appear that the benefit is due to the reduction in total metabolism and that the insufficient supply of insulin for the obese state is adequate when the total body mass is reduced.

Prospects of Acquiring Complications. Diabetics are just as prone to develop most of the common diseases as are members of the general population. They are more likely than their normal counterparts to be victims of certain *acute* disorders, notably furuncles, carbuncles, tuberculosis and malnutrition, if their diabetes is uncontrolled.

The prognosis will depend upon three integrated features: (a) the change in the character of the diabetes as a result of the complications, (b) the management of the complication and (c) the proper evaluation and institution of appropriate measures to combat the influence which diabetes has upon the complication and *vice versa*. Actually, when suitable treatment is available the outlook for the diabetic suffering from most of the acute complications is as good as for the nondiabetic. Diabetic coma, the specific acute complication of diabetes, has become an uncommon cause of death—less than 2 per cent of diabetic deaths in well equipped hospitals.

The complications which cause most concern are those characterized by *chronic degenerative changes*—vascular disease, notably disease of the coronary arteries and of the arteries of the extremities, diabetic retinitis, intercapillary glomerulosclerosis and the diabetic neuropathies.

Disease of the coronary arteries is the most common cause of death in diabetics at the Pennsylvania Hospital, accounting for 41 of 188 consecutive deaths between 1947 and 1957. Intercapillary glomerulosclerosis is a menace of increasing proportions (see p. 787). In fact, it was the most common cause of death in patients whose diabetes developed in childhood and who had survived fifteen or more years,[82] whereas deaths from diabetic gangrene have declined precipitously since the advent of extensive antibiotic therapy.

Evidence is steadily accumulating that the likelihood of the diabetic acquiring any or all of these distressing chronic complications increases with the duration of the diabetes and the increase bears a direct relation to poor control of the diabetes.

Life Expectancy. The proximity of the life expectancy for diabetic patients to the normal expectancy has progressed rapidly since the discovery of insulin. Actually, many diabetic patients outlive the normal life expectancy.

The child diabetic lived but a short time—a scant two years—in the preinsulin era. Contrast this with the outlook of today when the young diabetic may with assurance anticipate maturing, marrying and raising a family.

The prognosis for the intelligent and cooperative diabetic patient is excellent if the diabetes is identified early and treated diligently by a physician who has interest and training in this field of metabolism. Standards of therapy vary greatly. Life insurance policies are issued to selected diabetic patients who are known to be conservative and cooperative.

Despite this progress, statistics based on an analysis of the experience of the Joslin Clinic in Boston, by the Metropolitan Life Insurance Company,[83] indicate a considerable disparity between the life expectancy of diabetics in contrast with the general population (Table 11).

Statistically, the diabetic patient of ten years of age has a life expectancy of about seventeen years less than that of the general population. With increasing age the disparity decreases until at age seventy the difference is only 3.7 years.

A much greater disparity exists in the mortality rates, as indicated in Table 11. The death rates for children and young adults with diabetes were five to ten times the rates for the general population. Improvement in the ratio occurred

TABLE 11. EXPECTATION OF LIFE AND MORTALITY RATE AT SELECTED AGES AMONG DIABETICS AND AMONG WHITE PERSONS IN THE GENERAL POPULATION
Experience in 1947–51 for Diabetic Patients of Joslin Clinic First Observed in 1930–51 and for General Population of United States in 1949–51[83]

ATTAINED AGE	EXPECTATION OF LIFE, IN YEARS		MORTALITY RATE PER 1,000	
	Diabetics*	General Population	Diabetics*	General Population
10	44.3	61.5	2.6	.5
15	40.0	56.7	4.6	.8
20	36.1	51.9	8.0	1.2
25	32.8	47.2	13.1	1.3
30	30.1	42.5	15.2	1.5
35	27.2	37.9	12.6	2.0
40	23.7	33.3	12.2	3.2
45	20.2	28.9	16.1	5.1
50	16.9	24.7	21.6	7.9
55	13.8	20.8	32.2	12.2
60	11.3	17.2	49.8	18.7
65	9.2	13.9	64.9	27.4
70	7.2	10.9	86.3	41.9

* Excludes deaths within one week of first observation or hospital discharge.
Note: Analysis of Joslin Clinic experience by Metropolitan Life Insurance Company.

with increasing age, but in middle and later life the mortality rates for the diabetic population were still more than twice that of the general population.

PREVENTION

In view of the increasing incidence of diabetes, the prevention of this disease should concern everyone. The problem is especially vital to members of families in which diabetes is prevalent. It has to do with the sidetracking of a hereditary predisposition of an organ of biological inferiority. *Diabetic patients should not intermarry.* As surely as they do, their offspring, if they live long enough, will develop diabetes. The observations of Pincus and White[84] leave no doubt about this. A diabetic patient may, without fear of such a catastrophe, marry into a family whose record is clear of diabetes. The mendelian recessive character of diabetes provides this guarantee. Looking further into the future, the children of this marriage should also marry into nondiabetic families. Wilder suggests that members of diabetic families limit their families to one or two children.

Members of diabetic families are predisposed to diabetes by heredity and there can be no doubt that the appearance of this disorder will often be prevented if precipitating factors are not added to the hereditary diathesis. I refer especially to obesity. The correction and prevention of obesity are the greatest practical means available for the prevention of diabetes. Every member of every diabetic family should be made aware of this.

Physical exercise is an important preventive measure. It inhibits the development of obesity and it develops muscles which are carbohydrate-consuming; at the same time muscular exercise is an "insulin-sparer." Accumulations of fatty tissue, on the other hand, increase the total metabolism in quite a different way and in one that increases the need for insulin. This is not surprising, as much more insulin is utilized in the production of fat from carbohydrate than in glycogen formation from carbohydrate. Observe the diabetic patient who maintains a program of active daily exercise. His insulin requirement decreases. Observe the sedentary diabetic patient who gains considerably in weight. His need for insulin increases.

The importance of keeping the body weight at or a trifle below the normal standard after the age of thirty-seven years cannot be overemphasized (see p. 1069). Regulation of body weight in this manner and the limitation of the size of diabetic families are the most practical means of preventing diabetes. Extraordinary care in the management of the pregnant woman who has a family history of diabetes may possibly prevent the development of clinically apparent diabetes.

Some diabetics achieve families by adoption, but this probably does not prevent diabetes as it is a step that is usually taken as a consequence of sterility.

It has been suggested that diabetic patients be sterilized, or that members of diabetic families remain childless via contraceptive means, as measures to stamp out the disease. This would not solve the problem unless extended to include those relatives of diabetic patients who pass on the hereditary predisposition. If it were possible to identify such persons (which it is not) we should realize, as Joslin has estimated, that the relatives of the 4,350,000 people in the United States (who, it is believed, have or will have diabetes) number nearly one in four of the entire population.

FOOD REQUIREMENT AND GENERAL CONSIDERATIONS

Introduction. Every diabetic patient must give special attention to his diet for best results. The restrictions are not great. In fact, *uniformity of an adequate diet from day to day is the most important feature of the dietary therapy* for diabetes, rather than the severe restrictions as formerly practiced. The dietary needs will vary with the conditioning influences such as (1) change in occupation and physical activity, (2) obesity, indicating a reduced caloric intake but with a more liberal diet as the body weight approaches the desired level, and (3) acute complications during which a full quota of calories, protein and carbohydrate with an equally spaced distribution of the diet, throughout the twenty-four hours, permits better control of the diabetes with insulin.

In determining the diet, individualization, in terms of so many grams of protein, carbohydrate and fat and the total calories, is the *first* requisite. The *second* is filling of the diet prescription in menu form. This menu will indicate certain food exchanges (see p. 819), which permit a selection from a variety of foods without sacrificing uniformity of values. *Thirdly*, the patient is thoroughly trained in the use of standard household measures, viz., the teaspoon, tablespoon, cup, slice of bread, strip of bacon, etc., in accord with the food exchanges permitted in his specific diet.

This training is most effective if done by a dietitian who is especially qualified in simplifying the dietary program, in instructing the patient in the latitude of the selection of foods permitted, and in accurately completing the menus. Weighing of the food is usually not necessary in the treatment for uncomplicated diabetes, but it is a practice adhered to by some authorities.

Dietary Needs

Normal. Dietary needs are conditioned by age, sex, body weight and activity. The *protein* quota of 1.0 to 1.5 gm. per kg. of the estimated ideal weight is quite liberal for adults. Larger allowances per kilogram are given children (see p. 922) and during pregnancy and lactation (see p. 906). The normal quotas for *fat* vary from 1 to 2 gm. and the carbohydrate from 3 to 5 gm. per kg. of the desired body weight. Illustration: A male, a train conductor, twenty-five years of age, 6 feet in height, weighing 165 lb. (75 kg.), would require approximately 75 to 110 gm. of protein, 75 gm. of fat and 300 to 330 gm. of carbohydrate—the total approximating 2300 calories.

Diabetic. The patient whose diabetes is well controlled needs no more and no less food to accomplish the same result than the normal person but there is great urgency to restrict the calories for diabetic patients who are overweight, and a modest reduction of the carbohydrate for nearly all diabetics simplifies the control of the diabetes. Also, these patients often present variable degrees of malnutrition. The diabetes, for one or more reasons, may not be well controlled over long periods, permitting loss of nourishment in the form of glycosuria and at times ketonuria. Also, to allow the same quota of carbohydrate for a diabetic as for a normal person would increase the difficulty of maintaining good control of the diabetes.

Total Calories. The total calories are a most important consideration in planning the diabetic diet. One of the fundamental principles in the dietary treatment of the diabetic patient is to avoid overfeeding, and for the patient over thirty-five years of age the body weight, barring certain complications (p. 890), should be brought to 5 to 10 per cent below the standard weight for his age, height and sex. Thus thin patients add to their weight, obese patients are reduced, and patients of standard weight are subjected to a minor reduction in weight.

Changes in the total calories have a more far-reaching effect on the insulin requirement than have changes in the allowance of carbohydrate (see p. 834).

Approximately 80 per cent of adult diabetic patients are overweight when they first seek medical attention because of their diabetes. All authorities on diabetes agree that the *obese diabetic patient* should be reduced, yet the neglect of this important method of controlling the disease and avoiding the use of insulin is widespread. The untreated obese diabetic patient has a mild diabetes and, barring complications, control of the disorder can be achieved and maintained by reducing the caloric intake sufficiently to bring about a slow reduction in weight—about two pounds per week. All will agree that the reduction in weight, in itself, will greatly enhance life expectancy. As a further illustration, an obese patient, although admitted in coma with a blood sugar of 1450 mg. per 100 ml., had an inherently mild diabetes, as shown by the ease with which it was eventually controlled by restricting the caloric intake and reducing the body weight. The prompt elimination of a large dose of insulin—110 units daily—would be a hazardous undertaking in the case of a thin patient but in the obese subject who is relatively resistant to insulin this can be done without fear in the absence of acute complications. For the overweight patient, a diet low in calories will achieve a proper reduction in weight. As soon as the diabetes is controlled, the rate of reduction may be cut in half by gradually increasing the caloric intake. When the body weight reaches a trifle below the standard level, further increases in the diet are made to prevent continued loss of weight. Suitable adjustments are made in the early control phase and in the eventual long-term treatment period to regulate the rate of reduction and to achieve a stationary weight at a desirable level.

By using the formula for prescribing the diet, as outlined on page 815, the individual with a *body weight closely approximating that of the normal* will have a more liberal diet than the overweight patient. Drug therapy—insulin or oral therapy—will probably be needed. The *underweight patient* will need a diet adequate to promote a gain in weight and, because of the liberal diet and the increasing total body mass and total metabolism, insulin therapy in the past, has been essential. Such a patient having developed diabetes in mid or later life may possibly do well on oral therapy without insulin.

PROTEIN. We have been more liberal with protein in the past few years and have gained the impression that diabetic patients have a better sense of well-being when the protein intake exceeds, by a small margin, that ordinarily consumed by a normal person. As a result, *it is unusual to prescribe less than 100 gm. of protein for the adult male and less than 80 gm. for the adult female diabetic.*

The diabetic's need for protein is the same as that of the nondiabetic as long as the diabetes is well controlled. A protein deficit occurs if large amounts of sugar are lost in the urine. To correct this feature a liberal allowance of protein, in excess of the normal allowance, and the control of the diabetes are indicated. For the actual estimation of the protein quotas for the individual patient, see page 815.

Need for increased protein during growth and in the treatment for certain complications, notably hepatitis, pregnancy, cirrhosis of the liver and nephrosis, is recognized and appropriate amounts are prescribed.

Carbohydrate. The carbohydrate allowance varies with the severity of the diabetes. In the case of the overweight patient with mild diabetes, insulin and oral therapy can be avoided by the continued restrictions of total calories and carbohydrate. These restrictions are relaxed as the body weight decreases and it is not unusual to find these patients tolerating, eventually, a diet of nearly normal content—carbohydrate, protein, fat and total calories, without hyperglycemia or glycosuria. *It is desirable to have the long-term diet contain 225 to 300 gm. of carbohydrate.* This permits a wider selection of vitamin- and mineral-containing carbohydrate foods as well as sparing protein for tissue synthesis, unless it increases significantly the difficulty in controlling the diabetes.

For the underweight diabetic there is ordinarily no escape from insulin, or in suitable cases, tolbutamide therapy and, as these agents permit large increases in carbohydrate, liberal quotas of carbohydrate are allowed at once—as much as 200 gm.—with additions to 250 and infrequently to 300 gm. after the diabetes is controlled.

Fat. Fat is used to make up the calories not provided by the protein and carbohydrate. Each gram of protein and of carbohydrate can be considered as providing 4 calories, and each gram of fat 9 calories. Hence, the calculation of the fat allowance is a simple matter. Because of the lipemia and the higher cholesterolemia so commonly associated with diabetes, and the effect of fat on the body weight, we prefer to keep the fat content of the diet as low as is practicable. It is better to give higher carbohydrate quotas and control the diabetes with insulin or oral therapy, when necessary, and to keep the fat content of the diet lower than has formerly been the practice. Fat in excess of 100 gm. daily is rarely justified. It is highly probable that the degenerative changes in the vascular system will be less if the fat intake is kept down to 50 gm. daily as advocated by Rabinowitch.[85] A compromise—between 50 and 100 gm.—at this stage is justifiable. Such allowances will force the carbohydrate and protein quotas upward. This is permissible. Diets extremely low in fat—less than 40 gm. daily—are unpalatable, but with 50 to 75 gm. of fat there need be no sacrifice of palatability, essential fatty acids and fat soluble vitamins.

Distribution of Meals. Uniformity of distribution of the diet from day to day reduces the amplitude of the oscillations in the blood sugar concentrations and permits better control of the diabetes than when no two successive breakfasts are alike, or no two lunches or no two dinners. The diet is adjusted to the individual's needs and the distribution arrived at, as indicated below, is maintained from day to day until new circumstances warrant a change.

The distribution of the diet in the presence of acute complications is considered on pages 886 to 889.

Diet Plans. Convenience is served in the use of standard diet prescriptions and, for most patients with uncomplicated diabetes, such diets are satisfactory. Eleven dietary plans are presented in Table 15 (see p. 822) and on pages 823 to 833. The diet most closely approximating, in total calories, the diet prescription discussed on pages 822 and 833 is adopted for the individual patients and suitable changes to the more liberal or the more restricted diets are made if indicated by alterations in body weight.

Standardized diets are not applicable in dealing with acute complications, such as hepatitis, nephritis with nitrogen retention and duodenal ulcers. Diets for such patients must be more highly individualized and made to conform with the diet which experience has shown to be more effective in treatment for existing complications. Uniformity of the diet from day to day will permit adequate control of the diabetes, a factor which is usually of no small importance in fortifying the therapy for the complicating disorder.

The use of standard diet prescriptions has simplified greatly the dietetic aspects of the therapy for diabetes. It facilitates including adequate components in the diets of various levels, and patients, thoroughly instructed in the flexibilities permitted by the various food exchanges, may select appropriate foods from the family table or restaurant menu.

The foregoing plan of dietetic treatment adheres in principle to that advised by Allen and by Joslin, though we are more liberal with the protein and carbohydrate quotas but rely greatly on restricted fat and total calories in treating diabetic patients who are overweight.

The more liberal protein allowance adds to the "staying value" of a meal. Also, the appetite is more effectively satisfied. The carbohydrate allowance is higher than is recommended by Joslin and his associates. We favor this increase because it permits a lower fat intake and because it has been proved by Allen and observed many times by us that great increases in carbohydrate are permissible with but little change in the need for insulin, provided the total calories are not increased at the same time—appropriate reductions being made in the fat intake. Also, the high incidences of lipemia and hypercholesterolemia and the tendency to degenerative changes in the vascular system in diabetics encourage us to increase the carbohydrate and to decrease the fat to the limits of practicability.

Contrast with Other Diets. Diets of historical interest are commented upon in the Chapter on History. The diets of today vary greatly. We believe the diet prescriptions presented in this book are those which, in general, are used most widely.

In general, three types of diet are considered in present-day medical writings:

1. The more conservative diet with liberal protein, nearly normal carbohydrate and with the total calories regulated according to the dictates of the body weight. This measured diet is aimed, with suitable use of insulin or oral therapy, at restoring physiologic processes, as closely as is practicable, to normal. We think of this plan of therapy as the *Physiologic Plan.*

2. The high carbohydrate, low fat and low calorie diet advocated by Rabinowitch[85] is standing the test of time and has much in its favor, but it makes good control of the diabetes a relative impossibility in cases of unstable or juvenile type diabetes. An illustrative diet is as follows: protein, 70 gm.; carbohydrate, 400 gm.; fat, 50 gm. (2330 calories).

3. Free diets as recommended by Stolte are advocated by Tolstoi.[86] These are normal diets, not weighed or measured. Insulin is used to prevent symptoms but otherwise glycosuria and hyperglycemia are disregarded. This program fosters the maintenance of an unphysiologic state and one which, by permitting hyperglycemia over long periods, predisposes to early and more rapidly progressive degenerative changes. Diabetic neuropathies, increased susceptibility to tuberculosis and increased hazards during pregnancy are characteristically more prevalent and diabetic retinitis in its advanced form is especially common in patients with uncontrolled diabetes. It appears inescapable, from accumulating clinical data, that uncontrolled diabetes will exact a penalty which otherwise might be prevented in many and postponed in others.

Vitamins and Minerals. VITAMINS. There is no convincing evidence that vitamin therapy has a more specific benefit for the diabetic patient than it has for the nondiabetic. There is, however, considerable evidence that diabetic patients require more of the vitamin B complex, thiamine, nicotinic acid, B_{12}, and riboflavin than do normal persons.

Peripheral neuritis is a common complication of diabetes which yields to adequate therapy with thiamine, although the response is often a slow one. Thiamine, riboflavin and nicotinic acid are known to play essential parts in the enzymatic processes of carbohydrate metabolism and other components of the B complex are possibly just as essential. Thiamine deficiency results in a diminution of an essential co-carboxylase, diphosphothiamine, and the failure of the carbohydrate to be metabolized past the pyruvic acid phase which follows is detected by finding excessive amounts of pyruvic acid—one of the most active of all the intermediary metabolites—in the blood. This abnormal state is intensified by increasing the carbohydrate intake. Normal conditions are restored following the administration of thiamine and prolonged control of the diabetes.

A recommended practice of giving more than the normal requirement of vitamins to diabetic patients is based on the clinical improvement observed as a result of it and that by doing so neuropathic changes may be prevented.

Refinements in the industrial processing of foods have reduced their vitamin content. This is especially so in the commercial preparation of grains and vegetables and justifies using vitamin-enriched foods and, when advisable, the prescription of supplementary vitamins. Vitamin E has not influenced the insulin requirement favorably, in contradiction to publicity to this effect.

Minerals. *Sodium chloride* is provided in adequate amounts in the usual diet for uncomplicated diabetes. As ketosis appears and progresses unfavorably, the loss of sodium chloride may reach grave proportions. Sodium chloride administered early in the treatment of ketosis is an effective supplementary measure in preventing peripheral vascular collapse.

Calcium and *potassium* also are present in adequate amounts in the usual diet for the uncomplicated diabetic. Great losses of both of these minerals occur in ketosis. Decalcification of the bones is common in the elderly diabetic. The inclusion of a pint of whole milk or skim milk in the daily diet for the adult and a quart of whole milk for the child will prevent calcium and potassium depletion in the absence of complications. Special consideration is given to the potassium intake in ketotic patients (see p. 881), in whom a hypopotassemia may be fatal.

Choline, or a combination of choline, methionine and inositol, (methischol) is administered three or four times daily in cases in which there is enlargement of the liver due to deposits of fat. This measure speeds the benefit that will in any case follow adequate control of the diabetes.

DIET THERAPY

Introduction. The treatment of the diabetic patient embraces the control of the physiologic disturbances, in so far as this is practicable, and the guiding and reassuring of the patient in the readjustments which are inevitable with the onset or disclosure of a chronic and, to all intents and purposes, an incurable disease which still carries, to the uninformed, grim stigmata of the past. Reassurance and instruction, especially concerning the diabetes, are important until the patient understands that he will not be starved; that he will be relieved of his symptoms; that he can anticipate a nearly normal life expectancy; that he, himself, will be the helmsman in conducting the treatment—a most reassuring feature when he is qualified to be his own helmsman—and that he will not need to change his occupation, except in rare instances, or give up customary activities.

In short, diabetes, though it is a chronic disease, is controllable and the changes for the patient will be: improved health, the adoption of a more uniform plan of eating and exercising from day to day, and the administration of insulin, or oral therapy, if necessary.

Reassurance, in the early days of his diabetes, when he is apt to be needlessly concerned, is an important phase of the preparation of the patient for a lifetime plan of treatment. The psychologic aspect and the physiologic therapy are inseparable.

The treatment for diabetes is not a simple one and, while a certain degree of uniformity exists in the measures employed, no two patients will be treated in identically the same manner. The *objectives* are to provide relief from symptoms; to restore, as nearly as is practicable, a normal physiologic state with freedom from hyperglycemia, glycosuria, hyperlipemia and hypercholesterolemia; to promote normal development physically and mentally; to restore and maintain a high standard of nutrition and stabilize the body weight at a desirable level; to prevent complications and to reduce the risks to which patients with diabetes are exposed, e.g., infections, surgery, pregnancy and accidents; and to have these patients partake of varied activities which will culminate in an enjoyment of a full life. A due regard for the patient as a whole, and not only for his blood sugar level and glycosuria, is important.

Blood sugar values restored to and maintained within the normal range of fluctuation can have none other than a good result when wisely done. It is true that in some cases too strenuous efforts to maintain a normal blood sugar increase the risk of hypoglycemic reactions. However, the proper distribution of the diet and the correct selection and combination of insulins, tolbutamide therapy when indicated (see p. 854) and the exercise of good clinical judgment will go far in solving these problems. In most cases the glycosuria will subside with proper treatment and the immediate symptoms of diabetes will be abruptly stopped.

The means available for correcting the physiologic disturbances associated with diabetes are (1) dietary management, (2) insulin, (3) oral therapy, (4) training of the patient, (5) exercise, (6) general care, and (7) miscellaneous measures.

Treatment is most effective if the initial phase is carried out in a hospital with the patient on an ambulatory basis. A few days—usually four or five—suffice to interrupt improper dieting at home, to gain an acquaintance with the characteristics of the individual, to institute treatment under controlled conditions, to evaluate the diabetes and decide on the most suitable measures, to observe the initial response to these measures and—of greatest importance—to train the patient in diet management, drug therapy—insulin, tolbutamide, chlorpropamide or phenformin—testing the urine and special hygiene.

The initial treatment conducted at the physician's office is time-consuming and often doomed to failure. In the unusual instance, however, in which properly trained office personnel are available, the effort may succeed. We know of nothing, however, that has such a lasting impression on these patients as the hospital routine and training, and we know of no patient who regretted having had this experience.

Diet. Every diabetic patient should be diet conscious. He should be aware of the degree of flexibility of the diet permitted and he should understand why there should be quantitative uniformity in diet and regularity of mealtime from day to day. The objectives of the diet therapy for diabetics are: adequate *calories* to restore and maintain a near-normal body weight; a normal or slightly higher than normal *protein* intake with slight restriction in the *carbohydrate* with sufficient *fat* to provide the calories not provided by the protein and carbohydrate. There should be no shortchanging in minerals nor vitamins, and finally, when the optimum diet distribution is decided upon, this plan should be adhered to from day to day. To eat a large breakfast and small lunch one day and the reverse on the next would create undesirable fluctuations of the blood sugar.

DIET PRESCRIPTION IN THE ABSENCE OF ACUTE COMPLICATION. The initial diet is, at best, a trial diet and alterations are necessary, in most cases, as circumstances change. The dietary requirements will vary with sex, age, growth, body build and weight, activities, response to treatment, the severity of the diabetes—and whether the patient needs insulin or oral therapy or not—and complications. There is no permanently fixed diet for the individual but one which is subject to changes as circumstances dictate. However, the aim is to arrive at the diet which will meet all essential requirements and be relatively uniform from day to day.

Total Calories. The total caloric value of the diet is important when dealing with the dietary needs of the diabetic patient, and changes in the total caloric content of the diet have a far-reaching effect on the control of the diabetes. These features are exemplified especially in the treatment of the overweight patients, who comprise over 80 per cent of the new diabetic patients seen month after month by general practitioners. This is a fact that might easily be overlooked when it is realized that most medical writings on the subject of diabetes deal with patients who need tolbutamide or insulin. The most satisfactorily effective manner of controlling the diabetes in overweight patients is to reduce their weight by means of a reduced caloric intake. The untreated obese diabetic patient has a mild diabetes despite the degree of hyperglycemia and, barring acute complications, control of the diabetes can be maintained readily by reducing the caloric intake sufficiently to accomplish a slow reduction in weight.

The American Diabetes Association, through its Educational Committee, is fostering a uniform method of prescribing diets for diabetic patients. With some modification, the following plan conforms with their recommendations, except that here we employ measures to reduce the obese patient more rapidly and we allow more protein and more carbohydrate in the diets and hence, less fat.

(a) To estimate the approximate basic caloric requirement for twenty-four hours, multiply the ideal body weight (see Appendix) in pounds* by 10. Add 100 to 200 calories if the patient is a young tall male; deduct 100 to 200 calories if the patient is elderly, short, or female; or *if the patient is obese deduct 200 to 400 calories.* (b) For a patient with *ordinary light* activities the diet should usually provide 30 per cent more than the basal calories (see illustrative diets).

Example: Female patient fifty-five years of age, ideal weight 140 pounds, light activity:

Multiply ideal weight by 10 (140 × 10)	1400 calories
Correction for age and sex; deduct	100 calories
Basal calories	1300 calories
Add 30 per cent	390 calories
Maintenance diet (Total)	1690 calories

Protein. Multiply the ideal weight in pounds by ⅝ to determine the protein in grams—children will need higher quotas of protein (Chapter 16).

Carbohydrate. The carbohydrate allowance is influenced by the total calories permitted and the severity of the diabetes and, in particular, by whether or not insulin or tolbutamide therapy is needed. Accordingly, the plan of prescribing this dietary component is as follows:

(a) *Carbohydrate allowance—100 to 125 gm.—for the obese diabetic receiving a low caloric intake and neither insulin nor other hypoglycemic agent.* As the diabetes is controlled and the body weight is reduced, additions are made at varying intervals until the diet contains 225 to 300 gm. of carbohydrate, if these amounts do not cause hyperglycemia and glycosuria, in which case lesser amounts, 200 to 250 gm., are employed.

(b) *Carbohydrate allowance—250 gm.—for the patient who is underweight or normal weight and who needs insulin or an oral hypoglycemic agent, increases to 250 or 275 gm. are desirable.* A quota as high as 300 gm. is permitted if this liberal allowance does not appreciably increase the difficulty in controlling the diabetes.

Fat. The balance of the calories not provided by protein and carbohydrate are made up with fat, e.g., a diet containing 100 gm. protein 275 gm. carbo-

* Pounds are used in preference to kilograms. This is done without sacrifice of any benefit and because scales for weighing purposes on this continent record weights in pounds and because the computation of kilograms from pounds is avoided.

hydrate and 2200 calories will need 77 gm. of fat, viz.,

Protein	100 gm.	400 calories
Carbohydrate	275 gm.	1100 calories
	Total	1500 calories

Balance of calories to be made up with fat: 2200 − 1500 = 700 calories: 700 ÷ 9 = 77 gm. of fat.

The prescription of the diet may be simplified by merely deciding upon the total calories and adopting the standard diet outlined in Table 15 (see p. 822), in which the total calories most nearly approximate that of the prescribed diet.

ILLUSTRATIVE DIET PRESCRIPTIONS. *Obese patient,* female, aged fifty-five years, actual weight 180 pounds, ideal weight 136 pounds, light activity.

Multiply ideal weight by 10 (136 × 10)	1360 calories
Correction for age, sex, degree of obesity; deduct	400 calories
	960 calories
Add 30 per cent for light activity	288 calories
Total	1248 calories

As diet No. III (p. 825) approximates this total caloric value it may be selected without further calculation. It will be found to check closely. However, the diet prescription may be carried on to include protein and carbohydrate, viz.:

Protein	⅝ × 136	85 gm.
Carbohydrate		130 gm.

Fat = 1248 − 860 = 388 calories: 388 ÷ 9 = 43 gm.

Patient of normal weight, male, age thirty-two, actual weight 150 pounds, ideal weight 150 pounds, light activity and receiving insulin or tolbutamide.

Multiply ideal weight by 10 (150 × 10)	1500 calories
Correction for age and sex; add	200 calories
	1700 calories
Add 30 per cent for light activity	510 calories
Total	2210 calories

The total calories, as calculated, most closely approach that of Diet No. VIII (p. 830) hence this diet can be prescribed without further calculation. Or, if the entire diet prescription is computed it would be as follows:

Protein	⅝ × 150	93 gm.
Carbohydrate (250 to 275 gm.)		275 gm.

Fat = 2210 − 1472 = 438 calories: 438 ÷ 9 = 48 gm.

The difference between the diet calculated in this manner, and Diet No. VIII, or Diet No. VII, is not sufficient to be of great clinical significance.

Underweight patient, female, age eighteen, actual weight 96 pounds, ideal weight 132 pounds, quite active and requires insulin or oral therapy.

Multiply ideal weight by 10 (132 × 10)	1320 calories
Correction for age and sex; deduct	100 calories
	1220 calories
Correction for activity 75 per cent; add	915 calories
Total	2135 calories

The total calories as estimated most closely approximate those of Diet No. VII (p. 829). This diet may be employed without additional calculation. However, individual calculation of the other dietary components would indicate:

Protein	⅝ × 132	80 gm.
Carbohydrate		260 gm.

Fat = 2135 − 1360 = 775 calories; 775 ÷ 9 = 86 gm.

Adjustments in the diets are made as indications arise after the initial stages of therapy.

In the case of the obese patient the rate of the reduction of body weight may be slowed up to a pound or two per month as soon as the diabetes is controlled. Suitable increases in the total caloric allowance of the diet are made to secure this end. When the body weight reaches the standard level, which may require several months, further increases are made to prevent little if any further decrease in weight. Return to an obese state would restore the hazards which accompany it.

It is important that the intake of certain vital food factors should not be reduced beyond the minimal requirements. This involves the selection of protein of high biologic value—containing all the essential amino acids—for normal tissue synthesis and precursors of vitamins they supply. Also, as indicated on page 812, the diabetic patient may need more of the vitamin B complex than do normal persons.

DISTRIBUTION OF MEALS IN RELATION TO INSULIN THERAPY. Appropriate distribution of meals permits better control of the diabetes and decreases remarkably the risk of hypoglycemic reactions. The accomplishment of these desirable features and the allowance of an adequate diet with great flexibility in the choice of foods comprise our chief reason for adhering to a form of therapy that comes close to physiologic control of the diabetes. This is in preference to measures which permit unwarranted degrees of hyperglycemia and glycosuria.

These dietary considerations may appear confusing but they are based on well founded principles and have proved to be most satisfactory. Combinations of insulin therapy are common and by observing the simple plans of distributing the diet outlined, it will be observed that when the ideal program of insulin therapy is determined the distribution of the diet becomes automatic. In this manner decreases are made in meals preceding the period in which a hyperglycemia is likely and more liberal food intake is permitted preceding periods in which hypoglycemic reactions might otherwise occur.

1. For the diabetic receiving *no insulin* a portion is taken from the total diet for a bedtime nourishment. In the case of low caloric diets, e.g., Diet No. I (900 calories), this nourishment must necessarily be scant. In fact, a glass of skim milk—one milk exchange with the fat omitted—is all that is allowed on the diet referred to. But when 1100 calories are permitted, a bedtime nourishment of 1 graham cracker—½ of a bread exchange—is added as indicated in Diet No. II, page 824.

The diet, after the bedtime nourishment is deducted, is divided into three equal meals—for breakfast, lunch and supper, as indicated in Figure 13. The deduction of food from the main meals serves to decrease the peaks of demand for insulin and the evening nourishment aids in correcting and in preventing excessive hunger, a favorable feature when the diets are small, as is frequently the case when insulin is not needed.*

2. In cases in which *tolbutamide therapy* is employed, a bedtime nourishment—taken from the total diet before it is divided into three meals—is desirable for the same reasons given above, but also as a protective measure against possible hypoglycemic reactions during the night. This is a rare occurrence, but it can be prevented entirely.

3. With insulin therapy a simple plan of distributing the diet is to divide the total diet into three equal meals but from one or another meal a bread and a milk exchange (or other portion, provided it is the same on successive days)

* Except when the caloric value of the diet is very low, as in Diets No. I and No. II, the usual values for odd-time nourishments are: one milk and one bread exchange, e.g., one glass of milk and five saltine crackers.

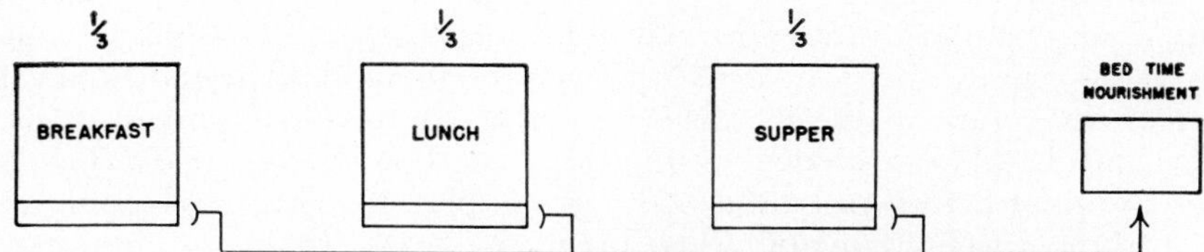

FIG. 13. Depicts the deduction of a nourishment from the total diet for a bedtime nourishment. This method of dividing the diet is employed:

A. When no insulin is needed (see Diets I, II, III and IV, on pages 823 to 826).

B. When a combination of regular and protamine zinc insulin—separately or mixed—is given before breakfast with a dose of regular insulin before supper (very unusual).

is taken for consumption at a time when it serves the purpose of preventing a hypoglycemia (Table 14, see p. 822).

In cases of labile diabetes, maximum protection is provided by taking an appropriate portion from each meal for a nourishment at 11 A.M., 3:30 to 4:30 P.M. and at bedtime.

When an *intermediate insulin*—globin, NPH (isophane) or lente—is given before breakfast, a late afternoon nourishment between 3:30 and 4:30 P.M. is prescribed. With the greatest degree of insulin activity before the evening meal, this is an important precautionary measure against a hypoglycemia at this time. Also, it permits a larger dose of insulin, the effect of which is more likely to carry over to the following morning than would be the case if the protective nourishment were not given. If an intermediate insulin only is given before breakfast, the afternoon (3:30 to 4:30 P.M.) nourishment is subtracted from the breakfast. This, by reducing the breakfast, aids in preventing a hyperglycemia during the forenoon, which would be likely because of the delay in the action of the insulin.

Occasional patients tend to have hypoglycemic reactions during the night while taking an intermediate insulin before breakfast. In these cases a nourishment given at bedtime is also desirable. A portion of the evening meal may be saved for this purpose or an "extra" allowance, though uniform from day to day, may be given at this time.

A small dose of one of the intermediate insulins is frequently given after supper, in which case a bedtime nourishment taken from the evening meal is protective against hypoglycemic reactions during the night.

A *long acting insulin*—protamine zinc or ultra-lente—given before breakfast has its greatest apparent effect between midnight and breakfast. Hypoglycemic reactions are guarded against by a bedtime nourishment. This may be "extra" in excess of the prescribed diet, but it is usually given in the form of a bread and milk exchange subtracted from the breakfast.

Simplified Method of Completing the Menu from a Prescribed Diet as Outlined for the Patient. The essentials in transposing the information contained in a diet prescription to a menu with the amount of each food for each meal are:

1. A prescription for a diet, e.g., protein 90 gm., carbohydrate 210 gm., and fat 55 gm. (1700 calories).

2. A familiarity with household measuring devices—*8-ounce measuring cup, a teaspoon and tablespoon.* Level and not heaped measures are referred to.

3. Special information about foods.

a. Diets for diabetics are such that no special "diabetic foods" are necessary—the same foods used for the family are best. Use in appropriate amounts milk, vegetables, meats, fats and fruits without added sugar. (Indeed, some of the diets high in carbohydrate may contain sugar, but this is an individual consideration and one to be settled by the physician.)

b. Seasoning of foods is the same as for the nondiabetic when the following agents are used: chopped parsley, mint, garlic, onion, celery, salt, nutmeg, mustard, cinnamon, pepper and other spices, lemon, saccharine and vinegar.

c. You may use freely, and without reducing your "diet account," coffee, tea, clear broth, bouillon (without fat), gelatin (unsweetened), rennet tablets, pickles (sour, or unsweetened dill), cranberries and rhubarb.

4. A working knowledge of the source of food components. *Carbohydrate* foods are fruits, cereals, breads, vegetables, etc. *Protein* foods are meat, eggs, milk, nuts, etc. *Fat* foods are butter, cream, margarine and olive oil.

These food components may overlap. For instance, while milk is considered a protein food it also contains fat and carbohydrate. Also, bread and cereals are carbohydrate foods but contain some protein. This overlapping has complicated diet problems in the past but with the adoption of the Exchange System it is now a simple matter to make an appropriate menu from a prescribed diet.

5. A familiarity with the Exchange System* which is summarized in Table 12.

MILK EXCHANGES—LIST 1

One exchange of milk contains 12 gm. carbohydrate, 8 gm. protein, 10 gm. fat and 170 calories.

Milk is one of our most important foods. You can use the milk on your meal plan to drink, in coffee, on cereal, or with other foods.

This list shows the different types of milk to use for one exchange:

TYPE OF MILK	GM.	AMOUNT TO USE
Whole milk (plain or homogenized)	240	1 cup
* Skim milk	240	1 cup
Evaporated milk (undiluted)	120	½ cup
Powdered whole milk	35	¼ cup
* Powdered skim milk (Non-fat dried milk)	35	¼ cup
Buttermilk (made from whole milk)	240	1 cup
* Buttermilk (made from skim milk)	240	1 cup

You can use one type of milk instead of another. For example, you may use one-half cup evaporated milk in place of one cup of whole milk.

* You may wish to use skim milk or buttermilk made from skim milk instead of whole milk. Skim milk and buttermilk have the same food values as whole milk except they contain less fat. Add 2 fat exchanges to your meal when you use one cup of skim milk or buttermilk made from skim milk.

VEGETABLE EXCHANGES—LIST 2

All vegetables contain sugar but some have more sugar than others. The vegetables have been divided into three groups according to the amount of sugar they have:

List 2A vegetables have the smallest amount of sugar.

List 2B vegetables contain more sugar.

List 4 contains some vegetables which have a large amount of sugar.

VEGETABLE EXCHANGES A

(Contain little carbohydrate, protein or calories)

You may eat as much of these vegetables raw as you wish, except tomatoes. (Limit tomatoes to one tomato or ½ cup tomato juice at a meal). If these vegetables are cooked, you can use as much as one cup at a time. When you want more, you can use another cup of these vegetables in exchange for a list 2B vegetable.

Asparagus
* Broccoli
Brussels sprouts
Cabbage
Cauliflower
Celery
* Chicory
Cucumbers
* Escarole
Eggplant

* GREENS
Beet greens
Chard
Collard
Dandelion
Kale
Mustard
Spinach
Turnip greens
Lettuce

Mushrooms
Okra
* Pepper
Radishes
Sauerkraut
String beans, young
Summer squash
* Tomatoes
* Watercress

* These vegetables contain significant amounts of vitamin A.

VEGETABLE EXCHANGES B

(Contain 7 grams carbohydrate, 2 grams protein and 35 calories)

These vegetables contain more sugar than the vegetables in List 2A. You may use these vegetables raw or cooked. One half cup constitutes one helping. One cup cooked vegetables from list 2A may be substituted for ½ cup, or 1 serving of a 2B vegetable. The approximate weight of one serving is 100 grams.

Beets
* Carrots
Onions
Peas, green

Pumpkin
Rutabagas
* Squash, winter
Turnip

* These vegetables are rich in vitamin A.

* Meal planning has been simplified by the introduction of the "Exchange System" through the cooperative efforts of the American Diabetes and American Dietetic Associations, and the Diabetes Branch, Public Health Service, Federal Security Agency. Copies with illustrative photographs of average helpings can be purchased from the American Dietetic Association, 620 N. Michigan Ave., Chicago 11, or from American Diabetes, Inc., 1 E. 45th St., New York 17.

TABLE 12. COMPOSITION OF FOOD EXCHANGES

LIST	FOOD	MEASURES	GM.	P	C	F	CAL.
1	Milk Exchange	½ pint	240	8	12	10	170
2a	Vegetable Exchange	as desired					
2b	Vegetable Exchange	½ cup	100	2	7	..	36
3	Fruit Exchange	varies	...	..	10	..	40
4	Bread Exchange	varies	...	2	15	..	68
5	Meat Exchange	1 oz.	30	7	..	5	73
6	Fat Exchange	1 tsp.	5	..	..	5	45

You may serve vegetables plain or with part of the meat or fat exchange for seasoning. You may wish to use the vegetables, milk, and meat exchanges in your meal plan together. In this way you can make soups, stews or other dishes.

For salads you may use mayonnaise or French dressing as your fat exchange. (For example, if you use 1 teaspoon of mayonnaise you would give up 1 fat exchange.)

FRUIT EXCHANGES—LIST 3

One exchange of fruit contains 10 grams carbohydrate and 40 calories

Each exchange of fruit shown below contains about the same amount of sugar. Your meal plan will tell you how many exchanges you can have each day. You may use your fruit fresh, dried, cooked, canned or frozen as long as no sugar has been added. Look at the label on the can or package to be sure it indicates "unsweetened" or "no sugar added."

This list shows the different amounts of fruits to use for one fruit exchange:

	MEAS.	GM.
Apple	1 small (2″ diam.)	80
Applesauce	½ cup	100
Apricots, fresh	2 medium	100
Apricots, dried	4 halves	20
Banana	½ small	50
Berries: Straw., * Rasp., Black	1 cup	150
* Blueberries	⅔ cup	100
Cantaloupe	¼ (6″ diam.)	200
Cherries	10 large	75
Dates	2	15
Figs, fresh	2 large	50
Figs, dried	1 small	15
* Grapefruit	½ small	125
* Grapefruit juice	½ cup	100
Grapes	12	75
Grape juice	¼ cup	60
Honeydew melon	⅛ (7″ diam.)	150
Mango	½ small	70
* Orange	1 small	100
* Orange juice	½ cup	100
Papaya	⅓ medium	100
Peach	1 medium	100
Pear	1 small	100
Pineapple	½ cup	80
Pineapple juice	⅓ cup	80
Plums	2 medium	100
Prunes, dried	2 medium	25
Raisins	2 tbsp.	15
* Tangerine	1 large	100
Watermelon	1 cup	175

For variety a fruit as a salad or with unsweetened gelatin may be served as a dessert.

* These fruits are rich sources of vitamin C; use at least one serving each day.

BREAD EXCHANGES—LIST 4

One bread exchange contains 15 grams carbohydrate, 2 grams protein and 70 calories.

For each bread exchange called for on your meal plan, choose any one item on the list below.

For example:

½ cup cooked cereal provides 1 Bread Exchange.

1 slice bread and 1 small potato provides 2 Bread Exchanges.

1 slice bread and ½ cup cooked rice and ⅓ cup corn provides 3 Bread Exchanges.

This list shows the different amounts of foods to use for one bread exchange.

	MEAS.	GM.
Bread	1 slice	25
Biscuit, roll	1 (2″ diam.)	35
Muffin	1 (2″ diam.)	35
Cornbread	1 (1½″ cube)	35
Flour	2½ tbsp.	20
Cereal, cooked	½ cup	100
Cereal, dry (flake & puffed)	¾ cup	100
Rice, grits, cooked	½ cup	100
Spaghetti, noodles, etc., cooked	½ cup	100
Crackers, graham (2½″ sq.)	2	20
Oyster	20 (½ cup)	20
Saltines (2″ sq.)	5	20
Soda (2½″ sq.)	3	20
Round, thin (1½″ diam.)	6–8	20
Vegetables		
Beans & peas, dried, cooked (lima, navy, split pea, cowpeas, etc.)	½ cup	90
Baked beans, no pork	¼ cup	50
Corn	⅓ cup	80
Parsnips	⅔ cup	125
Potatoes, white, baked, boiled	1 (2″ diam.)	100
Potatoes, white, mashed	½ cup	100
Potatoes, sweet, or yams	¼ cup	50
Sponge cake, plain	1 (1½″ cube)	25
Ice cream (Omit 2 fat exchanges)	¼ pint	70

Use these foods carefully because they contain considerable amounts of sugar.

Measure all the foods on the bread exchange list after they have been cooked.

Whole grain (dark) or enriched breads and cereals are good sources of iron and the B vitamins. Plan to use them often in your meal plan. They are better for you than white crackers, rice, or spaghetti that do not have the vitamins added.

MEAT EXCHANGES—LIST 5

One meat exchange contains 7 grams protein, 5 grams fat and 75 calories

You may have any kind of meat you wish. Cheese, eggs and peanut butter can be taken in place of meat for variety.

For each meat exchange called for on your meal plan choose any one item on the list below.

For example:

1 Egg provides 1 Meat Exchange.

1 ounce Cheese and 1 ounce Ham provides 2 Meat Exchanges.

1 Egg and ¼ cup Cottage Cheese and 1 slice Bologna provides 3 Meat Exchanges.

This list shows the different amounts of foods to use for one meat exchange:

	MEAS.	GM.
Meat & poultry (med. fat) . . . (beef, lamb, pork, liver, chicken, etc.)	1 oz.	30
Cold cuts (4½″ sq., ⅛″ thick)	1 slice	45
Frankfurter	1 (8–9/lb.)	50
Fish: Cod, mackerel, etc	1 oz.	30
Salmon, tuna, crab	¼ cup	30
Oysters, shrimp, clams	5 small	45
Sardines	3 medium	30
Cheese, cheddar, American	1 oz.	30
Cottage	¼ cup	45
Egg	1	50
Peanut butter	2 tbsp.	30

You may use the meat or fish, etc., that is prepared for the family as long as no fat or flour has been added. If you wish to fry the meat, you may do so with the fat you are allowed on your meal plan. Meat juices with the fat removed may be used with the meat or vegetables for added flavor.

FAT EXCHANGES—LIST 6

One fat exchange contains 5 grams fat and 45 calories

All fat foods are high in calories. Too much fat or too much of any food may cause you to gain weight. A person with diabetes should try to reach his ideal weight. If he weighs too much his diabetes will be harder to control.

Use the foods on this list only as allowed on your meal plan.

You may use your fat exchanges in preparing such foods as vegetables and meats. For example, if you use a teaspoon of fat to fry an egg give up one fat exchange.

For each fat exchange called for on your meal plan choose any one item on the list below.

For example:

1 teaspoon butter provides 1 Fat Exchange.

1 teaspoon margarine and 1 slice bacon provides 2 Fat Exchanges.

This list shows the different foods to use for one fat exchange.

	MEAS.	GM.
Butter or margarine	1 tsp.	5
Bacon, crisp	1 slice	10
Cream, light, 20%	2 tbsp.	30
Cream, heavy, 40%	1 tbsp.	15
Cream cheese	1 tbsp.	15
French dressing	1 tbsp.	15
Mayonnaise	1 tsp.	5
Oil or cooking fat	1 tsp.	5
Nuts	6 small	10
Olives	5 small	50
Avocado	⅛ (4″ diam.)	25

6. A familiarity with the means and advantages of a varied dietary. The recipes included in the patients' pamphlet as prepared by the American Diabetes and American Diabetic Associations are included in the prospect that that they will be helpful as examples in this respect.

Making the Menu. *Illustration:* Diet Prescription: Protein 90 gm.; carbohydrate 210 gm.; fat 55 gm.; and 1700 calories. (Standard Diet No. V, p. 827).

Step I: Divide the day's protein, fat and carbohydrate allowances into approximately three equal meals.* Example—

Protein	$90 \div 3 = 30$ gm.
Fat	$55 \div 3 = 18$ to 19 gm.
Carbohydrate	$210 \div 3 = 70$ gm.

Step II: Plan the menu for each meal.

Example: (a) List the foods desired for breakfast as designated in column A, Table 13.

(b) Insert the exchange from which each food is taken as in column B and for convenience add the list number of each as in column C.

Step III: Adjust the amounts (the number of exchanges) until they fill the total for each dietary component as in

* Unequal distribution of the diet is often indicated. This is discussed on pages 817 and 818 and illustrated in the standard diets on pages 823 to 833.

TABLE 13. ILLUSTRATIVE MENU FOR BREAKFAST

A	B	C	D	E
Eggs	Meat exchange	list #5	2	2 . . . . eggs
Bread	Bread exchange	list #4	3	3 slices . . . . . bread
Butter	Fat exchange	list #6	1	1 tsp. . . . . . . butter
Milk	Milk exchange	list #1	1	1 cup . . . . . . milk
Fruit	Fruit exchange	list #3	1½	1½ serving . . . . fruit

TABLE 14. ILLUSTRATION OF COMPLETED MENU

	NO. EXCHANGES	HOUSEHOLD MEASURE	WEIGHT GRAMS	P.	F.	C.
Breakfast						
Meat	2	2 eggs		14	10	—
Bread	3	3 sl.	75	6	—	45
Fat	1	1 tsp.	5	—	5	—
Milk, skim	1	1 c.	240	8	—	12
Fruit	1½	1½ serv.	See list 3	—	—	15
				28	15	72
Lunch or supper						
Meat	2	2 oz.	60	14	10	—
Bread	3	3 sl.	75	6	—	45
Fat	2	2 tsp.	10	—	10	—
Vegetable	2A	1 serv.	100	—	—	—
Vegetable	2B	1 serv.	100	2	—	7
Milk, skim	1	1 c.	240	8	—	12
Fruit	1	1 serv.	See list 3	—	—	10
Evening or main meal				30	20	74
Meat	3	3 oz.	90	21	15	—
Bread	3	3 sl.	75	6	—	45
Fat	1	1 tsp.	5	—	5	—
Vegetable	2A	1 serv.	100	—	—	—
Vegetable	2B	1 serv.	100	2	—	7
Fruit	1½	1½ serv.	See list 3	—	—	15
				29	20	67
		Day's Total		87	55	213

column D. This procedure is expedited by completing the *carbohydrate* quota first, then the *protein*, and lastly the *fat*. The foods and amount of each which are selected to use up the exchanges allowed are listed in column E. The completed menu is presented in Table 14.

Standard Diet Prescriptions. Diet prescriptions, as indicated in Table 15, aid in simplifying the treatment of diabetic patients. For uncomplicated diabetes they serve admirably but they should not be used at the expense of more intensive individualization, which may be highly desirable during the course of complicating diseases, e.g., duodenal ulcer, hepatitis, etc. The diet prescription may be suitable in such cases but the food components and the distribution of the diet are altered to meet the individual's needs, and appropriate changes are made in the insulin therapy to maintain good control of the diabetes.

TABLE 15. STANDARD DIET PRESCRIPTIONS

	PROTEIN	CARBOHYDRATE	FAT	CALORIES
I	75	100	22	900
II	80	120	33	1100
III	85	130	49	1300
IV	90	180	47	1500
V	90	210	55	1700
VI	90	230	69	1900
VII	95	260	75	2100
VIII	95	280	89	2300
IX	100	300	100	2500
X	110	320	109	2700
XI	120	335	120	2900

Eleven standard diet prescriptions are filled in this table. Diets III, IV, V and VI are suitable for the initial treatment in the majority of cases and for the more permanent programs diets VI, VII and VIII suffice for the majority of the adult patients. It will be noted that (a) the protein and carbohydrate allowances in the more permanent diets are more liberal than formerly used and (b) the fat content is kept below 100 grams except in the three high caloric diets.

Diet No. I—900 Calories

Protein 75 gm.; Fat 22 gm.; Carb. 100 gm.

Division of diet: approximately $\frac{1}{3}$ for each meal with a bedtime nourishment

NO. EXCHANGES	FOOD EXCHANGE	LIST NO.	SAMPLE MENU	HOUSEHOLD MEAS.	WT. GM.	P	F	C	CAL.
Breakfast									
2	Meat	5	Eggs	2		14	10	—	146
1	Bread	4	Bread	1 sl.	25	2	—	15	68
1	Fruit	3	Orange	1 sm.	100	—	—	10	40
$\frac{1}{4}$	Milk	1	Skim milk	$\frac{1}{4}$ c.	60	2	—	3	20
				Total		18	10	28	274
Lunch or supper									
3	Meat	5	*Roast beef (lean)	3 oz.	90	21	9	—	165
1	Bread	4	Bread	1 sl.	25	2	—	15	68
1	Vegetable	2A	String beans, young	$\frac{1}{2}$ c.	100	—	—	—	—
$\frac{1}{2}$	Milk	1	Skim milk	$\frac{1}{2}$ c.	120	4	—	6	40
1	Fruit	3	Peach	1 med.	100	—	—	10	40
				Total		27	9	31	313
Dinner or main meal									
2	Meat	5	Broiled liver	2 oz.	60	14	6	—	110
$\frac{1}{2}$	Bread	4	Bread	$\frac{1}{2}$ sl.	13	1	—	8	36
1	Vegetable	2A	Lettuce and cucumber		100	—	—	—	—
1	Milk	1	Skim milk	1 c.	240	8	—	12	80
1	Fruit	3	Strawberries	1 c.	150	—	—	10	40
				Total		23	6	30	266
Nourishment									
1	Milk	1	Skim milk	1 c.	240	8	—	12	80
				Day's total		76	25	101	933

* Visible fat removed.

Note: sm.—small; med.—medium; lg.—large; oz.—ounce; tbsp.—tablespoon; tsp.—teaspoon; c.—cup; sl.—slice.

This low calorie diet (900 calories) is used as a temporary measure to permit a reduction in the weight of the obese diabetic patient. A nourishment has been taken from the total diet for use at bedtime. Ordinarily patients receiving this diet are not taking insulin.

Diet No. II—1100 Calories

Protein 80 gm.; Fat 33 gm.; Carb. 120 gm.

Division of diet: approximately $\frac{1}{3}$ for each meal with a bedtime nourishment

NO. EXCHANGES	FOOD EXCHANGE	LIST NO.	SAMPLE MENU	HOUSEHOLD MEAS.	WT. GM.	P	F	C	CAL.
Breakfast									
2	Meat	5	Eggs	2		14	10	—	146
1	Bread	4	Bread	1 sl.	25	2	—	15	68
$\frac{3}{4}$	Milk	1	Skim milk	$\frac{3}{4}$ c.	180	6	—	9	60
1	Fruit	3	Cantaloupe	$\frac{1}{4}$ med.	200	—	—	10	40
				Total		22	10	34	314
Lunch or supper									
2	Meat	5	Cottage cheese	$\frac{1}{2}$ c.	90	14	10	—	146
1	Vegetable	2A	Tomato and lettuce	1	100	—	—	—	—
1	Bread	4	Muffin	1	35	2	—	15	68
$\frac{3}{4}$	Milk	1	Skim milk	$\frac{3}{4}$ c.	180	6	—	9	60
1	Fruit	3	Applesauce	$\frac{1}{2}$ c.	100	—	—	10	40
				Total		22	10	34	314
Dinner or main meal									
3	Meat	5	Roast lamb	3 oz.	90	21	15	—	219
1	Vegetable	2A	Spinach	$\frac{1}{2}$ c.	100	—	—	—	—
1	Vegetable	2B	Pickled beets	$\frac{1}{2}$ c.	100	2	—	7	36
1	Bread	4	Bread	1 sl.	25	2	—	15	68
1	Fruit	3	Apricots	2 med.	100	—	—	10	40
				Total		25	15	32	363
Nourishment									
1	Milk	1	Skim milk	1 c.	240	8	—	12	80
$\frac{1}{2}$	Bread	4	Graham cracker	1	10	1	—	8	36
				Total		9	—	20	116
				Day's Total		78	35	120	1107

For key to abbreviations see footnote, p. 823.

As in the case of the first diet (900 calories) this diet—1100 calories—is also employed to reduce body weight of obese diabetic patients. A nourishment, deducted from the total diet, is taken at bedtime. Ordinarily this diet is not supplemented with insulin therapy.

Diet No. III—1300 Calories
Protein 85 gm.; Fat 49 gm.; Carb. 130 gm.
Division of diet: approximately $\frac{1}{3}$ for each meal with a bedtime nourishment

NO. EXCHANGES	FOOD EXCHANGE	LIST NO.	SAMPLE MENU	HOUSEHOLD MEAS.	WT. GM.	P	F	C	CAL.
Breakfast									
2	Meat	5	Eggs	2		14	10	—	146
1	Bread	4	Bread	1 sl.	25	2	—	15	68
1	Milk	1	Skim milk	1 c.	240	8	—	12	80
1	Fruit	1	Grapefruit	$\frac{1}{2}$ sm.	125	—	—	10	40
1	Fat	6	Butter	1 tsp.	5	—	5	—	45
				Total		24	15	37	379
Lunch or supper									
2	Meat	2	Cheese	2 oz.	60	14	10	—	146
1	Milk	1	Skim milk	1 c.	240	8	—	12	80
1	Vegetable	2A	Asparagus and lettuce	$\frac{1}{2}$ c.	100	—	—	—	—
1	Bread	4	Bread	1 sl.	25	2	—	15	68
1	Fat	6	Mayonnaise	1 tsp.	5	—	5	—	45
1	Fruit	3	Peach	1 med.	100	—	—	10	40
				Total		24	15	37	379
Dinner or main meal									
3	Meat	5	Roast chicken	3 oz.	90	21	15	—	219
1	Vegetable	2A	Cabbage	$\frac{1}{2}$ c.	100	—	—	—	—
1	Vegetable	2B	Peas, green	$\frac{1}{2}$ c.	100	2	—	7	36
1	Bread	4	Potato	1 sm.	100	2	—	15	68
1	Fat	6	Butter	1 tsp.	5	—	5	—	45
$1\frac{1}{2}$	Fruit	3	Plums	3 med.	150	—	—	15	60
				Total		25	20	37	428
Nourishment									
1	Milk	1	Skim milk	1 c.	240	8	—	12	80
$\frac{1}{2}$	Bread	4	Saltines	2–3	10	1	—	8	36
				Total		9	—	20	116
				Day's Total		82	50	131	1302

For key to abbreviations see footnote, p. 823.
Diet No. III is employed to reduce the body weight of obese diabetic patients who, barring acute complications, are not receiving insulin.

Diet No. IV—1500 Calories

Protein 90 gm.; Fat 47 gm.; Carb. 180 gm.

Division: approx. $\frac{1}{3}$ for each meal with a bedtime nourishment

NO. EXCHANGES	FOOD EXCHANGE	LIST NO.	SAMPLE MENU	HOUSEHOLD MEAS.	WT. GM.	P	F	C	CAL.
Breakfast									
2	Meat	5	Eggs	2		14	10	—	146
2	Bread	4	Bread	1 sl.	25	2	—	15	68
			Oatmeal	$\frac{1}{2}$ c.	100	2	—	15	68
1	Milk	1	Milk, skim	1 c.	240	8	—	12	80
1	Fat	6	Butter	1 tsp.	5	—	5	—	45
1	Fruit	3	Grapefruit juice	$\frac{1}{2}$ c.	100	—	—	10	40
				Total		26	15	52	447
Lunch or supper									
2	Meat	5	Frankfurter	2	100	14	10	—	146
1	Milk	1	Milk, skim	1 c.	240	8	—	12	80
1	Vegetable	2A	Sauerkraut	$\frac{1}{2}$ c.	100	—	—	—	—
2	Bread	4	Rolls	2 sm.	70	4	—	30	136
1	Fat	6	Butter	1 tsp.	5	—	5	—	45
1	Fruit	3	Applesauce	$\frac{1}{2}$ c.	100	—	—	10	40
				Total		26	15	52	447
Dinner or main meal									
3	Meat	5	Roast lamb	3 oz.	90	21	15	—	219
1	Vegetable	2A	Chard	$\frac{1}{2}$ c.	100	—	—	—	—
1	Vegetable	2B	Carrot strips	$\frac{1}{2}$ c.	100	2	—	7	36
2	Bread	4	Potato	1 sm.	100	2	—	15	68
			Bread	1 sl.	25	2	—	15	68
$1\frac{1}{2}$	Fruit	3	Watermelon	$1\frac{1}{2}$ c.	260	—	—	15	60
				Total		27	15	52	451
Nourishment									
1	Milk	1	Milk, skim	1 c.	240	8	—	12	80
1	Bread	4	Graham crackers	2	20	2	—	15	68
				Total		10	—	27	148
				Day's Total		89	45	183	1493

For key to abbreviations see footnote, p. 823.

Diet No. IV is employed temporarily when a slow or slight reduction in weight is indicated. Insulin therapy may or may not be used in conjunction with this diet.

Diet No. V—1700 Calories
Protein 90 gm.; Fat 55 gm.; Carb. 210 gm.
Division: approx. $\frac{1}{3}$ of diet for each meal*

NO. EXCHANGES	FOOD EXCHANGE	LIST NO.	SAMPLE MENU	HOUSEHOLD MEAS.	WT. GM.	P	F	C	CAL.
Breakfast									
2	Meat	5	Eggs	2		14	10	—	146
1	Fat	6	Butter	1 tsp.	5	—	5	—	45
2	Fruit	3	Banana	1 sm.	100	—	—	20	80
2½	Bread	4	Bread	1½ sl.	38	3	—	23	104
			Wheaties	**¾ c.**	**20**	**2**	—	**15**	**68**
1	Milk	1	**Milk, skim**	**1 c.**	**240**	**8**	—	**12**	**80**
				Total		27	15	70	523
Lunch or supper									
3	Meat	5	Egg	1	—	7	5	—	73
			Tuna	½ c.	60	14	10	—	146
1	Milk	1	Milk, skim	1 c.	240	8	—	12	80
1	Vegetable	2A	Lettuce	¼ head	100	—	—	—	—
1	Vegetable	2B	Pickled beets	½ c.	100	2	—	7	36
2	Bread	4	Bread	2 sl.	50	4	—	30	136
1	Fat	6	Butter	1 tsp.	5	—	5	—	45
2	Fruit	3	Tangerine	2 lg.	200	—	—	20	80
				Total		35	20	69	596
Dinner or main meal									
2	Meat	5	Mackerel	2 oz.	60	14	10	—	146
1	Vegetable	2A	Spinach	½ c.	100	—	—	—	—
1	Vegetable	2B	Onions	½ c.	100	2	—	7	36
1	Fat	6	Oil	1 tsp.	5	—	5	—	45
2	Fruit	3	Apricots	4 med.	200	—	—	20	80
3	Bread	4	Potato	2 sm.	200	4	—	30	136
			Bread	**1 sl.**	**25**	**2**	—	**15**	**68**
1	Meat	5	**Egg**	**1**	—	**7**	**5**	—	**73**
				Total		29	20	72	584
				Day's Total		91	55	211	1703

* Though this diet is divided into approximately three equal meals, a milk and a bread exchange are indicated in bold type in the breakfast and a bread and meat exchange in the dinner menus. One or both of these designated nourishments can be deducted from the respective meal and given at other times of the day in keeping with the insulin therapy as outlined on pages 817 to 818. The same provision is made in the subsequent diets VI to XI.

For key to abbreviations see footnote, p. 823.

Diet No. VI—1900 Calories
Protein 90 gm.; Fat 69 gm.; Carb. 230 gm.
Division: approx. $\frac{1}{3}$ of diet for each meal*

NO. EXCHANGES	FOOD EXCHANGE	LIST NO.	SAMPLE MENU	HOUSEHOLD MEAS.	WT. GM.	P	F	C	CAL.
Breakfast									
2	Meat	5	Eggs	2	—	14	10	—	146
2	Fat	6	Butter	2 tsp.	10	—	10	—	90
2	Fruit	3	Orange juice	1 c.	200	—	—	20	80
3	Bread	4	Bread	2 sl.	50	4	—	30	136
			Bread	**1 sl.**	**25**	**2**	—	**15**	**68**
1	Milk	1	**Milk, skim**	**1 c.**	**240**	**8**	—	**12**	**80**
				Total		28	20	77	600
Lunch or supper									
2	Meat	5	Oysters	10	90	14	10	—	146
1	Milk	1	Milk, skim	1 c.	240	8	—	12	80
1	Vegetable	2A	Mixed vegetable salad	$\frac{1}{2}$ c.	100	—	—	—	—
3	Bread	4	Oyster crackers	$\frac{1}{2}$ c.	20	2	—	15	68
		4	Bread	2 sl.	50	4	—	30	136
3	Fat	6	Butter	3 tsp.	15	—	15	—	135
2	Fruit	3	Peach	4 halves	200	—	—	20	80
				Total		28	25	77	645
Dinner or main meal									
2	Meat	5	Steak	2 oz.	60	14	10	—	146
1	Vegetable	2A	Tomato, sliced	1	100	—	—	—	—
1	Vegetable	2B	Peas, green	$\frac{1}{2}$ c.	100	2	—	7	36
2	Fat	6	Butter	2 tsp.	10	—	10	—	90
1	Fruit	3	Pear	1 sm.	100	—	—	10	40
4	Bread	—	Bread	3 sl.	75	6	—	45	204
			Bread	**1 sl.**	**25**	**2**	—	**15**	**68**
1	Meat	5	**Cheese**	**1 oz.**	**30**	**7**	**5**	—	**73**
				Total		31	25	77	657
				Day's Total		87	70	231	1902

* See footnote, p. 827.
For key to abbreviations see footnote, p. 823.

Diet No. VII—2100 Calories
Protein 95 gm.; Fat 75 gm.; Carb. 260 gm.
Division: approx. ⅓ of diet for each meal*

NO. EXCHANGES	FOOD EXCHANGE	LIST NO.	SAMPLE MENU	HOUSEHOLD MEAS.	WT. GM.	P	F	C	CAL.
Breakfast									
2	Meat	5	Eggs	2	—	14	10	—	146
1	Fat	6	Butter	1 tsp.	5	—	5	—	45
1½	Fruit	3	Prunes	3 med.	38	—	—	15	60
4	Bread	4	Bread	3 sl.	75	6	—	45	204
			Bread	**1 sl.**	**25**	**2**	—	**15**	**68**
1	Milk	1	**Milk, whole**	**1 c.**	**240**	**8**	**10**	**12**	**170**
				Total		30	25	87	693
Lunch or supper									
2	Meat	5	Cold cuts	2 sl.	90	14	10	—	146
1	Milk	1	Milk, whole	1 c.	240	8	10	12	170
1	Vegetable	2A	Lettuce and cucumber	½ c.	100	—	—	—	—
1	Vegetable	2B	Carrots	½ c.	100	2	—	7	36
3	Bread	4	Bread	3 sl.	75	6	—	45	204
1	Fat	6	Butter	1 tsp.	5	—	5	—	45
2	Fruit	3	Grapes	24	150	—	—	20	80
				Total		30	25	84	681
Dinner or main meal									
3	Meat	5	Chicken	3 oz.	90	21	15	—	219
1	Vegetable	2A	String beans, young	½ c.	100	—	—	—	—
1	Fat	6	Butter	1 tsp.	5	—	5	—	45
1	Vegetable	2B	Winter squash	½ c.	100	2	—	7	36
2	Fruit	3	Pineapple	1 c.	160	—	—	20	80
4	Bread	4	Biscuits	3	105	6	—	45	204
			Bread	**1 sl.**	**25**	**2**	—	**15**	**68**
1	Meat	5	**Egg**	**1**	—	**7**	**5**	—	**73**
				Total		38	25	87	725
				Day's Total		98	75	258	2099

* See footnote, p. 827.
For key to abbreviations see footnote, p. 823.

Diet No. VIII—2300 Calories
Protein 95 gm.; Fat 89 gm.; Carb. 280 gm.
Division: approx. $\frac{1}{3}$ of diet for each meal*

NO. EXCHANGES	FOOD EXCHANGE	LIST NO.	SAMPLE MENU	HOUSEHOLD MEAS.	WT. GM.	P	F	C	CAL.
Breakfast									
2	Meat	5	Eggs	2	—	14	10	—	146
2	Fat	6	Butter	2 tsp.	10	—	10	—	90
2	Fruit	3	Orange, sliced	2 sm.	200	—	—	20	80
4	Bread	4	Bread	3 sl.	75	6	—	45	204
			Ralston	**$\frac{1}{2}$ c.**	**100**	**2**	—	**15**	**68**
1	Milk	1	**Milk, whole**	**1 c.**	**240**	**8**	**10**	**12**	**170**
				Total		30	30	92	758
Lunch or supper									
2	Meat	5	Crab meat	$\frac{1}{2}$ c.	60	14	10	—	146
1	Milk	1	Milk, whole	1 c.	240	8	10	12	170
1	Vegetable	2A	Tomato juice	$\frac{1}{2}$ c.	100	—	—	—	—
1	Vegetable	2B	Peas, green	$\frac{1}{2}$ c.	100	2	—	7	36
4	Bread	3	Bread	4 sl.	100	8	—	60	272
1	Fat	6	Butter	2 tsp.	10	—	10	—	90
$1\frac{1}{2}$	Fruit	3	Banana	$\frac{3}{4}$ sm.	75	—	—	15	60
				Total		32	30	94	774
Dinner or main meal									
2	Meat	5	Lamb chops	2 sm.	60	14	10	—	146
1	Vegetable	2A	Lettuce	$\frac{1}{4}$ head	100	—	—	—	—
1	Vegetable	2B	Beets	$\frac{1}{2}$ c.	100	2	—	7	36
3	Fat	6	Butter	2 tsp.	10	—	10	—	90
			French dressing	1 tbsp.	15	—	5	—	45
1	Fruit	3	Cherries	10 lg.	75	—	—	10	40
5	Bread	4	Bread	3 sl.	75	6	—	45	204
			Lima beans	$\frac{1}{2}$ c.	90	2	—	15	68
			Soda crackers	**3**	**20**	**2**	—	**15**	**68**
1	Meat	5	**Cheese**	**1 oz.**	**30**	**7**	**5**	—	**73**
				Total		33	30	92	770
				Day's Total		95	90	278	2302

* See footnote, p. 827.
For key to abbreviations see footnote, p. 823.

Diet No. IX—2500 Calories
Protein 100 gm.; Fat 100 gm.; Carb. 300 gm.
Division: approx. $\frac{1}{3}$ of diet for each meal*

NO. EXCHANGES	FOOD EXCHANGE	LIST NO.	SAMPLE MENU	HOUSEHOLD MEAS.	WT. GM.	P	F	C	CAL.
Breakfast									
2	Meat	5	Eggs	2	—	14	10	—	146
3	Fat	6	Butter	3 tsp.	15	—	15	—	135
2	Fruit	3	Orange juice	1 c.	200	—	—	20	80
$4\frac{1}{2}$	Bread	4	Bread	$3\frac{1}{2}$ sl.	87	7	—	53	240
			Maltex	**$\frac{1}{2}$ c.**	**100**	**2**	—	**15**	**68**
1	Milk	1	**Milk, whole**	**1 c.**	**240**	**8**	**10**	**12**	**170**
				Total		31	35	100	839
Lunch or supper									
2	Meat	5	Cold beef	2 oz.	60	14	10	—	146
1	Milk	1	Milk, whole	1 c.	240	8	10	12	170
1	Vegetable	2A	Escarole, raw	$\frac{1}{2}$ c.	100	—	—	—	—
1	Vegetable	2B	Carrots	$\frac{1}{2}$ c.	100	2	—	7	36
4	Bread	4	Bread	4 sl.	100	8	—	60	272
3	Fat	6	Butter	3 tsp.	15	—	15	—	135
2	Fruit	3	Applesauce	1 c.	200	—	—	20	80
				Total		32	35	99	839
Dinner or main meal									
$2\frac{1}{2}$	Meat	5	Roast pork	$2\frac{1}{2}$ oz.	75	17	12	—	176
1	Vegetable	2A	Cole slaw	$\frac{1}{2}$ c.	100	—	—	—	—
1	Vegetable	2B	Peas, green	$\frac{1}{2}$ c.	100	2	—	7	36
4	Bread	4	Biscuits	2	70	4	—	30	136
			Sweet potato	$\frac{1}{2}$ c.	100	4	—	30	136
3	Fat	6	Butter	3 tsp.	15	—	15	—	135
2	Fruit	3	Grapes	24	150	—	—	20	80
1	Meat	5	**Cottage cheese**	**$\frac{1}{4}$ c.**	—	**7**	**5**	—	**73**
1	Bread	4	**Saltines**	**5**	**20**	**2**	—	**15**	**68**
				Total		36	32	102	840
				Day's Total		99	102	301	2518

* See footnote, p. 827.
For key to abbreviations see footnote, p. 823.

Diet No. X—2700 Calories
Protein 110 gm.; Fat 109 gm.; Carb. 320 gm.
Division: approx. $\frac{1}{3}$ of diet for each meal*

NO. EXCHANGES	FOOD EXCHANGE	LIST NO.	SAMPLE MENU	HOUSEHOLD MEAS.	WT. GM.	P	F	C	CAL.
Breakfast									
2	Meat	5	Eggs	2	—	14	10	—	146
3	Fat	6	Butter	3 tsp.	15	—	15	—	135
2	Fruit	3	Grapefruit	1 sm.	250	—	—	20	80
5	Bread	4	Bread	4 sl.	100	8	—	60	272
			Cheerio	**$\frac{3}{4}$ c.**	**20**	**2**	—	**15**	**68**
1	Milk	1	**Milk, whole**	**1 c.**	**240**	**8**	**10**	**12**	**170**
				Total		32	35	107	871
Lunch or supper									
3	Meat	5	Tuna	$\frac{3}{4}$ c.	90	21	15	—	219
1	Milk	1	Milk, whole	1 c.	240	8	10	12	170
1	Vegetable	2A	Celery and lettuce	$\frac{1}{2}$ c.	100	—	—	—	—
1	Vegetable	2B	Onions	$\frac{1}{2}$ c.	100	2	—	7	36
4$\frac{1}{2}$	Bread	4	Bread	4 sl.	100	8	—	60	272
			Saltines	2–3	10	1	—	8	36
2	Fat	6	Butter	2 tsp.	10	—	10	—	90
2	Fruit	3	Plums	4	200	—	—	20	80
				Total		40	35	107	903
Dinner or main meal									
2	Meat	5	Lamb chops	2 sm.	60	14	10	—	146
1	Vegetable	2A	Lettuce and chives	$\frac{1}{2}$ c.	100	—	—	—	—
1	Vegetable	2B	Rutabaga	$\frac{1}{2}$ c.	100	2	—	7	36
5	Fat	6	Butter	5 tsp.	25	—	25	—	225
1	Fruit	3	Pineapple	$\frac{1}{2}$ c.	80	—	—	10	40
6	Bread	4	Bread	3 sl.	75	6	—	45	204
			Potato, mashed	1 c.	200	4	—	30	136
			Graham crackers	**2**	**20**	**2**	—	**15**	**68**
1	Meat	5	**Cottage cheese**	**$\frac{1}{4}$ c**	**45**	**7**	**5**	—	**73**
				Total		35	40	107	928
				Day's Total		107	110	321	2702

* See footnote, p. 827.
For key to abbreviations see footnote, p. 823.

Diet No. XI—2900 Calories
Protein 120 gm.; Fat 120 gm.; Carb. 335 gm.
Division: approx. $\frac{1}{3}$ of diet for each meal*

NO. EXCHANGES	FOOD EXCHANGE	LIST NO.	SAMPLE MENU	HOUSEHOLD MEAS.	WT. GM.	P	F	C	CAL.
Breakfast									
2	Meat	5	Eggs	2	—	14	10	—	146
3	Fat	6	Butter	3 tsp.	15	—	15	—	135
2	Fruit	3	Prunes	4	50	—	—	20	80
5	Bread	4	Bread	4 sl.	100	8	—	60	272
			Rice Krispies	**$\frac{3}{4}$ c.**	**20**	**2**	—	**15**	**68**
1$\frac{1}{2}$	Milk	1	**Milk, whole**	**1$\frac{1}{2}$ c.**	**360**	**12**	**15**	**18**	**255**
				Total		36	40	113	956
Lunch or supper									
3	Meat	5	Cold cuts	2 sl.	90	14	10	—	146
			Cheese, American	1 sl.	30	7	5	—	73
1	Milk	1	Milk, whole	1 c.	240	8	10	12	170
1	Vegetable	2A	Lettuce and cucumber		100	—	—	—	—
1	Vegetable	2B	Beets	$\frac{1}{2}$ c.	100	2	—	7	36
5	Bread	4	Bread	5 sl.	125	10	—	75	340
3	Fat	6	Butter	3 tsp.	15	—	15	—	135
2	Fruit	3	Banana	1 sm.	100	—	—	20	80
				Total		41	40	114	980
Dinner or main meal									
3	Meat	5	Liver	3 oz.	75	21	15	—	219
1	Vegetable	2A	Tomatoes	$\frac{1}{2}$ c.	100	—	—	—	—
1	Vegetable	2B	Onions	$\frac{1}{2}$ c.	100	2	—	7	36
4	Fat	6	Butter	4 tsp.	20	—	20	—	180
1	Fruit	3	Orange, sliced	1	100	—	—	10	40
6	Bread	4	Noodles	$\frac{1}{2}$ c.	100	2	—	15	68
			Bread	3 sl.	75	6	—	45	204
			Sponge cake	1$\frac{1}{2}$ cube	25	2	—	15	68
			Saltines	**5**	**20**	**2**	—	**15**	**68**
1	Meat	5	**Cheese**	**1 oz.**	**30**	**7**	**5**	—	**73**
				Total		42	40	107	956
				Day's Total		119	120	334	2892

* See footnote, p. 827.
For key to abbreviations see footnote, p. 823.

Maximum usefulness of the dietary plans will be obtained (1) when the prescription for the diet is arrived at as outlined on pages 814 to 817 and (2) when full advantage is taken of the flexibilities permitted by the various food exchanges. In the *illustrative* dietary plans (pages 823 to 833) a "food exchange" column is included to simplify the substitution of suitable foods for those indicated in the sample menu.

The standard diet prescriptions, Nos. I to IV inclusive—providing 900, 1100, 1300 and 1500 calories, respectively—are used in the treatment of overweight patients having mild diabetes. These patients do not need insulin and they are at liberty to save any part of any meal to be taken between meals or at bedtime if desired. It is inadvisable, on the other hand, to take only two large meals in the day or two very small meals and one large meal.

The more liberal diets—from 1700 to 2900 calories—are commonly used by patients taking insulin, in which case there are specific indications for a distribution of the diet which gives maximum advantage to the respective insulin therapy. This feature has been dealt with already in some detail (p. 817).

INSULIN THERAPY*

Salient Features Governing the Need for Insulin. Familiarity with the various insulin preparations and the rate, degree and duration of their respective activities is necessary for the proper selection and the most effective combinations of insulins for the individual patient. No two patients may require the same dose of insulin. It is only after the amount of insulin given is adjusted to conform with the individual's "need pattern" that the diabetes is controlled. Too often one hears the remark that one unit will "look after" a certain number of grams of glucose. The insulin need does not conform to any such exact equivalent, and the claim that it does indicates a failure to understand the multitude of influences which determine the amount of insulin a patient may need. In order to emphasize some fundamental dietary factors which affect the insulin need clinically, several illustrative studies are offered.

First, a diet of 80 gm. protein, 120 gm. fat and 150 gm. carbohydrate, giving a total value of 2000 calories (theoretical glucose equivalent or G.E. = 58 per cent of protein + 100 per cent of carbohydrate + 10 per cent of fat = 208 gm.) may be allowed. Let us assume that with this diet 60 units of insulin are necessary to control the diabetes. The dosage of insulin having been established, an abrupt change in the diet is made to 80 gm. protein, 280 gm. carbohydrate and 70 gm. fat (2000 calories and G.E. = 333 gm.). It will be observed that the glucose equivalent has been increased from 208 to 333 gm. but the total calories have been kept constant by reducing the fat content of the diet. If the insulin need fluctuated only with the amount of carbohydrate allowed in diet, an increase of 60 per cent —or a dosage of 96 units—would be needed to control the diabetes as efficiently as 60 units had done previously. This is not what happens. With the abrupt increase in the carbohydrate of the diet some glycosuria and hyperglycemia usually occur, *but* these changes are small and are readily overcome by the addition of only a few units of insulin. Why is this so? The reason is that the total calories were kept unchanged and the only reason why there was any increase in the insulin dosage at all is that carbohydrate has stronger glycosuric and hyperglycemic effects than the caloric equivalent of fat.[87,88]

A *second consideration* of equal clinical significance is illustrated. Had the initial diet (P. 80 gm., F. 120 gm., and C. 150 gm.—2000 calories) been changed by merely adding the 130 gm. of carbohydrate and the total calories (520) provided by it to make the new diet, P. 80 gm., F. 120 gm. and C. 280 gm. —2520 calories, the increase in the in-

* Insulin is measured in units. Three units depress the blood sugar of a fasting 2 kg. rabbit to 0.0045 mg. per cent. Pure crystalline zinc insulinate contains 22 units per milligram.

sulin need would far exceed that found necessary to control the diabetes when the carbohydrate increase was accompanied by a reduction in fat. Combining these two phenomena, it is observed that the *total calories profoundly affect the insulin dosage, and the carbohydrate allowance of the diet can be greatly increased with only minor changes in the insulin need resulting, provided the total calories are not increased also.*

A *third established fact, and one of importance in this respect,* can be illustrated if a diet of protein 80 gm., fat 120 gm., carbohydrate 150 gm.—2000 calories (theoretical glucose equivalent: 208 gm.) is replaced by a diet with approximately the same theoretical glucose equivalent but with a reduced total calories, e.g., protein 80 gm., fat 50 gm., carbohydrate 155 gm., 1400 calories (G.E.: 207 gm.). If the dietary influence on insulin need were confined to carbohydrate, no change in the insulin need would ensue, but instead there is a remarkable reduction in the insulin need. The initial reduction is due to the reduced calories. With progressive loss of weight and reduction in the total metabolism, there is also a progressive reduction in the need for insulin.

The foregoing phenomena, reproducible at will, indicate that:

1. Carbohydrate has a greater insulin demand than the caloric equivalent of fat.
2. The insulin need is governed to a large extent by the total caloric value of the diet.
3. The combination of a low calorie diet and a reduction in body weight exerts a profound insulin-sparing action.
4. The combination of a diet sufficiently high in calories to add to the body weight exerts an increase in the need for insulin which is progressive until the diet is reduced or until the body weight becomes stabilized. This effect on the insulin is by virtue of the large amount of food plus the increased total metabolism that accrues with a gain in body mass.
5. Similarly, complications affect the insulin requirement. All influences which increase the total metabolism with but one exception—physical exercise—increase the need for insulin. These are: increased caloric intake, obesity, infections, fevers, toxemias, pregnancy and thyrotoxicosis. Contrariwise, all influences which reduce the total metabolism with but one exception—the cessation of physical exercise—reduce the need for insulin. These are: reduction in caloric intake, reduction in weight, correction of infections, fevers and toxemias, termination of pregnancy and the control or cure of thyrotoxicosis.

The protein content of the diet is not subject to the great fluctuation observed in the fat and carbohydrate contents and also its effect on the insulin requirement is feeble in contrast to that of carbohydrate and total calories.

Insulin therapy is indicated *at once* in:

1. All diabetic children.
2. All underweight adults who have glycosuria and hyperglycemia.
3. All patients having acute complications, whether the underlying diabetes is mild or not, if there is glycosuria or hyperglycemia at any time in the twenty-four hours.
4. All cases of pregnancy complicating diabetes.
5. All patients with a history of a sudden onset of symptoms of diabetes within the three months prior to the consultation.

Insulin therapy is indicated in the treatment for diabetes when this disorder is not, or obviously will not be, controlled satisfactorily by suitable dietetic measures and exercise. Some authorities give insulin, in the initial days of treatment, to all diabetic patients. In favor of this plan is the more rapid control of the diabetes—not always desirable in patients in the "degenerative age group"—and the training of the patient in the administration of insulin while he is under competent supervision. It also emphasizes that many patients can discontinue insulin. The majority of diabetic patients have a mild diabetes and ultimately do not need insulin. This information has a good effect in neutralizing a general and erroneous belief that once one uses insulin he must always use it. Unfortunately, this is usually true for the thin patient having severe diabetes, but it is not true for obese patients who have mild diabetes.

All patients who have an acute onset of the diabetes, which may be mild or severe, should be given insulin with the hope that some may be cured.

The amount of insulin needed is not relative to the degree of hyperglycemia with any constancy, nor can it be calculated with any degree of exactness according to the amount of sugar in the urine. If glycosuria exists in the case of a patient taking insulin, more insulin is needed, but what 5 units will do in ridding the urine of sugar in one patient may require 25, or more, units in another.

It is a good working rule, barring acute complications which will be considered later, that *all untreated diabetic patients who are considerably overweight will not need insulin nor oral therapy* notwithstanding the presence of a high fasting blood sugar level on the first examination.

It is a good working rule, too, that *all children and underweight diabetic patients require insulin* even if the initial level for fasting blood sugar should not be high. The certainty that insulin will be needed by growing children and underweight adults is based on the knowledge that to promote normal health and physical growth, a gain in weight and a liberal diet, each of which increase the need for insulin, are necessary. The combination of a persistently elevated fasting blood sugar level and undernutrition makes insulin therapy imperative if good health is to be restored. It has been our practice at the Pennsylvania Hospital never to give insulin to overweight diabetic patients unless during some acute complication and unless there has been a recent sudden onset of the diabetes. The merit for the control of the diabetes should go to the dietetic measures and not to a preliminary and temporary course of insulin treatment. In this manner the patient can be deeply impressed by the value of a restricted diet. We have observed the effect of insulin on obese diabetic patients at other clinics and, for the purposes of study, have given insulin to similar patients. Knowing that the diabetes is inherently mild and that the reduction of a few pounds in weight would control it, one might expect that a small dose of insulin would suffice to accomplish the same result. *This is not so.* These patients are relatively resistant to insulin. Repeatedly, over 100 units of insulin a day were necessary to accomplish, in reducing the blood sugar level, what was as readily obtained by a slight reduction in weight. These patients have three means to control their diabetes without insulin—low caloric diet, a reduction in weight, and physical exercise. Various attempts have been made, especially by Himsworth,[89] to classify diabetic patients into insulin-resistant and insulin-sensitive groups. Most of the insulin-resistant patients were middle-aged or overweight. There seems to be a general lack of appreciation for the fact that the overweight insulin-resistant patient loses this resistance to insulin in direct proportion to the reduction of body weight. Any factor which reduces the total metabolism, with one exception (i.e., the cessation of physical exercise), aids in the control of the diabetes. Reduction in body mass seems to be the most effective of these factors.

One to several weeks are needed, as a rule, to control the diabetes in these overweight patients. All who are familiar with the effect of obesity on life expectancy agree that overweight should be corrected. In the diabetic this result, accomplished by appropriate dietary measures, carries a double benefit—it cures the obesity and controls the diabetes.

If, for any reason, the body weight is not reduced and the diabetes is not controlled, prolonged and needless hyperglycemia and glycosuria should not be allowed. Insulin or an oral hypoglycemic agent should be employed. This is a recognition of failure, however. The patient will lose weight without either of these agents, as he should, if he is convinced of the advantages that will accrue, and if he has the will power to do it. Hospitalization, training and reassurance are essential to successful treatment in most of these problem cases.

The obese patient's appetite is greater and a reduction in weight is more difficult to secure if he is given insulin. Fortunately, tolbutamide does not stimulate the appetite.

The Lente Insulins. Three relatively new insulin-zinc modifications, developed by Hallas-Møller and co-workers,[18,90] are designated as *semi-lente, lente* and *ultra-lente* insulins, so named because of their respective rates of activity—rapid, intermediate and long acting.

The range of insulin activity—onset, degree and duration—is modified by combining insulin with compounds (in this case zinc) which are insoluble at the *p*H of the blood—7.2. Prior to the discovery of the lente insulins, prolongation of the blood sugar lowering effect was attained by combining insulin with foreign proteins—protamine or globin—and the effect was prolonged, intensified and stabilized by the addition of zinc, 2 mg. per 1000 units. Smaller quantities of zinc, 0.5 to 1 mg. per 1000 units, added to the insulin without added protein substance resulted in a product which is slowly soluble at blood *p*H provided certain anions, phosphate and citrate, are absent.[18] The range of the activity which can be secured extends from that of rapidly acting insulins to longer than that of protamine zinc insulin depending upon the physical state of the precipitates produced—amorphous or crystalline. The amorphous suspension has a range of activity slightly longer than that of unmodified or crystalline insulin, whereas crystalline suspensions are effective as long as or longer than protamine zinc insulin.

The amount of "excess zinc" in these lente preparations is 2.0 mg. per 1000 units of insulin, which is five to ten times the concentration utilized in preparing zinc insulin crystals (USP) and is about equal to that which is present in protamine zinc insulin.

The zinc renders the insulin crystals relatively insoluble at the neutral point. Taking advantage of this effect two physical forms of insulin suspension were produced. In one the *p*H was adjusted until the amorphous precipitate which formed was such as to ensure relatively rapid absorption and provide an insulin effect for approximately twelve hours. This is *semi-lente* insulin (see Fig. 14). The other, with the *p*H adjusted in the range of 4.8 to 5.7, is very slowly soluble and, as a result, provides a long acting insulin effect—as long as thirty-six hours. This is *ultra-lente* insulin. A mixture comprising 30 per cent semi-lente and 70 per cent ultra-lente insulin has been shown to have an intermediate acting effect quite similar to that of globin and NPH insulin. This is *lente* insulin.

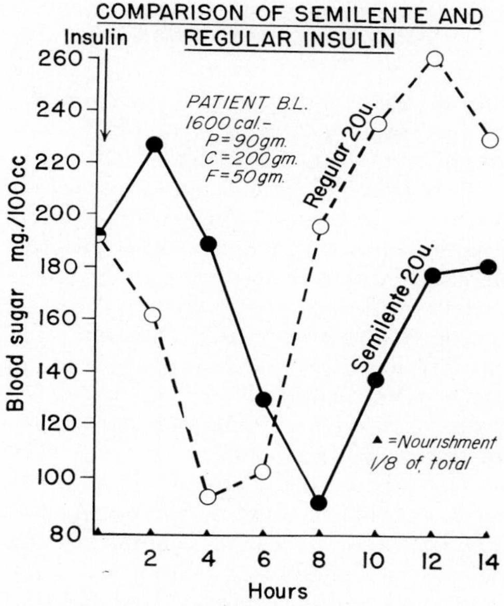

FIG. 14. The differences in the speed of action, period of greatest effect and duration of hypoglycemic action exerted by regular and semi-lente insulins studied under identical circumstances.

Lente insulin owes its intermediate effect to the additions of small quantities of zinc (0.5 to 1 mg. per 1000 units)

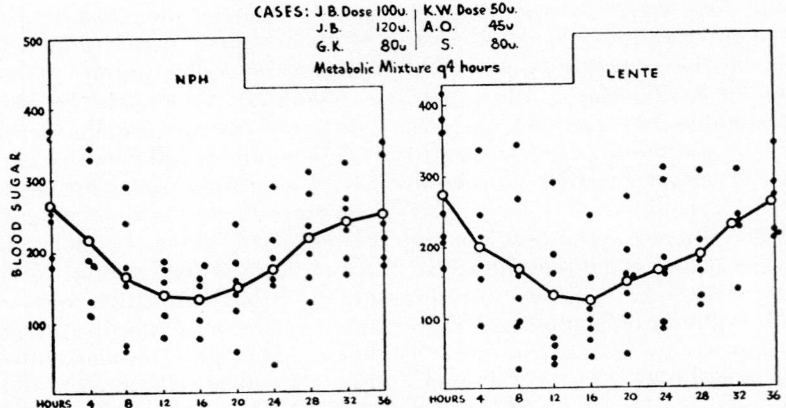

FIG. 15. Comparative blood sugar lowering effects of NPH and lente insulins in a composite controlled study (after Peck and associates).[91]

and a *p*H identical with that of the blood, provided certain anions, phosphate and citrate, are absent.

In clinical practice lente insulin is, with but minor adjustments, interchangeable with globin or NPH insulins. It is not unusual, however, to find that NPH insulin has a somewhat longer action than globin insulin and that lente insulin has a somewhat longer action than NPH insulin. The comparative effects of NPH and lente insulins are illustrated in Fig. 15.

The advantages claimed for lente insulin are that it contains no foreign protein and that it has, in general but not always, a somewhat longer action than NPH and globin insulins. The hope that the development of lipodystrophy as a complication of insulin therapy would not occur with lente insulin has not been substantiated. One patient developed an allergy to insulin while taking lente insulin.[91]

While these new insulins have not, in my experience, improved the control of the diabetes over that achieved with the appropriate use of the previously available insulins, neither have they been less efficient. As they contain no added protein, they offer a potential advantage for certain individuals.

Also, by "tailor made" adjustments in the relative amounts of semi-lente and ultra-lente mixtures, a larger number of patients can secure good control by one daily injection of insulin than was possible heretofore.

Choice of Insulin. There are eight insulins commercially available in this country—regular (or unmodified), crystalline, protamine zinc, globin, NPH, lente, semi-lente and ultra-lente.

The selection of the insulin therapy for optimum results is highly individualized. No one form of insulin is satisfactory for all patients. Assuming that the diet is appropriate and uniform from day to day, the aim has been to obtain an insulin which, when given alone and in a single injection, will control the hyperglycemia for twenty-four hours. None of the insulins yet available qualifies in this respect for most cases of unstable or for the "juvenile type" of diabetes. A single injection of a suitable mixture of insulins suffices in a considerable proportion of cases. For most of these patients our best results have been obtained with a mixture of an intermediate and a crystalline insulin before breakfast and a small dose of an intermediate insulin in the evening, but there is promise that probably many of these patients will get good results from a single injection of a mixture of semi- and ultra-lente insulins, the relative proportions of which are determined for each patient.

The complexity of insulin therapy may be simplified by classifying the relative insulins according to their speed, degree and duration of action into four groups, those having (1) a *rapid*, (2) an *intermediate*, (3) a *prolonged* action, and (4) combined effects.

Insulins with a rapid action of relatively short duration are crystalline insulin (zinc insulin crystals in solution), *regular* or *unmodified*, and *semi-lente insulin*. Each has the same antidiabetic properties and they are ordinarily interchangeable, but the crystalline insulin, because of its purity, and semi-lente, because it contains no foreign protein, are somewhat less likely to cause allergic reactions.

Crystalline insulin exerts an appreciable blood sugar lowering effect within one hour, when given subcutaneously, and has its maximum action between two and six hours[92] (see Fig. 16). In the patient with no acute complications, its action gradually subsides after the sixth hour until, usually, no discernible effect is noted after ten to twelve hours. Because of its short period of maximum activity, crystalline insulin does not control clinical diabetes when given as a single daily injection, but it is the ideal insulin during acute emergencies, e.g., diabetic ketosis, keto-acidosis and acute infections. To achieve greatest speed of effect, a portion of the initial dose is given intravenously to patients in diabetic ketosis.

Crystalline insulin has a zinc content of only 0.016 to 0.04 mg. per 1000 units and has no buffer protein added to it.

Insulins with an intermediate action. Three insulin preparations—*NPH*, *globin* and *lente insulins*—exert a slower blood sugar lowering effect than do the rapidly acting insulins, but they act more rapidly than the long acting insulins—protamine zinc insulin and ultralente insulin. Also, their effect is longer than that of rapidly acting insulin but shorter than that of protamine zinc or ultra-lente insulins. It is because of these properties that they are known as intermediately acting insulins.

NPH (N = neutral, P = protamine, H = Hagedorn) (isophane) *insulin* is widely used as a single insulin and as a mixture with crystalline insulin. Unlike protamine zinc insulin, it has little or no excess protamine. Because of this, crystalline insulin when added to NPH insulin does not combine with protamine and so does not lose its identity as a rapidly acting insulin. Hence, a mixture of NPH and crystalline insulins, when given in a single injection, combines the rapid and the intermediate actions of these two insulins. In treatment, adjustments in the dosage of each, made according to the needs of the individual patient, provide more uniform control of the hyperglycemia than is possible in

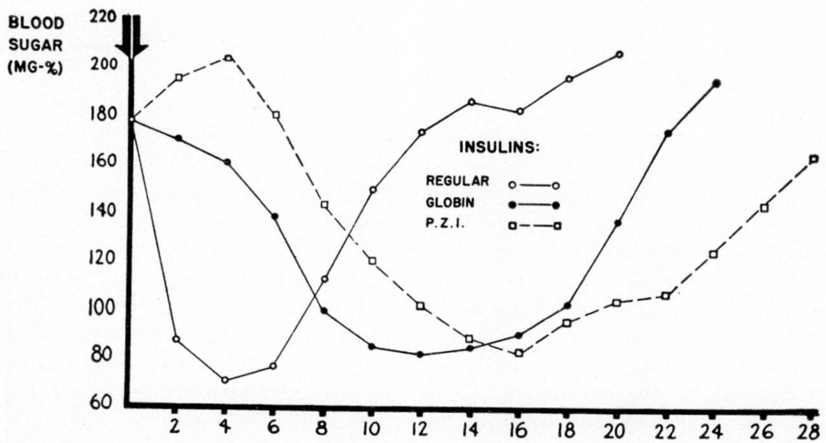

FIG. 16. The comparative effects of identical doses—60 units—of regular, globin and protamine zinc insulin when administered subcutaneously to a hyperglycemic patient who received 20 grams of carbohydrate by mouth at two-hour intervals during the observations.

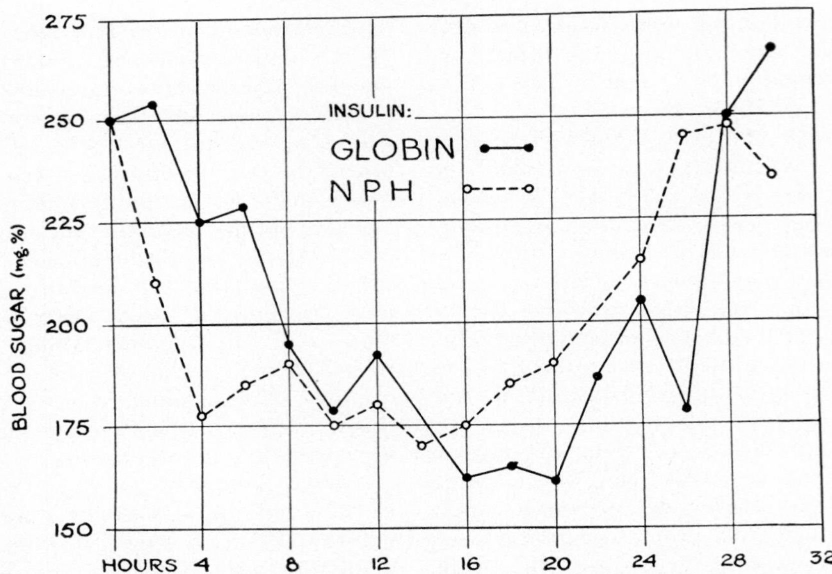

FIG. 17. The similarity of effect—degree and durations—of identical doses (30 units) of globin and NPH insulin is depicted. Each insulin was administered subcutaneously in the presence of a hyperglycemia, to a patient who received a nourishment—20 gm. of carbohydrate, 8 gm. of protein, and 8 gm. of fat—at two-hour intervals during the observations.

patients with moderately severe and severe diabetes with either insulin alone.

The degree of predictability of the effect obtained from mixing crystalline insulin with NPH insulin makes it a specially valuable insulin. When it is used in conjunction with suitable adjustments in diet, satisfactory results are obtained in a larger percentage of patients than from an injection of any other single insulin or other mixture of insulins except possibly a suitable combination of semi-lente and ultra-lente insulins. This does not mean that excellent results are not obtainable from mixtures of crystalline insulin with protamine zinc insulin or with globin or lente insulins.

The intermediate retarded effect of NPH insulin in correcting hyperglycemia is illustrated in Fig. 17. It has little effect on the level of blood sugar in the first four hours. The greatest effect is between eight to sixteen hours, and some effect persists as long as twenty-eight to thirty hours. In clinical practice the maximum effect of NPH insulin given before breakfast is usually manifested before the evening meal. There are exceptions in which the greatest apparent effect is delayed until late evening and occasionally until during the night.

The insulin therapy for patients with severe, unstable or juvenile diabetes which has given the best results comprises a mixture (mixed at the time of injection) of crystalline and NPH insulin given *twenty to thirty minutes before breakfast and a small dose of NPH insulin afer supper.* The occasional patient does better when the evening dose is given immediately before supper, although some have the best results when it is given at bedtime.

The crystalline insulin in the morning dose is increased until the forenoon glycosuria disappears; the morning dose of NPH insulin is increased until there is no glycosuria before supper; and the evening dose is increased cautiously until the overnight urine contains no sugar.

For clinical purposes the three intermediately acting insulins—NPH, globin and lente—are, with minor adjustments in timing and dosage, interchangeable. The effects of globin insulin are contrasted with those of identical doses of regular (unmodified) and protamine zinc insulin in Fig. 16. For practical purposes, the curves obtained with NPH and lente insulins vary but little from that obtained with globin insulin. In some patients NPH and lente insulin may have a somewhat longer effect, with maximum activity from eight to sixteen hours, in contrast to globin, which in general exerts its greatest effect between six and twelve hours.

Globin insulin is a clear solution which owes its intermediate action to the addition of 3.8 mg. of highly purified globin and 0.30 mg. of zinc, as a zinc salt, to each 100 units. I have not seen a patient who was allergic to globin insulin who was not also allergic to the insulin molecule and, hence, allergic to all insulin preparations. Globin insulin has a slight blood sugar lowering effect within two hours of its injection. Its greatest effect is between six and twelve hours, and it has little or no effect after twenty-four hours.

The larger the dose of globin insulin the more rapidly it reduces the blood sugar, and this effect is more protracted than when the doses are small. As with the other intermediately acting insulins, there is considerable individual variation in the rate of action and duration of effect.

Given before breakfast the greatest apparent effect usually occurs before supper, though sometimes the greatest apparent effect may be in the late evening or during the night.

Additions of 4 or 6 units on alternate days to the initial dose of 8 to 16 units are made until the specimen of urine voided before supper is free from sugar. At this point, 3 P.M. and fasting venous blood sugar values are determined. If the patient is free from hypoglycemic reactions, if the 3 P.M. blood sugar is between 80 and 130 mg. per ml., and if the fasting blood sugar does not exceed 130 mg. per 100 ml., the diabetes is under satisfactory control. Moderate reductions in the dose of insulin are advisable after a few days of good control of the diabetes, and a further decrease is usual when normal activities are resumed. Further minor adjustments are made as indications arise. Some patients prefer globin insulin solely because there is practically no danger of a hypoglycemia during the night, as exists with protamine zinc insulin.

Globin insulin affords satisfactory control of the diabetes when the dosage required is not large and when suitable adjustments in diet are made (see p. 818). Usually if more than 40 units are necessary, a single dose of globin insulin will not give good control "around the clock." There are exceptions to this rule.

If the 3 P.M. blood sugar value referred to above is between 80 and 130 mg. per 100 ml. and the fasting blood sugar is in excess of 200 mg. with early morning and forenoon glycosuria, it is clear that further increase in the morning dose of globin insulin should not be made because of the danger of hypoglycemia in the late afternoon, and yet the diabetes is not well controlled. A small dose—6 to 10 units—of globin insulin after supper or at bedtime might be added with complete success. Or, a combination of crystalline and protamine zinc insulin—a 2:1 mixture—given before breakfast might suffice; or a mixture of semi-lente and ultra-lente insulins, adjusting the ratio until it fits the need of the individual patient, might serve to achieve satisfactory results without resorting to a second dose.

Some patients (2 to 4 per cent of those needing insulin), because of allergic reactions or unsatisfactory response with protamine zinc insulin or one of its modifications, may have to be treated with globin or lente insulins. Formerly these patients had to resort to crystalline insulin alone—a regimen no longer necessary. One dose of either globin or lente insulin before breakfast may suffice. A small dose of the same insulin may be needed after supper to prevent undue hyperglycemia and glycosuria during the night. For the more unstable diabetes, crystalline insulin may also be necessary before breakfast. The effect is most predictable if the crystalline insulin is given as a separate injection, but a mixture with either globin or lente insulin may be deter-

TABLE 16. THE VARIOUS INSULINS AND THEIR RESPECTIVE EFFECTS

	INSULIN	TIME USUALLY ADMINISTERED	NUMBER OF DOSES EACH DAY	GREATEST RISK OF HYPOGLYCEMIA (TIME)	SPECIAL NOURISHMENT	SPECIMEN MOST LIKELY TO CONTAIN SUGAR	SPECIMEN MOST LIKELY TO BE FREE FROM SUGAR
I.	Intermediate effect: (1) Globin (2) NPH (3) Lente	If given alone—1 hour before breakfast	One	Before supper	3:30–4:30 P.M.	Before breakfast and before lunch	Before supper
II.	Rapidly acting, if it were given alone (1) Crystalline (2) Semi-lente	20 to 30 minutes before breakfast	One	Before lunch	11 A.M.	During evening and before breakfast	Before lunch
	Rapidly acting insulins are not used alone in the treatment of uncomplicated diabetes. When given with intermediate or long acting insulins the effects of the former, as well as the latter, are as indicated.						
III.	Combined rapidly acting and long acting insulins*	20 minutes before breakfast	One (mixed insulins)	Before lunch and between midnight and breakfast	11 A.M. and at bedtime	Before supper and late evening	Before lunch and before breakfast
IV.	Combined intermediate and rapidly acting in A.M. with intermediate acting after supper	20 minutes before breakfast and after supper or in some cases at bedtime	Two	Before each meal	11 A.M., 3:30–4:30 P.M. and at bedtime	Very variable in these cases of labile diabetes	Before each meal
V.	An intermediate and crystalline (mixed) and a separate dose of a long acting insulin	20 minutes before breakfast (two injections)	Two	Before each meal	11 A.M., 3:30–4:30 P.M. and at bedtime	Same as IV	Before each meal

Note: The characteristic effects of each insulin are emphasized, but cognizance must be taken of the composite effects of insulin mixtures and also of the fact that equal amounts of the same insulin may vary in their period of activity in different patients.

* We do not employ long acting insulins—protamine zinc and ultra-lente—except when given in combination with a rapidly acting insulin.

mined by trial and adjustments that will give satisfactory results. During acute complications, crystalline insulin is the preparation of choice.

Insulins with a prolonged action are *protamine zinc* and *ultra-lente*. These insulins are relatively insoluble and when injected subcutaneously are released very slowly. Consequently, the greatest effect on the level of the blood sugar becomes apparent between twelve and twenty-four hours, depending somewhat on the size of the dose. The activity range extends to thirty or more hours.

Protamine zinc insulin owes its retarded effect to the relative insolubility of insulin when bound to the protein protamine, whereas the protracted action of ultra-lente insulin is achieved by making a slowly soluble complex at blood *p*H by adding small amounts of zinc to insulin, without added protein, and in the absence of certain anions—citrates and phosphates.[18]

Protamine zinc insulin is slowly absorbed and hence its blood sugar lowering effect does not gain headway in the first two to four hours after the injection (Fig. 16). The slow absorption of this insulin provides its greatest advantage—a prolonged effect. The blood sugar depressing effect of a dose of protamine zinc insulin lasts for twenty-four to thirty-six hours. In spite of the overlapping effect of the waning dose with that of the newly injected dose, the combined effects are not adequate in most cases to prevent marked hyperglycemia and glycosuria during the forenoon.

Clinically, there appears to be no bona fide indication for protamine zinc insulin given as the sole insulin. If the diabetes is sufficiently mild to permit good results with a single dose of protamine zinc insulin given one hour, or longer, before breakfast, a single dose of an intermediate insulin is to be preferred. The latter has its maximum effect during the period in the twenty-four hours in which three meals are taken in rather close succession, and it has a waning effect during the night. In contrast, protamine zinc insulin exerts its greatest apparent effect during the night, when its effect is on the wane but when no food is taken. This maximum apparent effect and the risk of a hypoglycemia occur during the night, whether the insulin is taken before breakfast or before supper. Because of the slowness of the action of protamine zinc insulin, allowing undue hyperglycemia and glycosuria during the daytime and the risk of hypoglycemic reactions during the night, we have not used it as a single insulin for several years.

Advantage can be taken of the time action of protamine zinc insulin by giving it as a mixture with crystalline (or unmodified) insulin or in combination—but not mixed—with one of the other insulins (see p. 844).

Ultra-lente insulin has a blood sugar lowering effect which persists for more than thirty hours. Small doses have a shorter effect than large doses, and the duration of effect differs somewhat in different patients. Clinically, the great advantage of ultra-lente insulin is that it can be mixed with semi-lente insulin without disturbing the characteristic effect of either insulin. This mixture is available as a standardized insulin, i.e., lente insulin, which is composed of 70 per cent ultra-lente and 30 per cent semi-lente insulin. Varying degrees of retarded effect can be obtained, to meet the needs of the individual patient, by increasing the proportion of semi-lente insulin when a more rapid effect is desired and that of ultra-lente insulin when a more prolonged effect is needed.

There appears to be no indication for giving ultra-lente insulin as the sole insulin in the treatment of diabetes, for the same reason that protamine zinc insulin should not be used alone (see elsewhere on this page).

*Combined insulins.** The most widely used combination in this country is a mixture of *NPH* and *crystalline insulin.* This combination, given before break-

* The respective insulins are mixed in the syringe at the time of injection.

fast, is adjusted until a sufficiently rapid action from the crystalline insulin is obtained to achieve good control in the forenoon and until the intermediate effect of NPH secures this result in the afternoon and evening. If the effect of the latter does not carry through the night, a small dose of NPH insulin after supper is often desirable. This regimen has been the most effective, in my experience, in treating patients with severe and unstable diabetes. However, with increasing experience with suitable proportions of semi-lente and ultra-lente insulins, I believe they may be equally, if not more, satisfactory.

Globin and *crystalline insulin* are less widely used as mixtures. The effect of the rapidly acting insulin is somewhat less predictable than when it is mixed with NPH insulin. Nevertheless, equal parts of crystalline and globin insulin are quite satisfactory for some patients and for others different proportions adjusted on an individual basis may suffice to attain adequate control of the diabetes.

Protamine zinc and *crystalline insulins* given simultaneously as a mixture may be used in the attempt to reduce the number of injections to one daily. When other plans of therapy entail more than one injection per day, a single dose of a 2:1 mixture of crystalline and protamine zinc insulin gives equally satisfactory results in a small percentage of patients. Results are more predictable when these two insulins are injected separately, in which case the amount of protamine zinc insulin is invariably greater than that of the crystalline insulin. The relatively large amount of crystalline insulin in a mixture of these two insulins is attributable to the fact that protamine zinc insulin contains sufficient excess protamine to combine with added crystalline insulin up to approximately a 1:1 mixture. Hence, if a rapid effect is expected from crystalline insulin added to protamine zinc insulin, the ratio must be greater than 1:1. A ratio of 2:1 is the most widely effective mixture but a ratio of 3 of crystalline to 1 of protamine zinc insulin is used occasionally.

I rarely use this mixture now in view of the better results obtained with NPH and crystalline (mixed) and a small evening dose of the former when necessary, or with a single injection of a mixture of semi- and ultra-lente insulins.

Crystalline and *lente insulins* may be regulated in an approximate mixture to secure good results, but, in my experience, the outcome of this therapy has not been as uniformly satisfactory as combinations of NPH with crystalline insulin and ultra- with semi-lente insulins. The addition of crystalline insulin to lente insulin alters the *p*H of the latter. As the uniformity of predictability of the effect of lente insulin is predicated on its *p*H being identical with that of the blood, crystalline insulin added in varying amounts reduces somewhat the predictability of the results.

Semi-lente and *ultra-lente insulins* in proportions of 30 and 70 per cent, respectively, produce lente insulin, an intermediate insulin. When the action of lente insulin is not sufficiently rapid to prevent undue hyperglycemia in the forenoon, the ratio may be changed by adding semi-lente insulin as needed until the desired result is achieved. This plan of "mixture therapy" with a single daily injection holds promise of maintaining good control of the diabetes in a large percentage of patients.

Simplified and Recommended Plan of Insulin Therapy. Confusion in the management of insulin therapy can be kept at a minimum if a simple plan is adopted. The format of one general plan of insulin therapy is presented in Table 17.

A small percentage, possibly 10 per cent, of *patients who must take insulin* will achieve good control of the diabetes with a single dose of an intermediate acting insulin—globin, NPH or lente. The percentage would be much higher if patients who are given insulin but who could do well without it were included. For practical purposes, the effects of these three insulins are identical. The single dose is given, preferably, an hour before breakfast. Its favorable effect is enhanced if a bread and milk

TABLE 17. ILLUSTRATIVE SIMPLE AND EFFECTIVE SCHEMES OF INSULIN THERAPY IN THE ABSENCE OF ACUTE COMPLICATIONS

I. *Mild diabetes in obese patients*
No insulin

II. *Relatively mild diabetes*
One dose of an intermediate insulin 1 hour before breakfast, e.g., 14 units of globin or NPH or lente insulin

III. *Moderately severe but relatively stable diabetes*
A mixture of NPH and regular insulin ½ hour before breakfast, e.g., 12 units of regular insulin, to which are added 40 units of NPH insulin

IV. *Severe and labile diabetes*
A mixture of NPH and regular insulin 20 to 30 minutes before breakfast and a small dose of an intermediate insulin after supper, e.g., 16 units of regular insulin added to 60 units of NPH insulin ½ hour before breakfast and 10 units of NPH (or globin or lente) insulin after supper. A suitable mixture of semi- and ultra-lente insulins may be equally satisfactory in some cases and yet only one injection daily is required.

exchange is taken from the breakfast to be consumed between 3:30 and 4:30 P.M.

A somewhat larger percentage of patients need a rapidly acting insulin, as well as an insulin with an intermediate effect, before breakfast if a forenoon hyperglycemia of undue degree is to be avoided. The need is met by adding some crystalline insulin to NPH insulin and giving this mixture a half hour before breakfast.

For a still larger percentage of the young diabetics and the patients with labile or moderately severe and severe diabetes, the most effective plan, in my experience, is to give a mixture of NPH and crystalline insulins 20 to 30 minutes before breakfast and a small dose of NPH insulin after supper. The evening dose may in some cases be given at bedtime. The diet with this program is divided into three equal meals, but a bread and milk exchange is taken from breakfast for consumption between 3:30 and 4:30 P.M. and a similar amount is taken from supper for consumption at bedtime.

These simple plans of insulin therapy have proved most effective, though other plans may suffice equally well in individual patients.

Indeed, a mixture of semi-lente and ultra-lente insulins in which the proportions are adjusted to the individual's needs and which gives a combined rapid, intermediate and protracted action is quite effective in a considerable percentage of patients.

In determining the appropriate insulin regimen I am guided by the presence or absence of glycosuria in specimens voided before each meal and at bedtime. This plan has largely replaced that of collecting complete fractional specimens, i.e., 7 to 11 A.M.; 11 A.M. to 4 P.M.; 4 to 9 P.M., and 9 P.M. to 7 A.M. It is more practicable, in general, but in instances of unstable diabetes examination of complete fractions is preferred.

The patient is instructed to examine the single specimens before each meal and at bedtime at home, but the frequency of testing is individualized, every attempt being made to reduce the number of tests to a practicable minimum.

TABLE 18. FACTORS WHICH ALTER THE NEED FOR INSULIN

THOSE INCREASING NEED FOR INSULIN	THOSE DECREASING NEED FOR INSULIN
Gain in weight	Reduction in weight (therapeutic)
Increased diet	Reduced caloric intake
Cessation of exercise	Increased physical exercise
Pregnancy	Termination of pregnancy
Therapies:	Termination of the following therapies:
Thyroid	Thyroid
Epinephrine	Epinephrine
Corticoid therapy	Corticoid therapy
Deep roentgen ray	Deep roentgen ray
Toxemias	Correction of:
Hyperthyroidism	Hyperthyroidism
Sepsis	Acute infections
Acute infections	Burns
Fever	Ketosis
Ketosis	Fever
Ultraviolet ray burn	

Complications of Insulin Therapy

HYPOGLYCEMIA (INSULIN REACTION)*

Causes and Nature of Hypoglycemic Reactions in Diabetes. In general, too much insulin or too little food or both

* "Hypoglycemic reactions" or "insulin reactions" are the acceptable terms and are preferable to "insulin shock," which is misleading.

embrace the factors causing hypoglycemic reactions following insulin treatment.

The causes can be presented more specifically as follows:

1. Unusual exercise without reducing insulin or increasing the diet. Exercise, in all but very severe and untreated diabetes, has a blood-sugar lowering effect. As a result, the routine dose of insulin becomes excessive and insulin reactions are likely.

2. Failure to eat all the food allowed, or delaying meals too long after the insulin has been given.

3. Overdose of insulin because of error in measuring.

4. Vomiting.

5. Diarrhea.

6. Failure to anticipate gains in carbohydrate and total food tolerance, and a proportionate reduction in the need for insulin following (a) the control of the diabetes, (b) a reduction in weight, (c) eradication of infections and toxemia and (d) a reduction in diet.

7. Erroneous distribution of the insulin and diet.

8. A too rapid increase in the amount of insulin given.

9. The development of cachexia with poor glycogen storage as in malignant disease and in certain instances of tuberculosis. Underweight persons are more sensitive to insulin than those who are well nourished.

10. A change of the site of insulin injection from an insulin tumefaction to other areas may precipitate a hypoglycemia (p. 851).

Symptoms. The symptoms characterizing varying degrees of severity of hypoglycemic reactions are as follows:

MILD REACTIONS. Mild hypoglycemic reactions exhibit symptoms of a stimulated sympathetic nervous system: hunger, weakness, tremulousness, nervous instability, mild emotional disturbances, headache, mild mental confusion and depression, and a detached manner in answering questions.

MODERATELY SEVERE REACTION. As the more severe grades of hypoglycemia develop disturbances in the central nervous system and psychiatric manifestations occur—increased weakness, excessive perspiration with skin cold and clammy to the touch, numbness of tongue, lips or buccal mucosa, cardiac palpitation, difficulty in mental concentration, loss of memory, diplopia, staring expression, blurring of vision, difficulty in walking, impaired coordination, increased emotional instability and disorientation.

SEVERE REACTION. Severe hypoglycemic reactions include twitching of muscles, convulsions, unconsciousness, paraplegias, incontinence of urine and, in unusual cases, transient hemiplegia. Protracted coma for hours or days even after the blood sugar is restored to normal may rarely occur. Mental deterioration is a rare complication of prolonged severe hypoglycemic states. Fatalities due to insulin reactions are rare. They are most likely to occur in debilitated individuals with poor glycogen reserves and least likely in the robust and muscular patients with ample stores of glycogen.

Hypoglycemic reactions due to protamine zinc insulin may not be observed in the early stages. They occur most frequently between midnight and breakfast time. The patient may be found stuporous or in an unconscious state, drenched with perspiration. He may, on the other hand, feel weak on rising and have a "cloud over his mind" until he has eaten. Headache is particularly common during and following the correction of a hypoglycemia due to a long acting insulin. Also, retrograde amnesia is common. Patients may go about their duties in a dazed manner for varying periods before attracting attention or before taking food, and yet they may have no recollection of "driving home," of "crossing the street," of "the conclusion of an important meeting" or other happenings, many of which carry grave possibilities.

Diagnosis. A history indicating that the patient has diabetes and is receiving insulin treatment is helpful. This information is not always obtainable and, even if it is, the possibility of unconsciousness resulting from other causes makes a careful differential diagnosis important.

The patient in an insulin reaction may exhibit signs ranging from slight transitory moments of confusion to complete unconsciousness. The mode and time of onset of symptoms are important. The patient may appear "queer," a fixed expression is common and conversation may be without proper sequence. He may behave like an automaton. He appears confused and is emotionally upset over trivial matters or without apparent cause. He may become boisterous and resist examination and treatment. The onset of unconsciousness before mealtime should make one suspect hypoglycemia, while if it occurs between one and three hours after a hearty meal hypoglycemia is not likely to be the cause.

There is usually some pallor of the skin but, in general, the patient's appearance is not that of a person who has been ill, but that of one who has fainted. The skin is wet, the face, body and extremities are cold and clammy, and the underclothes are wet with perspiration. The body temperature may be slightly below normal. The pupils are dilated; the intraocular tension is not disturbed; the pulse rate is rapid with normal or increased force and the blood pressure either is normal or, as frequently occurs, is elevated. It falls below normal only when the patient is *in extremis*. The breathing is undisturbed. Marks from the injection of insulin are usually apparent on legs, arms or abdomen. The tendon reflexes are overactive and a Babinski sign may be elicited during but not immediately after recovery from the reaction.

The examination of the urine offers little of value in confirming the diagnosis. The absence of glycosuria is suggestive evidence, however, in the case of an unconscious patient known to have diabetes and known to take insulin. Furthermore, the absence of glycosuria and ketonuria is definite evidence against diabetic ketosis. On the other hand, the patient whose blood sugar goes quickly from a high to a low level may have sugar in the urine from a preceding hyperglycemic phase. Sugar in the first specimen obtained from the unconscious patient should not rule out the possibility of a hypoglycemia. After the bladder has been emptied, a second specimen should contain no sugar in case of a hypoglycemia.

A low blood sugar level, below 60 mg. per 100 ml., is the most important single evidence of an insulin reaction. One must make a diagnosis on clinical evidence, however, and begin treatment. The patient's welfare should not be jeopardized by delaying therapy until the blood sugar concentration is known.

Differential Diagnosis. The most frequent causes of unconsciousness likely to be confused with insulin reactions are alcoholism, diabetic coma (ketosis) and intracranial lesions. Trauma, poisonings, epilepsy, uremia, syphilis of the central nervous system, and rarely, hyperinsulinism, malaria and Addison's disease may simulate, in part, a hypoglycemia due to an overdose of insulin. Night sweats of tuberculous infections complicating diabetes are occasionally suggestive of, and may be confused with, an insulin reaction.

DIABETIC COMA (KETOSIS). The chief characteristics of diabetic coma are presented on page 848 and the characteristic clinical differences between diabetic coma and an insulin reaction are presented in Table 19. The blood sugar level is above normal, the *plasma acetone* is promptly detectable (see p. 875) and the carbon dioxide combining power of the blood plasma is reduced in ketosis.

If there is any doubt whether one is dealing with diabetic coma (ketosis) or an insulin reaction (hypoglycemia), the therapeutic test of giving glucose (dextrose), 20 cc. of a 50 per cent solution in distilled water, intravenously, should be made. This will do the ketotic patient no harm and it will restore the hypoglycemic individual to consciousness in most cases.

INTRACRANIAL LESIONS. The more common intracranial lesions that are likely

TABLE 19. A COMPARISON OF THE CLINICAL EVIDENCES OF HYPOGLYCEMIA AND DIABETIC COMA

	HYPOGLYCEMIA	DIABETIC COMA (KETOSIS)
Cause	Too much insulin or not enough food	Not enough insulin
General appearance	A well person who has fainted	Very ill
Breathing	Normal	Rapid and deep (air hunger)
Onset	Rapid (minutes)	Slow, at least 12 hours
Hunger	Great	Anorexia
Thirst	None	Great
Vomiting	Rare	Common
Eyes	Staring, and pupils dilated	Sunken
Disturbed vision	Diplopia and difficulty in focusing	Haziness
Headache	Common	Absent
Intraocular tension	Normal	Decreased
Skin	Wet (especially forehead)	Dry
Tissues	Normal	Dehydrated
Pulse	Full and rapid	Weak and rapid
Air hunger	Absent	Present
Blood pressure	Elevated or normal	Subnormal
Cardiac palpitation	Frequent	Absent
Constipation	None	Present
Muscular twitching	Common	Absent
Nervousness	Common	Absent
Babinski's sign	Common	Absent
Complicating infections	Absent	Common
Abdominal pain	Absent	Common
Urine sugar	None after residual urine is discarded	Present
Blood sugar	Below normal	Above normal
Acetonuria	Absent	Present
Ketonemia	Absent	Present
Response to treatment	Rapid (minutes)	Slow (hours)

to confuse one are: hemorrhage, thrombosis and emboli in cerebral vessels, tumors and trauma. A careful physical examination will reveal signs of arterial disease, localizing neurologic signs or evidence of trauma and there will be no marks of the insulin injection. The blood sugar level will be normal or moderately elevated and glycosuria is common when there is injury to the base of the brain.

Treatment of Hypoglycemia. The hypoglycemia should be corrected without delay. Mild reactions are readily remedied by a glassful (240 ml.) of orange juice, or four or six glucose lozenges* (8 or 12 gm.). All patients taking insulin should carry these lozenges or lumps of sugar with them. Cane sugar is somewhat slower than glucose in correcting a hypoglycemia. Honey, molasses, syrup and hard candy are all effective, but if these are not available other carbohydrate foods may be given if the patient is able to take food by mouth. Fruits, cereals, bread and crackers will correct mild reactions. Often it is necessary only to take a meal a trifle earlier than usual.

Dextrose, 20 ml. of a 50 per cent solution in distilled water, is given intravenously without delay to the patient who is unconscious or is having convulsions as a result of a hypoglycemia. Often consciousness is restored before the intravenous injection is completed. Should this measure fail to restore consciousness, a continuous intravenous administration of a 10 per cent solution of glucose (dextrose) in distilled water is begun. This measure is rarely necessary but in two instances when enormous doses of insulin were taken by mistake, I believe it was life-saving. Consciousness having been restored, intravenous treatment is no longer necessary, but when the reaction is due to protamine zinc insulin it is a good plan to give 10

* Obtainable from White Laboratories, Ambler, Pa.

or 20 gm. of carbohydrate half-hourly or hourly until the next meal is taken, or until glycosuria is provoked. In this manner one can prevent hypoglycemic reactions due to protamine zinc insulin which are likely to recur. A recurrence of the reaction is not as likely when the hypoglycemia follows overdosage with crystalline insulin.

If sterile glucose is unobtainable and if feedings by mouth are not practical, carbohydrate in liquid form may be administered *via* a tube passed through one nasal passage and into the stomach. Retention of food in the stomach may prevent absorption of carbohydrate, hence too much reliance should not be placed on oral or tube feedings if there is not a prompt (within ten or fifteen minutes) satisfactory clinical response.

The hypoglycemic individual absorbs considerable glucose if it is administered by rectum. Twenty grams of glucose or corn syrup dissolved in 8 ounces of warm water and given by the drip method has served well in emergencies.

Epinephrine, 0.5 to 1.0 cc. of a 1 in 1000 solution given subcutaneously, may cause a return of consciousness and allow food to be taken by mouth. It liberates glucose from hepatic glycogen. Little effect can be expected from epinephrine in the emaciated patient or in the patient who has a severe reaction from protamine zinc insulin in which the hepatic glycogen is heavily drawn upon before symptoms of a hypoglycemia appear. Epinephrine is most effective in the well-nourished patient and when the hypoglycemia is the result of an overdose of a rapidly acting insulin, unmodified or crystalline. The effect of the epinephrine in any case is only transitory. It should never be relied upon alone but should be supported by the administration of food.

It is well to advise patients with unstable diabetes who are subject to severe hypoglycemic reactions on slight deviation from their usual regimen to keep "on hand" 2 ampules of glucose (each containing 20 ml. of a 50 per cent solution) for emergency use by their physician.

Prevention of Insulin Reactions (Hypoglycemia). A recurrence of an insulin reaction may be prevented by reducing the appropriate dose of insulin on succeeding days. Should the hypoglycemia have followed unusual exercise, an omitted meal or vomiting, no reduction is indicated on the following day if normal conditions are restored.

Insulin reactions may be prevented in the following ways.

1. A small reduction of the insulin dosage, of 2 to 8 units or more, according to the dictates of experience, is made when unusual and strenuous exercise is planned. When the usual amount of insulin has been injected and extra exercise is taken, a moderate addition to the usual diet such as a banana, a glass of milk or a glass of orange juice is advisable. A regular daily plan of exercise, uniform in time and amount, will reduce the likelihood of reactions.

2. In event of vomiting, the amount of insulin is reduced to one-half the usual requirement if there is no glycosuria, keeping in mind that even if food is not ingested metabolism of the body tissues continues. Rarely indeed should a dose be completely omitted, though this is a common (and dangerous) practice. Each specimen of urine is examined separately and if heavy glycosuria should occur more insulin is given. This plan is also adopted in case of diarrhea. Close supervision of the diabetic patient who is vomiting or has diarrhea is essential as in one patient they may cause hypoglycemic reactions and in another ketosis.

3. Appropriate reductions are made in the insulin dosage after the diabetes is controlled. A gain in carbohydrate and total food tolerance occurs and the need for insulin decreases proportionately. A decrease of 4 to 8 units a day until glycosuria occurs is a good practice. At this point a small increase in the amount of insulin will usually suffice to adequately control the diabetes. Greater reductions should follow the reduction in body weight and eradication of ketosis, infections and toxemia.

4. Increasing the insulin too rapidly

is a cause of reactions. The increases should be small—2 or 4 units daily—as control of the diabetes is approached.

5. The timing and distribution of the insulin are arranged according to the plan presented on page 842. It is especially important, when a rapidly-acting insulin and protamine zinc insulin are given before breakfast, that the meal be not delayed more than fifteen minutes after the insulins are administered.

6. In cases with marked tendencies to develop hypoglycemia readily it is well to observe the distribution of the diet which will reduce to a minimum the risk of hypoglycemic reactions (see p. 817).

7. A small reduction—4 to 12 units—of insulin dosage or a moderate increase in the diet when the patient is discharged from the hospital is a wise precaution to offset the effect which the increased exercise has in precipitating low blood sugar levels. Final adjustments in the insulin dosage are made under "home conditions."

ALLERGIC REACTIONS TO INSULIN

Local reactions may occur about the site of the insulin injection and are manifested by swelling, redness, discomfort and itching. They are common when protamine zinc insulin is used and unusual when the rapidly acting, globin or lente insulins are given. Swollen and indurated areas about an inch or an inch and a half in diameter appear and become hot and tender. These local reactions first appear from two to twelve hours after the injection is given. The reaction is at its height from eighteen to twenty-four hours, after which the inflammatory reaction and the swelling gradually subside until there is no trace of them in three or four days. In the sensitive patient, there may be three or four of these "areas" in the various stages of progression and regression at one time. Fortunately, within three or four weeks this type of reaction subsides.

It is rare to encounter a patient who is allergic to insulin protein itself—identified by noting allergic reactions to all forms of insulin. Allergic sensitivity to the specific animal protein is somewhat more frequent and is identified, as an example, when relief follows the change from insulin of pork origin to that made from beef.* The most common of all allergic manifestations to insulin therapy are associated with sensitivity to protamine zinc insulin—alleviated spontaneously in most cases and, in the persistent cases, by changing to globin or to lente insulin. The addition of protamine (having no antigenic properties) to insulin (a true antigen) is believed to create a higher incidence of sensitivity to insulin than when insulin alone is injected into individuals having no detectable sensitivity to protamine solution (Kern and Langner).[93] Resumption of insulin therapy after a lapse of weeks to years is followed in a week to ten days by systemic reactions, urticaria, swelling of face and extremities in some patients having an allergic sensitivity to insulin.

By recrystallizing mixed beef and pork insulin several times Jorpes[94] was successful in retaining the activity of the insulin while eliminating impurities which were considered to be the causes of the allergic reactions.

It is rare to find a patient who is allergic to globin or to lente insulin, but if sensitivity to the insulin protein is present an allergic response may be expected following the injection of insulin of any brand or source.

Treatment for Allergic Reactions to Insulin. 1. It may be practicable to omit insulin in the obese patient with uncomplicated diabetes. Control of the diabetes by appropriate restriction in diet and reduction in weight or by an oral hypoglycemic agent will avoid untoward allergic reactions from insulin. It must be assumed, however, that every diabetic patient will sooner or later develop acute complications and will need insulin temporarily. It is therefore of great importance to establish his allergic status and determine which insulin, if any, he can take without risk of severe allergic reactions. If he has an allergic

* Beef insulin is available from Eli Lilly & Company.

sensitivity to all insulins desensitization is recommended, after which insulin is given with sufficient frequency to avoid a return of his sensitivity. In the case of the obese diabetic one injection per week will suffice, whereas daily injections will be needed for therapy in the thin diabetics.

2. No special treatment is needed for the common local reactions which subside spontaneously after a few weeks of continued insulin therapy.

3. Allergic reactions to protamine zinc insulin of sufficient severity to warrant more vigorous action usually subside by changing from protamine zinc insulin to globin or to lente insulin. Changing of the commercial brand of insulin—from one lot of insulin to another or from the product of one pharmaceutical company to that of another—has been beneficial on some occasions. This is attributable in most cases to changing the animal source of insulin. Semi-lente and ultra-lente insulins may be used, in appropriate proportions, in cases of sensitivity to protamine.

Generalized urticaria or constitutional reactions, especially edema of the face and mucous membranes, dyspnea, prostration, gastrointestinal symptoms and stiffness of joints following insulin administration are uncommon but present a genuine problem when they occur.

These reactions as well as the persistence of severe local reactions are treated as follows:

a. Epinephrine hydrochloride (Adrenalin) 1:1000, subcutaneously, 0.5 ml. for an adult and 0.2 ml. for a child. The dose is repeated as frequently as every half hour depending upon the severity of the reaction. In extreme emergencies prednisolone-21-phosphate may be given intravenously in doses of 20 mg.

b. Ephedrine sulfate is given by mouth, 25 mg. (3/8 gr.) for the adult and 8 mg. (1/8 gr.) for the child, at four-hour intervals until improvement occurs.

c. One of the antihistamine drugs is given orally at four-hour intervals until relief is secured and maintained.

FAT DYSTROPHIES—TUMEFACTIONS AND ATROPHY

Insulin Tumefactions. Local painless, indurated areas of fat hypertrophy sometimes occur where insulin is injected in the same area over long periods. The swelling (see Fig. 18, *B*) is "rubbery" to palpation and the skin is adherent to the subcutaneous tissue. Not infrequently the overlying skin is peculiarly insensitive to pain. For this reason patients, especially children, wish to have the insulin injected into this area, but as the induration interferes with absorption of the insulin, this practice should be forbidden.

Treatment consists of changing the site of injection in such a manner that one site will not be used a second time in any fortnight. The swelling gradually

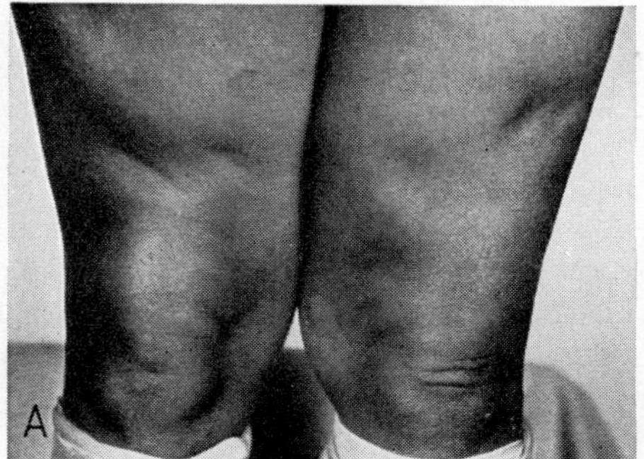

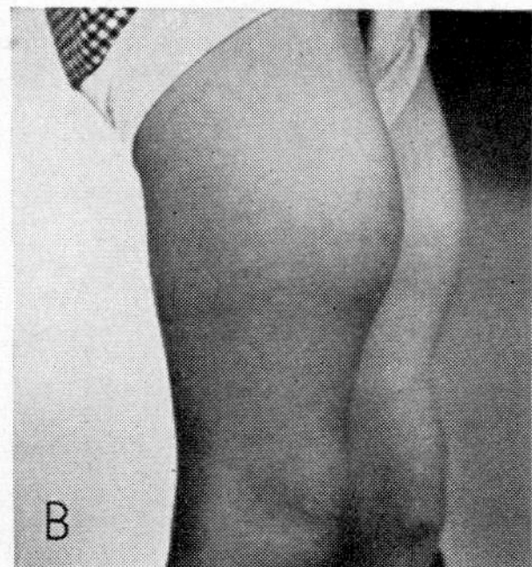

FIG. 18. *A*, Pitting of the skin caused by atrophy of the subcutaneous fat following many injections of insulin in the same area. (Courtesy of J. West Mitchell.) *B*, Swelling of the anterior aspect of both thighs caused by hypertrophic changes in the subcutaneous adipose tissue following many injections of insulin in the same areas. (Courtesy of L. L. Pennock.)

subsides. Injections of insulin elsewhere with a more rapid absorption may precipitate hypoglycemic reactions until suitable adjustments in the dosage are made.

Fat Atrophy Due to Insulin. Concave depressions in the cutaneous contour due to atrophy of subcutaneous fat and appearing in areas into which insulin has been injected over relatively long periods—several weeks to several years—are not uncommon in child diabetics of both sexes and of adult females—usually under thirty years of age (see Fig. 18 *A*).

The cause of the fat atrophy at the site of the insulin injection is unknown beyond the fact that it is related to insulin therapy. Many theories have been advanced—faulty technique of administration of insulin, impurities in the alcohol used for cleansing and sterilizing purposes, the preservative in insulin, local metabolic reactions, the low temperature of insulin when injected, local injury and androgen insufficiency. The sex and age occurrence suggests that the androgens may have a protective effect against this disorder. On the other hand, the paucity of subcutaneous fat in the adult male may be a factor. The condition is not restricted to insulin therapy, as repeated injections of other drugs are known to have caused it. Varying the sites of injection has been recommended on a preventive measure. Also, administration of insulin which is at room temperature has been observed to correct this abnormality. The pitting disappears slowly, requiring from two to four months and rarely one to two years, to subside completely.

INSULIN EDEMA

A filling out of the face, giving it a waxy appearance, smooth and free from wrinkling with a reduction of facial expression is seen in some patients following the rapid control of a severe diabetes with insulin. These patients are usually, but not always young females. One patient had not only the "insulin facies" but extensive edema of his extremities and disturbance of vision as well, during the first few weeks he received insulin. This patient had a complicating xanthoma diabeticorum with a blood cholesterol of 1666 mg. per 100 ml. and a severe diabetes. The water retention probably was exaggerated by the high carbohydrate diet which was allowed.

Ordinarily no special treatment is necessary for "insulin edema," though in this case the edema was so extensive that the salt was withdrawn from his diet and for a few days he was given ammonium chloride 1.3 gm. (grains 20) three times daily.

PRESBYOPIA DUE TO INSULIN

A transient presbyopia occurs in a considerable number of patients whose diabetes is rapidly controlled with insulin. This disturbance is attributed to a reduced elasticity of the lens and is probably the consequence of a disturbance of the adjusted osmotic pressure in the tissue of the lens and circulating fluids. The degree of change usually amounts to about 2 diopters, but in young patients, in whom the condition is most troublesome, changes of 8 diopters are sometimes observed. This disturbing complication has occurred in my experience for the most part in young adult patients. It is entirely apart from hypoglycemic reactions, and after two to four weeks of treatment the presbyopia precipitated by insulin therapy disappears entirely.

The patient should be advised that the disturbance is temporary. Glasses purchased at such a time, though satisfactory during the period of presbyopia, gradually become unsuitable with the control of the diabetes. Examinations preparatory to prescribing for glasses should be delayed until at least six weeks have elapsed subsequent to control of the diabetes. In isolated instances it may be desirable to secure suitable lenses for temporary use.

IDIOPATHIC INSULIN RESISTANCE

It has become customary to consider insulin needs above 200 units daily to indicate *idiopathic insulin resistance.* I would add that the large amounts of insulin should be needed for at least several months, and in the absence of any apparent acute disorder that might account for this need, an appreciable and spontaneous reduction in the need for insulin ultimately occurs. The unusual resistance to insulin ordinarily subsides within several months to two years, although Smelo[95] reported an instance in which the resistance prevailed for four and a half years.

Idiopathic insulin resistance is distinct from the condition or conditions which indefinitely call for insulin in amounts exceeding that necessary to control the diabetes precipitated by a pancreatectomy. These amounts range, usually, from 50 to 160 units. It was probably a wise accident that the arbitrary dosage which exceeds 200 units per day was chosen to identify idiopathic insulin resistance.

Glucose tolerance tests with and without insulin and insulin tolerance tests in a case reported by Yankelowitch and associates[96] showed insulin in moderate doses to be without apparent effect. An insulin neutralizing factor in the serum was detected by the Lowell[97] mouse and rat diaphragm glucose uptake and glycogen synthesis tests; the serum contained skin sensitizing antibodies and an antibody which agglutinated insulin-coated tannic acid treated red blood cells. No explanatory hormonal nor metabolic disturbance was found to account for the insulin requirement of 1500 units per day, nor did paper electrophoresis indicate increased gamma globulin values.

Severe degrees of idiopathic resistance to insulin are uncommon and their cause is unknown. One woman had an insulin need in 1947 which ranged between 400 and 2800 units daily. The only apparent complicating factor was a cholelithiasis with no acute manifestations. No abrupt change followed cholecystectomy. However, over several months the need for insulin decreased gradually; in August 1950 her diabetes was controlled by 176 units and in November 1957 by 230 units daily.

The foregoing is the pattern usually observed in these patients—the unexplained development of a reduced hypoglycemic response to insulin but with ultimate spontaneous restoration of insulin sensitivity.

The possible causes of this phenomenon include allergic reactions to insulin, extreme rapidity of degradation of insulin, formation of circulating insulin-blocking antibodies bound to the gamma globulin fraction (as demonstrated by Lowell[97]), skin sensitizing antibodies in the beta globulin fraction, formation of an insulin antagonist or hyperglycemic agent, overaction of physiologic opponents of insulin (notably the growth hormone and corticoids), poor absorption of insulin and a biochemical metabolic block in which there is an absence of the enzyme catalyzing a particular process.[98]

In observing the disappearance of I^{131} labeled insulin, Berson and Yalow[99] found that in individuals who had been receiving insulin the immediate insulin effect seemed to be lessened by a binding of the insulin to its antibody and that not until this binding capacity was exceeded did the insulin act in a normal manner.

It has been suggested that the insulin is excreted in the urine. If so, it is not in an active form; the injection into a mouse of appreciable quantities of urine voided by a patient after the injection of 2000 units of insulin had no hypoglycemic effect.

Downie[100] reported instances in which severe resistance to insulin was associated with the disappearance of insulin from the serum, but when the resistance to insulin had passed, insulin could again be demonstrated in the blood. He also recorded instances of insulin resistance in which no obvious disturbance of the insulin content of the serum was detectable, supporting the concept that not all cases of idiopathic insulin resistance have a common cause.

The short periods of resistance to insulin, as commonly observed during acute infections and ketosis, could possibly be acute episodes on the same basis as the long term periods of unexplained resistance to insulin, but this seems improbable.

Treatment of Insulin Resistance. Insulin is given in sufficient amounts and with sufficient frequency to avoid ketosis. When no cause is detected, it may be necessary to treat these patients identically as for an acute complication. It was necessary to give one patient regular insulin in doses as high as 475 units every four hours day and night over a prolonged period. Attempts to give fewer doses or smaller amounts resulted in the prompt appearance of ketosis. The ultimate favorable outcome that occurred in this case is the rule.

ACTH or hydrocortisone may reduce antibody formation and be helpful,[101] but when this abnormality is not present, these drugs may intensify rather than relieve the state of insulin resistance.[102,103]

Dimercaptopropanol (BAL), an SH compound, seemed to be helpful in two cases of insulin resistance reported by Butterfield.[104] Insulin resistance associated with an allergy to insulin was prevented by the use of recrystallized commercial insulin.[94]

Oral Drug Therapy. The sulfonylureas*, ** and phenformin, in contrast to universal diet therapy, are used selectively. Tolbutamide* has a milder blood sugar lowering effect than the other oral preparations, chlorpropamide** and phenformin.***

All patients in whom diabetes develops after forty years of age who are not appreciably overweight, who have no acute complications, and who formerly would have *required insulin to control the diabetes* are proper candidates for a trial with tolbutamide or chlorpropamide. These drugs may be given to the overweight patient but either should be considered a temporary measure and one to be discontinued when a suitable reduction in weight achieves control of the diabetes without it. Substitution of these oral therapies for diets aimed to correct obesity will probably be widespread; this practice is to be deprecated.

In more than two-thirds of the patients referred to the diabetes responds adequately to these drugs, which are ineffective, with rare exceptions, when the diabetes developed in youth. Both are ineffective in the presence of acute febrile complications and with rare exceptions when ketonuria develops readily; hence the need for adequate training in insulin therapy as, sooner or later, the diabetic, like the nondiabetic, will have acute complications to contend with.

Neither tolbutamide nor chlorpropamide controls, though it is claimed that they may stabilize diabetes acquired in childhood or in youth. In the presence of "adult acquired diabetes" it is well to be sure that the patient needs drug therapy before embarking on a treatment that may not be necessary. Even specialists in the treatment of diabetes have been surprised to find that in many patients past middle age no glycosuria nor hyperglycemia followed the withdrawal of insulin.

The prompt appearance of ketonuria during the first twelve hours after an appreciable reduction or discontinuance of insulin is, in most cases, an indication that these drugs will not be effective and that insulin should be promptly increased or resumed, in order to avoid unfavorable progression of the ketosis (see Fig. 19, Patient A). On the other hand, if no ketonuria appears when insulin is discontinued, as in the case of Patient B, Fig. 19, it is highly probable that this form of therapy will be adequate to control the diabetes.

The foregoing statements regarding the probable effectiveness of the sulfonylureas usually apply. However, occasionally patients taking unusually large amounts of insulin, e.g., 140 to 200 units, may have their need reduced to less than half by this form of therapy. In some instances the withdrawal of tolbutamide after several months does not result in a resumption of the need for the former large amounts. This has been

* Available commercially as Orinase (Upjohn), ** as Diabinese (Pfizer) and *** as DBI (U.S. Vitamin).

true in several patients even though an initial test reduction in insulin had promptly precipitated a ketosis. Similar results have been noted by Fabrykant.[28]

Apparent side effects of tolbutamide therapy are few, occurring in less than 3 per cent of cases. Skin rashes—urticarial, macular, eruptions or flushing—with pruritus are most common. If of mild degree, they tend to subside without interrupting the therapy. Leukopenia, disturbed bromsulfalein tests and elevated alkaline serum phosphatase values in mild and transitory forms have been observed but are rare.

Hypoglycemia, in my experience, is an uncommon complication of tolbutamide therapy. Possibly this is because I do not give more than 1.5 gm. daily and more often less than this amount for long-term treatment.

Changing from insulin to tolbutamide or chlorpropamide therapy is individualized. The following plans have proved satisfactory:

1. If the patient is taking in excess of 40 units of insulin, the dosage is reduced by 20 units, and when increasing glycosuria establishes with certainty the need for drug therapy, tolbutamide is given: 1 gm. with each meal the first day, 1 gm. with breakfast and lunch the second day, and 0.5 gm. with each meal thereafter until it can be determined whether smaller amounts will suffice. As the glycosuria subsides, the remaining dose of insulin is reduced by a second 20 units and then omitted entirely if glycosuria does not return.

On the other hand, if no appreciable decrease in glycosuria results when tolbutamide is substituted for 20 units of insulin, no further reduction in insulin is made, and if glycosuria persists for one week the former dosage of insulin is resumed and the tolbutamide is abandoned or prolonged. Combined therapy may be given a trial.

2. A patient taking 20 to 40 units of insulin is given half the usual dosage and tolbutamide is tried as indicated above.

3. If the usual dose of insulin is 20 units or less, it can be abruptly discontinued and the effect of tolbutamide observed.

4. In the case of the young patient with labile diabetes, tolbutamide may be tried in the hope that it will tend to stabilize the diabetes even if it does not reduce appreciably the need for insulin. In such cases no initial reduction in insulin is made and tolbutamide is begun in doses of 0.5 gm. with each meal. Appropriate reductions are made in the amounts of insulin, should the tolbutamide have an insulin sparing action.

If tolbutamide is given only to patients who would otherwise be obliged

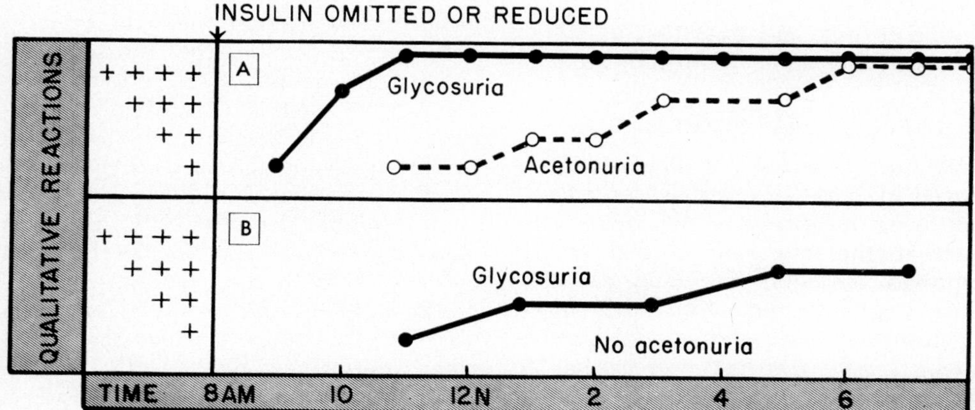

FIG. 19. A method of predicting the effectiveness of the sulfonylureas. Patient A: Increasing glycosuria and acetonuria following omission or appreciable reduction of insulin indicates that, in all likelihood, tolbutamide will be ineffective. Patient B: Glycosuria but no acetonuria is presumptive evidence that tolbutamide will be effective.

to take insulin, a considerable number must resume insulin within four to ten months without any apparent cause.[27] Chlorpropamide therapy is instituted in the same manner except that the initial dose is 0.5 gm. each morning. Less is used routinely if found to be adequate.

Phenformin may reduce the lability of the diabetes and reduce the need for insulin *in the juvenile type of diabetes.* The initial dose should be small—12.5 mg. or less with each meal. Small increases are made until maximum benefit is obtained without causing gastro-intestinal disturbances.

The instruction of patients regarding oral therapy is for the most part individualized but they should know that:

1. Sulfonylureas are effective in controlling the diabetes in the majority of older diabetics and are rarely effective in young diabetics.
2. They are not a form of insulin, nor do they act like insulin.
3. They are not a cure, immediate or projected, for diabetes.
4. They should not be taken when the diabetes may be satisfactorily controlled by diet alone.
5. They are ineffective during acute complications, notably acute infections, surgical procedures and ketosis.
6. Their favorable effects are transitory in some patients, being of four to six months' duration.
7. They do not reduce the need for attention to *diet* and *tests* for sugar, nor for tests for acetone when indicated.

EXERCISE AND GENERAL CARE

Physical exercise judiciously employed by patients who have no contraindicating conditions is of inestimable value in the treatment of diabetes. It improves the total food and carbohydrate tolerance and reduces the need for insulin. In the overweight patient having a mild diabetes, exercise has an insulin-like action, and a more gradual effect is the reduction of body weight. Exercise speeds the control of the diabetes in the overweight person. Patients quickly learn that glycosuria tends to occur when they are physically inactive and that it subsides when they are active.

In untreated undernourished patients having severe diabetes exercise is not helpful but actually accentuates the wasting processes characteristic of this disease and the blood sugar level is increased instead of lowered. But exercise becomes a helpful instead of a harmful agent when the diabetes is adequately treated by diet and insulin. Its blood sugar lowering effect is restored and all the advantages that accrue as the result of a good physical condition are added. The decrease in the need for insulin following discharge from the hospital is largely due to the effect of exercise.

For the patients for whom exercise would be advantageous a half hour's walk daily is prescribed. This includes climbing of hills, grades or steps; little energy is expended by walking on the level unless it is done briskly. Substitution of various forms of exercise is quite as important as substitutions in the diet. Irregularities in time and amount of exercise are permissible for the overweight diabetic person who does not require insulin. For the patient who has severe diabetes and is taking insulin, approximately the same amount of exercise at about the same time each day is desirable. Irregularities in exercise call for a reduction in the insulin or an increase in the diet on the days of unusually great exercise and *vice versa.*

Extra exercise in the forenoon increases the likelihood of a hypoglycemia before lunch if crystalline or semilente insulin is taken before breakfast. In the afternoon it increases the likelihood of reactions during the late afternoon if globin, lente or NPH insulin is taken before breakfast. In the afternoon and especially in the evening, extra exercise increases the prospects of hypoglycemic reactions during the night when protamine zinc or ultra-lente insulin is taken before breakfast or when an intermediate acting insulin is taken before or after supper. Reductions in the insulin or additional food at the appropriate times is indicated.

General care of the patient under treatment for diabetes mellitus embraces his mode and habits of living, diet customs, environment, occupation, vacations, social activities and personal hygiene.

The habit of securing adequate rest and sleep is important. Tobacco used in moderation has no apparent deleterious effect on the diabetic patient, though it is contraindicated if there is disease of the peripheral arteries or if there is a complicating disease of the coronary arteries. Alcohol may be injurious because of the added nourishment it provides. When used temperately and when the food value is allowed for by detracting a like amount from the diet, it has no serious effect but neither can it be considered beneficial. Patients who require insulin may be exposed to special hazards if they use alcohol.

Occupations requiring considerable physical exercise are to be desired over those which are sedentary. An occupation which allows the patients to live and eat at home is to be advised in preference to that which entails travelling. Patients with severe diabetes who require large doses of insulin should avoid occupations which necessitate their driving an automobile or working with power-driven machinery.

Social activities bring up innumerable problems. Irregularities in diet and in time of meals are common difficulties. Sensitive individuals often break diet rather than let their friends know they have diabetes. It may be wise to point out to certain patients the illustrious persons who have had and who have diabetes, in order to make them realize that diabetes is no disgrace. It is not wise to vary from the general principles of accurate treatment no matter how socially prominent the patient may be. They respect discipline who have little of it, even though they may resent it at first.

Though personal hygiene refers to habits, clothing and cleanliness, we are particularly interested in the special hygiene made necessary by diabetes, notably care of the feet.

The Training of the Patient. Patients should have a general knowledge of diabetes. Otherwise they give up treatment early and may think themselves cured. Each of my patients is required to read "A Modern Pilgrim's Progress for Diabetics"[105] and to be able to answer the questions outlined in it. They should be instructed regarding the incurability of diabetes and the effect which infection has upon it. They should be taught how to test the urine for sugar and acetone, how to prepare, weigh or measure their food, how to administer insulin, how to carry out the prescribed plan for tolbutamide therapy when indicated and how to care for their feet. It is important that every diabetic patient be made to realize with what speed acute complications may overtake him.

COMPLICATIONS

Introduction. *Chronic complications,* notably degenerative disturbances of the vascular and nervous systems and of the kidneys, present problems quite different from those of acute complications. They cause no appreciable change in the severity of the diabetes. The real problem is that these chronic complications are common and that once established they tend to progress. It is they, and not the diabetes *per se,* that incapacitate and threaten life. The measures recommended in dealing with the chronic degenerative disorders pertain to good control of the diabetes month after month and year after year, to suitable changes in diet, and to preventive and corrective procedures that may be indicated in the individual case. Nondegenerative disorders of a chronic nature which complicate diabetes are, in general, treated as in the nondiabetic.

Every diabetic patient will have an *acute complication* sooner or later. Whether it is an acute appendicitis, tonsillitis, carbuncle or other disturbance, the treatment that is satisfactory under usual conditions abruptly becomes inadequate. The anorexia so common during acute febrile episodes may lead the uninformed to omit insulin at such times. This mistake may lead to grave dangers.

Too much emphasis cannot be put on, *first,* the unfavorable effect which most acute complications have on diabetes. Even the patient who ordinarily does not need insulin may suddenly—within a matter of hours—present the indications for emergency insulin therapy. In the case of a patient with mild diabetes, diabetic coma developed during an acute infection, and he was in a perilous condition requiring 1750 units of insulin in the first twenty-four hours of treatment (see p. 810). The *second* feature of acute complications is that as the acute complication subsides, the severity of the diabetes is reduced and, in this case, satisfactory control of the disorder was maintained without insulin. *Thirdly,* good control of the diabetes is an important aid in overcoming the acute complication and it makes complete return to the pre-complication status of the diabetes more certain than if the diabetes is allowed to remain out of hand during the acute episode. *Fourthly,* the most severe case of diabetes can be controlled during these trying periods.

It is not true that the diabetes cannot be controlled during acute complications nor is it true that poor control of the diabetes does not alter the outlook in an unfavorable manner. It is not true that diabetic patients are unfavorable risks nor that they respond less well than nondiabetic patients to sulfa or antibiotic therapy. Recognizing these principles, the physician who is familiar with the need to alter the diet and its distribution and to adjust the insulin therapy, as the indications for these changes arise, will tide the diabetic patient through acute crises with little, if any, more risk than if the patient were not diabetic.

Degenerative Vascular Lesions

Prolongation of life expectancy of diabetics has been accompanied by a remarkable increase in the incidence of vascular disease. Reviews by Ricketts[106] and LeCompte[107] and observations by Bryfogle and Bradley[108] indicate the magnitude of this problem. They quote White and Waskow's series of 200 patients with diabetes since childhood and of twenty years' duration or more, of whom 92 per cent showed evidence of vascular disease. Also, Bell's series of 1559 autopsies revealed vascular disease as a causative or major contributing factor in 49.3 per cent of diabetics, in contrast with 24.5 per cent in nondiabetics. *Gangrene of an extremity, disease of the coronary arteries* and *renal arteriosclerosis* were the chief offenders in the diabetics. The average life span in the Naunyn era (1897–1914) was 44.5 years; in the Allen era (1914–1922) 46.7 years; in the latter part of the Banting era (1930–1936) 63.0 years in the Hagedorn era (1937–1943) 65.1 years, and in the Best era (1944–1951) 64.7 years.

Three distinct abnormalities, usually grouped under the heading of arteriosclerosis, are especially common in the diabetic population and appear at an earlier age than in nondiabetics. These are (a) *atherosclerosis*—essentially a disease of the intima, (b) *calcification of the arterial walls* (*Mönckeberg's sclerosis*) and (c) *arteriolarsclerosis.* All grades of involvement, from minimal to extensive changes of an advanced nature, are seen. These three subcategories of arteriosclerosis are apparently independent of each other—any one may occur singly or they may be combined in the same patient. However, whatever underlying processes are at work, all three are commonly associated with diabetes and especially diabetes that has not been well treated and is of long duration. These changes are apt to appear at an early age—in the twenties—and far outstrip, in progressiveness, similar changes seen in older nondiabetic individuals. The early start, the speed with which the degenerative processes progress and the advanced degree of the degenerative changes in the diabetic patient are in contrast with the later onset, the slow progress, and the lesser degree of the same disorder in nondiabetic individuals.

A most careful evaluation of the arteriosclerotic status will involve especially a most careful *history* dealing with symptoms and functional capacity, *retinoscopy, blood pressure determinations,* notation of the *degree of thickening of the palpable arteries,* the *extent of the cardiac borders,* preferably determined by fluoroscopy and recorded by roentgen ray pictures, *electrocardiogram evaluation of the circulation of the feet* (see p. 861), and a *roentgen ray search for calcified vessels.* A recording of the *blood cholesterol* (venous blood with patient in fasting state) may be of value for comparative purposes. The presence or absence of *albuminuria* should be noted and also the range of the *specific gravity of sugar-free urine.* The *blood urea nitrogen* concentration is determined if albuminuria or arterial hypertension is present.

Arteriosclerosis Obliterans (Atherosclerosis). The changes in the intima of the arteries which characterize this disorder make it the outstanding vascular complication of diabetes. Intimal plaques form on the side of the medium-sized arteries causing a localized narrowing of the lumen which predisposes to occlusion, especially of the coronary arteries and the arteries of the distal extremities, hence the term *arteriosclerosis obliterans.*

The obliterative nature of the atheromatous changes reduces the capacity of the vessel to deliver blood to the peripheral tissues in normal amounts. As the lumen of the artery is progressively infringed upon, eventually symptoms, notably anginal pains and intermittent claudication, are noted on occasions of increased physical activity. Still later, the patient becomes more and more conscious of the impaired circulation as indicated by coldness and disturbances in sensation in the feet, and finally with complete occlusion, localized death of tissue occurs as in the case of myocardial infarction or of gangrene of an extremity.

Atherosclerosis is not a static condition but one with periods of exacerbation and periods of quiescence. It comprises localized intimal thickening in which necrosis takes place and cholesterol and other lipids are laid down in the diseased site. These subsequently are dissolved out, leaving clefts. The resulting softened mass is the so-called *atheroma.* The atheroma is subject to cellular exudation, vascularization of the margins, organization and, in the advanced lesion, hemorrhage. Destruction of the media occurs in advanced cases and calcification of the plaque is common. Atherosclerosis bears a direct relationship to *obesity, to the duration of the diabetes and to hypercholesterolemia with poorly controlled diabetes.*

Mönckeberg's Sclerosis. Calcification of the media of the muscular arteries is the salient feature of Mönckeberg's sclerosis. It is not as common as atherosclerosis in diabetic patients but is seen more frequently and in more advanced stages in these patients than in nondiabetic individuals. It gives to the palpable artery a beaded contour of stony hardness—the so-called pipestem artery. Calcification of the media may occur in any artery but involvement of the vessels of the distal extremities is the most common.

Arteriolarsclerosis. In this form of arteriosclerosis hyaline material is laid down in the walls of the arterioles and occurs more frequently and at an earlier age and to more severe degree in diabetic than it does in nondiabetic subjects. Of diabetic patients over fifty years of age arteriolarsclerosis involving renal vessels is present about five times as frequently as in nondiabetic controls.

Intercapillary Glomerulosclerosis (Kimmelstiel-Wilson's Disease). The pathologic changes typical of this complication are presented on page 787. Clinically, the diagnosis is by presumption unless supported by a renal biopsy. The criteria are edema, hypertension and proteinuria. Diabetic retinopathy and anemia are common and with the loss of renal reserve, azotemia appears. Hypoproteinemia is usual in long standing cases but is not a diagnostic essential.

Renal disease, with intercapillary

glomerulosclerosis predominating, increases in contrast to cardiac disease as the age at death decreases.

Clinical progression of this disease gives the false impression of a decreasing severity of the diabetes. Such changes are not specific to renal disease, and if one considers the nutritional state of the patient and the continued proteinuria, the claim that the diabetes per se becomes milder is not substantiated.

TREATMENT FOR CHRONIC DEGENERATIVE VASCULAR COMPLICATIONS OF DIABETES

The chief aim is to restore disturbed physiologic processes to normal or as nearly to normal as is practicable. In so doing it is hoped that the tendency of the disorder to become worse will be allayed.

The measures employed are:

1. Gradual reduction of glycosuria and hyperglycemia guarding against risk of hypoglycemic reactions.

2. Reduction of hypercholesterolemia, excessive cholesterol esters, and lipemia by (a) correcting obesity, (b) allowing liberal carbohydrate—250 to 350 gm.—but reducing the fat intake to 50 gm. or less daily and (c) allowing a liberal quota of protein—usually in excess of 100 gm. daily.

Diseases of the Coronary Arteries Complicating Diabetes

Occlusion of the coronary arteries has far outstripped other causes of death in diabetic patients at the Pennsylvania Hospital. The frequency of this serious complication has been more frequent in the female than in the male diabetic patients. In contrast, in the nondiabetic population, this complication occurs in males and females between the ages of fifty-one and sixty in approximately a 5 to 1 ratio. There is an increasing incidence of diseases of the coronary arteries in diabetics and especially is this true for the female patients.

The main known factors at work in increasing the prevalence of disease of the coronary arteries in diabetic patients are: (1) the extended *duration of the diabetes*, the *degree of severity* and *poor control* of the diabetes, (2) the increased span of life for diabetics influencing unfavorably the incidence of disease of the coronary arteries, (3) *excessive concentration of cholesterol* and *other lipids* in the blood associated with a higher frequency of atherosclerotic changes and occlusive phenomena than when these chemical abnormalities are absent, (4) *arterial hypertension,* (5) *obesity,* (6) *excessive use of tobacco* and (7) *hypoglycemic reactions* predisposing to occlusion of the coronary arteries which have undergone marked atherosclerotic changes. It seems most probable that this is the result of an "alarm reaction" and bears a relationship to the increased amount of epinephrine in the circulation which occurs with the development of a hypoglycemia and which accelerates the clotting of blood.

There is no satisfactory yardstick with which to measure the efficacy of prophylactic measures in the individual case but it is my impression that benefit accrues from control of the diabetes, from reduction of hypercholesterolemia through the agency of liberal carbohydrate and protein and low fat allowances in the diet, from the correction of obesity and hypertension, from the restriction or complete elimination of the use of tobacco and by practicing great care in preventing hypoglycemic reactions.

Treatment. Insufficiency of the coronary circulation may be manifest by attacks of *angina pectoris,* the treatment for which comprises:

1. Gradual control of the diabetes—this takes several weeks if the risk that attends rapid control is to be avoided.

2. The correction of obesity. A low calorie diet is employed and when the weight has reached a satisfactory level, the diet is increased, using liberal protein and carbohydrate with low fat contents; e.g., protein 90 gm., carbohydrate 275 gm., and fat 59 gm. (1900 calories).

3. Vasodilators—nitroglycerin, 0.3 mg. ($\frac{1}{200}$ gr.) and aminophylline, 0.5 gm. ($7\frac{1}{2}$ gr.) are most commonly used for the alleviation of an attack of angina pectoris. Patients who are subject to at-

tacks of angina should never be without nitroglycerin, which may also be used as a prophylactic measure when the patient's "attack pattern" is known. To prevent recurrent attacks a tranquillizing agent is helpful and, in cases of mild hypertension, combined Rauwolfia and Veratrum veride therapy with restricted sodium intake has prophylactic value.

4. General measures are identical with those prescribed for nondiabetics, e.g., restriction of vigorous exercise and interdiction of tobacco.

5. In refractory cases in which the disorder is crippling, ablation of the thyroid function by administering radioactive iodine may be most helpful.

The treatment for *coronary occlusion* is the same as for the nondiabetic. Control of the diabetes, as in the case of other acute complications, with division of the diet into four equal nourishments equally spaced at six hour intervals (see p. 886), is important. Crystalline insulin also is given, if needed, at six hour intervals with precautions against causing a hypoglycemia.

Circulatory Disturbances in the Legs and Feet

Appraisal of the Circulation. The evaluation of the circulation is in reality the determination of the degree of patency of the lumen of the artery at its narrowest point and it is upon this feature that the prognosis and therapy depend.

Symptoms. Mild degrees of arteriosclerosis obliterans cause no symptoms, but as the condition progresses the sensation of *coldness* in the affected extremity becomes apparent. *A decrease in the muscular endurance,* impaired sensitivity to minor injuries and an accompanying partial anesthesia appear subsequently.

Intermittent claudication, first appearing after brisk walks for considerable distances, appears as a frequent symptom. A severe grade of arterial obstruction is present when this symptom is provoked by walking 20 to 30 yards at a slow pace. A short rapid walk will provoke intermittent claudication when a slow walk for a long distance may not be accompanied by this distressing symptom.

Pain—severe and persistent—*in the feet* and especially in the digits *while at rest,* and especially at night, indicates advanced vascular obstruction, provided neuropathic changes are not responsible. The onset of rest pain may be insidious and progress gradually or it may be sudden with the complete occlusion of an artery. Rest pain is common in the region of an ulcer or of a gangrenous area.

Pain due to an ischemic neuritis is of wider distribution and the discomfort is variable in nature and intensity and has burning or shooting characteristics.

The onset of pain in an extremity having a poor circulation may follow a minor injury to the foot. In this case the local reaction exerts a demand for circulation which the circulatory means at hand is unable to meet. The situation may be made worse by local vasoconstriction. This is a common occurrence preceding the appearance of gangrene, although gangrene may appear spontaneously with or without pain. Frequently a vesicle is the first local sign of gangrene.

Physical Signs. The dependent limb with advanced arteriosclerosis obliterans becomes bluish red. This discoloration fades proximally over the dorsum of the foot but in some cases it extends halfway to the knee or higher. The development of collateral circulation may prevent these color changes even though the large vessels are pulseless. It is significant that arteriosclerosis obliterans involves chiefly the larger vessels and it is not infrequent that the capacity for arteriolar dilatation is not greatly impaired. Marked pallor may follow the sudden occlusion of an artery of medium size.

Trophic changes in the skin, muscles and nails may be apparent on inspection. Ulceration and gangrene with or without apparent infection may be present. Evidences of a pyogenic infection, a lymphangitis and an *epidermophytosis* are important. Local injuries, and especially fissures that result from fungus infections, predispose to infection.

Gangrene involves the more prominent parts of the feet as a rule—the toes, the heel, the prominence of the metatarsophalangeal joints of the small and great toes, the dorsum of the foot and the malleolar regions.

Palpation. The tips of the toes are cold in advanced degrees of obliterative arteriosclerosis. A difference in temperature in the two feet is especially significant when both have been exposed to the same environmental temperature. Whether this coldness is due to a functional or organic obstruction is determined by studies of the skin temperature. It is important to detect impaired or absent pulsations in the dorsalis pedis, posterior tibial, popliteal and femoral arteries. Pulsations of the dorsalis pedis arteries may be absent because of congenital anomalies but if, in addition, the posterior tibial and popliteal pulsations are impaired or absent, arteriosclerosis obliterans is almost certain to be the cause. *The degree of pulsation, color changes, relation of pain to rest and to exercise and changes in temperature of the tips of the toes are the most important of the clinical clues in appraising the circulatory efficiency of a limb.* Poor tone of the muscles and impaired or intensified cutaneous sensitivities are among the less specific results of an impaired circulation.

The clinical evaluation of the state of the circulation is superior to special tests. The latter have an important place in supporting clinical findings, however. In general, *the circulation is good* if the patient does not complain of pain in the extremities, if there are no color changes, if there is good pulsation in the dorsalis pedis and posterior tibial arteries, and if the tips of the toes are warm. Warm toe tips in the absence of good pulsation of the peripheral arteries is a sign of good collateral circulation. Contrariwise, *the circulation in the limb is severely impaired* if rest pain and intermittent claudication are prominent, if the bluish red cyanosis (rubor) of the dependent foot gives way to a cadaveric pallor when the foot is elevated, if the tips of the toes and the foot are persistently cold and if there is absence of pulsations in the peripheral arteries of the foot—the dorsalis pedis and posterior tibial arteries.

Special Tests. The following studies are used selectively when needed to support clinical impressions. *Usually they are not necessary.*

ROENTGENOGRAPHY. Roentgenograms aid in determining the degree and position of calcified areas in the arterial wall. These studies should include not only the foot and leg but also the thigh, as obstructive lesions in the femoral arteries are frequent. Patchy, dense deposits of calcium causing a marked degree of obstruction may in some cases influence the selection of the site of amputation.

Roentgenograms are of value also in detecting osteomyelitis of the small bones of the feet and in assaying the degree of osteoporosis and destruction of bone in the rare case of neurotrophic foot (see p. 872).

SKIN-TEMPERATURE STUDIES. These studies tend to (1) confirm the clinical diagnosis and (2) afford information regarding the relative degree of functional arterial spasm and of organic arterial occlusion. The temperatures of the skin over the tips of the toes, the dorsum of the affected foot and various other levels are taken, the patient having been in a room the temperature of which is approximately 20° C. (68° F.) for one-half hour. These ratings are recorded and compared with those taken one hour after both arms and hands have been immersed in hot water, 43° to 45° C. This test, as advocated by Gibbon and Landis,[109] causes a definite reflex vasodilatation and a rise in temperature in the distal extremities from a normal temperature of about 24.7° C. on the toe and 30.2° C. on the sole of the foot, to 33.5° or 34.5° C. if the vascular supply is normal or if occlusion has been due to vascular spasm (Fig. 20). There is little or no rise in the skin temperature of the feet in the event of an advanced occlusion of the arteries due to organic changes. This test identifies the vascular spastic type of occlusion for which sympathectomy holds promise of success in contradistinction to the organic occlusive vascular disease, in which it would be not only valueless but dangerous. Satisfactory evaluation of the alterations in circulation is obtained by the induction of spinal anesthesia or by the injection of the peroneal nerve. Refinements in the execution of this test have detracted from its value and hence are not included.

PLANTAR ISCHEMIA TEST. This test, popularized by Samuels,[110] is carried out with the patient in the reclining position. The patient raises the foot being studied to an angle of 45 degrees, in which position he flexes and extends the foot rapidly for one minute. Obstructive arterial disease of a severe degree is indicated by blanching of the plantar surface of the foot when it is raised and exercised and a slow return of color when the foot is placed in a dependent position. There is little or no change in color if the arterial circulation is normal.

Other Tests. Oscillometric studies, arteriography, histamine flare test, intradermal saline wheal test and the fluorescein test are listed because they appear in medical writings frequently and not because of their clinical value. We do not employ them because they either add little or no information and are unnecessary, or mislead, or carry risk out of proportion to the information they might reveal. I do not mean to detract from the value of these tests as research procedures.

Differential Diagnosis. *Arteriosclerosis obliterans* as it is encountered in diabetes characteristically develops occlusive manifestations in patients over forty years of age; it involves especially the arteries of the lower extremities and the coronary arteries; thrombophlebitis is not a feature of the disorder; there is calcification of the arteries in 69 per cent; males constitute 83 per cent of those afflicted;[111] 34 per cent have an associated hypertension; 20 per cent of Allen's patients had diabetes; and elevated blood lipids is a common finding.

In contrast, thromboangiitis obliterans, with which arteriosclerosis obliterans might be confused, practically always occurs in male subjects under fifty years of age; 40 per cent have involvement of the upper extremity; 40 per cent have thrombophlebitic phenomena; there is no calcification of the arteries; diabetes is a rare complication; and the blood lipids are usually normal.

Diabetic neuropathy may co-exist with arteriosclerosis obliterans but numbness,

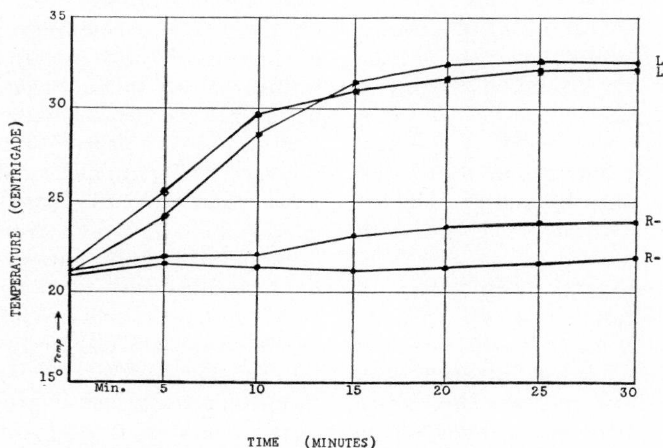

FIG. 20. Skin temperature vasodilatation test. The increase in temperature in the left foot upon immersion of the hands and arms in hot water indicates a high degree of spastic vasoconstriction. The absence of a similar response in the right foot is indicative of organic vascular occlusion.

lightning pains and ulcerations may be due to neurotrophic changes in the presence of warm toe tips and excellent pulsation of the peripheral arteries. Absent or sluggish tendon reflexes and an impaired vibratory sense over the distal extremities afford valuable clues in identifying the neurologic nature of the disorder in contrast to the predominantly vascular changes already presented.

There should be no difficulty in differentiating *gout, arthritis, sciatica, the burning feet of malnutrition states, erythromelalgia* and *thrombophlebitis* if the history is carefully taken and if the physical examination is complete.

Gangrene in an extremity of the diabetic patient occurs primarily because of the occlusive nature of arteriosclerosis obliterans (Fig. 11) and the resulting incompetency of the arterial circulation in meeting sudden or increased circulatory demands. The precipitating causes of gangrene are trauma, infection or extremes of temperature. Thrombotic or embolic phenomena in an atheromatous vessel also may be the exciting cause of gangrene. Any combination of events that will increase the need for circulation or that will obstruct the supply route may be sufficient to deprive the tissues of nutrition adequate to retain their viability.

The onset of gangrene may be sudden and painful, as occurs in the abrupt cutting off of the circulation by an arterial embolus. Or, there may be no pain and a vesicle may be the first ominous sign of local capillary damage to be followed by changes in color from the normal to a dark blue-gray or black in the underlying tissues. Infection, with its complicating hyperemia and lymphangitis, is a common complication. It may progress rapidly or slowly and the speed with which local death of tissues proceeds as a result of infection will depend on the degree of the devitalization of the tissue and the virulence of the infection. Infection tends to cause local inflammatory changes with an exudative lesion and accounts for more pain than is usually the case when infection is absent. In the latter instance the gangrenous area may be relatively painless and may become demarcated, hard, dry, mummified, shriveled and black.

In appraising the clinical state of a diabetic patient who has a gangrenous area special attention is given to the degree of concomitant degenerative changes, notably in the coronary, cerebral, renal and retinal circulations. These patients are usually over fifty years of age and have degenerative changes in their arteries of a degree seen in control nondiabetic subjects who are at least ten years older.

Prevention. More often than not arteriosclerosis obliterans is present to an advanced degree when these patients seek treatment. Nevertheless, there will be ample opportunity to practice prophylaxis, though it is not always as successful as desired. The preventive measures are:

1. CONTROL OF THE DIABETES.
2. CORRECTION OF HYPERCHOLESTEROLEMIA IF POSSIBLE (see p. 860).
3. SPECIAL CARE OF THE FEET.
4. SYMPTOMATIC RELIEF FROM PAIN.
5. LOCAL AND SYSTEMIC TREATMENT FOR ULCERS AND INFECTIONS. In addition to local therapy, bacterial cultures are taken from ulcerating areas and from discharging sinuses, and the sensitivities of the pathogenic organisms to the various antibiotic agents are determined. Too much emphasis cannot be placed on the value of complete bacteriologic evaluation of these infections. Lives and limbs will be saved if such studies are done in every case of bacterial infection. Furthermore, cultures of the blood are taken if the patient is febrile and has an increase in the number of leukocytes in the blood. Most staphylococcal infections in diabetic patients are resistant to penicillin.
6. PHYSICAL THERAPY. The circulation in the legs and feet may be improved by: (a) Sanders oscillating bed, (b) intermittent suction and pressure, (c) intermittent venous occlusion, (d) Buerger's exercises, (e) application of heat to hands and arms or abdomen, and (f) thermoregulated foot cradles which do not permit temperatures in excess of 90° F. (32.2° C.). *Applications of heat,*

without appropriate automatic thermoregulation, to the legs and feet are contraindicated. Probably no other single, exciting cause of gangrene outnumbers that of the unwise application of heat. Heat, under normal conditions, causes vasodilatation and hyperemia in the limb. With an impoverished circulation it does not exert this effect but rather tissue damage occurs, due to a local increase in the tissue metabolism without a commensurate increase in the circulation.

Sanders Oscillating Bed.[112] This is a satisfactory form of passive mechanical therapy. The rhythm with which the legs are raised and lowered is regulated to allow the feet to be dependent for long periods and elevated for short periods. The treatment may be continuous or intermittent, e.g., one hour three times daily depending upon the degree of relief from pain that is achieved. It is contraindicated in the presence of a bacterial infection with cellulitis.

Suction and Pressure.[113] This method* has suffered in popularity in recent years but is nevertheless helpful in some cases. It is contraindicated in the presence of collections of purulent material, acute bacterial infections and cellulitis. Suction amounting to 80 to 120 mm. of Hg is applied for twenty-five seconds alternating with a positive pressure of 40 to 80 mm. of Hg for five seconds. At the outset of the treatment pressures alternating from minus 80 to plus 40 mm. of Hg and progressing to minus 120 to plus 80 mm. are used according to the relief achieved. Treatments are given one to two hours daily, decreasing as improvement is established to three treatments, and finally one treatment per week.

Intermittent Venous Occlusion.[114] A cuff is fitted above the knee and is inflated to a pressure of 70 to 80 mm. of Hg, obstructing the venous return for one, two or three minutes, followed by a like period of release. When a reactive hyperemia occurs appreciable relief from intermittent claudication results. The treatment is continued for one to two hours daily. It is contraindicated in cases of venous insufficiency.

*Buerger's Exercises.** The great advantage of this form of therapy is that it can be carried out by the patient without intricate apparatus at home and for long periods. The patient, lying on his back, raises one or both feet at an angle of 45 degrees, and allows them to rest on an adjustable board until the feet are blanched or until the foot becomes painful. This usually requires about one minute if foot exercises are conducted in this position and somewhat longer, up to three minutes, if the feet are passive. The patient then assumes the sitting position with the legs hanging over the edge of the bed until a reactionary hyperemia develops or until pain is experienced in the legs or feet. After two to five minutes in this position a rest period for about three minutes is allowed in the horizontal position. This cycle may be repeated several times daily at first and increased gradually until the exercises last from one-half to one hour daily. Improvement is slow but worth while.

Application of Heat. In cases of vasospasm an appreciable increase in the temperature of the feet follows the application of heat—hot water bath or electric pad—*to the hands and arms, or heat applied to the abdomen.* This is a simple therapy that patients can carry out. Also this method enhances the value of the suction and pressure therapy when the two treatments are given simultaneously.

Thermoregulated Foot Cradles. Foot cradles without thermostatic controls are dangerous devices and should not be used. However, great relief is frequently secured by having the feet and legs in a foot cradle, the temperature of which is maintained at 90° F. (32.2° C.).

* Equipment is manufactured by The Burdick Corporation, Milton, Wis.

* A Buerger board which is adjustable to different angles is made simply by having two boards, each ¾ inch thick, 30 inches long and 12 inches wide, hinged at one end, with a supporting prop between, which is adjustable to fit on various cleats according to the angle desired.

7. VASODILATOR DRUGS. Some drugs may be effective in a case in which others give no benefit. In any case, most benefit may be anticipated when the element of vasospasm is great, and least, or no benefit, when organic arterial obstruction is of a severe grade.

Nicotinic acid, 50 to 200 mg. four times daily in conjunction with papaverine hydrochloride, 0.1 gm. (gr. 1½) three times daily, both given by mouth, is sometimes surprisingly helpful. Other vasodilators, as a group, give disappointing results but the occasional benefit, in addition to that served by physical methods mentioned above, makes it advisable to list the products from which benefits have been claimed. These are tetra ethyl-ammonium chloride (etamon), Dibenamine hydrochloride, Depropanex (tissue extract) and diethyl oxide (ether). *Regitine, Ilidar* and *Arlidin* have gained some popularity. Like that of other peripheral vasodilator drugs, their effectiveness is enhanced by warm, and reduced by cold, atmospheres.

8. OTHER MEASURES. The *ligation of the femoral veins* has in several instances in my experience given abrupt relief from intractable pains and the relief was attended with an increase in the warmth of the skin in the affected extremities. This is not a widely used procedure but the response is so striking, even in severe grades of arteriosclerosis obliterans, that it deserves consideration when conservative measures fail and amputation seems to be the last resort in the attempt to alleviate pain. The beneficial response is apparently due to a slowing of the venous return and to an increase of blood in the impoverished area.

Exercise. Mild forms of exercise are helpful. Patients with intermittent claudication must, however, be instructed to walk slowly. Buerger's exercises are recommended. The pain of nocturnal ischemia is not infrequently relieved by elevating the head of the bed 6 to 8 inches.

Occupation. Occupation and other activities which present special risk of injury to the feet should be given up in the face of advanced occlusive arterial disease of the legs and feet.

Sympathectomy. In carefully selected cases, in the face of failure of conservative methods to relieve pain, particularly that of intractable intermittent claudication, and in cases in which the element of vasospasm is considerable, a lumbar sympathectomy may be indicated. It is not an emergency procedure. Other measures—exercises, omission of tobacco, application of heat to body and vasodilator drugs—should be given a thorough trial.

Care of the Feet in the Prevention of Gangrene. *Calluses* and *corns* carry special risks and are to be dealt with by a well informed chiropodist and orthopedist. Mild manifestation of *epidermophytosis* is usually controlled promptly by applying a thin film of fungicidal foot powder, containing zinc undecylenate, undecylenic acid and talc* over the affected areas and between the apparently unaffected toes after each bathing until the condition is controlled and, thereafter, once weekly.

When *fissures* are present the following preparation is applied daily:

℞		
	Salicylic acid	3.5 gm.
	Benzoic acid	7.0 gm.
	Castor oil	30.0 ml.
	95% ethyl alcohol	180.0 ml.

With correction of the fissure, treatment with foot powder is begun, or resumed.

For the *severe cases* with acute vesicular or bullous eruptions and with secondary infections, the feet are soaked in a 1:8000 solution of potassium permanganate for thirty minutes three times daily, for not more than one week. As the acute phase subsides the prescription (salicylic acid, benzoic acid, castor oil and ethyl alcohol) included above, or a stronger keratolytic agent such as one-half strength Whitfield's ointment, or the daily application of Castellani's paint, is used until it appears advisable to change to the foot powder for long-term therapy and prevention.

*Available commercially as Desenex Powder.

Untreated epidermophytosis provides portals of entry for secondary infection which is often sufficient to tip the balance unfavorably when the local circulation is adequate in the absence of infection but insufficient to meet the increased circulatory demands that attend an infectious process.

Treatment for Gangrene. The therapy for gangrene due to occlusive vascular disease in a diabetic is conducted in cooperation with a surgeon who is especially skilled in the management of these patients.

Many factors may influence therapy but the most important are (1) the degree of efficiency of the circulation and (2) the presence of infection. Conservative nonoperative treatment is justifiable if the area of gangrene is well demarcated and superficial, if the tips of the toes are warm and there is good pulsation in the dorsalis pedis and the posterior tibial arteries, when the extremity retains normal color on elevation and when in the dependent position. The active therapy comprises: (1) Control of the diabetes but not so strictly that hypoglycemic reactions are likely. (2) Eradication of infection. After release of the confined pus, a culture is grown, and the sensitivity of the pathogenic organism to the various antibiotic agents is determined. Suitable doses of the appropriate antibiotic agent are given. (3) If crusts of dried exudates are present with evidence of trichophyton infection, the affected foot is soaked in a solution of potassium permanganate 1:8000, the temperature of which should not be lower than 86° F. (30° C.) and not higher than 95° F. (35° C.) for one-half hour three times daily. (4) Subsequent to the foregoing local treatments, local applications of Furacin have been valuable. Dressings of zinc peroxide are of special value if there is extensive necrosis. The same benefit has been claimed from the use of trypsin. Acute infection indicates complete rest of the affected part, and as a result most of the measures that are of use prophylactically are to be avoided when infection is present. (5) Ligation of the femoral veins has yielded gratifying results in a few carefully selected cases in which pain was predominant and in which indolent gangrenous ulcers were at a standstill. (6) Exercise promotes collateral circulation and healing and avoids some of the hazards of bed rest, notably decreased blood flow, wasting of muscles and loss of tissue turgor. Hence, walking is prescribed in progressively longer periods except when contraindicated by severe debility, acute cardiac difficulties, high fever, thrombophlebitis (before the inflammation subsides) and recent gangrene that is actively spreading.[115]

AMPUTATION. The incidence of amputations has decreased as a result of sulfonamide and antibiotic therapies. Furthermore, when amputation is decided upon, removal of the foot at the transmetatarsal site is done with less prospect of subsequent higher amputations than was formerly the case. The occlusive vascular disease is not confined to the legs. The vessels of the heart, brain and kidneys have not escaped. Despite these considerations, with the skill of the surgeon, the advances in anesthesiology and the newer drug therapies, these patients with widespread vascular disease do wonderfully well when subjected to surgery.

The indications for amputation are:

1. Extensive penetrating gangrene with no improvement under conservative treatment and in a limb which is extremely impoverished of circulation.

2. Deep extensive and extending infection and especially with an extensive osteomyelitis which is intractable to conservative measures. A phalanx may be safely removed if the osteomyelitis is limited to this area.

3. Intractable pain with evidence of extreme grades of organic vascular occlusion—care being taken not to be misled by a peripheral neuritis.

Site. The level at which the amputation will be done is decided upon after a careful appraisal of the local circulation. The site selected should be high enough to be in a relatively well vascularized zone. If in the process of re-

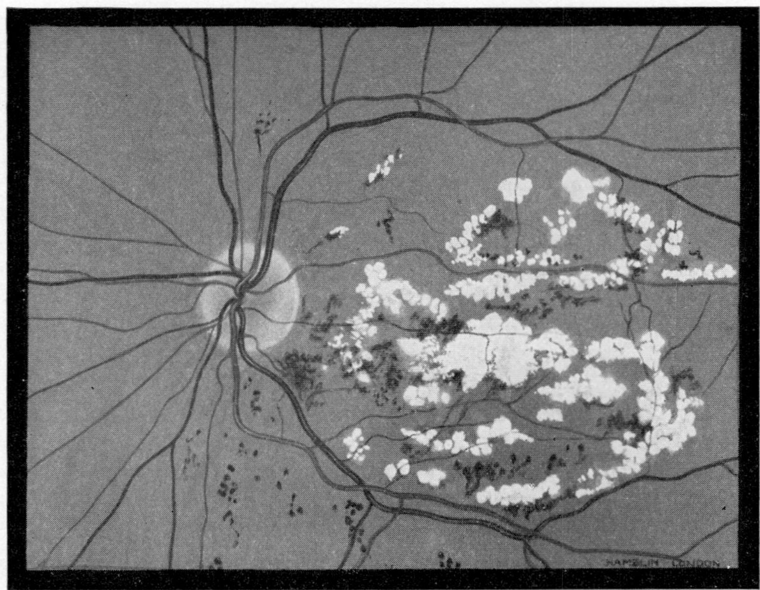

FIG. 21. Diabetic retinitis. Note the deep round hemorrhagic areas, the waxy exudates and decreased caliber of the arterioles.

moving a limb the surgeon finds more extensive occlusive disease and less bleeding than he thinks might promise good postoperative progress, a higher site is immediately selected. In general, it is wise, in case of doubt, to elect the higher of two contemplated sites. Roentgen ray films may show a marked degree of arterial obstruction just above the knee. The amputation in such a case would be above the obstruction unless the evidences of an efficient collateral circulation are marked.

Anesthetic. The choice of anesthetic is made by a competent anesthetist. Generally, spinal anesthesia is used for amputations. However, if there is an extreme degree of infection and necrosis and the patient shows marked evidences of a toxemia, the circulation of the limb is entirely obliterated by placing a tourniquet above the knee sufficiently tight to stop the arterial circulation, and the limb is refrigerated by packing it in ice to a point several inches above the tourniquet.[116] After several days, with the pronounced clinical improvement that is usual, the leg is amputated above the level of the tourniquet. With refrigeration no other anesthetic agent is used. In properly selected cases the foregoing procedure is an excellent one. Ordinarily the procedure of amputation causes little difficulty in maintaining control of the diabetes but, when necessary, the same measures are used as are employed with other surgical procedures as outlined on page 897.

Ocular Lesions

Ocular changes attributable to diabetes have a degenerative basis and patients with degenerative ocular changes present a high incidence of arterial disease—hypertension and diseases of the coronary and peripheral arteries, chronic renal disease and hypercholesterolemia. The degree of severity of the ocular lesions has a definite and direct relationship to the duration of the diabetes and to its control. Sixty per cent of patients who have diabetes for more than ten years show retinal hemorrhages[117] (see Fig. 21). Poor control of the diabetes is not always evident, however, as some patients exhibit advanced degenerative changes and yet have a mild diabetes that has not been appreciably out of hand.

The retinal abnormalities are the most

frequent of the serious ocular complications. They comprise:

Vascular Changes. 1. Round microaneurysmal dilatations (Fig. 21), in the inner nuclear layer, of the venous ends of the retinal capillaries provide the earliest distinctive ocular changes in diabetes. They are rarely seen in other conditions. Unlike hemorrhages, they do not change in appearance from week to week. They are seen in nearly all cases of advanced intercapillary glomerulosclerosis. They are not necessarily related to arterial hypertension.

2. Superficial hemorrhages which tend to be flame-shaped occur in the nerve fiber layer and are of arterial origin and are related, in some cases, to the degree of arterial hypertension.

3. Engorgement of the retinal veins which, as the disorder progresses, become tortuous with evidences of beading.

4. Narrowing of the arterioles, with evidences of sclerosis.

Exudates. 1. Waxy exudates, which appear to be the result of hyalinization of the deep retinal hemorrhages.

2. Cotton wool exudates.

3. Lipid deposits.

Proliferative Changes. *In retinitis proliferans* there is a laying down of new tissues most probably in the attempt to correct previous damage. As a result dense white areas of new tissue with newly formed blood vessels are to be seen, most frequently in the region of the macula. Vision is impaired to complete blindness, depending on the areas involved. Contraction of the scar tissue may cause separation of the retina. Also, spontaneous hemorrhage may precipitate a hemorrhagic glaucoma. Headache is associated with acute glaucoma.

Other Ocular Complications of Diabetes. 1. *Cataracts* occurring with other degenerative phenomena in the adult diabetic are indistinguishable from the senile cataract of the nondiabetic. If a cataract develops in a diabetic child, as they infrequently do, it is directly related to the diabetes and to poor control of this disorder.

2. *Corneal wrinkling* is demonstrable with a slit lamp and a corneal microscope.

3. *Transitory changes in refraction* occur for a short period after a hyperglycemia is corrected (see p. 852).

4. *Argyll Robertson pupil* in nonsyphilitic diabetic subjects is a manifestation of neuropathic changes (see p. 871).

5. *Xanthelasma.* Patches of lipid deposits in the eyelids are an innocent complication of diabetes, although they are not distinctive of this disease.

6. *Tobacco amblyopia* has been observed in two diabetic patients. Improvement followed the withdrawal of tobacco and the control of a mild diabetes in each instance.

Treatment. Treatment for ocular complications of diabetes includes:

1. Control of the diabetes.

2. The use of a diet liberal in protein, not less than 100 gm. for the male nor less than 90 gm. for the female diabetic and including liberal amounts of carbohydrate (225 to 300 gm.) and small amounts of fat (below 75 gm. daily).

3. Ascorbic acid, 200 mg. daily, with rutin, 20 to 200 mg. three times daily according to the degree of capillary fragility as determined by the Göthlin index test, may be tried in cases of retinal hemorrhages, but I have not been convinced of its value. Large doses of nicotinic acid, 100 to 400 mg., as tolerated, four times daily, are of value in some cases of retinitis.

4. Cataracts are treated as in the nondiabetic subject.

5. Transitory refractive errors due to a reduction of hyperglycemia are managed as outlined on page 852.

6. Neurologic changes involving the eyes as part of a diabetic neuropathy are treated vigorously and in the same manner as other neurologic abnormalities (see p. 873).

7. Xanthelasmic patches ordinarily should not be interfered with. If removed they almost invariably recur.

8. Hypophysectomy has been done in the attempt to retard the rapid progression of advanced vascular disease in the

diabetic.[118] It is conjectural whether progression of the advanced stage of vascular disease will be retarded, although the marked improvement in the retinopathy of a young diabetic woman after the development of hypopituitarism due to postpartum pituitary necrosis (Sheehan's syndrome) is encouraging (Poulsen).[119] One is impressed with the probability not only that control of the diabetes is necessary but also that some more subtle yet formidable influence is to be identified and corrected before good results in these tragic cases can be expected.

Adrenalectomy, bilateral, has more in its favor than hypophysectomy as a means of coping with diabetic retinopathy. Remission of vascular degeneration, as evidenced in two patients by minor reversals in retinal changes, decrease in blood pressure to normal, decrease in proteinuria and nitrogen retention and the disappearance of edema ensued after adrenalectomy.[120,121] Progression of the disorder appeared to be halted in three other patients. One patient died of adrenal insufficiency, and in two cases progression of renal failure continued unabated after adrenalectomy. Both of these patients died subsequently, one of a cerebral vascular accident after four and a half months, and the other of pulmonary and myocardial infarctions four months after operation. Great interest is centered on the possible benefits from hypophysectomy and adrenalectomy, but it would appear that until those who are leading the way in these enterprises have had the opportunity to observe a larger number of cases over a significant period, these procedures should be looked upon as high level clinical research problems, the outcome of which is not clear.

Neurologic Disturbances Complicating Diabetes

Neurologic disturbances are among the most common complications of diabetes, occurring in approximately 60 per cent of adult patients. The cause or causes of these disorders are not entirely clear, but accumulated evidences indicate that disturbances in nutrition which accompany loss of weight in the presence of a long-standing and poorly controlled diabetes are the usual precipitating factors. Although uncontrolled diabetes and loss of weight are usual forerunners of these disturbances, this is not always so. In fact, findings typical of the milder forms of so-called diabetic neuropathy have been observed in patients before the diabetes developed. Also, patients who have not lost weight and whose diabetes has been under excellent control for long periods may experience a mildly progressive neuropathy indistinguishable from that ordinarily accepted as diabetic in origin. It would appear that there is an underlying disturbance which tends to be intensified by *poor control of the diabetes and loss of weight* but that these features are not essential to its development. It is true, however, that this type of neuropathy is seen for the most part but not exclusively in diabetic patients. Acute infections and vitamin deficiencies may play a part but it appears that these, with the possible exception of vitamin B_{12} deficiency, are modifying circumstances rather than essential features. The neurologic abnormalities are degenerative in nature and it is not surprising that the other major degenerative disorders are frequently found in varying grades of development in subjects with neurologic disturbances. I refer especially to diabetic retinitis, disease of the coronary arteries, the kidneys and peripheral vascular disease.

The various neurologic disorders associated with diabetes are, in all likelihood, part of the same process, but observed at different phases and under different circumstances they present features so variable that their separation into several categories is not surprising.

For detection of a diabetic neuropathy in its early stages studies of the vibratory sense are valuable. Disturbances are recognized clinically by (1) decreased acuity or a complete inability to detect the vibrations of a tuning fork and (2) increased perception time. Barach[122] and Collens[123] have attracted attention to the value of this examination. We can support their claims and emphasize that the common error of attributing symptoms of neurologic origin to disturbances in circulation can be eliminated if proper investigation of each possibility is carried out.

For the detection of an impaired vibration sense a tuning fork of an aluminum alloy with a frequency of 128 serves admirably. Impaired vibration sense in the upper extremity occurs but not nearly as frequently nor to as great a degree as is observed in the legs and feet.

The degenerative changes which account for the blocking of the transmission of the vibratory impulses occur in the peripheral nerves.[124]

The vibration sense normally is less acute in older age groups; it is variable under normal circumstances. Findings indistinguishable from those found in diabetes are observed in patients with tabes dorsalis and with primary or pernicious anemia.

Chronic Neuropathies. 1. The *early* or *mild* and often ill defined form of diabetic neuropathy—the most common form—is gradual in onset and the symptoms, most frequently encountered and associated with loss of weight and uncontrolled diabetes for long periods, are: vague pains, aches, shooting pains, cramps, numbness, tingling and burning, lightning stinging or needling sensations, stiffness and formication, most frequently occurring in the legs and feet but occurring infrequently in the upper extremities and in the trunk. *These symptoms tend to be worse at night and upon exposure to cold.* The increasing intensity of symptoms at night provides a clue in differentiating neurologic disturbances from a circulatory insufficiency. Tendon reflexes are frequently impaired or absent. Tenderness of the calf muscles is common and some impairment in the vibratory sense is usual in the legs and feet in this relatively early phase.

This disorder may remain relatively stationary for long periods in some patients, but characteristically it subsides readily with the control of the diabetes and with appropriate supplementary therapy.

2. The *moderately severe* stage of diabetic neuropathy is characterized by greater disturbances in the tendon reflexes and in the vibratory sense. The symptoms have been present for a prolonged period and areas of cutaneous paresthesia are often detectable. We include also in this group those cases with abnormalities of the autonomic nervous system which respond satisfactorily to therapy in contrast to those which do not and which are classified in the severe or refractory group. Falling in this moderately severe group are some cases of intermittent nocturnal diarrhea, or intermittent diarrhea and constipation, stubborn constipation of relatively recent onset, delayed emptying of the stomach, impotence, vasomotor instability causing giddiness on rising from the recumbent to the erect position, and absent sense of bladder filling. These patients tend to be underweight, and indeed it is quite likely that malnutrition plays a contributory part in the production and maintenance of this clinical state.

Involvement of the autonomic nervous system is detected in patients having disturbances of the gastrointestinal and the genitourinary tracts. The absence of free hydrochloric acid from the gastric secretions is a prevalent but not an essential finding. Incontinence of feces has been noted. Epigastric pain, indistinguishable from the gastric crises of tabes, is occasionally encountered. Roentgenologic studies indicate disturbed motility in the gastrointestinal tract with, in some cases, a scattered barium pattern as seen in severe deficiency states. Unlike the steatorrhea of pancreatic insufficiency, the diarrhea of diabetic neuropathy is not influenced by the oral administration of pancreatic extracts.

Involvement of the sympathetic nervous system leads to reduction or elimination of perspiration in the involved areas, reduced vasomotor and pilomotor function and to dependent edema secondary to the altered permeability of the capillaries. Reduced functioning of the sebaceous glands may account for the atrophic and shiny changes which the skin of the extremities undergoes. The protein content of the spinal fluid is usually but not always elevated during acute episodes.

Orthostatic hypotension occasionally occurs as a result of neurocirculatory abnormalities in patients exhibiting characteristics of diabetic neuropathy. Dizziness, weakness on physical exertion and, in the more severe grades of the disorder, syncope occur in association with the decrease in blood pressure which follows the change from the supine to the standing position.

Disturbances in the genitourinary tract identifiable with diabetic neuropathies include disturbances in sphincter control due to degenerative changes in the pudendal nerves, permitting dribbling, paralysis of the bladder with the "cord bladder" syndrome—painless distention of the bladder with retention of urine, an impaired sense of bladder filling and a predisposition to infection in the genitourinary tract. Sexual impotence is a common complication. This may exist with or without a loss of libido. Loss of ejaculatory power may exist without loss of potentia but a combination of these disorders is the rule, with atony of the bladder an additional but less frequent complication.

3. *The late, severe and relatively refractory neuropathies in the diabetic patient* are uncommon in contrast with the frequent occurrence of the milder forms. The most frequent complaints when *peripheral nerves* are involved are: loss of weight, general weakness and disturbed sensation in the feet varying from numbness, tingling, pins and needles sensation and a feeling that "his feet do not belong to him" to a complete loss of sensation with painless ulcerations. Foot- or wrist-drop is an uncommon feature but unsteadiness of gait is not infrequent.

Involvement of the peripheral nerves and the fasciculi propii of the spinal cord causes disturbances in the tendon reflexes. There may be complete absence of all reflexes, but *diminished or absent Achilles reflexes* are especially frequent, as is a depression of the peripheral superficial sensibilities. *Reduced pupillary responses* to light even to the degree observed in the Argyll Robertson pupil have been observed.

Cases of *neurotropic feet* in which there is complete loss of sensation and great destruction of bone are not as uncommon as formerly supposed. Chronic ulcerations of the feet may be mistaken for diabetic gangrene on the basis of arteriosclerosis obliterans, but in the cases I have seen the tips of the toes have been warm and there has been excellent pulsation of the peripheral arteries of the feet. Destruction of bone and the extrusion of bony fragments through a sinus at the base of an ulcer may occur. Shortening and stubbiness of the foot develops as a result of marked destruction of bone.

There are evidences that, in some cases, this destruction of bone is due to a secondary infectious process, but in others the disorder appears to be on a purely neurotrophic basis.[64]

In cases of extreme degree, irreparable organic changes in the nervous system have been noted.

TREATMENT FOR DIABETIC NEUROPATHY. Vitamin B_{12} has been, in my experience, the most promptly effective measure in correcting these neuropathic disorders. It is given intramuscularly in doses of 500 micrograms daily for one week and thereafter, while indicated, three times per week. The part played by vitamin B_{12} in the treatment for diabetic neuropathies is controversial. It is agreed that if prompt benefit does not accrue, the drug should be discontinued. The relief from night pains and from swaying or giddiness on walking has been so prompt as to leave no uncertainty about the specific relief which this drug provides. Also, a return of the vibratory sense is noted within a few days and a more gradual correction of impotence has been observed, but this result is not the rule.

A diet low in calories, unless fortified with vitamins, may increase the intensity of the neurologic manifestations. This is avoided by giving a diet of sufficiently high caloric value to prevent a reduction in weight for the time being, by controlling the diabetes and by employing vitamin B_{12}.

Acute Peripheral Neuritis. This distressing complication is infrequent in contrast to the common chronic neuropathies. Sciatica serves to illustrate this group. The onset of peripheral neuritis is usually rapid with severe pain throughout the distribution of the involved nerve, intensified by motion, with exquisite tenderness on pressure over the nerve, and with tender muscles. Involvement of the muscular function varies from a mild degree of weakness to actual paralysis as seen in foot- or wrist-drop. Atrophic changes occur in prolonged cases. Absent tendon reflexes in the involved zones, e.g., the Achilles reflex in cases of sciatica, is characteristic. When directly attributable to the disturbed physiology associated with diabetes, the duration of attacks varies from three to twelve weeks.

TREATMENT. Therapy for acute peripheral neuritis in the diabetic is identical with that for the nondiabetic with the added features of (1) *prompt control of the diabetes* and (2) the prevention of a loss in weight. The reduction of body weight tends to intensify the symptoms, and great care should be taken to maintain the existing weight, even in the obese patient, until the neuritis is corrected.

Thiamine hydrochloride, 50 mg., is administered intramuscularly daily until relief is secured, and vitamin B_{12}, 500 micrograms, is given intramuscularly daily for one week, and thereafter three times weekly.

Other features of treatment are *rest in bed,* and infrared heat treatments over the involved areas for at least one-half hour several times daily.

Acetylsalicylic acid, 0.6 gm. (10 gr.) three times during the day, and an enteric-coated tablet of sodium salicylate, 0.6 gm. (10 gr.) before retiring, are recommended. When the pain is severe *codeine sulfate,* 0.03 gm. (0.5 gr.), may be used to supplement the salicylates.

Diabetic Ketosis, Keto-Acidosis and Coma

Introduction. The term "diabetic coma" is used loosely in clinical circles. Modifying slightly the terminology recommended by Danowski[125] for the purpose of comparison, and taking into consideration the phase in which ketosis *per se* is predominant and that in which acidosis is superimposed, the term *ketosis* is given in those cases in which the total serum CO_2 content is between 15.1 and 20.0 mEq. per liter and *keto-acidosis* in those with values below 15.0 mEq. per liter.

The results of bedside determinations of the degree of ketonemia affords an excellent and, I consider, a more generally reliable classification for clinical purposes. A grade 4 reaction for acetone in the undiluted plasma is indicative of a relatively *mild ketosis;* a grade 4 reaction in the undiluted plasma and also in the first dilution 1:1 with water or normal saline is indicative of *moderately severe ketosis.* When, in addition to these reactions, a grade 4 response is obtained in a second dilution in which 50 per cent solution of plasma further is diluted 1:1 (yielding a solution 25 per cent of which is plasma), it indicates a profound ketosis and the term of *keto-acidosis* becomes applicable. The usefulness of this classification as a guide to therapy is presented on page 879.

Diabetic coma is one of the greatest of medical emergencies. It does not develop while the diabetes is under good control. It is recognizable and may be readily corrected in its early stages. Deaths from diabetic coma have been reduced dramatically but they still occur because of ignorance, delay and neglect.

Nature of Diabetic Coma and Its Diagnosis. Fundamentally, the course of events which leads to diabetic coma (see Fig. 22) proceeds from an insuf-

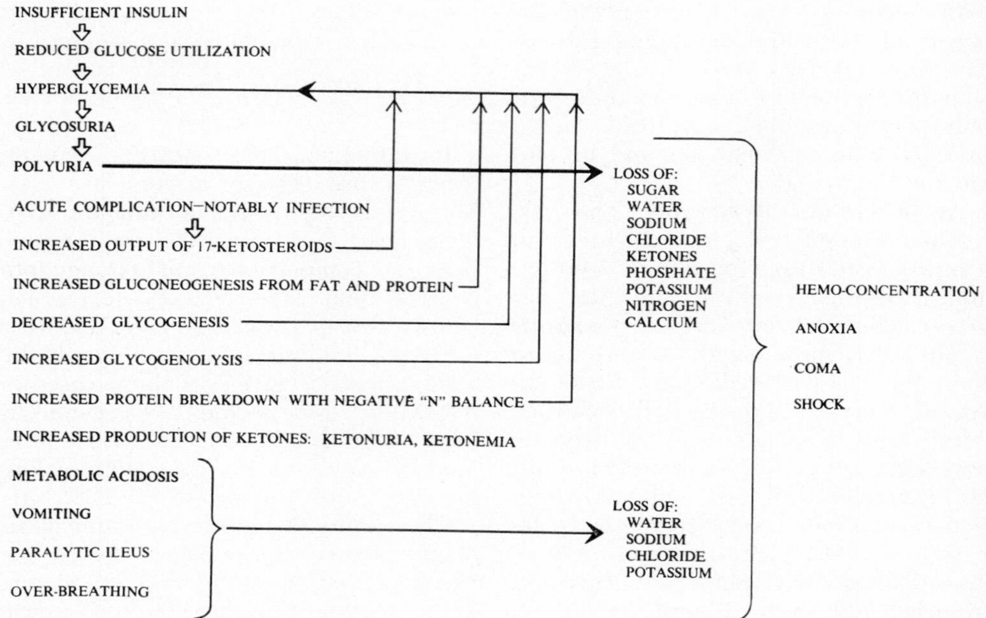

FIG. 22. The major disturbances in diabetic coma, the chronologic order in which they appear and the influences which they exert on the development of ketosis and ketoacidosis.

ficiency of insulin and the reduced utilization of carbohydrate which results. These abnormalities may persist for long periods without any indication of ketosis. They do, however, set the stage and sensitize the subjects to the circumstances which tend to precipitate ketosis and coma.

The insufficient supply of insulin becomes increasingly apparent when it fails to meet the increased demand during acute complications. It is this failure that initiates the series of abnormalities associated with ketosis and keto-acidosis. Glycosuria and hyperglycemia, if not present, develop and, if present, become intensified during acute complications. It is unusual for a patient with known diabetes and under treatment to develop ketosis without the abrupt withdrawal of insulin or the presence of an acute complication being the precipitating factor. Acute complications are not essential to the development of ketosis, however. A child or thin adult may have a diabetes of such severe degree that, barring treatment with insulin, keto-acidosis may develop very gradually—over days and weeks—without an acute complication. The slowness of the development of ketosis and coma under these circumstances is in contrast with the speed—from hours to a day or two—with which they develop when the demands are magnified by an acute infection.

Characteristically and preliminary to the actual ketotic phase, the degrees of hyperglycemia and glycosuria are increased—the forerunners to the development of ketosis. Concomitant with, and as a result of, the increased glycosuria, a diuresis occurs. The amounts of fluid presented to the kidneys are so great that they overwhelm the reabsorptive capacity of the renal tubules and the escape from the body economy of large quantities of water, sugar and, as the disorder progresses, electrolytes (sodium, chloride, phosphate, potassium, magnesium and calcium), nitrogen and ketones occurs.

Increased adrenal cortical activity, as indicated by increased excretion of 11-oxysteroids and 17-ketosteroids, occurs early in the development of diabetic ketosis. This has the unfavorable effect of neutralizing somewhat the effect of insulin, of intensifying glycogenolysis and of increasing the breakdown of body proteins with increased loss of potassium.

As the result of these combined effects, increased amounts of glucose are set free, increasing the degrees of hyperglycemia, glycosuria, polyuria and loss of electrolytes. Added to this effect is the increased production of sugar from fat and protein (increased gluconeogenesis), and as glycogen formation ceases and glycogenolysis is stepped up, increasing amounts of sugar now unavailable to the body economy because of the presenting circumstances are excreted. Body proteins are forfeited for their carbohydrate potential, but the glucose thus obtained, not being utilized, adds to the hyperglycemia. Because of this gluconeogenesis from protein and because protein intake is prohibited by anorexia, nausea and vomiting, a marked negative nitrogen balance ensues.

Concomitant with the increasing inability to utilize carbohydrate, the metabolism of fat is increased. Shortly the acetyl CoA, which is in excess of available oxaloacetate, is converted to ketones—acetoacetic and beta-hydroxybutyric acids and acetone.

Profound changes occur in the anion-cation exchange as the anions, notably ketones and inorganic phosphate, accumulate and displace bicarbonate. The metabolic acidosis which ensues is, in effect, the result of disturbances in the system of buffers (carbonic acid, bicarbonate, proteins, phosphates, electrolyte transfers between cells and extracellular fluids, and the osmotic activities of electrolytes within the cells), which normally maintain, by virtue of renal and respiratory regulation, the hydrogen ion concentration in the blood.[126]

The metabolic acidosis is enhanced by impaired renal function and sodium depletion. Air hunger (Kussmaul breathing) which follows is an attempt to restore the hydrogen ion concentration to normal.

Dehydration and hemoconcentration follow the development of deficits in water precipitated by nausea, vomiting, reduced intake, increased respirations and diuresis. With progression of the disorder, the ketone bodies are produced at a rate which exceeds the ability of the body to complete their oxidation, and the excess, in the early stages, is as a rule excreted in the urine. As this process progresses, 1 plus reactions for acetone in the urine are replaced by 2 plus, 3 plus, and finally 4 plus reactions. The kidneys and, to a minor extent, the lungs can carry off, for variable periods, the excess ketones from the blood, but barring relief, finally ketone production exceeds the functional capacity of the excretory mechanisms and ketones accumulate in the blood. At first, this stage is detectable by the appearance of traces of acetone in the blood plasma but, if not corrected, 2 plus, 3 plus, and finally 4 plus qualitative reactions for plasma acetone are observed. Usually, it is not until 4 plus reactions for acetone in the urine are observed for variable periods that amounts of acetone increase in the plasma to a sufficient concentration to be detected by the usual tests employed. Hence, in general, a *3 or 4 plus reaction for acetone in the plasma indicates a much more advanced degree of ketosis than do similar reactions obtained on examination of the urine.* On the other hand, renal disease may inhibit the excretion of acetone, in which case 1, 2 or 3 plus reactions for acetone in the urine may prevail, while 4 plus reactions are obtained on testing the plasma. A mild degree of ketonuria is not to be regarded with complacency in the case of a seriously ill diabetic. Examination of the plasma for acetone will give positive evidence of the degree of ketosis, and the CO_2 combining power will reflect the changes due to ketosis plus the acidosis of renal origin.

The diabetic patient having 4 plus

reactions for glycosuria and a 4 plus reaction for plasma acetone fulfills the chemical criteria necessary to make the diagnosis of diabetic coma. The diagnosis can be made at the bedside. Urine for testing is obtained by catheter if necessary and 10 ml. of oxalated blood allowed to stand for a few minutes will provide plasma, of which only one drop is needed in the test for acetone (see p. 796).

The diagnosis can be established without elaborate equipment or technical assistance and—of most importance—therapy can be started at once. Hence the chances of recovery from diabetic coma are greatly enhanced if the diagnosis is made in the home and not delayed until the patient is admitted to the hospital.

Prior to and in the early stages of ketosis important disturbances in the patients' fluid and electrolyte balances have been taking place. These later considerations account for the intense dehydration, hemoconcentration, increased specific gravity of the whole blood, low, and at times imperceptible, blood pressure, vascular collapse with evidences of the resulting renal incompetence as indicated in the gravely ill patient by oliguria with albumin and granular casts, or in some instances by anuria with the development of the uremic state, if correction is delayed. If the shocklike state is prolonged, changes in the renal tubules characteristic of a lower nephron nephrosis may occur. In these rare cases the excessive administration of fluids is fraught with great danger.

Second only in importance to an *early diagnosis* and *insulin therapy* are the halting and correction of these secondary and dangerous processes. *Administration of salty broth, orally, as soon as the diagnosis is made is beneficial.*

Precipitating Causes of Diabetic Coma. The patient who disregards—by ignorance or indifference—dietary restrictions and overeats, with the result that the diabetes is out of control, is a candidate for a rapidly developing ketosis in the event of infections, even of a minor nature, gastrointestinal disturbances (vomiting or diarrhea), surgical complications and the omission of insulin. The abrupt withdrawal of insulin, without appropriate precautions when instituting tolbutamide therapy (see p. 855) is a new means of precipitating diabetic ketosis. It is remarkable how frequently the diabetic patient, because of anorexia during an acute complication, omits insulin. This omission, with or without the advice of a physician, is the most common accelerator of ketosis. In such cases the anorexia is frequently due to ketosis in its early stages and all that remains to speed the quickest possible development of coma is the withdrawal of insulin therapy. The anorexic diabetic patient is a potential emergency at all times. Such patients who exhibit strongly positive reactions for glycosuria and acetonuria and whose plasmas give a 2 plus or 1 plus reaction for acetone are in the pre-coma state.

The anorexia of the diabetic patient suffering from an acute clinical condition is intensified by nausea and, with the onset of vomiting and its unfavorable influence on the fluid balance, sodium and potassium depletion, the dehydration and vascular collapse in these patients are quickened.

Sodium chloride, administered as salty broth in the anorexic phase, may halt and will certainly postpone the downward progress. We have repeatedly observed that this simple measure alleviates nausea, and vomiting often ceases when salty broth is ingested. Failing an early diagnosis or early treatment, or both, the ketosis gains headway slowly without acute complications, but very rapidly—a matter of hours—in the presence of acute infection and toxemia.

Physical Findings. The patient in the diabetic coma appears desperately ill. The cheeks are flushed. Air hunger, as evidenced by an increased rate and depth of respirations, is pronounced. Replacement of this Kussmaul breathing by feeble, rapid and gasping respirations is an ominous sign. The odor of acetone is noted on the breath. General dehydration is pronounced. The skin is dry. This is important in differentiating coma due to ketosis from unconsciousness due to an insulin reaction, in which the skin is characteristically moist. In some cases of ketosis and in nearly all of keto-acidosis the intraocular tension is reduced, the eyes are sunken, the mucous membranes of the nasal passages, lips and mouth are dry. The tongue is dry and has a dirty brownish coating. The pharynx is dry and beefy red, and stringy dried secretions may be seen in the mouth and dried deposits are observed on the teeth.

The blood pressure is low. The pulse rate is rapid and lacks normal force, and the heart sounds may be distant. Occasionally a pleural friction rub is heard. The extremities are cold and the body temperature is usually subnormal but rises above normal in the presence of infection shortly after treatment has been instituted. Patients in uncomplicated coma are afebrile. Fever in a ketotic patient should suggest a complicating infection. The abdomen may be tender, especially in the epigastrium, and frequently there is guarding by the abdominal muscles. These findings with leukocytosis and vomiting may suggest an acute surgical condition. Distention of the abdomen, especially in the epigastric area, is common. The tendon reflexes tend to be sluggish. In examining these patients, the detection of complications may be difficult. The history is usually incomplete, and the unconscious patient can tell no more than can be observed. It is easy to overlook an otitis media, mastoiditis or an early pneumonia. Furuncles, carbuncles, infections of the respiratory tract, surgical conditions in the abdomen or pelvis, infections of the urinary tract, gangrene and septicemia are among the more common complications which precipitate ketosis.

Differential Diagnosis. The conditions likely to be confused with diabetic coma are intracranial hemorrhage and severe insulin reactions (hypoglycemia). Trauma to the head, uremia, drug poisoning and meningitis deserve special consideration as glycosuria is frequently encountered in these conditions.

HYPOGLYCEMIA. The hazard of treating an insulin reaction as a diabetic ketosis is obvious. It is best to withhold insulin until the effect of intravenous dextrose is observed in any case in which the differential diagnosis between these two conditions is doubtful. *The absence of detectable ketonemia excludes the possibility of ketosis.*

The chief differentiating points between unconsciousness due to hypoglycemia and to ketosis are presented in Table 19. The most important of these are: the quickness of onset of unconsciousness in the insulin reaction as against the gradual onset in coma. Furthermore the hypoglycemic patient has a wet skin, no evidence of dehydration, normal breathing, usually no vomiting, no reduction of intraocular tension, a normal or elevated blood pressure, no abdominal tenderness or rigidity, no sugar in the urine,* and the blood sugar level is below normal in contrast to the hyperglycemia of the patient in diabetic coma. Immediate response to glucose given intravenously is the rule in cases of hypoglycemia.

INTRACRANIAL HEMORRHAGE. Glycosuria is common following intracranial hemorrhage. The onset is sudden. Asymmetries in contour, muscle tone and reflexes, if present, are helpful in making a diagnosis. The patient in coma as a result of intracranial hemorrhage is not dehydrated. The skin is moist, the intraocular tension is not decreased, and the blood pressure is usually elevated. The spinal fluid may contain gross blood. Compared with diabetic coma the degree of unconsciousness is marked in contrast to the moderate elevation of the blood sugar; there is little or no acetonuria; no 4 plus reaction for plasma acetone is demonstrable, and the carbon dioxide combining power of the blood is not greatly depressed.

* The first specimen of urine from the hypoglycemic patient may contain sugar which was secreted several hours previously but the bladder being emptied, a second specimen will be aglycosuric.

UREMIA. The patient in uremia is less dehydrated than the patient in diabetic coma. There is an ammoniacal odor on the breath, an enlarged heart, an elevated blood pressure and usually no glycosuria. No acetone is demonstrable in the blood and the blood sugar is not elevated.

Findings common to both uremia and diabetic coma are: unconsciousness, reduced carbon dioxide combining power, elevated blood urea nitrogen values, and moderate dryness of the skin.

There should be no difficulty in differentiating between diabetic coma and other forms of unconsciousness if a history is carefully obtained and physical and laboratory examinations are conducted.

Prognosis. The prognosis is good if the patient is young, if he is only drowsy or semiconscious, if the blood pressure is not greatly reduced, if there is no complicating infection, and if the carbon dioxide combining power of the blood plasma is not below 6.6 mM/L (15 volumes per cent)* and if the plasma acetone is present in less than *4 plus reactions* when the plasma is diluted with equal parts of saline.

The prognosis is grave if the patient has been completely unconscious for more than twelve hours, if he is over forty years of age, if the systolic blood pressure is below 50 mm. Hg, if a severe complicating infection is present, especially a septicemia, if the carbon dioxide combining power is below 5.8 mM/L (12 volumes per cent), if the plasma after 2 serial dilutions with equal parts of normal saline still gives *4 plus reactions* for acetone, if there is anuria with a marked retention of nitrogen in the blood, if there is concomitant arteriosclerotic heart disease, and, in general, if the level of the blood sugar is extremely high—above 1000 mg. per 100 cc.

Age is one of the most important prognostic factors. The mortality of Wilder's patients in diabetic coma in the first four decades of life was 4 per cent, and in the next four decades it was 40 per cent.

The *degree and duration of unconsciousness* are also important. In Dillon and Dyer's[127] series the mortality of patients who could be aroused was 28 per cent. The mortality of the completely unconscious was 81 per cent.

The *degree of disturbance in kidney function* is also a prognostic index. In 268 cases of coma reported by Dillon and Dyer the mortality was 22 per cent in those patients in whom the blood urea nitrogen value was 20 mg. per 100 cc. or less, but in those in whom this value was exceeded the mortality was 62.4 per cent.

Infection, its nature and severity, influences greatly the outcome of a case of diabetic coma. Its early detection and identification are essential if suitable antibiotic therapies are to be utilized with greatest benefit. Finally, the mortality rate is less than 2 per cent when adequate facilities are available and wisely employed.

Patients in profound coma with chemical derangements, as in the case of a patient with a CO_2 combining power of 0.45 mM/L (1 volume per cent) and grade 4 reactions for acetone in the plasma when the latter had been diluted by 75 per cent with saline, require much greater quantities of insulin and the outlook is more grave than in the milder case illustrated in Figure 23. In the latter, although the reaction for plasma acetone was grade 4 in undiluted plasma, it was grade 2 in the first dilution, i.e., with 50 per cent of normal saline solution. The latter patient needed only 160 units in the first twenty-four hours of therapy, as compared with 905 units in the first case.

Prevention. Diabetic coma is preventable, but to achieve this goal patients must be trained concerning (1) the factors which precipitate coma, (2) the speed with which coma may develop and (3) the manner in which the early symptoms are manifested. Also, one must make an earlier diagnosis,

* The formula by which the CO_2 combining power is changed from volumes per cent to millimols is: $\text{mM/L} = \frac{\text{Vol. \%} \times 10}{22.4}$.

avoid causing ketosis when attempting to change from insulin to oral therapy, or provide adequate therapy if this complication is to be prevented or corrected with minimum risk if it is already established.

Patients should be aware of the upheaval that can come with great rapidity with an acute infection. It is remarkable how many patients test the urine regularly for sugar only until they feel ill. Following in rapid succession come anorexia, nausea and often vomiting.

The patient should know that in the anorexic phase insulin must not be omitted if strongly positive reactions for glycosuria are present. The pre-coma state should be suspected under these circumstances. In case this suspicion is confirmed by a 4 plus reaction for glycosuria and acetonuria and a 1 or 2 plus reaction for plasma acetone,* small frequently administered doses (every four hours) of crystalline insulin are indicated. The amounts are regulated according to the changes in the degree of glycosuria. In these instances the administration of salty broth by mouth will usually alleviate the nausea and permit frequent administration of carbohydrate by mouth which, with the accompanying insulin therapy, will quickly correct the early ketosis.

In the event that the acute complication which is precipitating the ketosis is not correctable promptly—within a matter of hours—the danger of ketosis can be reduced and the control of the diabetes can be more exactly regulated by prescribing the diet in four equal feedings—one every six hours—and crystalline insulin—at least one third of the former total insulin dosage before each feeding, making adjustments according to the effect on the glycosuria in the respective six-hour fractions. We have used and advocated this principle of treatment for many years.[128]

A liquid diet divided into four equal feedings which has been found to be satisfactory is presented in Diet XIII (see p. 889). When regular foods are tolerated a diet, as illustrated in Diet XII (see p. 888), may be employed until the routine diet and insulin may be resumed after the acute complication has subsided.

Treatment. Therapy is directed at the fundamental faults by giving insulin frequently and in adequate amounts, by restoring fluids and electrolytes until normal values prevail, and by providing adequate carbohydrate to permit a reduction in fat metabolism and to replenish depleted glycogen stores. Other, but secondary, therapeutic measures are included in the following outline of treatment for diabetic coma employed at the Pennsylvania Hospital.

INSULIN. For patients in *relatively mild ketosis* (Fig. 23)—with a 4 plus reaction for ketosis in the undiluted plasma but a lesser degree of ketonemia in plasma diluted 1:1 with water—the initial dose of crystalline insulin for the adult is 100 units. Of this, 40 units are given intravenously and 60 units subcutaneously. Fifty units of insulin are given at four or six hour intervals until the ketonemia is corrected. Recovery on this regimen is prompt.

In cases of *moderately severe ketosis* with a 4 plus reaction for plasma acetone in the undiluted plasma and in the 1:1 but not in the 1:3 dilution of plasma with normal saline, an initial dose of 200 units of insulin is given. If the second dilution (1:3) gives a 4 plus reaction, indicating a *profound ketosis,* 300 units are given as the initial dose with 50 units at one-half hour intervals until a marked improvement in the degree of ketonemia occurs. If shock is a prominent feature, the possibility of delayed absorption of insulin may be avoided by giving one half or two thirds of the insulin intravenously until the peripheral vascular collapse is corrected.

It is not unusual to find little detectable improvement, chemically, in the first

* Chemically pure acetone when added to nitro-prusside, as in the Rothera-Wishart and Acetest tests (see p. 796), yields no color reaction. When in solution with water or plasma, however, color changes indicating the qualitative and quantitative presence of acetone occur.

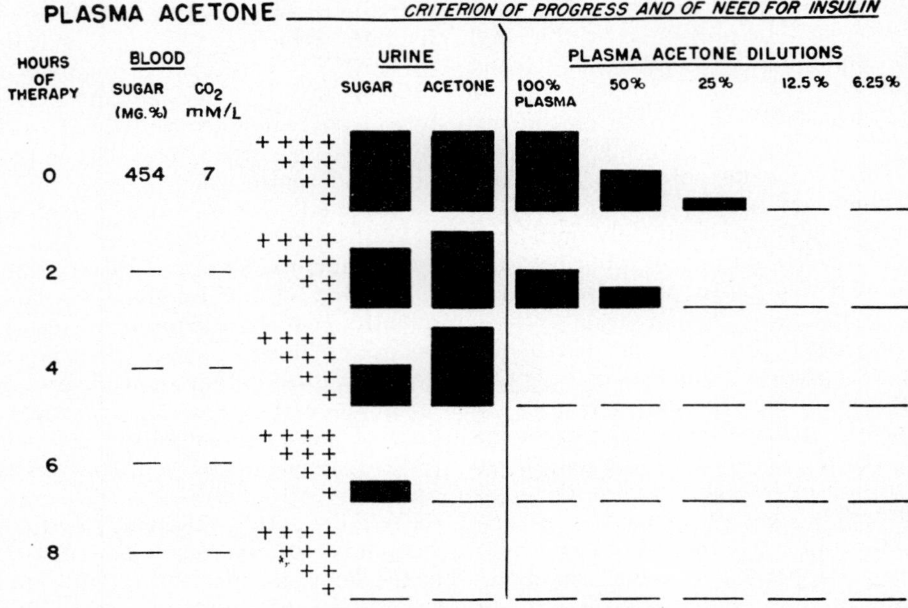

FIG. 23. A relatively mild case of diabetic coma is depicted. Note the criteria for the diagnosis of coma and the grade 2 reaction for acetone in the plasma on the first dilution—an indication for a relatively small dosage of insulin for the first 24 hours of treatment which was confirmed when only 160 units corrected the ketosis.

four hours of treatment, but it is unusual for no improvement to be noted by the end of six hours.

As the amount of acetone in the plasma decreases, the patient's sensitivity to insulin increases, and as the plasma acetone decreases to 1 plus, nourishment and insulin can be given at six-hour intervals with return, at the end of twenty-four hours, barring other acute complications, to the pre-coma plan of treatment. Some patients may require huge doses of insulin—even thousands of units—in the first twenty-four hours. In this event there is more likely to be a cumulative action with a great danger of hypoglycemic reactions immediately following the correction of the ketosis. In such cases, I stop the giving of insulin until glycosuria returns and then shift to the six-hour interval dosage and nourishments.

Determination of the blood sugar level at two-hour intervals—until the patient is out of danger—will serve to identify the occasional patient whose blood sugar decreases below 250 mg. per ml. while a moderate degree of ketonemia persists. Increased amounts of carbohydrate to prevent a hypoglycemia and aid in eradicating the undue degree of ketonemia are indicated. *Knowledge of the level of the blood sugar is of value in guarding against hypoglycemia but is not nearly as reliable a guide to the magnitude of the need for insulin in the early phases of treatment for diabetic coma as is the degree of ketonemia.*

FLUIDS AND ELECTROLYTES. Two liters of normal saline, or of 0.45 per cent saline, are given rapidly, and further quantities of fluids are given more slowly but are continued as long as the specific gravity of the whole blood exceeds 1.055 and as long as the hematocrit reading exceeds 50 per cent. Following these guides, it will be found that some patients need no more than 3 liters of fluid intravenously, whereas occasional

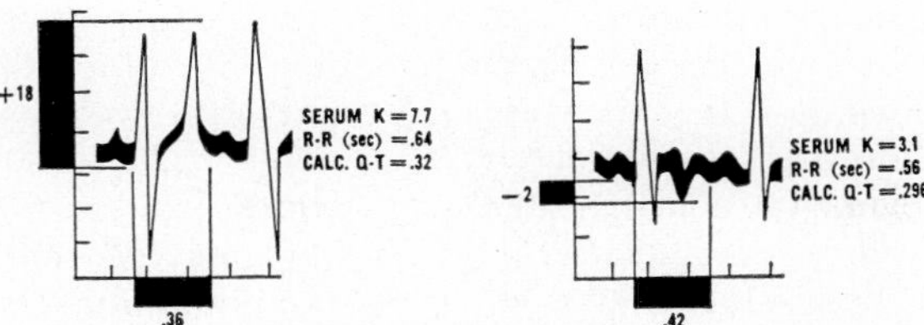

FIG. 24. The influences of the concentration of potassium in the blood on electrocardiographic records are illustrated in precordial lead CR_3 (after Nadler *et al.*).

patients need huge quantities. After the initial 2 liters of saline, adequate volumes of water are provided, the correction of the electrolyte depletion is properly slowed up, and the increasing disparity between the chloride and sodium concentrations in the blood will be reduced by giving 0.45 per cent saline in 5 per cent glucose solution, if oral administration of liquids is still impracticable. One of my patients received more than 8 liters of fluid intravenously in the first twelve hours and yet showed no indication of overhydration. Routinely, except in the case of an oliguric or anuric patient, I administer potassium phosphate or potassium chloride orally, 1 gm. every four hours for five doses, beginning after four or six hours of therapy.

Frequent electrocardiographic tracings may serve as guides to the need for potassium. The characteristics indicating excessive concentrations of potassium in the serum are shown in the left tracing of Figure 24, namely, the increased amplitude of the T wave with a narrow base. This finding is common at the outset of treatment and is a contraindication to the administrations of potassium at that time. As therapy proceeds, the T wave flattens and the Q-T interval becomes prolonged. In the right tracing in Figure 24, the T wave has become inverted with prolongation of the Q-T interval. These are indications for giving potassium. Excessive potassium is reflected in peaked T wave, loss of P wave and disruption of the QRS complex.

In the event of prolonged hypopotassemia, as may occur in patients who have been in coma for unusually long periods, I have used successfully the plan of potassium therapy outlined by Welt (see Chapter 4, p. 324). No attempt is made to correct the potassium deficit until the dehydration has been corrected and urine flow is established. Oral administration of not more than 20 mM. per hour is desirable, but when this is impracticable the first replacement may be limited to 60 to 100 mM., administered intravenously at approximately 20 mM. per hour, the infusate containing 50 mM. per liter.

Great danger may attend the attempt to correct hypopotassemia rapidly by intravenous infusion.[124] There is no need to do this. Actually the serum potassium value is not a reliable index of potassium deficit. The safest plan appears to be to give potassium as indicated above, not with the expectation that it will correct the deficit quickly but that it will protect against the dangers of an increasing hypopotassemia until it is safe to complete the correction of the deficit when oral administration of potassium becomes practicable.

ALKALI. Alkali is usually not needed in the treatment for diabetic coma, but in cases of very low CO_2 combining power and in cases of extreme hyperpnea, an amount sufficient to raise the CO_2 combining power not beyond 13 mM. (30 volumes per cent) is given. As treatment continues, base is released in large quantities from combination with the ketoacids, and an alkalosis is easily precipitated by unwarranted amounts of a solution of sodium racemic lactate. The administration of alkali deprives one of the CO_2 content of the serum as an index of improvement. However, the degree of ketonemia is a more reliable guide of the degree of ketosis than is the CO_2 value.

GLUCOSE. Glucose given early in the treatment will, I believe, do no harm, neither do I believe it will serve any useful purpose while marked degrees of hyperglycemia prevail. Ordinarily, 1,000 cc. of 5 per cent solution of glucose (or fructose) is given, beginning at the end of six hours of therapy, *if at that time the patient is unable to retain nourishment by mouth.* As a result of this rule, only a small percentage of patients in diabetic coma need glucose intravenously.

GASTRIC LAVAGE. This measure is not carried out as a routine but only when indicated by abdominal pain, distention of the stomach, and excessive vomiting. The semicomatose patient may wince when the abdomen is palpated. This reaction is due to distention of the stomach, resulting from a paralytic ileus or to sodium chloride depletion or to both. In such cases gastric lavage is done, and 8 ounces (240 cc.) of physiologic saline solution are allowed to remain in the stomach.

ENEMA. An enema is essential in these severely dehydrated patients, but it may be postponed until the patient's clinical condition is considerably improved.

Treatment for Diabetic Coma. The working diagnosis of diabetic coma is made when 4 plus glycosuria and 4 plus plasma acetone—4 plus reactions for acetonuria are usually, but not consistently, present—are found in the case of an acutely ill patient. When these findings are present:

1. Begin immediate administration of:
   Insulin (crystalline)—40 units intravenously*
   60 units subcutaneously

   In moderately severe ketosis, 200 units, and in profound coma 300 units are given as the initial dose.

   Fluids and chlorides—2000 ml. normal saline (0.9 per cent), or 0.45 per cent saline are given intravenously—20 to 30 ml. per minute. If shock is a prominent feature, dextran may be added to the saline, or the simultaneous administration of plasma and l-norepinephrine (Levophed) may be life-saving;† nothing is given per os.
2. Studies—Secure immediately:
   a. Blood (venous) for sugar content, acetone, hematocrit, CO_2 combining power, specific gravity (whole blood), and urea determinations.
   b. Urine for culture and routine complete analysis. Collect all urine. Record intake and output of fluids.
3. The resident will alert the laboratory for emergency studies. Also, arrangement should be made for full-time service of a resident and nurse until the patient's life is out of danger.
4. Test blood for acetone, and urine at two-hour intervals‡ for sugar and acetone until the ketosis is corrected.
5. Secure samples of blood at four-hour intervals, day and night, for CO_2, sugar, potassium, specific gravity (whole blood), and hematocrit until the patient is conscious and retaining nourishment by mouth. Subsequent studies as conditions indicate.
6. Secure an electrocardiogram as early as is practicable and repeat at four-hour intervals for twenty-four

* With the exception of this initial dose, insulin is administered subcutaneously unless peripheral vascular collapse is a feature, in which case two thirds of the dose is given intravenously and one third subcutaneously.

† Heat should not be applied to patients in diabetic coma as the peripheral vasodilation which it causes may intensify the shocklike state. Normal room temperatures are quite satisfactory.

‡ A retention catheter may be used for this purpose when necessary. Utmost care should be taken to avoid introducing infection. As a prophylactic measure against infection in the genitourinary tract and elsewhere, Gantrisin, 1.0 gm., is given orally four times daily as soon as is practicable, provided the patient is secreting urine. Appropriate antibiotic therapy is given.

hours. More frequent tracings are indicated to guide therapy in cases of hypokalemia.

7. Treatment during critical phase subsequent to the preliminary measures outlined in 1.

Immediately upon receiving confirmative reports on the blood sugar value and the plasma CO_2 combining power, begin:

Insulin (crystalline), 50 units subcutaneously at one-half hour intervals in cases of severe ketosis, at two hour intervals in moderately severe and at four or six hour intervals in mild cases (see p. 879), until an appreciable reduction of the plasma acetone or increase in the CO_2 combining power is noted. Increases above these amounts will rarely be necessary, but if no decrease in plasma acetone or increase in CO_2 combining power of the blood plasma has occurred after six hours* of therapy each succeeding dose may be increased by 25 units, or more, until such changes are noted. Dangers of a rapidly developing hypoglycemia will be avoided by giving glucose (1 liter of 5 per cent solution) intravenously after six hours of therapy (see Par. 10) or carbohydrates orally, if practicable.

8. When to reduce insulin.

An appreciable reduction of the plasma acetone and an appreciable increase of the CO_2 combining power of the blood plasma coincide with a lessening of the resistance to insulin. The possibility of a rapidly developing hypoglycemia should be guarded against.

The reduction of plasma acetone to a trace is, if the clinical condition of the patient permits, indication for insulin and diet at six-hour intervals (see Par. 13).

* It is not unusual to find little change in the blood findings in the first four hours but by the end of six hours improvement should be noted unless unusual circumstances are present.

9. Fluids and salts.

Loss of electrolytes and fluids to a marked degree occurs in the development of diabetic coma indicating the intravenous administration of saline solution, 2000 cc. within the first two hours of treatment. Further fluid—hypotonic saline (0.45 per cent) or a mixture of normal saline and 5 per cent solution of glucose or in severe cases a mixture of 5 per cent glucose and Ringer's lactate solution—is given freely while the specific gravity of the whole blood remains above 1.055, while the hematocrit values remain above 50 per cent and the systolic blood pressure remains below 90 mm. Hg. As soon as the patient's condition permits, broths and carbohydrate-containing fluids—strained cereal, gruel, ginger ale (non-effervescent), sweetened tea and, later, fruit juices—may be given. Potassium phosphate or chloride, 1 gm. every four hours, orally, for five doses, is given routinely to the adult patient after four hours of therapy, *provided urine is being excreted freely*. Relatively smaller amounts are given to children. If oral administration of potassium is impracticable and if hypokalemia is present, an intravenous infusion of potassium phosphate or chloride as buffered solution, containing 50 mM. per liter of 5 per cent glucose in water, is given at a rate of 20 mM. per hour. The electrocardiogram is of value in checking response and indications for added amounts. However, it may mislead, and clinical appraisal may indicate that satisfactory progress is being made.

Plasma expanders—dextran in normal saline, plasma or other colloid solutions—may be given to protect against salt depletion shock but are specifically indicated if there are evidences of peripheral vascular collapse. Neo-Synephrine (phenylnephrine HCl) or Levophed (l-norepinephrine) may be life-saving in cases of shock.

10. Carbohydrate.

    Glucose, 1000 cc. of a 5 per cent solution is given intravenously beginning six hours after the first dose of insulin, if at this time liquids given orally are not retained. This is repeated in six hours if the patient is not taking or retaining nourishment by mouth.

11. Alkali.

    The administration of alkali usually is not necessary. However, an amount of $NaHCO_3$ or racemic sodium lactate sufficient to raise the CO_2 combining power to a relatively innocent level—13 mM/L (30 volumes per cent)—will relieve air hunger rapidly. Larger amounts are contraindicated. The foregoing amount of alkali is permissible, also, for the critically ill patient having a plasma CO_2 combining power below 6.6 mM/L (15 volumes per cent).

12. Gastric lavage—enema.

    The stomach should be emptied of its contents in cases of abdominal distention, abdominal pain, or vomiting. Eight ounces of warm normal saline solution are left in the stomach. An enema is indicated in nearly every case of coma. It may be delayed until improvement in the patient's condition is noted.

13. Diet.

    When evidences of acute ketosis have subsided, a liquid diet is allowed for twelve to twenty-four hours and thereafter a regular diet of the same values: for example, protein 110 gm., fat 65 gm., and carbohydrate 250 gm. (2000 calories). The diet is given in four equal feedings, one every six hours; and finally, with complete recovery from the attack the diet and insulin regimens as for the uncomplicated diabetic patient are resumed.

Although the part of the foregoing plan that deals with hydration and restoration of acid-base equilibrium may be satisfactory in most cases of diabetic coma, it is highly desirable, as indicated by Welt (see p. 324) that the therapy be directed toward correcting the distorted values in the specific patient at hand.

Acute Infections

Acute infections are the most common of the acute complications. They impair the effectiveness of insulin and tend to precipitate a high degree of hyperglycemia and diabetic ketosis progressing to coma with great speed, that is, in a matter of hours. The effect of fever alone, and fever plus infection, on the duration and degree of the blood-sugar-lowering effect of insulin in contrast with the effect when no fever nor infection nor leukocytosis are present is depicted in Figure 25. For these

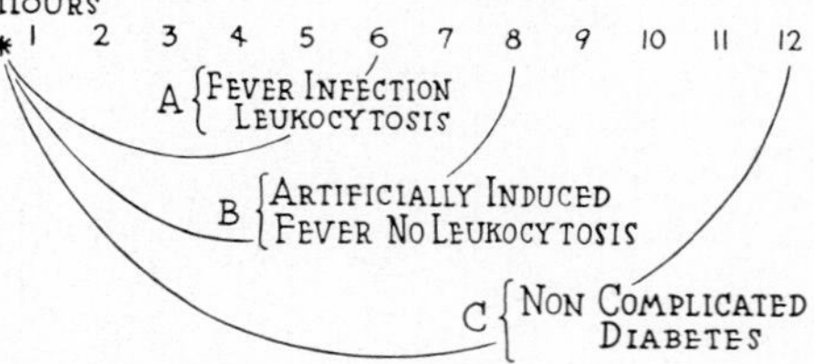

FIG. 25. The speed of action, the degree and duration of effect of identical and large doses of rapidly acting insulin on the degree of hyperglycemia of diabetic patients: A, in the presence of acute infection, fever and leukocytosis; B, in the presence of infection or leukocytosis; and C, in the absence of acute complications.

reasons and the fact that recovery from infections is retarded if the diabetes is not adequately controlled, special attention toward the prevention of infection and a special alertness when infection is already present are important.

Diabetes is more difficult to control during acute infections and it is for this reason that changes in the distribution of the diet and insulin are usually made—changes which permit more certain and prompt control of a diabetes.

Patients with uncontrolled diabetes have a subnormal resistance to infectious organisms, especially to the tubercle bacillus and *Staphylococcus aureus*. Furthermore, staphylococcal infections in diabetics are usually resistant to penicillin.

All of the reasons why acute infections affect the diabetes so unfavorably are not known but infections which increase the need for insulin most markedly are those causing *fever* and *leukocytosis*, and the behavior of the diabetes is frequently a reliable index, favorable or unfavorable, of the trend of an infectious process. Infections not causing fever have little effect on the insulin need and those which cause no leukocytosis cause relatively little increase in the need for insulin. Viral infections and tuberculosis are examples of the latter. If secondary pyogenic organisms get a foothold, as in the case of an acute sinusitis complicating a simple coryza of viral origin, or a mixed infection in a case of pulmonary tuberculosis, a change in the need for insulin is likely to be prompt.

Increases in tissue metabolism, derangement of enzymatic processes, increased proteolytic activities in the blood in patients having a fever and leukocytosis and increased amounts of gamma globulin detected in electrophoretic studies[130,131] may explain the behavior of the need for insulin.

Patients who have mild diabetes and ordinarily do not need insulin will almost always require insulin if an acute infection is contracted. There are a few patients who have no detectable evidences of diabetes under normal circumstances but who have manifest diabetes during the course of an acute infection, notably infections due to *Staphylococcus aureus* and especially carbuncles.

Prevention. Preventive measures comprise immunization when practicable, control of the diabetes, an adequate diet, hygienic care of the skin and special care of the feet.

Treatment. GENERAL CONSIDERATIONS.

1. Cognizance of the effect which infections exert on the diabetes and on the need for insulin.
2. Specific measures directed toward eradicating the infection—drainage, antibiotic or sulfa therapy, and antitoxin when indicated.
3. Insulin therapy—who should receive insulin, the brand of insulin, the amounts and the distribution.
4. Diet therapy—alterations in diet and in its distribution.
5. Special measures—surgery, roentgen ray irradiation, intravenous therapies.

SPECIFIC CONSIDERATIONS. The high degree of specificity with which antibiotic drugs overcome bacterial infection makes the early identification of the offending organism or organisms and their respective sensitivities to the various antibiotic agents of great importance. *Best results will follow if material for a culture is secured at once before any antibiotic agent is given.* The material for culture growth may be from a carbuncle, furuncle, abscess, discharging sinus, an ulcer, the urine, the blood, the spinal fluid, etc. Too often carbuncles which have been doing badly and threatening life are caused by organisms which are resistant to the antibiotic that the patient has been receiving.

Other specific measures should not be overlooked; e.g., adequate drainage in cases of pent-up purulent material.

Insulin Therapy. Insulin is given to every patient, no matter what the degree of severity of his diabetes, if his fasting blood sugar level exceeds 120 mg. per 100 cc. or if the postprandial value exceeds 160 mg. per 100 cc.

Crystalline insulin is used exclusively in preference to longer acting insulins during the course of moderately severe and severe infections. In many cases, however, the disturbance is so slight that small to moderate increases in the amount of insulin given will suffice.

The action of crystalline insulin is prompt and the fact that its action is of short duration makes it simple to manipulate when both the blood sugar level and the insulin requirement may be subject to rapid alterations.

The following method of distributing the insulin[128] has been employed at the

TABLE 20. AN ILLUSTRATIVE GUIDE TO INSULIN THERAPY IN THE CASE OF AN ACUTE INFECTION

TIME	1 P.M.	7 P.M.	1 A.M.	7 A.M.	1 P.M.	7 P.M.	1 A.M.	7 A.M.	1 P.M.
Glycosuria	4+	4+	3+	2+	0	1+	0	0	0
Acetonuria	2+	1+	1+	0	0	0	0	0	0
Plasma acetone	0	0	0	0	0	0	0	0	0
Blood sugar mg./%	320							135	
Insulin	25	40	30	25	25	20	20	20	15

Pennsylvania Hospital for the past twenty-five years with favorable results: During the course of moderately severe infections the insulin is given in four divided doses, at evenly spaced intervals. The diet is similarly divided so that the patient receives the same amount of carbohydrate, fat and protein after each injection of insulin. It is convenient to give meals and insulin at 7 A.M., 1 P.M., 7 P.M., and 1 A.M. This program permits relatively uniform control of the blood sugar level during the most severe complications. The degree of glycosuria before each feeding and the level of the blood sugar (see Table 20) serve as guides in adjusting the dosage of insulin.

Occasionally, in cases of severe infections in which large amounts of insulin, several hundreds of units daily, are given, it has been a temporary expedient to divide the insulin into six doses and the diet into six equal nourishments, both given at four-hour intervals. As the critical phase passes, the injection of insulin and a nourishment are given every six hours.

The regulation of the insulin dosage in the case of a patient taking 80 units of insulin prior to admission for treatment for a carbuncle is illustrated in Table 20.

In the unusual case in which meals and insulin are given at four-hour intervals, collections of urine are made for the same periods; likewise when meals and insulin are given every six hours, the urine is collected each six-hour period. The bladder is emptied before each feeding and the degree of glycosuria is determined.

The degree of, or the absence of, glycosuria is a suitable guide in changing the dosage of insulin, but occasional blood sugar determinations are of value. Of great value is the testing of the plasma for acetone. The patient is in no danger from ketosis if there is no detectable acetone in the plasma. For the technique of performing this test, see page 796. If the patient's condition is not progressing favorably and the infection is of a serious nature and there is acetone in the urine, a test for acetone in the plasma is advisable at least twice daily. The appearance of ketonemia indicates larger amounts of insulin and of carbohydrate.

The change from the pre-complication insulin regimen is illustrated in Table 21. It provides a simple plan of crudely estimating a safe initial program of insulin therapy, following which the amounts of insulin given are altered as indicated according to the degree of, or absence of, glycosuria. The initial dose of insulin for the patient having a mild diabetes can safely be 12 units. For those receiving insulin routinely the initial dose will not be excessive if it equals one third of the former dose. The insulin is increased at each injection until the diabetes is brought under relatively good control. It is well to maintain a fairly firm rein on the diabetes. When the time to reduce the insulin dosage arrives it is preferable to reduce and *not to omit* a dose. Nothing will upset diabetic control more quickly than omitting a dose of insulin when a reduction in the amount given is all that is needed. As the infection subsides the insulin is reduced steadily to prevent hypoglycemic reactions. The need for great reductions is often necessary following the prompt correction of an infection. In such cases there is no danger in making big reductions until the pre-complication dosage of insulin is nearly approximated.

The pre-complication regimen is resumed after one or two days have elapsed without fever. This can be done abruptly.

TABLE 21. A GUIDE IN CHANGING THE RESPECTIVE INSULIN PROGRAMS IN THE EVENT OF ACUTE COMPLICATIONS

PRIOR TO COMPLICATION	DURING COMPLICATION—THE INITIAL DOSE—CRYSTALLINE INSULIN
(1) No insulin	12
(2) Single doses of 30 units or less of P. Z. insulin, Globin or NPH insulin.	15
(3) Combined insulin therapies totaling 90 units.	30
(4) Combined insulin therapies—total 120 units.	40
(5) Combined insulin therapies—total 150 units.	50

Note: The initial dose is one third of the former daily dose. Subsequent doses will be adjusted according to the degree of glycosuria in each succeeding six-hour urine fraction.

Diet Therapy. As has been indicated, the diet is divided into four equal feedings during acute illnesses—except in rare cases when six equal feedings, one every four hours—are given as illustrated in Diets XII and XIII.

The diet requires some modification from the usual form. It is important to maintain an adequate protein allowance—a minimum of 0.5 gm. per pound of the normal body weight. Liquids fortified with concentrated protein foods are desirable if the usual protein foods are unpalatable. Convalescence is speeded by giving liberal allowances of protein—up to 0.66 gm. per pound of body weight. This protein quota is especially desirable in dealing with prolonged infections or open wounds such as ulcers from which much protein is lost. Liquid nourishment may be all that the acutely ill patient can take and this should consist largely of fruit juices, skim milk, cream, gruels and ginger ale with glucose.

A sample diet prescription is as follows: Protein 110 gm., Carbohydrate 250 gm., Fat 50 gm., Total calories 2000.

This diet is presented in menu form as a liquid diet (page 889) and a diet of normal foods (page 888). In each instance the diet is divided into four equal meals suitable for use in most cases of acute complications. Following the recovery from the acute complication the pre-complication diet is resumed simultaneously with resumption of the former plan of insulin therapy.

Parenteral Nourishment. When a patient cannot take feedings by mouth or by gavage, an intravenous program of feeding is used, being patterned on the six-hour schedule outlined above. No method in present use can supply adequate nutrition by this route, and caution must be exercised to use it no longer than necessity dictates and to prevent the excessive administration of sodium chloride.

We have found the basic formula, for parenteral feedings, as recommended by the National Research Council,[132] to be eminently satisfactory:*

An intravenous infusion of 750 cc. is started every six hours and crystalline

* To meet the requirements for the nutrition of a patient who will be unable to take any food or fluids for some days and therefore should receive a nutrient which will provide an adequate amount of some protein substitute.

Water	3,000 cc.
Casein hydrolysate	100 Gm.
Glucose	200 Gm.
Salt	10 Gm.

This will require 2 liters of 5 per cent casein hydrolysate, 5 per cent glucose solution, and 1 liter of 10 per cent glucose solution, a total of 3,000 cc. Since the casein hydrolysate is neutralized, it will contain 5 gm. of salt per liter. Other convenient formulae can be devised by which the volume can be kept below 3,000 cc.

Diet No. XII. "House Diet"—Four Equal Meals
(Protein 110 gm.; Fat 65 gm.; Carb. 250 gm.—2000 Calories)

NO. EXCHANGES	FOOD EXCHANGE	LIST NO.	SAMPLE MENU	HOUSEHOLD MEAS.	WT. GM.	P	F	C	CAL.
6:00 A.M.									
2	Bread	4	Bread	1 sl.	25	2	—	15	68
			Oatmeal	½ c.	100	2	—	15	68
2	Meat	5	Eggs	2	—	14	10	—	146
1⅓	Milk	1	Milk, skim	1 c.	240	8	—	12	80
		1	Milk, skim, powder	1 tbsp.	12	2	—	4	24
1	Fat	6	Butter	1 tsp.	5	—	5	—	45
1½	Fruit	3	Banana	¾ sm.	75	—	—	15	60
				Total		28	15	61	491
12:00 NOON (Repeat at 6:00 P.M. with suitable exchanges)									
2	Meat	5	Beef, roast, lean	2 oz.	60	14	6	—	110
2	Bread	4	Bread	1 sl.	25	2	—	15	68
			Lima beans	½ c.	90	2	—	15	68
1	Vegetable	2A	Lettuce and tomato	1 serv.	100	—	—	—	—
1	Vegetable	2B	Carrots	½ c.	100	2	—	7	36
1	Milk	1	Milk, skim	1 c.	240	8	—	12	80
2	Fat	6	Butter	2 tsp.	10	—	10	—	90
1½	Fruit	3	Pear	1 med.	150	—	—	15	60
				Total		28	16	64	512
12:00 MIDNIGHT									
1⅓	Milk	1	Milk, skim	1 c.	240	8	—	12	80
			Milk, skim, powder	1 tbsp.	12	2	—	4	24
2	Meat	5	Cottage cheese	½ c.	90	14	10	—	146
1	Bread	4	Saltines	5	20	2	—	15	68
1	Fat	6	Butter	1 tsp.	5	—	5	—	45
3	Fruit	3	Grape juice	¾ c.	180	—	—	30	120
				Total		26	15	61	483
				Day's Total		110	62	250	1998

This diet, equally divided into four nourishments, illustrates that employed for treatment during acute complications when a dose of regular insulin is given at six-hour intervals (see p. 886).

Diet No. XIII. Liquid Diet—Four Equal Meals
(Protein 110 gm.; Fat 65 gm.; Carb. 250 gm.—2000 Calories)

NO. EXCHANGES	FOOD EXCHANGE	LIST NO.	SAMPLE MENU	HOUSEHOLD MEAS.	WT. GM.	P	F	C	CAL.
6:00 A.M.									
1	Bread	4	Oatmeal in	½ c.	20	2	—	15	68
1	Milk	1	Milk, whole	1 c.	240	8	10	12	170
			Lactose or sugar or dexin	2 tbsp.	20	—	—	20	80
2	Meat	5	Eggs, coddled	2	—	14	10	—	146
1½	Fruit	3	Pineapple juice	½ c.	120	—	—	15	60
				Total		24	20	62	524
12:00 NOON (Repeat at 6:00 P.M. with suitable exchanges)									
			Soup (thin with broth)						
2	Meat	5	Meat puree	2 oz.	60	14	6	—	110
1	Bread	4	Potato, mashed	½ c.	100	2	—	15	68
1	Vegetable	2B	Peas puree	½ c.	100	2	—	7	36
1½	Fruit	3	Grapefruit juice	¾ c.	150	—	—	15	60
1	Milk	1	Milk, whole	1 c.	240	8	10	12	170
			Lactose or sugar or dexin	4 tsp.	15	—	—	15	60
				Total		26	16	64	504
12:00 MIDNIGHT									
			Milk drink						
2⅓	Milk	1	Milk, skim	1 pt.	480	16	—	24	160
	Milk	1	Milk, skim, powder	1 tbsp.	12	2	—	4	24
2	Meat	5	Eggs	2	—	14	10	—	146
			Lactose or sugar or dexin	1 tbsp.	10	—	—	10	40
1	Fat	6	Light cream	2 tbsp.	30	—	5	—	45
2	Fruit	3	Grape juice	½ c.	120	—	—	20	80
				Total		32	15	58	495
				Day's Total		108	67	248	2027

This liquid diet is designed for patients with acute complications and who are unable to eat regular food. The division into four equal meals, one every six hours, in conjunction with four doses of regular insulin facilitates the control of the diabetes during emergency periods (see p. 886).

insulin is injected subcutaneously as each infusion is begun.

The quantity of fluids given is adjusted to promote and maintain normal hydration. Mild degrees of glycosuria are permitted as a safeguard against a hypoglycemia but sufficient amounts of insulin and carbohydrate are given to prevent appreciable degrees of acetonuria. Blood sugar values are likely to be misleading while glucose is being administered by vein.

The dosage of insulin is regulated in such cases also according to the degree of glycosuria. For an unconscious or incontinent patient an indwelling catheter is introduced into the bladder, under appropriate precautions, in order that the samples of urine may be secured. Gantrisin is employed, in doses of 1 gm. four times daily, as a prophylactic agent against infection in the urinary tract while the catheter is in place. This therapy is fortified by the daily administration of vitamins, ascorbic acid—at least 100 mg., thiamine 2 mg., riboflavin 2 mg., and nicotinic acid amide 20 mg. These vitamins may be added to the intravenous infusion.

Tuberculosis

Diabetic patients are especially susceptible to tuberculous infections. Pulmonary tuberculosis was about twice as common in 3106 diabetics as in a comparable nondiabetic group.[133] It was three times as common in those taking more than 40 units of insulin daily as in those taking less or no insulin, and tuberculosis was about twice as common in diabetic patients who were below the standard weight in contrast with those above standard weight. Boucot and associates[133] found 5.3 per cent "active tuberculosis among 430 diabetics under 40 and 1.7 per cent in 2653 diabetics over 40 years of age." Attacks of diabetic coma predispose to the development of pulmonary tuberculosis.

Early diagnosis of tuberculosis in diabetic subjects depends upon the detection of (1) increased pulse rate, (2) mild degree of fever, (3) rapid sedimentation rate, (4) the absence of clinical improvement with control of the diabetes, and—by far the most important—(5) the roentgen ray evidence of the disease. *Roentgenography* will reveal early tuberculous lesions which fail to give detectable physical signs. Every diabetic patient should have a roentgen ray examination of the lungs and every young diabetic patient, especially if the diabetes is not controlled, should have such an examination annually. Every patient with the rapidly forming "true diabetic cataract" should be carefully examined for tuberculosis. Four of ten such patients reported by Himsworth[89] had pulmonary tuberculosis. Both conditions are prone to occur in young patients with uncontrolled and severe diabetes.

Pathology. The extension of the tuberculous process in the untreated diabetic patient is rapid. It is usually far advanced before it is recognized clinically. The fulminating course of the disease is attributable to the extension of the characteristically deep seated lesions, pneumonic in type, spreading toward the hilum of the lung with little tendency to fibrosis or pleural involvement. Caseation proceeds promptly and rapidly with early cavitation but minimal amounts of sputum and, as might well be expected, if the disease is not recognized and energetically treated the prognosis is grave. Incipient tuberculosis is practically unknown in diabetic patients.

Prevention. Patients are cautioned against contact with persons known to have tuberculosis. It is highly desirable for every diabetic, and especially if he is underweight, to have a roentgen ray film of his chest once yearly. Good hygienic measures aid in preventing tuberculous infections.

Treatment. In general, the treatment for tuberculous infection in the diabetic is the same as in the nondiabetic. The diet is sufficiently liberal to prevent a reduction in weight during acute episodes of the disease. It is preferable to keep the body weight 5 to 10 per cent above the normal standard (see Appendix).

Tuberculous infections may not alter the need for insulin greatly. Additions to the usual insulin frequently suffice to control the diabetes but in some, especially those with secondary infections, it is necessary to employ the four-equal-meal schedule—a meal every six hours with an appropriate amount of insulin before each (see p. 886). It is important that the diabetes be continuously controlled. Repeatedly we have observed patients do badly at times when the diabetes was out of hand. Occasionally, as the tuberculous process progresses the need for insulin becomes less.

The acute nature of "diabetic tuberculosis" makes it particularly sensitive to modern antimicrobial drugs—streptomycin (SM), para-aminosalicylic acid (PAS) and isoniazid (INH).

Therapies are not static. At present the treatment of choice for tuberculosis is isoniazid, 10 mg. per kg. per day, given in three divided doses with PAS, 8 to 12 gm. per day, divided into four doses and given after food. In view of the predisposition of diabetics to neuropathic disorders, pyridoxine, 50 to 100 mg. daily while taking isoniazid, is recommended. Single drug therapy is contraindicated, and the antimicrobial measures are continued for 18 months to 2 years as with the nondiabetic.

The outlook for diabetic patients suffering from tuberculosis is quite as good as that for the nondiabetic having this disease, provided the diagnosis is made early and provided the diabetes is properly controlled.

Cancer

Cancer appears more frequently in the diabetic population than in the population at large, and this trend is becoming increasingly apparent as more diabetic patients live longer in "the cancer age." In the majority the onset of malignant disease occurs after the diabetes is established. Of 243 of Joslin's fatal cases there was carcinoma of the breast in 35, of the pancreas 33, of the uterus 27, of the stomach 17, of the urinary bladder 15, and of the liver 14. Carcinoma of the pancreas comprised 12 per cent of the total in contrast to 2.5 per cent in 5300 cases of cancer reported by Hoffman. Diabetic subjects are, therefore, more likely to develop cancer of the pancreas than are nondiabetic patients. Endometrial malignancies are especially common in diabetics.

Some cases of carcinoma of the pancreas cause diabetes. This is not common, however, probably because of the independent blood supply to the islets of Langerhans and because cancer usually involves the head of the pancreas—that portion containing the fewest islets.

Skin Disorders Complicating Diabetes Mellitus

The most troublesome skin disorders complicating diabetes are bacterial infections, notably carbuncles and furuncles; fungus infections, especially intertriginous moniliasis, and pruritus of multiple causes. Less common are xanthomatous lesions—xanthoma diabeticorum, necrobiasis lipoidica diabeticorum and xanthelasma—dermal changes secondary to arterial disease, especially cellulitis, gangrene and atrophy, and neurotrophic disorders, notably trophic ulcers.

The foregoing and other acute complications are presented according to their relative frequencies in Table 22.

Carbuncles. Carbuncles are among the most serious and yet are among the preventable complications of diabetes. Fortunately they are not common. The mortality rate, formerly approximately 20 per cent, has been greatly reduced by appropriate antibiotic therapy. Neglect of the diabetes and obesity, meddlesome local therapy, septicemia, and failure to determine and act upon the sensitivity of the offending organisms to antibiotic drugs doubtless will prevent the complete elimination of mortality from these infections.

It is not known why diabetic patients are prone to develop staphylococcal infections. It is not due directly to the hyperglycemia but it has been sug-

TABLE 22. DIABETIC COMPLICATIONS IN 3564 CONSECUTIVE PATIENTS ADMITTED TO THE PUBLIC WARDS OF THE PENNSYLVANIA HOSPITAL FOR ACUTE COMPLICATIONS OF DIABETES

Complication	Number
Cardiac disease	648
Hypertensive and arteriosclerotic, exclusive of myocardial infarction	
Cutaneous infections	358
Infections of respiratory tract	292
Infections of urinary tract	263
Myocardial infarction	184
Gangrene, lower extremity	175
Gynecologic conditions	138
Cerebral vascular disease	130
Diabetic ketosis (coma)	100
Fractures	85
Diabetic neuropathy	81
Cholecystitis	72
Gastrointestinal tract cancer	59
Osteomyelitis	29
Embolism	26
Thrombophlebitis	24
Peritonitis	20
Hyperthyroidism	19
Pancreatitis	18
Cancer of respiratory tract	16
Miscellaneous	827
Total	3564

gested that the sugar content of the skin is an important factor. It has been found that the sugar content of normal skin averaged 59 per cent (61 mg.) of the average normal blood sugar of 103 mg. per 100 ml., whereas in diabetic patients with skin diseases the sugar content was higher than in diabetic patients without skin disorders, being on the average 69 per cent of the blood sugar level. Also in contrast with the large quantity of glycogen in normal skin, almost none is found in the skin of patients with untreated diabetes. Appropriate treatment of diabetes reduces the glucose and increases the glycogen content of the skin.

Overweight patients who have a mild but neglected diabetes and who are uncleanly in their habits and personal hygiene are especially likely to contract furuncles and carbuncles. Carbuncles may occur anywhere on the surface of the body, but are especially prone to affect the vulva in the female and the neck in the male.

The occasional patient, though having an apparent diabetes during the course of the infection, has no demonstrable sign of the disease a few months after the infection has subsided.

PREVENTION. Control of the diabetes, correction of obesity, cleanliness of the skin and clothing, avoiding shaving the back of the neck, and early and appropriate treatment for minor infections of the skin comprise the outstanding prophylactic measures.

TREATMENT. A diabetic with a carbuncle should be treated in a hospital. Carbuncles are still serious infections. The diet and insulin are employed as outlined for other acute infections (see p. 886). Determination of the sensitivity of the causative organism to the various antibiotics is of utmost importance and will be instrumental in saving lives. Newly discovered antibiotic drugs to which the organisms have had no opportunity to develop a resistance may be especially effective. Liberal amounts of the specific antibiotics are recommended. Hot compresses and release of confined pus are the only surgical measures employed. Extensive surgical interference is contraindicated.

Furuncles. Furuncles, also staphylococcal infections, occurring in diabetic patients should be looked upon as potential carbuncles and treated as such. They may occur singly, but more frequently they are multiple and widespread. They tend to recur in crops.

Freshly laundered underclothes and bed linen daily aid in preventing the spread of the infection. Furthermore, the infected area should be protected from the rubbing of underclothes by a dressing held in place by a bandage or liquid adhesive. Adhesive tape should never be applied to the skin in these cases.

Eradication of foci of infection occasionally gives dramatic results in preventing recurring furuncles. Antibiotic therapy, as recommended in the treatment for carbuncles, and strict control of the diabetes are essential.

Pruritus. Pruritus is the most common symptom affecting the skin of the diabetic patient. It is especially common in females, affecting the pudenda, the intense itching of which makes many patients seek treatment.

The itching is caused (1) by the irritation of the skin set up by dried urine, which contains sugar, and (2) by Monilia, which find in the sugar-laden urine an ideal medium in which to multiply. Minute injuries resulting from rubbing or scratching may be portals of entry for infecting organisms, notably the staphylococcus. Furuncles, carbuncles and erysipelas are contracted in this manner.

TREATMENT. The treatment consists of local and general measures.

Local. Cleanliness of the genitalia is essential. Gentle bathing of the parts with a cold solution of boric acid (saturated) after each voiding of urine is helpful. This is followed by daubing the affected areas with toilet lanolin or a bland ointment, such as nupercaine, having mild anesthetic properties. If, as not infrequently occurs, there is an associated vaginitis a douche composed of a saturated solution of boric acid or sodium perborate, 1 dram in a quart of water, twice daily, is indicated.

General. Control of the diabetes deprives the fungi of the glucose medium, and with correction of the glycosuria the cause of the local irritation is corrected in most cases.

The nervousness and fatigue, due largely to disturbed rest, tending to intensify the symptoms and sometimes responsible for generalized pruritus, are usually alleviated by sedation and analgesics.

Xanthochromia. Xanthochromia, or xanthosis, is a yellowish tinting of the skin especially noticeable in the palms of the hands, the soles of the feet and the nasolabial folds. Associated with rubeosis—a rosy coloration of the skin of the face occurring in young patients with neglected diabetes—xanthochromia gives a "peaches and cream" complexion. It is due to an impaired destruction or impaired excretion of certain lipochromes, the most conspicuous of which is carotene, derived from pigment-containing foods, notably carrots, sweet potatoes, corn, butter and egg yolk. An accumulation of the lipochrome in the blood, xanthemia, is a prerequisite to the xanthochromic discoloration of the skin. Fruits and vegetables rich in lipochrome have been extensively employed in diets for diabetic patients. Hence an increased supply superimposed on a faulty utilization, destruction or excretion of the pigment makes the diabetic patient a susceptible subject to this disorder. The recent trend toward normal diets for diabetic patients and better facilities to control the diabetes has reduced the frequency of xanthochromia.

It appears that xanthosis occurs in diabetes as the result of the disturbance of carbohydrate metabolism. Contrasted with normal subjects, diabetic children showed a marked delay in reducing an artificially increased blood carotin content to normal.

Xanthochromia may be confused with jaundice. The sclerae are not icteroid, however, the bilirubin content of the blood is normal, and there is no bile in the urine.

TREATMENT. Beyond its cosmetic effect, which is not marked, xanthochromia is an innocent condition. It causes no symptoms but occasional embarrassment. The xanthochromia subsides slowly. Its disappearance may be hastened by temporarily reducing foods rich in lipochromes, notably eggs, sweet potatoes, corn, butter and carrots. Care should be taken not to interfere with the vitamin and mineral intake. Yeast concentrates and vitamins A and D may be administered. Skim milk will provide calcium.

Xanthelasma. Xanthelasma occurs in nondiabetic as well as in diabetic patients, though it occurs much more frequently in the latter. It consists of a collection of slightly raised yellow, fatty, flattened tumors, and occurs about the inner canthus of the eyelids. It is usually bilateral. The condition is more prevalent in females than in males. No treatment beyond that of controlling the diabetes and maintaining a normal blood cholesterol is indicated. The tumors do not disappear unless excised

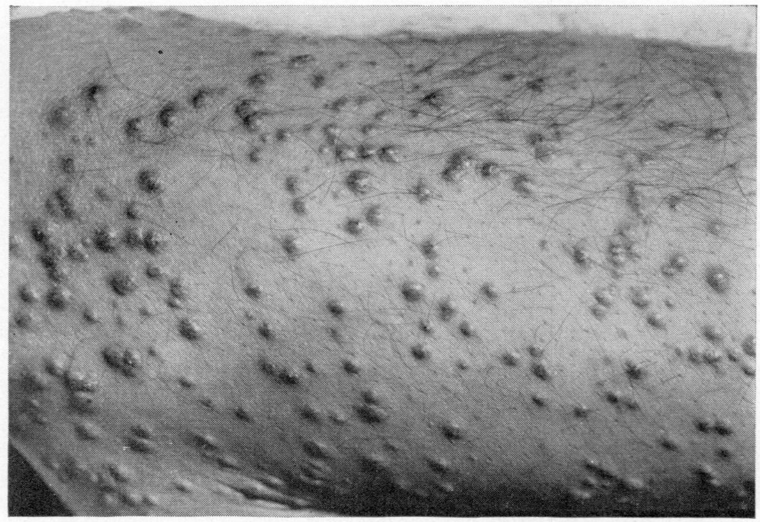

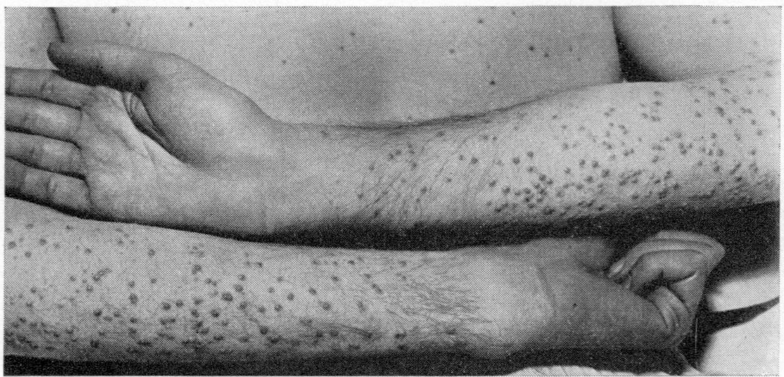

FIG. 26. Nodular cutaneous eruption in a case of xanthoma diabeticorum.

or otherwise removed. This may be indicated for cosmetic reasons. If excised, however, they almost invariably recur. Otherwise, the condition is innocent.

Xanthoma Diabeticorum. This rare complication of diabetes is manifested by discrete cutaneous nodules (Fig. 26), 1 to 3 mm. in diameter, appearing symmetrically for the most part about the elbows, knees and buttocks, though the forearms, dorsum of the hands, the toes, neck and back are affected but to a much less degree. The eruption does not occur on the face. The nodules have a yellowish center with a reddish periphery, are hard, like kernels of wheat, and are not tender. Xanthomatous nodules may also occur on the tongue. Xanthoma diabeticorum is a manifestation of uncontrolled diabetes with hyperlipemia. The patient, of whom the photograph in Figure 26 was taken, had an initial blood cholesterol level of 1666 mg. per 100 ml. (cholesterol ester 340 mg.) and a blood sugar concentration of 488 mg. per 100 ml. This patient also exhibited a classic example of lipemia retinalis, and his blood plasma had the appearance of cream.

TREATMENT. Control of the diabetes is essential. The diet, until the disorder is corrected, should contain but little fat (30 to 40 gm.) and a liberal carbohydrate quota (300 to 340 gm.). The patient, aged twenty-five years, being 181 cm. (6 feet and ¾ inch) in height and weighing 72 kg. (158 lb.), was given a diet of protein 110 gm., carbohydrate 350 gm. and fat 40 gm. (2200 calories). He required 44 units of protamine zinc and 24 units of crystalline insulin each morning. On this regimen the diabetes was controlled, the lipemia retinalis disappeared promptly, the cutaneous nodules lost their firmness, the affected areas became flattened, and within two months all evidences of the disorder, including xanthomatous nodules on the tongue, had disappeared.

Though the lesions disappear under treatment, they tend to recur if the diabetes is neglected. Subsequent to the control of the diabetes it is permissible to increase the fat and reduce the carbohydrate contents of the diet to amounts employed in the treatment of uncomplicated diabetes.

Necrobiosis Lipoidica Diabeticorum. These discrete, clearly defined, reddish cutaneous papules, from 1 to 3 mm. in diameter, occur four times as frequently in the female with neglected diabetes as in the male. The condition is rarely seen in nondiabetic individuals. The lesion does not fade on pressure. It increases in size and progresses slowly from the reddish papule with a smooth glistening and firm surface. Eventually atrophic changes with ulceration in the center take place. At this stage the lesion may be several centimeters in diameter surrounded by a reddish or violaceous region of infiltration.

A single lesion of necrobiosis lipoidica diabeticorum may appear, but more frequently there are multiple lesions in various stages of development and located for the most part on the legs below the knees. Histologically, necrobiotic changes in the collagenous tissues and obliterative changes in the smaller blood vessels are characteristic.

The cause of this disorder is unknown. Local injury may play a part. In most cases it occurs in patients with neglected diabetes, and the majority of patients in whom this disorder appears are between ten and forty years of age.

Prevention as well as treatment lies in the control of the diabetes. Diets low in fat and containing liberal carbohydrate quotas (250 to 350 gm.) are indicated. No effective local treatment for this disorder has been found.

A comprehensive review of this subject has been presented by Hildebrand et al.[134]

Hirsutism. Hirsutism appears as a fine lanugo hair on the back and arms of undernourished young patients whose diabetes is not controlled. It occurs especially in those with a fair complexion. This type of hirsutism is corrected by control of the diabetes and by improved nutrition.

Achard and Thier (1921) attracted attention to the *diabète des femmes barbes.* They described the syndrome of hirsutism, amenorrhea and obesity due to hyperplasia or tumor growth of the adrenal cortex. The prevalence of hirsutism in diabetic women suggests that an increased functional activity of the adrenal cortex, either primary or secondary to hypophyseal dysfunction, is a common occurrence in diabetes. Adrenal cortical tumors, on the other hand, are uncommon and infrequently cause diabetes. The literature on this subject was reviewed by Duncan and Fetter,[135] who found that the incidence of adrenal cortical tumors causing hirsutism and diabetes is very low indeed.

Control of the diabetes is indicated. Removal of adrenal tumors is advisable. Measures should be taken to prevent an acute adrenal insufficiency which may follow the operation.

Hirsutism similar to that seen in cases of adrenal cortical tumors occurs in pituitary basophilism. The treatment is directed toward reducing the functional effect of the tumor either by irradiation or removal. Most cases of hirsutism seen in a diabetic clinic are probably the result of previous excessive adrenal cortical activity which is no longer present.

Local Necrosis Following the Injection of Contaminated Insulin. One patient was admitted to the Pennsylvania Hospital because of large (3 to 5 cm.) areas of necrosis appearing at the site of each "insulin injection." These reactions occurred immediately after the injection and after using insulin for eight years without any untoward reactions. On investigation it was discovered that the insulin in the bottle had been partially replaced by concentrated ammonium hydroxide with homicidal intent.

Dermatitis Gangrenosa. A rare condition of gangrene involving the skin of the trunk or extremities has been described by Riven.[136] Large vesicles occurred on the back, thighs, and legs with subsequent gangrene of the underlying areas. The patient had fever, and staphylococci were recovered from the vesicle fluid.

Dupuytren's Contracture. This disorder, involving the palmar fascia in one or both hands, of slow progression and appearing for the most part in mild to moderate forms, is a common complication in male diabetic patients. Surgical correction is usually not necessary.

Disturbances in Sexual Characteristics Complicating Diabetes

Female. Delayed development of secondary sexual characteristics, disturbance or absence of menstruation and an early menopause are frequent in women with untreated diabetes. Fertility is reduced, though the incidence of conception has increased during the insulin era. Libido is frequently reduced. It is rarely increased. Abortions are more prevalent in the diabetic than in the nondiabetic women.

With control of the diabetes catamenia commences at a normal age. Catamenia is restored within a few months if amenorrhea has occurred as a result of the diabetes. A restoration of sexual desire is usual and the likelihood of conception is increased.

Male. The chief sexual disturbance in the male resulting from diabetes is impotence. There is apparently no disturbance in fertility. Formerly impotence was rarely corrected by control of the diabetes, but when this disturbance is due to a diabetic neuropathy and in its early stages, recovery may, but usually does not, follow treatment with vitamin B_{12}. Most male diabetics have decreased potentia, and loss of libido is more common in diabetic than in nondiabetic men.

Diseases of the Liver

Despite the important part played by the liver in carbohydrate metabolism, disease of this organ is an uncommon complication of diabetes. In uncontrolled diabetes enlargement of the liver is not infrequent, however. This is noted especially in children and is due to infiltration of fat, and in some cases to accumulation of water in the intercellular spaces. Tests of liver function usually show normal responses.

The hepatomegaly of diabetes is corrected by controlling this metabolic disorder. The new insulins have greatly simplified the control of the diabetes even in the young patients. As a consequence they have aided in correcting and preventing hepatomegaly. Experimentally the feeding of raw pancreas, and the administration of lecithin, choline or betaine, and lipocaic have prevented and corrected hepatomegaly in depancreatized animals. Resort to these measures is not necessary clinically. Uniform control of the diabetes suffices.

Bell[137] observed, on autopsy material, that diabetes was five times as frequent in males with cirrhosis of the liver as it was in the general male population. This increase was not observed in females with this form of hepatic disease.

Cholecystitis and Cholelithiasis

Cholecystitis and cholelithiasis are so frequent in obese but otherwise normal patients that it is not surprising to find them to be common in the middle-aged diabetic population, the majority of whom are overweight. Warren[138] found that 31 per cent of 453 diabetic patients who were over thirty years of age and who came to autopsy had gallstones. In contrast, he found gallstones in 21 per cent in the same age group of 500 nondiabetic patients.

Extension of infection from the gallbladder via the biliary passages, lymphatics, contiguity and blood stream to the pancreas has been considered as a cause of secondary diabetes.

Treatment. A chronic cholecystitis occurring in the diabetic patient should be treated conservatively if practicable.

Cholelithiasis associated with colic is an indication for surgical intervention. Furthermore, since the diabetic patient withstands a chronic infection poorly, surgical drainage or removal of the gallbladder is advised when gallstones are observed roentgenologically, in the symptom-free patient. The risk, in biliary tract disease, as well as in surgery of the biliary tract, is not to be considered greater in the diabetic than in the nondiabetic person.

Surgery and Diabetes

Insulin therapy has made it possible to give diabetic patients the benefits of surgery with prospects of results closely approaching those achieved with nondiabetic subjects.

The diabetes is controlled prior to elective operations but in emergencies diabetes is not a contraindication to surgical procedures provided a moderate or severe degree of ketosis is not present; i.e., a 2 plus or greater reaction for acetone in the plasma or a CO_2 combining power of the plasma below 15 mM/L (35 volumes per cent).

Procedure of Therapy. Our procedure in preparing these patients for operation has been as follows:

1. ELECTIVE SURGERY. Patients undergoing elective surgery are kept on their usual routine of therapy until the day of operation.

2. NONELECTIVE, NONEMERGENCY SURGERY. In nonelective surgery when a delay of two or three days is permissible, the diabetes is controlled using the four equal meals, one every six hours, and each preceded by a dose of crystalline insulin. This is identical with the plan of therapy for acute infections (see p. 886).

3. EMERGENCY SURGERY. When immediate surgery is necessary and (a) the diabetes is not complicated by ketosis, no delay is indicated, but (b) when the patient has ketosis with a 2 to 3 plus reaction for acetone in the plasma or a CO_2 combining power below 15 mM/L (35 volumes per cent), a delay of four to six hours will be adequate, with liberal doses of insulin given subcutaneously and glucose and normal saline given intravenously, to restore the carbohydrate metabolism, acid-base equilibrium and water balance sufficiently to proceed with the operation. (c) Patients in diabetic coma should not be subjected to surgery beyond minor remedial measures; e.g., myringotomy for the drainage of an abscess, the opening of an airway, the arrest of hemorrhage, or other measures to forestall an immediate disaster.

THE DAY OF OPERATION. Procedures for this day are modified by the urgency and nature of the operation, the severity of the diabetes, the clinical condition of the patient, the anesthesia, the necessity in some cases for an empty stomach, and the prospective ability of the patient to take food orally after the operation.

In dealing with the diabetes there are two main objectives: (1) Avoid ketosis, and (2) avoid hypoglycemic reactions.

Management of the diabetes is integrated with the other needs of the patient as indicated by our usual program, which is as follows:

1. NOURISHMENT, FLUIDS AND SODIUM CHLORIDE. The six-hour schedule of giving nourishment is adhered to. The nourishment before operation is given as 1 liter of 5 or 10 per cent solution of glucose. Following operation the basic plan is to give 750 ml. of a 5 or 10 per cent solution of glucose or 10 per cent invert sugar intravenously, slowly, in each six-hour period. A new bottle is started every six hours. Every third administration is given as a 5 per cent solution of glucose in normal saline. If nourishment is given in this manner for more than one or two days, casein hydrolysate is added—the equivalent of 25 gm. of protein per day.

On some occasions more fluids are indicated, in which case 1 liter is given in place of a 750 ml. administration. Contrariwise, in cases of surgical shock with anuria and a lower nephron nephrosis resulting, the amount of fluid

DIAGRAMS to ILLUSTRATE PLANS for MANAGEMENT of DIABETES on OPERATIVE DAY

For Incision and Drainage, Vein Ligation and Similar "Minor" Procedures

	3AM	6AM	9AM	12N	3PM	6PM	9PM	12M
FEEDINGS								
I.V. GLUCOSE								
INSULIN								
OPERATION								

For Amputation, Setting of Fractures

	3AM	6AM	9AM	12N	3PM	6PM	9PM	12M
FEEDINGS			LIQUID					
I.V. GLUCOSE					1000 ml.			
INSULIN			REDUCED DOSE					
OPERATION								

For Amputation, TRANSURETHRAL PROSTATECTOMY

	3AM	6AM	9AM	12N	3PM	6PM	9PM	12M
FEEDINGS								
I.V. GLUCOSE			1000 ml.					
INSULIN								
OPERATION								

GASTRECTOMY and THYROIDECTOMY and CHOLECYSTECTOMY

	3AM	6AM	9AM	12N	3PM	6PM	9PM	12M
FEEDINGS								
I.V. GLUCOSE	750 ml.		750 ml.		750 ml.		750 ml.	
INSULIN								
OPERATION								

FIG. 27. Four plans of therapy for diabetic patients subjected to surgery of varying degrees of complexity are depicted diagrammatically. (After Alexander, J. B., Loomis, A. H., and Lee, C. T., Jr.: M. Clin. North America, Sept., 1949.)

would be reduced to approximately 1200 ml. daily until the anuria or oliguria is corrected.

2. INSULIN. *Crystalline insulin is used and is given subcutaneously.* Ordinarily, one fourth of the previous day's total dose of insulin is given prior to the preoperative administration of glucose. This is not a fixed rule. It may be advisable to give less if there is any fear of a hypoglycemia, or if the operation is prolonged the risk of a hypoglycemia can be eliminated by giving glucose intravenously during the latter stages of the operation.

Postoperatively the amounts of insulin, a dose every six hours, are regulated according to the degree of glycosuria. Mild degrees of glycosuria are preferable during the first two or three postoperative days.

Simple operative procedures—the ligation of veins, incisions and drainage, and dental extractions—and, indeed, many amputations may be performed without any change in the four-meal schedule, the operation being simply inserted between feedings.

Four illustrative plans of therapy in operative cases are presented in Figure 27. It will be observed that nourishments are given at intervals of six hours.

The normal distribution of meals—usually three meals and a bedtime nourishment—and insulin are resumed when the patient is afebrile and can take regular food. The transition from the six-hour schedule to the normal regimen is performed in the same manner as that following an acute infection (see p. 886).

Choice of Anesthesia. The choice of anesthesia properly rests with a well qualified anesthesiologist.

Ordinarily, *regional anesthesia*—block, spinal, etc.—is the method of choice. Nausea and vomiting are infrequent and many patients can take their diets earlier in the postoperative period than when a general anesthesia is used. Improved circulation by the incidental sympathetic block is of value in surgery of the extremities.

Premedication for regional or general anesthesia is individualized. Morphine, if used, is given in minimal doses. It causes nausea and vomiting in a considerable number of patients, and a moderate elevation of the blood sugar is caused by this drug. A combination of a short acting barbiturate (Seconal or Nembutal, 100 mg.), Demerol, 100 mg., and scopolamine, 0.4 mg., produces satisfactory tranquility in the average adult.

Of the general anesthetics, *ether* has been observed to increase the blood sugar by 100 to 200 per cent and *cyclopropane* by about 30 per cent. These alterations are readily controlled by insulin therapy, and diabetic patients should not be deprived of these agents if the anesthesiologist feels that one or the other is the drug of choice for a particular patient.

Pentothal, which increases the blood sugar but a trifle, is a valuable adjunct to *nitrous oxide* anesthesia, and this combination, with curare if necessary to produce relaxation, has received widespread adoption.

Infections of the Urinary Tract

Infections of the urinary tract are frequent and serious complications of diabetes. They may present few symptoms, and their presence should be carefully sought for in every case. They occur frequently in patients whose diabetes is neglected.

Pyelonephritis is a common complication of diabetes. It is, however, an infrequent cause of death in contrast to degenerative and malignant diseases (Table 23). Diabetic patients, and especially diabetic women, are predisposed to infections in the urinary tract. Bowen and Kutzman[139] found normal urinary tracts in only seven of eighty-four unselected diabetic women. Pyelonephritis is four and one half times more common as a cause of death among diabetic than it is among nondiabetic patients,[140] and of 307 deaths of diabetic patients it was the sixth commonest cause. Pyelonephritis was the cause of twenty-one of these deaths.[141] A peculiar form of pyelonephritis—a necrotizing renal papillitis—is associated mostly with diabetes. A specific total necrosis of the renal pyramids occurs with, or without, abscess formation, and involvement of both kidneys is frequent. This serious complication occurred in 25 per cent of the cases of acute pyelonephritis and accounted for the most severe forms of the disease.[142]

TABLE 23. CAUSES OF DEATH IN 3564 CONSECUTIVE DIABETIC PATIENTS ADMITTED TO THE PUBLIC WARDS OF THE PENNSYLVANIA HOSPITAL BETWEEN 1947 AND 1957 BECAUSE OF ACUTE COMPLICATIONS

Cause	Number
Myocardial infarction	80
Cerebral artery disease	46
Malignant tumors	25
Pneumonia	19
Diabetic keto-acidosis	12
Renal disease	12
Embolism	9
Cirrhosis of the liver	7
Pulmonary tuberculosis	3
Pyelonephritis	3
Gas gangrene	2
Miscellaneous	40
Total	258

A sugar-laden urine is probably a better medium for organisms than urine containing no sugar. This feature and the higher frequency of bladder catheterization in diabetic subjects who have been in coma combine to increase the likelihood of pyelonephritis in these patients.

Clinically, pyelonephritis is characterized by the sudden onset of recurring attacks of fever, chills and backache. The urine sediment contains pus and myriads of organisms, and albumin is present.

The studies recommended comprise, first and most important, the identification of the organism by culture of the urine and the determination of its sensitivity to the various antibiotic agents. Though the colon bacillus is the most common offender, other organisms may be present. Ten cases of infections of the urinary tract in which neomycin was the only antibiotic agent to which the infecting organism was sensitive illustrate the need for highly specialized selective study and therapy.[142]

Diabetic patients are predisposed to tuberculous infections. The importance of identifying a renal tuberculosis while the infection is confined to one kidney is obvious.

Second, the appraisal of physical abnormalities by a urologist comprises a phenolsulfonphthalein excretion test, a pyelogram—the dye being administered intravenously—and if found essential to establish the diagnosis, a retrograde pyelogram is recommended.

The treatment for pyelonephritis should be prompt and conservatively aggressive. The diabetes is controlled as in the case of other acute infections (see p. 886). The degree of glycosuria is reduced in some cases by sugar-consuming organisms in the urinary tract. This is a minor matter.

The medical therapy will be dictated by the type or organism and the remedial agents to which it is sensitive. In the event sulfonamides are used, as is frequently the case, it is important that at least one specimen of urine per twenty-four hours be alkaline in reaction and at least 1500 ml. of urine be excreted in this period. It is easier to secure one alkaline specimen by giving a single large dose of bicarbonate of soda daily than it is to keep the urine alkaline by giving multiple smaller doses. Gantrisin has gained popularity for its effect in sterilizing the urinary tract of gram-negative organisms and the absence of renal complications attending its use.

Surgical measures that are indicated should be carried out without fail if the patient's clinical condition permits. The diabetes is not a deterrent to such corrective measures.

HEMOCHROMATOSIS (BRONZE DIABETES)

Primary or idiopathic hemochromatosis is a cause, not a result of diabetes mellitus. It is a rare, chronic, and slowly progressive inborn error of cellular iron metabolism, the first case of which was described by Trousseau in 1865. The outstanding characteristics of hemochromatosis are (1) an abnormal deposition of pigments, especially hemosiderin, an iron-containing pigment, in the skin and viscera, (2) cirrhosis of the liver and pancreas and (3) diabetes mellitus. Pigmentation of the skin is absent in approximately 20 per cent of cases. Progressive cirrhotic changes take place in the various organs. The liver and pancreas are the first organs affected and are the sites of the more extensive cirrhotic changes. Diabetes mellitus is present in most, but not all, cases. It occurs as a complication of hemochromatosis and is an index of the damage done to the islet cells of the pancreas. Diabetes is usually a late manifestation of the disease.

Hemochromatosis occurs in the great majority of instances in patients between the ages of forty-five and fifty-five years. The condition is practically unknown before the age of twenty years but from this age to forty-five years there is a consistent increase in its incidence. A decline in the incidence occurs between the ages of fifty-five and seventy years. Females are rarely affected before the fifth decade of life. The disorder affects males from twenty to twenty-five times as frequently as females (see Table 24). The disease is uncommon. Sheldon[143] was able to collect only 311 authentic cases of hemochromatosis in the entire medical writings on this subject. Only thirty-four cases of hemochromatosis were ob-

TABLE 24. THE AGE AND SEX INCIDENCE IN 290 CASES OF HEMOCHROMATOSIS*

AGE GROUP	20 TO 25	26 TO 30	31 TO 35	36 TO 40	41 TO 45	46 TO 50	51 TO 55	56 TO 60	61 TO 65	66 TO 70	71 TO 75
No. of cases (male)	2	7	13	37	48	59	56	34	9	8	4
No. of cases (female)	..	1	1	..	..	2	5	1	3	1	
	2	8	14	37	48	61	61	35	12	9	4

* After Sheldon.[143]

served at the Mayo clinic in seventeen years (1923–1940).

Etiology. Von Recklinghausen, in 1889, identified two pigments derived from hemoglobin, (1) hemosiderin, an iron-containing compound, loosely bound with fat and protein, which turns black when brought in contact with ammonium sulfide, and (2) hemofuscin, which contains no iron but stains readily with basic aniline dyes and is believed to be related to the melanins. In hemochromatosis, hemosiderin is retained and deposited chiefly in the connective tissue of the glandular organs, the lymph nodes, striated muscles, reticuloendothelial system, alveolar epithelium, cartilage and the synovia. Cirrhotic changes progress in direct proportion to the amount of hemosiderin deposited in the organs. Necrosis of the pigment-containing cells is followed by the cirrhotic process.

Dry[144] and Sheldon[143] believed that the disease is an inborn constitutional abnormality of iron metabolism. Sheldon stated, "This hypothesis of an inborn error of metabolism appears to be the only one which will encompass the enormous array of facts provided by the clinical, pathological, and chemical aspects of the disease." Hemochromatosis has been observed to occur as the result of a familial and hereditary predisposition. Whatever the cause, there is an abnormal retention of iron. The total iron content of the body reaches 25 to 50 gm. in hemochromatosis in contrast to approximately 3 gm. in the normal person. Finch et al.[145] believed that the excessive deposits of iron responsible for hemochromatosis are the result of excessive absorption or parenteral administration of iron.

Hemochromatosis is distinct from hemosiderosis in which iron pigments, resulting from the excessive destruction of erythrocytes, are deposited in the tissues. In the latter condition there is irrefutable evidence to indicate that such iron pigments are used again in the formation of blood, whereas in hemochromatosis the hemosiderin is not used again and, furthermore, there is no apparent abnormal destruction of red blood cells in hemochromatosis.

There is convincing evidence that minute quantities of iron in excess of body needs are retained and accumulate over a period of many years. Eventually this retention of iron brings about the clinical characteristics of hemochromatosis. This retention may be due to an inherited abnormal avidity of the tissues for iron with an inability of the cells to rid themselves of the ferrous compounds.

A secondary type of hemochromatosis has been identified and attributed to multiple transfusions of blood. However, in some instances only small amounts of blood were given and in others there had been no transfusion. Patients with severe anemias kept alive by transfusions live longer than formerly, and it has been suggested that the anemia, not the transfusions, is the aggravating factor. Anoxia, hyperactive erythroplasia and viral hepatitis have been considered as possible mechanisms by which secondary hemochromatosis develops. It differs from the primary or idiopathic form of the disease in that it develops much more rapidly; the deposits of iron in the liver are great in proportion to the degree of cirrhotic changes in contrast to advanced cirrhosis in the primary form, and it lacks the predisposition to cancer of the liver in contrast to the high incidence of this outcome in the primary form. Approximately 10 per cent of patients with primary hemochromatosis eventually develop hepatic carcinoma.

Pathology. Hemosiderin and to a less extent hemofuscin are found in excess of normal throughout the organs and tissues of the body with the exception of the brain and nervous system.

Hemosiderin is deposited in the propria of the sweat glands and in the deeper strata of the malpighian layer of the skin, and hemofuscin is seen in the sweat glands and in the walls of the small blood vessels. The liver is reddish, rusty or of an ochre tint. It is enlarged and the capsule is thickened. The surface is firm and nodular (hobnail appearance), and there are massive accumulations of hemosiderin and lesser amounts of hemofuscin. The hemosiderin predominates in the extracellular areas but is present also in large amounts in the cells of the liver, in the fibrous tissue, in the Kupffer cells, in the liver capsule, and in the walls of the blood vessels.

The *pancreas* is also heavily pigmented with hemosiderin and some hemofuscin, giving it a reddish or rusty color. It is enlarged, firm and cirrhotic. The normal architecture of the pancreas is largely replaced by fibrous tissue, and there is degeneration and actual loss of acinar and islet tissues. Acute necrosis of the pancreas is, in rare instances, the cause of death.

Melanin, normally present in the deeper layers of the epidermis, is present in excessive quantities. Deposits of hemosiderin are found also in the spleen, lymph nodes, pituitary, thyroid and salivary glands, and in the myocardium. Involvement of the hypophysis may be related to the loss of libido and the testicular atrophy, although in some cases destructive cirrhotic changes in the adrenal cortex account for these changes. Hemofuscin is found in the cells of glandular organs, in connective tissue, in smooth muscle, and particularly in the walls of the medium-sized and small arteries.

Pigmentation of the skin and mucous membranes and the enlargement of the liver are the most constant physical findings in this disease. The liver is quite firm, not tender, and is usually smooth but may be rough (hobnail) if the disorder is well advanced. In late stages of the disease the liver is small and cannot be palpated. The spleen is palpable in about 60 per cent of cases. Ascites appears frequently as a late manifestation.

Laboratory Investigations. A moderate hypochromic anemia, hyperglycemia, glycosuria, and reduced serum albumin with a reversal of the albumin-globulin ratio are common findings. Icterus, though an unusual complication, may be present and cause an elevation of the serum bilirubin. Hypercholesterolemia with xanthomatous eruptions is sometimes present.

Dry[144] found no significant departure from normal in the iron balance studies in cases of hemochromatosis, indicating that the average daily retention is exceedingly small but must be greatly prolonged to account for the large quantities of iron in the tissues.

Hemochromatosis was observed in a patient who did not have glycosuria or iron-containing pigment in the skin.[146] The skin, however, was blue-bronze in color due to excessive deposits of melanin. The absence of glycosuria and of iron-containing pigment in the skin with the presence of cutaneous xanthomatosis and with hypercholesterolemia and hyperbilirubinemia, caused considerable difficulty in making a correct diagnosis. The true nature of the condition was established by examination of a section of liver removed during a peritoneoscopic examination. Evidences of adrenal cortical hormone and male sex hormone deficiencies were obtained during life. The possibility was suggested that a reduced carbohydrate tolerance or actual diabetes which might otherwise have been present might have been mitigated by the hypocortico-adrenalism.

Chemical examination of the tissues revealed enormous quantities of iron in the liver, pancreas and retroperitoneal lymph nodes, but relatively little iron was found in the heart and skeletal musculature. Death was due to the unusual complication of acute necrosis of the pancreas.

Diagnosis and Symptomatology. The diagnosis is easily made when the outstanding characteristics—*pigmentation of the skin, diabetes mellitus* and *cirrhosis of the liver*—are present. The urinary sediment may contain hemosiderin but the identification of the pigment in a section of skin is diagnostic. A specimen of liver secured by a special "biopsy needle" or during a peritoneoscopic examination and found to contain large deposits of iron serves to establish the diagnosis with certainty and especially in puzzling cases.

The disorders which are likely to be confused with hemochromatosis are argyria and Addison's disease. Pigmentation is the only characteristic which these three conditions have in common. An adequate history and careful physical examination should establish the correct diagnosis. Hemochromatosis and Addison's disease occasionally occur in the same patient.

The *pigmentation* of the skin is visible in approximately 80 per cent of cases. It occurs as the first sign of the disease in about a quarter of the cases and gives the skin a bronzed, bluish-metallic, leaden or slate color. This color involves the entire body but is more obvious in parts normally pigmented, about the genitalia and perineum, and in the folds of the skin, scars and on exposed portions—the face, the extensor surfaces of the forearms, and the dorsum of the hands. Pronounced pigmentation may be due to increased melanin in the malpighian layer of the skin without any iron-containing pigment being present. Pigmentation of the buccal mucosa occurs in about 16 per cent of cases. The conjunctiva may also be pigmented. Pigmentation has been observed to decrease during insulin therapy. Some patients have intense itching of the skin.

Diabetes mellitus, with characteristic symptoms, is a usual result of hemochromatosis. Though the symptoms of diabetes were the first noted in 25.7 per cent of Sheldon's collected cases, diabetes is usually a late manifestation of the disease. Death within twelve months usually followed the onset of diabetes. The diabetes may now be controlled but it may in rare instances become exceedingly severe and the patient may pass through a state of increasing insulin resistance to one in which insulin is completely ineffective.

Twenty-six of the thirty cases of hemochromatosis observed by Butt and Wilder[147] had diabetes as demonstrated by laboratory methods, and diabetes was present in 78 per cent of Sheldon's cases.

Asthenia is a common symptom of hemochromatosis. It may be secondary to disturbances in the function of the pituitary and adrenal glands, to the cirrhosis of the liver, or to the diabetes if this complication is not controlled.

Cirrhosis of the liver and the symptoms which it causes, notably lassitude, discomfort in the epigastrium, the sensation of heaviness in the abdomen, distention of the abdomen due to ascites and enlargement of the liver are usually present. In the final stages of the disease the liver is usually small. Hematemesis, purpura, icterus, diarrhea, dyspepsia, vomiting, lanugo-like hair appearing on the scalp and loss of normal hair are among the infrequent manifestations of this disease.

Tuberculosis, hypogonadism, hypocortico-adrenalism and carcinoma of the liver are not infrequent complications of hemochromatosis.

Prognosis and Treatment. Hemochromatosis is a chronic disease, the clinical manifestations of which appear gradually, over periods of months and years. Hepatic decompensation has replaced diabetic coma as the most common cause of death; cardiac and endocrine disorders are frequent contributing causes. Control of the diabetes has prolonged life, and indeed in some cases insulin treatment seems to have interrupted the progressiveness of the hemochromatosis.

The **treatment** for hemochromatosis comprises (1) treatment of cirrhosis of the liver and (2) control of the diabetes.

The diabetes is controlled as outlined elsewhere in this chapter. The diet should contain large amounts of carbohydrate (300 to 400 gm. a day) and adequate protein (at least 1.25 gm. per kilogram of the normal body weight). Insulin therapy is usually necessary. The amount given is increased until the diabetes is controlled. Usually moderate amounts suffice but occasionally the insulin may be remarkably ineffective. Huge doses may then be necessary.

Concentrated vitamin preparations, especially those of A and B_1 (thiamine) supplement the diet. Abstinence from alcohol is advisable, as are the curtailment of activities, restriction of the sodium chloride intake (if ascites is present), the administration of diuretics, and, when necessary, abdominal paracentesis.

Restriction of the iron intake is futile as it would require many years to make any impression on the quantities of stored ferrous compounds.

PREGNANCY COMPLICATING DIABETES

Introduction. In the pre-insulin era pregnancy was infrequent in diabetic patients; if conception did occur, gestation rarely proceeded to full term with a viable baby and without grave risks to the mother. But with insulin therapy and all that it permits, pregnancy is no longer uncommon. It carries little, if any, greater risk to the life of the diabetic mother than to nondiabetic controls, and the frequency with which full-term viable babies are secured has increased greatly. Although mothers come through pregnancy without the former risk to life, they are predisposed to ketosis, hypertensive and renal disease, hydramnios and irritability of the uterus. Notwithstanding the progress that has been made, diabetes, because of the degenerative changes associated with it and notably arterial and renal disease, exerts far-reaching effects on the course of pregnancy. In these cases, pregnancy is not a contract to be entered upon lightly, but barring exceptional hazards that may be associated with a diabetes of over twenty years' duration with premature arterial disease, the outcome is likely to be satisfactory. A satisfactory outcome depends considerably on the control of the diabetes, the adequacy of the diet, timing of and selection of the method of terminating the pregnancy, and special care for the newly born.

The Diabetic Mother. MENSTRUAL IRREGULARITIES. Delayed development of secondary sexual characteristics, amenorrhea, irregular menstruation, meno- and metrorrhagia, and an early menopause are frequent in women with untreated or poorly controlled diabetes. However, with good control of the diabetes, catamenia usually occurs at a normal age or returns after a few months of amenorrhea, if the latter has been due to uncontrolled diabetes.

FERTILITY. Poorly controlled diabetes militates against conception, but with better management of the diabetic patient fertility is improved. Despite this improvement, diabetic women become somewhat less fertile earlier than nondiabetics. Nutritional deficiencies associated with uncontrolled diabetes are probably a big factor in the production of sterility.

ABORTION AND MISCARRIAGE. *Abortion and miscarriage are directly proportional to the lack of control of the diabetes.*

STILLBIRTHS AND TOXEMIA. Stillbirths are, despite insulin therapy, six times more common in diabetic than in nondiabetic women. Factors that operate to produce this are the tendency of the babies of diabetic women to be overweight, "diabetic postmaturity," premature vascular aging of the mother and the increased frequency of hydramnios. Calcification of the pelvic arteries, though not common, increases the likelihood of stillbirths. There is no corroborative proof that hormone imbalance is a causative factor in toxemias of pregnancy. Toxemia was not notably increased, occurring in only six of 163 pregnancies, in the experience of Reis and his associates.[148] No hormone therapy was employed. Diabetic patients are predisposed to toxemia by the prevalence of arteriosclerosis.

Vascular diseases are the most common abnormalities affecting diabetic mothers. White[149] found evidences of vascular disease (coronary artery disease, calcified vessels, retinopathies or nephritis) in 70 per cent of patients whose diabetes began in childhood and was of twenty years' duration or more. Because of the serious vascular disease present in diabetic patients whose disease is of long standing, pregnancy is inadvisable after thirty years of age. Diabetic women tend to be gynecologically older than their stated age.

Chemical abnormalities of diabetic pregnancies are a low renal threshold for dextrose and a disturbance of water balance. The former, which is physiologic in pregnancy and has been reported in excess of 10 per cent of all pregnancies, can result in the excretion of large amounts of glucose in the urine while the blood sugar levels remain within normal range. When less than 100 gm. of glucose are utilized daily, ketosis may result. The disturbance of water balance is shown by an excessive gain in weight, followed by edema, hydramnios and fetal edema.

MORTALITY. *Maternal.* In the pre-insulin era, the maternal mortality was between 25 and 30 per cent, but now with the diabetes properly controlled, it is no higher than the 0.6 per cent which occurs in nondiabetic controls. *There is no excuse for diabetes, in itself, being responsible for a maternal death.*

Fetal. Abortions, miscarriages and stillbirths remain higher in diabetic than nondiabetic pregnancies. Furthermore, the fetal and neonatal mortalities have been found to be as high during the five years preceding the onset of diabetes as after the disease developed.[150] Surveys indicate fetal losses as high as 70 per cent and as low as 11 per cent. However, the circumstances under which these data were collected varied considerably.[151] White[152] has reported a fetal survival rate of 82 per cent in 433 consecutive diabetic pregnancies. Her best results were attributed to normal or corrected hormonal values and the poorest to abnormal balance of sex hormones.

The Diagnosis of Diabetes Complicated by Pregnancy. When a pregnant woman develops diabetes, the diagnosis may be complicated because of the great frequency with which renal glycosuria occurs in normal pregnant women. The diagnosis of renal glycosuria as opposed to that of diabetes can be established by simultaneous determinations of the sugar in the blood and urine (see p. 804). In questionable cases, glucose tolerance tests in each trimester are indicated. A pregnant woman showing glycosuria, even with a normal glucose tolerance curve, but having a family history of diabetes should be watched for the development of diabetes. Formerly pregnancy was believed to reduce the carbohydrate tolerance in normal pregnancies, but this has not been confirmed by either intravenously[153] or orally[154] administered glucose. Elevated glucose tolerance curves are frequent in pregnancies (in nondiabetics) which produce large babies.[155]

The Effect of Pregnancy on the Diabetes. The effect of pregnancy on the diabetes is unpredictable. In some, the insulin requirement remains unchanged and in others it decreases, but in the majority it increases.

In general, if the diabetes is well controlled, the need for insulin (1) increases slightly in some and decreases in others during the first trimester, (2) remains relatively stationary in the second trimester—the qualitative developmental phase for the child, and (3) increases in the third trimester—during the phase of quantitative growth with an over-all increase in the total metabolism.

Occasionally the mother's diabetes appears to improve in the last trimester. This improvement probably is due to insulin provided by the fetus because, following delivery, the insulin need increases. Much more common is the progressive increase in the insulin requirement during the last three months of pregnancy. This is an expected response to the increase in total metabolism accompanying the increase in the size of the baby. An abrupt reduction in the need for insulin usually follows termination of the pregnancy.

Diabetes, if adequately controlled during gestation, is not made worse by pregnancy.

Management of the Pregnant Diabetic Patient. GENERAL MEASURES. The regimen is, in general, the same for the pregnant diabetic woman as for the nonpregnant. Good general hygiene and a reasonable amount of outdoor exercise are encouraged. The patient must be under close scrutiny by both the internist and the obstetrician throughout the pregnancy. She should be seen every two weeks during the first two trimesters and every week during the last trimester.

DIET. In general, the diet should be adequate to prevent undernutrition during pregnancy and, as there is considerable evidence that diabetic patients need more vitamins than is usually the case, special care is taken to prevent vitamin deficiencies (see p. 812).

Total Calories. These are calculated as for the nonpregnant diabetic—multiply the ideal body weight (see p. 810) in pounds by 10 and in case of pregnancy add 100 calories. The correction for activity will be varied according to the behavior of the body weight but for the initial diet 30 per cent of the basal diet is added. Example: Patient twenty-eight years of age, ideal weight 136 pounds:

Multiply ideal weight by 10 (136 × 10)	1360
Correction for age and pregnancy, add	100
Basal calories	1460
Add 30 per cent for activity	438
Total calories	1898

For the obese patient, a severe reduction regimen is delayed until the pregnancy is terminated.

Protein. Multiply the ideal weight in pounds by ⅞ to determine the protein in grams. In the illustrative case above this would be $\frac{7}{8} \times 136 = 119$ gm.

Failures have been appreciably reduced since the adoption of high protein diets.

Carbohydrate. We prefer a liberal quota of carbohydrate, e.g., *250 gm. or more,* if the liberal allowance does not make control of the diabetes appreciably more difficult. The calories not provided by protein and carbohydrate are supplied by fat, e.g.,

Protein 119 × 4	476 calories
Carbohydrate 250 × 4	1000 calories
Calories from protein and carbohydrate	1476

Fat = 1898 − 1476 = 422; 422 ÷ 9 = 47 gm

Dietary Supplements. One quart of whole or skim milk is included in each day's diet to care for the need for calcium. Also, supplemental vitamins* are prescribed to meet the increased demands of pregnancy (see Chap. 6).

INSULIN. We give insulin to every pregnant diabetic patient. The amount, brand and distribution are determined as for the nonpregnant patient with unstable diabetes (see p. 845), but special care is taken to keep the fasting and postprandial blood sugar values within normal ranges or as close to this ideal as is practicable. One to three injections of insulin daily may be required.

In cases in which the insulin requirement increases during the final trimester —the usual occurrence—a marked reduction in the need for insulin follows delivery. Contrariwise, when the severity of the diabetes appears to be alleviated and the need for insulin decreases during the last three months of gestation, delivery is followed by an increased severity of the diabetes, and insulin must be given in increased

* One therapeutic vitamin capsule daily will provide adequate amounts of vitamins A, D, thiamine HCl, riboflavin and niacinamide. Ascorbic acid is prescribed separately. The supplemental administration of vitamins E and K has been recommended.

amounts to control the diabetes and to avert ketosis.

TOLBUTAMIDE. We have not given tolbutamide to pregnant diabetic patients who for the most part have a "juvenile type" or unstable diabetes. It is in this group that tolbutamide is least effective, though its successful use has been observed by others.

Management of Complications. NAUSEA AND VOMITING. The nausea and vomiting of pregnancy have rarely been troublesome in our experience. Frequent feedings supplemented by glucose administered intravenously may be necessary to prevent ketosis. In this event a temporary schedule of four, or six, feedings in each twenty-four hours with crystalline insulin before each is employed as in dealing with other acute complications (see p. 886). This program is usually not needed, but when it is, the normal or usual regimen is restored as promptly as is practicable.

CORRECTION OF HORMONAL IMBALANCE. The relative merits of hormonal therapy, high protein diets with supplements and early delivery by cesarean section are not clear.

I have had no cause to regret abandonment of hormone therapy for the past three years.

White[156] advocates daily intramuscular injections of estrogenic hormone to prevent the elevation of serum chorionic gonadotropin, and progesterone is given to prevent excessive destruction of estrogen.

A less expensive therapy has been recommended by Smith,[157] comprising the oral administration of diethylstilbestrol. Unfortunately, the laboratory procedures necessary for the detection of a hormonal imbalance, viz., serum level of estrogen and chorionic gonadotropin, and urinary excretion of pregnandiol, are expensive and not available in most laboratories. Furthermore, the cost of the estrogen (diethylstilbestrol) and progesterone (proluton) in the doses recommended is often prohibitive.

The value of hormone therapy is controversial. Results equally good without it have been reported. It would appear that meticulous care of the diabetic is the important feature; e.g., prior to 1953 there had been a fetal mortality of 50 per cent of babies born of diabetic women. A "diabetic team" was organized in 1953, and it is attributed to the cooperative functioning of the internist and obstetrician that the survival was increased to 95 per cent.[158]

SODIUM RESTRICTION. A moderate restriction of the daily salt intake, not more than a total of 3 gm. if edema is present, and 200 mg. of sodium if the retention of salt and water assumes more than a mild degree is exercised. In addition, courses of *ammonium chloride* —4 to 8 gm. daily for three days—are given as needed with rest periods of two or three days between courses. Chlorothiazide (Diuril), 250 mg. four times daily, may yield spectacular results.

TERMINATION OF PREGNANCY. If the mother has had one or more previous successful and uncomplicated full term pregnancies, and especially if they occurred subsequent to the development of diabetes, there is no need to induce premature delivery. If, however, full term deliveries have been complicated by large babies, toxemia or stillbirths, the induction of labor at the thirty-sixth to thirty-eighth week is advisable.

X-ray examination of the fetus for ossification of the femoral epiphysis is done to prevent delivery of an unduly premature or immature infant. This is not a routine practice.

Cesarean sections at the thirty-sixth to the thirty-eighth week, the time being selected by the obstetrician, is advisable in all (1) primiparae, (2) pre-eclamptic patients with increasing blood pressure, edema and albuminuria, (3) those who have had previous abortions or stillbirths and no successful full-term pregnancies, and (4) if the baby appears to be unusually large.

The risk attending a cesarean section is extremely small. Furthermore, the management of the diabetes is subjected to less disturbance by this method of terminating the pregnancy than if normal labor is permitted.

TREATMENT DURING LABOR AND DELIVERY. During labor, when the normal route of delivery is permitted, and in the case of cesarean section, nourishment is provided during the period when food is not taken by mouth by the intravenous administration of 10 per cent invert sugar (5 per cent glucose and 5 per cent fructose) in distilled water, 750 ml. being started every six hours. One liter of the same solution given at eight-hour intervals is equally satisfactory.

The insulin is reduced on the day of delivery to one third of the predelivery dosage. This amount is divided into four equal doses of crystalline insulin, one of which is given subcutaneously every six hours, the administration coinciding with the beginning of each intravenous infusion of invert sugar. The amount of insulin is increased or decreased according to the degree of glycosuria, or its absence, in specimens obtained at six-hour intervals. Exact control of the diabetes is not important during the short period involved. The aim is to steer a course which will permit neither ketosis nor hypoglycemia. Mild degrees of ketosis—causing ketonuria but no detectable ketonemia—are harmless. Four equal meals with four doses of insulin, as in cases of other acute complications (see p. 886), are given for two to four days, after which period a return to the prepregnancy diet and insulin, with suitable adjustments of the latter, are prescribed.

ANESTHESIA. Regional anesthesia, caudal or spinal, is preferable for vaginal deliveries because the infants are often premature or react as though they are immature. Fetal anoxia during delivery is least with this type of anesthesia. Spinal anesthesia is used for cesarean sections.

LACTATION. Diabetic women lactate poorly even though the diet is ample. Supplementary feedings are needed if the mother nurses her baby, a procedure which is not advocated. The deficiency of milk may be due to a decrease in the lactogenic hormone. The diabetic mother who nurses her baby needs less insulin than she did before she became pregnant. Since lactose in the urine may be mistaken for glucose—though this will not be the case if enzymatic tests are employed (see p. 793)—frequent blood sugar determinations are needed to guide the insulin dosage in the lactating mother.

POSTPARTUM COMPLICATIONS. Eclampsia may develop in the postpartum period. It is treated, as in the nondiabetic, with intravenous injections of dextrose solution and of concentrated human albumen (salt-free), oxygen therapy, intramuscular injections of 50 per cent magnesium sulfate solution, and sedatives. Hydralazine (Apresoline) has some degree of specificity in the treatment of postpartum eclampsia. Chlorothiazide (Diuril) therapy has promise in such cases. Hypertensive crises may be readily controlled with mecamylamine (Inversine) but with cognizance of the increased risk of hypoglycemia when a ganglion blocking agent is employed.

Pyelitis and pyelonephritis are the most common causes of postpartum fever in the diabetic patient. Sulfonamides, streptomycin or other antibiotics to which the organism is sensitive are indicated as in the nondiabetic. Puerperal fever, a rare complication, is also treated as in the nondiabetic. While infection persists, the insulin dosage is increased as need be, and the patient should be placed on the regimen for patients with acute complications (see p. 886).

Care of the Newborn Infant of the Diabetic Mother. The infant born to a diabetic mother needs the specialized care of a pediatrician.

The immediate danger is asphyxia with a complicating atelectasis, both of which occur more often in infants born of diabetic than of normal mothers. Ketosis, hypoglycemia or trauma to the cerebral cortex from a long labor associated with a large baby may contribute to the production of asphyxia. Special care in removing mucus from the infant's mouth and throat by suction and postural drainage, and the use of an incubator, in which the temperature is 29° C. (84.2° F.) and the atmosphere contains an appropriate amount of oxygen, will reduce the danger of asphyxia.

Hypoglycemia of severe degree is an uncommon hazard to the newborn. When it occurs it is presumably due to compensatory overactivity of the fetal pancreas resulting from inadequate control of the mother's diabetes during the final trimester of the pregnancy. This islet cell hyperactivity, in the occasional case, appears to be responsible for the mother's reduced need for insulin. When it occurs, or when increased suckling action of the infant suggests a hypoglycemia, a few drops of 50 per cent aqueous solution of glucose are given through a medicine dropper every thirty minutes for two hours after birth. After this period, breast milk, ½ to 1 ounce, may be alternated with a similar amount of 5 per cent glucose every two hours throughout the first three days of life. This is a modification of the feeding plan recommended by Reis and associates.[148] After three days have elapsed, the hyperplastic islet function will have become adjusted to the change in the demands made upon it.

A high percentage of the deaths of babies of diabetic mothers which occur after the second or third day show typical pathologic changes of *hyaline membrane disease.* Immaturity at birth and cesarean section contribute to the incidence of this disease.

FETAL ANOMALIES. Congenital defects are said to be unduly frequent in babies born of diabetic mothers. White[156] reported congenital defects in 80 per cent of infants of diabetic mothers, in contrast to the normal expected incidence of 1.8 per cent. Congenital defects in our infants have not exceeded the incidence seen in infants of nondiabetic mothers, an experience also of Reis.[148]

LARGE BABIES. Babies born to diabetic mothers are often unusually large. The overweight is due to *fat, edema* and *splanchnomegaly,* the last being most marked in the liver, spleen and heart. Atelectasis, persistence of fetal glomeruli and hyperplasia of the islets of Langerhans are relatively common. Miller and Wilson[159] have likewise reported cardiac hypertrophy, excessive erythropoiesis in the liver, and hyperplasia of the islets of Langerhans in babies born to diabetic mothers. These findings were most frequent in the large babies.

Outlook for the Child. If the infant of the diabetic mother is born alive, its chances of survival are nearly as good as those of infants born of normal mothers. The mortality during the first year of life of babies born to diabetic mothers is the same—5 per cent—as that for babies born of nondiabetic mothers (White).

Diabetes is transmitted as a recessive mendelian trait. Hence, the child cannot inherit the disease from the mother alone. Unless the father has diabetes also or carries a recessive factor for diabetes, the child will not develop the disease, although the predisposition to the disease may be passed on to the third generation.

Summary. Although good control of the diabetes in the pregnant woman has reduced the maternal mortality to almost nil, the incidence of abortions, miscarriages and stillbirths remains higher than in nondiabetic women. The high fetal mortality is attributable to the large size of the baby, poor control of the mother's diabetes, "diabetic postmaturity" of the infant and premature vascular aging of the mother.

The outstanding dangers to the newborn are asphyxia with pulmonary atelectasis, hyaline membrane disease and hypoglycemia. There is accumulating evidence that hormonal imbalance does not play as important a role in the pregnant diabetic as was formerly thought to be the case.

During pregnancy, there is usually an increase in the insulin requirement, slight but not always, in the first trimester but rather marked in the third trimester. An abrupt reduction in the need for insulin follows delivery. With adequate control of the maternal diabetes during the last trimester, overactivity of the islets of Langerhans of the fetal pancreas is probably prevented, the risk of hypoglycemia in the newborn baby thereby is decreased, and the incidence of stillbirths is reduced. Cesarean section in selected cases has increased greatly the infant survival.

References

1. Stetten, D., Jr.: Proc. Am. Diabetes A., *7:*67, 1947.
2. Joslin, E. P.: J.A.M.A., *139:*1, 1949.
3. Marks, H. H.: Diabetes, *5:*313, 1956.
4. Duncan, G. G.: Bull. New York Acad. Med., *34* (No. 2):73, 1958.
5. Allen, F. M., Stillman, E. and Fitz, R.: Monogr. Rockefeller Inst. Med. Res., *11:*1, 1919.
6. Allen, F. M.: J.A.M.A., *63:*939, 1914.
7. Banting, F. G., Best, C. H., Collip, J. B., Campbell, W. R. and Fletcher, A. A.: Canad. M.A.J., *12:*141, 1922.
8. Young, F. G.: Lancet, *2:*372, 1937.
9. Hagedorn, H. C., Jensen, B., Krarup, N. B. and Woodstrup, I.: J.A.M.A., *106:*177, 1936.
10. Scott, D. A. and Fisher, A. M.: Proc. Am. Soc. Biol. Chem., *8:*88, 1936.
11. Abel, J. J., Geiling, E. M. K., Rouiller, C. A., Bell, F. K. and Wintersteiner, O.: J. Pharmacol. & Exper. Therap., *31:*65, 1927.
12. Reiner, L., Searle, D. S. and Lang, E. H.: J. Pharmacol. & Exper. Therap., *67:* 330, 1939.
13. Krayenbühl, C. and Rosenberg, T.: Rep. Steno. Memorial Hosp., *1:*60, 1946.
14. Lukens, F. D. W. and Dohan, F. C.: Science, *92:*222, 1940.
15. Haist, R. E., Campbell, J. and Best, C. H.: New England J. Med., *223:* 607, 1940.
16. Stetten, D., Jr.: Proc. Am. Diabetes A., *7:*67, 1947.
17. Field, J. B. and Stetten, D., Jr.: Diabetes, *6:*391, 1957.
18. Hallas-Møller, K., Petersen, K. and Schlichtkrull, J.: Ugesk. laeger., *113:* 176, 1951.
19. Janbon, M., Chaptal, J., Vedel, A. and Schaap, J.: Montpellier med., *21/22:* 441, 1942.
20. Loubatieres, A.: Compt. rend. Soc. de biol., *138:*766, 830, 1944; Arch. Int. Physiol., *54:*174, 1946.
21. Conference on Carbutamide. Canad. M.A.J., *74:*957, 1956.
22. Report on Tolbutamide. Deutsche med. Wchnschr., *81:*823, 887, 1956.
23. Symposium on Clinical and Experimental Effects of Sulfonyl Ureas in Diabetes Mellitus. Metabolism, *5* (No. 6, Part II):721, 1956.
24. Third Conference on Carbutamide. Diabetes, *6* (No. 1):1, 1957.
25. Symposium on Sulfonyl Urea Compounds. Ann. New York Acad. Sc., *71:*1, 1957.
26. Houssay, B. A., Penhos, J. C., Urgoiti, E., Teodosio, N., Apelbaum, J. and Bowkett, J.: Ann. New York Acad. Sc., *71:*25, 1957.
27. Duncan, G. G., Lee, C. T. and Young, J. K.: Ann. New York Acad. Sc., *71:* 233, 1957.
28. Fabrykant, M.: Metabolism, unpublished data.
29. Marks, H. H.: M. Clin. North America, *31:*369, 1947.
30. Wilkerson, H. L. C. and Krall, L. P.: J.A.M.A., *135:*209, 1947.
31. Spiegelman, M. and Marks, H. H.: Am. J. Pub. Health, *36:*26, 1946.
32. Blotner, H.: J.A.M.A., *131:*1109, 1946.
33. Danowski, T. S.: Diabetes Mellitus. Baltimore, Williams & Wilkins, 1957, p. 122.
34. Perrott, G. St. J., Tibbitts, C. and Britten, R. H.: Pub. Health Rep., *54:*1663, 1939.
35. Mosenthal, H. O. and Bolduan, E.: Am. J. M. Sc., *186:*605, 1933.
36. Dublin, L. I. and Marks, H. H.: Mortality Among Insured Overweights in Recent Years. Tr. 60th Ann. Meet. A. Life Ins. Med. Dir. Am., Oct. 11–22, 1951.
37. Rockey, E. W.: Ann. Surg., *118:*603, 1943.
38. White, P. and Pincus, G.: In Joslin, E. P.: Treatment of Diabetes Mellitus, 8th ed. Philadelphia, Lea & Febiger, 1946.
39. von Mering, J. and Minkowski, O.: Arch. f. exper. Path. u. Pharmakol., *26:*371, 1889–1890.
40. Allen, F. M.: J. Metab. Research, *1:*165, 1922.
41. Jacobs, H. R.: Proc. Soc. Exper. Biol. & Med., *37:*407, 1937.
42. Dohan, F. C. and Lukens, F. D. W.: Endocrinology, *42:*244, 1948.
43. Griffiths, M.: J. Biol. Chem., *172:*853, 1948.
44. Copp, E. F. F. and Barclay, A. J.: J. Metab. Research, *4:*445, 1923.
45. Lukens, R. D. W., Dohan, P. C. and Wolcott, N. W.: Endocrinology, *32:* 475, 1943.
46. Haist, R. E.: Physiol. Rev., *24:*409, 1944.
47. Scott, D. A. and Fisher, A. M.: J. Clin. Invest. *17:*725, 1938.
48. Houssay, B. A.: New England J. Med., *214:*961, 1936.
49. Young, F. G.: Brit. M.J., *2:*393, 1939.
50. Haist, R. E., Campbell, J. and Best, C. H.: New England J. Med., *223:* 607, 1940.
51. Lukens, F. D. W. and Dohan, F. C.: Science, *92:*222, 1940.

52. Danowski, T. S.: Diabetes Mellitus. Baltimore, Williams & Wilkins, 1957, p. 389.
53. Conn, J. W., Louis, L. H. and Johnston, M. W.: Science, *109:*279, 1949.
54. Houssay, B. A.: Endocrinology, *35:*158, 1944.
55. Root, H. F. and Bloor, W. R.: Am. Rev. Tuberc., *39:*714, 1939.
56. Best, C. H., Lucas, C. C. and Ridout, H. J.: Ann. New York Acad. Sc., *57:*646, 1954.
57. Becker, B.: Ann. Int. Med., *37:*273, 1952.
58. Becker, B., Maengwyn-Davies, G. D., Rosen, D., Friedenwald, J. S. and Winter, F. C.: Diabetes, *3:*175, 1954.
59. Givner, I.: Diabetes, *4:*284, 1955.
60. Kimmelstiel, P. and Wilson, C.: Am. J. Path., *12:*83, 1936.
61. Hamilton, J. D.: Diabetes, *2:*180, 1953.
62. Bell, E. T.: Renal Diseases. Philadelphia, Lea & Febiger, 1946, p. 376.
63. Mallory, G. K., Crane, A. R. and Edwards, J. E.: Arch. Path., *30:*330, 1940.
64. Beidleman, B. and Duncan, G. G.: Am. J. Med., *12:*43, 1952.
65. Dunn, J. S. and McLetchie, N. G. B.: Lancet, *245:*384, 1943.
66. Bailey, C. C. and Bailey, O. T.: J.A.M.A., *122:*1165, 1943.
67. Conn, J. W., Lewis, R. H. and Johnson, M. W.: Proc. Am. Diabetes A., *8:*213, 1948.
68. Conn, J. W. and Hinerman, D. L.: Am. J. Path., *24:*429, 1948.
69. Benedict, S. R.: J.A.M.A., *57:*1193, 1911.
70. Smith, M.: J. Lab. & Clin. Med., *7:*364, 1922.
71. Stadie, W. C., Lukens, F. D. W. and Zapp, J. A., Jr.: J. Biol. Chem., *132:* 423, 1940.
72. Parkhurst, L. W. and Betsch, W. F.: M. Clin. North America, *39:*1571, 1955.
73. Fajans, S. S. and Conn, J. W.: Diabetes, *3* (No. 4):296, 1954.
74. West, K. M.: Diabetes, *6:*168, 1957.
75. Langner, P. H., Romansky, M. J. and Rohin, E. D.: Am. J. M. Sc., *212:*466, 1946.
76. Cori, C. F. and Cori, G. T.: Ann. Rev. Biochem., *3:*151, 1934.
77. Allen, F. M.: J.A.M.A., *63:*939, 1914.
78. Duncan, G. G.: Diabetes Mellitus and Obesity. Philadelphia, Lea & Febiger, 1935, p. 79.
79. Fetter, F., Durkin, J. K. and Duncan, G. G.: Am. J. M. Sc., *195:*781, 1938.
80. Durkin, J. K. and Fetter, F.: M. Clin. North America, *23:*1499, 1939.
81. Newburgh, L. H. and Conn, J. W.: J.A.M.A., *112:*7, 1939.
82. White, P.: Seminar on the Degenerative Lesions of Metabolism. U. S. Public Health Service, 1947.
83. Statistical Bulletin. Metropolitan Life Insurance Co., *38* (Nov.) 1957.
84. Pincus, G. and White, P.: Am. J. M. Sc., *186:*1, 1933.
85. Rabinowitch, I. M.: Canad. M.A.J., *23:* 489, 1930; *33:*136, 1935.
86. Tolstoi, E.: In Soskin, S.: Progress in Clinical Endocrinology. New York, Grune & Stratton, 1950, p. 292.
87. Allen, F. M.: J. Metab. Research, *3:*61, 1923.
88. Sherill, J. W.: J. Metab. Research, *3:*13, 1923.
89. Himsworth, H. P.: Lancet, *1:*127, 1936.
90. Jersild, M.: The First Congress of the International Diabetes Federation, Leyden, July, 1952.
91. Peck, F. B., Sr., Kirtley, W. R., Dyke, R. W. and Ernst, C. E.: Diabetes, *3:*261, 1954.
92. Duncan, G. G., Cuttle, T. D. and Jewesburg, E. C. O.: Bull. Ayer Clin. Lab., *3:*293, 1939.
93. Kern, R. A. and Langner, P. H., Jr.: J.A.M.A., *113:*198, 1939.
94. Jorpes, J. E.: Arch. Int. Med., *83:*363, 1949.
95. Smelo, L. S.: South. M. J., *40:*333, 1947.
96. Yankelowitch, T., Massry, S. and Gitter, S.: Diabetes, *5:*457, 1956.
97. Lowell, F. C.: J. Clin. Invest., *23:*233, 1944.
98. Haldane, J. B. S.: The Scientific Basis of Medicine. London, Athlone Press, 1954, vol. III, p. 45.
99. Berson, S. A. and Yalow, R. S.: Diabetes, *6:*402, 1957.
100. Downie, E.: Ann. Int. Med., *46:*126, 1957.
101. Kay, M., McGarry, E. and Rosenfeld, I.: Diabetes, *4:*133, 1955.
102. Loveless, M. H. and Cann, J. R.: J. Immunol., *74:*329, 1955.
103. Kleeberg, J., Diengott, D. and Gottfried, J.: J. Clin. Endocrinol., *16:*680, 1956.
104. Butterfield, W. J. H.: Lancet, *1:*489, 1955.
105. Duncan, G. G.: A Modern Pilgrim's Progress for Diabetics. Philadelphia, W. B. Saunders Company, 1956.
106. Ricketts, H. T.: Am. J. Med., *19:*933, 1955.
107. LeCompte, P. M.: J. Chron. Dis., *2*·178, 1953.
108. Bryfogle, J. W. and Bradley, R. F.: Diabetes, *6:*159, 1957.
109. Gibbon, J. H. and Landis, E. M.: J. Clin. Invest., *11:*1019, 1932.
110. Samuels, S.: Diagnosis and Treatment of the Peripheral Arteries. New York, Oxford Publications, 1936.
111. Allen, E. V., Barker, N. E. and Hines, E. A., Jr.: Peripheral Vascular Diseases. Philadelphia, W. B. Saunders Company, 1946, p. 353.
112. Sanders, C. E.: J.A.M.A., *106:*916, 1936.

113. Herrmann, L. G. and Reid, M. R.: Arch. Surg., *29:*697, 1934.
114. Collens, W. S. and Wilensky, N. D.: J.A.M.A., *107:*1960, 1936.
115. Foley, W. T.: Circulation, *15:*689, 1957.
116. Allen, F. M.: Tr. A. Am. Physicians, *52:* 189, 1937.
117. Waite, J. H. and Beetham, W. P.: New England J. Med., *212:*367, 429, 1935.
118. Kinsell, L. W., Lawrence, L., Balch, H. E. and Weyand, R. D.: Diabetes, *3:*358, 1954.
119. Poulsen, J. E.: Diabetes, *2:*7, 1953.
120. Wortham, J. T. and Headstream, J. W.: Diabetes, *3:*367, 1954.
121. Selye, H. and Horava, A.: Third Annual Report on Stress. Montreal, Acta, Inc., 1953, p. 195.
122. Barach, J. H.: Arch. Int. Med., *79:*602, 1947.
123. Collens, W. W.: Am. J. Med., *1:*636, 638, 1946.
124. Bailey, A. A.: Diabetes, *4:*32, 1955.
125. Danowski, T. S.: Diabetes Mellitus. Baltimore, Williams & Wilkins, 1957, p. 309.
126. Greenman, J. H., Danowski, T. S., Johnson, S. Y.: J. Clin. Endocrinol., *10:* 519, 1950.
127. Dillon, E. S. and Dyer, W. W.: Ann. Int. Med., *11:*602, 1937.
128. Duncan, G. G., Fetter, F. and Durkin, J.: Surgery, *1:*939, 1937.
129. Vander Veer, J. B. and Fisher, G. R.: M. Clin. North America, *39:*1587, 1955.
130. Sehon, A. H., Kaye, M., McGarry, E. and Rose, B.: J. Lab. & Clin. Med., *45:*765, 1955.
131. Colwell, A. R. and Weiger, R. W.: J. Lab. & Clin. Med., *47:*844, 1956.
132. National Research Council on Convalescence and Rehabilitation, Report No. 1, Feb. 1944.
133. Boucot, K. R., Cooper, D. A., Richardson, R., Dillon, E. S. and Meier, P.: Amer. Rev. Tuberc., *65:* (Part 2) 1, 1952.
134. Hildebrand, A. G., Montgomery, H. and Rynearson, E. H.: Arch. Int. Med., *66:*851, 1940.
135. Duncan, G. G. and Fetter, F.: M. Clin. North America, *18:*261, 1934.
136. Riven, S. S.: Am. J. M. Sc., *189:*550, 1935.
137. Bell, E. T.: Diabetes, *4:*435, 1955.
138. Warren, S.: Pathology of Diabetes. 2nd ed. Philadelphia, Lea & Febiger, 1938, p. 246.
139. Bowen, B. D. and Kutzman, N.: Ann. Int. Med.: *17:*427, 1942.
140. Robbins, S. L. and Tucker, A. W.: New England J. Med., *231:*865, 1944.
141. Robbins, S. L.: Bull. New England M. Center, *10:*78, 1948.
142. Duncan, G. G., Wolgamot, J. R., Clancy, C. F. and Beidleman, B.: J.A.M.A., *145:*75, 1951.
143. Sheldon, J. H.: Hemochromatosis. London, Oxford University Press, 1935, p. 11.
144. Dry, T. J.: Proc. Staff Meet., Mayo Clin., *8:*56, 1933.
145. Finch, C. A., Hegsted, M., Kinney, T. D., Thomas, E. D., Rath, C. E., Haskins, D., Finch, F. and Fluharty, R. G.: J. Hematology, *5:*983, 1950.
146. Cantarow, A. and Bucher, C. J.: Arch. Int. Med., *67:*333, 1941.
147. Wilder, R. M.: Clinical Diabetes Mellitus. Philadelphia, W. B. Saunders Co., 1940, p. 325.
148. Reis, R. A., De Costa, E. J. and Allweis, M. D.: Amer. J. Obst. & Gynec., *60:* 1023, 1950.
149. White, P.: Proc. Am. Diabetes A., *6:*259, 1946.
150. Miller, H. D., Hurwitz, D. and Kuder, K.: J.A.M.A., *124:*271, 1944.
151. Danowski, T. S.: Diabetes Mellitus. Baltimore, Williams & Wilkins, 1957, p. 467.
152. White, P.: Am. J. Med., *7:*609, 1949.
153. Johnson, D. G. and Bonsnes, R. W.: J. Clin. Invest., *27:*745, 1948.
154. Cobley, J. F. C. C. and Lancaster, H. O.: M. J. Australia, *1:*171, 1955.
155. Lund, C. J. and Weese, W. H.: Am. J. Obst. & Gynec., *65:*815, 1953.
156. Joslin, E. P., Root, H. F., White, P. and Marble, A.: Treatment of Diabetes Mellitus. Philadelphia, Lea & Febiger, 1952.
157. Smith, O. W.: Am. J. Obst. & Gynec., *56:*821, 1948.
158. Guest, G.: Panel on Diabetes and Pregnancy. *Diabetes, 5:*308, 1956.
159. Miller, H. C. and Wilson, H. W.: J. Pediat., *23:*251, 1943.

CHAPTER 16

By PRISCILLA WHITE, M.D.

Juvenile Diabetes

Incidence. TOTAL. Juvenile diabetes is not a common form of diabetes, nor is diabetes a common disease among children. Juvenile diabetics, defined as patients in whom the onset of diabetes occurred before 15 years of age, comprise 5 per cent of all diabetics. Only one child in 2500 contracts diabetes before the age of 15 years. In spite of this seemingly low incidence, the problems presented by these patients are not only of great pathognomonic but also of great numerical magnitude. In the United States today some 100,000 persons are surviving the childhood form of this disease.

SEX, AGE AND RACE. The sex incidence among juvenile patients is nearly equal, whereas in older decades females predominate. Girls, coincidental with their earlier maturity, contract diabetes at a slightly earlier age than do boys. The peak of age incidence for Joslin Clinic diabetic children is 12 years: for girls 11 years and for boys 13 years. Three peaks in the age at onset of diabetes occur in childhood, namely, at 3, 6 and 12. Jewish children comprise 8 per cent of Joslin Clinic cases.

Etiology. The juvenile diabetic patient whose family history may be rechecked for many years and whose past history may be recalled with great accuracy has contributed much to our knowledge of the etiology of diabetes.

INHERITANCE. Every individual who develops diabetes does so because of an inherited predisposition to the disease. It was the juvenile patient who first emphasized the importance of the hereditary nature of diabetes. At onset of the disease 20 per cent of the children report diabetic relatives. After twenty years of diabetes, however, 57 per cent have found other diabetics in their families.

The evidence in favor of the hereditary transmission of diabetes is as follows: first, the incidence of diabetes in similar twin mates, which is 50 per cent; second, the statistically significant excess of diabetes in the close blood relatives of diabetics (in their parents and siblings this amounted to 7 times the incidence in the control populations); third, the demonstration of mendelian ratios of the recessive type in cases reporting in sequence; fourth, the demonstration of mendelian ratios of the recessive type in families tested with glucose tolerance tests.

Secondary factors permitting the expression of the gene are presupposed because the clinical signs and symptoms of diabetes are not evident at birth or soon thereafter.

INFECTIONS. Acute infections have not appeared to play a frequent rôle in the etiology of our diabetic children. Whereas 10 per cent of 504 cases reviewed with great care had an infection of severity in the year of onset, 90 per cent had none. The experience of Grishaw, West and Smith[1] is similar. They report an incidence of infection in 20 per cent of their cases in the year of onset. John[2] and Lande,[3] found a relatively high incidence of infections prior to the onset of the disease, and Danowski[4] reports 42 per cent. The relative frequency of infections in the year of onset in the 504 children studied carefully in this respect is shown in Table 1.

TABLE 1. INFECTIONS IN THE YEAR OF ONSET OF 504 DIABETIC CHILDREN

Pertussis	12	Tonsillitis	5	Adenitis	2
Measles	10	Mumps	3	Appendicitis	1
Chickenpox	8	Influenza	3	Diphtheria	1
Scarlet fever	7	Jaundice	2	Rheumatic fever	1
Coryza	7				

TRAUMA, PSYCHOSOMATIC DISTURBANCE, OBESITY. Trauma, important from the medicolegal point of view, did not precede diabetes onset in more than 0.1 per cent of the cases. The relationship may be considered coincidental rather than causal. Psychosomatic disturbances were the exception rather than the rule prior to the onset of diabetes. Only 5 per cent of the children at onset of diabetes had exceeded their expected weight for age. Since growth peculiarities, especially large size, have been found to characterize the offspring of diabetic mothers, the birth weights of juvenile diabetics have been recorded and show no significant deviation from normal.

ENDOCRINE OVERACTIVITY. An appraisal of the diabetic child at onset of the disease was made to determine the presence or absence of disturbance of normal endocrine balance. This has included, in addition to the physical examination, an x-ray examination for bone age, basal metabolism tests, and in a few cases the determination of serum follicle-stimulating hormone and urinary 17-ketosteroids.

Overheight was found in 86 per cent of Joslin Clinic diabetic children measured within three months of the onset of the disease.

At the time of onset the average bone development was found by Bogan and Morrison[5] to be eighteen months in advance of the chronologic age, and the dental development was found by Robinson[6] to be twelve months in advance. The basal metabolism was on the average +12 per cent. In a study by Wagner, White and Bogan,[7] the development of hips and breasts, appearance of pubic and axillary hair and age at onset of menarche occurred earlier in short-term diabetics than in the normal controls or in long-term diabetics.

CONGENITAL DEFECTS. Congenital anomalies were reported by Wagner, White and Bogan to occur more often in the diabetic than in the control children. These anomalies were usually minor, as follows: Dupuytren contracture, curved fifth finger, brachydactylia, brachycephalus, ear nodule on the lateral aspect of the auricle.

CORRELATION OF EXPERIMENTAL AND CLINICAL DATA. Pancreatectomy, anterior pituitary extract, adrenal cortical extract, possibly thyroid and androgen, alloxan and alloxan-like derivatives, uric acid, glucose, quinoline, dithiocarbonate and fluoroacetate have produced diabetes experimentally. Hemosiderin has been thought to cause diabetes found in cases of hemochromatosis. No clinical counterpart to hemosiderin diabetes is found in our diabetic children. Boulin and Uhry,[8] however, report two cases, and hemochromatosis is not unknown in childhood. Alloxan diabetes in the human patient awaits chemical proof. Congenital hypoinsulinism, corresponding to ablation of the pancreas, is suggested by the small size of the pancreas and poor islet development found at postmortem examination. Gene linkage of anomalies is thus suggested. Thyroid or androgen diabetes in children is not borne out any more than in the adult by physical or laboratory examination. A mechanism through the adrenal is suggested by the severity of diabetes and the elevation of 17-ketosteroid excretion. A mechanism through the anterior pituitary is suggested by the high elevation of serum FSH, urinary 17-ketosteroid and basal metabolic rate. Advanced bone and gonad development and the early appearance of body hirsutism further suggest increased activity of the pituitary gland. The theory is therefore postulated that the gene induces hyperactivity of the pituitary, which then produces the diabetes complex by reducing insulin output and increasing gluconeogenesis.

The theory of increased insulin destruction appears to be less applicable to the child than to the adult diabetic.

Histopathology. PANCREATIC. Significant variations in the relative rate of growth of islet tissue have been observed. Under 2 years of age the rate of islet growth parallels that of the pancreas as a whole. Between the ages of 4 and 12 years the relative rate of islet growth falls to about one half the rate of the entire pancreas. In adolescence the rates of growth become equal again. After the age of 3 the number of islets remains constant. The lag in islet growth appears to coincide with the peaks of age of onset of the disease. The weight of the pancreas averages 2.6 grams at birth and increases to an average of 66 grams at 21 years of age. Warren and LeCompte[9] have reported changes in the islets of 47 juveniles as follows: few islets 16, hydropic degeneration 7, lymphocytic infiltration 6, fibrosis 8, pyknotic nuclei 3, hyalinization 4, hypertrophy 1, sclerosis 5. Warren and LeCompte have emphasized that, as in the adult, the chief characteristic is the wide variety of lesions observed in a single pancreas, suggesting an agent destroying islets and permitting regeneration.

GENERAL PATHOLOGIC CHANGES. In juvenile diabetes these have varied in four therapeutic eras as follows: preinsulin, early, mid- and late insulin eras. The preinsulin changes were the chemical rather than the histologic ones of diabetic coma. Cerebrocapillary dilatation, perivascular edema, degeneration of the central nervous system and toxic tubular nephritis were observed. Fatty infiltration of the liver was a constant finding and lipid histiocytosis of the reticuloendothelial system was reported.

In the early insulin era, 1922 to 1930, juvenile diabetics examined by Warren had survived on the average about two years of diabetes. The abnormal distribution of glycogen and fat was the most striking change observed by the pathologist. Fatty infiltration of Kupffer's cells of the liver, of the spleen pulp, of the intima of the aorta and of the skin was shown along with depletion of fat in the central nervous system. Abnormal deposition of glycogen was found in liver cell nuclei, in Henle's loops, in the convoluted renal tubules and in the heart. Depletion of glycogen was observed in the skin, muscle and cytoplasm of the liver cells. Atherosclerosis was found in 30 per cent. With the more skillful use of insulin the above changes became less conspicuous, and the postmortem examinations in the mid-insulin era, 1930 to 1940, showed the ravages of sepsis including pyelonephritis and metastatic abscesses of the liver, heart, lung, spleen and brain. In the diabetic child, as in the general population, chemotherapy and antibiotics have altered the course of fatal sepsis. In this era the fatal cases which were studied had survived five years of diabetes. All showed evidence of atherosclerosis.

In the late insulin era, 1940 to 1957, the duration of diabetes in fatal cases coming to autopsy at the New England Deaconess Hospital exceeded fifteen years. All were in the third or fourth decade of life and all showed intercapillary glomerulosclerosis with or without pyelonephritis.

Although in youth the predominant damage is to renal vessels, widespread involvement of coronary, cerebral and other vessels occurs with advancing age and duration of the disease.

Symptoms and Signs. The characteristic symptoms of diabetes are invariably present in the child. Those most frequently reported are polyuria, polydipsia, polyphagia, loss of weight, loss of appetite, pruritus, furunculosis, alternating near and far vision, pains in the legs, muscle cramps, change in disposition and school failure. The signs are those of loss of weight and dehydration in the typically tall child with advanced bone and dental development.

Diagnosis. Errors in the diagnosis of diabetes in childhood arise from the fact that glycosuria is very common in children. Children may thus be treated with dietary restriction and insulin before an accurate diagnosis is established. The diagnostic levels for true glucose in this clinic are as follows: 110 mg. fasting, 150 mg. postprandial, venous, and 180 mg. postprandial, capillary blood.

Glucose tolerance tests are used if the diagnosis of diabetes is not established by random blood and urine analysis. The preparation of the child for a glucose tolerance test is as important as preparation of the patient for a basal metabolism test or for x-ray examinations. Fever, bed rest, sodium restriction, past restrictions of total calories or of carbohydrate and past administration of insulin favor hyperglycemia. Repeated administration of glucose, excess sodium and exercise favor relative hypoglycemia. At the time of the test the child must be afebrile. The diet of the week prior to the test should be of normal composition. Insulin should not have been administered during this same period. The patient should be at rest during the test.

In the oral test the dose of glucose used if the patient is under 3 years of age is 3 grams per kilogram of body weight. For all other juvenile patients who weigh less than 100 pounds the normal test dose is 1.8 grams per kilogram of body weight. To children weighing over 100 pounds, the adult quantity, 100 grams of glucose, is given. Obese children who have abnormal curves when they have received glucose according to actual body weight are retested with that quantity of glucose which is based upon their ideal weight for height and age. For practical purposes we use 1 gram of glucose per pound of body weight. Danowski[4] recommends 2.5 grams for children under 18 months and 2 grams for those 18 months to 2 years. The blood sugar is then obtained fasting, after one half, one and two hours for venous curves, and preferably an additional hour for capillary curves. The diagnosis, as with the adult patient, is based upon the peak rather than upon the fall of the curve. If the Exton-Rose test is employed, the quantity of glucose is again calculated on the basis of body weight. The total quantity is divided into equal parts, one administered fasting, the other one half hour later.

Unclassified glycosuria, renal glycosuria and potential diabetes designate the same types of glycosurias as they do in the adult population. Of some importance in the juvenile population are the meliturias with excretion of sugars other than glucose—namely, pentose, levulose, lactose and galactose. Renal glycosuria has been demonstrated in 12 Joslin Clinic diabetic children, essential levulosuria in 2 and essential pentosuria in 6 (5 males and 1 female, all Jewish). Lactosuria has not been sought. It is a physiologic finding in the nursling. Galactosuria may be found in children with digestive disturbances.

Natural Course of Diabetes. Acute (24 hours), rapid (1 week) and gradual (1 month) types of onset occur more often in the child than in the adult, the onset of whose diabetes is most often indefinite. The early course of diabetes in the child is often virulent. The first recognition of the disease may be in coma. In these children, as it was in Young's[10,11] pituitary diabetic dogs, the sign of nascent diabetes is ketosis.

In spite of the virulent nature of juvenile diabetes at its onset and regardless of the type of management, a favorable phase occurs. During this period of remission, insulin requirement drops and a low level of 4 units may be reached in 33 per cent of cases. Undoubtedly insulin therapy could be omitted temporarily.

Many factors influence the intensification of juvenile diabetes. For the most part they are not preventable. These factors include linear growth, common infections and the onset of puberty. Ketoacidosis and excessive gain in weight also alter the favorable course.

Intensification of juvenile diabetes progresses at variable rates, but by the third year few diabetic children have escaped a degree of intensification which suggests total diabetes. The total diabetic state was revealed in the early insulin era by nearly uncontrollable nocturnal hyperglycemia, in the era of longer acting insulins by the disproportionately greater requirement of long acting insulins compared with the continued small requirement for shorter, quicker acting insulins and the change from the original requirement of 0.25 unit per pound to 0.5 unit per pound of body weight.

Chemical assays support this concept. Wrenshall[12] has shown almost no extractable insulin in the pancreases of long-term juvenile diabetics and Bornstein[13] found no assayable insulin in the blood of diabetic children. The response of juveniles to test doses of the sulfonylurea oral substitutes parallels these earlier experiences. Three hundred of our juvenile diabetics were tested with from 1 to 3 grams of tolbutamide or carbutamide. No differences were found between the two drugs, but the duration of diabetes was inversely related to favorable response. Fasted children tested within 6 months of diabetes onset showed a 20 per cent or more fall of blood sugar by 4 hours in 90 per cent; when the duration of diabetes varied from 6 months to 1 year, this fall occurred in 60 per cent; 1 to 2 years of diabetes, in 40 per cent; 2 to 3 years of diabetes, 30 per cent; after 3 years, 10 per cent; after 5 years, 6 per cent.[14]

The pathologic changes in the pancreas correspond to these clinical and chemical observations. Fresh cases of diabetes show acute responses such as islet lymphocytic infiltration in a pancreas of normal size. Long-term cases show scars in pancreases disproportionately small for age and, finally, may show no islets and a few scattered beta cells. No insulin granules can be shown by special staining techniques.

The restoration of normal carbohydrate metabolism, the synthesis of protein and fat, and the maintenance of the hormonal balance among those hormones concerned with carbohydrate metabolism become difficult. Patients totally diabetic are completely dependent upon exogenous insulin, which is unaffected by tissue sugar level. Juvenile patients, therefore, constantly exhibit periods of insulin excess and insulin lack.

GROWTH AND DEVELOPMENT. Linear growth of juvenile patients is for the most part satisfactory. Based on twenty-year survivors, the median height finally attained by the males was 68 inches and by the females 63 inches, comparable to general experience.

The weight after age 20 was maintained at a normal or more often a subnormal level in nearly 90 per cent (51 per cent of the males and 45 per cent of the females were five or more pounds below weight). Only 14 per cent of females and 13 per cent of males were five or more pounds above weight for height.

Although very few American girls have not menstruated before age 14, only 28 per cent of these patients had matured at that age. The median age for their first menses was 15. However, there was no evidence of hypo-ovarianism in their later life. Sterility was no problem.

COMPLICATIONS. The further natural course of diabetes is shown by the tendency to develop complications. The most important complications of diabetes in childhood include (1) ketoacidosis, (2) infections, abscesses or carbuncles, osteomyelitis and pulmonary tuberculosis, (3) neuropathies and (4) the vascular lesions. Specific skin lesions, xanthosis, xanthoma diabeticorum and necrobiosis lipoidica diabeticorum may occur. Hepatomegaly may develop and cataracts may be observed.

The relative frequency of these complications varies with the duration of diabetes. Thus in the first five years of diabetes the following occur most commonly: ketosis, sepsis, cataracts, hepatomegaly and the three skin lesions, xanthosis, necrobiosis lipoidica diabeticorum and xanthoma diabeticorum. Between the fifth and the fifteenth year are seen the neuropathies, and after 15 years the vascular lesions appear.

Diabetic Coma. The incidence of diabetic coma (defined as a CO_2 content of the blood of 9 mEq. or below) is relatively great. Nearly 40 per cent of the coma admissions of the Joslin Clinic are childhood diabetics, although the children comprise but 10 per cent of all of our diabetics. The intercurrence of infections, omission of insulin and overeating are the inciting causes. Similar irregularities in the diabetic adult do not precipitate coma as easily as they do in the child. Upon a quantitative basis, the adult has greater stores of protective glycogen. The child's deficiency of glycogen has been demonstrated experimentally by Mirsky and Nelson[15] who administered phlorhizin, 15 to 20 grams, to diabetic children and produced hypoglycemia and ketonuria. This did not occur in the adult.

The incidence of severe ketoacidosis in juveniles with many possible years of exposure was measured in 1072 of our children who in January 1956 had survived 20 or more years of diabetes. It was 52 per cent for females and 39 per cent for males, 12 per cent having had multiple attacks.

Pyogenic Infections. Formerly pyogenic infections were as lethal in young diabetics as ketoacidosis. The most frequent infections are those of the skin and of the urinary tract. Osteomyelitis, common in adult diabetes, is relatively rare in childhood. The incidence of skin infections, pyelonephritis and osteomyelitis in males and females respectively in 1072 twenty-year survivors was 30, 2 and 0.8 per cent and 33, 12 and 0.5 per cent.

Tuberculosis. In the association of diabetes and tuberculosis, diabetes increases susceptibility to tuberculosis but tuberculosis does not increase susceptibility to diabetes. In our juvenile population diabetes antedated tuberculosis in all cases.

The incidence of tuberculosis in juvenile diabetes is 12 times and in adolescent diabetes 20 times that of the general population. Among 1072 twenty-year survivors the incidence of tuberculosis was 4 per cent.

The outcome of the Mantoux test does not seem to indicate increased susceptibility. Thirteen per cent of the children tested between 5.0 and 9.9 years of age showed positive reactions, 39 per cent between 10.0 and 14.9, and 22 per cent between 15.0 and 19.9 years. Acquired immunity gave no protection. Forty-two per cent of juveniles in the first decade have tracheobronchial adenitis. The incidence of tuberculosis increases after diabetic coma. This is not surprising, since the tubercle bacillus multiplies when dehydration occurs and when the *p*H is between 6.4 and 7.8. Growth is further favored by protein catabolites and by glucose. Its virulence is increased in acid media and phagocytosis is interfered with when fat is stored in excess in the reticuloendothelial system.

Cataracts. The typical juvenile diabetic cataract may be recognized at the diagnosis of diabetes. Many of these do not progress or progress extraordinarily slowly. By the fourth and fifth decades senile cataracts occur.

Hepatomegaly. Hepatomegaly was seen commonly in the juvenile diabetic before the use of long acting insulins. These livers were so large they frequently extended into the true pelvis and contained large quantities of lipid material. However, as biopsies were done mostly on patients prepared for a surgical procedure, biopsy results have frequently shown the presence of glycogen and fat in quantities greater than normal. Long acting and intermediate insulins prevent and correct this complication.

Xanthosis Diabeticorum. Xanthosis diabeticorum has been common in juveniles because they select the vegetables high in carotene, carrots, peas and tomatoes being the favorite three. With the large liver the diagnosis of hepatitis was formerly made.

Xanthoma diabeticorum has been more common in children than in adults. It was seen when with rapidly acting insulin the control of fat metabolism was more difficult. Today these lesions are exceptional.

Failure of Growth. The complications seen most frequently between the fifth and fifteenth year of the duration of diabetes were formerly the failure of growth and pulmonary tuberculosis. Growth failure was seen more commonly in the young diabetic male than in the young diabetic female, and the incidence was formerly as high as 10 per cent of diabetic children. However, long acting insulins have nearly brought about the disappearance of this complication. Some children today are still treated with forms of rapidly acting insulins alone.

Neuropathy. Among 1072 twenty-year survivors neuropathy occurred in 26 per cent of the females and 20 per cent of the males. Acroneuritis was the form observed most commonly, with gastrointestinal neuropathies in second place. Such malignant neuropathies as Argyll Robertson pupils, tabetic bladders and Charcot joints occurred infrequently, in only 0.3 per cent, 0.3 per cent and 0.5 per cent, respectively.

Vascular Damage. In incidence, disability and mortality, vascular damage is by far the most important complication. At 35 years' duration nearly all juvenile diabetics show lesions; 94 per cent have calcified arteries, 93 per cent retinopathy, 59 per cent neovascularization, 53 per cent hypertension and 44 per cent nephropathy. These lesions were not observed in the first five years of diabetes and were rarely found in the first ten years, but by fifteen years, 19 per cent of those examined had retinopathy, 14 per cent calcified arteries, 7 per cent proteinuria, 4.5 per cent hypertension and 3 per cent retinitis proliferans.

The lesions were rare under age 20 but were prevalent by age 30 (63 per cent had retinopathy, 46 per cent calcified arteries, 29 per cent retinitis proliferans, 34 per cent albuminuria and 40 per cent hypertension). Although the incidence of the disabilities arising from the vascular lesions for the entire series of living and fatal cases is appreciable (uremia in 9 per cent, blindness in 6, myocardial infarction in 6, cerebrovascular accident in 2 and gangrene in 0.5 per cent), there is increasing evidence that certain numbers of these patients show a stationary status of their vascular lesions. This favorable course can be evaluated best in the retina.

Although it is evident from the foregoing that all of the vessels of these young patients are involved in all types of sclerosing processes, the significant, progressive and lethal lesions involve the arterioles, capillaries and venules. These small vessels can be observed at the microscopic level in the bulbar conjunctiva. Such examinations have been made upon this group by Ditzel[16] and have shown two types of patterns. One is characterized by the loss of venular tone and by venular dilatation. The second is characterized by increased arteriolar constriction. The changes are followed by intravascular aggregation of erythrocytes, by perivascular edema and by hyaline deposition. Long-term diabetics show these abnormal responses, and untreated and uncontrolled cases to an exaggerated degree. It is significant that these changes were also observed in children of diabetic mothers, 16 per cent in those with normal glycemia, 51 per cent in those with hyperglycemia.

MANAGEMENT OF JUVENILE DIABETES

Insulin. From the foregoing, the fundamental principle for the management of juvenile diabetes becomes evident—regulation of insulin and diet to enhance both physiologic and chemical control.

CHOICE OF INSULINS. The choice rests among regular quickly acting insulin, the intermediate acting insulins (globin, NPH, lente and 2:1 and 3:1 mixtures of regular and protamine) and the one slowly acting insulin (protamine zinc insulin). The time-action curves of these insulins are reviewed here. The three properties which concern us are onset, intensity and duration of the hypoglycemic action.

Regular insulin acts quickly. By the subcutaneous route it commences its hypoglycemic action within an hour of administration, reaching its peak in 3 to 4 hours and lasting 6 to 8 hours. Of the intermediate acting insulins, globin starts its action within an hour, NPH and lente within 2 hours; all reach a maximum effect 8 to 10 hours after administration and last approximately 24 hours (globin the shortest, NPH between, and lente the longest). Approximating the time-action curves of the intermediate acting insulins are the 2:1 and 3:1 mixtures of regular and protamine insulin. After mixture they are respectively 1 unit of regular to 2 of protamine and 1 of regular and 1 of protamine.

The one long acting insulin, protamine zinc, has little hypoglycemic effect for 6 to 8 hours, maximum effect 12 to 24 hours (nearer 24) and lasts for 36 hours, with weak action up to 72 hours. One more property of protamine zinc insulin should be emphasized, the ability to adsorb regular insulin. This is due to the excess of protamine which has been added and explains why in mixtures the effect is reversed.

The effect of the size of the dose of insulin upon the time-action curve is of great therapeutic importance. Increase in the dose of regular insulin increases the depth to which the blood sugar falls. Increase in the dose of protamine zinc increases duration of action. Increases in doses of intermediate insulins increase intensity and duration of action. The principle is not perfect. Massive doses of regular insulin given to patients in ketoacidosis prolong the action of regular insulin. For the most part, the intermediate acting insulins are the most effective in the daily management of juvenile patients.

Special situations occur for the use of regular insulin in preference to intermediate or long acting insulins. These include diabetic coma, and supplementary use during infections or following surgery. It is possibly a better choice for patients with epilepsy. It is more effective in patients with a low kidney threshold, and some pediatricians prefer to treat infants for the first year or two with quickly acting insulin. Its prolonged use in the juvenile is not wise. It would be successful if given by the clock, but in the hands of patients the frequency of injection may be twice in 24 hours or even once, so that the hours of controlled diabetes are few. It was during the era of regular insulin when growth failure, hepatomegaly and skin complications were frequent complications of diabetes.

Among the intermediate acting insulins, the first choice for allergic children is lente. In the juvenile population globin and lente have one common objection—they are slightly more painful than NPH. The 2:1 mixture of protamine and regular has had wide use. The 3:1 mixture is limited almost exclusively to the young population, under age 5, in whom the requirement for rapidly acting insulin is high and for long acting insulin low. Protamine zinc insulin today is specifically indicated for the occasional patient in whom the control of nocturnal hyperglycemia is most difficult. Usually a split schedule of intermediate acting insulin is desirable, but when this is not feasible, protamine alone or in combination with regular insulin may prove to be effective.

Special insulins are reserved for patients with allergies, although they may have to be desensitized. U-500 regular insulin is used exclusively in the rare refractory cases of juvenile diabetes in which the requirement is from 200 up to several thousand units daily.

REGULATION OF INSULIN. The prescription of insulin for initial stabilization of newly contracted cases of juvenile diabetes, exhibiting no signs of ketoacidosis, is based upon age or weight rather than upon the degree of hyperglycemia or glycosuria: one quarter of a unit per pound; or at one year, 5 units; at 5 years, 10 units; at 10 years, 20 units; and at 15 years, 30 units.

A mathematical rule for the regulation of insulin has been recommended by Hartmann and is calculated as follows: The total glucose of the diet is estimated. From this is subtracted the quantity of glucose which was excreted in 24 hours. When this figure is divided by the dose of insulin received, one can determine how much glucose 1 unit of insulin utilized in this particular patient. The units necessary on this basis to eliminate the excreted glucose can then be added.

There are two concepts concerning the regulation of the dose of insulin, one to correct glycosuria and the other to anticipate it. With intermediate and long acting insulins, anticipation appears more logical. The depot of insulin with its constant blood sugar lowering action should be remembered. In regulation, tests three times during the day are the most valuable. The second of two voided specimens pinpoints the metabolic behavior and is closer to the blood sugar level. When insulins are administered, as they are usually, before breakfast, the poor pre-lunch test indicates that the patient needs a dose of regular acting insulin before breakfast and with intermediate insulins this can be mixed. A poor test before the evening meal indicates that the patient has not received enough intermediate acting insulin. If the specimen before the evening meal has become sugar-free but the pre-breakfast specimen contains significant quantities of glucose, a dose of intermediate acting insulin may be added at bedtime. The pre-breakfast test becomes the guide for regulating the bedtime dose of insulin. Control is satisfactory if the patient is excreting less than 5 per cent of his carbohydrate intake, and for the majority of dietary prescriptions today this will place the loss at between 5 and 10 grams.

Variations in this prescription may be necessary. Sometimes regular insulin should be mixed with the bedtime dose of intermediate. Often one has to prescribe these mixtures earlier before the evening meal in order to prevent glycosuria in the period from supper to bedtime.

With juvenile patients the changes in dosage of insulin are best made daily. With very young children the changes should be only a unit at a time, with the average 4 units, but with patients with a high insulin requirement, doses may be changed by larger increments.

COMPLICATIONS. Complications of insulin therapy in childhood are hypoglycemia, atrophy, induration, allergy, abscesses, presbyopia and edema.

Hypoglycemia. Hypoglycemia, if mild, may be corrected by glucose-containing substances administered orally; if moderately severe, by glucose administered intravenously. Hypoglycemic encephalopathy is an entity observed, almost without exception, when insulin has been administered to patients already hypoglycemic. This severest manifestation of hypoglycemia deserves aggressive treatment: glucose by constant venoclysis, 150 to 300 grams in 24 hours, adrenalin or cortisone, transfusions of fresh whole blood, anticonvulsants, therapeutic lumbar puncture and oxygen under positive pressure.

Insulin Atrophies. Insulin atrophies plague the patients. These are limited almost exclusively to women and children, and their importance is cosmetic. The prognosis for recovery is good. They often disappear in from two to eight years. For the few patients who fail to recover, intramuscular instead of subcutaneous injections may be tried.

Dietary Treatment. The caloric prescription must be adequate to maintain rates of growth normal for the individual child. Calories may be prescribed by one of several rules: (1) by age alone: at year 1, 1000 calories, 100 calories added for each growth year; (2) by weight and age: 100 calories/kg. at age 1; 80 calories/kg. at age 5; 60 calories/kg. at age 10; 40 calories/kg. at age 15; (3) by height: 35 calories per inch; (4) by theoretical basal metabolism plus 80 per cent. These diets should be increased by 20 per cent for unusual activity. Such rules should be modified for individual needs.

Because of obesity among adolescent girls, at 13 their dietary prescription may be reduced to 30 calories/kg. of ideal body weight for height and age.

Although the division of the diet into its component parts, carbohydrate, protein and fat, has lost some of its significance with the concept of the common metabolic pool and the common metabolic pathway, such division is useful in practical therapy. The normal partition, derived from the formula of milk, is carbohydrate 50 per cent, protein 15 per cent and fat 35 per cent of the total calories. In the diets of the juvenile patients of the Joslin Clinic the carbohydrate does not exceed 40 per cent of the total calories, the fat is usually 40 per cent and the protein 20 per cent. The range of carbohydrate has varied from 100 to 200 grams. Diets high in carbohydrate are avoided, because they favor the development of wide fluctuations of blood glucose levels and extreme degrees of postprandial hyperglycemia.

For rapid calculation, the carbohydrate in grams is 10 per cent of the figure for the total calories, and the protein and fat are approximately half the figure of the carbohydrate. Thus, according to our rule for age, the child of nine requires 1800 calories; 10 per cent of that figure gives carbohydrate 180, halved for protein and fat gives 90 (or 1890 calories). The maximum carbohydrate prescribed is 225 grams. After age 13 the protein and fat portions of the diet are increased for diabetic boys.

Not only the quantity but the quality of diets remains important, the carbohydrate low in concentration, the protein of high quality, fats unsaturated.

Supplementary doses of vitamins are added, for although the diabetic diet is liberal in all vitamins except vitamin D, faulty utilization may occur. Freston and Loughlin[17] reported the vitamin deficiencies at Camp Nyda to be 27 per cent in 93 children. The report of Mosenthal and Loughlin[18] showed vitamin A deficiency in 68 per cent, B in 25 per cent and C in 4 per cent. Hypercarotinemia was present in 28 per cent. At the Clara Barton Birthplace Camp, 130 children were tested for vitamin C in 1938 and no subnormal values were found. During years of depression we found clinical signs of vitamin A deficiency; during war restriction, vitamin B deficiencies were found to predominate. Dark adaptation was normal in a small group of our children tested; none has given a history of night blindness, but characteristic skin lesions occur. Faulty utilization of vitamin A has been suspected because of hypercarotinemia and hepatomegaly. Since vitamin A is formed in the liver by the splitting of carotene, lack may be inferred.

The calcium content of our diets exceeds 1 gram. If adequacy can be measured by low incidence of osteoporosis, our diets are adequate. Bone atrophy has been exceptional since 1926. Serum determinations for calcium and phosphorus show the former to be normal, the latter usually slightly below normal.

EMERGENCY DIETS. The diet during acute infections may be reduced to carbohydrate 150, protein 50 and fat 50 grams, consisting of eggnogs, milk and fruit juices. A simple rule is an alternate glass of fruit juice or eggnog every two hours for seven feedings. The surgical patient should receive 75 to 100 grams of glucose parenterally, preferably as a 5 per cent solution.

For other plans for treatment, see Barach,[19] Boyd,[20] Escudero,[21] Wilder,[22] Stolte,[23] Lichtenstein,[24] Colwell *et al.*,[25] Jackson and McIntosh,[26] and Danowski.[4]

Exercise. The third part of the treatment is of great importance, namely, exercise, the timing of which should be somewhat different from that of the child without diabetes, postmeal exercise being favored over premeal exercise periods. The explanation for the favorable effect of exercise upon diabetes is that it actually simulates the action of insulin. Thus, muscle extracts have been found to accelerate the hexokinase effect, and exercise has been found to increase the volume of distribution of certain sugars.

The follow-up of juvenile patients is extremely important. New patients may require weekly visits, whereas after the first year visits at intervals of three months are desirable.

Readjustments of treatment are made on the majority of our children at summer camp units where the activity is normal. Group psychology is helpful in solving the problems of the children.

Psychologic Problems. Because of the unusual medical responsibility imposed by the details of treatment, menu planning, chemical testing and administration of therapy hypodermically; because of the stress produced by the sudden development of critical situations, insulin reactions or acidosis; and because of their knowledge of the future possibilities, parents may develop certain faulty attitudes and these in turn affect the child's adjustment to diabetes. These parental attitudes are largely of four types: overanxiety, overindulgence, perfectionism, or indifference. The overanxious parent may precipitate anx-

TABLE 2. SAMPLE DIETS

EGG	MEAT	BACON	VEGETABLES 3%	VEGETABLES 6%	OATMEAL	BUTTER	CREAM	MILK	ORANGE	POTATO	BREAD
Carbohydrate 121; Protein 52; Fat 59; 1223 Cal.											
1					15	5		240	100		
	30		75	38		7.5		240	100		15
	30		75	38		7.5		240	100		15
May split cereal portion into 60 cereal + 10 gm. bread			Forenoon: 1 Uneeda			Afternoon: 2 Uneedas or 100 Orange			Bedtime: 2 Uneedas or 100 Orange		
Carbohydrate 140; Protein 61; Fat 71; 1443 Cal.											
1					15	5		240	100		15
	30		75	38		10		180	100		15
	30		75	38		10		180	100		15
Forenoon: 1 Uneeda			Afternoon: 2 Uneedas + 180 milk					Bedtime: 2 Uneedas + 180 milk			
Carbohydrate 163; Protein 72; Fat 97; 1633 Cal.											
1					15	5		240	100		15
	45		75	38		10		180	100		30
	45		75	38		10		180	100		30
Forenoon: 2 Uneedas			Afternoon: 2 Uneedas + 180 milk					Bedtime: 2 Uneedas + 180 milk			
Carbohydrate 183; Protein 83; Fat 88; 1856 Cal.											
1		15			15	5		240	100		30
	60		150	75		10		240	150		30
	60		150	75		10		180	150		30
School Recess: 100 orange			Afternoon: 2 Uneedas + 120 milk					Bedtime: 2 Uneedas + 180 milk			
Carbohydrate 202; Protein 92; Fat 98; 2058 Cal.											
1		15			15	10		240	100		30
	60		150	75		10		240	200		30
	90		150	75		10		240	150	75	30
School Recess: 2 Uneedas			Afternoon: 2 Uneedas + 120 milk					Bedtime: 2 Uneedas + butter or peanut butter			

iety states, dependence or defiance in the child; the overly indulgent, exploitation; the perfectionist, deception and rebellion; the indifferent, depression or, more rarely, rebellion.

Self-management, when the child is ready, should be encouraged as well as diabetic undercentralization. The exploration for and the development of aptitudes are important. Regular emotional support will help in the solution of the child's problems. Reassurance for normal social, recreational and economic future life should be given repeatedly. The anticipation of pleasing projects at frequent intervals, such as every three months, is a must for the child with chronic disease. Expertness in dietetics is a specific need for the solution of the adolescent's social life, as is a substitute for food hunger in the form of extra affection for the very young diabetic. Summer camp programs dispel the feeling of being different and, finally, the value of the group therapy should be explored.

SUMMER CAMPS. The first camp for diabetic children was started by the late Dr. Wendt in Detroit. Our own camp program had its simple beginning when a Deaconess nurse took one child to her home in Maine for the summer. The result was excellent and in the subsequent year, 1927, she was persuaded to take five children and gradually expanded her work, until the time when her own health failed. In 1932 our first group of children was sent to the Clara Barton Camp in North Oxford. Ninety children can be cared for at one time for three-, six- or nine-week periods. This camp is supported equally by The Association of Universalist Women, The Diabetes Camp, Home and Hospital Fund and the children themselves. In 1948 the Elliott P. Joslin Camp for diabetic boys was established in Charlton, Massachusetts. Here, also, ninety children can be cared for at one time for three,- six- or nine-week periods. For other camps, see Joslin[27] and A.D.A. Forecast.[28]

Summer camps for diabetic children supplement hospital and office management. Group psychology is beneficial. Patients may be taught at their own age level. Close contact with resident doctors, nurses, dietitians and laboratory technicians increases the children's knowledge and understanding of their disease. Treatment may be carried out under ideal conditions of normal physical activities.

The physical setup at the Clara Barton and Elliott P. Joslin Camps includes cabins, administration building with dining room, infirmary and laboratory, as well as a recreation unit. The medical personnel include the resident physician, three nurses, three laboratory technicians and a dietitian for each camp. The physical activity is that of a regular camp. However, diets are weighed, daily quantitative and qualitative urine tests are done, and serial blood sugars are estimated once or twice weekly.

Behavior Problems. Close adherence to the prescribed routine is the rule in the first year of treatment. The child may have pride in hypodermic injections, testing outfits, etc. After the first year, the routine of treatment palls. Indiscretions occur. Up to the time of adolescence the child may be coaxed back to routine, but in adolescence medical rejection parallels parental rejection. The diabetic routine does not favor the social success of the patient. Unity of behavior pattern and fastidiousness conflict with the prescribed diabetic treatment. Complete break in the control of diabetes occurs only too often. With the normal diabetic child the rejection rarely lasts more than two years, but if the rejection is long and bizarre, psychiatric study is indicated. Abnormal electroencephalograms suggesting psychomotor behavior should be investigated. Self-induced hypoglycemia or coma, pseudo cures and repeated hospitalization require psychiatric evaluation. Incorrectly kept (perfect) urine charts, the substitution of water for a specimen of urine, the substitution of an obliging normal friend's urine for the patient's own, while annoying to the physician, should not be considered abnormal behavior for the juvenile diabetic. Such acts do not require a psychiatric consultation.

Intelligence of the Diabetic Child. Intelligence tests were made by Louise Cone on 169 of our diabetic children; they were found to be higher by 10 on the average than a control series whose median age was the same. Brown and Thompson,[29] and McGavin, Schultz, Peden and Bowen,[30] on the other hand, have not found evidence of mental superiority.

Physical Examination. The physical examination of the diabetic child after several years' duration of the disease, compared with normal children, reveals that the diabetic has a wider range of height and weight, short and obese children occurring less frequently in the control population studied and reported by Wagner, White and Bogan. Fischer, Mackler and Marks[31] report similar deviations of height and weight for a diabetic group.

The skin, except for xanthosis, shows no common difference. The teeth have less evidence of caries; hardly more than physiologic caries of the sixth and twelfth molars was observed. Pyorrhea, usually of only slight degree, occurs more frequently in the diabetics than in the nondiabetics. Systolic heart murmurs are heard more often. These are functional, not organic. The liver is palpable more often, and there is more evidence of congenital anomalies of the mesenchymatous tissue, such as ear nodules, clubbed fingers, curved fingers and webbed toes.

Of the secondary sex characteristics, the early ones are often precipitated and the late ones postponed. The measurement of the follicle-stimulating hormone and of 17-ketosteroid shows the same behavior, especially in reference to the latter, the excretion of which is high at onset of diabetes and later falls to subnormal values. The follicle-stimulating hormone is elevated at onset, falls to low values and then may rise again.

Standards for Control. Perhaps the most debated question in the management of the juvenile diabetic today concerns the degree of chemical control. Three schools of thought regarding control of diabetes exist: first, that which advocates perfect chemical control; second, that which advocates good but not quite perfect chemical control; third, that which advocates clinical but not chemical control of the disease. The proponents of perfect and good control of diabetes maintain that the degenerative complications are precipitated by chemically uncontrolled diabetes, whereas those who favor clinical over chemical control of diabetes believe that the degenerative complications of diabetes are caused by diabetes *per se* rather than by its poor control. The standard for control which is taught at the Joslin Clinic is the following: that the glycosuria in 24 hours should not exceed 5 per cent of the carbohydrate intake; that blood sugar levels should be normal before meals and the cholesterol normal for children (below 200 mg.); that the urine should be free from ketone bodies; that the rate of growth should be normal and the child able to carry on the activities appropriate to his age.

DIAGNOSIS, COURSE, PREVENTION AND TREATMENT OF THE COMPLICATIONS OF JUVENILE DIABETES

Ketoacidosis. The relative and actual frequency of ketoacidosis in childhood type diabetes, previously described, indicates its importance in this group. The course, though more rapid than in adults, is relatively slow. The symptoms of insatiable thirst and difficult breathing are always present and are usually accompanied by weakness, nausea, vomiting, abdominal pain and drowsiness. Hyperpnea and acetone odor of the breath are unfailing signs as well as evidences of dehydration and medical shock. Abdominal rigidity, so-called pseudoperitonitis of diabetic coma, causes confusion in differential diagnosis.

In the juvenile patient, as in the adult patient, the diagnosis of diabetic coma is determined by the level of the carbon dioxide content of the blood. When this falls to 9 mEq. or below, in the Joslin

Clinic the case is classified as diabetic coma. This is an arbitrary figure, selected because until the discovery of insulin few patients whose reserve fell to this level recovered. In the juvenile population those who are most susceptible to coma are the adolescents. Eighty per cent of the juvenile comas are in adolescents, 66 per cent in females. Short duration cases under 5 years constitute 44 per cent.

Laboratory findings include, in addition to lowering of the CO_2: hyperglycemia range in juveniles from 180 to 2200^{+} mg.; rising NPN; fall of sodium and chloride; normal protein, albumin and globulin; elevation of cholesterol; increase of calcium; variable potassium and inorganic phosphorus; increased, normal or low magnesium; leucocytosis; and increase in oxysteroids. The urine contains sugar, acetone, albumin and casts. The level for acetone in the serum is high.

The objectives in the correction of metabolic upheaval include (1) abolition of hyperglycemia and glycosuria, (2) deposition of glycogen, (3) elimination of ketosis, (4) restoration of body fluid, Ph and BH CO_3, and (5) repair of electrolyte pattern. Although insulin functions in each objective, its action must be supplemented with other measures.

INSULIN TREATMENT. The age of the patient is frequently a guide for the dose of insulin to be employed. Thus, the average dose in the first 24 hours of treatment for Joslin Clinic patients under age 1 was 65 units; for patients between the ages of 1 and 5, 80 units; between ages 5 to 10, 110 units; between ages 10 to 14, 220 units; between ages 15 to 19, 250 units; and above the age of 20, 360 units. When the blood sugar was between 500 and 750 mg., the dose of insulin was 250 units, and when the blood sugar was between 750 and 1000 mg., the average dose for these patients was 500 units. As the severity of coma becomes more marked, as measured by the state of consciousness, the intravenous administration of insulin should be combined with the subcutaneous administration and the frequency of the dose increased to half hour intervals. The percentage of the fall of blood sugar is a guide for the rate of administration. Thus, regardless of the original level, when the blood sugar has fallen to 50 per cent of the admitting level, enough insulin has been given for several hours to come. However, the dangers of overtreatment are far less than the dangers of undertreatment.

Hydration is gauged by the volume of the urinary output. It is considered adequate when the output is 50 cc. per hour. Normal saline appears to be effective for most cases.

For electrolyte repair, potassium is used if the blood level falls below 3 mEq. or electrocardiographic changes occur or gastric dilation persists or the clinical picture of flaccidity and respiratory failure develops.

Sodium lactate (1/6 M) is used, especially if nephritis complicates ketoacidosis. Hartmann uses sodium lactate 60 to 90 cc. per kg. and Ringer's solution 40 cc. per kg. Guest favors bicarbonate. Butler recommends the multiple hypotonic electrolyte solution of Talbot and Crawford, 3.5 liters per square meter. This solution contains per liter Na 40 mEq., K 35.5 mEq., Cl. 40 mEq., lactate 20 mEq., phosphorus 15 mEq., and glucose 0 to 80 grams. Thorn and Forsham recommend adding 500 cc. of 1/6 molar lactate (1.9 per cent) or bicarbonate (1.3 per cent) to each liter of 0.85 per cent sodium chloride solution, and to correct or prevent hypokalemia potassium hydrogen phosphate 2 gm., potassium dehydrogen phosphate 0.4 gm., distilled water to 50 cc. added to a liter of the solution used.

Glucose is used only if the level of blood glucose is low, since its use favors water intoxication and hypokalemia.

Carbohydrate as orange, oatmeal or milk, 5 grams per hour, is given when vomiting is controlled; antibiotics are often necessary.

Shock may be treated with Levophed, and hypochloremic anuria with 10 per cent salt solution.

Unless the patient is in marked shock, gastric lavage should be a routine procedure. In spite of restlessness and obvious pain, opiates and sedatives should be avoided. During convalescence the first day's diet consists of a soft solid diet of 150 grams carbohydrate, 50 of protein and 50 of fat.

DIFFERENTIAL DIABETIC DIAGNOSIS. In the juvenile patient the following must be differentiated from ketoacidosis: surgical abdomen coexistent with ketoacidosis, uremia, diphtheria, pneumonia, hypoglycemia, salicylic acid poisoning, fractured skull and lead poisoning. The complications in the convalescence from ketoacidosis include: hypoglycemia, rebound into acidosis, anuria, shock, aspiration pneumonia, urinary tract infection, arterial thromboses and infection.

PREVENTION. Prevention of ketoacidosis should be taught by careful chemical control. Thus, parents can be taught a quantitative determination of sugar for the 24-hour period, daily qualitative tests, spot tests for acetone, the daily regulation of insulin, the important rule never to omit insulin on a day of illness, continuous reassurance through follow-up, and stress for the hope for curability of diabetes. In other words, "Live today in expectation of the cure tomorrow."

PROGNOSIS. Among childhood cases of coma at the Joslin Clinic, the case recovery was 98 per cent and the patient recovery 97 per cent. There were no deaths under age 10, two under age 15. Multiple attacks of diabetic coma carry added risk. Twenty-six of our juvenile patients had from three to ten attacks, and in this group the death rate was 60 per cent. The subsequent course of the juveniles who had had diabetic coma showed the following: tuberculosis in 5 per cent, retinopathy in 25 per cent, nephropathy in 20 per cent. Seventy-five per cent were alive at the time of the most recent follow-up.

Infections. Prior to the discovery of chemotherapy the average duration of life in juvenile diabetics was some seven years followed by death from septicemia. Perhaps because of difficulty in early diagnosis the especially malignant necrotizing papillitis may defy our therapeutic programs and terminate fatally. Even today, delayed development of antibody to staphylococcus toxin in diabetic children was observed by Bates and Weiss,[32] who compared 14 normal children with diabetics given 7 or 8 weekly injections of unmodified staphylococcus toxin. There was no effect upon the diabetes, but there was a delay in the development of the antibody after intradermal injection of staphylococcus toxin in diabetic children. Not only was there slower production of alpha antistaphylolysin, but the maximum titers attained after several weeks of immunization were lower than those of a similar group of normal children. Lack of control of diabetes retarded and diminished the production of antihemolysin.

The rules for the management of infections in diabetes are the same as those for the general population. However, *Staphylococcus albus* is more often pathogenic. Simple therapeutic rules are as follows: penicillin for gram-positive and erythromycin for resistant gram-positive cocci; Gantrisin for gram-negative organisms and streptomycin for resistant gram-negative organism; for marked resistance, the combination of Aureomycin, Terramycin and Chloromycetin.

Cataracts. Cataracts have been identified in 1.5 per cent of our juvenile diabetics. Not all of the children have been examined routinely with the slit lamp. Most of these cataracts occur early in the course of the disease, even at the time of the diagnosis of diabetes; often they are observed in patients whose disease is of less than three years' duration. They are rarely first diagnosed after five years of diabetes. Opacities in the posterior subcapsular area and showers of fine cholesterol crystals can be demonstrated. The treatment is surgical when the vision is sufficiently impaired.

O'Brien[33] reports cataracts in 14 per cent of 260 cases examined. Wachs[34] reports reversal of the cataract, a case in a 16-year-old diabetic. Boyd, Jackson and Allen[35] report posterior subcapsular opacities in one third of 69 diabetics related to episodes of poor control of diabetes. In contrast to this latter view, Karlstrom[36] reports 38 children treated with the free diet without cataracts.

Our own experience with these patients who have developed cataracts correlates them with poor control of the disease. A common history is of unrecognized diabetes, active symptoms of diabetes for a year, recognition of diabetes in coma and signs of vitamin B deficiency. Recently, it has become apparent that after twenty years of diabetes, susceptibility to senile cataract formation occurs.

Retinopathy. The earliest of the vascular lesions to be recognized clinically in the juvenile patient is retinopathy. In the juvenile patient marked changes occur in the capillary, venule and arteriole. The capillary changes include microaneurysms, looping and new formation. Seen almost simultaneously is the earliest of the venular changes, dilatation and darkened color, later sacculation and rupture. Occlusion may occur.

In the arterioles A-V nicking, tortuosity, silver-wire and obliteration are evident, but these changes are less striking than the capillary and venular ones.

Sheathing of vessels may be evident and hemorrhages of many types—punctate, small and round, blotchy, preretinal, vitreous and at any time superimposed renal nerve-fibre or striate.

Exudate at first is punctate; the waxy character is clearer as the lesion increases in size, and suggests coalescence. Cotton-wool exudate may be superimposed. The white exudate is sometimes evident; at other times it may appear yellow. Dense white scars traverse the retina, leading to separation.

Hemorrhagic glaucoma may intervene and phthisis of the bulba result.

Prevention of retinopathy and its stationary status is sought by chemical control of diabetes.

Nephropathy. Diabetic nephropathy is a mixed lesion consisting of intercapillary glomerulosclerosis, arteriolarsclerosis, arteriosclerosis and pyelonephritis. The clinical picture of nephropathy is revealed by the appearance of proteinuria which is transitory at first, then becomes constant. Diabetic retinopathy usually precedes proteinuria. Soon renal retinopathy appears. Proteinuria occurs rarely before the fifteenth year of diabetes and rarely before twenty years of age. Edema develops gradually, as does hypertension, which is usually of moderate degree. The total protein falls, the A/G ratio is reversed, the cholesterol levels increase and lipoprotein in the SF 12:20 range increases. The urine contains doubly refractile bodies but few cells or casts. Anemia becomes progressively severe, renal acidosis is common, low salt syndrome develops; congestive heart failure occurs, distressing encephalopathies intervene and uremia is almost inevitable.

The management of nephropathies must be planned for the phase or phases present. The nephrotic stage is best controlled with diets high in protein, low in sodium. The acid ash diet is useful. Ammonium chloride and/or potassium chloride, nitrate mercurial, xanthines or magnesium sulfate is indicated; Amigen, acacia and salt-poor albumin may be tried. The anemias, largely intractable, are benefited temporarily by transfusions of packed red cells; copper, cobalt or iron is usually given, too.

The salt-losing phase must be managed carefully. Dietary sodium chloride or normal salt solution may be adequate.

The acidosis may be treated with sodium lactate if acute and with ammonium citrate if chronic.

When uremia develops, the sodium may be restricted further to 0.5 gram daily and protein to 0.5 gram per kilo.

Congestive heart failure requires digitalization, rest and restriction of fluid to 2000 cc.

Encephalopathies may require lumbar puncture, magnesium sulfate, hypotensive drugs or anticonvulsants.

Exchange resins, splanchnicectomy and rice diets have not been successful in our hands. The chronicity of the lesions makes the artificial kidney, replacement transfusions, intestinal and peritoneal lavage useless procedures. The use of heparin to alter lipoproteins may be explored further. Adrenalectomy —surgical, x-ray or medical—appears too radical.

Calcification. Next to retinopathy, calcification of arteries is the most common vascular lesion in juvenile diabetes. Between the fifteenth and nineteenth year of disease, 25 to 35 per cent of juveniles carefully studied show this lesion. It has not been observed under ten years of age or prior to the fifth year of diabetes. The youngest patient in our group to show the lesion was eleven years of age. The shortest duration occurred in two cases, both of which showed calcification by x-ray at eight years' duration.

Following the areas of lowest vascular reserve the lesion appears first in the ankle, then the leg, pelvis and abdominal aorta. Lichtenstein[24] believes patients treated with higher carbohydrate diets do not tend to develop this lesion. Such has not been our experience.

Gangrene is an infrequent complication in diabetes with onset in childhood.

Mortality. Cardiorenalvascular lesions have replaced nearly all other causes of death. The changing status with respect to causes of death is shown by the near disappearance of coma, sepsis and tuberculosis, formerly the chief cause of death.

References

1. Grishaw, W. H., West, H. F. and Smith, B.: Arch. Int. Med., *64:*787, 1939.
2. John, H. J.: Ann. Int. Med., *8:*198, 1934.
3. Lande: Klin. Wchnschr., *10:*359, 1931.
4. Danowski, T. S.: Diabetes Mellitus, with Emphasis on Children and Young Adults. Baltimore, Williams and Wilkins Co., 1957.
5. Bogan, I. K. and Morrison, G.: Am. J. M. Sc., *174:*313, 1927.
6. Robinson, H.: Personal communication.
7. Wagner, R., White, P. and Bogan, I. K.: Am. J. Dis. Child., *63:*667, 1942. Also White, P.: Diabetes in Childhood and Adolescence. Philadelphia, Lea & Febiger, 1932.
8. Boulin, R. and Uhry, P.: Acta gastroenterol. belge., *12:*540, 1949.
9. Warren, S. and LeCompte, P. M.: Pathology of Diabetes Mellitus. 3rd ed. Philadelphia, Lea & Febiger, 1952, Chap. XI.
10. Young, F. G.: Lancet, *2:*372, 1937.
11. Young, F. G.: Biochem. J., *32:*513, 1938.
12. Wrenshall, G. A., Bogoch, A. and Ritchie, R. C.: Diabetes, *1:*87, 1952.
13. Bornstein, J. and Lawrence, R. D.: Brit. M. J., *1:*732, 1951.
14. Camerini-Davalos, R., Marble, A., White, P., Belmonte, M. and Sargeant, H. L.: New England J. Med., *256:*817, 1957.
15. Mirsky, I. A. and Nelson, W. E.: J.A.M.A., *67:*100, 1944.
16. Ditzel, J. and White, P.: J. Chron. Dis., *3:*205, 1956.
17. Freston, J. M. and Loughlin, W. C.: New York J. Med., *42:*1833, 1942.
18. Mosenthal, H. O. and Loughlin, W. C.: Arch. Int. Med., *73:*391, 1944.
19. Barach, J. H.: Am. J. Digest. Dis., *11:*350, 1944.
20. Jackson, R. L., Boyd, J. D. and Smith, T. E.: Am. J. Dis. Child., *59:*332, 1940.
21. Escudero, P.: Inst. Nac. Nutricion, Buenos Aires, Recop. Tirab. Acnt., *5:*200, 1940.
22. Wilder, R. M.: Clinical Diabetes and Hyperinsulinism. Philadelphia, W. B. Saunders Co., 1940.
23. Stolte, K.: Med. Klin., *28:*831, 1931.
24. Lichtenstein, A.: Nord. med. Wchnschr., *10:*1329, 1935.
25. Colwell, A. R., Izzo, J. L. and Stryker, W. A.: Arch. Int. Med., *69:*931, 1942.
26. Jackson, R. L. and McIntosh, C. B.: Proc. Cent. Soc. Clin. Res., *17:*74, 1944.
27. Joslin, E. P.: New England J. Med., *234:* 442, 476, 1946.
28. A. D. A. Forecast, *4:*6, 1951.
29. Brown, G. D. and Thompson, W. H.: Am. J. Dis. Child., *59:*238, 1940.
30. McGavin, A. P., Schultz, E., Peden, G. W. and Bowen, B. D.: New England J. Med., *223:*119, 1940.
31. Fischer, A. E., Mackler, H. S. and Marks, H. H.: Am. J. Dis. Child., *64:*413, 1942.
32. Bates, G. and Weiss, C.: Am. J. Dis. Child., *62:*346, 1941.
33. O'Brien, C. S. and Allen, J. H.: J.A.M.A., *120:*190, 1942.
34. Wachs: Am. J. Ophth., *25:*336, 1942.
35. Boyd, J. D., Jackson, R. L. and Allen, J. H.: J.A.M.A., *118:*694, 1942.
36. Karlstrom: Sveno Ratak Tidning, *38:*2623, 1941.

CHAPTER 17

By RULON W. RAWSON, M.D., AND
MARTIN SONENBERG, M.D., Ph.D.

Diseases of the Thyroid

INTRODUCTION

During the past two decades increasing interest in the physiology of the thyroid has resulted in a better understanding of the various diseases of this gland and in several improved forms of therapy. These advances have resulted not only from the efforts of investigators in all of the disciplinary specialties of medicine, but also from the efforts of investigators in apparently quite unrelated fields such as physical chemistry and physics.

The radioactive isotope method of studying the metabolism of iodine is probably one of the most important tools made available during the last two decades. With this technique many of the original concepts of the physiology of the thyroid gland have been confirmed and expanded, and newer phenomena have been discovered. Studies with the goitrogenic agents, i.e., thiouracil, potassium thiocyanate, etc., have made it possible to elucidate certain mechanisms in the synthesis and metabolism of thyroid hormones. Recent studies done with pituitary, adrenal and gonadal hormones have improved our knowledge of the physiology of the thyroid gland and have indicated directions for future studies.

Notwithstanding the important advances made by a large group of modern investigators who have had available the newer tools of study, we must not lose sight of the important contributions made by a small group of investigators some of whom are now deceased and others who have retired from active academic life. These senior investigators' keen clinical observations led to accurate definitions of the effects of excess and lack of thyroid hormone and other disorders of the thyroid in the human. We hope that with all of our modern tools of study we do not neglect those qualities which made the clinical observations of our teachers so important to the study of diseases of the thyroid.

We plan to correlate clinical manifestations of the various diseases of the thyroid to normal and morbid physiology as we interpret it today. Where there exist serious disagreements in the literature, we shall present both sides. There may, however, be instances in which we will support the theories that we favor as of now.

ANATOMY OF THE THYROID

Comparative Anatomy. The thyroid is first present as a discrete structure in some chordates. In certain protochordates the endostyle has been regarded as the homologue of the thyroid, and endocrine activity has been ascribed to it. Gorbman, however, has found that the endostyle of the ascidians *Perophora annectens, Styela montereyensis* and *Ciona intestinalis* and of amphioxus does not concentrate radioiodine.[1] The iodine instead was concentrated in the stolonic septum in as great a concentration as is stored in the vertebrate thyroid. In the ammocoetes of the free living lamprey certain cells of the endostyle do concentrate radioiodine.[1] In this animal the homology between the endostyle and the thyroid of the adult form is well established from morphologic data.

The administration of neither iodine nor thyroxine will accelerate metamorphosis in the cyclostomes (of which the lamprey is an example), so the question of a hormonal function in the endostyle of these forms is still uncertain.[2] In all vertebrates the thyroid is present. In many species of fish, however, the thyroid is present as a diffuse layer of follicles.

From a functional standpoint, the thyroid is necessary for metamorphosis in certain vertebrates and to cause metamorphosis in one form that normally lives its entire life in the larval stage (axolotl). The thyroid does not seem to affect O_2 consumption in fish, although Smith and Matthews[3] have reported that thyroxine increases the O_2 consumption in the grunt. The thyroid is necessary for metamorphosis in amphibians such as the frog.[4] It appears to play a role in molting in reptiles[5] and is an important controlling factor in plumage growth in birds.[6] In mammals the thyroid affects both growth and general body metabolism.

Recently it has been demonstrated that certain analogues of thyroxine have a much greater effect on metamorphosis but much less calorigenic effect on mammals than does thyroxine. For example, triiodothyropropionic acid is 300 times more active than thyroxine in promoting metamorphosis in the tadpole but when tested in the rat for calorigenic activity is only one tenth as active as thyroxine.

Embryology. The thyroid gland is first represented in a human embryo of five to six primitive segments by a mid-ventral outpouching of the pharynx in the region of the first and second pharyngeal pouches. This anlage becomes elongated and enlarges laterally, the pharyngeal region contracting to become a narrow stalk—the thyroglossal duct—which finally separates from the pharynx, leaving a dimple represented in the adult by the foramen caecum at the base of the tongue. The thyroglossal duct persists in the adult of a few species, but in man it atrophies completely. Occasionally, it may fail to atrophy and occurs as a cystic mass in the midline of the neck, anywhere from the base of the tongue to the hyoid bone. The normal thyroid continues to grow and simultaneously migrates caudally.

Histologically, the thyroid anlage shows differentiation into discrete cords of cells by the 8 mm. stage. By the fourteenth week of pregnancy, the thyroid has developed well-differentiated glandular structures with empty lumina. In the fourteenth week these glands become filled with a homogeneous protein material known as colloid. At the same time, a certain amount of function of the thyroid becomes evident as demonstrated by the ability of the gland to concentrate radioiodine.[7]

Two associated structures, the ultimobranchial bodies and the internal epithelial body, both derivatives of the fourth pharyngeal pouches, migrate downward and become associated with the thyroid. It has been suggested that the ultimobranchial bodies are usually without thyroid function in mammals. Kingsbury,[8] on the other hand, believes that these structures disappear. In certain species (Echidna) the ultimobranchial bodies persist as discrete glands similar to the thyroid. The fate of the inferior epithelial body is obscure but it seems to disappear in the substance of the thyroid.

The embryologic journey of the thyroid throws some light on occasional clinical problems encountered in man. The origin of the thyroid from a position cephalad to its final location explains lingual and pretracheal thyroids. The thyroglossal cysts are likewise easily understood. Aberrant thyroid tissue in the mediastinum may represent abnormal caudal descent of the thyroid, although in most instances it represents downward growth of a nodular goiter. The lateral aberrant thyroid of which Lahey[9] and Graham[10] write, may represent truly aberrant tissue. However, the frequent demonstration of microscopic carcinoma in the thyroids of most of these patients[11] with so-called lateral aberrant thyroid tissue suggest that they usually are metastases from a low-grade, well differentiated thyroid carcinoma.

Gross Anatomy. In the adult human, the thyroid is found as two lobes joined by an isthmus, attached to the anterior surface of the trachea. There is usually a pyramidal lobe arising just to the left of the midline and pointing upward, which represents the thyroidal vestige of the thyroglossal duct. The total gland in adults weighs between 15 and 20 gm. but will vary with the birthplace of the subject, his iodine intake and his intake of goitrogenic foods. Rice[12] found that in Minnesota, which is in a goitrous area, the average adult thyroid weighs 30 gm.

Microscopic Anatomy. Microscopically, the thyroid, as intimated above, is composed primarily of small (Wilson[13] has calculated the mean acinar diameter as 300 microns) spheroidal structures, lined with an epithelium, one cell in thickness and filled with homogeneous, highly refractile material. This latter substance is known as colloid and is a protein, thyroglobulin, with a molecular weight of 680,000.[14] The cells lining these structures, which are variously known as follicles, acini and alveoli, are outfitted with mitochondria and Golgi bodies. Both of these minute structures have been studied intensively, and their size seems to be correlated with the functional state of the gland. The size and, more particularly, the height of these cells is an excellent index of the functional activity of the thyroid.[15] The acini are incompletely separated by fibrous septa radiating from a thin fibrous capsule which covers the entire gland. The thyroid is endowed with an abundant blood supply said to be comparatively greater than that of any other organ except the adrenal. Most of the blood to the thyroid in man is derived from two superior thyroidal arteries which arise from the external carotids and two inferior thyroidal arteries arising either directly from the subclavian or from the thyrocervical trunk. Modell[16] investigated the blood supply microscopically and found arteriovenous anastomoses and peculiar muscular cushions at the place where arteries branch. He attributed a blood flow regulating property to these cushions. The nervous supply to the thyroid was investigated by Nonidez,[17] who found abundant innervation of the vascular system in the thyroid but could find no anatomic evidence for direct nervous control of the cells of the acini. Attempts to demonstrate the effect on thyroid hormone secretion resulting from stimulation or denervation of the nerves leading to the thyroid have been equivocal. Friedgood and Cannon[18] reported that continuous stimulation of the cervical sympathetics anastomosed to the phrenic nerve produced nervousness, exophthalmos and the symptoms of hyperthyroidism. They suggested that these effects appeared to be mediated via the anterior pituitary with secretion of thyroid stimulating hormone as the direct factor stimulating the thyroid. Evidence suggests that the direct nervous supply controls only the arteries and veins in the thyroid.

THE NORMAL PHYSIOLOGY OF THE THYROID

The Function of the Thyroid Follicle. In essence, the function of the thyroid follicle is to remove adequate iodine from the blood, combine it with an organic molecule, probably a complex protein, and both store this protein and eventually break it down for future release (see Fig. 1). Since iodine is an integral part of the thyroid hormone and plays a major role in regulating thyroid activity, we plan to separate the events occurring in the physiology of the thyroid on the basis of the routes through the body traveled by iodine.

Pre-Thyroid Iodine Metabolism. Iodine, present in both food and water in varying concentrations, ultimately represents the principal source of the iodine contained in thyroid hormone. Iodine is readily absorbed from the gastrointestinal tract as inorganic iodide. Tracer experiments with radioactive iodine have shown that the absorption is essentially complete within sixty minutes after oral administration.[19] Iodine is excreted as iodide primarily through the kidneys. Several balance experiments were reported some time ago in which exhaustive efforts were made to determine all the ingested and all the excreted iodine. With careful attention to the smallest detail, it was possible to account for 90 to 95 per cent of the iodine ingested. The net result suggested that under normal situations well over half of the iodine was excreted in the urine. A variable proportion, from 3[20] to 27 per cent,[21] was found to be excreted in the feces. The excretion of iodine in the sweat may vary considerably depending on the amount of perspiration. In one experiment reported by Scheffer,[20] 42 per cent of the iodine accounted for in the excreta was found in the sweat. Iodine has also been demonstrated in milk and in saliva, although under ordinary circumstances these routes of elimination account for a very minor amount of the total iodine excreted.[20,21,22]

More accurate determinations of the routes of excretion of iodine have been made utilizing radioactive isotopes. It has been found that in the normal human, aproximately 60 per cent of a single dose of radioactive iodine is excreted in the urine within three days.[23,24] One to 3 per cent of the dose is found in the stool within this same period of time. The concentration of iodine in saliva and gastric secretions has been reported to be 4 to 100 times as great as in serum but ordinarily does not represent a means of loss of the radioiodine.[25] In patients with myxedema, fixation of radioiodine by the thyroid does not occur, and thus a more complete accounting of the ingested radioactivity may be made.[23,24] In these patients from 90 to 100 per cent of the ingested radioiodine may be recovered in the urine within a period of six to seven days. It appears

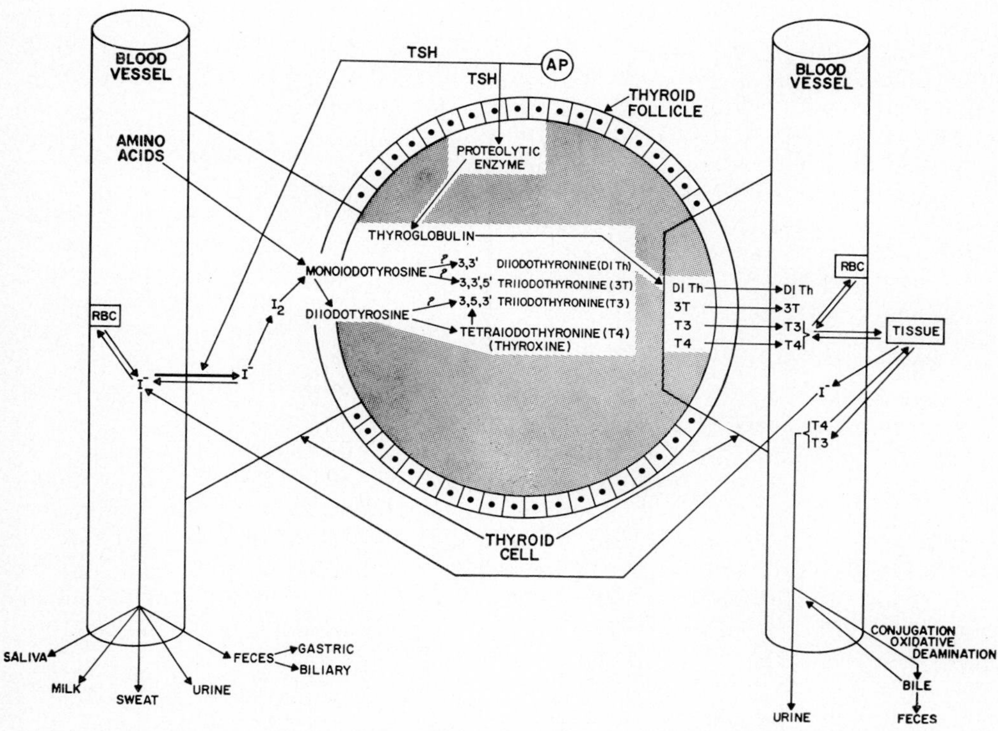

FIG. 1. Diagrammatic representation of iodine metabolism as it is presumed to occur under normal conditions.

that the kidney of a normal human clears iodide at the rate of approximately 33 cc. of serum per minute.[26] The concentration of iodine in the bile is generally quite high and usually is in the form of organic compounds of iodine which will be referred to later.

The initial fixation or trapping of iodide by the thyroid is apparently accomplished in two fashions. It appears that the thyroidal iodide is in some state of equilibrium with the serum iodide. It is impossible to evaluate quantitatively the equilibrium ratio if at the same time iodide is fixed in the thyroid by organic combination. The organic binding of iodine may be prevented, however, by the administration of antithyroid drugs of the thiouracil group which interfere with the oxidation of iodide. Such drugs do not disturb the thyroid's capacity to trap iodide. Vanderlaan and Vanderlaan[27] have demonstrated that when rats are given an adequate dose of propyl thiouracil followed by a tracer dose of radioiodine, the iodine is concentrated by the thyroid to an extent approximately 25 times greater than in blood. In rats previously made goitrous by the administration of propyl thiouracil this ratio was 250 to 1. Childs et al.[28] have shown that in patients with Graves' disease, the iodide trap concentrates about 350 times more iodide than does the serum. They observed that the concentration of I^{131} in the blocked thyroid parallelled that in the serum and that the administration of large "carriers" of iodide resulted in rates of loss of I^{131} from the serum which were almost identical with the curves of rate of loss of I^{131} from the thyroid.

That the trapping of iodide is a dynamic process probably dependent on certain intracellular enzymes is suggested in the observations made by Freinkel and Ingbar[29] and by Slingerland[30] who have studied the effects of temperature, oxygen concentration, *p*H, and various enzyme inhibitors on the capacity of thyroid slices to concentrate iodide in the presence of propyl thiouracil or tapazole. In these studies it was found that aerobic conditions were necessary for the concentration of iodide. The ability of the thyroid slices to concentrate iodide was markedly diminished by extremes of temperature or of *p*H. Many compounds which react with sulfhydryl groups were found to diminish the iodide concentrating function of thyroid slices. It was also found that compounds which depressed the iodide concentrating capacity of these thyroid preparations did not necessarily depress the respiration of the slice—though most of them did.

The details of how iodide trapped in the thyroid is converted to thyroglobulin or the various thyroid hormones which can be recovered from thyroglobulin have not been defined.

Intrathyroidal Iodine Metabolism. In the normal thyroid almost all of the thyroid iodine is contained in a protein molecule, thyroglobulin. Thyroglobulin has been characterized as a glycoprotein with a molecular weight estimated to be 680,000. Because of the large size of this molecule it is found normally only within the thyroid follicles as a colloid. It occurs in the circulation only after the cell membranes of the thyroid follicle have been damaged. The essential role of thyroglobulin is that of storing the thyroid hormones which are not diffusible.

Presumably the first step in the conversion of accumulated inorganic iodide to organic iodine by the thyroid involves the oxidation of iodide to free iodine or hypoiodite. This is presumptive since free iodine has never been isolated from the thyroid gland. Fawcett and Kirkwood[31] have, however, with chromatographic techniques obtained suggestive evidence for the presence of free iodine in the thyroids of rats under the influence of certain sulfonamides. It would appear that this oxidation of iodine occurs very rapidly and that the oxidized form of iodine reacts immediately with proteins or amino acids to form organic iodine.

Evidence for this presumed oxidation of iodide being an enzymatic process is meager. It is known that thyroid slices are capable of synthesizing labelled iodinated compounds from radioactive iodide. Previously, the integrity of the cell was considered crucial for this reaction. Recently, however, homogenates and cell-free preparations of thyroid have been reported by Fawcett and Kirkwood[32] to produce organically bound iodine. These same investigators have also reported that the addition of a cell-free preparation of thyroid tissue to iodide ion, cupric ion and tyrosine resulted in the iodination of tyrosine. It has been postulated that thiouracil and related drugs which inhibit the iodination of tyrosine exert their antithyroid effects by preventing the action of peroxidase, an enzyme known to occur in the thyroid and to be absent from the thyroids of animals under treatment with such drugs.

Since hydrolysis of thyroglobulin with alkali results in the release of diiodotyrosine and thyroxine, the presumption has been that these compounds are formed and then converted into the heavy protein molecule, thyroglobulin. Until recently, it was commonly accepted that thyroxine was the only hormone synthesized by the thyroid. Kendall first isolated thyroxine from the thyroid in 1915.[33] Its chemical structure was elucidated in 1927,[34] and it was synthesized in 1928 by Harington and associates.[35] Harington postulated early that the *in vivo* synthesis of thyroxine occurred as the result of the coupling of two molecules of diiodotyrosine. The yield from these methods has been greater than 25 per cent.

Recent studies done with radioactive iodine and various chromatographic methods of separation have resulted in the isolation of new and previously unsuspected iodinated amino acids and iodinated thyronines from the thyroid. Monoiodotyrosine has been found in direct extracts of thyroid tissue and thyroid hydrolysates. By specific activity measurements monoiodotyrosine would appear to be the natural precursor of diiodotyrosine. Trace amounts of monoiodohistidine have also been recovered from hydrolysates of thyroid tissue. This iodinated amino acid appears to play no physiologic role nor to be utilized in the synthesis of thyroid hormones.

Recent reviews of Roche[36] and by Michel[37] describe a series of imaginative and methodical studies by which three new iodinated thyronines or thyroid hormones have been recovered not only from the thyroid but also from the circulation. The first of these compounds to be identified as a new thyroid hormone was 3:5:3′ triiodothyronine. It was isolated from the serum by Gross and Pitt-Rivers[38,39,40] and from the thyroid by Roche, Lissitzky and Michel,[41] who also isolated and identified 3:3′ diiodothyronine and 3:3′:5′ triiodothyronine from thyroglobulin and from the serum of animals which had received radioactive iodine.[36]

There are several possibilities for the conversion of free iodine or hypoiodite to thyroxine and other iodinated thyronines. The most favored theory is that iodine reacts with tyrosine to form monoiodotyrosine and then diiodotyrosine. A coupling of two diiodotyrosine molecules would result in the formation of thyroxine. A coupling of two molecules of monoiodotyrosine would result in the synthesis of 3:3′ diiodothyronine. A condensation of one monoiodotyrosine and one diiodotyrosine would result in one or the other molecules of triiodothyronine. Theoretically thyronine may be iodinated to yield tetraiodothyronine, thyroxine, directly or consecutively from the mono-, di- and tri-iodo derivatives of thyronine.

Measurements of specific activity at varying intervals after the administration of I^{131} to laboratory animals strongly suggest that monoiodotyrosine and diiodotyrosine are precursors of thyroxine. Furthermore, it has been demonstrated chemically that diiodotyrosine can be oxidized directly to thyroxine by hydrogen peroxide in alkaline solution.

There are, however, many who find it difficult to accept the rearrangement of two molecules of diiodotyrosine to give a molecule of thyroxine. It has been suggested that the thyroid gland might elaborate an iodine-free thyroglobulin which might then be iodinated to a greater or lesser extent, depending upon the supply of iodine as well as upon other physiologic conditions.

If the hormonogenesis did prove to occur through a direct iodination of thyronine in the protein molecule, the presence of monoiodotyrosine and of diiodotyrosine in the thyroid would probably indicate a carrier function of these molecules. This suggested function is consistent with the observation of Roche et al.[36] that the thyroid has a dehalogenase which is capable of deiodinating monoiodotyrosine and diiodotyrosine—but is not capable of deiodinating any iodinated thyronines. Notwithstanding the arguments in favor of the direct iodination of thyronine, it must be pointed out that thyronine has not yet been isolated from thyroglobulin.

The thyroid hormones, following their synthesis, are stored within the follicle as thyroglobulin, a molecule which is too large to be transported across the intact acinar cell wall. This heavy protein has been recovered from the serum only after trauma to the acinar wall as occurs following heavy isotopic irradiation. Normally thyroglobulin is hydrolyzed by a protein whose presence and function were first demonstrated by de Robertis and associates.[42] More recently MacQuillan et al.[43] have isolated this protease system, a cathepsin with certain enzymatic properties which are similar to those of pepsin. Weiss[44] has postulated that there are two enzymes in this system—one a protease, the other a peptidase. It has been suggested, though not adequately proved, that such protease systems are activated by the thyrotrophic hormone of the pituitary. Certainly the rapid release of iodine from the thyroid following the administration of TSH is consistent with this theory.

The Metabolism of Thyroid Hormone. Only recently has it been possible to follow the fate of physiologic amounts of thyroid hormone. This has been made possible by the synthesis of various analogues of thyroxine and triiodothyronine, of high specific activity labeled with I^{131}. Although the data support the position that thyroxine is a thyroid hormone, it may well be that there are several thyroid hormones.

The thyroid secretes thyroxine into the circulation. Of this there is little doubt.[45–48] However, other iodinated compounds have been characterized in blood only after patients have been treated with radioiodine, thus permitting the small amounts of these substances to be identified by virtue of their radioactivity. One such compound in euthyroid people and patients with Graves' disease[38,49] or cancer of the thyroid is presumably[50] triiodothyronine. This substance may not only be secreted from the thyroid[51] but produced by the peripheral metabolism of thyroxine even in the thyroidectomized organism.[52] This has been demonstrated also in kidney slices.[53] The conversion of thyroxine to triiodothyronine has been reported[54] to be blocked with the butyl ester of 3,5-diiodo-4-OH-benzoic acid.

Other compounds which have been identified in blood are thyroglobulin after destructive doses of radioactive iodine to normal and cancerous thyroids[55–57] as well as a new iodine component, "compound X," in the serum of patients with functioning thyroid cancer.[58] This latter compound has a greater proportion of monoiodotyrosine than has thyroglobulin[57,58] as well as an electrophoretic mobility in serum greater than that of thyroxine or thyroglobulin. The other iodinated amino acids, monoiodotyrosine and diiodotyrosine, which normally occur in the thyroid, do not normally appear in the blood.

It has been known for some time that the thyroid hormone which circulates in blood is bound to proteins and is precipitated by reagents which precipitate proteins. In recent years the nature of this protein binding has been elucidated somewhat. Thyroxine is bound to a specific globulin which on zone electrophoresis occurs between the alpha-1 and alpha-2 globulin[59–67] and by Cohn fractionation occurs in Fractions IV-b and IV-9.[68] Thyroxine is bound more strongly than triiodothyronine,[64,69] which may account for the rapid disappearance of the latter substance from the circulation. This thyroxine-binding protein has a limited capacity to bind thyroxine and is completely saturated at serum thyroxine levels which are 2 to 3 times normal.[63,66] When this alpha globulin is saturated, additional amounts of thyroxine are bound to albumin.[63] There has been only one report[70] of a qualitative difference in transport mechanism, and this was an unusual instance of thyroxine binding by human gamma globulin. Most differences in the transport mechanisms of normal and abnormal patients are quantitative.[65] There is an increase in the thyroxine-binding protein in the sera of pregnant women[67] and a decrease in nephrosis.[69,71] The latter is increased in nephrotic patients treated with adrenocortical steroids.[72] The physiologic significance of the *in vitro* uptake of radioactive thyroxine and triiodothyronine by red blood cells and red blood stroma[73,74] is not clear.

The levorotatory isomer is undoubtedly more active than d-thyroxine. Foster et al.[75] found l-thyroxine twice as effective as the racemic mixture in increasing the O_2 consumption of guinea pigs. Pitt-Rivers and Lerman[76] concluded from comparative studies that l-thyroxine is ten times as active as d-thyroxine measured by the rise in BMR in subjects with myxedema. There is a relatively long latent period after the intravenous administration of thyroxine before any observable effects occur. Boothby and Baldes[77] noted that there was no effect on the BMR of myxedematous subjects for 24 hours. However, Logan and Lien[78] have reported a noticeable effect on the BMR of guinea pigs as early as four hours after administering thyroxine. After thyroxine therapy has been discontinued in myxedematous patients, the BMR and clinical status do not revert to pretreatment levels for 30 to 50 days.

Studies have been made with thyroglobulin and thyroxine labeled with radioiodine. Following the intravenous injections of tracer amounts of labeled thyroxine or labeled triiodothyronine the blood showed disappearance rates fitting the curves of a double exponential of the form $Q = Q_1e^{-\gamma t} + Q_2e^{-\gamma t}$.[79,80] The first rate of disappearance from the blood was very rapid and was thought probably due to the diffusion of the thyroxine from blood plasma into the extracellular fluid. The second slow disappearance rate was presumed to represent the combined catabolism and excretion of thyroxine. The initial volume of distribution of the labeled thyroxine was roughly equivalent to the blood plasma volume, and the second volume of distribution approximated the extracellular fluid volume.[79–81] The largest proportion of the thyroxine is apparently catabolized in the tissues by deiodination, although a certain amount is excreted in the urine mainly as diiodotyrosine. Salter[82] has reported a concentration of protein-bound iodine in lymph which is somewhat less than that in blood.

After man is injected with an intravenous dose of radioactive thyroxine, 30 per cent of the radioactivity appears in the urine and thyroid after 24 hours.[81] After the intravenous administration of radioactive thyroxine the biologic half life was approximately seven days in euthyroid persons;[83,84] a more rapid rate of disappearance occurred in exophthalmic goiter[85,86] and a slower rate in myxedema.[86] The daily turnover of thyroid hormone for the euthyroid person[87] is similar to the minimum oral dose, 150 micrograms, of l-thyroxine necessary to maintain the myxedematous human.[77,88] In the nonthyrotoxic person there is close agreement between the rates of thyroid hormone degradation and synthesis.[89]

Although thyroxine occurs in many tissues in the body, a major tissue involved in the metabolic alteration of this hormone is the liver.[90–92] After the administration of labeled thyroxine or triiodothyronine to the experimental animal[93–96] or its perfusion through the liver,[97] the glycuronide of these thyroid hormones may be detected in the bile. The biliary excretion of radioiodine is increased in experimental hyperthyroidism after the administration of labeled thyroxine and decreased in hypothyroidism.[98] There is an active enterohepatic circulation of thyroxine,[99-101] for the glycuronide of the thyroid hormones is apparently deconjugated and free hormone absorbed from the intestine. Even when all the formed thyroid hormone passes through the liver[102] there is no manifestation of thyroid hormone insufficiency. The fecal radioiodine represents material secreted not only through the bile, but through the gut wall itself. The liver and bile may be a mechanism whereby excess thyroxine is eliminated from the organism,[100] although the conjugation of thyroid hormone in the liver may be considered a normal physiologic mechanism.

Elmer and Scheps[103] investigated large quantities of urine from euthyroid and hyperthyroid patients. In all euthyroid patients they found less than 2 per cent of the urine iodine as "thyroxine" iodine. This percentage they point out, however, merely represents the solubility of inorganic iodide in butanol, so they concluded that normally no thyroxine was excreted in the urine. They obtained similar results from analysis of the urine from hyperthyroid patients. Mitolo[104] investigated the form in which iodine occurs in the urine and claimed to have demonstrated from 1 to 9 micrograms of "thyroxine" iodine per liter of urine. More recently, the nature of urine iodine was investigated,[48] and a similar but variable proportion of the urine iodine was found in the thyroxine fraction. That this iodine was thyroxine was confirmed by paper chromatographic separation and recrystallization techniques. A larger (3 to 68 per cent of the total urinary iodine) proportion of diiodotyrosine-like iodine was found in the urine. The precise nature of this fraction was unknown but probably represented organic iodine compounds.

Although much is known about the factors which control the secretion of thyroid hormone into the circulation, there are less data about the factors that influence the peripheral disposition of the hormone and so-called "tissue sensitivity." In acute experiments it has been found that cold[105,106] and epinephrine[107] induce a fall in the PBI—protein-bound iodine—presumably because of increased peripheral utilization of thyroid hormone. In myxedematous or panhypopituitary patients, ACTH or the corticosteroids have no effect on the degradation rate of administered labeled thyroxine.[108]

Although monoiodotyrosine and diiodotyrosine do not normally occur in the serum, these substances have been reported[109] in the serum of certain patients with familial goiter. When radioactive iodotyrosines are administered to normal persons, the substances disappear rapidly from the circulation and the radioiodine in the urine occurs predominantly as iodide.[110] In certain patients with familial goiter radioactive iodotyrosines are excreted as such without significant radioiodide,[109] presumably because of a thyroid and general somatic failure of dehalogenation.[111]

THE RELATIONSHIP OF THE PITUITARY AND OTHER ENDOCRINE ORGANS TO THYROID FUNCTION

Pituitary. A relationship between the pituitary and the thyroid has been suspected since 1851 when Nièpce[112] observed that humans with endemic goiter or cretinism had enlarged anterior pituitary glands. In 1888 Rogowitsch[113] observed in rabbits that total thyroidectomy results in changes in the anterior pituitary, i.e., the appearance of certain large granular cells and of increased vacuolization. In 1912 Cushing[114] noted that the thyroids of dogs involuted following hypophysectomy. In 1926 Foster and Smith[115] demonstrated that hypophysectomy results in a fall in metabolic rate which can be reversed by daily transplants of anterior pituitary or by the administration of desiccated thyroid.

Following early experiments[116] in hypophysectomized tadpoles and rats it was shown that pituitary transplants and extracts, when injected, repair the atrophied thyroid. A large number of investigators reported that there exists in the anterior pituitary a thyroid stimulating hormone (TSH) which has been variously labelled as thyrotrophin, thyrotrophic hormone or thyrotropic hormone.

There have been many attempts to extract from animal pituitaries a pure and potent preparation containing only thyrotrophic hormone. As yet, however, it appears that pure crystalline TSH has not been prepared. Reviews of this subject have been prepared by White[117] and by Albert.[118] TSH is most likely a protein with a molecular weight of about 10,000.

Since the exact nature of thyrotrophic hormone is unknown, its quantitation is dependent upon bioassay techniques. These methods of assay are dependent upon either direct action of TSH on the thyroid gland or secondary effects subsequent to release of thyroid hormone. Of primary importance in such assays is the sensitivity of various species to the hormone. The day-old chick, the guinea pig and the tadpole have very sensitive thyroids. Notwithstanding the fact that the thyroids of hypophysectomized rats are much more sensitive to TSH than are the thyroids of intact rats, this assay preparation is considerably less sensitive than one can develop in animals listed above. Methods dependent upon direct action of the hormone on the thyroid are: (1) increase in weight of the thyroid in the chick,[119] (2) increase of the mean cell height in thyroid of the chick or guinea pig[120] and (3) loss of iodine from the thyroids of chicks.[121] A method dependent upon secondary effects subsequent to release of thyroid hormone is the acceleration of tadpole metamorphosis.[122]

Recently several newer and sensitive methods of assay for TSH have been described. It has been reported[123] that thyrotrophic activity equivalent to 0.0001 U.S.P. unit can be detected by following the increase of I^{131} in the blood of guinea pigs previously given tracer doses of I^{131} and thyroxine and that the intracardiac injection of TSH results in a quantitative increase in the concentration of P^{32} in the thyroid. This method of assay is reported to detect as little as 0.00025 U.S.P. units of TSH activity. More recently,[124] with *in vivo* techniques of following the release of radioactive iodine from the chick thyroid, one can detect between 5 and 40 U.S.P. milliunits of TSH. This test[125] requires chicks which concentrate more than 15 per cent of a dose of I^{131} and the administration at different sites of thyroxine and propyl thiouracil during the testing period.

One study[126] indicates that TSH when administered to intact chicks causes, within six hours, a significant decrease of thyroid iodine. This purging of thyroid iodine is maximum within twenty-four hours after administering the pituitary hormone. A significant increase in mean cell height of the thyroid was not evident until eighteen hours after injecting TSH and was maximum at thirty hours. Keating et al.[121] demonstrated a decrease in thyroid radioiodine and an increase in mean cell height twenty-four hours after injecting TSH but no increase in avidity for I^{131} until twenty-four hours after the second daily injection of TSH. Thus it appears that the primary action of TSH is to mobilize and promote secretion of the thyroid's hormonal iodine. De Robertis[42] has suggested that this effect is due to the activation of a proteolytic enzyme which breaks down the thyroglobulin molecule to thyroxine, a molecule small enough to be transported across the thyroid cell. This thesis is supported by recent reports. MacQuillan et al.[43] have isolated a proteolytic enzyme from the thyroid which exerts a proteolytic effect on hemoglobin. Weiss[44] has isolated a protease and a peptidase from the thyroid, both of which are presumed to play a role in the hydrolysis of thyroglobulin. Alpers et al.[127] have demonstrated proteolytic activity in the thyroid which hydrolyzes thyroglobulin. A direct action of TSH on these enzymes *in vitro* has not been demonstrated consistently. We cannot as yet say that the increase in thyroid cell mass as well as the increased avidity for iodine in the thyroid treated with TSH are secondary only to the purging of the thyroid hormonal iodine.

Several investigators[128,129] have demonstrated that TSH, when administered to guinea pigs, results in a picture very similar to classic Graves' disease, i.e., a diffuse hyperplasia of the thyroid, with an increased rate of oxygen consumption, exophthalmos, muscle weakness and histologic changes in the muscles similar to those described in Graves' disease. Very early these observations led to the hypothesis that Graves' disease is due to an increased secretion of thyrotrophic hormone. Rawson and Starr[15] have not been able to demonstrate active TSH in the urine of patients with untreated Graves' disease. However, in studies done with *in vitro* techniques in which thyroid tissue and other tissues were bathed in media containing TSH it was demonstrated[130] that the TSH is inactivated by thyroid tissue and to a lesser degree by thymic and lymph nodal tissues. No other tissues studied had this effect on the thyroid-stimulating effect of the pituitary extract. Furthermore, it was found that thyroid tissue is incapable of inactivating gonadotrophic hormone.

In view of the fact that this inactivated TSH could be reactivated by thiouracil, a strong reducing agent, in the same fashion that TSH inactivated by elemental iodine, an oxidizing agent, can be reactivated by thiouracil and other reducing agents, we have postulated that TSH exerts its action on the thyroid through reduction. TSH possibly acts as a hydrogen donor to the thyroid cell.[126]

It has been observed that the administration of excessive amounts of thyroid hormone to rats results in an involution of the thyroid not unlike that seen in hypophysectomized animals. This has been explained on the basis of a depression of the pituitary's capacity for producing and secreting TSH. We have not been able to demonstrate an absence of TSH from the pituitaries of rats subjected to an excessive administration of thyroid hormone. Another possible explanation, however, is that the increased level of thyroid hormone inhibits the action of TSH on the thyroid cell. This phenomenon has been noted by Cortell and Rawson[131] in hypophysectomized rats treated with thyroxine and TSH.

Other Endocrine Organs. Evidence suggests that other endocrine organs are also closely related to the function of the thyroid. Starr and Patton[132] reported in 1934 that the thyroids of mature guinea pigs responded to TSH with a greater stimulation when the hormone was administered during the luteal phase of the estrous cycle than it did in the estrogenic phase. Gassner[133] has found in rats on a diet deficient in iodine that estrone and diethylstilbestrol not only increased the involutional action of iodine but that they also increased the storage of iodine by the thyroid. Money and associates[134] have observed that several gonadal steroids affect the uptake of radioiodine by the rat thyroid.

Soffer[135] and Money[134] have both observed that, whereas adrenalin when administered to rats produces a decreased pickup of I^{131} by the thyroid, the same stimulus when administered to adrenalectomized rats causes a marked increase in the collection of I^{131}. Money has pursued these studies in rats on an iodine-deficient diet receiving ACTH or various adrenal steroids. He has observed that ACTH, cortisone, Compound A, Compound L and desoxycorticosterone, if administered in large enough amounts, cause a decreased concentration of I^{131}.

Forsham, Thorn, Prunty and Hills[136] have induced remissions in patients with Graves' disease by administering ACTH. Wolfson et al.[137] have observed decreased thyroid function in patients given cortisone or ACTH over a long period of time.

It has been observed that total thyroidectomy and its resultant myxedematous state result in a failure of ovulation and persistent graafian follicles without the development of corpora lutea.[138]

Total thyroidectomy or the induction

of hypothyroidism by the administration of thiouracil in the rat results in a decreased adrenal size as well as in a decreased tolerance for stress.[139] It has been observed also that the administration of the thyroid hormone to intact rats in excess results in hyperplasia of the adrenal.[140]

The Effects of Environment on the Thyroid. Several investigators[141,143] have reported that the exposure of laboratory animals to cold stimulates the thyroid. In two of these studies the stimulus was quantitated by demonstrating an increased mean cell height of the thyroid, and in another study an increased collection and turnover of radioactive iodine was observed. It might be postulated that this stimulus was excited by an effect of the cold on some temperature control center in the midbrain. Support for this thesis comes from the fact that stalk-sectioned animals do not demonstrate any change in the thyroid on exposure to cold.[144] Since it has been demonstrated that animals in the cold require more thyroxine to prevent the goitrogenic effect of thiouracil than do those exposed to warmer temperatures,[145] the effects of cold might be explained on the basis of an increased need for thyroid hormone by the peripheral tissues, with the stimulus mediated via the midbrain and pituitary. This effect of cold on the thyroid has also been demonstrated in the thyroids of newly hatched chicks.[146] When the eggs were incubated at temperatures of 96.8° F., the thyroids of the newly hatched chicks weighed 7.38 mg., whereas the thyroids of chicks hatched from eggs which had been incubated at 102.2° F. weighed 2.19 mg.

The effect of general body irradiation on the uptake of radioiodine by the thyroid has recently been investigated.[147–149] With the smaller doses, 800 to 1000 r, there was observed at two hours an increased uptake of I^{131} which lasted for one day, following which there occurred a decreased uptake of I^{131}. Animals exposed to the larger doses of x-ray manifested increased uptakes of I^{131}. The decreased uptake of I^{131} observed initially might be attributed to an increased output of adrenal steroids. The increased uptake, on the other hand, might be attributed to starvation as a result of x-ray sickness. At any rate, it has been demonstrated that the thyroids of starved animals have an increased avidity for radioiodine.[141]

Exposure of mice to darkness stimulates the thyroid, as evidenced by increases in the growth of the thyroid and in its avidity for I^{131}.[150] On the other hand, continuous exposure to light results in a suppression of growth and function of the thyroid.[150]

Many of the changes in the thyroid induced by environmental stimuli might be attributed to the effects of adrenal steroids on the body economy. This decrease in thyroid function with increased adrenocortical function has been demonstrated[151] after exposure to low atmospheric pressure. Forced muscular exercise, which resulted in depression of the thyroid's avidity for I^{131}, was followed by an increased urinary excretion of iodide.[152] The stress of a major surgical procedure increased[153,154] the hormonal radioiodine in patients who received a previous tracer dose. The PBI was often acutely elevated in patients subjected to psychologic stress.[155]

Pharmacologic Agents Affecting the Thyroid. It has long been accepted that an iodine deficiency results in the development of goiters. This is discussed in the section on nodular goiters. The occurrence of sporadic goiters in areas not deficient in iodine has been, until recently, unexplained. A possible explanation of their etiology may be found in the demonstration of a wide variety of normally occurring goitrogenic agents. The first experimental demonstration of a positive goitrogen resulted from the investigations of Chesney et al.[156] who, while studying experimental syphilis in rabbits, observed large hyperplastic goiters and demonstrated that these goiters were associated with low rates of oxygen consumption and could be prevented by the administration of iodine. However, if iodine was administered after the development of large goiters, their animals developed a rather severe hyperthyroidism which occasionally was lethal. They also showed that the positive goitrogen in these experiments was in the cabbage in the rabbit's diet. Marine et al.[157] confirmed their observations and suggested that the goitrogen in cabbage was a nitrile which was abundant in the cabbage being used. One of the most important studies done with the positive naturally occurring goitrogens is that of Greer et al.,[158] who have demonstrated in humans that certain foods, i.e., turnips and the brassica group of foods, have the capacity to interfere with the utilization of I^{131} by the human thyroid. From turnips they have isolated and identified L-5-vinyl-2-thio-oxazolidone as the active thyroid inhibitor, which suggests that there exist in natural foods agents which may account for the development of goiters in our nonendemic goiter regions.

Further evidence for positive goitrogens was discovered in 1941 by MacKenzie et al.,[159] who reported that rats receiving sulfaguanidine developed large goiters. Shortly thereafter Richter and Clisby,[160] while studying rat poisons, observed that animals receiving thiocarbamide developed large hyperplastic goiters. Kennedy and Purves[161] observed that rats maintained on a rapeseed diet developed large goiters which were associated with low rates of oxygen consumption and thyroidectomy cells in the anterior pituitary. Subsequent studies demonstrated that the goitrogenic agent in rapeseed was allyl thiourea.

These demonstrations of positive goitrogens excited extensive studies of related chemical agents and resulted in the discovery that there exists a large variety of natural and synthetic goitrogenic agents. Reports by the MacKenzies[162] and by Astwood[163] which appeared in 1943 illustrated that most of the sulfonamides, thiourea and thiouracil had marked goitrogenic activity which could not be prevented by the administration of iodine. Potassium thiocyanate, a less active goitrogen, did not produce goiters if iodine was administered concomitantly; an intact and functioning pituitary was necessary to the development of such goiters; and the prolonged administration of these drugs resulted in a fall in oxygen consumption to myxedematous levels. It was postulated that the goiters occurred as the result of increased secretion of TSH by the anterior pituitary secondary to the hypothyroidism.[163]

The explanation that the goiters observed in rats maintained on thiouracil are due to a compensatory increased secretion of TSH by the pituitary is plausible. However, it is probable that at least one other factor is involved in the production of such goiters. Rats given thiouracil showed a significant increase in cell height within 24 hours after the drug was administered in the food or drinking water. Hence, we suggest the hypothesis that thiouracil augments the action of TSH. Thiouracil markedly increases the response of the thyroid to TSH in chicks. Propylthiouracil, one of the most active goitrogens tested in the rat, was found to have the greatest capacity for augmenting the action of TSH.[164] Furthermore, Albert et al.[164,165] have demonstrated with *in vitro* studies that these goitrogenic agents which are also strong reducing agents are capable of reactivating TSH following inactivation by elemental iodine, an oxidizing agent.

Since these classic original observations, a long list (Table 1, p. 944) of agents with varying chemical structures have been found to exert an effect on the thyroid, mostly of an inhibitory nature. Most of the thyroid inhibitors, have been found to be goitrogenic to varying degrees. The thiocarbamides constitute the largest series of agents studied. A second group is made up of aniline derivatives, which with some modification lead to the third group, the aromatic phenols. Inorganic chemicals constitute the fourth and fifth groups, namely inorganic anions and metals, respectively. A sixth or miscellaneous group includes thyroid-inhibiting or goitrogenic compounds which do not fit into any of the above groups.

The thiocarbamides, i.e., thiouracil,

2-mercaptoimidazole, etc., have been demonstrated to interfere with thyroid function by preventing the oxidation of iodide, thus preventing the utilization of iodine in the synthesis of thyroid hormone.[166] It was observed that, whereas the thyroids under the influence of thiouracil or related agents were able to concentrate only small amounts of iodine,[167] iodine was present as iodide and never incorporated into diiodotyrosine or into thyroxine.[27] It has been suggested that these agents exert this effect by inhibiting an oxidative enzyme necessary for the oxidation of iodide.[168,169] It is not readily appreciated that some drugs employed clinically fall into the group of thiocarbamides. Claims have been made from laboratory studies that barbiturates[170–172] and regitin[172] have a direct antithyroid effect. Other agents which might be included among the thiocarbamide derivatives and have wide clinical use, like penicillin,[173] have no effect on the thyroid.

A theory with experimental support has been presented that the aromatics (sulfonamides, para-aminobenzoic acid, resorcinol, etc.) and possibly iodides in excess compete with tyrosine for the oxidized iodine in the thyroid gland.[174] This interference with the iodination of tyrosine interferes with the synthesis of thyroid hormone and is followed by chemical hypothyroidism. It is of interest that the aromatic phenol, dinitrophenol, although it causes a fall in PBI,[175,176] does not lead to increased pituitary thyrotrophin[175] or have a goitrogenic action.

It has been demonstrated that thiocyanate interferes with the trapping of iodide by thyroid slices.[177] The goiters produced by thiocyanate are incapable of concentrating even iodide if the drug level is above a critical level.[178] It has also been demonstrated *in vivo* that thiocyanate discharges stored iodide from the thyroid under the control of thiouracil.[179] Studies reported by one group[180,181] have demonstrated that several monovalent anions, i.e., perchlorate, chlorate, hypochlorite, periodate, iodate, biiodate and nitrate, share with thiocyanate[178] the properties of blocking the iodide trap of the thyroid and of discharging iodide from the gland. These agents have also been found to have certain goitrogenic properties. Potassium perchlorate has been shown to be an effective agent in controlling the overactive thyroid of Graves' disease.[182]

Another well-known inhibitor to the thyroid is iodide. This halogen is well-known to the clinician as an effective inhibitor in controlling the hyperthyroidism of Graves' disease. Its effects are quite different from those produced by thiouracil or other goitrogenic agents, since iodide results in an involution of the hyperplastic goiter of this malady and in a storage of thyroglobulin in the thyroid follicles. By following the histologic changes in serial biopsies taken before any therapy and after control of the hyperthyroidism with thiouracil, and in the same thyroids which were removed after continued treatment with thiouracil and added iodides, it has been shown that this involutional or therapeutic effect of iodide can be separated from the nutritive role of iodide. In this study[183] the pretreatment biopsies showed the classic thyroid hyperplasia of Graves' disease, which was not decreased in the biopsies taken after treatment with thiouracil had restored the patients to euthyroidism. However, the addition of iodides caused an involution of the thyroid. Since the thyroglobulin iodine values in the operatively removed thyroid were very low, i.e., 2.7 mg. per 100 gm. of tissue, it can be said that the involutional effect of iodide occurred notwithstanding the fact that thiouracil was given in a dose great enough to prevent the utilization of iodine in the synthesis of thyroid hormone.

It has been suggested[184] that iodides exert their therapeutic effects by preventing the trapping of iodide and also that iodide works much like the aromatic goitrogens by competing with tyrosine for any oxidized iodine.[31] Notwithstanding the experimental evidence presented by both of these groups, it must be pointed out that the hyperplastic thyroids of Graves' disease after successful

TABLE 1. PHARMACOLOGIC AGENTS AFFECTING THE THYROID

INORGANIC ANIONS	METALS	THIOCARBAMIDE DERIVATIVES	ANILINE DERIVATIVES	AROMATIC PHENOLS	MISCELLANEOUS
iodide fluoride thiocyanate nitrate chlorate biiodate hypochlorite iodate periodate perchlorate	antimony cobalt	thiourea thiosemicarbazone 2-mercapto-imidazole 2-thiohydantoin ergothioneine aminothiazole L-5-vinyl-2-thio-oxazolidone 2-mercaptothiazole 2-thiouracil 5-iodo-2-thiouracil thiopyridone-2 thiopiperidone-2 promizole regitine barbiturates	p-aminobenzoic acid p-aminosalicylic acid phenothiazine amphenone "B" sulfonamides antistine phenylbutazone chlorpromazine	resorcinol p-hydroxypropiophenone hesperidine methyl chalcone dinitrophenol	nitrogen mustard disulfiram colchicine

treatment with iodide alone contain even greater than normal amounts of iodinated thyroglobulin.[185] Wolff and Chaikoff[186,187] showed that the level of inorganic iodine in the blood controls, in part, the synthesis of thyroid hormone. When rats were given I^{127} sufficient to produce a concentration of 35 micrograms per cent or more and I^{131} was then administered, a certain amount of the I^{131} was concentrated in the thyroid. This was shown to be inorganic and rapidly disappeared from the thyroid. None of the I^{131} was incorporated into thyroid hormone, as occurs with normal plasma levels of inorganic iodide. Additional experiments carried out over a longer period of time showed that after two days or so the thyroid regained its ability to synthesize thyroid hormone regardless of the level of iodide in the blood. Stanley[188] has examined the effect of large carrier doses of I^{127} on the synthesis of thyroid hormone in normal and hyperthyroid humans and suggests that a high level of serum iodide inhibits the synthesis of thyroid hormone. Stanley has shown that the level of iodide in the plasma necessary to suppress the synthesis of thyroid hormone is lower in hyperthyroid patients with a normal thyroid.

It has also been suggested[120,189] that this therapeutic effect of iodide in Graves' disease is due to an inhibitory action on the reaction that occurs between thyroid cell and thyrotrophic hormone. Evidence for this thesis comes from the observations that (1) iodide inhibits the action of TSH on the thyroid of hypophysectomized rats; (2) the *in vitro* inactivation of TSH by explants of thyroid tissue is inhibited by adding iodide to the medium; and (3) whereas the urine of untreated thyrotoxic patients contains no active thyrotrophic hormone, a thyroid-stimulating factor is demonstrated in the urine of thyrotoxic patients shortly after instituting treatment with iodine.

This thesis may be further supported by the observation[190] that pituitary preparations rich in thyrotrophic hormone labeled by esterification with S^{35} labeled sulfate are concentrated in the thyroids of rats to a significantly greater degree when the animals are receiving an iodine-deficient diet than when the animals are receiving adequate or excess amounts of iodides.

Of the other halogens, chloride and bromide are without inhibitory effect on the thyroid. There is some evidence, however, that fluoride[191] might exert some inhibitory effect on the thyroid without having a goitrogenic action.

Among the inorganic chemicals which might affect the thyroid are the cations, cobalt and antimony. Although cobalt chloride seems to have been goitrogenic in anemic patients[192,193] its administration to normal children,[194] mice, rats or pregnant women[195] did not induce disturbances in thyroid function. Antimony, on the other hand, was reported[196] to induce glandular hyperplasia in the thyroid which could be prevented by the simultaneous administration of thyroxine.

Other drugs used clinically and checked for antithyroid activity and found to have none include the tetracycline antibiotics[197,198] and reserpine.[199] Nitrogen mustard[200] and phenylbutazone[201] may have some antithyroid properties.

ACTIONS OF THYROID HORMONE

Relation to Structure. "Thyroid hormone" has been used as a generic term to indicate any substance that will relieve human myxedema when properly administered.[202] As such, this definition would not require that this substance be thyroidal in origin or have a specific physical and chemical constitution. However, almost all contain iodine substituted in an inner aromatic ring of a chemical grouping named thyronine.[203] Some bromine substituted thyronines have hormonal activity[204,205] as well as the diphenyl thioether analogue of thyroxine.[206] At present, various forms of the thyroid hormone exist including thyroglobulin, various degradation products of thyroglobulin, thyroxine recovered from thyroglobulin[207] or synthesized chemically,[208] other substituted thyronines,[209] various crystalline products from the hydrolysis of iodinated proteins,[210] and the circulating and active form of the thyroid hormone. Thyroglobulin is reported[211] to have greater calorigenic activity than thyroxine or than can be accounted for by the thyroxine iodine of thyroglobulin. One cannot justly claim that the substance with the greatest biologic activity per mole is indeed the thyroid hormone. It has been reported[212] that thyroxine polypeptides obtained from tryptic digests of thyroglobulin have a greater biologic effect than thyroxine.

With the study of the structural analogues of thyroxine, some insight has been gained as to what portions of the structure of thyroxine are necessary for its physiologic action[213–215] and what substitutions make for the most effective antithyroxine agents. The two

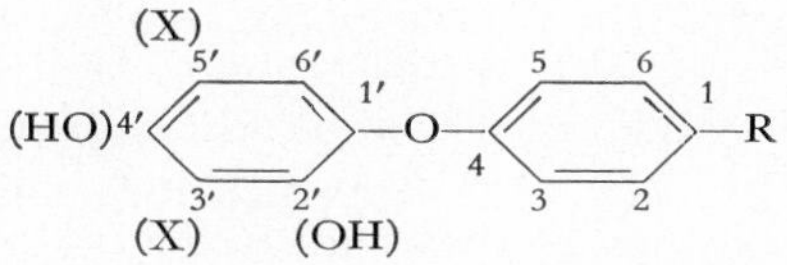

(X)
5′ 6′ 5 6
(HO)4′ 1′ —O— 4 1 —R
3′ 2′ 3 2
(X) (OH)

halogens at 3′ and 5′ appear necessary only for maximal activity, iodine being more effective than bromine or chlorine.[204,216–219] The side chain (R) at position 1 of the inner ring must be a polar group such as $CHNH_2COOH, NH_2$, $—CH = CH\ COOH$, $—CH_2CH_2COOH$ and $—COOH$, although tetraiodothyroacetic acid and triiodothyroacetic acid have only a tenth of the activity of triiodothyronine in the prevention of goiter.[220] It has been suggested that the acetic acid analogues of thyroxine and triiodothyronine, namely tetraiodothyroacetic acid[221] and triiodothyroacetic acid,[222] can make a myxedematous person euthyroid, and there may be some dissociation between the effect on cholesterol and the clinical signs and symptoms. Such a variety suggests that a simple compound itself may be active, because most of these compounds have only one reactive group.

In general, the diiodothyronine framework provides the optimum starting point for maximal hormonal activity. In mammalian studies, thyroxine itself (where R is alanine, all four X's are I, and the hydroxyl is in the 4′ position) has until now consistently proved the most active single compound. Recently, triiodothyronine, which is similar to thyroxine except that there is an iodine atom absent at the 5′ position, has been found to be three to five times more active than thyroxine in increasing oxygen consumption[40,223–228] and in its antigoitrogenic effects.[226]

Most compounds which were active thyroxine antagonists[229–231] contained iodine in the 2 and 6 positions counting from the oxygen bridge. 2′, 6′-Diiodothyronine exhibited thyroxine inhibition as well.[232] The alkyl esters of 3, 5-diiodo-4-OH benzoic acid[233] as well as the monoiodo derivative[234] also formed a series of potent antithyroxine agents, with the butyl ester most effective.[235] The simplest substances tested having antithyroxine activity are those which contain predominantly the diiodophenoxy group.[230,236,237] It is interesting that on the basis of studies with radioactive thyroxine and the butyl ester of 3, 5-diiodo-4-OH-benzoic acid, the site of action of this thyroxine analogue was considered to be in the blocking of the conversion of thyroxine to triiodothyronine.[238,239] Also, the physiologic effect of triiodothyronine was enhanced and its excretion diminished by this analogue.[238] The block to thyroidal uptake of I^{131} by this thyroxine analogue appeared to be by no other mechanism than the breakdown of this compound to iodide, which then exerted the same effect as inorganic iodide.[240]

Thyronine[241] and a thyroxine-free peptone[242] have been reported effective against thyrotoxicosis and experimental hyperthyroidism. Dibromotyrosine and diiodotyrosine have also been claimed[243–245] to depress various aspects of thyroid function, but this has been questioned.[246] 3-Fluorotyrosine[247,248] and 3-fluoro-4-hydroxyphenyl-acetic acid[249] have also been studied. The latter may exert some noncompetitive effects.[250] Although the metabolic response of rats to thyroxine or desiccated thyroid is lowered by methylthiouracil[251] and animals made hypothyroid by thiouracil are less responsive metabolically to thyroxine,[252] one gains no insight into the structure of thyroid hormone from such studies. This may well represent a toxic effect of the thiouracil derivative rather than a peripheral antagonism to thyroxine.[253]

The principal generalization which can be made[229,250] is that the configuration

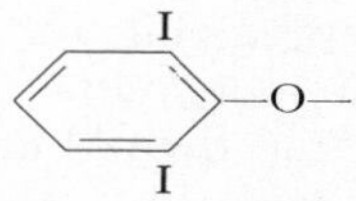

I
—O—
I

has exhibited antithyroxine activity with a wide variety of different groups substituted on each end.

Fundamental Actions. The extreme variety of effects noted after the administration of thyroid hormone may well reflect a primary action of this hormonal substance at one biochemical site. All the changes noted may then be the consequence of this fundamental action. The ubiquitous nature of thyroid hormone effects may be appreciated from the number and types of enzymes affected.

In general, the oxidizing enzymes are usually decreased after thyroidectomy and increased after administering a thyroid hormone. Thyroid hormone also seems to increase the activity of the carbohydrases, amidases, transferases and proteolytic enzymes. The esterases, however, show no consistent change in concentration with either thyroidectomy or thyroid administration.

Since diffuse changes are induced after concentrations of thyroxine in body fluids of 10^{-7} M, it has been tempting to consider this hormone as acting either as a catalyst on "the fundamental reaction" or in a more general fashion as a coenzyme for many reactions. Of course, the concentration at any histologic or biochemical site may well be many times in excess of this figure. This "reaction" is as yet unidentified, although many suggestions have been offered. Perhaps all oxygen consumption and indirectly the various metabolic processes are regulated by the effect of thyroxine on cytochrome c.[254] However, it is difficult to feel secure in the specificity of action of thyroxine on cytochrome c when adrenalectomy, like thyroidectomy, will produce a fall in total body cytochrome c.[255] Until the relationship of this iron-containing enzyme to the other enzymes is established, it is presumptious to conclude that thyroxine affects certain enzymes like xanthine oxidase, cholinesterase and lipase via its effect on cytochrome c.

More recently the hypothesis has been presented[256] that thyroxine may exert its metabolic effects by "uncoupling" a specific oxidative phosphorylation occurring at a rate-limiting step. The decrease in metabolic efficiency which would accompany such a process might be more than offset by the enhanced rate of oxidation, which would yield, in a given period, more total utilizable energy. Indeed, it has been found that thyroxine *in vitro* depresses the ratio of esterified, i.e., high-energy, phosphorus to oxygen of tissue preparations.[218,257–260] Not only thyroxine but also what may be the active thyroid hormone, triiodothyronine, will dissociate phosphorylation from respiration and even depress the respiration absolutely.[261] Other substituted phenols[262] as well as diiodothyronine[263] and iodine,[263] but not iodide, had a similar action. Oxidative phosphorylation may be the pivotal area for the action of thyroid hormone, for the association of the tricarboxylic acid cycle and cell respiration through phosphorylation is less tenuous.[264] The crucial role of enzymes in the effect of thyroxine on phosphorylation is given further support in the observed reduction by enzyme poisons of the elevated P^{32} turnover following treatment with thyroid hormone.[265] That the ubiquitous high-energy phosphorus compounds may control to some extent many phases of metabolism may be appreciated from the study[266] in which decreased oxygen consumption because of swelling mitochondria was in turn attributed to a decrease in adenosine triphosphate which was present in the hyperthyroid state.

In general, it may be stated that except for the aforementioned demonstration of an *in vitro* effect of thyroxine on oxidative phosphorylation, there has been no *in vitro* response to thyroxine, triiodothyronine or thyroglobulin which has been consistent and reproducible enough to isolate the site of action of thyroid hormone.

Thyroid and Nitrogen Metabolism. Many aspects of nitrogen metabolism are affected by the administration of thyroid hormone. Frequently, one may have to accept the over-all observation on the nitrogen balance without being able to evaluate the indirect contributions of altered metabolic rate, appetite or absorption from gut. It would appear, for example, that the subnormal growth of cretins is related to some extent to the decreased food intake associated with the decreased metabolic rate.

Total nitrogen balance was studied[267] in normal patients treated with thyroid hormone, and it was found that the negative nitrogen balance could be accounted for on the basis of increased urea excretion. Among nitrogen products, thyroid hormone is considered[268] to act on "deposit" protein, the protein of extracellular fluid, which is in excess in myxedema. When myxedematous patients are treated with thyroid hormone, the increased nitrogen excretion is associated with a sodium diuresis, whereas normal subjects excreted an excess of potassium with their nitrogen diuresis.[269] This lends support to the concept that the protein which is mobilized in myxedema is extracellular.

In experimental animals that were thyroparathyroidectomized, there was a higher level of blood urea than in control rats[270] and an increased nitrogen excretion.[271] The surgical procedure and reduced food intake put the animals into a negative nitrogen balance which became positive when the food intake assumed normal proportions.[272] With paired feeding, normal and thyroidectomized rats had almost identical nitrogen balances.[272] In hyperthyroid rats there were increases in the urinary nitrogen, ammonia, uric acid and creatinine.[273] In hyperthyroid animals on a high carbohydrate diet and in thyroidectomized animals[274] on a constant diet, there was a greater excretion of nitrogen in urine than in control situations. The administration of thyroxine normalized the urinary nitrogen excretion.

The increase in plasma amino acids which follows evisceration is decreased by thyroidectomy and increased by thyroxine.[275] This emphasizes the catabolic role of thyroxine in nitrogen metabolism rather than its role in promoting deamination or urea synthesis. Whether the thyroid hormone is primarily anabolic or catabolic may depend to a large extent on the dose at which it is administered as well as on the metabolic state of the organism at the time of administration of this hormone.

Thyroxine does not lead to a negative nitrogen balance in adrenalectomized rats.[276,277] In experimental burns, where there is a marked negative nitrogen balance, there is no reduction of the urinary nitrogen after thyroidectomy.[278,279] The adrenal rather than the thyroid appears to be the crucial gland in the negative nitrogen balance of burns.[278,279] Vitamin B_{12} reduced the negative nitrogen balance of rats made hyperthyroid with thyroxine[280] suggesting that B_{12} spares proteins and that this vitamin may be involved in the action of thyroid hormone.

It has been found that thyroid hormone will promote the utilization of proteins entering the organism, as measured by the ability to increase the liver nitrogen of previously starved rats[281] and using N^{15}-labeled glycine, the rate of protein catabolism is decreased in thyroidectomized rats, whereas the rate of amino acid catabolism in the same animals was increased to such an extent that a negative nitrogen balance ensued.[271] The rate of synthesis of protein from amino acids in thyroidectomized and control animals was the same. In humans, with the aid of N^{15} glycine, it has been found that the rate of protein synthesis is decreased in myxedema and can be restored with triiodothyronine.[282] The administration of the latter hormone to normal individuals will lead to a decreased rate of protein synthesis.

In rats made hyperthyroid and given heavy water, there was a larger concentration of deuterium in the proteins of liver than in control animals.[283] Thyroxine inhibited glutamic acid oxidation by rat kidney cortex.[284] Liver slices from thyroidectomized rats liberated less nitrogen and formed less amino nitrogen than those from normal rats.[285] These net rates, of course, need not apply in human beings, but in human myxedema the blood globulin, including alpha-2 globulin, is increased and accordingly the total blood protein is moderately elevated,[286,287] while the administration of thyroxine decreases the plasma proteins at the expense of the globulins.[287] In myxedema the spinal fluid protein is likewise higher than normal.[288] In general, there is a decrease in the turnover rate for serum albumin in myxedematous patients which is normalized by treatment with thyroid hormone.[289]

Thyroidectomy of rats at birth leads to a decrease in muscle mass as well as to a deficient amount of myosin.[290] It has been shown[291] that thyroidectomized rats have a carcass containing less protein and more fat than control rats. The liver and kidney weights were reduced in such animals as well as the total and relative protein contents of both organs.[272] However, in contradistinction to thyroidectomy, liver protein in thiouracil-treated rats is increased above that of *ad libitum* fed controls. Thyroxine, on the other hand, will increase both liver weight and liver protein.[292]

The thyroid hormone is intimately involved in creatine and creatinine metabolism.[293] There is a creatinuria and associated decrease in creatinine excretion in Graves' disease. This metabolic defect is corrected when the Graves' disease is treated with iodides.[294] Patients with hyperthyroidism show a decreased tolerance for creatine, insofar as such patients excrete more of an administered dose of creatine than do normal individuals.[295–297] There is faulty conversion of creatine to creatinine in hyperthyroid patients, and an increased transformation of creatine to its anhydride in hypothyroid patients.[298] For this reason there is an elevated serum creatine in hyperthyroidism and a decreased creatine in hypothyroidism.[299]

In experimental animals, the relationship of the thyroid to creatine metabolism is similar to that noted in man. Experimental hyperthyroidism in rats results in a profound creatinuria.[300] The creatine and phosphocreatine content of the muscles of the rabbit are increased after thyroidectomy and decreased after the administration of thyroid substance.[301] It has been suggested[302] that this disorder in creatine metabolism may be nonspecific, inasmuch as insulin and adrenalin as well as thyroid hormone will cause a decrease in creatine content of heart and skeletal muscle. However, the creatinuria induced by adrenalin is not manifested in thyroidectomized animals.[303] Thyroxine or thyrotrophic hormone, when administered to the intact animal, causes a loss of stored creatine with no increase in the rate of creatine synthesis.[298]

The role of the thyroid in nucleic acid metabolism has only recently been investigated. Thyroxine increases both the pentosenucleic acid as well as the deoxypentosenucleic acid of rat kidney,[304,305] whereas thyroidectomy decreases these same purine and pyrimidine derivatives.[306] Oddly enough, thiouracil has an effect similar to that of thyroxine,[306] suggesting that this thiopyrimidine has an additional action beyond its ability to decrease the production of thyroid hormone. Human beings receiving thyroxine do not show any change in the level of their blood uric acid, although they may show a decrease in urinary uric acid.[307] In another study, urinary uric acid was unchanged by the administration of thyroxine or triiodothyronine.[308] In thyroidectomized human beings, there is no increased excretion of uric acid.[307]

The metabolism of other nitrogenous products seems to be related to the thyroid. In patients made hyperthyroid with thyroxine, there is a decrease in blood glutathione levels, whereas in hypothyroidism induced by methylthiouracil there is an increase in the level of this tripeptide.[309] There is no correlation in patients between ergothioneine levels in blood and thyroid activity.[310] It appears that thyroidectomized animals synthesize less acetylcholine, whereas hyperthyroid animals produce more of this compound.[311,312] However, since the formation of acetylcholine from pyruvate and choline requires the presence of coenzyme A, it has also been suggested[311] that the decreased acetylcholine synthesis in thyroidectomized animals is only a reflection of decreased coenzyme A formation.

Thyroid and Carbohydrate Metabolism. The effect of thyroid hormone on digestion and absorption of carbohydrate and on glucose degradation and utilization has been studied by few investigators.

Geyelin[313] observed an elevated blood sugar and glycosuria in certain patients with hyperthyroidism. Furthermore, unusually high blood sugar values have been noted in hyperthyroid patients[314] after the oral ingestion of carbohydrate. However, Lozner et al.[315] did not find "diabetic" type glucose tolerance curves in hyperthyroid patients if the glucose was administered intravenously. The presumption seems to be that glucose is more readily absorbed in the hyperthyroid patient. Althausen[316] demonstrated that not only glucose but also galactose and xylose are more readily absorbed from the gut of hyperthyroid rats. Moseley and Chornack[317] however, found no significant differences in the rate of absorption of galactose from the small bowel in normal and thyrotoxic patients. Nevertheless, it is a clinical observation that diabetes is frequently first found when hyperthyroidism develops and, in a patient with established diabetes, the subsequent development of hyperthyroidism aggravates the diabetes. This could be due to the thyroid hormone acting to impair the utilization of glucose, to inadequate formation of glycogen in the liver, or to an increase in the total metabolic activity. The first possibility was ruled out by Mirsky and Broh-Kahn who found that the blood sugar of eviscerated hyperthyroid rats actually fell faster than it did in normal rats.[314] Richardson et al.[318] found by an ingenious application of metabolism determination in fasting subjects that hyperthyroid patients had a normal liver glycogen content. The diminished storage of glycogen in hyperthyroid rats given glucose found by Coggeshall and Greene[319] is most likely due to increased utilization of the injected sugar. The most probable cause of the aggravation of diabetes by hyperthyroidism is the increase in caloric needs that hyperthyroidism dictates. Houssay[320] has noted that in partially pancreatectomized dogs the administration of thyroid produces a diabetes-like state—a metathyroid diabetes. When diabetic dogs were thyroidectomized with radioiodine, the loss of the thyroid did not appear to influence the diabetes.[321]

Pentose excretion in the rat is increased with thyroid feeding and decreased after treatment with thiouracil.[322]

There is some evidence that the thyroid affects intermediary carbohydrate metabolism. For example, in experimental hyperthyroidism an elevation of the pyruvic acid in blood was found.[323] The blood lactic acid fell after thyroidectomy in dogs, and the rise in blood lactate produced by adrenalin was less than normal in thyroidectomized dogs.[324]

The thyroid also affects acetylation of p-aminobenzoic acid. In normal subjects given 500 mg. of p-aminobenzoic acid, approximately 88 per cent was acetylated. Liver disease and hypothyroidism did not affect this, but the fraction acetylated was below normal in hyperthyroid subjects.[325]

Thyroid and Fat Metabolism. It has been long known that in man hypothyroidism is quite regularly accompanied by hypercholesterolemia. In addition, the level of neutral fat and phospholipid is elevated in hypothyroidism.[326–328] Hyperthyroidism is irregularly accompanied by a fall in the level of these fatty substances of blood. The level of fat in the diet plays a major role in the development of hypercholesterolemia in the rat, for starvation or a severely limited food intake can prevent hypercholesterolemia induced by hypothyroidism.[329] Contrariwise, a high-fat diet protects animals against the lethal effect of large doses of thyroxine.[330] Furthermore, the administration of thyroid will lower the level of cholesterol in the serum of rats fed a high-cholesterol and high-fat diet.[331]

The fall in blood cholesterol is associated with the increase in BMR in patients treated with desiccated thyroid, thyroxine or triiodothyronine. This association is not observed upon administration of triiodothyroacetic acid,[332] a derivative of triiodothyronine. Triiodothyroacetic acid may induce a decrease in blood cholesterol in myxedema patients without the associated increase in BMR. No change in the blood lipids of myxedema was noted when TSH was administered.[333] Lipoproteins of S_f 10-20 size have been reported to be increased in amount in the serum of hypothyroid subjects.[334] Both in myxedematous patients and in persons with normal thyroid function, the administration of thyroid extract may induce a fall in the lipoproteins S_f 10-20 size.[335,336]

A partial understanding of the mechanisms whereby thyroid hormone controls fat metabolism has recently been achieved. The synthesis of phospholipids in the liver has been shown to be increased in rats treated with thyroxine and decreased in rats given thiouracil.[337] Phospholipid turnover in the thymus has been reported to be decreased by desiccated thyroid, although nucleic acid turnover was increased.[338] The same investigators also found that thyroid increased phospholipid and nucleic acid turnover in liver. The excretion of cholesterol in the bile is controlled in part by the thyroid and plays a role in regulation of the level of cholesterol in serum. The biliary excretion of cholesterol is regularly reduced in hypothyroid rats and increased in hyperthyroid rats.[339–341] Cholic acid excretion in the bile is apparently lowered in both hypothyroid and hyperthyroid rats.[342] In experiments with both deuterium and tritium labeling the synthesis of cholesterol was found to be increased in hyperthyroid rats and decreased in hypothyroid rats.[343–345] The turnover time of visceral cholesterol paralleled that of cholesterol synthesis. Exposure of hypothyroid rats to a cold environment had no effect on the rate of cholesterol synthesis.[343] In contrast to the effect of thyroid on nitrogen metabolism, there appears to be a consistent gradation of effect of thyroid on fat metabolism from hypothyroidism to euthyroidism to hyperthyroidism. There are equivocal data on the level of cerebrosides in blood in hypo- and hyperthyroidism.[346] The urinary 17-ketosteroids are normal in thyrotoxicosis[347] but decreased in myxedema.

In human myxedema the electrophoretic pattern of serum is essentially normal except for an elevation of the beta-globulin,[348] which decreases with correction of the hypothyroidism.[349]

The role of the thyroid in atherosclerosis has been extensively investigated in animals and in man. A recent study of eight patients who had been hypothyroid for an average of seven years and who had elevated serum cholesterols showed at autopsy an essentially "normal" amount of atherosclerosis.[350] In dogs, thiouracil feeding *per se* appears to have no effect on the development of atherosclerosis but does potentiate the atherosclerosis induced by the feeding of cholesterol.[351] On the other hand, even with a low fat diet, arteriosclerosis has been noted[352] in thyroidectomized and hypophysectomized dogs.

Desiccated thyroid, on the other hand, protects against the development of atherosclerosis in the chicken subsequent to the feeding of cholesterol.[353] Thyroxine has been reported[354] to suppress the marked hyperlipemia produced in chicks with estrogens. In rabbits after atherosclerosis had been induced by the feeding of cholesterol, a normal diet, 2,4-dinitrophenol and thyroxine did not accelerate regression of these lesions.[355] Whether the suppressive action on the hyperlipemia of ducks[354] or euthyroid humans[356,357] is due to a direct effect on intermediary fat metabolism or a suppressive action on the fat mobilizing factor of the pituitary[358] is not yet clear.

Electrolyte and Water Metabolism. Thyroid hormone appears to be involved in the metabolism of a rather large number of mineral elements.

Studies of the effect of the thyroid on sodium and potassium are confined almost exclusively to man and are subject to some dispute.[268] Boothby and his associates found no consistent effect of intravenous thyroxine on either sodium or potassium. Byrom,[269] however, in a later study reported that in the hypothyroid or normal man, thyroxine (in a massive dose) caused a loss of both these elements. In the hypothyroid subjects the loss of sodium was much greater than that of potassium, whereas in the normal subjects more potassium was lost. He suggested that this meant that the fluid accumulated by the myxedematous patient was largely extracellular but that in the normal subject an intense thyroxine effect could cause loss of intracellular water and salts. More recently, two studies have been reported with thyroxine and triiodothyronine, and both studies failed to reveal a consistent effect on the over-all balance of sodium or potassium.[308,359] Using radioactive sodium, Na^{24}, it has been noted[360] that the sodium space is equal in normal and athyreotic monkeys.

Thyroid hormone has a profound effect on water. In myxedematous patients given thyroxine or triiodothyronine, there is a marked diuresis. One report shows an increase in the level of sodium and chloride in serum, suggesting that enough water was excreted to cause a relative concentration of extracellular fluid.[308] Similar effects have been noted with TSH[361] in myxedema where the trophic factor also induced an increase in the extracellular fluid space and the total body water, followed by a contraction of the extracellular fluid space with diuresis.

The effect of thyroid hormone on calcium metabolism is not entirely clear. This is hardly surprising, since calcium intake, renal function, vitamin D, nitrogen balance, activity, etc., exert such marked effects on calcium metabolism that smaller effects can easily be masked. It was first noted that in hyperthyroid patients an increase in urinary calcium could be detected.[362] Later it was shown that in rabbits the administration of desiccated thyroid caused a loss of calcium.[363] Several studies in man have shown that patients with hyperthyroidism, if kept on a rather low calcium intake, excrete more calcium than do normal subjects.[364–366] These same investigators showed that hypothyroid human subjects tended to excrete less calcium than did normal subjects.[367] In patients with hyperthyroidism who showed hypercalciuria (four of six), treatment of the hyperthyroidism with thiouracil caused a fall in urinary calcium to normal values.[368] There may actually be a hypercalcemia associated with this hypercalciuria.[369] However, in two more recent studies with both thyroxine and triiodothyronine no consistent effect was seen on calcium excretion or balance.[308,359] There was in no instance any change in the level of calcium in the blood as a result of change in thyroid activity.

Recent studies[370] with radioactive calcium, Ca^{45}, reveal a decrease in the specific activity of calcium in the serum and urine of hyperthyroid patients. In myxedema this ratio fell more slowly than in normal persons. This suggests that thyroid function modifies the size of the calcium compartments and the rate of flow to and from these compartments. The compartment sizes and flow rates are greatest in hyperthyroidism and least in myxedema. In thyrotoxicosis, bone formation as well as bone destruction are proceeding at rates above normal. A recent report of pathologic examination of vertebrae from patients with active hyperthyroidism showed excess destruction in all cases. The earlier clinical reports on the effects of hyperthyroidism on the skeleton are well reviewed in this article.[371]

Phosphorus metabolism is markedly affected by the thyroid. Either thyroxine or triiodothyronine causes a loss of phosphorus in both urine and stool.[308,359,365–367] If one attempts to account for the phosphorus loss on the basis of nitrogen loss (using the ratio of these two as found in normal muscle), there is a considerable excess in phosphorus excretion.[308] The source of this phosphorus is not clear. Thyroid has no effect on the level of phosphorus in the blood, however.[372]

No consistent effect of thyroxine or triiodothyronine on chloride excretion in urine or stool in man has been found.[308] However, earlier investigators found that the feeding of desiccated thyroid to cats caused a decreased urinary excretion of chloride in spite of diuresis.[373] According to another report, thyroxine or desiccated thyroid caused an increase in urinary chloride.[374] The adrenal may play a role in these responses, since Gaunt has found that in rats thyroxine increases the diuresis after a water load. Previous adrenalectomy abolished this effect of thyroid.[375] A study of chloride excretion in the sweat of normal and hyperthyroid subjects may help in explaining these differences. The chloride content of sweat was decreased in hyperthyroid subjects; the more severe the hyperthyroidism, the less chloride was found in the sweat.[376] The chloride concentration in the serum of patients with myxedema is the same as that of euthyroid persons.[377]

Iron metabolism appears to be influenced by thyroid function. In rabbits thyroidectomy caused a rise of 15 per cent to 25 per cent in the serum iron and a slight fall in tissue iron. Thyroxine caused a reversion of these levels to normal.[378] In man the serum iron has been reported by one group to be high in hyperthyroidism, and has been reported by another group to increase in patients with hyperthyroidism after treatment.[379,380]

Two groups of investigators have reported that the level of bound magnesium in the serum is elevated in hyperthyroidism and below normal in myxedema.[381,382] A more recent report shows that nondiffusible magnesium of plasma is unchanged in patients with definite alterations in thyroid function.[383]

Table 2 summarizes the effect of hyperthyroidism on certain electrolytes.

Thyroid and Vitamin Metabolism. A vast literature on this subject was re-

TABLE 2. EFFECT OF HYPERTHYROIDISM

	ON CONCENTRATION IN SERUM	ON TOTAL EXCRETION
Sodium	No change	Increased
Potassium	No change	Increased
Calcium	No change	Increased
Magnesium (Bound)	Increased	?
Chloride	No change	?
Phosphorus	No change	Increased

viewed in 1943;[384] the reader is directed to this reference.

VITAMIN A. The thyroid is necessary for the conversion of carotene to vitamin A, and carotene does not prevent the development of signs of vitamin A deficiency in hypothyroid animals.[385–389] In myxedematous subjects treatment with desiccated thyroid was said to decrease blood carotene and increase blood vitamin A.[390] In cows and goats, thyroxine appears to decrease the carotene content of stool, and thiouracil increases it.[391] Thyroid feeding may have improved absorption of carotene or increased its conversion to vitamin A.

The effect of vitamin A on the thyroid is less well understood. It has been reported that vitamin A deficiency does not affect iodine uptake by the thyroid but does diminish incorporation of iodine into thyroxine.[388] On the other hand, a very extensive investigation showed that either vitamin A lack or vitamin A excess increased radioiodine uptake by the thyroid.[392]

Vitamin A has also been reported to protect animals against the rise in O_2 consumption caused by desiccated thyroid[393] and vitamin A in large dosage decreased the TSH content of rat pituitary.[394]

There is conflicting evidence on the relationship between vitamin A and thyroxine with respect to amphibian metamorphosis; some data suggest an antagonism between the two substances.[395–398]

VITAMIN B. Thiamine requirements and the urinary excretion of thiamine appear to be increased in hyperthyroidism.[399–401] Pigeons in which a thiamine deficiency had been induced have been reported to show a reduction in the calorigenic effect of thyroxine.[402] Riboflavin deficiency has been reported in hypothyroid rabbits and in myxedematous patients.[403,404] A lack of riboflavin has been reported to alter the histologic picture of the thyroid without altering its weight.[405] In hyperthyroid rats there is an increased need for riboflavin.[406] Thyroidectomy or the administration of thiouracil appeared to lower the N′ methyl nicotinamide excretion, whereas this defect was corrected by thyroxine.[407] It was suggested that thyroxine might participate in the methylation of nicotinic acid.

Vitamin B_6, in large dosage, has been reported to cause hypofunction of the thyroid of rabbits.[408] Vitamin B_6-deficient rats have a lower oxygen consumption than normally fed controls but the same oxygen consumption as pair fed controls.[409] Signs of vitamin B_6 deficiency were unaffected by hypothyroidism.

The administration to rats of large amounts of iodocasein causes loss of body weight and eventual death. Vitamin B_{12} appears partially to protect rats from these effects.[410–413] However, vitamin B_{12} does not inhibit the increase in O_2 consumption secondary to thyroprotein feeding.[414] The diet may affect the antagonism between B_{12} and thyroxine, for it was observed in animals on a soy flour diet and was not seen with rats on a wheat flour diet.[415] Other reports indicate that B_{12} does not protect against thyroxine administration, but a fraction of liver does.[410,416,417] Dried penicillin mycelia and Aureomycin mash, but none of the B vitamins, have been reported to be antagonistic to the effects of fed desiccated thyroid.[418] Vitamin B_{12} itself apparently has no effect on the rat thyroid as measured by radioiodine uptake.[419,420] In mice, vitamin B_{12} will increase the growth rate, and iodinated casein abolishes this effect.[421] Vitamin B_{12} will inhibit in rats the growth-depressing effect of thiouracil, although it has no effect on the reduction in I^{131} thyroidal uptake caused by thiouracil.[419] Thyroidal hypertrophy of the B_{12}-supplemented rats has been reported to be less than in those given thiouracil alone.[419] Of some interest is the fact that dinitrophenol, an agent which lowers the PBI, may cause a retardation in body and testis weight, which is reversed by liver fractions.[417]

Citrovorum factor was said to be excreted in excessive quantity in the urine of hyperthyroid rats.[422] If the rats were also deficient in folic acid, there was no change in excretion of citrovorum factor after the feeding of thyroid.

VITAMIN C. Considerable work has been reported on vitamin C deficiency and the thyroid, but in general it is contradictory or inconclusive. Even the effect of scurvy on the thyroid is not clear, for both marked changes and no changes have been reported.[423–431] The effect of TSH on the normal and scorbutic guinea pig is also not clear. It has been recently reviewed.[431]

Both thyroxine and triiodothyronine catalyze the cupric-ascorbic acid oxidation system and are roughly equally effective.[432]

Effect of Thyroid on Oxygen Consumption. The remarkable effect of thyroid hormone on oxygen consumption was first demonstrated many years ago by Magnus-Levy[433] and was very well quantitated in normal and hyperthyroid human subjects.[434–436]

The decay curves of the effect of thyroxine in patients with myxedema have been carefully investigated.[437] When triiodothyronine was identified in plasma, synthesized[38,438,439] and shown to have physiologic activity,[223] further interest was generated. Experiments in man and rats have shown that triiodothyronine is roughly three to four times as potent in elevating oxygen consumption as is thyroxine.[359,440–443] There are marked differences between these two compounds, however, in onset of action and duration of action. A single dose of thyroxine, given intravenously, requires about 10 days before its peak effect on BMR is seen. After this the basal oxygen consumption falls off in exponential fashion, with a half time of about 15 days. Recently, it was noted that in guinea pigs a rise in oxygen consumption could be seen four hours after the administration of thyroxine.[78] Triiodothyronine, administered in a single dose intravenously, has its peak effect in 24 to 36 hours and thereafter declines in exponential fashion, with a half time of about eight days. A careful study of comparative effects of different amounts of these two agents disclosed that the ratio of total increase in oxygen consumption $\frac{T_3\Delta O_2}{T_4\Delta O_2}$ was four or five for low doses and actually less than one for high doses.[442]

There is a recent report that in rats thyroxine caused less increase in O_2 consumption in females than in males and that castration increased the sensitivity of females to the calorigenic action of thyroxine.[444] Both in rats[445] and humans[446] there is a decrease in the rate of oxygen consumption with age.

One aspect of oxygen consumption has been used as a test of thyroid hormone. In this test survival time of animals placed in a closed vessel has been measured. Thyroxine or triiodothyronine caused a definite decrease in survival time.[447] Much work has been done on the respiration of tissues from normal, thyroxine-treated and thyroidectomized animals. Muscle, kidney, liver[448] and cardiac muscle[449–451] show an increased O_2 utilization after thyroxine treatment and decreased O_2 consumption after thyroidectomy.

Although thyroidectomy[452] and myxedema[453] have been reported to be associated with a decreased cerebral oxygen consumption, others[454,455] have denied this. In hyperthyroidism, there is normal oxygen consumption by the brain of man,[456] although rats demonstrated a transitory increase.[457] Net splanchnic oxygen consumption in hyperthyroid patients was increased even more than basal oxygen consumption.[458] There is some discrepancy in the results, but in general most tissues are affected with the exception of the brain, spleen and gonads.[450]

THYROID AND THE CARDIOVASCULAR RENAL SYSTEM

The administration of desiccated thyroid increases the cardiac output. In hyperthyroid patients the cardiac output is elevated, and in myxedematous patients it is below normal.[453,458,459] Hyperthyroidism appears to increase the mean and systolic pressures in the right ventricle, although the diastolic pressure remains normal. Therefore a normal pulmonary vascular resistance is present.[458] The blood flow to the skin is decreased in myxedema. The blood flow through the skin and musculature is increased in hyperthyroidism.[460,462] The hepatic blood flow in hyperthyroidism is little changed.[463] The cerebral blood flow in myxedema is markedly decreased as a result of an increase in cerebrovascular resistance.[453] Hyperthyroidism results in no appreciable change from normal in renal blood flow, however, and the treatment of hyperthyroidism does not change the renal blood flow.[463] Myxedema, on the other hand, causes a marked reduction in renal blood flow which is restored to normal by treatment with desiccated thyroid.[463] Many aspects of renal function are depressed by myxedema, e.g., urea clearance, excretion of indigo carmine, glomerular filtration rate and tubular secretory capacity.[463] Furthermore, the administration of thyroid increases the maximal tubular excretory capacity for Diodrast in dogs and man.[463,464] The blood volume is decreased in myxedema[465] and increased in hyperthyroidism.[466] There may be a direct effect of thyroid hormone on the heart over and above that increase in the heart rate necessary to maintain an increased cardiac output.[467] Meyer and Jost[468] suggest that thyroxine or thyroglobulin had less effect on heart rate per unit increase in metabolism than did whole thyroid.

Whether or not there is a direct action of the thyroid hormone on the heart has been seriously doubted. It has been suggested that the cardiac symptoms and even heart disease seen in some patients with long-standing hyperthyroidism are secondary to the hypermetabolism produced by the hyperthyroidism. Recent studies have suggested a direct action of the thyroid hormone on the heart. Rasmussen[469] reported that induced hyperthyroidism resulted in cardiac changes which could not be correlated with the rate of metabolism. Barker,[470] who has studied the effects of various thyroid hormones on cellular metabolism, has noted, with these methods of study, that the heart is the first tissue to respond to the systemic administration of triiodothyronine.

Notwithstanding the above evidence for a direct action of the thyroid hormones on the heart, the most common severe cardiac problems in patients with hyperthyroidism are usually observed in those with previous heart disease.

Whether hyperthyroidism in the absence of heart disease can cause congestive failure in the human is disputed. The multiplicity of problems in a patient who has been hyperthyroid for years makes it difficult to assign a definite and single cause to the effects seen.

TABLE 3. EFFECT OF HYPERTHYROIDISM AND MYXEDEMA ON ORGAN BLOOD FLOW

ORGAN	EFFECT OF MYXEDEMA	EFFECT OF HYPERTHYROIDISM
Brain	Decreased	No change
Kidneys	Decreased	No change
Skin	Decreased	Increased
Muscle		Increased
Liver		No change
Lungs		Increased

Table 3 summarizes the effects of over- and underactivity of the thyroid on the blood flow to some of the organs.

GROWTH AND THYROID HORMONE

Since the relationship between the thyroid and cretinism has been known, it has been apparent that the thyroid is necessary for normal growth. An extension of the effect of the thyroid on growth was made in an important contribution by Gudernatsch[4] in 1912 when he fed thyroid glands to tadpoles and markedly accelerated metamorphosis. The converse was shown by Smith[116] and by Allen,[471] who found that thyroidectomy or hypophysectomy would prevent tadpole metamorphosis. The affect of thyroid administration in the axolotl, fish and eels is well established.[472] The axolotl is particularly remarkable because this amphibian ordinarily spends its entire life in the larval form. If thyroxine is given, it will metamorphose into a terrestrial salamander.

Thyroidectomy also prevents normal growth in sheep and goats,[473] rats[474] and rabbits.[475] Thyroidectomy in monkeys resulted in a myxedematous condition similar to that observed in humans.[476] Fleischmann[477] finds that in the adult monkey complete thyroidectomy results in little apparent change in the animal and that the blood cholesterol is unchanged. Thyroidectomy in the immature animal leads to retardation of growth. Karnofsky and Cronkite[478] have noted that the administration of thyroxine to rats markedly accelerates the time of eruption of incisor teeth. Dziewiatkowski[174] has investigated the effect of thiouracil and of thyroxine on the incorporation of S^{35} administered as Na_2So_4. Pretreatment with thyroxine either decreased or had no effect on the uptake of S^{35} by cartilage. Thyroxine, however, reversed the effect of thiouracil on S^{35} uptake in cartilage. Thyroxine also increased the rate of disappearance of S^{35} from cartilage once it had been incorporated in the cartilage. Thiouracil decreased the rate of disappearance of the labeled sulfur. Simpson et al.[479] found that in hypophysectomized rats, the administration of growth hormone permitted normal growth regardless of the presence or absence of the thyroid, adrenals or gonads. Thyroxine, on the other hand, when administered in relatively large dosage caused early skeletal maturity with closure of the epiphyses before adult size was obtained. Schlesinger and Fisher[480] report three cases of juvenile thyrotoxicosis which resulted in increased skeletal growth. It appears that the thyroid hormone is necessary for growth in most vertebrates studied and is also necessary for metamorphosis.

THYROID AND CENTRAL NERVOUS SYSTEM

The "nervousness" in patients with Graves' disease has been noted since the disease was first recognized. Similarly, the apathy and sluggishness of cretins has been known for centuries. Furthermore, various psychoses are occasionally associated with hyperthyroidism and with myxedema.[481,482] However, Brody and Man[483] were unable to find a significant deviation from normal in the protein-bound blood iodine levels in a large group of schizophrenic patients. Cohen[484] investigated the oxygen consumption of the brain of hyperthyroid rats in a Warburg tissue respirometer. He found that initially the O_2 consumption was above normal, but in two hours it fell to a normal value. Most investigators have been unable to detect a change in the rate of O_2 consumption by brain slices upon the addition of thyroxine to the media.[485] Electroencephalograms done on athyreotic patients typically revealed diminished voltage, absent alpha waves, no change after light stimulus and a slow frequency[486] with a reversion toward normal after treatment with desiccated thyroid.[453] Scheinberg et al.[453] also report the findings in athyreotic patients of cerebral oxygen and glucose consumption as measured by the techniques of Kety. In myxedematous patients there was a 38 per cent decrease in cerebral blood flow and a 28 per cent decrease in cerebral O_2 and glucose consumption. There was dramatic increase of 91 per cent above normal in the cerebral vascular resistance in myxedema. All those values returned toward normal upon treatment with desiccated thyroid. These findings suggest that the mental aberrations in myxedema may be a result of a decreased cerebral metabolism. "Myxedematous Madness" is, for example, the title of a recent paper on mental changes in this condition.[487] In this paper fourteen myxedematous patients who had been admitted to a psychiatric hospital for care of various psychoses are described. Most of these patients had delusions of persecution and hallucinations. Some presented a picture of dementia, some were maniacal and others had depressions. The problems for which they were institutionalized were corrected upon restoration to a euthyroid state. Scheinberg[456] also measured cerebral blood flow, O_2 and glucose consumption in hyperthyroid patients and found these values to be in the normal range in all nine patients studied.

Lambert et al.[488] have measured the efficiency of the peripheral nerves in myxedema as revealed by quantitative analysis of the components entering into the ankle jerk. They found that the rate of contraction of the muscle after tapping of the Achilles tendon and the time involved in the nervous transmission of the reflex were in the normal range in myxedematous subjects. Apparently there is no change in nerve conduction in this disease. There was however, a marked delay in the time required for relaxation of the muscle. This appeared to represent a defect in muscle function. Treatment with desiccated thyroid restored the time for muscle relaxation to normal.

THE GASTROINTESTINAL TRACT

Severely thyrotoxic patients may have diarrhea, and myxedematous patients usually suffer with constipation. The constipation of athyreosis may be attributed to decreased peristalsis of the entire gastrointestinal tract, and the diarrhea of hyperthyroidism may be attributed to increased peristaltic activity. In both myxedema and hyperthyroidism there is a significant incidence of achlorhydria. In myxedema, a 53 per cent incidence of absolute achlorhydria has been reported. In Graves' disease, it has been found that 38 per cent of a large group of cases had achlorhydria.[489] This phenomenon is easily explained in myxedema as being secondary to the generally decreased body metabolism. It is less easily explained in hyperthyroidism unless there is an insensitivity of the stomach to vagal stimulation similar to the reported insensitivity of hearts to vagal stimulation in experimental hyperthyroidism. Experimental thyroidectomy reduces the time required to produce a perforating peptic ulcer in guinea pigs treated with histamine.[490] It has also been observed that, whereas thyroxine does not protect against the development of fatal peptic ulceration, desiccated thyroid does.[491]

Notwithstanding the fact that the liver of severely thyrotoxic patients has been reported to have certain impaired functions, there are no known specific effects of thyroxine on the liver except for a loss of glycogen observed in experimental hyperthyroidism.

It has been reported that thyroidectomy is followed by a fall in hemoglobin but that the administration of thyroxine causes only a slight increase in the hemoglobin level. The administration of thyroxine has been reported to cause a fall in lymphocytes.[492] It has also been reported that the addition of thyroxine to a mixture of fibrinogen and thrombin delays coagulation. This effect is attributed to an inactivation of thrombin by thyroxine.[493]

IODINE DETERMINATIONS AND THE SIGNIFICANCE OF THE BLOOD IODINE

The high iodine content of the thyroid hormone and the apparent lack of iodine in any other compound normally present in the mammalian organism make the importance of iodine determinations as a measure of the thyroid hormone quite clear. Such is the importance of iodine that several comprehensive and detailed books have been published dealing exclusively with the physiologic role of iodine. The reader is referred to Salter's *The Endocrine Function of Iodine*[494] and Elmer's *Iodine Metabolism and Thyroid Function*[495] for reviews of this subject. The normal iodine content of the blood in the human is approximately from 4 to 8 micrograms per 100 cc. of blood. Commonly only that iodine which is precipitated along with proteins is measured, and it is then referred to as the "protein-bound iodine" or the "serum-precipitable iodine." Since this concentration is so small (less than one part in ten million, under normal circumstances), its measurement has been fraught with considerable difficulty. Iodine analyses were first introduced by the methods of Rabourdin[496] and Chatin.[177] These were cumbersome, required large amounts of blood (500 and 1000 cc.) and unless performed by professional chemists were rather unreliable. Kendall's method[497] of alkaline ashing of the serum or gland with a colorimetric procedure using the starch iodine and iodate-iodide reaction was a considerable improvement. However, the final color reaction was not as sensitive as desired. A major advance was made when Sandell and Kolthoff[498] discovered that iodine in extremely small concentration markedly accelerated the reduction of the ceric ion by the arsenious ion. This effect under certain rigidly controlled conditions could be quantitated. Chaney[499] developed a very useful still for the distillation of iodine, and later Barker[500] introduced certain modifications so that the method has become rather widely used and normal values generally agreed upon. Man et al.[501] have described a somewhat different procedure and have evaluated it in terms of reproducibility and accuracy in a large number of analyses. Barker[502] has described a simplified method of analysis which dispenses with the distillation step and substitutes an ashing procedure for destruction of the organic material. A recent simplification by Zak[503] employing chloric acid has produced a more efficient method without sacrifice of accuracy. Precipitation of proteins is now generally accomplished with the Somogyi reagent, which is essentially precipitation with zinc hydroxide or by the use of trichloracetic acid. Iodine analyses of thyroid glands which usually contain approximately 0.1 per cent iodine are perhaps best accomplished by a method such as Kendall's alkaline ash procedure.[497] Radioiodine has been of considerable help in evaluating the methods and in correcting for loss in the procedure. Iodine analysis of blood is still a difficult and time-consuming procedure requiring skilled technicians. Usually a room devoted solely to iodine analysis and remote from any source of elemental iodine is necessary. Many compounds in medical use contain iodine and may give spuriously high blood iodine values. There are also compounds in use containing mercury which will give falsely low values for blood iodine through interference with the final cerate arsenite reaction. Danowski[504] has demonstrated that the long continued administration of iodide will result in a spurious elevation of the protein-bound iodine (PBI). A partial list (Table 4) of such compounds and their effect on the protein-bound blood iodine and the total blood iodine are given below.

There is no question as to the value of blood iodine determinations in establishing a diagnosis of hypothyroidism or hyperthyroidism. What is measured is an approximation of the level of circulating thyroid hormone. It is possible and even probable that sensitivity of the tissues to the thyroid hormone is a real factor in the development of clinical hyperthyroidism or hypothyroidism. This can, of course, be evaluated in part by determination of the basal metabolic rate. Skanse[505] attempted an evaluation of the efficiency of the serum protein-bound iodine as a diagnostic measure in hyperthyroidism and felt that approximately 88 per cent of the cases of hyperthyroidism were correctly diagnosed by the PBI alone. This was in contrast to the BMR, which was consistent with the diagnosis in approximately 60 per cent of the cases. This is an extremely difficult study to conduct for one is always utilizing in making the diagnosis the guides one wishes to evaluate. In our clinic it is felt that the PBI is an accurate guide to the diagnosis of hyperthyroidism in approximately 80 to 90 per cent of the cases. It is probably about equally accurate in myxedema.

Until recently, it was felt that all the blood iodine which was precipitable was hormonal iodine and thus a reflection of thyroid function. As indicated earlier, it is now apparent that several organic iodine compounds occur in blood which either originate in the thyroid or are the result of administered organic iodine. Because of this it has been found[506] that the organic iodine which is soluble in butanol, i.e., butanol-extractable iodine, is a more precise reflection of blood hormonal iodine than the PBI.

Obviously, if several laboratory procedures are combined, there will be a greater correlation with the number of cases in which the diagnosis has been established clinically. Thus, the butanol-extractable radioiodine, the BEI^{131}, has been found to be predominantly thyroxine[507] and is approximately 80 per cent of the PBI^{131} in the blood of patients without thyroid malignancy.[508] In the latter instance, the BEI^{131} may represent as little as 20 per cent of the PBI^{131}.[508] The BEI^{131} has been found[508,589] to be a reliable index of thyroid function.

The determination of the blood iodine has been used not only to evaluate thyroid function but to assist in the management of patients being treated with various forms of thyroid hormone. Desiccated thyroid[510,511] and thyroxine[512,513] will increase the PBI while triiodothyronine either will have no effect or will decrease the PBI. With the latter agent, obviously determination of blood iodine is of little aid in following replacement therapy.

THE USE OF RADIOIODINE IN STUDYING THYROID PATHOLOGY

In employing radioactive iodine as an aid in the diagnosis of thyroid pathology certain properties of the isotope and limitations of its use should be emphasized. This isotope of iodine has strong gamma and beta rays. The former permits detection at some distance from the source of radiation, namely, by a detector outside the body. The latter, as well as the former, contributes to the radiation delivered to the thyroid and other tissues.

TABLE 4. THE EFFECT OF VARIOUS IODINE-CONTAINING COMPOUNDS ON THE LEVEL OF SERUM IODINE AND PBI

COMPOUND	INCREASES PBI	INCREASES INORGANIC I	DECREASES APPARENT PBI	TIME OF DISAPPEARANCE OF DRUG FROM BLOOD
Iodides				
Lugol's solution	x*	x		10 ± days
Syrup hydriotic acid	x*	x		10 ± days
Saturated solution potassium iodide	x*	x		10 ± days
Dyes used to visualize the bronchial tree				
Lipiodol	x			months
Dyes used to visualize the gallbladder				
Priodax	x			months or years
Dyes used to visualize the urinary tract				
Diodrast	x			10 to 20 hours
Neoiopax	x			10 to 20 hours
Amebacides				
Diiodoquin	x			4 to 6 days
Thyroid hormone				
Desiccated thyroid	x			1 to 2 weeks
Thyroxine	x			1 to 2 weeks
Triiodothyronine			x	1 to 3 days
Mercurial diuretics				
Salyrgan			x	1 to 2 days
Thiomerin			x	1 to 2 days

* The elevation in the PBI occurs only after long continued administration of large amounts of iodide.

Note: Many cough syrups, "tonics" and some vitamin preparations contain iodine in one form or another.

It has been estimated, for example, that a 10 microcurie tracer dose in a normal person will deliver approximately 15 rads to the thyroid, an amount of radiation considered to be "the maximum permissible safe dose" throughout the course of an entire year. Frequently, it is necessary to give 20 times this amount of radiation to a person in order to obtain more detailed information. It has actually been claimed[514] that remissions or striking changes in laboratory values have been noted after the administration of as little as 240 microcuries of radioactive iodine to hyperthyroid persons. Therefore, diagnostic procedures employing radioactive iodine carry a calculated risk, one that may be justified if the data obtained will benefit the patient.

Although we speak of radioactive iodine as a "label" for the nonradioactive iodine in the body, it must be emphasized that radioiodine need not label all the different forms of iodine in the body in the same manner, i.e., there may be differences in specific activity, as will become apparent in the subsequent discussion. We are only measuring the isotope unless radioactive iodine determinations are combined with other chemical separation and analytic procedures for various forms of stable iodine. Inasmuch as we are measuring all forms of radioactive iodine when we determine radioiodine in body tissues, we do not have sufficient data to dissect out the complex set of reactions involved in the metabolism of iodine discussed in the earlier sections. Since it would appear that certain diseases of the thyroid involve only an isolated biochemical defect, it behooves the thyroid investigator to devise more elaborate techniques to determine these abnormalities. Thus, a decrease in circulating hormone may be the consequence of inadequate iodine intake, impaired iodide trapping, faulty conversion of iodide to an organic form, disordered thyroglobulin synthesis or proteolysis, secretion of abnormal organic iodine products into the circulation, accelerated degradation of thyroid hormone, poor thyroid hormone transport in the blood, etc. Most of these defects have already been demonstrated with a greater or lesser amount of convincing data.

Many tests have been devised, each with the hope of improving the accuracy of diagnosing morbid thyroid physiology. Unfortunately, any one procedure may focus on one or a limited number of processes in iodine metabolism but exclude others, although some procedures may correlate better than others with the patient's clinical status. Just as any one symptom, sign or laboratory determination is not sufficient to make a precise clinical diagnosis, so it may be necessary to have several determinations with radioiodine to establish an accurate diagnosis of thyroid function. In addition to the more frequently employed radioiodine tests listed in Table 5, other tests have been suggested which are not tabulated because they are more involved or have not been sufficiently employed by several groups of investigators to establish their applicability as a routine laboratory procedure. These include the thyroid secretion rate,[83,89,515] the extrarenal disposal rate,[26,516] thyroid organification of I^{131},[517,518] the saliva/plasma ratio of I^{131} and others.

On theoretic grounds it would seem more appropriate to measure the output of thyroid hormone, for that is, in the last analysis, the function of the gland. McConahey[519] has shown that there is a marked difference between the level of protein-bound blood radioiodine two to three days after the administration of a tracer dose of radioiodine in hyperthyroid, euthyroid and hypothyroid patients. The level of PBI^{131} three days after administration of the I^{131} was the highest in hyperthyroid patients, virtually nil in myxedema patients and intermediate in euthyroid patients. Clark et al.[520] have modified this procedure to measure the total and protein-bound radioactivity in the blood 24 hours after the administration of a tracer dose of radioiodine. The bound radioactivity divided by the total radioactivity gives what he terms a "conversion ratio." This is then a measure of both the amount of iodide remaining in the blood and the amount converted to hormone 24 hours after the dose of radioiodine. As such, it would seem to be, and indeed Clark presents data supporting this thesis, a good index of thyroid activity. However, the absolute amount of radioiodine secreted into the blood as labeled hormone is a function of both the rate of secretion of hormone and the amount of hormone in the gland. If, for example, one thyroid containing 10 milligrams of iodine is secreting 0.5 mg. of iodine into the blood per day (as thyroid hormone), the patient will probably be hyperthyroid. If 50 per cent of a tracer dose of radioiodine is concentrated in this gland and is assumed to label the gland's iodine uniformly, then approximately $\frac{0.5}{10.0} \times 100$ or 5 per cent of the gland's iodine will be discharged per day. This is then 5 per cent of 50 per cent or 2.5 per cent of the dose of radioactivity that will be discharged from the gland per day into the blood stream. Another patient, however, may have only 2 mg. of iodine in his thyroid and secrete 0.2 mg. iodine as hormone into the blood stream per day. This is probably the approximate amount secreted per day by a euthyroid patient. If this patient concentrates 25 per cent of the administered dose of radioiodine, by calculations similar to those described above it will be seen that he too will secrete 2.5 per cent of the dose of radioiodine into the blood stream per day, and the absolute amount of PBI^{131} will be identical in the two patients.

It is difficult to arrive at an accurate evaluation of the accuracy of any of these procedures in diagnosing hyperthyroidism or hypothyroidism. In general, however, it would appear that they are accurate in approximately 90 per cent of the cases.[505,506,521,522] Because of some of the "failures" of radioiodine tests to correlate well with clinical diagnosis and because of the possibility that some of the factors which influence the radioiodine may be controlled or understood by either the patient or the physician, these will be mentioned. The prolonged administration of large doses of an antithyroid drug, like propylthiouracil or methimazole, may lead, even in the euthyroid person, to a goiter and increased uptake of radioiodine. The latter may be accompanied by a decreased urinary excretion of radioiodine, an elevated conversion ratio and an elevated protein-bound I^{131}. This consequence of prolonged block of stable iodine from entering the thyroid would suggest hyperthyroidism. The clinical status as well as the protein-bound iodine and other laboratory tests would quickly disclose this error. Conversely, a Graves' disease patient treated with several hundred milligrams of iodine daily over a long period of time might demonstrate all the clinical stigmata of the disease, including an elevated PBI, BMR and radioiodine uptake but with a level of PBI^{131} or conversion ratio characteristic of a euthyroid person. The actual number of micrograms of thyroid hormone secreted daily might indeed be increased, as occurs in Graves' disease, but this could occur in association with a smaller fraction of the I^{131} being converted to PBI^{131} because of the large iodine stores in the gland. Another Graves' disease patient of some duration, previously treated with surgery or radioactive iodine, might have so little thyroid tissue remaining that the uptake would not be in the hyperthyroid range. Such a patient would, however, have a high level of PBI^{131} or conversion ratio together with the associated signs, symptoms and laboratory findings of Graves' disease.

In addition to the antithyroid drugs mentioned which may alter the radioiodine tests as indicated, exogenous thyroid hormone may interfere with these procedures. A euthyroid person may actually take some form of thyroid hormone to the point of toxicity with a consequent decrease in the thyroid uptake of radioiodine. The discrepancy between an increased metabolic rate and a decreased uptake of radioiodine by the thyroid may actually suggest thyrotoxicosis factitia.

TABLE 5. VARIOUS INDICES OF THYROID FUNCTION IN COMMON UNTREATED THYROID DISEASE USING RADIOIODINE*

Diagnosis	Thyroid Plasma I^{131} Clearance (cc/min.)	Uptake in Thyroid (%)			PBI^{131} in Serum (%/L) (24–48 hrs.)	Conversion Ratio (24–48 hrs.)	24 or 48-hr. Urinary Excretion of I^{131} (%)
		1 hr.	6 hrs.	24 or 48 hrs.			
Euthyroid	5-40	5-20	8-25	15-40	0.01-0.20	<0.40	37-75
Hyperthyroid	40-1500	15-75	33-90	40-90	0.1-3.0	0.5-1.0	6-52
Hypothyroid	0-4	↓	2-7	↓	↓	<0.1	53-80
Subacute Thyroiditis Acute Phase	↓	?↓	?↓	0-20	—	↓	↑
Subacute Thyroiditis Subsiding	N or ↑	?↑	?↑	N or ↑	—	—	N
Hashimoto's Disease	N	N	N	N	—	—	N
Riedel's Disease	↓	?N	?N	N	—	—	N
Non-Toxic Nodular Goiter	N	5-15	5-28	10-60	N	N	N
Endemic Goiter Euthyroid	?↑	↑	?↑	50-70	?↑	?↑	?↓
Congenital Goiter A	?N	?↑	?↑	?↑	↓	↓	↑
Congenital Goiter B	↑	↑	↑	90+	±0.4	↑	↓
Congenital Goiter C	↑	↑	↑	90+	↑	↑	↓

N = Normal ↑ = Elevated ↓ = Depressed — = Unknown
* Modified from Rall.[543]

Other forms of iodine in addition to thyroid hormone may interfere with the radioiodine test. These include the various forms of organic iodine compounds used in diagnostic radiology. The length of time that these agents may affect radioiodine uptake studies varies from a few hours with an agent like Diodrast, which is completely cleared by an intact kidney with normal blood flow, to several years when Lipiodol may be retained after bronchography or myelography. Iodine which may distort the radioiodine test is also found in various expectorants, vitamin preparations and composite weight reducing diets. Tincture of iodine employed topically, as well as the amebicide diiodoquin, will also affect adversely uptake studies with radioactive iodine.

Since, in a gross way, the thyroid and kidney normally are in "competition" for the disposition of a given dose of iodine, the thyroidal uptake and the urinary excretion of radioactive iodine are inversely related. An increase in one parameter is accompanied by a decrease in the other. For this reason, the interpretation of thyroidal uptake studies should take cognizance of the status of renal function. In the presence of renal disease[523] the amount of stable iodine which is not excreted by the kidney will affect the thyroidal uptake as well. Thus, with an adequate dietary intake of stable iodine, there may be a decreased thyroidal uptake of radioiodine even with a decrease in the urinary excretion of the isotope in the first two days. The depressed uptake is a reflection of greater stable iodine localization so that there is no alteration in the production of thyroid hormone. If only small amounts of stable iodine are retained in the presence of renal disease, as might occur with inadequate intake of iodine, the uptake of radioiodine by the thyroid might increase even though there was no associated increase in the manufacture of thyroid hormone.

In nephrosis, with the decrease in circulating hormonal iodine, there may be an increase in radioactive iodine uptake by the thyroid[524] as well as a probable elevation in PBI^{131}.

In patients with impaired liver function, 40 per cent have been reported to have an increased thyroidal uptake of radioiodine.[525]

There are many drugs which have been reported to affect the thyroidal metabolism of radioactive iodine so that care should be taken in interpreting the results of radioiodine studies in patients receiving pharmacologic agents for whatever purpose. Most of these agents depress I^{131} uptake. This group includes ACTH and cortisone,[526,527] para-aminosalicylic acid,[528,529] phenylbutazone[201] and possibly cobalt.[192,193]

In addition to the use of routine radioiodine determinations as an estimate of thyroid function, such tests may be combined with another agent to help resolve a difficult clinical dilemma. The administration of some form of thyroid hormone in large doses for approximately eight days will decrease the uptake below 20 per cent in most euthyroid patients and will have little effect on those who are hyperthyroid.[530,531] This may help distinguish thyrotoxic patients from euthyroid patients with equivocal symptoms, signs and laboratory data. Thyroid stimulating hormone in one or more doses may fail to increase the uptake of I^{131} in patients with minimal or potential hypothyroidism[532] who have adequate thyroid function by conventional tests.

The use of radioiodine to obtain a graphic record of uptake with a "scintiscanner" has been suggested as a method of predicting accurately thyroid weight.[533,534] Others[535] have not been very successful in this approach and have questioned some of the assumptions upon which the empirical equation has been based. Radioiodine has been employed not only to identify[536–538] a lingual thyroid but has actually been used successfully in its treatment.[536–538] Substernal thyroids,[539] occasional functional metastases of thyroid cancer and possibly struma ovarii may be localized with I^{131}. In recent years it has been reported[540] that radioiodine may be useful in predicting which thyroid nodules are more likely to be malignant. "Hot" nodules with an increased uptake of radioiodine are less likely to be malignant; the reverse is true of "cold" nodules where there is a decreased accumulation of radioiodine.[540]

Although the thyroid uptake decreases progressively with age,[541,542] this is not thought to be clinically significant. Women in all age groups show a slightly higher uptake than men,[541] but again this is not felt to be important clinically. Season has no effect on I^{131} tests of thyroid function.[542]

HYPOTHYROIDISM

Hypothyroidism may be defined as a symptom complex caused by a deficiency of thyroid hormone and resulting in a lowered rate of all metabolic processes. Because of the variety of hypothyroid states which are seen in the clinic, we are presenting a classification which we find to be of value in the study and management of patients who present themselves with any of these disease syndromes.

HYPOTHYROIDISM

- I. Cretinism (congenital hypothyroidism)
  - A. Athyreotic (sporadic)
  - B. Goitrous (endemic)
- II. Myxedema of children (juvenile myxedema)
- III. Myxedema of adults (Gull's disease)
  - A. Primary hypothyroidism
    - 1. Spontaneous
    - 2. Induced
      - (a) Surgical
      - (b) I^{131}
      - (c) Cibare
      - (d) Medicamentare
  - B. Secondary or pituitary myxedema

Cretinism

The first clinical descriptions of cretinism came from Switzerland and the Bavarian or Austrian Alps where goiter has long been endemic. Von Hohenheim, who was better known as Paracelsus[544] in the sixteenth century, wrote an heretical essay concerning a group of foolish people with goiters. Platter[544] described a group of simple-minded infants who had large tongues, eyes which were wide apart and large goiters. Hoeffer[544] was impressed by the feeblemindedness of these children and by their goiters. He called attention to the way that they sat close to the oven. He prophetically proposed that the cause of the cretinism was to be found in the diet which he described as "foods giving much excrement and little nourishment." Curling[545] in 1850 first reported two cases of cretinism, one aged 10 and one six months, who at necropsy were found to have no thyroid tissue. In 1871 Fagge[546] reported four patients with sporadic cretinism who did not have goiters.

Etiology. The incidence of cretinism is many times greater in the old endemic goiter regions than it is in nongoitrous regions. In addition to the common environment of families which may lead to a high incidence of cretinism, there would appear to be sporadic nonendemic goitrous cretinism which may be transmitted genetically.[547] The infrequent[548–553] occurrence of multiple cretinism with or without goiter in a family suggests a common hereditary or environmental factor, perhaps a goitrogen[554] or a microbial agent. Perhaps the failure to treat myxedema in the mother may lead to numerous congenital and developmental defects in children,[550] one of which may be cretinism. That the disorder is not genetically determined in all circumstances but may be secondary to certain unknown environmental factors *in utero* is suggested by the presence of cretinism in only one of monozygotic twins.[556] One such possibility is an intrauterine thyroiditis, or infection involving the thyroid and liver which would lead to the syndrome of myxedema and jaundice.[557,558]

Goiters occur more commonly in endemic cretins than in sporadic cretins. If one attributes the goiter and the hypothyroid state to common etiologic factors, one must postulate an iodine deficiency state or the existence of certain positive goitrogens in the maternal diet during pregnancy. Hypothyroidism and compensatory thyroid growth with goiter may occur as a result of a congenital deficiency in those enzymes necessary to the iodination of thyroid hormone.[548]

Pathology. The pathology of cretinism is essentially that of myxedema, which will be discussed later. In addition to the pathologic changes observed in myxedema in the adult, there are certain changes which represent the need for thyroid hormone for normal development. These are most obvious in the skeletal and nervous systems. Delayed ossification of bones, delayed union of the epiphyses, and delayed dentition are observed. Lotmar[559] and others[560] have described a hypoplasia of the brain. The brain of a cretin who had been under observation for six years before death exhibited infiltrative changes in the vessel walls of the cerebellum and the dentate nucleus.[561]

Endemic cretins oftentimes have goiters which may be quite large. The histologic patterns of such goiters are not unlike those observed in experimental animals which have been exposed to goitrogenic agents for some time. The thyroids of two brothers studied by Lerman et al. presented a variety of histologic patterns which included the involutional changes of a colloid goiter and other patterns which could be compared to the various stages of differentiation observed in fetal thyroids.[562] In addition, some areas which showed a papillary structure were observed. The thyroids of sporadic cretins may be completely absent, or there may be nothing but extensive fibrosis at the site of the thyroid.

Since cretinism may well represent an inborn error of metabolism, many possibilities for a defect in the synthesis of thyroid hormone would exist. The thyroid may fail to concentrate iodide,[563] or once having accumulated iodide, may be unable to oxidize it and iodinate tyrosine residues.[564] It might be that the organic binding by the gland is enhanced but the enzymatically controlled hormone synthesis from iodinated tyrosine is impaired.[564] An organic iodine compound may be synthesized and released to the circulation which is not thyroxine or triiodothyronine.[565,566]

History and Physical Findings. The clinical picture of cretinism is a classic one which is readily recognized after the picture is fully developed. Unfortunately, this classic picture does not usually present itself until the latter part of the first year. In some instances the symptoms are so insidious as to be unnoticed until the second or third year.

In the typical athyreotic cretin the weight at birth is usually eight pounds or more. The abdomen and umbilicus are generally protuberant as the result of a laxity of the abdominal musculature. The base of the skull is short, and there is a persistence of the cartilaginous junction between the pre- and postsphenoid bones which normally ossifies in the eighth month of fetal life. In addition to the incomplete growth[567] associated with cretinism there are actually deformities of the vertebral bodies[568–570] as a consequence of retardation of bone age. There is almost complete lack of epiphyseal growth and a great delay in the development of centers of ossification. Furthermore, due to a delay in the ossification of the membranous bones, the frontal suture is unusually wide, and the anterior fontanel is exceptionally large.[571] As the picture develops, the facies is one of the most characteristic features. It is a round, stupid face with a yellowish color. The eyelids are puffy, and the palpebral fissures are narrowed but horizontal in contrast to the slant observed in Mongoloids. The nose is flat and thick, and the lips are thick with an open mouth from which there protrudes a large thick tongue. The voice is flat and harsh. The neck is short and thick. A goiter is observed in many endemic cretins. The skin is dry and cool and presents a picture of a nonpitting edema.[183] The hair is fine, lifeless, dry and often quite sparse, although hirsutism has been reported[572,573] as an accompaniment of myxedema in infants. As the disease progresses without treatment, the above symptoms progress, and the feeble-mindedness of the child becomes even more apparent. Dentition is late, and growth is retarded. In untreated cretins who have reached the age of 8 or 10 years, the measurement[571] from umbilicus to soles of the feet is often less than that from umbilicus to crown.

The intensity of the clinical picture varies from one individual to another depending on the degree of thyroid function. The thyroids of certain goitrous children may be capable of minimal function, enough to prevent the most extreme picture.

Diagnosis. The diagnosis of cretinism can be verified by determining the basal metabolic rate, which has to be done in a respiratory chamber. Unfortunately, such apparatus is available only in the larger medical centers. The most accurate laboratory determination presently available in many medical centers is the serum protein-bound iodine. Tracer studies with radioactive iodine may be of diagnostic value. There may be no pick-up of radioactive iodine by the thyroid, or as in the case of goitrous cretins, there may be normal or greater than normal collection of radioiodine.[574] This iodine, however, is usually present as iodide and may be discharged by the administration of thiocyanate.[548] The demonstration of delayed ossification in membranous or long bones,[570,575,576] together with an elevated blood cholesterol, may be sufficient to confirm a diagnosis of cretinism. It has been reported that the serum level of thyrotrophic hormone is elevated in infantile and juvenile hypothyroidism.[577]

Cretinism must be differentiated from Mongolism and from juvenile or acquired myxedema. The Mongoloid has finer features and lacks the coarse skin of the cretin. The eyes of the Mongoloid are slanted, whereas the puffy eyes of cretinism with their narrow palpebral fissures are horizontal. Furthermore, the Mongoloid is far more active than the cretin.

The child with juvenile or acquired myxedema can be differentiated from the cretin by the history of normal growth and development, normal dentition and absence of feeble-mindedness. Although children having acquired juvenile myxedema are slow in their responses, they do not show signs of impaired mental development.

Treatment. The most crucial point in the treatment of cretinism is its early diagnosis and the early institution of adequate replacement with thyroid hormone. If cretinism is recognized when the child is a few months old and adequate thyroid hormone is administered without omission throughout life, there is a fair chance for the child to develop normally. Treatment with desiccated thyroid, thyroxine or triiodothyronine may be employed. The dosage can be adequately adjusted by following the height and weight. As long as the growth and weight curves are within the normal range and the child shows no signs of hyperthyroidism, the dose can be considered within the physiologic needs. In addition to the levels of blood iodine,[578,579] the skeletal maturation by x-ray[580] may be used as a guide to treatment.

One complication of thyroid hormone therapy in cretinism is accelerated ossification.[580] In the more severe types which are not recognized until late, treatment with thyroid may produce changes which are undesirable, e.g., a vigorous, active and possibly intractable child whose cerebral cortex is incapable of learning.

Myxedema

Primary Myxedema. The syndrome of myxedema or of hypothyroidism in adults escaped the attention or recognition of physicians until Gull[182] reported "On a Cretinoid State Supervening in Adult Life in Women." Four years later Ord[581] reported five adult cases having this picture of severe hypothyroidism and first proposed the term "myxedema." The term was based on reports that the swollen skin of these patients contained many times the normal amount of mucin. In the following decade the disease aroused such interest that in 1883 the Clinical Society of London appointed a committee to study the disease. This committee presented in 1888 a report on myxedema which is one of the medical classics. The Reverdins[582] and Kocher[583] in 1882 and 1883 called attention to symptoms like those of myxedema which occurred in certain patients who had been subjected to total thyroidectomy and which did not occur if thyroid tissue was left in the neck.

Today spontaneous myxedema is not rare. Means[584] states that over a 10-year period 59 cases of myxedema were admitted to the medical wards of the Massachusetts General Hospital, in contrast to 467 cases of diabetes mellitus. The disease occurs about seven to eight times more frequently in females than in males.

Etiology. The immediate cause of the signs and symptoms of myxedema is a deficiency in the secretion of thyroid hormone. Certainly in a good percentage of cases the thyroid is found to have atrophied or to have been replaced by fibrous tissue. The cause of the atrophy is not clear. We also see myxedema occurring with goiter. Such situations may result from the administration of thyroid-inhibiting drugs, i.e., thiocyanate or thiouracil, or from the ingestion of foods which have goitrogenic properties. Recently a corticogenic hypothyroidism has been reported to have occurred in patients who had been subjected to prolonged treatment with ACTH or cortisone.[138] The goiters occur presumably as the result of a compensatory increased secretion of TSH.[585,586] Some cases of myxedema with or without an associated goiter have been reported[587–589] following the prolonged administration of iodides. Myxedema may also follow acute nonsuppurative thyroiditis or chronic thyroiditis, i.e., Hashimoto's struma or Riedel's struma. Postpartum shock has also been implicated[590] in the etiology of myxedema.

The incidence of myxedema following surgical thyroidectomy for Graves' disease or following treatment of this disease with radioactive iodine depends to a great extent on the amount of tissue removed or on the dose of I^{131} administered. However, it is of interest, though uncommon, that myxedema does follow in certain cases of Graves' disease which have not been subjected to any destructive treatment (surgery or radiation). The thyroid of one patient such as this showed the picture of a lymphadenoid goiter. Whitesell and Black[591] have reported that the incidence of postoperative myxedema in patients with Graves' disease subsequent to subtotal thyroidectomy is correlated with the degree of lymphoid infiltration in the thyroids. Finally, we do see states of secondary or "pituitary myxedema" occurring in people whose pituitaries have ceased to function. Some of these patients present a picture which on first observation is very similar to that of classic myxedema.

Pathology. Adequate descriptions concerning the pathology of untreated myxedema have to be sought in the older literature. This may be attributed to the fact that most patients are now diagnosed and adequately treated with thyroid.

Most commonly the thyroids are considerably smaller than normal, and on histologic examination the gland is usually replaced by fibrous tissue with some lymphocytic infiltration.[584,592] In some instances there may be found rare thyroid follicles which are atrophic. One patient who developed myxedema and a large vascular goiter had a biopsy of his thyroid which showed an extreme hyperplasia.[593]

The pituitary of one myxedematous patient was described by Fry[594] to contain an increased number of chromophobe cells, fibrous changes and colloid, while in another pituitary[592] the eosinophilic cells were increased.

The skin shows hyperkeratosis of the epidermis with hyperkeratotic plugging in the hair follicles and sweat ducts, irregular atrophy of epidermis, edema of the corium, separation of the collagen and elastic fibers and the constant presence of a mucinous staining material.[595] The heart has been described as enlarged and having muscle fibers widely separated by edema fluid.[584,592] Although arteriosclerosis has been described in myxedematous patients coming to necropsy, and some believe that the hypercholesterolemia of hypothyroidism[596] is one causative factor in the development of arteriosclerosis, we cannot definitely attribute such vascular changes to the myxedema. The central nervous system was described in 1917 by Mott[597] as showing disappearance of Nissl's granules. Untreated cases usually contain serous fluid in the serous cavities. Atrophy and lipid depletion of the adrenal cortex have been reported.[592] There are myxomatous changes in cardiac and striated muscles as well as in the corium of the skin.[592] The infiltration is considered[598] to be mucoprotein containing hyaluronic acid and chondroitin sulfate.

The symptoms of myxedema can be directly attributed to a lack of thyroid hormone and a subsequent lowering of the metabolic rate. In those patients whose thyroids have been destroyed by natural processes or by radical surgery or irradiation, it is easy to understand that they are incapable of utilizing ingested iodine in the synthesis of thyroid hormone. However, why the thyroids of goitrous patients with myxedema are incapable of producing thyroid hormone is not yet clear. In the sera of some such patients, monoiodotyrosine and diiodotyrosine as well as triiodothyronine and thyroxine may be found. It has been suggested[599] that a hyperplastic goiter and the hypothyroid state are the consequence of a continual and abnormal loss of hormone precursors from the thyroid. Regardless of mechanism, it has now been well demonstrated that these patients are incapable of synthesizing thyroid hormone. They excrete most of the inorganic iodide without utilizing it in the synthesis of thyroxine, and by direct analysis of their blood they are found to have protein-bound iodine levels of 2 gamma per cent or less.

Symptomatology and Physical Findings. The onset of symptoms and signs of the disease is usually insidious. The patient may be unable to date the onset of change, and his friends and family are likewise unaware of any change that they would not attribute to old age or possibly to the menopause. However, as the level of circulating thyroid hormone decreases and the BMR falls, the patient may first become aware of a decreased tolerance for the cold and some decrease in sweating. Then the patient begins to develop the facies of myxedema. The hair has less life, does not take a good curl, is fine and dry in texture and becomes thinner, as has been noted[600] in thyroidectomized animals. The face is expressionless at rest and placid, round and moderately edematous in appearance. This is particularly true of the eyelids, which are puffy to the point that it appears necessary to raise the eyebrows to keep the eyes open. The features are moderately coarse. The color is pale with a lemon tint. Oftentimes there is a slight malar flush. The nose and mouth are thickened. The tongue is characteristically thick and often smooth and red.

The voice is one of the most characteristic features of the disease and classically may be recognized over the telephone. It can be described as husky, leathery, froglike and lacking in inflections.

The skin is swollen but does not pit on pressure. It is rough, inelastic and dry, and there is characteristic hyperkeratinization of the elbows and knees.[601] Xanthomatoses may erupt in myxedema.[602] Many so-called neurotic excoriations are due to a hypothyroid pruritus and can be improved by treating with thyroid hormone.[603]

Though these patients are often intelligent, they have a slow reaction time and they complain of an impaired memory. Their intellectual functions, as represented by Rorschach tests, suffer some impairment and fall between those of the neurotics and patients who have organic brain damage.[604] They oftentimes are apathetic and lethargic, although anxiety is not uncommon in hypothyroidism. Marked personality changes, which are reversible with treatment, may occur in myxedema.[605] The disordered cerebral function which occurs in myxedema gives rise to no characteristic psychiatric reaction.[606] Most of the mental aberrations, even when presenting as a frank psychosis, are corrected by administering thyroid hormone and raising the metabolic rate. The reflexes are characteristic, with a normal rate of contraction and a very prolonged rate of relaxation.[489] This is easily demonstrated in the ankle jerk.

Various types of ear, nose and throat disorders, including frank deafness,[607,608] may be associated with hypometabolism. Hypothyroidism was reported to be the cause of headaches[609] as well as atypical facial neuralgia.[610] In all, prompt relief was obtained by treatment with thyroid hormone.

Constipation is common. Ascites may be seen in patients whose disease is of severe and long duration.[611,612] Menorrhagia or polymenorrhea[613] is usually the first symptom related to the menstrual cycle that will be noted by a woman with myxedema. The periods may also become irregular. Not infrequently these patients will be subjected to dilatation and curettage for severe menorrhagia. If untreated for a long period of time, a woman with myxedema may be amenorrheic. Libido is usually decreased in both males and females.

Hypertension may be found in a certain group of patients with myxedema. The heart is frequently enlarged[214] and has a pericardial effusion.[615,616] The cardiac changes associated with myxedema, i.e., enlarged heart, pericardial effusion, electrocardiographic abnormalities and cardiac failure, may all be reversed with treatment.[617-619]

The tolerance of myxedematous patients for morphine and related drugs is extremely poor. One of our patients went into an alarming and almost fatal coma following the administration of 10 mg. of morphine sulfate for the pain of a pathologic fracture.

Many types of nonspecific arthralgias and myalgias seem to be associated with myxedema and are readily relieved with thyroid hormone.

Diagnosis. Laboratory studies which are of value in developing a diagnosis of myxedema are those which measure: (1) the total body metabolism, (2) cholesterol metabolism, (3) the level of circulating thyroid hormone and (4) the capacity of the thyroid to concentrate iodine.

The basal metabolic rate is a laboratory test which in some centers is considered old fashioned. However, it is one which has stood the test of time and is of genuine value. Indeed, it gives us information that no other tests give, i.e., the sum total of oxygen consumption in the entire organism. Furthermore, it is a practical test that can be done properly in inexpensively equipped hospital and office laboratories. Patients with myxedema or developing myxedema practically always have basal metabolic rates below the level of minus 25. Occasional exceptions to this are patients with cardiac decompensation or large serous effusions, which alter the standard body surfaces, or with complicating diseases such as a pheochromocytoma. A good basal test in a patient with well developed myxedema will usually be minus 40 to minus 50. It is exceptionally rare to see a false low test. However, we have seen such when the machine used contained old soda lime.

The blood cholesterol is also a well established test which can be carried out with accuracy in most hospital laboratories. The normal levels, by most techniques, vary between 180 and 225 mg. per 100 cc. of blood. In myxedema it is usually elevated and may reach levels as high as 700. Usually the level obtained in classic myxedema is in the neighborhood of 300. We have, however, seen patients with classic myxedema who had normal or low blood cholesterol levels. Usually on checking the dietary histories of such patients we have found that their intake of fat and protein had been deficient. As a rule, however, such patients are observed to have an increase in blood cholesterol to levels consistent with myxedema after a week or two of adequate hospital diet. In addition to the increase in total cholesterol in hypothyroidism there is also an increase in total lipids, phospholipids and beta but not alpha lipoproteins.[620] Associated with the lipemia and hypercholesterolemia there is a proportionally greater carotinemia.[621]

The serum protein-bound iodine is the most direct method for measuring circulating thyroid hormone. Normal values vary between 4.0 and 8.0 micrograms per 100 cc. of blood. In classic myxedema we find levels below 2.0 micrograms per 100 cc. We have observed levels as low as 0.0. It should be pointed out that the ingestion of any of a large number of iodinated compounds may give spuriously high values for the PBI. A partial list of such compounds is given in Table 4.

Radioiodine tracer techniques are of real value in determining whether a thyroid is present, and, if so, whether it is capable of utilizing iodine in synthesizing thyroid hormone. These techniques are discussed in a separate section. Athyreotic myxedematous patients concentrate practically no radioiodine in the neck region and excrete in the urine at a slower rate than do normals between 70 and 95 per cent of an administered dose.

In patients with low thyroid reserve or equivocal hypothyroidism, it may be necessary to demonstrate an impaired response of thyroidal uptake of I^{131} to TSH.[532] We have observed patients with ascites and polyserositis complicating myxedema who failed to excrete more than 50 per cent of the administered iodine in the urine. We have also observed this in one patient who developed myxedema and a large goiter following prolonged treatment with potassium thiocyanate.[593] This patient retained in his hyperplastic thyroid most of the administered radioiodine. This situation does not always hold in patients having this type of struma medicamentare and myxedema.

There are a few miscellaneous laboratory findings which will suggest the diagnosis of myxedema. Examination of the blood frequently shows an anemia and a relative lymphocytosis. Not infrequently there is an achlorhydria. Occasionally a pericardial effusion is noted. The electrocardiogram shows decreased voltage and lowering to flattening of the T waves and small P waves. Such hearts beat feebly and have a diminished volume output.[622] In such patients the heart size decreases and the electrocardiographic changes return toward normal upon the administration of thyroid. The urinary excretion of 17-ketosteroids is lowered in most patients with myxedema.[623]

Other abnormalities in myxedema have been established with more elaborate laboratory procedures. Myxedema is associated with a decreased cerebral vascular flow[624] with consequent decrease in glucose consumption[453] as well as an abnormal electroencephalogram.[486,625] The gross energy metabolism of the brain, as reflected by oxygen utilization, may be independent of the action of the thyroid hormone.[626] There is an excess of magnesium in myxedema, which is excreted when the patient is treated with triiodothyronine.[627] The glomerular filtration rate and renal blood flow are decreased in myxedema.[622,628] As a consequence, there is a decrease in the renal clearance of I^{131}, since the latter is a linear function of the glomerular filtration rate.[629] The bone marrow demonstrates a hypoplasia of all the myeloid elements without any increase in fat but with excess hyperemia[630] Protein synthesis as measured by N^{15} glycine is decreased[282] while the degradation rate of human serum albumin is decreased[289] in myxedema. There is frequently an increase in the total proteins with an increase in the globulins and M-2 mucoproteins.[631] The increase in the beta globulin fraction in myxedema[632] may account for the increased erythrocyte sedimentation rate which is not due to the anemia or hypercholesterolemia.

Differential Diagnosis. Myxedema must be differentiated from chronic glomerulonephritis with edema and from nephrosis. Such patients present not only a lemon-tinted pallor and puffiness of the face but also frequently a low basal metabolic rate. The edema in these diseases is pitting, whereas in myxedema there is practically no pitting. Careful examination of the urine and studies of kidney function should give an accurate diagnosis.

In Addison's disease subjective symptoms may be confused with those of myxedema. Furthermore, a low basal metabolic rate, a diminished amount of urinary 17-ketosteroids and a reduced uptake of I^{131} by the thyroid may occur or may reflect secondary adrenocortical failure.[633] Even a hyponatremia has been reported[634] in primary myxedema. The hypotension, pigmentation, low blood sodium and chlorides, and an absent response to ACTH which occur in Addison's disease distinguish it from myxedema.

Pernicious anemia may also have to be differentiated from myxedema because of the lemon-tinted pallor, the anemia (in myxedema there may even be a macrocytic and hyperchromic anemia), and the achlorhydria which occur in both diseases. In pernicious anemia the BMR should not be below minus 25. A normal protein-bound iodine and normal uptake of I^{131} should rule out myxedema. However, the two diseases may occur together[635] and require treatment with both liver and thyroid.

Myxedema may have to be differentiated from euthyroid or nonmyexedematous hypometabolism.[636,637] In the latter condition, although the basal metabolic rate may be as low as that seen in myxedema, the radioiodine uptake and turnover, PBI and cholesterol are all normal. There is no improvement with desiccated thyroid in euthyroid hypometabolism, but there is a response of the BMR and clinical status with triiodothyronine alone or in combination with thyroxine.[636,637]

It is of importance to differentiate pituitary or secondary myxedema from primary myxedema or Gull's disease. Pituitary or secondary myxedema is a term used to describe those patients whose primary trouble is in a failure of anterior pituitary function and whose clinical picture is one of myxedema. There may be a solitary deficiency of thyrotrophin[638,639] or a deficiency of the latter hormone in association with one or more of the other anterior pituitary hormones. The clinical picture may be indistinguishable from primary myxedema unless it is associated with other pituitary deficiencies. Under such circumstances one observes impaired gonadal and adrenal function as well as thyroid function. Of help with the latter group are the decreased urinary gonadotrophins, 17-ketosteroids and corticosteroids. Adrenal insufficiency may also be reflected in the decreased blood chlorides and sodium. The most deciding factor in the differentiation of pituitary myxedema from primary myxedema, whether the former is associated with other pituitary deficiencies or not, is the response to administered TSH. In secondary myxedema there is an in-increased uptake of I^{131} by the thyroid[640–643] or an increase in the protein-bound iodine of blood[643,644] after treatment with TSH.

Treatment. Myxedema is treated by the administration of thyroid hormone. This is obviously replacement therapy. It is not curative.

The object of treatment is to return the patient to a euthyroid state or to rid him of all symptoms of myxedema on the minimal dose of thyroid. The yardstick for this objective of treatment may be the basal metabolic rate, or it may be some chemical determination, such as the serum protein-bound iodine or the blood cholesterol. The clinical picture must also be followed carefully and the point of maximum well-being should be sought. The latter is of importance since the mean normal BMR or blood iodine or blood cholesterol may be greater or less than is physiologic for the patient in question.

Three main types of thyroid hormone preparations are available for the treatment of myxedema. These are desiccated thyroid, l-thyroxine, and l-triiodothyronine. The effect of desiccated thyroid on the BMR in classic myxedema can almost be quantitated. Means[584] states that a daily ration of 30 mg. of U.S.P. thyroid keeps the level at approximately minus 20; 60 mg. at minus 10; 100 mg. at minus 5. Those[645] who use the PBI as a guide in therapy with desiccated thyroid estimate that there is a one microgram rise in the PBI with each grain of desiccated thyroid.

In older patients with myxedema whose disease has produced changes in the heart or in patients with complicating heart disease, we prefer to begin treatment cautiously with a dose no greater than 30 mg. daily. The dose may be gradually increased to the point of maximum well-being or, if each increment of dose is well tolerated, to the level of euthyroidism. If there are no complicating factors which make it desirable to begin treatment gradually, we prefer beginning treatment with a dose of 100 mg. daily. On this dose the response to treatment is characterized by an acceleration in every metabolic process. The first change is a marked diuresis which occurs in the first two or three days. With this diuresis a loss of weight begins. The blood cholesterol and the plasma protein fall to normal levels. Within 10 to 14 days of this dose of thyroid, the BMR rises to a normal level, and the picture of myxedema disappears. The myxedema facies usually disappears rather rapidly. The skin and hair are slow in recovering. The tolerance for cold improves. The voice returns to normal within about 14 days. The patient becomes brighter, the hearing improves, appetite improves, constipation is corrected, and menstruation becomes normal in premenopausal women. During the first week or two of treatment the patient may complain of pains deep in the leg muscles. The mechanism of this is not known. Angina pain occurs in some patients and may require cutting the dose or even stopping treatment for a while. Although the myxedematous patient is sensitive to thyroid hormone, after restoration of the euthyroid state the tolerance to thyroid is similar to that of a euthyroid person.[646]

The increased use of l-thyroxine in recent years has been attributed to the advantage of administering a fixed quantity of a chemically identifiable material. This agent has the same effects as desiccated thyroid in its ability to depress uptake of radioactive iodine in normal glands, reduce nontoxic goiters and maintain the euthyroid state in myxedema patients.[647,648] There is a decrease in the cholesterol and an increase in the BMR and PBI with l-thyroxine[647] as with desiccated thyroid. There seems to be good absorption of this thyroid hormone administered orally.[648,649] It has been suggested[650] that there may develop a resistance to thyroxine, but this may be no more than the increased tolerance to thyroid hormone when the myxedema patient is restored to the euthyroid state.[646]

Recently with the discovery and synthesis of a new thyroid hormone, 1-triiodothyronine, this agent has been used very effectively in the treatment of myxedema.[308,440,651–658] In general, this agent is three to five times more effective than 1-thyroxine on a weight basis in terms of a daily maintenance dose.[651,652,654,655,657] Whereas 1-thyroxine, after intravenous administration, produces its maximum response in 8.9 days, 1-triiodothyronine gives its maximum response after a similar route of administration in 2.1 days.[658] Whereas treatment with desiccated thyroid or 1-thyroxine produces an increase in the PBI, treatment with 1-triiodothyronine induces no rise in the PBI.[652,654] Thus, this laboratory procedure cannot be used as a guide to therapy with triiodothyronine. In general, it would appear that 60 to 100 mg. of desiccated thyroid is equivalent in terms of the daily maintenance dose of myxedema to 100 micrograms of 1-thyroxine or 20 to 30 micrograms of 1-triiodothyronine.[653,657]

There is no effect of cortisone on the clinical or laboratory features of hypothyroidism save for some quickening of the mental processes.[659]

Complications and Prognosis. Patients adequately treated with thyroid hormone can expect to live in a physiologic and clinical state of euthyroidism. Evidence of the effectiveness of this type of treatment is found in Murray's report in 1920[660] of the first patient treated for myxedema. He administered thyroid to this patient from 1891 to 1919 when she finally died at the age of 74, having lived a healthy and normal life for 28 years after the diagnosis of myxedema had first been made. In 1946 Burgess[661] published a final report on a patient who had taken thyroid in treatment for myxedema from 1892 to 1943. She died at the age of 94. Notwithstanding a moderately severe arteriosclerosis and hypertension, she had lived in a healthy and euthyroid state for 51 years on this type of replacement therapy.

Despite the fact that therapy is so effective, some patients are seen for the first time in myxedema coma. This condition is characterized by extremely low body temperatures[662,663] and is frequently resistant to treatment, terminating fatally.[662–666]

It has been reported[555] that untreated myxedema during pregnancy may lead to numerous congenital and developmental defects in the children.

HYPERTHYROIDISM

Introduction. One of the most common maladies of the thyroid is associated with a clinical picture which is usually attributed to increased secretion of thyroid hormone. It is most commonly known as "toxic goiter," "exophthalmic goiter," "Graves' disease," or "von Basedow's disease." Since some major features of the disease cannot be explained by an increased secretion of thyroid hormone, we prefer not to use the term "toxic goiter," and because not all patients have exophthalmos, we find the "exophthalmic goiter," an unsatisfactory one. Thus, we prefer to label this disease entity with an eponym, *"Graves' disease."* We might be criticized for not using the term "Parry's disease" since Parry's description of the disease appeared in 1825,[667] ten years earlier than Graves'[668] first report appeared. However, Parry, who was a scholarly and distinguished student of medicine, did not choose to publish his observations of patients presenting this malady, notwithstanding the facts that he observed his first patient with this symptom complex in 1786 and that in 1813 when he saw three such patients he wrote in his records that he suspected some connection between the cardiac symptoms and the goiters presented by these patients. It was Parry's son who collected and published these and other observations of his distinguished father in 1825 three years after his father's death.

Although the major features of the disease, as recorded by most early clinicians who wrote about it, were palpitation, tachycardia and goiter, Basedow's classic description of the disease which appeared in 1840 is the most complete description that we have found in the older literature of the disease as we know it today.[669] In his original report Basedow not only emphasized the occurrence of exophthalmos, goiter and tachycardia, but he also described the nervous restlessness, excessive perspiration, air hunger, diarrhea, amenorrhea and emaciation of this malady. It is of interest that he also described a brawny nonedematous swelling of the legs which suggests that some of his patients had localized myxedema. Such a careful description of this malady certainly justifies the eponym used by most continental writers, i.e., "Basedow's Disease." Charcot[670] was the first to emphasize the nervous symptoms of hyperthyroidism. Plummer[671] was the first observer who differentiated between the clinical manifestations of "exophthalmic goiter" or "Graves' disease" and "adenomatous goiter with hyperthyroidism."

Graves' disease is a constitutional disease, which in its full-blown classic picture is characterized by exophthalmos, a large hyperplastic goiter and changes in most systems of the body, many of which can be attributed to increased levels of circulating thyroid hormone.

Etiology. The etiology of this disease is quite unknown. Since the disease is not reportable, we know neither its incidence nor its geographic distribution. We have the impression, however, that its distribution is not the same as that of endemic goiter.

Although the disease may occur at any age, it appears most commonly between the third and fifth decades. It is more common among females than among males (in Chicago and Boston about four times more frequently in females than in males[672]). A significant familial tendency of the disease is encountered not infrequently. Boas and Ober[673] who studied one family found 11 cases which occurred in three generations. Ingbar and Freinkel[674,675] have observed an abnormality in the disposal of thyroxine in patients with Graves' disease and their kin which might point to a familial metabolic defect in patients who acquire this disease.

Ingbar and Freinkel[674] have studied the fate and turnover of labelled l-thyroxine in euthyroidism, in treated and untreated myxedematous subjects and in patients with Graves' disease. They have found that the turnover rate of labelled thyroxine in 11 euthyroid subjects averaged 6.6, in untreated myxedema 7.5, and in treated myxedema 6.9 days. Patients with untreated Graves' disease had a rapid turnover rate of 2.2 to 4.3 days with a mean of 3.1 days. This accelerated turnover rate of thyroxine was observed as long as one year after correction of the hyperthyroidism, i.e., mean 4.2 days. The same investigators[675] have also observed a similar rapid turnover rate of thyroxine in many of the blood relatives of their patients who had had Graves' disease.

Iversen[676] and Meulengracht[677] noted that, following the occupation of Denmark by the German army, there was a significant increase in the incidence of this malady throughout that country. In conversation with these and other physicians from Denmark, we have been assured that they experienced no hunger. One asks whether or not this epidemic can be related to the psychic traumata which naturally came with the defeat and occupation of their country. Certainly, as one sees more Graves' disease, one is impressed with the fact that a large percentage of patients give a history of psychic traumata to which they frequently relate the onset of disease. Some give a history of an infection or of physical trauma following which the symptoms of the malady developed. It is impossible to state whether these various situations of stress are of etiologic importance or whether they occurred during the course of the disease and were accentuated because of the disease. Notwithstanding the reasonable doubt which we have about these stress situations, we do think of them as trigger phenomena which cause an increased release of TSH through

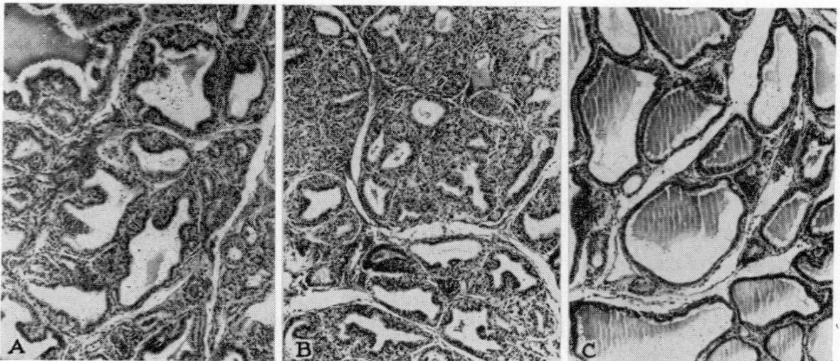

FIG. 2. Microscopic anatomy of thyroid in Graves' disease. (All sections taken from same thyroid during various stages of treatment.)

A. Biopsy before beginning treatment. B.M.R. plus 40%. Note hyperplasia. Mean cell height 15.3 micra.

B. Biopsy after treatment with thiouracil had caused fall in B.M.R. to plus 8%. Note hyperplasia. Mean cell height 17.3 micra.

C. Section of thyroid removed after ten days of treatment with thiouracil and sodium iodide. Note involution. Mean cell height 10.3 micra. Thyroglobin iodine of this gland was 2.3 mg. per 100 gm. of wet tissue.

some hypothalmic pituitary pathway and subsequent stimulation of the thyroid.

Hertz and Means[678] observed a series of patients who developed the classic picture of this syndrome after having been on a weight-reducing diet with or without administered thyroid. We have not been able to elicit any specific dietary deficiencies in such patients. Similar studies were reported by Stephens,[679] who studied the effect of dietary intake on the guinea pig's response to thyrotrophic hormone. He observed that animals which were on a weight-reducing diet were much more sensitive to TSH than were those animals receiving enough food to maintain normal growth and gain of weight.

In view of the observations made by Ingbar and Freinkel,[674,675] it would be most interesting to determine the effect of starvation or of specific dietary deprivation on the turnover and metabolism of l-thyroxine in both laboratory animals and human subjects.

Pathology (Anatomic and Functional). The most striking pathologic changes in this disease are observed in the thyroid gland. In patients with classic Graves' disease, the thyroid is uniformly and more or less symmetrically enlarged. It varies in size from two to several times the normal. It is vascular and friable. A marked hypertrophy and hyperplasia of the thyroid acinar cells with intrafollicular papillary projections are seen (Fig. 2). There is a loss of intrafollicular colloid which in the extreme case is complete. Another feature of the thyroids of Graves' disease is a significant amount of lymphoid tissue. This may vary from a diffuse appearance of lymphocytes to the development of lymph follicles with germinal centers. Whereas this histologic structure was the usual picture before Plummer introduced preoperative treatment with iodine, it became the unusual picture until we began removing the thyroids of these patients following treatment with thiouracil and no iodine.

The thyroids which are not examined until after adequate treatment with iodine, with or without the thiouracil drugs, are quite different; they are firm and are much less vascular and on microscopic examination they are characterized by involution. The cells are of almost normal size. The papillary projections have almost disappeared, and the acini are filled with a deep staining colloid (Fig. 2). In some instances the effects of iodine are so great as to produce a hyperinvolution. Here the microscopic picture can be likened to that of a colloid goiter.

Such hyperplastic thyroids characteristically utilize iodine and synthesize and secrete thyroid hormone into the circulation at an increased rate, as evidenced by the elevated blood levels of protein-bound iodine and the increased metabolic rates of this disease. Those factors which contribute to this set of circumstances are not clear, but in animals similar changes can be produced in the thyroid by administering thyrotrophic hormone. Furthermore, we are unable to produce a hyperplasia of the thyroid with any goitrogenic agents unless the pituitary is intact. These and other experimental studies, to be discussed later, are indirect evidence in support of the thesis that thyrotrophic hormone is produced in excess by the pituitary to produce this disease.

Although the most dramatic anatomic and physiologic changes of this malady are found in the thyroid, the structural and functional changes are by no means limited to this organ. Indeed, some of the most interesting and challenging pathologic changes are observed in several other tissues of the body. The pathologic changes within the orbit are not well defined. Indeed, opportunities for studying these changes have developed only in recent years since Naffziger described a method of treating severe or so-called "malignant" exophthalmos by surgical decompression of the orbit. Naffziger and co-workers[680,681] reported that the orbital muscles of the unfortunate patients whose exophthalmos had advanced to the point of requiring this extreme form of treatment had swollen from three to eight times the normal size, and thus increased the intraorbital tension. Microscopically the muscles which were biopsied showed edema, round cell infiltration, an increase in fibrous tissue, hyalinization, fragmentation and destruction. Naffziger attributes the exophthalmos of Graves' disease to increased muscle mass and to orbital edema. Rundle and Pochin[682] described the eyes of seventeen patients who had died of Graves' disease. In these studies they demonstrated an increased content of fat in the orbits which they postulated to be the cause of protrusion of the eyes. The discrepancies between these two groups of workers probably stem from the fact that they were studying the same disease but in different stages of development and with different techniques. It is quite possible that the proptosis of the eyes in patients suffering with the severe exophthalmos of this disease is due to orbital fat, edema, increased muscle mass, and possibly a loss of the tensile strength of the orbital muscles with a subsequent loss of resistance to an increased intraorbital pressure. The stare and lid lag of this disease, which usually disappear following correction of the hyperthyroidism, cannot be related to the above findings but must be attributed to a spasm of the palpebral muscles—a spasm of the levator palpebrae superioris, a striated muscle which is innervated by the oculomotor nerve.[683] Mulvaney,[684] on the other hand, attributes the stare and lid lag to a spasm of Landström's muscle, which is a smooth muscle innervated by sympathetics.

True exophthalmos has not been produced by the administration of thyroid hormone. Notwithstanding the apparent decrease in lid lag and stare following correction of the hyperthyroidism in these patients, the proptosis is not improved. Indeed, by measurement the proptosis actually increases following thyroidectomy.[685] On the basis of studies done on animals it has been postulated that the exophthalmos is due to an action of thyrotrophic hormone.[129,130,686,687] All of these investigators have produced experimental exophthalmos by administering pituitary extracts rich in thyrotrophic hormone. Since all of these preparations were crude and impure extracts containing TSH, we are unable to ascribe these changes to thyrotrophic hormone *per se*. Furthermore, sheep pituitary extracts produce exophthalmos very readily in the Fundulus, whereas extracts of beef pituitaries equally rich in thyrotrophic activity have minimal exophthalmic activity. Dobyns and associates[688,689] have pursued this observation and have demonstrated that the exophthalmos-producing substance (EPS) of the anterior pituitary can be separated from the thyrotrophic hormone. They have demonstrated that the EPS in a dose as small as 15 micrograms is capable of inducing a measurable exophthalmos in the Atlantic "minnow" *Fundulus heteroclitus,* Linn. They have also reported that with similar methods of assay an exophthalmos-producing substance can be demonstrated in the serum of patients with severe exophthalmos.

Askanazy[690] was the first to note fatty infiltration, loss of striations and degenerations of the muscle fibers. Dudgeon and Urquhart[691] described an infiltration of plasma cells and endothelial cells with an atrophy of the muscle fibers of skeletal muscles. These anatomic changes of Graves' disease may explain the muscle weakness which is so common in patients with this malady. They are quite likely, also, related to the creatinuria and decreased tolerance for creatine which are so commonly found in these patients. Although the administration of thyroid hormone in toxic amounts to rats will produce a loss in skeletal muscle mass, the microscopic changes described above have not been described in animals subjected to treatment with thyroid hormone. They have, however, been demonstrated[130] in the skeletal muscles of intact and thyroidectomized guinea pigs after treatment with pituitary extracts rich in thyrotrophic hormone. Thus the muscle changes and symptoms may be quite unrelated to the degree of hyperthyroidism seen in these patients.

Changes in the heart are inconsistent. Hypertrophy of the heart muscle is not uncommon. Although some authors[692,693] have reported finding fibrosis and lymphocytes in the myocardium of patients dying of this disease, others[694,695] have failed to find any characteristic changes in the heart.

The livers of 107 patients who died from Graves' disease have revealed a high incidence of fatty infiltration and focal and central necrosis.[696] Atrophic changes were noted in about half of these patients. The mechanism by which these changes occur is not clear. Experimentally some of these changes can be produced by administering large doses of thyroid. Likewise, fatty livers followed by some round cell infiltration and fibrosis have been observed in intact and thyroidectomized guinea pigs after treatment for varying periods with pituitary extracts rich in thyrotrophic hormone.[130]

A persistent or enlarged thymus and enlarged lymph nodes have been described in patients who came to autopsy after dying from Graves' disease. Warthin[697] was so impressed by the thymico-lymphadenopathy of Graves' disease that he labelled it the "Graves' constitution." Halstead[698] advocated irradiation of the thymus or thymectomy for symptoms persisting after thyroidectomy. We are unable to explain the reasons for the thymico-lymphadenopathy of this disease but having observed that the only tissues which, when explanted and bathed in physiologic media containing a pituitary extract, inactivate thyrotrophic hormone are thyroid, thymus and lymph nodes, we have postulated that the thymus and lymph nodes are target glands of TSH, as is the thyroid. If such is the case, the thymicolymphadenopathy of Graves' disease might be explained on the basis of an increased secretion and action of TSH.

There is some evidence which suggests an adrenal insufficiency in this disease. LeCompte[699] reported in 1949 that the width of adrenal cortices of patients who died of Graves' disease was less than that of controls who did not manifest any signs of disease of the thyroid or of people who died of lymphosarcoma or lymphatic leukemia. Also, patients having Graves' disease when given ACTH manifest minimal to no eosinopenia.[137,526] This apparent decreased responsiveness of the adrenals to ACTH in Graves' disease may be related to the rapid rate of disappearance of hydrocortisone from the blood of patients with Graves' disease as demonstrated by Peterson et al.[700]

There have been no significant pathologic changes described in the gonads of patients with this disease. Notwithstanding the fact that we have postulated an increased secretion of or sensitivity to pituitary thyrotrophic hormone, there are no significant anatomic changes in the pituitaries of patients dying of this disease. Relatively short periods of treatment with desiccated thyroid, thyroxine or triiodothyronine suppress the uptake of radioactive iodine in normal humans, but do not suppress the hyperfunctioning thyroids of Graves' disease.[701] Werner interprets these observations as evidence against any pituitary control of the thyroid in Graves' disease. This interpretation might be a reasonable one if we had conclusive evidence for a fine balance between the thyroid and the pituitary's secretion of TSH and if we could assume a normal responsiveness on the part of the pituitary or of the hypothalamus in this diseased state. Having observed a limited number of patients with Graves' disease whose thyroids were suppressed by treatment with desiccated thyroid or thyroxine in relatively large doses over a period of months, we would suggest that the balance between thyroid and pituitary is not as sensitive as we had previously postulated. The thyroids of Graves' disease can at least in some instances be suppressed by adequate treatment with the thyroid hormones.

Further evidence against the thesis that this disease is due to an increased secretion of thyrotrophic hormone is the observation[15] that such patients do not excrete in the urine any active thyrotrophic hormone, whereas totally thyroidectomized patients excrete greater amounts than do normal young men. On the other hand, thyrotrophic hormone, when exposed to explants of rabbit thyroid tissue, is inactivated.[131] Furthermore, explants of thyroids taken from patients with Graves' disease, after a maximum response to treatment with iodine, inactivate twice as much TSH as do similar explants of normal human thyroid tissue taken as biopsy specimens at parathyroid operations.[702] We would suggest, therefore, that the failure to recover thyrotrophic hormone from the body fluids of patients with Graves' disease is due to an increased metabolism of TSH by the thyroid and other tissues.

On the basis of these observations, we have postulated that Graves' disease is in part due to an increased sensitivity of the thyroid to thyrotrophic hormone and possibly to an increased secretion of TSH. Thus, we might attribute to an increased secretion of thyroid hormone the anatomic and functional changes of this disease: increased metabolic rate, weight loss, increased cardiac output, nervousness and hepatic damage. Those changes which we might attribute to thyrotrophic hormone are: thyroid hyperplasia and hyperfunction, enlarged thymus and lymph nodes, muscle changes and weakness, and exophthalmos.

Symptomatology and Physical Findings. The presenting symptoms may vary from none to those of fulminating thyrotoxicosis with many systems of the body affected. Those patients who admit to no symptoms may even insist that they feel better than they have at any time previously. Such patients are usually males who actually feel exhilarated by the increased levels of thyroid hormone and who usually consult the physician primarily to satisfy a friend or relative who has noted prominence of the eyes, a goiter or increased excitability. Others whose disease is manifest primarily by the ophthalmic symptoms, may first consult an ophthalmologist because of symptoms referable to the eyes. Some older patients may present themselves primarily because of symptoms of cardiac failure. We have seen one male patient who presented himself to the clinic with gynecomastia, fearing that he had a cancer of the breast.

Although it is not common, we do see patients with fulminating Graves' disease in whom all of the symptoms and findings of the disease have developed within a few days. We observed a 40-

year-old woman who developed a full-blown picture of moderately severe Graves' disease while in the hospital recovering from a panhysterectomy. On the other hand, we may see patients who have had the disease with exacerbations and remissions for many years, who finally present themselves because of some complication such as heart failure or even impending thyrotoxic crisis. The most commonly seen picture, however, is that of a woman who presents a fairly classic picture of the disease which has been developing over a period of eight or nine months.

The symptoms described in the presenting complaint or those elicited in a careful review of systems illustrate the many and varied actions of the thyroid hormones with changes in practically every system of the body.

Notwithstanding the fact that many patients experience some exhilaration in the early stages of the disease, most of them, by the time they consult a physician, complain of nervousness and increased excitability. They may be more emotional and irritable than previously. Frequently, they complain of tremors on lifting a cup of coffee or other small objects. On examination, such patients usually have a tremor of the outstretched hand. This tremor is a fine and rapid one. Some of the older patients may exhibit a coarse but rapid tremor. The excitability of these patients, when considered along with the stare and lid retraction, impresses one with a picture of fear or even anger.

Some of the most common symptoms of this malady are those related to the cardiovascular system. They may vary from a palpitation which is most noticeable with excitement to the symptoms of frank cardiac failure. Although the blood pressure is not characteristically elevated, the pulse pressure is usually increased. This elevation in pulse pressure as a rule can be related to a slight increase in systolic pressure and a slight decrease in diastolic pressure. The heart size is not characteristically increased. The heart sounds may be normal except for the rapid rate, which usually is 90 or more per minute. In males it is not as rapid as in females. An apical systolic murmur of mild to moderate intensity is common. Rarely a diastolic murmur is heard at the apex which disappears on correction of the hyperthyroidism. One very characteristic sign of hyperthyroidism is a systolic scratch heard over the second to third interspace just to the left of the sternum. This scratch is usually heard at the end of inspiration, though it may also be heard at the end of expiration. Bounding carotids may be seen and the pulse is usually quite full and rapid.

Some patients present themselves primarily because of a goiter. Women complain of it because of its undesirable cosmetic effects. Men, if they complain of it, usually say that it has increased in size enough to make their collars intolerably tight. On physical examination, the thyroid of a patient with Graves' disease is invariably enlarged to some extent. This enlargement may vary from two to many times its normal size. The gland is more or less symmetrical, though the right lobe is often larger than the left. The trachea as a rule is not displaced. The gland is meaty in consistency. The pyramidal lobe, which as a rule is found on the left side of the trachea, is enlarged. Characteristically, the gland is very vascular, and a bruit is heard over the upper or lower poles of either lobe. In the more vascular glands a thrill may be felt over either the upper or lower poles. The gland of a patient who recently has been treated with iodides is firm and rubbery in consistency. The thyroid may be nodular, with discrete nodules palpable, if the Graves' disease is of long duration; particularly if the patient has received iodides, involution of some areas may have occurred to produce the nodules; or Graves' disease may develop in a goiter which is nodular.

The patient with classic Graves' disease will usually complain of some *intolerance for heat.* If he does not, he frequently will state that he has greater tolerance for cold than previously. Such symptoms may be so subtle that the patient simply reports that he needs fewer bed clothes than he previously required or that in rooms where other occupants are quite comfortable, he wishes to have the windows and doors opened. Such patients complain of increased sweating.

The skin is often warmer than normal. Indeed, if one finds a cool skin in a patient suspected of this malady, the diagnosis becomes doubtful. The skin is often moist and characteristically of a velvety texture. Vitiligo is frequently found on the skin. This change is more prominent on the hands or other exposed surfaces. These patients usually state that they have had the vitiligo for many years before the onset of the present malady. Occasionally, women who have this disease complain of thinning of the hair. Loss of hair over the lower third of the legs is common.

A *loss of weight,* notwithstanding a normal or increased caloric intake, is almost a cardinal symptom of hyperthyroidism. Rarely, dietary intakes are so great as to protect against any loss of weight. The weight loss is readily explained on the basis of the increased metabolic rate. Frank diarrhea is not common. However, most patients with Graves' disease admit to a change in bowel habits; that is, they may have two stools instead of one per day and stools which are softer than normal. It is of interest that peptic ulcers are most uncommon in patients with hyperthyroidism. There are no characteristic findings in the gastrointestinal tract. However, an extremely ill patient, with hyperthyroidism of long standing, may show evidence of liver damage.

Weakness is also characteristic and may be the primary complaint. The weakness can be demonstrated by having the patient in the sitting position hold his leg in the extended position. As a rule a patient with Graves' disease is unable to hold his leg in this position for longer than one minute and a half. Rarely, weakness is so profound that the patient has difficulty in lifting himself off the bed. Such weakness is an ominous sign and demands prompt and effective treatment. Wasting of various muscle groups, a characteristic finding, is often most striking in the temporal muscles or in the muscles of the shoulder girdle or of the legs. The tendon reflexes are usually hyperactive.

Polyuria and increased thirst which disappear on control of the hyperthyroidism are common. There are no other urinary manifestations which can be related to this malady.

Oligomenorrhea is the usual complaint in premenopausal women with this disease. Rarely, amenorrhea is a major complaint which is corrected after the hyperthyroidism has been adequately controlled. There is no evidence that the fertility of such patients is significantly altered.

Male patients with this malady seldom note a change in gonadal function. A few patients, however, complain of impotence. On the other hand, it has been reported in the lay press that a recently discovered portrait of Casanova, the great lover, demonstrated some exophthalmos and other signs suggesting that this accomplished gentleman had Graves' disease. Gynecomastia is quite common in males suffering with this malady. Indeed, we have the impression that if one looks for it, one will find it more frequently than not in those males who have exophthalmos as a major component of their Graves' disease. Such gynecomastia is usually characterized by a thickening of the subareolar tissue which on palpation oftentimes is tender. The gynecomastia may be so exaggerated that the patients' breasts are not unlike those of a pubescent girl. Some female patients have reported that with the onset of moderately severe exophthalmos, their breasts had so increased in size that they had to wear larger brassieres.

The ophthalmic symptoms in the majority of these patients are not distressing. Often the average patient will state that a member of the family or friend has noted a prominence of his eyes. The only complaints may be of increased tearing on awakening or on exposure to cold or wind. Examination of the eyes reveals dilated pupils with a widening of the palpebral fissures and rather infrequent or irregular blinking. The widened palpebral fissures give the appearance of a stare which has been likened to the facies of fright or even rage. Although there frequently is a true exophthalmos, one may be deceived by the lid retraction and may interpret it as a proptosis. This stare, which is usually benefited by controlling the hyperthyroidism, has given the impression that thyroidectomy corrects the exophthalmos of hyperthyroidism. There is usually a lag of the upper lid on looking downward and a lag of the globe behind the lids on looking upward.

The generalized lymphadenopathy which usually accompanies Graves' disease leads to palpable lymph nodes in the cervical area in many cases. Axillary, inguinal and epitrochlear lymph nodes may also be palpable. A palpable spleen is not common.

"Ophthalmopathic" Graves' Disease. Although the classic case of Graves' disease presents both a goiter with hyperthyroidism and exophthalmos, there are some patients who present only the picture of goiter and hyperthyroidism. Their eye signs may be completely lacking, or they may be limited to lid retraction and lid lag. On the other end of the spectrum we find an unfortunate group of patients who present the ophthalmopathy of this malady. We have seen patients who during the period of follow-up have developed at different times all of the above phases of the disease. For that reason we prefer not dividing these stages into separate categories. However, the ophthalmic phase of the disease when it occurs is so troublesome that we feel justified in discussing it more extensively.

Patients who develop the ophthalmic component of this disease often first seek help from the ophthalmologist. In other cases the eye symptoms do not become seriously troublesome until after thyroidectomy or after too rapid control of the hyperthyroidism by means of antithyroid drugs or with radioactive iodine. Eye problems do not develop in some patients until several years after surgical correction of the previously existing hyperthyroidism. Those patients whose disease first declared itself with eye symptoms may observe first an apparently unilateral exophthalmos. Others, in whom the disease is more progressive, complain of increased tearing, blurring of vision and diplopia which may not be noticed except on looking upward or to one side or the other. They may complain of a pulling sensation behind the eyes. Such patients may present a frightening picture of moderate to severe proptosis (exophthalmometric measurements of 25 to 30 mm., normal being 14 to 17 mm.), edema of both upper and lower lids, chemosis, with edema and injection at the site of insertion of the lateral recti, and a decreased resilience of the eyes. Sometimes the proptosis is so great that these patients are unable to close their eyes, and corneal ulcerations develop. Such patients frequently have little or no goiter and are euthyroid or only slightly toxic. Rarely the exophthalmos in such patients progresses so rapidly that loss of the eye occurs unless adequate therapeutic measures are promptly instituted.

Localized myxedema is a strange lesion which complicates Graves' disease infrequently. We have never seen it except in patients who had moderately severe to very severe exophthalmos. It usually occurs over the lower third of the lower legs. Although it may encircle the entire leg, it most commonly involves the outer half of the lower third of the leg. It may also occur over the distal aspect of the forearm. We have studied one patient who had localized myxedema involving the forearms, wrists and hands and most of both lower legs and feet. Localized myxedema may present itself as a barely perceptible nonpitting swelling which has a purplish-reddish color. In the more severe cases there is a prominent area of nonpitting painless swelling which has a purplish color. Usually the covering skin is tight and smooth. Rarely the skin covering such areas of localized myxedema is so thick as to suggest the diagnosis of elephantiasis.

The mechanisms by which this complication occurs are not known. The term localized myxedema has been given this lesion by virtue of the fact that mucin-like substances have been demonstrated in tissue samples taken from such lesions. Control of the hyperthyroidism does not improve the localized myxedema. Indeed, it may make it worse.

Hyperfunctioning Adenomatous Goiters. In 1912 Plummer,[703] in discussing a paper by Marine, described a group of patients with hyperthyroidism and adenomatous goiters. Plummer[671] and Haines[704] have suggested that the disease picture in patients with hyperthyroidism secondary to an adenomatous goiter differs from that of a patient with Graves' disease.

The former disease is more frequently characterized by cardiovascular symptoms. Exophthalmos does not occur. Muscle weakness is absent, and the response of these patients to iodine is less rapid and complete than in patients with Graves' disease. Cope et al.[705] reported a group of patients with hyperthyroidism who had large single nodules and practically no palpable tissue in the remaining thyroid. Cure of these patients was obtained by simple removal of the nodule. Radioiodine tracer studies[705] done in such patients have revealed that the iodine is concentrated exclusively in the adenoma, none being concentrated in the remaining tissue. Treatment of these patients with iodine is not very effective. Treatment with thiouracil derivatives often is quite effective in controlling the hyperthyroidism of this malady and makes the surgical removal of such goiters a safe procedure. However, there are many examples of patients with hyperthyroidism arising from adenomatous goiters who did not respond well to prolonged treatment with agents such as propyl thiouracil or methimazole even in large doses. If the hyperthyroidism can be readily brought under control with any of the thiouracil derivatives and if the patient is otherwise in good condition, surgical removal of the diseased gland is a reasonable and effective manner of treating this disease. More recently, we have favored treating these patients with radioactive iodine, notwithstanding the fact that the dose of I^{131} deposited per gland necessary to control this disease is greater than that required in the treatment of Graves' disease.

Diagnosis of Graves' Disease. No diagnosis is easier to make than that of Graves' disease in a tremulous, thin, nervous patient with exophthalmos and goiter. On the other hand, the tense, anxious woman in whom many symptoms are suggestive and most tests equivocal presents an extremely difficult problem that even our modern diagnostic procedures do not always solve. Graves' disease must be suspected, first of all, in any patient with an enlarged thyroid. If the pyramidal lobe is enlarged, it is particularly suggestive. The symptomatology is so varied that almost every organ system may be involved. One must suspect Graves' disease if any of the following symptoms are present: (1) intolerance to heat or increased sweating, (2) recent weight loss in spite of adequate or increased food intake, (3) "nervousness" or hyperactivity, (4) diarrhea, (5) muscular weakness, (6) tremor of the hands.

This situation was called to our attention most dramatically when three consecutive patients with Graves' disease came to our thyroid clinic with the following stories. A house painter had a single complaint that a tremor of the hands, of such severity as to make it impossible for him to work, had developed. The next patient was a salesman who thought he had cancer of the bowel because of an intractable diarrhea. The third patient was a woman who complained of marked loss of weight and peculiar heart action that made her certain that her heart would stop. The cardiac arrhythmia turned out to be a mixed paroxysmal auricular tachycardia and fibrillation. All three patients were unaware of any thyroid enlargement and were convinced that their troubles stemmed from disease of the "nerves," "bowels" or "heart," respectively.

The differential diagnosis of Graves' disease must include at least the following: (1) psychoneurosis, (2) hypertensive cardiovascular disease, (3) cardiac decompensation from any cause, (4) cancer either in an occult location or involving the gastrointestinal tract to produce diarrhea, (5) chronic ulcerative colitis, (6) myasthenia gravis, (7) sprue, (8) chronic alcoholism and (9) pheochromocytoma.

The differentiation of Graves' disease from a psychoneurosis with neurocirculatory asthenia is perhaps the most common and the most difficult problem. Frequently the multitude of complaints that the patient with the neurosis presents is suggestive. Commonly there is no increase of appetite or weight loss that the patient with Graves' disease notes. The BMR may be elevated to as much as plus 40 per cent in a neurotic patient and, contrariwise, may be within normal limits in a patient with Graves' disease, although usually the reverse situation will be encountered.

Hypertensive cardiovascular disease may occasionally present a difficult problem in differentiation from Graves' disease. In the latter condition, elevation of the systolic blood pressure is frequent, and co-existence of the two diseases is not uncommon. Unfortunately, hypertension alone may give rise to a spuriously elevated BMR. Furthermore, the patient may be tense and may have a tremor. If the thyroid gland is enlarged, the diagnosis becomes a problem. Again, the radioiodine tracer and the protein-bound iodine studies (PBI) are of most help in establishing the presence or absence of hyperfunction of the thyroid. It must be remembered, however, that if the patient has renal damage resulting in the diminished excretion of radioiodine, the tracer result is liable to give spurious values. The problem is somewhat similar in a patient with congestive heart failure, as this condition may also cause an elevation of the BMR and, furthermore, is frequently accompanied by decreasing renal function.

Cancer of the gastrointestinal tract occasionally is mistaken for Graves' disease. The loss of weight is usually the symptom that causes confusion. However, if the cancer involves the colon and produces diarrhea, the physician may be directed even more forcefully toward the thyroid. Usually a careful history and physical examination with the appropriate x-ray procedures will reveal the true nature of the patient's condition.

Chronic ulcerative colitis, causing diarrhea and loss of weight in a tense anxious patient, may simulate Graves' disease. A careful history will usually disclose blood in the stools, and laboratory and x-ray examination may prove adequate to establish the correct diagnosis.

Myasthenia gravis is occasionally confused with Graves' disease. Diplopia and muscle weakness are common to both diseases. Furthermore, myasthenia gravis occurs in approximately 3 per cent of the cases of Graves' disease. The dramatic improvement in patients with myasthenia gravis given Prostigmine is dagnostic. The additional thyroid enlargement, an elevated BMR and serum protein-bound iodine usually will establish the diagnosis of Graves' disease.

Sprue, for the same reasons as those in chronic ulcerative colitis, may simulate Graves' disease. Furthermore, some patients with sprue have minimal exophthalmos and a definite lid lag. In addition, a small percentage of patients with sprue may not have typical bulky, fatty stools and have no complaints directed toward the gastrointestinal tract except a mild diarrhea.

Chronic alcoholism may result in symptoms that suggest Graves' disease. This may be particularly confusing when the patient for emotional reasons attempts to conceal his alcoholic intake. The weight loss, perspiration and tremor of the hands can be particularly suggestive of Graves' disease. If the patient's alcoholism has resulted in portal cirrhosis, the diagnosis may be complicated even more by the fact that nearly half of a group of patients with portal cirrhosis were found to concentrate in their thyroids more than 50 per cent of a tracer dose of radioactive iodine. Such patients, however, were found to have normal levels of serum protein-bound iodine.

Pheochromocytomas may simulate Graves' disease because of the signs associated with an increased level of circulating adrenalin, i.e., nervousness, palpitation and loss of weight. These patients usually have elevated basal metabolic rates. A normal serum protein-bound iodine level with a normal uptake of radioiodine will rule out hyperthyroidism in such patients. The demonstration of an increase in blood pressure following the administration of histamine or a fall in blood pressure following the administration of agents such as benzodioxane or regitine gives strong support to the diagnosis of pheochromocytoma. Recently it has been demonstrated that patients with pheochromocytoma characteristically excrete markedly increased amounts of catecholamines in the urine.[706]

Although in many instances the diagnosis of Graves' disease can be made without any question purely on the basis of clinical history and physical findings, there are several laboratory studies which are diagnostic or helpful in determining the severity of the disease.

The basal metabolic rate is a well-established laboratory test which reflects the organism's response to the increased levels of circulating thyroid hormone. In the classic case of Graves' disease, the BMR is usually elevated to levels of plus 30 to plus 60. Rarely do we see true basal rates above plus 80. It must be pointed out that the first BMR determined on a nervous but euthyroid patient is frequently elevated. Bartels[707] has advocated determining the metabolic rate on frightened patients after heavy sedation.

The blood cholesterol is usually normal or slightly below normal (140 to 225 mg. per 100 cc.) in this disease. We have, however, seen patients whose symptoms were predominantly ophthalmic who had elevated blood cholesterol levels.

The serum protein-bound iodine (PBI) is elevated in patients having a true hyperthyroidism. Levels in most clinics above 8.0 micrograms per 100 cc. are diagnostic of hyperthyroidism. Spuriously elevated levels are often obtained in patients who have taken iodine-containing compounds.

Tracer studies with radioactive iodine usually reveal an increased concentration and retention of the isotope in the thyroid or a decreased excretion of the tracer.

A decreased tolerance for creatine has been standardized and utilized as a diagnostic test in this disease.[296] Euthyroid humans excrete less than 30 per cent of a standard dose of creatine, but patients with Graves' disease excrete 50 per cent or more.

A relative to absolute lymphocytosis is usual with a normal to slightly depressed total white blood count.

Occasionally laboratory studies and the clinical picture are equivocal. In such patients a therapeutic test with iodides or with one of the thiouracil derivatives may be of diagnostic help.

Treatment of Graves' Disease. The first effective treatment of Graves' disease was surgical resection of all but a small portion of the thyroid gland. European surgeons gained considerable technical skill in surgery of the thyroid on nontoxic endemic goiters, and in the 1890's both Kocher[583] and the Reverdins[582] accumulated series of over one hundred thyroidectomies. In Graves' disease, however, not only was the surgical technique more difficult because of the vascularity of these thyroids, but the general condition of the patient was usually so poor that the mortality was almost prohibitive. Two-stage thyroidectomies with removal of one lobe at a time, ligation of the thyroid arteries and the injection of boiling water were frequently used in an effort to lower the mortality. Since the surgical mortality was so high and no effective medical treatment was available, it was natural that irradiation should be tried as a means of inhibiting the excessive secretion of the thyroid gland. For some years, x-ray treatment of Graves' disease was quite popular and was said to produce complete remissions in about 35 per cent of cases[708] and partial remission in another one third of the cases so treated.

The great improvement in surgical mortality and morbidity effected by the preoperative treatment with iodides, however, caused x-ray therapy to fall out of favor. Now it is rarely used.

Although iodine was suggested for "simple" goiter as early as 1820 by Coindet,[709] its use in hyperthyroidism was considered dangerous. General acceptance of iodine as a preoperative treatment did not occur until Plummer's convincing demonstration of its effectiveness in 1923.[710] The usefulness of this method of treatment is illustrated by a reduction in hospital mortality from 4 per cent before the use of iodine to less than 1 per cent one year after its routine use was adopted at the Mayo Clinic.[711] There was some hope in the 1920's that iodine offered an effective medical treatment for Graves' disease. Unfortunately, in most cases of Graves' disease iodine produced only a temporary remission. The effect of iodine administration usually is noted by the patient in twenty-four to forty-eight hours, and objective improvement occurs in two to three days. In approximately ten to twenty days the patient will have experienced the maximal improvement, which usually does not result in euthyroidism. The dose of iodine necessary to induce this remission has been found to be at least 6 mg. per day.[712] Ordinarily, however, a daily dose of from 50 to 350 mg. of iodine is given. The rate of fall of the BMR in a patient with Graves' disease given iodine is identical with the rate of fall in BMR of a patient with myxedema when desiccated thyroid administration is discontinued.[713] It would appear that iodine in some unknown manner prevents the release of thyroid hormone in patients with Graves' disease, although it does not prevent the synthesis of the hormone.

The therapeutic effect of iodine on the thyroid of Graves' disease has been separated from the nutritive effect of iodine in the normal thyroid economy. Thyroid biopsies were taken from four patients before any therapy and again after the administration of thiouracil had resulted in a normal BMR. Mean cell heights of those biopsy specimens were compared with those of the thyroids which were removed following continued treatment with thiouracil and added iodine. The thiouracil was administered in doses great enough to prevent the retention of iodine in the thyroid as evidenced by radioiodine studies and by analyses of the thyroids for thyroglobulin iodine. The mean cell heights before treatment averaged 12.9 micra, after treatment with thiouracil 14.1 micra, and after the treatment with thiouracil and iodine 8.0 micra.[714] Thyroglobulin iodine values averaged 2.7 mg. per 100 grams of thyroid tissue (wet weight), as opposed to 30 mg. per cent in normal thyroids and 36.6 per cent in thyroids of patients with Graves' disease treated with iodine only. We believe that the involuting action of iodine in this disease is due to an inhibition of the action of TSH on the thyroid cell.

In 1943 physiologists and pharmacologists introduced certain goitrogenic or antithyroid drugs.[59,162,163] These drugs, very effective in the treatment of Graves' disease, inhibit the synthesis of thyroid hormones. Thiouracil was the first such drug introduced. Because of the relative high incidence of toxic reactions it produced, related drugs were soon synthesized and tested. It appears that thiouracil produced agranulocytosis in approximately 1.7 per cent and fever in 4.9 per cent of the patients so treated.[715] In approximately 10 per cent of the cases it was necessary to discontinue thiouracil therapy because of toxic reactions.[716] Methylthiouracil and propylthiouracil were soon discovered to be equally effective, and the latter drug is now employed in most institutions. The over-all incidence of reactions to this drug appears to be about 1 per cent.[716] At first it was hoped that these drugs might prove curative in the sense that their administration for a few months would be followed by complete recovery of the patient. It soon became apparent that a substantial proportion of the patients who enjoyed a satisfactory remission of their Graves' disease while the drugs were being taken had a recurrence of hyperthyroidism when the drugs were discontinued. Reports[717] indicate that if these drugs have controlled the patient's hyperthyroidism for a year and if the drug is then withdrawn, relapse of the disease may be expected in approximately 50 per cent of the patients. The results are better in young females with moderately enlarged thyroids than in males, older women or patients with large goiters. Since the antithyroid drugs act to prevent further synthesis of thyroid hormone, it is evident that hyperthyroidism will continue as long as several months, until any stored hormone in the thyroid has been secreted and then metabolized or excreted. Rarely it takes less than three weeks. Patients with very large nodular goiters and hyperthyroidism have been reported to be insensitive to these goitrogenic drugs, but generally their control by this method is merely time-consuming. It may take as long as one year before a satisfactory remission has been achieved.

It was noted very soon that the thyroid glands of patients treated with thiouracil were quite vascular and friable, complicating their surgical removal rather markedly. The concomitant administration of iodine for the last ten to fourteen days prior to surgery, however, produced a decrease in vascularity and increase in firmness of the thyroid so that surgery was rendered less difficult. In many large centers Graves' disease is now routinely treated with one of the thiouracil compounds until the basal metabolic rate has fallen to normal levels and the patient has gained weight. Then iodine is added for about two weeks, following which the patient is subjected to subtotal thyroidectomy. This has resulted in a mortality of less than 0.1 per cent in some of the best medical centers. One of the newer antithyroid drugs which is quite potent and seems to have a low incidence of toxic reactions is 2-methyl-mercaptoimidazole. Although propylthiouracil is usually effective in dosages of 200 to 600 mg. per day, 2-methyl-mercaptoimidazole seems to be effective in a daily dosage of 20 to 40 mg.[716,718]

Potassium perchlorate is another goitrogenic inhibitor of the thyroid which interferes with the synthesis of thyroid hormone. This agent inhibits the thyroid by suppressing the natural iodide trap of the thyroid.[180] A patient under the influence of this agent is unable to concentrate iodide in the thyroid and is thereby prevented from forming new thyroid hormone. This agent, like the thiouracil derivatives, has its greatest usage in the preoperative preparation of the thyrotoxic patient for thyroidectomy. This drug is prescribed in doses of 200 mg. every eight hours.

In 1938, through the use of the newly discovered and perfected cyclotron, radioactive isotopes of iodine were prepared and their metabolism was studied. The first isotopes used were I^{128}, with a half-life of 25 minutes, and I^{130} with a half-life of 12.6 hours. Later I^{131}, with a half-life of 8 days, was prepared in the cyclotron by the deuteron bombardment of tellurium.

Chapman and his associates[720] recently reviewed their 10 year experiences of treating hyperthyroidism with radioactive iodine. Of 400 patients treated with I^{131}, 8 per cent developed myxedema. Fifty patients required two or more therapeutic doses of I^{131}, and 19 were better but still thyrotoxic six months after the first treatment. In patients who responded, the average interval between treatment and the development of a normal basal metabolic rate was two months. The average interval between treatment and the occurrence of myxedema was four months. However, some patients did not develop myxedema until several years after this form of treatment.

In our clinic it has been the practice to administer a dose of I^{131} which will deposit 150 microcuries of the isotope in each estimated gram of the thyroid. Thus, a typical patient with Graves' disease would be treated as follows:

Tracer dose I^{131} = 70% uptake in thyroid

Estimated thyroid weight = 40 Gm.

$$\text{Therapy dose} = \frac{40 \times 150}{0.70} = 8600\ \mu c$$

or 8.6 millicuries

In an analysis[721] of 116 patients who had been treated according to this practice, we found that 23 per cent were hypothyroid and 16 per cent remained hyperthyroid after one such therapeutic dose of I^{131}. Further analysis of these patients, most of whom had had blood levels determined 48 hours after administration of tracer or therapeutic doses of radioiodine, demonstrated considerable variation in the rates at which the I^{131} left the thyroid, presumably as thyroid hormone. Indeed, it was found that the half-life of I^{131} in the thyroids of these patients varied between 14 and 20 days. We are now taking this factor into consideration in planning therapeutic doses. Following a tracer study which includes blood levels at 48 hours, we are calculating the therapeutic dose from the following formula, which was derived from the data on 43 patients who became euthyroid after a single dose of I^{131}:

$$Y = 110 + 27B$$

where Y = microcuries to be deposited per gram of thyroid tissue at 48 hours, and B = concentration of I^{131} in whole blood 48 hours after the dose (per cent per liter).

For calculation of a therapeutic dose from tracer data, the following is the complete equation:

$$D = \frac{100(110 + 27B) \times G}{U}$$

where D = dose to be given (in microcuries), G = weight of thyroid (in grams), and U = percentage uptake of tracer dose in 48 hours.

Another method of treatment with I^{131} consists of the use of several smaller (3 to 6.5 mc.) doses given over a period of months.[521] With this technique 92 per cent of 103 patients with Graves' disease were rendered euthyroid and 4 cases of permanent hypothyroidism developed.

The complications and disadvantage of I^{131} in the treatment of hyperthyroidism are:

(1) Expense of equipment and trained personnel. Moderately expensive Geiger-Mueller counters and scintillation autoscalers are required, and a physicist should be part of the team.

(2) Myxedema is produced in from 4 to almost 20 per cent of the cases, depending on the techniques used. Generally this is not regarded as a serious problem because replacement therapy is completely effective and inexpensive.

(3) The time required for remission in the hyperthyroidism after the administration of I^{131} may be undesirable. This time interval varies from five to twelve weeks depending mainly upon the store of thyroid hormone in the thyroid gland. Also, if multiple small doses of I^{131} are used, it may require several months for complete remission. In a severely hyperthyroid patient with a complicating disease, such as congestive heart failure, this may be undesirable.

(4) Transient exacerbation of the hyperthyroidism subsequent to the administration of the radioiodine may be noted.[722] If this occurs, the most probable explanation would seem to be that the intense radiation delivered by the I^{131} damages the gland, permitting thyroid hormone to escape. Subsequent to treatment with radioiodine no more exacerbations of the hyperthyroidism occur than might be expected in the course of the disease. In patients with coronary sclerosis or carcinoma of the thyroid treated with thyroidectomizing doses of radioiodine the development of increased serum protein-bound iodine is in most instances unequivocal. In these cases most of the iodine discharged into the circulation is not thyroxine but behaves like thyroglobulin.[723]

(5) The possible carcinogenic effects of ionizing radiation, particularly with respect to cancer of the skin and of bone, are well known. So far, no one has reported cancer of the thyroid subsequent to the use of radioiodine. The isotope has, however, been in general use for only ten years, so it will require at least ten to twenty years' more observation before relevant data will become available. Quimby and Werner[724] investigated patients previously treated with x-ray to the thyroid and queried radiologists who had used this for treatment of Graves' disease. Although they were able to find several cases of cancer of the skin and a few cases of cancer of the esophagus and trachea which developed subsequent to the x-ray treatment of Graves' disease, they were unable to find any cases of cancer of the thyroid. Long-continued exposure to low doses of ionizing radiation appears to be most carcinogenic. The rather brief and intense radiation the thyroid receives from radioiodine is somewhat different and is perhaps less dangerous. A disadvantage upon which adequate data are available is the simultaneous occurrence of Graves' disease and cancer of the thyroid. Pemberton in a large series of cases found this association to occur in about 0.5 per cent.[725] Similar data are reported by Cope et al.[726] If one administers radioiodine, one cannot examine the thyroid pathologically, and this small fraction of patients with cancer will be undiagnosed. It is conceivable, although unlikely, that the radiation would in some cases destroy the cancer.

With these disadvantages and complications in mind, some fairly general criteria have been proposed for the selection of patients to be treated with radioiodine. The feeling of several groups, with which the authors agree, is that the following patients only should be treated with radioiodine:[521,722,727]

(1) Patients with Graves' disease recurrent after one or more thyroidectomies. The chance of relapse after another thyroidectomy is quite high, and the technical problems of surgery are such that the occurrence of parathyroid insufficiency or vocal cord paralysis is much greater than with the first operation.

(2) Patients with Graves' disease and other complicating diseases, i.e., cancer of the breast, rheumatic heart disease, etc., for whom either the life expectancy is so short that the future development of cancer of the thyroid is extremely remote, or else the complicating disease makes surgical thyroidectomy much more hazardous than usual.

(3) Patients with Graves' disease who are in the older age group. In those under the age of 45 with Graves' disease, the question of treatment with radioiodine is open to some dispute. Probably in our present state of knowledge it is desirable to treat most of these patients with propylthiouracil, iodine and subtotal thyroidectomy. There seems little reason, however, to subject a patient who is beyond middle age to thyroidectomy, and we prefer to treat such patients with radioiodine.

The treatment of severe exophthalmos in Graves' disease is the most difficult complication to treat successfully. Means[584] stresses the importance of avoiding surgical thyroidectomy in such patients, for in his experience the most severe cases of exophthalmos are seen soon after thyroidectomy. Many physicians treat such patients with desiccated thyroid, particularly if the BMR is minimally elevated. They frequently tolerate well large doses (250 to 600 mg. per day) of desiccated thyroid and appear to improve. Exophthalmos is so unpredictable and its course when untreated so erratic that it is difficult to evaluate the results of treatment. Local treatment directed toward the eyes consists of sleeping with the head of the bed elevated and dressings over the eyes at night to keep them closed. The prevention of corneal ulcers and blindness is frequently the most difficult problem. Dehydrating procedures with salt restriction and mercurial diuretics may be employed. Occasionally it is necessary to decompress the orbit. Poppen[728] reports considerable success with his technique. It has been suggested that x-radiation of the pituitary might be of benefit in some patients with severe exophthalmos. The evidence presented thus far, we feel, is inconclusive. We have, however, seen some patients with severe exophthalmos who were benefited following the administration of small doses of x-ray to the retro-orbital tissues. It is possible that the benefit attributed to x-ray directed at the pituitary occurred as a result of x-radiation to the retro-orbital tissues. It has been reported that ACTH is of benefit in the treatment of these patients. We have seen a few patients who responded dramatically to treatment with ACTH, cortisone or prednisone. In our experience, however, most patients have not been benefited by this treatment.

Treatment of Thyroid Storm. A patient in thyroid crisis presents one of the most serious of medical emergencies. Before the antithyroid drugs were available, this emergency was not an uncommon postoperative problem which we believe can now be avoided by insisting that no patient should come to thyroidectomy until appropriate treatment with the antithyroid drugs has resulted in euthyroidism and adequate gain in weight.

During the past decade one of us has had occasion to treat seven patients who were admitted to the wards in thyroid storm. The following program was carried out in all of them. Patients were placed in cool oxygen tents, were given morphine in doses of 15 mg. as often as needed to control restlessness, and were sponged with ice water and alcohol at least once every hour. Antithyroid therapy was instituted as follows: Thiouracil or methylthiouracil was administered in doses of 600 mg. at once and then 200 mg. every six hours. Potassium or sodium iodide was administered in doses of 300 to 2000 mg. one hour after each dose of thiouracil.

Five of these patients were also treated with aqueous adrenal cortical extract in doses comparable to those usually given in the treatment of an Addisonian crisis. The results in these five were dramatic, with a fall in temperature shortly after we first administered the adrenal extract, and they all survived. Those two patients who were not treated with adrenal extract died. In another patient we have had opportunity to compare the effects of cortisone and hydrocortisone with those of aqueous adrenal extract. In this patient we saw no effects from cortisone or hydrocortisone but did note a response upon administering watery extract of the adrenal cortex. On the basis of our results in this small series of cases, we would suggest that this program of therapy be followed in the management of thyroid storm.

NONTOXIC GOITER

Under this heading we shall discuss nodular goiter, benign tumors and malignant neoplasms of the thyroid.

Nodular Goiter

"Simple," "colloid," "endemic," "nodular goiter" and "nontoxic goiter" are all terms which have been given to an entity which is characterized by a goiter which is not associated with hyperfunction and often occurs endemically in mountainous and other areas which are poor in iodine. None of the terms listed is satisfactory. Although we frequently use the term "simple goiter," we consider this type of goiter anything but simple. The term colloid goiter is adequate to describe many of these thyroids. However, many of them present, in addition to the colloid changes, encapsulated nodules, many of which are benign neoplasms of one variety or another. Furthermore, the colloid goiter represents only one stage in the development of these goiters.

"Endemic goiter" is a less satisfactory term of description than it was before the general use of iodine in those areas known to be deficient in iodine. Now we see such goiters occurring sporadically in seacoastal communities as well as in the inland communities.

"Nodular goiter" is a descriptive term

which does not tell any more about the etiology, pathology or physiology of these goiters than do any of the other terms suggested. However, until we have a better classification, we shall continue to use the terms "nodular goiter" and "nontoxic goiter" because they do not commit us to any anatomic nor etiologic declaration.

Since we subscribe to the theory that nontoxic goiters and benign neoplasms of the thyroid represent various stages and degrees of the same disease process, we shall discuss these problems together.

Etiology. The fact that the incidence of goiter is not uniform among people living in the same community and exposed to similar environmental factors suggests that there are multiple factors which contribute to the development of such nontoxic goiters. Enlargements of the thyroid are much more common in women than in men. This increased incidence of goiter among women may be due to the repeated brief stimulation of the thyroid just prior to each menstrual period and to the more sustained stimulus to the gland experienced during each pregnancy.

Probably the most important factor in the production of a nontoxic goiter is an iodine deficiency. It has been estimated that the daily ration of iodine necessary to prevent an iodine-want goiter is at least 100 micrograms daily. In many parts of the world the dietary intake of iodine falls short of this minimal need. During puberty and pregnancy the basic needs for iodine are probably greatest. It has also been suggested that the stresses of infection or of trauma may increase the organism's demands for thyroid hormone and thus the need for iodine. Where endemicity of goiter is great, the iodine is usually low. In the United States this is notably true in the Great Lakes region, in the Pacific Northwest and on the western slopes of the Rocky Mountains. There is a similar correlation to be demonstrated in the foothills of the Himalayan Mountains, in the Alps and in mountainous western Argentina. In the United States the incidence of goiter is lowest in the northeastern seaboard states and those extreme southern states from the Atlantic coast along the Gulf through Texas.

Experimental support of the theory that an iodine want results in the development of goiters comes from the observations that goiters develop in rats maintained on iodine-deficient diets.[729,730] Also, the widespread use of iodized salt in the "goiter belt" has resulted in a significant decrease in the incidence of goiter in communities which previously had a very high incidence of nontoxic goiter.[731] Two patients seen recently lived in the "goiter belt" and developed goiters after following a low salt diet for more than a year. They had had iodized salt as their only source of iodine, and they had been deprived of that. Careful studies with modern tools of investigation of patients being instructed to follow low salt diets might well provide us with more accurate and precise information on the needs for iodine in man.

The sequence of events in the development of nontoxic goiters was first described by Marine in 1924.[732] He described a cycle which occurs as the result of an iodine deficiency, and the thyroid will go through such a cycle as many times as an iodine deficiency ensues.

Studies done in our laboratory with the positive goitrogens have illustrated a similar cycle.[733] Money has administered thiouracil to Sprague-Dawley rats over periods which varied between ten days and twenty-four months. He sacrificed groups of rats every month and examined their thyroids histologically. His findings may be summarized as follows: Thyroids removed within the first month of treatment showed simple but extreme hyperplasia. After three to four months there were observed intra-acinar growths which were composed of solidly packed cells in a trabecular fashion not unlike the structure observed in trabecular adenomas of the human thyroid. In animals sacrificed during the fifth month there were intrafollicular budding growths which presented microfollicular patterns of organization. These were similar to the earliest signs of differentiation and follicular development observed in human microfollicular adenomas. After seven to eight months he observed discrete lesions with a papillary structure and, following sixteen to eighteen months of treatment with thiouracil, hemorrhagic cysts were seen in these thyroids. After twenty to twenty-four months there were large colloid-containing follicles lined by flat and inactive epithelium, surrounded by areas of simple hyperplasia. These observations support the thesis advanced by Wegelin[734] that hyperplasia of the thyroid is a precursor to neoplasia. We have isolated observations which suggest that the sequence of events in the development of human nodular goiters are similar to those occurring in the rat.

Taylor has made a series of observations in patients of various ages who came from communities in which goiter is endemic. In his selected patients a sequence of thyroidal events has been described which is quite similar to that noted by Money in his rats.[735]

The colloid goiters, we believe, represent a state of exhaustion in tissue which is no longer capable of reacting with thyrotrophic hormone. Notwithstanding the fact that most cellular adenomas seen in such goiters are incapable of function, we suspect that they occurred as a result of a prolonged growth stimulus from the pituitary. Oftentimes, patients with such goiters have an associated hypothyroidism. In other instances such thyroids, by virtue of their mass, though functioning at a lower than normal level, are capable of secreting enough hormone to maintain a state of euthyroidism.

In recent years Greenwald has vigorously challenged the theory that nontoxic goiters are due to an inadequate intake of iodine[736] and has suggested that such goiters might be due to some unidentified infectious process.

Although we find it impossible to deny that an inadequate intake of iodine plays an important role in the development of nontoxic goiter, the frequency with which we have seen goiters in people who had had a generous intake of iodine has made us consider other causes. Stanbury[599] has reported on selected patients with familial goiters whom he found to be capable of trapping iodine but incapable of utilizing the iodine in hormonogenesis, presumably because of some defect in the enzyme systems necessary to the oxidation of iodine. Stanbury and associates[110] have also studied one goitrous patient who released and excreted monoiodotyrosine but was congenitally unable to synthesize thyroxine or other iodinated thyronines.

Many observers[160–162] have demonstrated that there are foods and chemical compounds such as thiouracil which have a positive goitrogenic action regardless of an adequate intake of iodine. However, tracer studies with I^{131} in experimental animals and in humans would indicate that these agents act to prevent the utilization of iodine in thyroid hormonogenesis. Certain foods, notably turnips, are capable of impairing the accumulation of radioiodine by normal human thyroids.[737] The active factor in this vegetable has been identified as 1,5,-vinyl-2-thio-oxazolidone. Cabbage has also been demonstrated to be goitrogenic in rabbits.[156] Recently we have had opportuntiy to examine a very hyperplastic thyroid in an infant who had been fed soy bean milk for one year because of a sensitivity to cow's milk. This child's goiter, which was so large as to necessitate a tracheostomy, disappeared on stopping the feeding of soy bean milk.

Recently, interest in calcium carbonate as a goitrogen has been reawakened by the careful clinical observations and biologic experiments made by Taylor,[738] whose rats, maintained on calcium carbonate, developed goiters which were avid for iodine. Such goiters could be prevented by the administration of iodine. The dose of iodine necessary to exert this prophylactic effect was greater, however, than that necessary to prevent the development of an iodine-want goiter.

Pathology (Anatomical and Functional). Grossly, these goiters may present a variety of patterns. On the basis of a few observations made in patients whose goiters were of recent origin, we believe that they all show, in the early stages, a uniform and diffuse hypertrophy and hyperplasia. They may be only twice normal size, or they may be considerably larger. They are vascular and friable. In this stage of development they show on microscopic examination a decrease to complete loss of colloid and hypertrophy and hyperplasia of the acinar cells.

Greatest experience has been obtained from studies of goiters of long standing which have been removed for cosmetic reasons or because of obstructive symptoms. Such goiters are usually quite large. They may be smooth or they may be nodular. On cross-section the tissue may be uniform and pale pink in color. Frequently the nodules are encapsulated. Oftentimes such old nodules contain bloody fluid or they may even be calcified. Microscopic studies of these goiters usually reveal the pattern of a colloid goiter with its large distended follicles containing a well-stained colloid and lined by flat epithelium.

Some of these goiters are asymmetric but on close examination do not differ greatly in over-all pattern from those described above. They are a source of concern, however, because they simulate thyroids which contain a single nodule. Single nodules may, however, exist in colloid goiters or they may be found in glands which, aside from the nodule, are perfectly normal in structure and function.

Because of the similarity of many of these tumors to various stages of development in the fetal thyroid, many pathologists have classified several of these tumors as "fetal adenomas." This nomenclature probably stems from the thesis proposed by Wölfler;[739] in 1880 he suggested that these tumors were derived from embryonal or fetal rests.

We prefer an anglicized modification of the classification proposed by Wegelin[740] because it is descriptive and can be adapted to emphasize the relationship of structure to function. Under this system of classification the least differentiated tumor which presents cords of solidly packed cells and resembles the least differentiated embryonal thyroid, we label a trabecular adenoma. By autoradiographic techniques these tumors do not manifest any capacity to concentrate radioiodine (Fig. 3).

The first stage of differentiation in the embryonic thyroid is very similar to a group of adenomas which are characterized by loosely packed cords of cells apparently surrounding a lumen like the walls of a tubule. This group of tumors we classify as tubular adenomas. By the autoradiographic techniques these tumors are generally incapable of concentrating I^{131}. However, they may contain some small follicles which in rare instances apparently are capable of concentrating some labelled iodine (Fig. 4).

The next stage of differentiation is represented by the microfollicular adenoma (Fig. 5). It is characterized by small uniformly-sized and shaped follicles which are lined by cuboidal cells and contain some faintly staining colloid. These tumors are usually capable of concentrating significant amounts of radioiodine.

The macrofollicular adenoma is a partially encapsulated nodule which contains large colloid-filled follicles, lined by flat epithelium. The structural pattern of such nodules is not unlike that of large colloid goiters. Some of these tumors are capable of concentrating radioiodine. However, the majority are quite incapable of function. Follicles of such colloid nodules have greater diameters than do those of normal or hyperfunctioning thyroid tissue[741] (Fig. 6).

Other tumors include two types of hyperplastic adenomas. Dobyns[742] has studied a group of these tumors which, by autoradiographic techniques, were incapable of concentrating any I^{131}. The

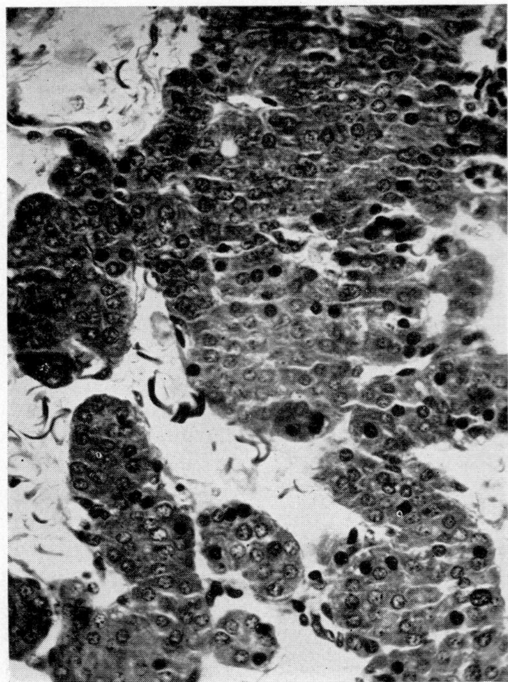

FIG. 3. Trabecular structure observed in nodule of large nodular goiter.

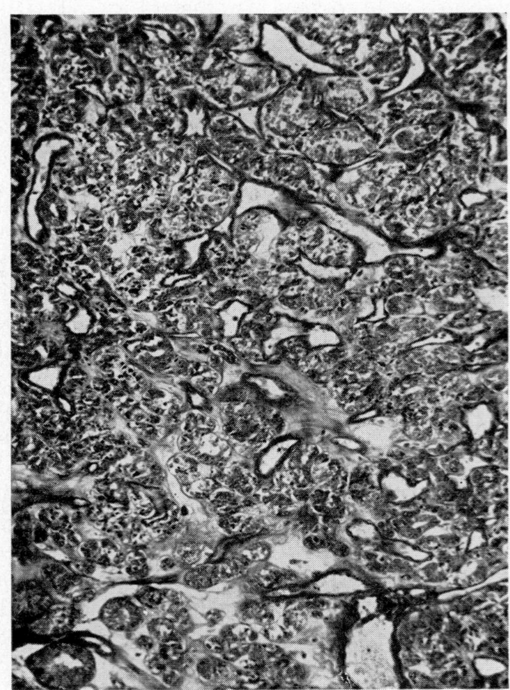

FIG. 4. Tubular structure observed in nodule of nodular goiter.

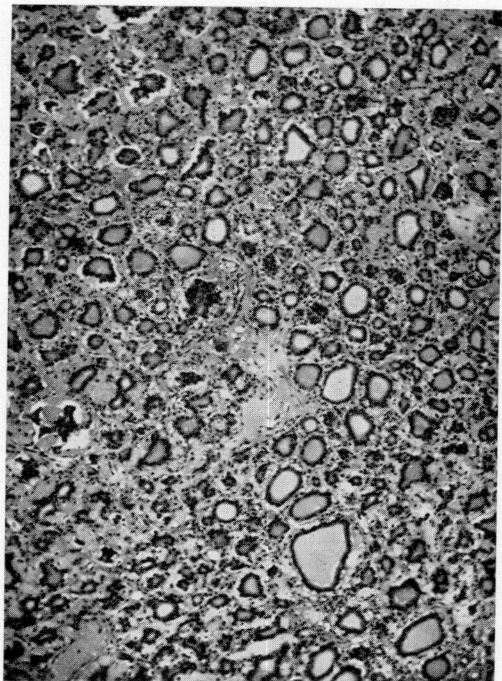

FIG. 5. Microfollicular structure observed in nodule of nodular goiter.

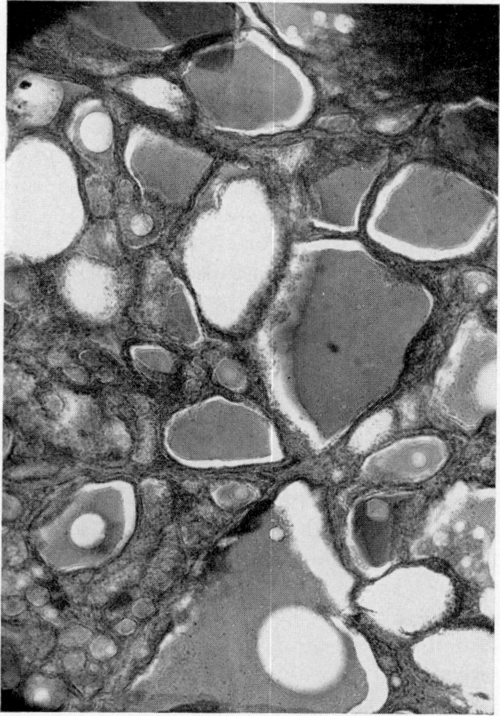

FIG. 6. Macrofollicular structure observed in large recurrent nodular goiter (note areas of secondary hyperplasia).

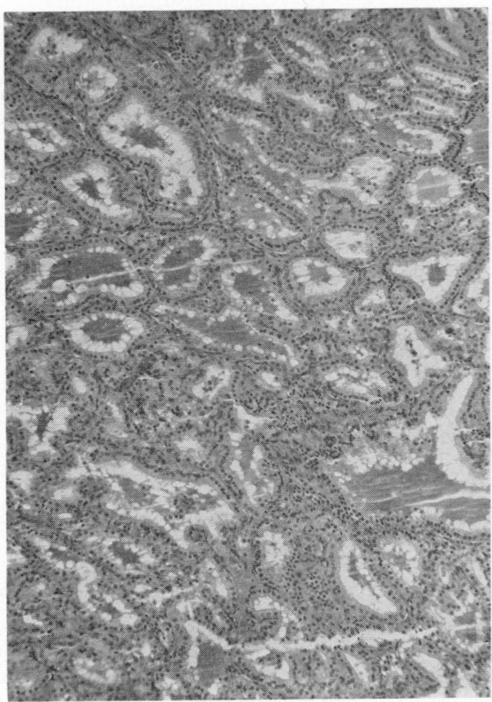

FIG. 7. Hyperplastic adenoma observed in single nodule of a mildly thyrotoxic woman.

cell height measurements of such tumors were irregularly hyperplastic. Another group of hyperplastic tumors (Fig. 7), which by cell height measurements were uniformly hyperplastic, Dobyns found capable of collecting maximum amounts of I^{131}. He found that thyroid tissue surrounding such adenomas is in a resting state incapable of collecting I^{131} and anatomically composed of acinar tissue with flat epithelium. Some of these latter hyperplastic tumors have been associated with hyperthyroidism which was corrected by simple removal of the adenoma.

Symptomatology. Such goiters frequently are asymptomatic. They may, however, on occasion be associated with subtle or frank symptoms of hypothyroidism. The goiters themselves may vary in size according to the organism's need for thyroid hormone. For example, just prior to each menstrual period such a goiter in a woman may show a slight increase in size but regress after the period. During a pregnancy such goiters, if not supported by exogenous thyroid, may enlarge significantly but partially regress during the postpartum period. As the goiter gradually increases in size and the shoulders become more rounded with increasing age, the goiter is likely to descend beneath the manubrium into the superior mediastinum, where it may interfere with the blood flow from the neck and cause distention of the neck veins. In the case of an unusually large goiter the picture of a superior vena cava syndrome may be seen. Large goiters may cause such compression on the trachea or on the esophagus as to cause respiratory embarrassment or dysphagia. Goiters which are asymmetric may displace the trachea with varying degrees of respiratory embarrassment. Hemorrhages into cysts or distended follicles may be associated with sudden pain and swelling and the mechanical symptoms that one would expect from an increased mass in the neck.

Some of these adenomas which are capable of function or hyperfunction may acquire enough function to produce insidious symptoms of low grade hyperthyroidism. In such instances the symptoms causing the patient to seek medical help are usually cardiovascular in nature.

Previously, it was often suggested that cellular adenomas in such nodular goiters might become cancerous. The opinion today is that cancers do not develop in such adenomas but that cancers which are found in such goiters were cancerous lesions from the beginning of their growth. However, in a multinodular goiter one is less likely to find a cancer than in a goiter which presents only one palpable nodule.

Treatment. The treatment of nontoxic or nodular goiters depends on an appraisal of the causation and on an appraisal of the individual patient. The development of simple goiter before or during puberty suggests an increased need for thyroid hormone, an increased stimulus to the thyroid which calls for replacement measures to prevent the further development and evolution of a goiter, i.e., iodides or thyroid hormone. The most common method of increasing the daily intake of iodine is that of adding iodides to the table salt. In certain areas of this country 0.01 per cent by weight of potassium iodide is added to purified salt. Thus, the average person who ordinarily ingests from 6 to 9 gm. of salt daily will receive from 600 to 900 micrograms of iodide daily. This is above the minimal daily requirement of 100 micrograms suggested by Marine. This method of replacing a natural iodine deficit is mandatory in only a few states. In such instances one may also prescribe solutions of potassium iodide.

Recently several groups have been following the effects of administered desiccated thyroid, l-thyroxine or l-triiodothyronine on nontoxic nodular goiters. In our own experience, this form of treatment has been associated with variable results. We have observed softening in the consistency of the gland and even significant regression of some nodular thyroids. The majority of such goiters, in our experience, have not regressed significantly on administration of such preparations of thyroid hormones.

Surgical removal of such nontoxic nodular goiters is indicated for the relief of obstructive symptoms, mainly for relief of obstruction to either the trachea or the major vessels of the neck. Surgical removal of a nodular goiter is only the first stage in the treatment of a patient, since the same factors which led to the development of goiter are still operative and are enhanced by removal of a major source of the patient's natural thyroid hormone. These factors, unless corrected by the administration of adequate amounts of thyroid hormone, may result in myxedema and in the regrowth of goitrous tissue. Many patients may request removal of their goiters purely for cosmetic reasons. If there are no medical contraindications and if the same considerations for adequate replacement therapy are made, we do not object to removal of goiters which are symptomatic only by virtue of the pressure that they exert on a patient's vanity.

Malignant Tumors of the Thyroid

Cancer of the thyroid is not ordinarily considered one of the diseases of metabolism. Indeed, all cancers have been generally considered as autonomous growths which could not be brought under any physiologic control. Studies now in progress would indicate that a large group of cancers of the thyroid can be made to respond to certain metabolic stimuli and needs. In view of these newer developments, we are including a discussion on cancer of the thyroid in this chapter.

Cancer of the thyroid is not a common disease. Analysis of two large series of autopsies done in general hospitals indicates that cancer of the thyroid is a rare cause of death.[743,744] The relationship of cancer to single or multiple nodules in the thyroid is a controversial and as yet unresolved issue. Most observers[745–761] conclude that there is an increased incidence of malignancy in nodular goiters and imply that such nodules, particularly solitary nodules,

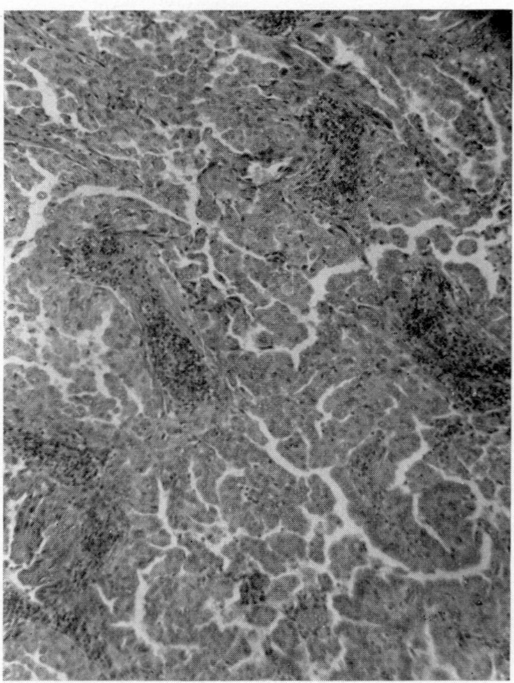

FIG. 8. Papillary carcinoma.

should be removed. The incidence of cancer in solitary nodules varies from 5 per cent to 24 per cent; cancer is found in multinodular thyroids in 3 per cent to 19 per cent of cases. Others[762–769] have conceded a high incidence of cancer in nodular thyroids but counter that patients treated surgically represent a selected group. They state that in an unselected series of nontoxic nodular goiters there would be no increased incidence of cancer. They add that nodular thyroid is a common condition, whereas cancer of the thyroid is comparatively uncommon. However, the incidence of cancer in nodular thyroids in routine necropsies when the disease was not suspected clinically was similar to that noted in surgically removed nodular thyroids.[757] Little can be brought to bear from experimental tumorgenesis[770] to help resolve this difficult clinical dilemma. Our present position represents something of a compromise and individualization in view of the large number of nodules seen.

There are several factors which should be considered in deciding whether a nodular thyroid should be removed surgically. The chances of a nodule in the thyroid being a cancer are much greater if the patient is under the age of 30 years. If, with tracer techniques, the nodule can be demonstrated to concentrate no radioactive iodine,[540] it is more likely to be cancerous and justifies early removal. If treatment with thyroid hormone does not result in a significant decrease in the size of the nodule, the likelihood of this nodule being cancerous is increased. Evidence of recent growth, extreme hardness and cervical lymphadenopathy call for surgical removal. If at the time of surgery a definitive diagnosis of cancer is made by the pathologist, adequate removal of cancerous tissue should be undertaken.

There would appear to be a significant experience[771–773] which indicates that prior irradiation about the head, neck and upper thorax predisposes to thyroid cancer. Although there are more than 95 cases reported,[772] it will require more extensive studies to resolve this issue.

Cancers of the thyroid can be subdivided into several varieties. Although none of the systems of classification is ideal, we prefer that suggested by Dr. Frank Foote of our institution because it can be correlated with the clinical course and even with the functional patterns of some of these tumors.

Papillary cancers are the most common malignant tumors found in the thyroid. They occur characteristically in young people. However, we have seen them in all ages from six years to the eighth decade. They occur in females about twice as often as in males. They are often small and may be found only on seeking an explanation for enlarged lymph nodes. Histologically these tumors present a picture of papillary cords with a delicately vascularized connective tissue lined by one to many layers of cuboidal and columnar cells. Colloid is characteristically absent from a pure papillary cancer of the thyroid (Fig. 8).

These cancers frequently metastasize to the cervical and upper mediastinal lymph nodes. When they spread beyond the confines of the neck it is usually to the chest. In this setting the x-ray of the chest reveals miliary nodules fanning out from the hilum. Such x-ray findings are often confused with those of miliary tuberculosis, sarcoidosis or silicosis (Fig. 8a). Skeletal metastases from this type of cancer occur, but rather infrequently. The prognosis of this type of cancer is excellent. If it is detected early and adequately treated, there is an excellent chance for a cure. Even those patients who have pulmonary or skeletal metastases may live for many years.

The *follicular* and *alveolar carcinomas* are less frequent than the papillary lesions. They occur characteristically in middle age but have been seen in children as well as in old age. They occur in males as often as in females. They frequently are large enough to occupy one full lobe of the thyroid and may on first examination appear to be a benign nodule. However, they are usually firm to hard on palpation. Histologically they present a follicular pattern with small but frequently irregular follicles lined by high cuboidal epithelium. These follicles often contain some colloid (Fig. 9). In some areas less differentiation with even a tubular structure is observed. These tumors metastasize to the regional lymph nodes, skeletal system and the lungs. Often patients with these tumors come to the clinic because of symptoms of skeletal metastases. In others a single firm to

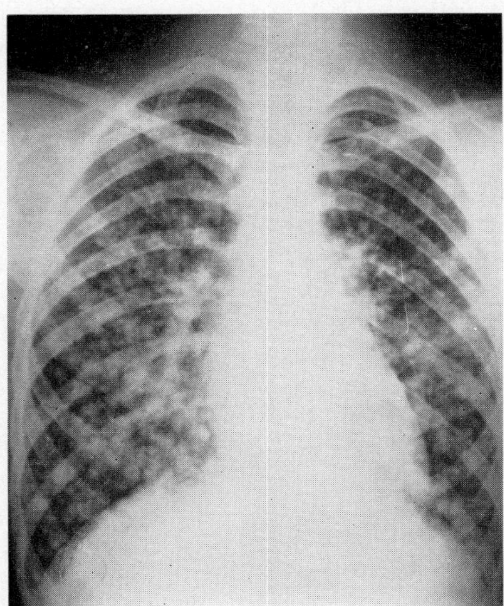

FIG. 8a. Chest x-ray of 15-year old boy with mixed papillary and follicular carcinoma of the thyroid. Note the miliary pattern of metastases.

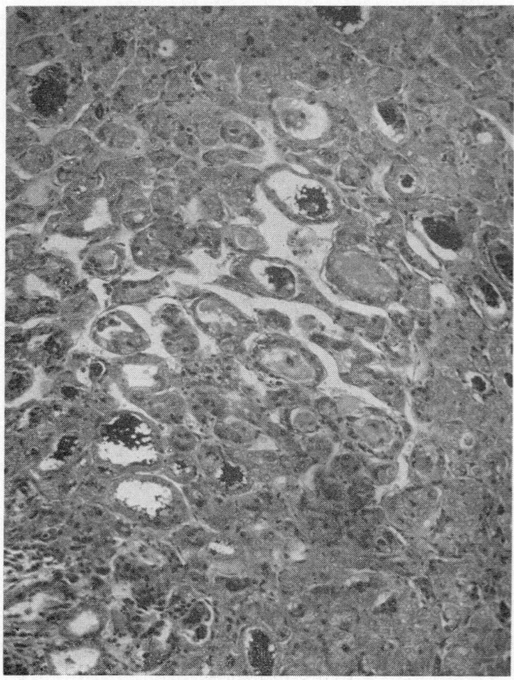

FIG. 9. Alveolar and follicular carcinoma.

hard nodule is found in the thyroid on routine examination.

Although patients having skeletal metastases from these tumors may live for several years, the disease is a lethal one and does not have as good a prognosis as does papillary cancer of the thyroid.

The *solid adenocarcinomas* are the second most common cancer of the thyroid observed at Memorial Hospital. They occur with equal frequency in males and females, usually in middle age. These tumors are large, bulky and hard, and they usually involve more than one lobe of the thyroid. On histologic examination they present a solid trabecular pattern of closely packed cells with much nuclear variation as to size and staining qualities (Fig. 10). These tumors are quite malignant and invasive. They metastasize most commonly to the skeleton and to the lungs. The survival rate of patients with these tumors is much less than that of the two tumors previously described.

Hürthle cell carcinomas do not occur frequently. There is some question[774,775] as to whether to classify these as benign or malignant lesions because of the prolonged clinical course. There is little doubt that there is a malignant variant of this disease which may metastasize to skeleton, cervical lymph nodes or lungs and actually may be the cause of death in a certain number of patients.[776-779] It has been suggested[778] that the Hürthle cell tumor is not a specific tumor type but may occur to the virtual exclusion of other cell types in any thyroid lesion and is, *per se*, of no diagnostic significance. This tumor is usually a single moderately-sized nodule localized to one lobe of the thyroid. Histologically, it is characterized by the presence of bright, almost opaque, pink-staining cells which are usually columnar and stratified in plexiform groups which are separated by a rich thin-walled capillary blood supply (Fig. 11).

The *giant* and *spindle cell cancers* of the thyroid are comparatively infrequent. They occur usually in older patients who give a history of having had goiters for many years. These cancers are rapid-growing and may produce

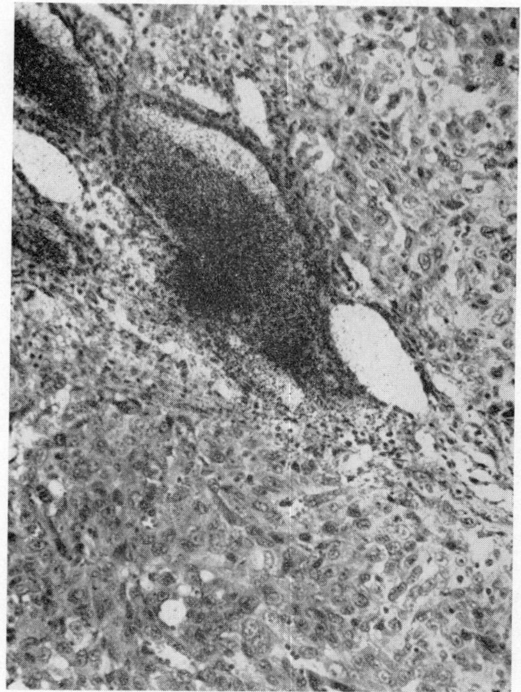

FIG. 10. Solid adenocarcinoma. Black shadow represents pickup of radioactive iodine in isolated follicles within this solid adenocarcinoma.

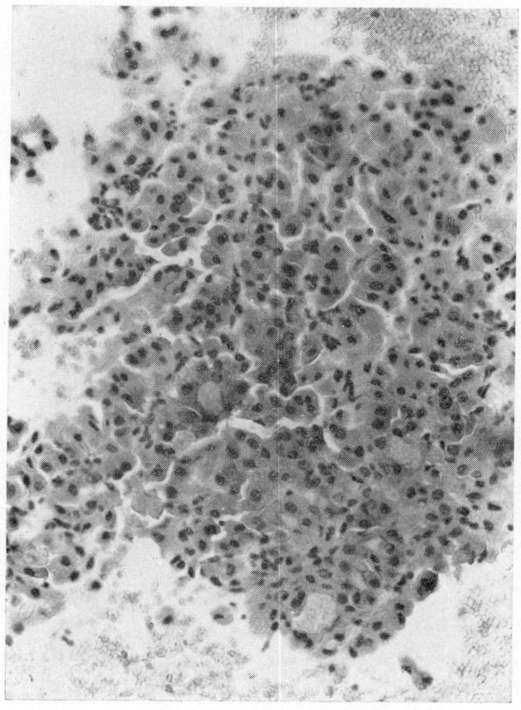

FIG. 11. Hürthle cell carcinoma.

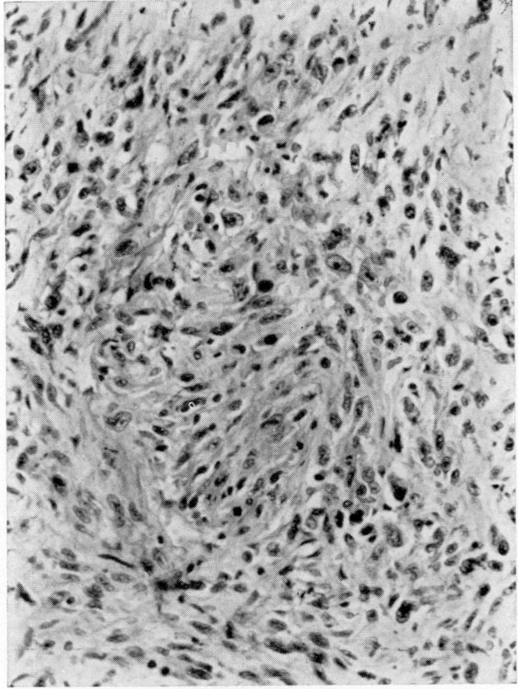

FIG. 12. Giant and spindle cell carcinoma.

obstructive symptoms early. The skin over the tumor may be red and warm. The tumor, which is hard, may also be tender. On opening such a tumor at operation a yellowish necrotic material resembling pus often is found. Histologically this tumor is a solid, highly anaplastic growth. Spindle cells and giant cells predominate. There may be, however, residual areas of atypical gland formation (Fig. 12). These tumors are the most malignant that occur in the thyroid. We have seen very few patients with this type of cancer who survived longer than six months after the diagnosis was made.

More unusual types of thyroid cancer include reticulum cell sarcoma[780] and malignant lymphoma.[781] Secondary malignant tumors of the thyroid have been reported[782] to occur in 4 per cent of patients dying of other cancers.

Functional Studies of Thyroid Cancer

During recent years the capacity of these tumors to concentrate radioiodine has been studied by many investigators. Fitzgerald and Foote,[783,784] using autoradiographic techniques, found 60 out of 150 different specimens of thyroid cancer which picked up measurable amounts of radioactive iodine (Table 6).

TABLE 6. POSITIVE AUTOGRAPHS IN THYROID CANCER

TYPE	NUMBER OF CASES	NUMBER POSITIVE	PER CENT POSITIVE
Papillary	49	12	24
Alveolar and follicular	56	38	68
Solid	17	6	35
Hürthle cell	13	3	23
Giant and spindle cell	10	0	0
Anaplastic	3	0	0
Unclassified	2	1	50
Total	150	60	40

In general, it can be concluded from this study that the concentration of radioiodine by cancers of the thyroid occurs primarily in those tumors bearing colloid-filled follicles and only rarely in tumors which do not contain colloid. In no instance was a functioning tumor found which concentrated as much radioiodine as did the adjacent normal thyroid tissue.

Although the correlation between histologic type of cancer and the localization of radioactive iodine is useful, two limitations must be considered. Many patients have tumors with more than one histologic type. In addition, even those tumors bearing colloid-filled follicles which concentrate radioactive iodine do not have a uniform distribution of the radioactive isotope. Some thyroid follicles show[785] no activity, whereas neighboring follicles with similar morphology do concentrate radioactive iodine. This may be related to the previous nonradioactive iodine stores of each follicle, or perhaps thyroid follicles have some phasic function. There would appear to be factors other than histologic structure which are significant.

From a functional point of view, the localization of radioactive iodine in malignant thyroid tissue has certain similarities to its localization in normal thyroid tissue. In the first report,[786] of storage of radioactive iodine in a metastasis from thyroid carcinoma, it was noted that carrier potassium ioxide did not wash out the isotope fixed by the metastatic tissue. It was observed[787] that radioactive iodine was fixed only by that tissue which resembled normal thyroid tissue. The incorporation of radioactive iodine into an organic molecule seems to be a property of both malignant and normal thyroid tissue which is functional. However, quantitative measurements of radioiodine retention in thyroid carcinoma after thyroid ablation in nonmyxedematous patients[788,789] reveal a rapid turnover. This may be a property of tumor tissue. Although thyrotoxic persons may also demonstrate a rapid turnover rate, they also demonstrate hyperthyroidism, whereas thyroid cancer patients are most often euthyroid. This may also reflect smaller iodine stores in thyroid carcinoma which has not had as long a period to collect stable iodine as does normal thyroid tissue. Perhaps the smaller follicles which are frequently seen in functioning thyroid carcinoma have a more rapid turnover of iodine.

It has been reported that the administration of thyroxine or triiodothyronine does not reduce the discharge of radioactive iodine from thyroid tumors.[789] This would suggest that the localizing property of thyroid tumors for radioiodine is not influenced by alterations in the pituitary function as might occur after the administration of thyroid hormones. Studies with thyroidectomy and thiouracil would seem to contradict this.

That the radioactive iodine which is present in thyroid cancer is not present as iodine is suggested by the observation[789] that potassium perchlorate, a substance which blocks iodide trapping, has no effect on the rate of radioiodine discharge. The presence of an abnormal iodinated compound in the serum of patients with functional cancers of the thyroid,[788,790] gives support to the theory that there is a difference in the metabolism of iodine between normal and neoplastic thyroid tissue.

It has been reported[791] that thiouracil does not inhibit the collection of radioactive iodine by certain functioning cancers of the thyroid to the same degree that it does in normal thyroid tissue. However, in hyperthyroidism due to functional thyroid metastases, thiouracil has been demonstrated to suppress thyroid hormone formation and to produce a euthyroid state.[792,793]

Most observers feel that thyroid ablation increases the likelihood of thyroid metastases retaining the radioactive isotope. This appears rational if one considers[794] thyroid carcinoma less efficient than normal thyroid tissue in concentrating radioactive iodine. Removal of normal thyroid tissue should also serve to reduce the amount of circulating thyroid hormone and hence decrease its antagonistic effect on the secretion of pituitary thyrotrophin. In addition, if the thyroid is one of the tissues which is efficient in inactivating thyrotrophin, thyroidectomy should permit more thyrotrophin to act on the tumor and promote radioiodine uptake. Whether the mechanism is understood or not, thyroidectomy increases the uptake of radioactive iodine by metastatic carcinoma of the thyroid. To date at Memorial Center, 32 of 61 patients have shown an increased uptake in thyroid cancer following thyroidectomy.

If the increased uptake of I^{131} by metastatic thyroid cancer after thyroidectomy is mediated by an increased secretion or action of thyrotrophin on metastases, then administered thyrotrophin should also have a similar effect. This appears to be so[795–801] in some cases. When TSH preparations were given daily for eight days, an increased uptake of radioiodine was noted in six of 16 cases.[795]

Further support for the partial regulation of radioiodine concentration in tumor tissue by thyrotrophin comes from observations[795,797,802–805] made with antithyroid drugs. These drugs presumably serve to increase the radioactive iodine uptake in several ways. They reduce thyroid hormone production by blocking the conversion of inorganic iodide to thyroid hormone. In addition, the antithyroid drugs have been demonstrated to potentiate the action of TSH. Under both circumstances there is an increased TSH action.

We have observed a significant increase in uptake by metastatic thyroid cancer in 35 of 56 patients treated with antithyroid drugs. Of 66 patients who have been thyroidectomized or treated with antithyroid drugs or both, 39 have shown an increased uptake of radioiodine in their metastatic thyroid cancer. Only seven patients have been treated with radioactive iodine without previously having had total thyroidectomy and/or treatment with antithyroid drugs.

The *treatment* of thyroid cancer is its removal by surgeons who are competent in this field. If the disease is extensive and cannot be removed, palliative surgery with removal of compressing masses and even tracheostomy may be desirable. We do not believe that cancer of the thyroid, which is localized to the neck and can be removed by a competent and experienced surgeon, should be treated with radioactive iodine.

Treatment with radioactive iodine of the metastatic tumors of the thyroid should not be attempted until a maximum pick-up of radioiodine has been obtained. Furthermore, this form of treatment should not be undertaken unless a cancericidal dose of radioiodine can be administered without causing serious damage to other vital tissues of the body.[806,807]

THYROIDITIS

Acute Thyroiditis

Acute thyroiditis, also referred to as acute diffuse thyroiditis, acute nonsuppurative thyroiditis or pseudo-tubercular thyroiditis, is an inflammatory disease characterized by fever, malaise and mostly a firm, very tender enlargement of the thyroid gland. Although the histologic picture observed in these thyroids is one suggesting an inflammatory process, no causative bacterial organism has, to our knowledge, been isolated. It is presumed by some that the disease is of virus origin, but this theory is not yet substantiated. Its viral etiology is supported by the report[808] of thyroiditis following cat scratches with an evident vaccination-like lesion and failure of antibiotics. The experimental production of thyroiditis in guinea pigs with radioactive iodine[809] suggests that generalized trauma, not only microbiologic, may be etiologically related. It has also been suggested[810,811] that there is a causal relationship between thyroiditis and thyrotoxicosis. If this were true, however, one would expect to see more cases of thyroiditis, a relatively uncommon disease.

We have recently seen[723] 10 cases of acute thyroiditis. Of these 10 patients, six were women. The ages varied between 29 and 50 years. All complained of pain and tenderness in the thyroid region. Four complained of dysphagia. In most of these patients the pain was worse on one side than on the other. In some the pain subsided on the first side before the other side became involved. Pain referred to the ears or to the face was not uncommon. Malaise, often severe, was complained of by all. Several complained of chills and profuse sweats. Four patients reported having had upper respiratory infections just prior to the onset of thyroiditis.

The thyroid gland was enlarged two to three times the normal size, was usually somewhat irregular and was firm in all of our cases. The thyroids in all cases were extremely tender. A few patients had palpable tender pretracheal nodes.

All patients had fever which varied from low grade elevations of about 100° F. to spiking temperature courses with peaks as high as 105° F. In four patients the total white count was elevated, the maximum being 13.8 thousand; in others it was normal. Six patients had a lymphocytosis. The erythrocyte sedimentation rate was uniformly elevated and ranged from 30 to 50 millimeters per hour.

None of the patients was judged clinically to be hyperthyroid. The basal metabolic rate was elevated in only two patients. The serum protein-bound iodine was measured in six patients. It was normal in two patients and slightly elevated in four, the maximum level being 9.4 micrograms per 100 cc. Tracer studies with I^{131} were done in all of these patients. The uptake of I^{131} by the thyroid was 2.3 per cent of the dose or less in all but one patient, who was beginning to recover at the time she received the tracer.

Surgical biopsies of the thyroid were taken from two patients. In both glands there was a diffuse inflammatory reaction with mononuclear cell infiltration predominating, moderate proliferation of fibrous tissue and giant cell formation. An occasional microscopic abscess was seen in both cases, but there was no gross suppuration (Fig. 13).

The diagnosis of this disease is quite readily made. It may have to be differentiated from a suppurative thyroiditis which usually becomes fluctuant and is usually associated with a definite neutrophilic leukocytosis. It may have to be differentiated from a hemorrhage into an adenoma which is characterized by the acute and abrupt onset of pain in one localized nodule of the thyroid without fever or other signs of infection. The pain and even redness are often

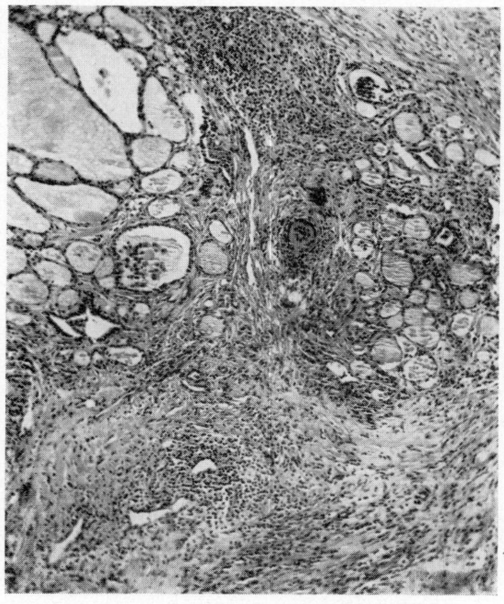

FIG. 13. Acute thyroiditis.

seen in patients with a giant and spindle cell carcinoma. Patients bearing this form of cancer usually give a history of rapid asymmetric growth of an old nodule in the thyroid without systemic signs of infection.

The course of this disease is a self-limited one. However, the symptoms may last as long as 18 months. Furthermore, there may be recurring episodes of the total picture. Seldom is the disease followed by a state of hypothyroidism.

In recent years it has become quite apparent that this disease can be effectively treated with several agents. It is not influenced by sulfonamides or any known antibiotic agents.[812] ACTH and cortisone[813,818–821] are especially effective in producing prompt and dramatic relief, often within 24 hours. Irradiation in a dose of 600 to 800 r may suffice to effect a resolution in a few weeks,[813,822–825] and the pain and tenderness may subside in a few days. It is interesting that both thiouracil[826–829] and TSH[723] are purported to have a beneficial effect on the course of acute thyroiditis. These latter two agents, as well as ACTH, cortisone and irradiation, are known to affect thyroid function in the absence of thyroiditis, and the question is raised as to whether this disease is indeed infectious or represents an acute functional disorder of the thyroid. Most of the data support an infectious nature of the disease, except for the lack of response to any known antibiotic agent. It would be surprising to see an infectious process respond to agents like thiouracil or TSH. The latter hormone, when administered intramuscularly for one to five days, not only resulted in a marked improvement in symptoms but also produced a significant increase in iodine-concentrating capacity where this was previously depressed. It is not clear what effect, if any, TSH or thiouracil might have on an infectious process.

Suppurative Thyroiditis

Suppurative thyroiditis or acute pyogenic thyroiditis[830] is a rare problem and usually represents a blood- or lymphatic-borne localized bacterial infection of the thyroid. It is characterized by pain and tenderness in the thyroid which is associated with dysphagia and pain on swallowing. Locally there is observed a tender firm mass which later becomes fluctuant. The skin over the mass may be reddened. It is associated with fever, a neutrophilic leukocytosis and an elevated sedimentation rate.

This process can be differentiated from acute nonsuppurative thyroiditis by its purely local nature. It may be confused with a giant and spindle cell carcinoma which even on incision may be found to contain necrotic material which on first appearance looks like pus. The differentiation should be made by absence of fever, leukocytosis and other signs of infection in the patient harboring the giant and spindle cell carcinoma.

Treatment of this malady is surgical drainage and antibiotic therapy. Subsequent partial thyroidectomy may be necessary. At the time of the incision, in addition to culture, a biopsy should be taken from the abscess wall to rule out the diagnosis of a giant cell cancer.

Chronic thyroiditis is a term given probably without adequate justification to two disease entities, one a disease described by Hashimoto[831] and the other a picture described by Riedel.[832]

Hashimoto's Struma. Hashimoto's struma, or lymphadenoid goiter, is a progressive disease of the thyroid nearly always occurring in middle-aged females,[833,834] although cases have been reported in the male[835,836] and in children.[837,838] Its etiology is unknown.

The relationship of Hashimoto's struma to neoplasms has been suggested.[839,840] In seven of eight cases of malignant lymphoma of the thyroid there was also evidence of Hashimoto's struma.[841] It may be associated with systemic disorders as manifested by abnormalities in serum globulin and its reflection in elevated thymol turbidity, cephalin flocculation and serum colloidal gold tests.[842–845] Shaw and Smith[846] have described a patient who showed not only the picture of lymphadenoid goiter but similar lymphocytic changes in the adrenals. The experimental production of struma lymphomatosa in rats on a deficient diet[847] or after prolonged treatment with thiouracil[848] suggests that this disease represents a compensatory hyperplasia in an exhausted thyroid. The hyperglobulinemia[842] with the abnormal serum flocculation tests may be the consequence of the hypothyroidism which frequently accompanies Hashimoto's struma.[834,835,849–851,854] This may also be a reflection of an increased amount of antibodies to thyroid tissue or thyroglobulin which is liberated into the circulation as a result of the disease process.[852]

Grossly, the thyroids bearing this disease are enlarged, firm, friable and avascular. The border tends to be scalloped with pseudopodia, which are more definite on the lower border. Its cut surface is gray and lobulated. The microscopic picture of such thyroids is characterized by marked lymphoid infiltration and varying degrees of fibrous infiltration, which is most marked in the interacinar tissues and is often associated with a peculiar atrophy of the neighboring acini. The cells which form many of these atrophic acini are large and acidophilic with small hyperchromatic nuclei. Colloid is diminished in amount and is often absent. Large hyperplastic lymph follicles with germinative centers are commonly present (Fig. 14).

The symptoms of this disease are insidious, usually beginning with a gradual enlargement of the thyroid. Pain is noted on occasion. There is no fever. Occasionally these patients complain of nervousness and loss of weight. There is no leukocytosis. However, there may be a relative to absolute lymphocytosis. The basal metabolic rate tends to be below normal. The protein-bound iodine may be normal or decreased, and the radioactive iodine uptake in the thyroid may be low, normal or elevated.[80,849,853] As mentioned,[842–845] the serum flocculation tests are abnormal.

Opinions vary as to the management of this disease. Although the diagnosis

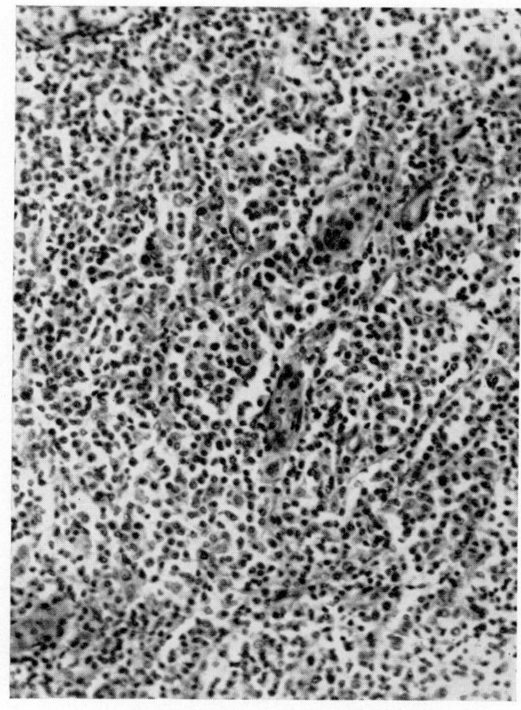

FIG. 14. Hashimoto's struma.

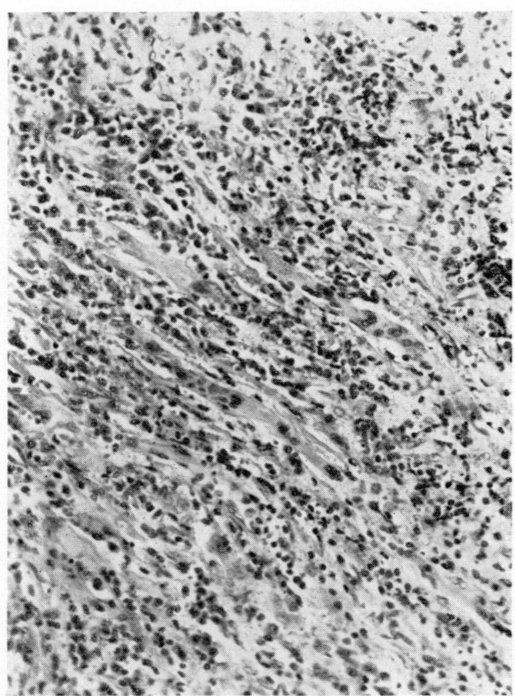

FIG. 15. Riedel's struma.

may be suggested by the combination of firm gland, hypometabolism and positive serum flocculation tests, it frequently is necessary to resort to needle biopsy or open surgical biopsy in order to distinguish this gland from cancer. If the diagnosis of Hashimoto's struma can be assured, it may be desirable to treat first with thyroid hormone, for which there have been claims[833,834,837,844,849,854] of successful treatment. If there is little response of the goiter to medical treatment, x-ray[833,854] may be necessary. When obstructive or pressure symptoms are present, a partial thyroidectomy[833,850] may be necessary.

Riedel's Struma. Riedel's struma, or ligneous thyroiditis, is an infrequently occurring, chronic, proliferative, fibrosing process involving the thyroid. It may extend to involve the trachea, the muscles and fascia.

Its etiology is unknown. Ewing suggested[855] that Riedel's struma and Hashimoto's struma are different stages of the same disease entity. Others[856,857] have strongly disagreed with this concept. They point out that Hashimoto's struma is a disease primarily of women and that, although Riedel's struma occurs more frequently in women, it does occur in a significant number of men. Against the argument that Riedel's struma is an end result of Hashimoto's struma, they point out that the mean age of a significant series of cases of Riedel's struma was less than the mean age of a comparable group of patients with Hashimoto's struma. Means[584] includes in his monograph a case report on one patient who was operated upon twice for chronic thyroiditis. The sections of thyroid taken at the first operation showed a classic lymphadenoid struma. At the second operation, which was performed two months later, the findings "were more characteristic of Riedel's than Hashimoto's struma."

Goetsch[858,859] feels that the irritative factors in this type of thyroiditis are the same as in toxic diffuse goiter. At first there is circumscription, isolation and destruction of numerous irritative foci and hyperfunctioning parenchyma by lymphoid and plasma cells. This process may terminate in virtually complete destruction of thyroid parenchyma and replacement by fibrous tissue. It may be nature's method for curing hyperthyroidism. Others[860] do not feel that the process is this specific and consider it a foreign body type of reaction with chronic inflammatory changes.

Grossly, the thyroid is enlarged, stony hard and firmly adherent to adjacent structures, but not to the skin. Often the gland is asymmetric, with greater enlargement on one side than on the other. Microscopically it is characterized by a marked diffuse sclerosis of the affected portions of the gland and varying numbers of persistent acini which appear compressed together by the surrounding dense fibrous stroma. The cells of persistent follicles are not remarkable and show no acidophilic degeneration nor any other signs of atrophy. Lymphocytes are accumulated focally but do not appear as lymph follicles. Although the histologic picture is often suggestive of an inflammatory process, no causative organisms have been found (Fig. 15).

Symptoms develop insidiously. There is gradual and slow enlargement of the thyroid which is usually painless. Tenderness and pain on swallowing do occur, but rarely. Subjective symptoms usually are those of pressure, which may be great enough to produce tracheal obstruction. There are practically no systemic symptoms. Temperature and pulse are usually normal.

This process must be distinguished from carcinoma and can usually be differentiated only by adequate histologic study.

Treatment consists of subtotal thyroidectomy for relief of pressure.

References

1. Gorbman, A. and Creaser, C. W.: J. Exper. Zool., *89:*391, 1942.
2. Stokes, M.: Proc. Soc. Exper. Biol. & Med., *42:*810, 1939.
3. Smith, D. C. and Matthews, S. A.: Am. J. Physiol., *153:*215, 1948.
4. Gudernatsch, J.: Roux Arch. Entw. Mech., *35:*457, 1912.
5. Noble, G. K. and Bradley, H. T.: Hemidactulus brookii. Biol. Bull., *64:*284, 1933.
6. Zawadowsky, B.: Endokrinologie, *10:*23, 1932.
7. Chapman, E.: J. Clin. Endocrinol., *8:* 717, 1948.
8. Kingsbury, B. F.: Am. J. Anat., *18:*329, 1915.
9. Lahey, F. H. and Ficarra, B. J.: Surg., Gynec. & Obst., *82:*705, 1946.
10. Graham, A.: Tr. Am. A. St. Goiter, p. 252, 1942–1946.
11. Rosencraft, P. and Foote, F. W., Jr.: Tr. Am. Goiter A., p. 150, 1948.
12. Rice, C. O.: Arch. Surg., *36:*96, 1938.
13. Wilson, G. E.: Anat. Rec., *42:*243, 1929.
14. Heidelberger, M. and Pederson, K. O.: J. Gen. Physiol., *19:*95, 1935.
15. Rawson, R. W. and Starr, P.: Arch. Int. Med., *61:*726, 1938.
16. Modell, W.: Anat. Rec., *55:*251, 1933.
17. Nonidez, J. F.: Am. J. Anat., *57:*135, 1935.
18. Friedgood, H. B. and Cannon, W. B.: Endocrinology, *26:*142, 1940.
19. Hertz, S., Roberts, A. and Evans, R. D.: Proc. Soc. Exper. Biol. & Med., *38* 510, 1938.
20. Scheffer, L.: Biochem. Ztschr., *259:*II, 1933.
21. Cole, V. and Curtis, G. M.: J. Nutrition, *10:*493, 1935.
22. Fellenberg, Th. von.: Ergebn. d. Physiol., *25:*176, 1926.
23. Hamilton, J. G. and Soley, M.: Am. J. Physiol., *127:*557, 1939.
24. Hamilton, J. G. and Soley, M.: Am. J. Physiol., *131:*135, 1940.
25. Schiff, L., Stevens, C. D., Molle, W. E., Steinberg, H., Klumpe, C. W. and Stewart, P.: J. Nat. Cancer Inst., *7:* 349, 1947.
26. McConahey, W. M., Keating, F. R. and Power, M. H.: J. Clin. Invest., *30:*778, 1951.
27. Vander Laan, J. E. and Vander Laan, W. P.: Endocrinology, *40:*403, 1947.
28. Childs, D. S., Keating, F. R., Rall, J. E., Williams, M. and Power, M. H.: J. Clin. Invest., *29:*726, 1950.
29. Freinkel, N. and Ingbar, S. H.: Tr. Am. Goiter A., p. 25, 1954.
30. Slingerland, D. W.: Tr. Am. Goiter A., p. 49, 1954.
31. Fawcett, D. M. and Kirkwood, S.: J. Biol. Chem., *204:*787, 1953.
32. Fawcett, D. M. and Kirkwood, S.: J. Biol. Chem., *205:*795, 1953.
33. Kendall, E. C.: J. Biol. Chem., *20:*501, 1915.
34. Harington, C. R. and Barger, G.: Biochem. J., *21:*169, 1927.
35. Harington, C. R. and Randall, S. S.: Biochem. J., *23:*373, 1929.
36. Roche, J. and Michel, R.: Recent Progress in Hormone Research, *12:*1, 1956.
37. Michel, R.: Am. J. Med., *20:*670, 1956.

38. Gross, J. and Pitt-Rivers, R.: Lancet, *261:*766, 1951.
39. Gross, J. and Pitt-Rivers, R.: Lancet, *262:*439, 1952.
40. Gross, J. and Pitt-Rivers, R.: Lancet, *262:*593, 1952.
41. Roche, J., Lissitzky, S. and Michel, R.: Compt. rend. Soc. de biol., *234:*1228, 1952.
42. De Robertis, E.: Ann. New York Acad. Sc., *50:*317, 1949.
43. MacQuillan, M. T.: Ph.D. Thesis, Melbourne, Australia, Univ. of Melbourne, 1952.
44. Weiss, B.: J. Biol. Chem., *205:*193, 1953.
45. Laidlaw, J. C.: Nature, *164:*927, 1949.
46. Taurog, A. and Chaikoff, I. L.: J. Biol. Chem., *176:*699, 1948.
47. Gross, J., Leblond, C. P., Franklin, A. E. and Quastel, J. H.: Science, *111:*605, 1950.
48. Rall, J. E.: J. Clin. Endocrinol., *10:*996, 1950.
49. Benua, R. S., Dobyns, B. M. and Ninmer, A.: J. Clin. Endocrinol., *15:*1367, 1955.
50. Robbins, J., Rall, J. E. and Rawson, R. W.: J. Clin. Endocrinol., *15:*1315, 1955.
51. Roche, J. and Michel, R.: Acta endocrinol., *17:*385, 1954.
52. Gross, J. and Leblond, C. P.: Proc. Soc. Exper. Biol. & Med., *76:*686, 1951.
53. Larson, F. C., Tomita, K. and Albright, E. C.: Endocrinology, *57:*338, 1955.
54. Wilkinson, J. H., Sprott, W. E., Bowden, C. H. and MacLagan, N. F.: Biochem. J., *56:*215, 1954.
55. Tong, W., Taurog, A. and Chaikoff, I. L.: J. Biol. Chem., *195:*407, 1952.
56. Robbins, J.: J. Biol. Chem., *208:*377, 1954.
57. Robbins, J., Petermann, M. L. and Rall, J. E.: J. Biol. Chem., *208:*387, 1954.
58. Tata, J. R., Rall, J. E. and Rawson, R. W.: J. Clin. Endocrinol., *16:*1554, 1956.
59. Gordon, A. H., Gross, J., O'Connor, D. and Pitt-Rivers, R.: Nature, *169:*19, 1952.
60. Deiss, W. P., Albright, E. C. and Larson, F. C.: J. Clin. Invest., *31:*1000, 1952.
61. Deiss, W. P., Albright, E. C. and Larson, F. C.: Proc. Soc. Exper. Biol. & Med., *84:*513, 1953.
62. Larson, F. C., Deiss, W. P. and Albright, E. C.: J. Clin. Invest., *33:*230, 1954.
63. Robbins, J. and Rall, J. E.: J. Clin. Invest., *34:*1324, 1955.
64. Robbins, J. and Rall, J. E.: J. Clin. Invest., *34:*1331, 1955.
65. Dingledine, W. S., Pitt-Rivers, R. and Stanbury, J. B.: J. Clin. Endocrinol., *15:*724, 1955.
66. Albright, E. C., Larson, F. C. and Deiss, W. P.: J. Clin. Invest., *34:*44, 1955.
67. Dowling, J. T., Freinkel, N. and Ingbar, S. H.: J. Clin. Endocrinol., *16:*280, 1956.
68. Freinkel, N., Dowling, J. T. and Ingbar, S. H.: J. Clin. Invest., *34:*1698, 1955.
69. Recant, L. and Riggs, D. S.: J. Clin. Invest., *31:*789, 1952.
70. Robbins, J., Rall, J. E. and Rawson, R. W.: J. Clin. Endocrinol., *16:*573, 1956.
71. Rasmussen, H.: J. Clin. Invest., *35:*792, 1956.
72. Sherer, M. G. and Diefring, B. N.: J. Clin. Endocrinol., *16:*643, 1956.
73. Crispell, K. R., Kahana, S. and Hyer, H.: J. Clin. Invest., *35:*121, 1956.
74. Crispell, K. R. and Coleman, J.: J. Clin. Invest., *35:*475, 1956.
75. Foster, G. L., Palmer, W. W. and Leland, J. P.: J. Biol. Chem., *155:*467, 1936.
76. Pitt-Rivers, R. and Lerman, J.: J. Endocrinol., *5:*223, 1948.
77. Boothby, W. M. and Baldes, E. J.: Proc. Staff Meet. Mayo Clin., *1:*166, 1926.
78. Logan, R. E. and Lien, A.: Fed. Proc., *10:*85, 1951.
79. Albert, A. and Keating, F. R.: J. Clin. Endocrinol., *9:*1406, 1949.
80. Albert, A., Rall, J. E., Keating, F. R., Power, M. H. and Williams, M.: J. Clin. Endocrinol., *9:*1392, 1949.
81. Myant, N. B. and Pochin, E. E.: Clin. Sc., *9:*421, 1950.
82. Salter, W. T.: Ann. New York Acad. Sc., *50:*358, 1949.
83. Berson, S. A. and Yalow, R. S.: J. Clin. Invest., *33:*1533, 1954.
84. Sterling, K., Lashof, J. C. and Man, E. B.: J. Clin. Invest., *33:*1031, 1954.
85. Benua, R. S., Albert, A. and Keating, F. R.: J. Clin. Endocrinol., *12:*1461, 1952.
86. Sterling, K. and Chodos, R. B.: J. Clin. Invest., *35:*806, 1956.
87. Hamolsky, M. W., Freedberg, A. S., Kurland, G. S. and Wolsky, L.: J. Clin. Invest., *32:*453, 1953.
88. Hart, F. D. and MacLagan, N. F.: Brit. M. J., *1:*512, 1950.
89. Ingbar, S. H. and Freinkel, N.: J. Clin. Invest., *34:*808, 1955.
90. Hamolsky, M. W. and Gierlach, Z. S.: Proc. Soc. Exper. Biol. & Med., *80:*288, 1952.
91. Lipner, H. J., Barker, S. B. and Winnick, T.: Endocrinology, *51:*406, 1952.
92. Lee, N. D. and Williams, R. H.: Endocrinology, *54:*5, 1954.
93. Taurog, A., Briggs, F. N. and Chaikoff, I. L.: J. Biol. Chem., *194:*655, 1952.
94. Roche, J., Michel, R. and Tata, J. R.: Biochim. & Biophys. Acta, *11:*543, 1953.
95. Roche, J., Michel, O., Michel, R. and Tata, J. R.: Biochim. & Biophys. Acta, *13:*471, 1954.

96. Klitgaard, H. M., Lipner, H. J., Barker, S. B. and Winnick, T.: Endocrinology, *52:*79, 1953.
97. Briggs, F. N., Brauer, R. W., Taurog, A. and Chaikoff, I. L.: Am. J. Physiol., *172:*561, 1952.
98. Klitgaard, H. M.: Proc. Soc. Exper. Biol. & Med., *82:*578, 1953.
99. Albert, A. and Keating, F. R.: Endocrinology, *51:*427, 1952.
100. Briggs, F. N., Taurog, A. and Chaikoff, I. L.: Endocrinology, *52:*559, 1953.
101. Johnson, P. C. and Beierwaltes, W. H.: J. Lab. & Clin. Med., *41:*676, 1953.
102. Rupp, J. J.: Endocrinology, *51:*306, 1952.
103. Elmer, A. W. and Scheps, M.: Compt. rend. Soc. de Biol., *115:*968, 1954.
104. Mitolo, M.: Endocrinol. e pat. constit., *11:*197, 1936.
105. Rand, C. G., Riggs, D. S. and Talbot, N. B.: Endocrinology, *51:*562, 1952.
106. Bondy, P. K. and Hagewood, M. A.: Proc. Soc. Exper. Biol. & Med., *81:* 328, 1952.
107. Eskelson, C. D., Firschein, H. E. and Jensen, H.: Proc. Soc. Exper. Biol. & Med., *85:*637, 1954.
108. Ingbar, S. H. and Freinkel, N.: J. Clin. Invest., *34:*1375, 1955.
109. Stanbury, J. B., Meijer, J. W. A. and Kassenaar, A. A. H.: J. Clin. Endocrinol., *16:*848, 1956.
110. Stanbury, J. B., Kassenaar, A. A. H., Meijer, J. W. A. and Terpstra, J.: J. Clin. Endocrinol., *16:*735, 1956.
111. Querido, A., Stanbury, J. B., Kassenaar, A. A. H. and Meijer, J. W. A.: J. Clin. Endocrinol., *16:*1096, 1956.
112. Nièpce, B.: Traité du goitre et du crétinisme. Paris, Ballière, 1851.
113. Rogowitsch, N.: Beitr. zu path. Anat. u. z. allg. Path., *4:*453, 1888.
114. Cushing, H.: The Pituitary Body and Its Disorders. Philadelphia, J. B. Lippincott Co., 1912.
115. Foster, G. L. and Smith, P. E.: J.A.M.A., *87:*2151, 1926.
116. Smith, P. E.: Anat. Rec., *11:*57, 1916.
117. White, A.: Physiol. Rev., *26:*574, 1946.
118. Albert, A.: Ann. New York Acad. Sc., *50:*466, 1949.
119. Reineke, E. P. and Turner, C. W.: Res. Bull. Missouri Agric. Sch., *355:*1, 1942.
120. Rawson, R. W. and Salter, W. T.: Endocrinology, *27:*155, 1940.
121. Keating, F. R., Rawson, R. W., Peacock, W. and Evans, R. D.: Endocrinology, *36:*137, 1945.
122. D'Angelo, S. A., Paschkis, K. E., Cantarow, A. and Gordon, A. S.: J. Clin. Endocrinol., *11:*761, 1951.
123. Adams, D. D. and Purves, H. D.: Endocrinology, *56:*17, 1955.
124. Greenspan, F. S., Kriss, J. P., Moses, L. E. and Lew, W.: Endocrinology, *58:*767, 1956.
125. Bates, R. W. and Cornfield, J.: Endocrinology, *60:*225, 1957.
126. Rawson, R. W.: Ann. New York Acad. Sc., *50:*491, 1949.
127. Alpers, J. B., Robbins, J. and Rall, J. E.: Endocrinology, *56:*110, 1955.
128. Friedgood, H. B.: Bull. Johns Hopkins, Hosp., *54:*48, 1954.
129. Dobyns, B. M.: Surg. Gynec. & Obst., *82:*290, 1946.
130. Rawson, R. W., Sterne, G. D. and Aub, J. C.: Endocrinology, *30:*240, 1942.
131. Cortell, R. and Rawson, R. W.: Endocrinology, *35:*488, 1944.
132. Starr, P. and Patton, H.: Endocrinology, *18:*113, 1934.
133. Gassner, F. X., Barret, H. W. and Gustavson, R. G.: Tr. Am. Goiter A., p. 156, 1947.
134. Money, W. L., Kirschner, L., Kraintz, L., Merrill, P. and Rawson, R. W.: Tr. Am. Goiter A., p. 213, 1950.
135. Soffer, L. J., Gabrilove, J. L. and Dorrance, W. R.: Proc. Soc. Exper. Biol. & Med., *76:*763, 1951.
136. Forsham, P. H., Thorn, G. W., Prunty, E. T. G. and Hills, A. G.: J. Clin. Endocrinol., *8:*15, 1948.
137. Wolfson, W. Q., Beierwaltes, W. H., Robinson, W. D., Duff, I. F., Jones, J. R., Knorpp, C. T., Siemienski, J. S. and Eyea, M.: Proc. 2nd Clin. ACTH Conf., *2:*95, 1951.
138. Chu, J. F.: Endocrinology, *34:*90, 1944.
139. Zarrow, M. X. and Money, W. L.: Endocrinology, *44:*345, 1949.
140. Long, C. N.: Endocrinology, *30:*870, 1942.
141. Catz, B., El-Rawi, I. and Geiger, E.: Am. J. Physiol., *172:*291, 1953.
142. Starr, P. and Roskelley, R.: Am. J. Physiol., *130:*549, 1940.
143. Uotila, U.: Endocrinology, *25:*605, 1939.
144. Uotila, U.: Endocrinology, *26:*129, 1940.
145. Dempsey, E. W. and Astwood, E. B.: Endocrinology, *32:*509, 1943.
146. Hoffman, E. and Shaffner, C. S.: Poultry Science, *29:*365, 1950.
147. Botkin, A. L., Praytor, E. H., Austing, M. E. and Jensen, H.: Endocrinology, *50:*550, 1952.
148. Hursh, J. B., van Valkenburg, P. A. and Mohney, J. B.: Radiology, *57:*411, 1951.
149. Mole, R. H. and Batt, O. D.: Proc. Roy. Soc. Med., *46:*250, 1953.
150. Puntriano, G. and Meites, J.: Endocrinology, *48:*217, 1951.
151. Verzar, F., Sailer, E. and Vidovic, V.: J. Endocrinol., *8:*308, 1952.
152. Bogoroch, R. and Timiras, P.: Endocrinology, *49:*548, 1951.
153. Shipley, R. A. and MacIntyre, F. H.: J. Clin. Endocrinol. *14:*309, 1954.
154. Goldenberg, I. S., Lutwak, L., Rosenbaum, P. J. and Hayes, M. A.: Surg. Gynec. & Obst., *102:*129, 1956.

155. Hetzel, B. S., de La Haba, D. S. and Hinkle, L. E., Jr.: Tr. Am. Goiter A., p. 242, 1952.
156. Chesney, A. M., Clawson, T. A. and Webster, B.: Bull. Johns Hopkins Hosp., *43:*261, 1928.
157. Marine, D., Baumann, E. J., Spense, A. W. and Cipra, A.: Proc. Soc. Exper. Biol. & Med., *29:*772, 1932.
158. Astwood, E. B., Greer, M. A. and Ettlinger, M. G.: Science, *109:*631, 1949.
159. MacKenzie, J. B., MacKenzie, C. G. and McCollum, E. V.: Science, *94:*518, 1941.
160. Richter, C. P. and Clisby, K. H.: Arch. Pathol., *33:*46, 1942.
161. Kennedy, T. H. and Purves, H. D.: Brit. J. Exper. Pathol., *22:*241, 1941.
162. MacKenzie, C. G. and MacKenzie, J. B.: Endocrinology, *32:*185, 1943.
163. Astwood, E. B.: J. Pharmacol. & Exper. Therap., *78:*79, 1943.
164. Albert, A., Rawson, R. W., Merrill, P., Lennon, B. and Riddell, C.: J. Biol. Chem., *166:*637, 1946.
165. Albert, A., Rawson, R. W., Riddell, C., Merrill, P. and Lennon, B.: Endocrinology, *40:*361, 1947.
166. Astwood, E. B.: Ann. New York Acad. Science, *50:*419, 1949.
167. Rawson, R. W., Tannheimer, J. F. and Peacock, W.: Endocrinology, *34:*245, 1944.
168. Tierney, N. A. and Peters, J. P.: J. Clin. Invest., *22:*595, 1943.
169. Kelley, B. and Day, H. G.: J. Biol. Chem., *175:*863, 1948.
170. Schwarz, F., der Kinderen, P. J., van Haaften, J. L., and Koopman, L. E.: Acta endocrinol., *19:*411, 1955.
171. Wase, A. W., Repplinger, E. and Foster, W. C.: Endocrinology, *53:*630, 1953.
172. Mayer, S. W., Kelly, F. H. and Morton, M. E.: J. Pharm. & Exper. Therap., *117:*197, 1956.
173. Libby, D. A. and Meites, J.: Science, *120:*354, 1954.
174. Dziewiatkowski, D. D.: J. Biol. Chem., *189:*717, 1951.
175. Goldberg, R. C. and Chaikoff, I. L.: Endocrinology, *49:*613, 1951.
176. Castor, C. W. and Beierwaltes, W.: J. Clin. Endocrinol., *16:*1026, 1956.
177. Chatin, A.: Compt. rend. Acad. Sc., *31:*529, 1851.
178. Wolff, J., Chaikoff, I. L., Taurog, A. and Rubin, L.: Endocrinology, *39:*2, 1946.
179. Stanley, M. M. and Astwood, E. B.: Endocrinology, *42:*107, 1948.
180. Wyngaarden, J. B., Stanbury, J. B. and Rapp, B.: Endocrinology, *52:*568, 1953.
181. Wyngaarden, J. B., Wright, B. M. and Ways, P.: Endocrinology, *50:*537, 1952.
182. Gull, W. W.: Tr. Clin. Soc. Lond., *7:*180, 1874.
183. Butterworth, T.: A.M.A. Arch. Dermat., *70:*565, 1954.
184. Wolff, J. and Chaikoff, I. L.: J. Biol. Chem., *172:*855, 1948.
185. Gutman, A. G., Benedict, E. M., Baxter, B. and Palmer, W. W.: J. Biol. Chem., *97:*303, 1932.
186. Wolff, J. and Chaikoff, I. L.: Endocrinology, *43:*174, 1948.
187. Wolff, J., Chaikoff, I. L., Goldberg, R. C. and Meier, J. R.: Endocrinology, *45:*504, 1949.
188. Stanley, M. M.: J. Clin. Endocrinol., *9:*941, 1949.
189. Rawson, R. W. and Money, W. L.: Rec. Progress in Hormone Research, *4:*397, 1949.
190. Sonenberg, M. and Money, W. L.: Rec. Progress in Hormone Research, *11:*43, 1955.
191. Ogilvie, A. L.: J. Dent. Res., *32:*386, 1953.
192. Gross, R. T., Kriss, J. P. and Spaet, T. H.: Pediatrics, *15:*284, 1955.
193. Kriss, J. P., Carnes, W. H. and Gross, R. T.: J.A.M.A., *157:*117, 1955.
194. Jaimet, C. H. and Thode, H. G.: J.A.M.A., *158:*1353, 1955.
195. Holly, R. G.: J.A.M.A., *158:*1349, 1955.
196. Westrick, M. L.: Proc. Soc. Exper. Biol. & Med., *82:*56, 1953.
197. Grant, W. C.: Science, *120:*724, 1954.
198. Telkka, A. and Kuusisto, A. W.: Acta endocrinol., *16:*365, 1954.
199. Goodman, J. R., Florsheim, W. H. and Tempereau, C. E.: Proc. Soc. Exper. Biol. & Med., *90:*196, 1955.
200. Skowron, S. and Jordan, M.: Bull. Intern. acad. polon. sci. classe méd., p. 111, Jan.–June 1949.
201. Green, T. W., White, W. E., Engelman, E. P. and Krupp, M. A.: Proc. Soc. Exper. Biol. & Med., *82:*155, 1953.
202. Salter, W. T.: The Hormones, New York, Academic Press, 1950, vol. II. p. 190.
203. Harington, C. R.: Biochem. J., *20:*300, 1926.
204. Lerman, J. and Harington, C. R.: J. Clin. Endocrinol., *9:*1099, 1949.
205. Compston, N. and Pitt-Rivers, R.: Lancet, *270:*22, 1956.
206. Lerman, J., Harington, C. R. and Means, J. H.: J. Clin. Endocrinol., *12:*1306, 1952.
207. Kendall, E. C.: J.A.M.A., *64:*2042, 1915.
208. Harington, C. R. and Barger, G.: Biochem. J., *21:*169, 1927.
209. Anderson, A. B., Harington, C. R. and Lyon, D. M.: Lancet, *224:*1081, 1933.
210. Salter, W. T. and Lerman, J.: Tr. A. Am. Physicians, *53:*202, 1938.
211. Kroc, R. L., Phillips, G. E., Stasilli, N. R. and Malament, S.: J. Clin. Endocrinol., *14:*56, 1954.
212. Abelin, I. and Huber, P.: Acta endocrinol., *6:*1, 1951.

213. Frieden, E. and Winzler, R. J.: J. Biol. Chem., *176:*155, 1948.
214. Gaddum, J. H.: J. Physiol., *64:*246, 1927.
215. Niemann, C. and Redemann, C. E.: J. Am. Chem. Soc., *63:*1549, 1941.
216. Abderhalden, E. and Wertheimer, E.: Ztschr. f. d. ges. exper. Med., *63:*557, 1928.
217. Barker, S. B., Kiely, C. E., Jr., Klitgaard, H. M., Dirks, H. B., Jr., Wang, S. C. and Wawzonek, S.: Endocrinology, *48:*70, 1951.
218. Leblond, C. P. and Grad, B.: J. Pharmacol. & Exper. Therap., *94:*125, 1948.
219. Richards, C. E., Brady, R. O. and Riggs, D. S.: J. Clin. Endocrinol., *9:*1107, 1949.
220. Pitt-Rivers, R.: Lancet, *265:*234, 1953.
221. Goolden, A. W. G.: Lancet, *270:*890, 1956.
222. Trotter, W. R.: Lancet, *269:*374, 1955.
223. Gross, J. and Pitt-Rivers, R.: Biochem. J., *53:*652, 1953.
224. Rall, J. E., Pearson, O. H., Robbins, J., Poppell, H. F. and West, C. D.: Tr. A. Am. Physicians, *66:*86, 1953.
225. Tomich, E. G. and Woollett, E. A.: Lancet, *264:*726, 1953.
226. Heming, A. E. and Holtkamp, D. E.: Proc. Soc. Exper. Biol. & Med., *83:*875, 1953.
227. Blackburn, C. M., McConahey, W. M., Keating, F. R. and Albert, A.: J. Clin. Invest., *33:*819, 1954.
228. Frawley, T. F., McClintock, J. C., Beebe, R. T. and Marthy, G. L.: J.A.M.A., *160:*646, 1956.
229. Frieden, E. and Winzler, R. L.: J. Biol. Chem., *179:*423, 1949.
230. MacLagan, N. F., Sheahan, M. M. and Wilkinson, J. H.: Nature, *164:*699, 1949.
231. Woolley, D. W.: J. Biol. Chem., *164:*11, 1946.
232. Cortell, R. E.: J. Clin. Endocrinol., *9:*955, 1949.
223. Gross, J. and Pitt-Rivers, R.: Biochem. J., MacLagan, N. F.: Biochem. J., *49:*710, 1951.
234. Sprott, W. E., Wilkinson, J. H. and MacLagan, N. F.: Endocrinology, *9:*xxxii, 1953.
235. Sheahan, M. M., Wilkinson, J. H. and MacLagan, N. F.: Biochem. J., *48:*188, 1951.
236. Wilkinson, J. H., Sheahan, M. M. and MacLagan, N. F.: Biochem. J., *49:*714, 1951.
237. Wilkinson, J. H., Sheahan, M. M. and MacLagan, N. F.: Biochem. J., *54:*491, 1953.
238. MacLagan, N. F., Sprott, W. E. and Wilkinson, J. H.: Lancet, *263:*915, 1952.
239. Wilkinson, J. H. and MacLagan, N. F.: J. Endocrinol., *9:*xliv, 1953.
240. Brayne, M. K. and MacLagan, N. F.: J. Endocrinol., *9:*90, 1953.
241. Raab, W.: Wien. Arch. inn. Med., *23:*321, 1932.
242. Abelin, I.: Biochem. Ztschr., *286:*160, 1936.
243. Abelin, I. and Kipfer, H.: Arch. internat. pharmacodyn., *82:*99, 1950.
244. Abelin, I. and Parhon, C. I., Jr.: Klin. Wochnschr., *12:*1167, 1933.
245. Roth, P.: Bull. musée nat'l. hist. nat., Paris, *13:*611, 1941.
246. Barker, S. B., Kiely, C. E., Jr., Dirks, H. B., Jr., Klitgaard, H. M., Wang, S. C., and Wawzonek, S.: J. Pharmacol. & Exper. Therap., *99:*202, 1950.
247. Kraft, K.: Hoppe-Seyler's Ztschr. f. physiol. Chem., *245:*58, 1936.
248. Litzka, G.: Arch. Exper. Pathol. u. Pharmakol., *183:*436, 1936.
249. May, R.: Deut. med. Wochnschr., *74:*374, 1949.
250. Barker, S. B.: Physiol. Rev., *31:*205, 1951.
251. Abelin, I.: Arch. internat. pharmacodyn. *75:*187, 1947.
252. Barker, S. B., Kiely, C. E., Jr. and Lipner, H. J.: Endocrinology, *45:*624, 1949.
253. Borell, U. and Holmgren, H.: Endocrinology, *42:*427, 1948.
254. Drabkin, D. L.: J. Biol. Chem., *182:*335, 1950.
255. Drabkin, D. L.: J. Biol. Chem., *182:*351, 1950.
256. Lardy, H. A.: Biology of Phosphorus. East Lansing, Michigan State College Press, 1951.
257. Hoch, F. L. and Lipmann, F.: Fed. Proc., *12:*218, 1953.
258. Martius, C. and Hess, B.: Arch. Biochem. & Biophys., *33:*486, 1951.
259. Martius, C. and Hess, B.: Arch. Exper. Pathol. u. Pharmakol., *216:*45, 1952.
260. Niemeyer, H., Crane, R. K., Kennedy, E. P. and Lipmann, F.: Fed. Proc., *10:*229, 1951.
261. Maley, G. F. and Lardy, H. A.: J. Biol. Chem., *204:*435, 1953.
262. Judah, J. D.: Biochem. J., *49:*271, 1955.
263. Klemperer, H. G.: Biochem. J., *60:*122, 1951.
264. Lehninger, A.: Harvey Lectures, *49:*176, 1953–1954.
265. Goldstein, M. S.: J. Biol. Chem., *199:*923, 1952.
266. Aebi, H.: Helv. physiol. & pharmacol. acta, *10:*C43–5, 1952.
267. Ord, W. M. and White, E.: Brit. M. J., *2:*217, 1893.
268. Boothby, W. M., Sandiford, I., Sandiford, K. and Sloss, J.: Tr. A. Am. Physicians, *40:*195, 1925.
269. Byrom, F. B.: Clin. Sc., *1:*273, 1933–34.

270. Persike, E. C.: Endocrinology, *42:*356, 1948.
271. Hoberman, H. D. and Graff, J.: Yale J. Biol. & Med., *23:*195, 1950.
272. Leathem, J. H.: Symposium on Protein Metabolism, Hormones, and Growth. New Brunswick, N. J., Rutgers University Press, 1952, p. 17.
273. Sure, B., Ford, Z. W., Jr., Theis, R. M. and Goldfischer, M.: Endocrinology, *28:*806, 1941.
274. Rupp, J., Paschkis, K. E. and Cantarow, A.: Endocrinology, *44:*449, 1949.
275. Bondy, P. K.: Endocrinology, *45:*605, 1949.
276. Hoffmann, F., Cori, O. and Cori, A. T.: Acta physiol. latino-am., *1:*84, 1951.
277. Pasqualetti, A. T.: Farm. Chilena, *24:*450, 1950.
278. Sellers, E. A., You, S. S. and You, R. W.: Endocrinology, *47:*148, 1950.
279. You, S. S., You, R. W. and Sellers, E. A.: Endocrinology, *47:*146, 1950.
280. Rupp, J., Paschkis, K. E. and Cantarow, A.: Proc. Soc. Exper. Biol. & Med., *76:*432, 1951.
281. Solganils, R. I.: Biokhimiya, *17:*649, 1952.
282. Crispell, K. R., Parson, W. and Hollifield, G.: J. Clin. Invest., *35:*164, 1956.
283. Karp, A. and Stetten, DeW., Jr.: J. Biol. Chem., *179:*819, 1949.
284. Feldott, G. and Lardy, H. A.: Fed. Proc., *10:*182, 1951.
285. Kline, D. L.: Endocrinology, *45:*596, 1949.
286. Deusch, G.: Deutsches Arch. klin. Med., *134:*342, 1920.
287. Villar Caso, J., Zofmann, A. E. and Rivero Fontan, J. L.: Rev. españ. enferm. ap. digest., *10:*446, 1951.
288. Thompson, W. O., Thompson, P. K., Silveus, E. and Dailey, M. E.: Arch. Int. Med., *44:*368, 1929.
289. Schwartz, E.: J. Lab. & Clin. Med., *45:*340, 1955.
290. Scow, R. O.: Am. J. Physiol., *173:*199, 1953.
291. Scow, R. O.: Endocrinology, *49:*522, 1951.
292. Sternheimer, R.: Endocrinology, *25:*899, 1939.
293. Shaffer, P. A.: Am. J. Physiol., *23:*1, 1908–9.
294. Palmer, W. W., Carson, D. A. and Sloan, L. W.: J. Clin. Invest., *6:*597, 1929.
295. Peters, J. H., Schwartz, R., Mermelstein, H., Nefores, M. N. and Mansuy, M. M.: J. Clin. Invest., *30:*799, 1951.
296. Richardson, H. B. and Shorr, E.: Tr. A. Am. Physicians, *50:*156, 1935.
297. Tierney, N. A. and Peters, J. P.: J. Clin. Invest., *22:*595, 1943.
298. Wilkins, L. and Fleischmann, W.: J. Clin. Invest., *25:*360, 1946.
299. Griffiths, W. L.: Lancet, *2:*467, 1951.
300. Mukherjee, R. and Mitchell, H. H.: J. Nutrition, *37:*303, 1949.
301. Wang, E.: Acta med. scandinav. (Suppl.), *105:*1, 1939.
302. Abelin, I.: Helvet. physiol. et pharmacol. acta, *9:*74, 1951.
303. Comsa, J.: Compt. rend. Soc. Biol., *140:* 613, 1946.
304. Mandel, L., Jacob, M. and Mandel, P.: Compt. rend. Soc. Biol., *145:*1231, 1951.
305. Mandel, P., Mandel, L. and Jacob, M.: Compt. rend. Soc. Biol., *232:*1513, 1951.
306. Mandel, L., Jacob, M. and Mandel, P.: Experientia, *8:*426, 1952.
307. Capra, P.: Arch. sc. med., *93:*353, 1952.
308. Rawson, R. W., Rall, J. E., Pearson, O. H., Robbins, J., Poppell, H. F., and West, C. D.: Am. J. M. Sc., *226:*405, 1953.
309. Capra, P.: Arch. sc. med., *88:*536, 1946.
310. Larson, F. and Albright, E. C.: Am. J. M. Sc., *222:*26, 1951.
311. Cohen, A. G. N. and Minz, B.: Arch. sc. physiol., *4:*145, 1950.
312. Jimenez, F. V.: Tesis quim. Univ. Chile, *2:*1, 1950.
313. Geyelin, H. R.: Arch. Int. Med., *16:* 975, 1915.
314. Mirsky, I. A. and Broh-Kahn, R. H.: Am. J. Physiol., *117:*6, 1936.
315. Lozner, E. L., Winkler, A. W., Taylor, F. H. and Peters, J. P.: J. Clin. Invest., *20:*507, 1941.
316. Althausen, T. L.: J.A.M.A., *115:*101, 1940.
317. Mosely, V. and Chornack, F. W.: J. Clin. Invest., *26:*11, 1947.
318. Richardson, H. B., Levine, S. Z. and Dubois, E. F.: J. Biol. Chem., *67:*737, 1926.
319. Coggeshall, H. C. and Greene, J. A.: Am. J. Physiol., *105:*103, 1933.
320. Houssay, B. A.: Endocrinology, *35:*158, 1944.
321. Neal, W. B., Jr., Dragstedt, L. R., Rogers, G. R. and McKeague, G.: Am. J. Physiol., *168:*29, 1952.
322. Roe, J. H. and Coover, M. O.: Proc. Soc. Exper. Biol. & Med., *75:*818, 1950.
323. Rabbi, A. and Rossi, C. A.: Boll. soc. ital. biol. sper., *26:*1114, 1950.
324. Pittoni, A. and Barbieri, E.: Boll. soc. ital. biol. sper., *28:*1745, 1952.
325. Gershberg, H. and Kuhl, W. J., Jr.: J. Clin. Invest., *29:*1625, 1950.
326. Foldes, F. F. and Murphy, A. J.: Proc. Soc. Exper. Biol. & Med., *62:*218, 1946.
327. Peters, J. P. and Man, E. B.: J. Clin. Invest., *22:*715, 1943.
328. Peters, J. P. and Man, E. B.: J. Clin. Invest., *29:*1, 1950.

329. Entenman, C., Chaikoff, I. L. and Reichert, F. L.: Endocrinology, *30:*794, 1942.
330. Greenberg, S. N. and Deuel, H. J., Jr.: J. Nutrition, *42:*279, 1950.
331. Weiss, S. B., Marx, L. and Marx, W.: Endocrinology, *50:*192, 1952.
332. Trotter, W. R.: Lancet, *270:*885, 1956.
333. Kyle, L. H., Welham, W. C., Doolan, P. D. and Schaaf, M.: J. Clin. Endocrinol., *14:*1029, 1954.
334. Gofman, J. W., Jones, H. B., Lindgren, F. T., Lyon, T. P., Elliott, H. A., and Strisower, B.: Circulation, *2:*161, 1950.
335. Strisower, B., Gofman, J. W., Galioni, E., Almada, A. A. and Simon, A.: Metabolism, *3:*218, 1954.
336. Strisower, B., Gofman, J. W., Galioni, E., Rubinger, J. H., O'Brien, G. W. and Simon, A.: J. Clin. Endocrinol., *15:*73, 1955.
337. Flock, E. V., Bollman, J. L. and Berkson, J.: Am. J. Physiol., *155:*402, 1948.
338. Fraenkel-Conrat, J. and Li, C. H.: Endocrinology, *44:*487, 1949.
339. Rosenman, R. H., Friedman, M. and Byers, S. O.: Science, *114:*210, 1951.
340. Rosenman, R. H., Byers, S. O. and Friedman, M.: J. Clin. Endocrinol., *12:*1287, 1952.
341. Friedman, M., Byers, S. O. and Rosenman, R. H.: Circulation, *5:*657, 1952.
342. Thompson, J. C. and Vars, H. M.: Proc. Soc. Exper. Biol. & Med., *83:*246, 1953.
343. Marx, W., Gustin, S. T. and Levi, C.: Proc. Soc. Exper. Biol. & Med., *83:* 143, 1953.
344. Rosenman, R. H., Friedman, M. and Byers, S. O.: Circulation, *5:*589, 1952.
345. Byers, S. O., Rosenman, R. H., Friedman, M. and Biggs, M. W.: J. Exper. Med., *96:*513, 1952.
346. DeCandia, S. and Nava, G.: Folia endocrinol., *3:*817, 1950.
347. Kinnunen, O. and Kauppinen, M.: Acta endocrinol., *8:*380, 1951.
348. Malmros, H. and Swahn, B.: Acta med. scandinav., *145:*361, 1953.
349. Gräsbeck, R. and Lamberg, B. A.: Acta endocrinol., *19:*82, 1955.
350. Blumgart, H. L., Freedberg, A. S. and Kurland, G. S.: Am. J. Med., *14:*665, 1953.
351. Steiner, A., Kendall, F. E. and Bevans, M.: Am. Heart J., *38:*34, 1949.
352. Lindsay, S., Feinberg, H., Chaikoff, I. L., Entenman, C. and Reichert, F. L.: Arch. Pathol., *54:*573, 1952.
353. Dauber, D., Horlick, L. and Katz, L. N.: Am. Heart J., *38:*25, 1949.
354. Hertz, R., Schricker, J. A. and Tullner, W. W.: Endocrinology, *49:*168, 1951.
355. Bainborough, A. R. and McMillan, G. C.: Arch. Pathol., *54:*204, 1952.
356. Priddle, W. W.: Ann. Int. Med., *35:* 836, 1951.
357. Soffer, A., Yu, P. N. G., Epstein, M. A. and Olsan, E. S.: Am. J. M. Sc., *222:*427, 1951.
358. Iversen, K. and Asboe-Hansen, G.: Acta endocrinol., *11:*111, 1952.
359. Asper, S. P., Jr., Selenkow, H. A. and Plamondon, C. A.: Bull. Johns Hopkins Hosp., *93:*164, 1953.
360. Pickering, D., Fisher, D. A. and Scott, K. G.: Am. J. Dis. Child., *86:*157, 1953.
361. Wiener, R., Tannaccone, A., Eisenberg, J., Griboff, S. I., Ludwig, A. W. and Soffer, L. J.: J. Clin. Endocrinol., *15:* 1131, 1955.
362. Koppen, H.: Neurol., *11:*219, 1892.
363. Parhon, M.: Mém. de la soc. de Biol., *72:*620, 1912.
364. Aub, J. C., Bauer, W., Heath, C. and Ropes, M.: J. Clin. Invest., *7:*97, 1929.
365. Robertson, J. D.: Lancet, *241:*129, 1941.
366. Robertson, J. D.: Lancet, *242:*672, 1942.
367. Robertson, J. D.: Lancet, *241:*216, 1941.
368. Green, J. and Lyall, A.: Lancet, *260:* 828, 1951.
369. Rose, E. and Boles, R. S., Jr.: M. Clin. North America, *37:*1715, 1953.
370. Krane, S. M., Brownell, G. L., Stanbury, J. B. and Corrigan, H.: J. Clin. Invest., *35:*874, 1956.
371. Follis, R. H., Jr.: Bull. Johns Hopkins Hosp., *92:*405, 1953.
372. Engfeldt, B. and Hjertquist, S.: Acta endocrinol., *15:*109, 1954.
373. Radcliffe, C. E.: Endocrinology, *32:*415, 1943.
374. Fujimaki, Y. and Hildebrandt, F.: Arch. exper. Pathol. u. Pharmakol., *102:*226, 1924.
375. Gaunt, R., Corsden, M. and Liling, M.: Endocrinology, *35:*105, 1944.
376. Koivusalo, M. and Pekkarinen, A.: Acta endocrinol., *13:*138, 1953.
377. Aikawa, J. K.: Ann. Int. Med., *44:*30, 1956.
378. Prina, C.: Arch. sc. med., *91:*478, 1951.
379. Forattini, C. and Selmi, W.: Folia endocrinol., *3:*869, 1950.
380. Sicuteri, F. and Minnini, G.: Arch. studio fisiopatol. e. clin. ricambio, *14:*35, 1950.
381. Dine, R. F. and Lavietes, P. H.: J. Clin. Invest., *21:*781, 1942.
382. Soffer, L. J., Cohn, C., Grossman, E. B., Jacobs, M. and Sobotka, H.: J. Clin. Invest., *20:*429, 1941.
383. Cosgrove, J. B. R. and Perry, W. F.: Canad. J. Research, *E 27:*10, 1949.
384. Drill, V. A.: Physiol. Rev., *23:*355, 1943.
385. Drill, V. A. and Truat, A. P.: Endocrinology, *40:*259, 1947.
386. Johnson, R. M. and Baumann, C. A.: J. Biol. Chem., *171:*513, 1947.

387. Kelley, B. and Day, H. G.: J. Biol. Chem., *175:*863, 1948.
388. Weise, C. E., Mehl, J. W. and Deuel, H. J.: J. Biol. Chem., *175:*21, 1948.
389. Bieri, J. G. and Schultze, M. O.: Arch. Biochem., *34:*280, 1951.
390. Concha, E., Atria, A. and Sabah, D.: Rev. med. Chile, *78:*791, 1950.
391. Chanda, R., Clapham, H. M., McNaught, M. L. and Owen, E. C.: Biochem. J., *50:*95, 1951.
392. Money, W. L., Fager, J., Lucas, V. and Rawson, R. W.: J. Clin. Endocrinol., *11:*747, 1951.
393. Sadhu, D. P. and Brody, S.: Am. J. Physiol., *149:*400, 1947.
394. Sadhu, D. P.: Am. J. Physiol., *152:*263, 1948.
395. Eufinger, H. and Gottlieb, J.: Klin. Wchnschr., *12:*1397, 1933.
396. Fleischmann, W. and Kann, S.: Wien. klin. Wchnschr., *47:*1488, 1936.
397. Logaras, G. and Drummon, J. C.: Biochem. J., *32:*964, 1938.
398. Weslaw, W. and Wrobleski, B.: Ztschr. ges. exper. Med., *105:*497, 1939.
399. Cowgill, G. R. and Palmieri, M. L.: Am. J. Physiol., *105:*146, 1933.
400. Himwich, H. E., Goldfarb, W. and Cowgill, G. R.: Am. J. Physiol., *99:*689, 1932.
401. Schneider, E. and Burger, A.: Klin. Wchnschr., *17:*905, 1938.
402. Rubino, F.: Boll. soc. ital. biol. sper., *26:*1018, 1950.
403. Green, J. A.: Am. J. M. Sc., *195:*618, 1938.
404. Kinde, N. N.: Proc. Soc. Exper. Biol. & Med., *23:*812, 1926.
405. Bologna, U. and Piccioni, V.: Ricerca science, *21:*1820, 1950.
406. Drill, V. A. and Overman, R. R.: Am. J. Physiol., *135:*474, 1942.
407. Calvo, J. M., Boehme, C. C. and Goemine, J.: Bol. soc. biol. Santiago, Chile, *6:*88, 1949.
408. Capretti, G. and Magnani, B.: Giorn. clin. med., *32:*417, 1951.
409. Beaton, J. R., Beare, J. L., Beaton, G. H., White, J. M. and McHenry, E. W.: J. Nutrition, *51:*599, 1953.
410. Bolene, C., Ross, O. B. and MacVicar, R.: Proc. Soc. Exper. Biol. & Med., *75:*610, 1950.
411. Emerson, G. A.: Proc. Soc. Exper. Biol. & Med., *70:*392, 1949.
412. Sure, B. and Easterling, L.: J. Nutrition, *42:*221, 1950.
413. Graham, C. E., Reichstein, I. P., Watson, W. J. and Hier, S. W.: Proc. Soc. Exper. Biol. & Med., *80:*657, 1952.
414. Meites, J. and Shay, J. C.: Proc. Soc. Exper. Biol. & Med., *76:*196, 1951.
415. Prinzie, A.: Ann. endocrinol., *12:*250, 1951.
416. Ershoff, B. H.: Proc. Soc. Exper. Biol. & Med., *71:*209, 1949.
417. Ershoff, B. H.: Metabolism, *2:*175, 1953.
418. Ershoff, B. H.: Arch. Biochem., *28:*359, 1950.
419. Meites, J.: Proc. Soc. Exper. Biol. & Med., *75:*193, 1950.
420. Wayne, E. J., MacGregor, A. G. and Miller, H.: Lancet, *248:*327, 1950.
421. Meites, J.: Proc. Soc. Exper. Biol. & Med., *82:*626, 1953.
422. Drysdale, G. R., Betheil, J. J., Lardy, H. A. and Baumann, C. A.: Arch. Biochem., *33:*1, 1951.
423. Abercrombie, W. F.: Am. J. Pathol., *11:* 469, 1935.
424. Bessesen, D. H.: Am. J. Physiol., *63:*245, 1923.
425. Harris, K. D. and Smith, E. A.: Am. J. Physiol., *84:*599, 1928.
426. Löwy, E.: Ztschr. ges. exper. Med., *38:* 407, 1923. Quoted from Drill, V. A.: Physiol. Rev., *23:*355, 1943.
427. McCarrison, R.: Indian J. M. Res., *7:*633, 1920.
428. Rondoni, P. and Montagnani, M.: Sperimentale, *68:*659, 1915.
429. Schulze, E. and Linnemann, H.: Arch. exper. Pathol. u. Pharmakol., *189:*448, 1938.
430. Uotila, U.: Virchow's Arch. pathol. Anat. u. Physiol., *301:*535, 1938.
431. Weisenfeld, S. and Rawson, R. W.: Tr. Am. Goiter A., p. 259, 1952.
432. Gemmill, C. L.: Am. J. Physiol., *172:* 286, 1953.
433. Magnus-Levy, A.: Berlin klin. Wchnschr., *32:*650, 1895.
434. Benedict, F. G., Emmes, L. E., Roth, P. and Smith, H. M.: J. Biol. Chem., *18:* 139, 1914.
435. Boothby, W. M., Berkson, J. and Plummer, W. A.: Ann. Int. Med., *11:*1014, 1937.
436. Means, J. H.: J. Biol. Chem., *21:*263, 1915.
437. Boothby, W. M. and Beldes, E. J.: Proc. Staff Meet., Mayo Clinic, *1:*166, 1926.
438. Gross, J. and Pitt-Rivers, R.: Biochem. J., *53:*645, 1953.
439. Roche, J., Lissitzky, S. and Michel, R.: Biochim. et biophys. Acta, *11:*220, 1953.
440. Gross, J., Pitt-Rivers, R. and Trotter, W. R.: Lancet, *262:*1044, 1952.
441. Heming, A. E. and Holtkamp, D. E.: J. Clin. Endocrinol., *13:*880, 1953.
442. McConahey, W. M., Blackburn, C. M., Keating, F. R. and Albert, A.: Tr. Am. Goiter A., p. 3, 1953.
443. Deltour, G. and Karamourtzounis, J.: Ann. endocrinol., *14:*82, 1953.
444. Prueter, R. D., Warson, M. D. and Ferguson, J. K. W.: Canad. J. M. Sc., *31:* 99, 1953.
445. Grad, B.: Am. J. Physiol., *174:*481, 1953.

446. McGavack, T. and Seegers, W.: J. Am. Geriat. Soc., *4:*535, 1956.
447. Smith, A. U., Emmens, C. W. and Parkes, A. S.: J. Endocrinol., *5:*186, 1946–1948.
448. Brophy, D. and McEachern, D.: Proc. Soc. Exper. Biol. & Med., *70:*120, 1949.
449. Barker, S. B. and Klitgaard, H. M.: Am. J. Physiol., *170:*81, 1952.
450. Barker, S. B. and Schwartz, H. S.: Proc. Soc. Exper. Biol. & Med., *83:*500, 1953.
451. Ulrick, W. C. and Whitehorn, W. V.: Am. J. Physiol., *171:*407, 1952.
452. Méhes, G. and Pintéa, L.: Acta phys. Acad. Sc., Hung., *2:*207, 1951.
453. Scheinberg, P., Stead, E. A., Brannon, E. S. and Warren, J. V.: J. Clin. Invest., *29:*1139, 1950.
454. Fazekas, J. F., Graves, F. B. and Alman, R. W.: Endocrinology, *48:*169, 1951.
455. Hoexter, F. M.: Endocrinology, *54:*1, 1954.
456. Scheinberg, P.: J. Clin. Invest., *29:*1010, 1950.
457. Cohen, R. A.: Proc. Soc. Exper. Biol. & Med., *32:*1446, 1935.
458. Myers, J. D., Brannon, E. S. and Holland, B. C.: J. Clin. Invest., *29:*1069, 1950.
459. Fullerton, C. W. and Harrop, C. A.: Bull. Johns Hopkins Hosp., *46:*203, 1930.
460. Stewart, H. J. and Evans, W. F.: Am. Heart J., *20:*714, 1940.
461. Stewart, H. J. and Evans, W. F.: Arch. Int. Med., *69:*808, 1942.
462. Eichna, L. W. and Wilkins, R. W.: Bull. Johns Hopkins Hosp., *68:*512, 1941.
463. Corcoran, A. C. and Page, I. H.: J. Clin. Endocrinol., *7:*801, 1948.
464. Eiler, J. J., Althausen, T. L. and Stockholm, M.: Am. J. Physiol., *140:*699, 1944.
465. Thompson, W. O.: J. Clin. Invest., *2:*477, 1926.
466. Blumgart, H. L., Cowgill, S. L. and Gillihan, D. R.: J. Clin. Invest., *9:*69, 1930.
467. Leblond, C. P. and Hoff, H. E.: Am. J. Physiol., *141:*32, 1944.
468. Meyer, A. and Jost, M.: Endocrinology, *24:*806, 1939.
469. Rasmussen, H.: Acta med. scandinav., Supp. 115, p. 1–202, 1941.
470. Barker, S. B.: Tr. Am. Goiter A., p. 16, 1956.
471. Allen, B. M.: Quart. Rev. Biol., *4:*325, 1929.
472. Goldsmith, E. D., Nigrelli, R. F., Gordon, A. S., Charipper, H. A. and Gordon, M.: Endocrinology, *35:*132, 1944.
473. Simpson, S.: Quart. J. Exper. Physiol., *6:*119, 1913.
474. Hammett, F. S.: Am. J. Physiol., *68:*1, 1924.
475. Tatum, A. L.: J. Exper. Med., *17:*634, 1913.
476. Horsley, V. A.: Proc. Roy. Soc. Lond., *38:*5, 1884.
477. Fleischmann, W.: Quart. Rev. Biol., *22:* 119, 1947.
478. Karnofsky, D. and Cronkite, E. P.: Proc. Soc. Exper. Biol. & Med., *40:*568, 1939.
479. Simpson, M. E., Osling, C. W. and Evans, H. M.: Yale J. Biol. & Med., *23:*2, 1950.
480. Schlesinger, B. and Fisher, O. D.: Lancet, *261:*289, 1951.
481. Dunlap, H. F. and Moersch, F. P.: Am. J. Psychiatry, *91:*1215, 1935.
482. Jamieson, G. R. and Wall, J. H.: Psychiatric Quart., *10:*464, 1936.
483. Brody, E. B. and Man, E. B.: Am. J. Psychiatry, *107:*357, 1950.
484. Cohen, R. A.: Proc. Soc. Exper. Biol. & Med., *32:*1446, 1935.
485. Harington, C. R.: Proc. Roy. Soc. Lond., sB, *132:*223, 1944.
486. Bertrand, J., Deloy, J. and Guillian, J.: Compt. rend. Soc. Biol., *129:*395, 1938.
487. Asher, R.: Brit. M. J., *2:*555, 1949.
488. Lambert, E. H., Underdahl, L. O., Beckett, S. and Mederos, L. O.: J. Clin. Endocrinol., *11:*1186, 1951.
489. Lerman, J. and Means, J. H.: J. Clin. Invest., *11:*167, 1932.
490. Watman, R. N. and Nasset, E. S.: Am. J. Physiol., *157:*216, 1949.
491. Watman, R. N. and Nasset, E. S.: Am. J. Physiol., *166:*131, 1951.
492. Majumdar, A. C.: Indian J. Physiol. & Allied Science, *4:*50, 1950.
493. Allegretti, N., Buta, S. and Milkovic, S.: Arkiv. kemi., *22:*207, 1950.
494. Salter, W. T.: The Endocrine Function of Iodine. Cambridge, Mass., Harvard University Press, 1940.
495. Elmer, A. W.: Iodine Metabolism and Thyroid Function. London, Oxford University Press, 1938.
496. Rabourdin: Compt. rend. Acad. Sc., *31:* 784, 1850.
497. Kendall, E. C.: J. Biol. Chem., *19:*251, 1914.
498. Sandell, E. B. and Kolthoff, I. M.: Mikrochim. acta, *1–2:*9, 1937.
499. Chaney, A.: J. Indust. & Engin. Chem., anal. ed., *12:*179, 1940.
500. Barker, S. B.: J. Biol. Chem., *172:*715, 1948.
501. Kydd, D. M., Man, E. B. and Peters, J. P.: J. Clin. Invest., *29:*1033, 1950.
502. Barker, S. B. and Humphrey, M. J.: Tr. Am. Goiter A., p. 13, 1950.
503. Zak, B., Koen, A. M. and Boyle, A. J.: Am. J. Clin. Pathol., *23:*603, 1953.
504. Danowski, T. S., Johnston, S. Y. and Greenman, J. H.: J. Clin. Endocrinol., *10:*519, 1950.
505. Skanse, B.: Radioactive Iodine in the Diagnosis of Thyroid Disease, Doctoral Thesis subm. in Sweden, 1949.

506. Chesky, V. E., Dreese, W. C., Duboczky, B. O., Hall, B. S. and Hellwig, C. A.: Am. J. Clin. Pathol., *23:*41, 1953.
507. Ingbar, S. H., Freinkel, N., Hoeprich, P. D. and Athens, J. W.: J. Clin. Invest., *33:*388, 1954.
508. Schultz, A. L., Sandhaus, E., Demorest, H. L. and Zieve, L.: J. Clin. Endocrinol., *14:*1062, 1954.
509. Durham, J. R., Cooke, R. E., Lancaster, J. W. and Man, E. B.: A.M.A. Am. J. Dis. Child., *87:*468, 1954.
510. Danowski, T. S., Huff, S. J., Tarail, R., Wirth, P., Peters, J. H., Mateer, F. M. and Garver, K.: J. Clin. Endocrinol., *12:*1572, 1952.
511. Wilson, H. T. and Maier, E. C.: J. Lab. & Clin. Med., *43:*422, 1954.
512. Starr, P. and Liebhold-Schueck, R.: Proc. Soc. Exper. Biol. & Med., *83:*52, 1953.
513. Starr, P. and Liebhold-Schueck, R.: Arch. Int. Med., *92:*880, 1953.
514. Werner, S. C., Hamilton, H. B. and Nemeth, M. R.: Radiology, *59:*720, 1952.
515. Hickey, F. C. and Brownell, G. L.: J. Clin. Endocrinol., *14:*1423, 1954.
516. Keating, F. R., Power, M. H., Berkson, J. and Haines, S. F.: J. Clin. Invest., *26:* 1138, 1947.
517. Vander Laan, W. P.: The Thyroid. Brookhaven Symposia in Biology. No. 7, p. 30, June, 1954.
518. Berson, S. A. and Yalow, R. S.: J. Clin. Invest., *34:*186, 1955.
519. McConahey, W. M., Keating, F. R. and Power, M. H.: J. Clin. Invest., *28:* 191, 1949.
520. Clark, D. E., Moe, R. H. and Adams, E. E.: Surgery, *26:*331, 1949.
521. Werner, S. C., Quimby, E. H. and Schmidt, C.: J. Clin. Endocrinol., *9:* 342, 1949.
522. Astwood, E. B. and Stanley, M. M.: West. J. Surg., *55:*625, 1947.
523. Perry, W. R. and Hughes, J. F. S.: J. Clin. Invest., *31:*457, 1952.
524. Recant, L. and Riggs, D. S.: J. Clin. Invest., *31:*789, 1952.
525. Mueller, R., Brausch, C. P., Hirsch, E. Z., Benua, R. S. and Dobyns, B. M.: J. Clin. Endocrinol., *14:*1287, 1954.
526. Hill, S. R., Reiss, R. S., Forsham, P. H. and Thorn, G. W.: J. Clin. Endocrinol., *10:*1375, 1950.
527. Berson, S. A. and Yalow, R. S.: J. Clin. Endocrinol., *12:*407, 1952.
528. Balint, J. A., Fraser, R. and Hanno, M. G. W.: Brit. M. J., *1:*1234, 1954.
529. MacGregor, A. G. and Somner, A. R.: Lancet, *267:*931, 1954.
530. Greer, M. A. and Smith, G. E.: J. Clin. Endocrinol., *14:*1374, 1954.
531. Werner, S. C. and Spooner, M.: Bull. New York Acad. Sc., *31:*137, 1955.
532. Jeffries, W. McK., Levy, R. P., Palmer, W. G., Storaasli, J. P. and Kelly, L. W., Jr.: New England J. Med., *249:* 876, 1953.
533. Allen, H. C., Jr. and Goodwin, W. E., Radiology, *58:*68, 1952.
534. Goodwin, W. E., Cassen, B. and Bauer, F. K.: Radiology, *61:*88, 1953.
535. Kelly, F. J.: J. Clin. Endocrinol., *14:* 326, 1954.
536. Richardson, J. R. and Lineback, M.: Laryngoscope, *62:*934, 1952.
537. Springer, K. C.: A.M.A. Arch. Otolaryng., *61:*386, 1955.
538. Einhorn, J. and Larsson, L. G.: Acta radiol., *45:*405, 1956.
539. Hummon, J. F. and Magalotti, M. F.: Am. J. Roentgenol., *75:*1144, 1956.
540. Perlmutter, M., Slater, S. L. and Attie, J.: J. Clin. Endocrinol., *14:*672, 1954.
541. Quimby, E. H., Werner, S. C. and Schmidt, C.: Proc. Soc. Exper. Biol. & Med., *75:*537, 1950.
542. Ackermann, P. G. and Iversen, K.: J. Gerontol., *8:*458, 1953.
543. Rall, J. E.: Am. J. Med., *20:*719, 1956.
544. Major, R. H.: Classic Description of Disease. 2nd ed. Springfield, Illinois, Charles C Thomas, 1939, p. 275.
545. Curling, T. B.: Med.-Chir. Tr., *33:*303, 1850.
546. Fagge, C. H.: Med.-Chir. Tr., *54:*155, 1871.
547. Hutchison, J. H. and McGirr, E. M.: Lancet, *270:*1035, 1956.
548. Stanbury, J. B. and Hedge, A. N.: Tr. Am. Goiter A., p. 389, 1950.
549. Hubble, D.: Lancet, *264:*1112, 1953.
550. Nabney, J. B.: Lancet, *267:*1107, 1954.
551. Sexton, D. L. and Mack, R.: J. Clin. Endocrinol., *14:*747, 1954.
552. Ainger, L. E. and Kelley, V. C.: J. Clin. Endocrinol., *15:*469, 1955.
553. Wilkins, L., Clayton, G. W. and Berthrong, M.: Pediatrics, *13:*235, 1954.
554. Morris, D.: Lancet, *264:*1284, 1953.
555. Hodges, R. E., Hamilton, H. E. and Keettel, W. C.: Arch. Int. Med., *90:* 863, 1952.
556. Pickering, D. E. and Koulischer, N.: A.M.A. Am. J. Dis. Child., *92:*63, 1956.
557. Akerrén, Y.: Acta paediat. *43:*411, 1954.
558. Christensen, J. F.: Acta paediat., *45:* 367, 1956.
559. Lotmar, F.: Ztschr. f. d. ges. Neurol. u. Psychiat., *146:*1, 1933.
560. Eayrs, J. T.: Nature, *172:*403, 1953.
561. Marie, P., Tretiakoff, C. and Stumfer, E.: Encephale, *15:*601, 1920.
562. Lerman, J., Jones, H. W. and Calkins, E.: Ann. Int. Med., *25:*677, 1946.
563. Reilly, W. A. and Bayer, D. I.: J. Pediat., *40:*714, 1952.
564. Stanbury, J. B., Ohela, K. and Pitt-Rivers, R.: J. Clin. Endocrinol., *15:* 54, 1955.

565. McGirr, E. M. and Hutchison, J. H.: Lancet, *264:*1117, 1953.
566. Hutchison, J. H. and McGirr, E. M.: J. Clin. Endocrinol., *14:*869, 1954.
567. Beierwaltes, W. H.: J. Clin. Endocrinol., *14:*1551, 1954.
568. Evans, P. R.: J. Pediat., *41:*706, 1952.
569. Andersen, H.: Acta paediat., *44* (Suppl. 103): 102, 1955.
570. Andersen, H.: Acta endocrinol., *18:*560, 1955.
571. McGavack, T. H.: The Thyroid. St. Louis, C. V. Mosby Co., 1951, p. 352.
572. Perloff, W. H.: J.A.M.A., *157:*651, 1955.
573. Ravera, J. J., Cervino, J. M. and Mussio Fournier, J. C.: J. Clin. Endocrinol., *16:*817, 1956.
574. Silverman, S. H. and Wilkins, L.: Pediatrics, *12:*288, 1953.
575. Engeset, A., Imerslund, O. and Blystad, W.: Acta radiol., *36:*1, 1951.
576. Lusted, L. B. and Pickering, D. E.: Radiology, *66:*708, 1956.
577. Andersen, H., Asboe-Hansen, G., Quaade, F. and Wichmann, R.: Acta paediat., *44* (Suppl. 103): 96, 1955.
578. Cooke, R. E. and Man, E. B.: Pediatrics, *17:*617, 1956.
579. Fisher, D. A., Hammond, G. D. and Pickering, D. E.: A.M.A. Am. J. Dis. Child., *90:*6, 1955.
580. Colver, T. and Lodge, T.: Brit. M. J.: *1:*89, 1952.
581. Ord, W. M.: Med.-Chir. Tr., *56:*57, 1878.
582. Reverdin, J. L. and Reverdin, A.: Rév. méd. de la Suisse. Rom., *3:*169, 1883.
583. Kocher, T.: Arch. f. klin. Chir., *29:*254, 1883.
584. Means, J. H.: Thyroid and Its Diseases. 2nd ed. Philadelphia, J. B. Lippincott Co., 1948.
585. Querido, A. and Lameyer, L. D.: Proc. Roy. Soc. Med., Lond., *49:*209, 1956.
586. Gilliland, I. C.: Proc. Roy. Soc. Med., Lond., *49:*212, 1956.
587. Morgans, M. E. and Trotter, W. R.: Lancet, *265:*1335, 1953.
588. Bell, G. O.: Tr. Am. Goiter A., p. 28, 1952.
589. Hydovitz, J. D. and Rose, E.: J. Clin. Endocrinol., *16:*1109, 1956.
590. Fraser, R. and Garrod, O.: Brit. M. J.: *2:*1484, 1955.
591. Whitesell, F. B. and Black, B. M.: Tr. Am. Goiter A., p. 403, 1949.
592. Berkheiser, S. W.: J. Clin. Endocrinol., *15:*44, 1955.
593. Rawson, R. W., Hertz, S. and Means, J. H.: Ann. Int. Med., *19:*829, 1943.
594. Fry, H. J. B.: Quart. J. Med., *8:*284, 1914.
595. Reuter, M. J.: Arch. Dermat. & Syph., *24:*55, 1931.
596. Steiner, A. and Kendall, F. E.: Arch. Pathol., *42:*433, 1946.
597. Mott, F. W. P.: Proc. Roy. Soc. Med., Lond., *10:*51, 1917.
598. Brewer, D. B.: J. Pathol. & Bact., *63:* 503, 1951.
599. Stanbury, J. B., Kassenaar, A. A. H., Meijer, J. W. A. and Terpstra, J.: J. Clin. Endocrinol., *15:*1216, 1955.
600. Baker, B. L.: Ann. New York Acad. Sc., *53:*690, 1951.
601. Ber, A.: Acta endocrinol., *16:*305, 1954.
602. Curtis, A. C. and Blaylock, H. C.: Arch. Dermat. & Syph., *66:*460, 1952.
603. Goldblatt, S.: Acta dermat.-venereol., *35:* 167, 1955.
604. Reitan, R. M.: Arch. Neurol. & Psychiat., *69:*436, 1953.
605. Miller, R.: J. Lab. & Clin. Med., *40:* 267, 1952.
606. Reiss, M., Hemphill, R. E., Maggs, R., Smith, S. and Haigh, C. P.: Brit. M. J., *1:*1181, 1951.
607. Hollender, A. R.: A.M.A. Arch. Otolaryng., *63:*135, 1956.
608. Howarth, A. E. and Lloyd, H. E. D.: Brit. M. J., *2:*431, 1956.
609. Jones, A. C., Jr.: A.M.A. Arch. Otolaryng., *62:*583, 1955.
610. Watts, F. B.: Ann. Int. Med., *35:*186, 1951.
611. Tracey, M. L. and Donovan, E. J.: J.A.M.A., *146:*1511, 1951.
612. Madenberg, F., Byfield, G. V. and Baker, L. A.: A.M.A. Arch. Int. Med., *93:* 787, 1954.
613. Benson, R. C. and Dailey, M. E.: Surg. Gynec. & Obst., *100:*19, 1955.
614. Lerman, J., Clark, R. J. and Means, J. H.: Ann. Int. Med., *8:*82, 1934.
615. Schmidt, S.: Brit. J. Radiol., *25:*389, 1952.
616. Marks, P. A. and Roof, B. S.: Ann. Int. Med., *39:*230, 1953.
617. Ellis, L. B., Mebane, J. G., Maresh, G., Hultgren, H. N. and Bloomfield, R. A.: Am. Heart J., *43:*341, 1952.
618. Weyher, R. F.: J.A.M.A., *153:*639, 1953.
619. Calvert, R. J., Smith, E. and Andrews, L. G.: Brit. M. J., *2:*891, 1954.
620. Jones, R. J., Cohen, L. and Gorbus, H.: Am. J. Med., *19:*71, 1955.
621. Josephs, H. W.: J. Pediat., *41:*784, 1952.
622. Davies, C. E., Mackinnon, J. and Platts, M. M.: Brit. M. J., *2:*595, 1952.
623. Beierwaltes, W. H. and Bishop, R. C.: J. Clin. Endocrinol., *14:*928, 1954.
624. Sensenbach, W., Madison, L., Eisenberg, S. and Ochs, H.: J. Clin. Invest., *33:* 1434, 1954.
625. Browning, T. B., Atkins, R. W. and Weiner, H.: A.M.A. Arch. Int. Med., *93:*938, 1954.
626. Sokoloff, L., Wechsler, R. L., Mangold, R., Balls, K. and Kety, S. S.: J. Clin. Invest., *32:*202, 1953.
627. Tapley, D. F.: Bull. Johns Hopkins Hosp., *96:*274, 1955.

628. Yount, E. and Little, J. M.: J. Clin. Endocrinol., *15:*343, 1955.
629. Hlad, C. J., Jr. and Bricker, N. S.: J. Clin. Endocrinol., *14:*1539, 1954.
630. Axelrod, A. R. and Berman, L.: Blood, *6:*436, 1951.
631. Mustacchi, P., Petermann, M. L. and Rall, J. E.: J. Clin. Endocrinol., *14:* 729, 1954.
632. McAlpine, S. G.: Lancet, *269:*58, 1955.
633. Paull, A. M. and Phillips, R. W.: J. Clin. Endocrinol., *14:*554, 1954.
634. Curtis, R. H.: Ann. Int. Med., *44:*376, 1956.
635. Leonard, M. E., Falconer, E. H. and Ellenhorn, M. J.: Ann. Int. Med., *34:* 1251, 1951.
636. Kurland, G. S., Hamolsky, M. W. and Freedberg, A. S.: J. Clin. Endocrinol., *15:*1354, 1955.
637. Freedberg, A. S., Kurland, G. S. and Hamolsky, M. W.: New England J. Med., *253:*57, 1955.
638. Schuman, C. R.: J. Clin. Endocrinol., *13:* 795, 1953.
639. Sampson, M. C., Rose, E. and Herbert, E.: Am. J. Med., *17:*871, 1954.
640. Querido, A. and Stanbury, J. B.: Tr. Am. Goiter A., 1950, p. 96.
641. Perloff, W. H., Levy, L. M. and Despopoulos, A.: J. Clin. Endocrinol., *11:* 1495, 1951.
642. Schneeberg, N. G., Perloff, W. H. and Levy, L. M.: J. Clin. Endocrinol., *14:* 223, 1954.
643. Skanse, B.: Acta endocrinol., *13:*358, 1953.
644. Lamberg, B. A., Wahlberg, P. and Forsius, P. J.: Acta med. scandinav., *153:* 411, 1956.
645. Wilson, H. T. and Maier, E. C.: J. Lab. & Clin. Med., *43:*422, 1954.
646. Goldsmith, R. and Stanbury, J. B.: J. Clin. Endocrinol., *15:*568, 1955.
647. Robertson, J. D. and Kirkpatrick, H. F. W.: Brit. M. J., *1:*624, 1952.
648. Papper, S., Burrows, B. A., Ingbar, S. H., Sisson, J. H. and Ross, J. F.: New England J. Med., *247:*897, 1952.
649. Starr, P. and Liebhold-Schueck, R.: J.A.M.A., *155:*732, 1954.
650. Müller, C.: Acta endocrinol., *21:*370, 1956.
651. Lerman, J.: J. Clin. Endocrinol., *13:* 1341, 1953.
652. Asper, S. P., Jr., Selenkow, H. A. and Plamondon, C. A.: Bull. Johns Hopkins Hosp., *93:*164, 1953.
653. Zondek, H., Leszynsky, H. E. and Zondek, G. W.: Acta endocrinol., *18:*117, 1955.
654. Starr, P. and Liebhold-Schueck, R.: Ann. Int. Med., *42:*595, 1955.
655. Selenkow, H. A. and Asper, S. P., Jr.: J. Clin. Endocrinol., *15:*285, 1955.
656. Frawley, T. F., McClintock, J. C., Beebe, R. T. and Marthy, G. L.: J.A.M.A., *160:*646, 1956.
657. McGavack, T. H. and Reckendorf, H. K.: Am. J. Med., *20:*774, 1956.
658. McConahey, W. M., Blackburn, C. M., Keating, F. R. and Albert, A.: Tr. Am. Goiter A., p. 3, 1953.
659. Summers, V. K.: Brit. M. J., *2:*430, 1956.
660. Murray, G. R.: Brit. M. J., *1:*359, 1920.
661. Burgess, A. M.: Ann. Int. Med., *25:*146, 1946.
662. Summers, V. K.: Brit. M. J., *2:*366, 1953.
663. Malden, M.: Brit. M. J., *2:*764, 1955.
664. Levin, M. E. and Daughaday, W. H.: Am. J. Med., *18:*1017, 1955.
665. LeMarquand, H. S., Hausmann, W. and Hemsted, E. H.: Brit. M. J., *1:*704, 1953.
666. LeMarquand, H. S., Hausmann, W. and Hemsted, E. H.: Brit. M. J., *2:*773, 1955.
667. Parry, C. H.: Collections from the Unpublished Medical Writings of Dr. C. H. Parry, *2:*111, London, 1825.
668. Graves, R. J.: London M. & Surg. J., Part II:516, 1835.
669. von Basedow, C. A.: Wchnschr. f. d. ges. Heilk., *6:*197, 1840.
670. Charcot, J. M.: Gaz. hebd. de méd., *6:* 216, 1859.
671. Plummer, S. H.: Tr. A. Am. Physicians, *43:*159, 1928.
672. Thompson, W. O. and Means, J. H.: J.A.M.A., *99:*1483, 1932.
673. Boas, N. F. and Ober, W. B.: J. Clin. Endocrinol., *6:*575, 1946.
674. Ingbar, S. H. and Freinkel, N.: J. Clin. Invest., *34:*914, 1955.
675. Ingbar, S. H., Freinkel, N., Dowling, J. T. and Kumagai, L. F.: J. Clin. Invest., *35:*714, 1956.
676. Iversen, K.: Temporary Rise in the Frequency of Thyrotoxicosis in Denmark, 1941–1943. Copenhagen, Rosengelde and Bagger, 1948.
677. Meulengracht, E.: Acta med. scandinav., *121:*466, 1945.
678. Hertz, S. and Means, J. H.: Tr. Am. Goiter A., p. 136, 1936.
679. Stephens, D. J. and Allen, W. M.: Endocrinology, *28:*580, 1941.
680. Naffziger, H. C.: Arch. Ophth., *9:*1, 1933.
681. Naffziger, H. C. and Jones, O. W., Jr.: J.A.M.A., *99:*638, 1932.
682. Rundle, F. F. and Pochin, E. E.: Clin. Sc., *5:*51, 1944.
683. Pochin, E. E.: Clin. Sc., *4:*91, 1939.
684. Mulvaney, J. H.: Am. J. Ophth., (Part I), *27:*589, 1944.
685. Soley, M. H.: Arch. Int. Med., *70:*206, 1942.
686. Smelzer, G. K.: Am. J. Ophth., *20:*1189, 1937.
687. Albert, A.: Endocrinology, *37:*389, 1945.

688. Dobyns, B. M. and Steelman, S. L.: Endocrinology, *52:*705, 1953.
689. Dobyns, B. M. and Wilson, L. A.: Tr. Am. Goiter A., p. 291, 1954.
690. Askanazy, M.: Deutsches Arch. f. klin. Med., *61:*118, 1898.
691. Dudgeon, L. S. and Urquhart, A. L.: Brain, *49:*182, 1926.
692. Goodall, J. S. and Rogers, L.: Lancet, *212:*486, 1927.
693. Wilson, L. B.: Collected Papers, Mayo Clinic, *7:*438, 1915.
694. White, P. D.: Heart Disease. New York, The Macmillan Co., 1948, p. 409.
695. Pemberton, J. and Willius, F. A.: Tr. South Surg. A., *44:*247, 1931.
696. Beaver, D. C. and Pemberton, J.: Ann. Int. Med., *7:*687, 1933.
697. Warthin, A. S.: Proc. Inter-State Post-Grad. M. A. North America, p. 383, 1929.
698. Halsted, W. S.: Bull. Johns Hopkins Hosp., *25:*223, 1914.
699. LeCompte, P. M.: J. Clin. Endocrinol., *9:*158, 1949.
700. Peterson, R. E. and Wyngaarden, J. B.: J. Clin. Invest., *34:*957, 1955.
701. Werner, S. C.: Bull. New York Acad. Med., *29:*523, 1953.
702. Rawson, R. W., Graham, R. M. and Riddell, C. B.: Ann. Int. Med., *19:*405, 1943.
703. Plummer, H. S.: Discussion of a paper by D. Marine, J.A.M.A., *59:*325, 1912.
704. Haines, S. F.: West. J. Surg., *47:*155, 1939.
705. Cope, O., Rawson, R. W. and McArthur, J. W.: Surg. Gynec. & Obst., *84:*415, 1947.
706. Cahill, G. F.: Bull. New York Acad. Med., *29:*749, 1953.
707. Bartels, E. C.: Tr. Am. Goiter A., p. 3, 1950.
708. Means, J. H. and Holmes, G. W.: Arch. Int. Med., *31:*303, 1923.
709. Coindet, J. R.: Ann. de Chim. et Phys., Paris, *15:*49, 1820.
710. Plummer, H. S.: J.A.M.A., *80:*1955, 1923.
711. Boothby, W. M.: Arch. Int. Med., *56:*136, 1935.
712. Thompson, W. O., Cohen, A. C., Thompson, P. K., Thorp, E. G. and Braily, A. G.: Arch. Int. Med., *45:*430, 1930.
713. Means, J. H. and Lerman, J.: Ann. Int. Med., *12:*811, 1938.
714. Rawson, R. W., Moore, F. D., Peacock, W., Means, J. H., Cope, O. and Riddell, C. B.: J. Clin. Invest., *24:*869, 1945.
715. Moore, F. D.: J.A.M.A., *130:*315, 1946.
716. Bartels, E. C. and Sjogren, R. W.: J. Clin. Endocrinol., *11:*1057, 1951.
717. Williams, R. H., Clute, H. M., Anglem, T. J. and Kenney, F. R.: J. Clin. Endocrinol., *6:*23, 1946.
718. McGavack, T. H., Chevally, J., Shearman, A. M., Drekter, I. J. and Stern, S.: J. Clin. Endocrinol., *10:*813, 1950.
719. Hertz, S., Roberts, A., Means, J. H. and Evans, R. D.: Am. J. Physiol., *128:*565, 1940.
720. Chapman, E. M., Maloof, F., Maisterrena, J. and Martin, J. M.: J. Clin. Endocrinol., *14:*45, 1954.
721. Rall, J. E., Sonenberg, M., Robbins, J., Lazerson, R. and Rawson, R. W.: J. Clin. Endocrinol., *13:*1369, 1953.
722. Haines, S. F.: J. Clin. Endocrinol., *8:*813, 1948.
723. Robbins, J., Rall, J. E., Trunnell, J. B. and Rawson, R. W.: J. Clin. Endocrinol., *11:*1106, 1951.
724. Quimby, E. H. and Werner, S. C.: J.A.M.A., *140:*1046, 1949.
725. Pemberton, J. and Black, B. M.: Tr. Am. Goiter A., 1948, p. 163.
726. Cope, O., Dobyns, B. M., Hamlin, E. and Hopkirk, J.: Tr. Am. Goiter A., 1949, p. 256.
727. Blomfield, G. W., Jones, J. C., MacGregor, A. G., Miller, H. and Wayne, E. J.: Brit. M. J., *2:*373, 1951.
728. Poppen, J. L.: Tr. Am. Goiter A., 1950, p. 305.
729. Levine, H., Remington, R. E. and von Kolnitz, H.: J. Nutrition, *6:*325, 1933a; J. Nutrition, *6:*347, 1933b.
730. McClendon, J. F. and Foster, W. C.: Fed. Proc., *6:*413, 1947; J. Clin. Endocrinol., *7:*714, 1947.
731. Kimball, O. P.: J.A.M.A., *130:*80, 1946.
732. Marine, D.: Medicine, *3:*453, 1924.
733. Money, W. L. and Rawson, R. W.: Cancer, *3:*321, 1950.
734. Wegelin, C.: Cancer Review, *3:*453, 1928.
735. Taylor, S.: J. Clin. Endocrinol., *13:*1232, 1953.
736. Greenwald, I.: Bull. Hist. Med., *17:*229, 1945; J. Clin. Endocrinol., *6:*708, 1946.
737. Greer, M. A.: Physiol. Rev., *30:*513, 1950.
738. Taylor, S.: Tr. Am. Goiter A., 1954, p. 347.
739. Wölfler, A.: Arch. f. klin. Chir., *29:*1, 1883.
740. Wegelin, D.: Handbuch der speziellen pathologischen Anatomie und Histologie, Vol. VIII. Drüsen mit innerer Sekretion. Henke, F. und Lubarsh, O. (editors). Berlin, Julius Springer, 1926, p. 415.
741. Taylor, S.: Am. J. Med., *20:*698, 1956.
742. Dobyns, B. M.: Am. J. Med., *20:*684, 1956.
743. Vander Laan, W. P.: New England J. Med., *237:*221, 1947.
744. Rogers, W. F., Jr., Asper, S. P., Jr. and Williams, R. H.: New England J. Med., *237:*569, 1947.
745. Cole, W. H., Slaughter, D. P. and Rossiter, L. J.: J.A.M.A., *127:*883, 1945.

746. Fisher, F. R. and Fisher, R.: Am. J. Surg., *82:*202, 1951.
747. Beahrs, O. H., Pemberton, J. and Black, B. M.: J. Clin. Endocrinol., *11:*1157, 1951.
748. Hermanson, L., Gargill, S. L. and Lesses, M. F.: J. Clin. Endocrinol., *12:*112, 1952.
749. Hendrick, J. W. and Reed, E. P.: Tr. Am. Goiter A., 1951, p. 403.
750. Cerise, E. J., Randall, S. and Ochsner, A.: Surgery, *31:*552, 1952.
751. Beal, J. M., Scholnick, G. L. and Stevens, G. A.: Arch. Surg., *65:*879, 1952.
752. Hinton, J. W. and Slattery, L. R.: S. Clin. North America, *33:*351, 1953.
753. Majarakis, J. D., Slaughter, D. P. and Cole, W. H.: J. Clin. Endocrinol. *13:* 1530, 1953.
754. Horn, R. C., Jr. and Dull, J. A.: Ann. Surg., *139:*35, 1954.
755. Vander, J. B., Gaston, E. A. and Dawber, T. R.: New England J. Med., *251:* 970, 1954.
756. Cloud, D. T. and Branch, C. D.: A.M.A. Arch. Surg., *71:*366, 1955.
757. Mortensen, J. D., Bennett, W. A. and Woolner, L. B.: Surg. Forum, *5:*659, 1955.
758. Miller, J. M.: New England J. Med., *252:* 247, 1955.
759. Horn, R. C., Jr.: S. Clin. North America, *35:*1669, 1955.
760. Alhadeff, R., Scott, F. and Taylor, S.: Brit. J. Surg., *43:*617, 1956.
761. Shallow, T. A., Wagner, F. B., Jr. and Colcher, R. E.: Surgery, *39:*252, 1956.
762. Kearns, J. F. and Davis, H., Jr.: A.M.A. Arch. Surg., *64:*622, 1952.
763. Dargent, M. and Guinet, P.: Brit. M. J., *2:*1122, 1952.
764. Crile, G., Jr.: New England J. Med., *249:* 585, 1953.
765. Sokal, J. E.: New England J. Med., *249:* 393, 1953.
766. Sokal, J. E.: J.A.M.A., *154:*1321, 1954.
767. Sokal, J. E.: Surg. Gynec. & Obst., *99:* 108, 1954.
768. Zimmerman, L. M. and Wagner, D. A.: Tr. Am. Goiter A., p. 287, 1953.
769. Perlmutter, M. and Slater, S. L.: New England J. Med., *255:*65, 1956.
770. Sonnenberg, M.: Am. J. Med., *20:*710, 1956.
771. Duffy, B. J., Jr. and Fitzgerald, P. J.: Cancer, *3:*1018, 1950.
772. Winship, T.: Tr. Am. Goiter A., p. 364, 1951.
773. Clark, D. E.: J.A.M.A., *159:*1007, 1955.
774. Chesky, V. E.: Am. Surgeon, *21:*419, 1955.
775. Chesky, V. E., Dreese, W. C. and Hellwig, C. A.: J. Clin. Endocrinol., *11:* 1535, 1951.
776. Frazell, E. L. and Duffy, B. J., Jr.: Cancer, *4:*952, 1951.
777. Goldenberg, I. S.: Arch. Surg., *67:*495, 1953.
778. Horn, R. C., Jr.: Cancer, *7:*234, 1954.
779. Gardner, L. W.: A.M.A. Arch. Pathol., *59:*372, 1955.
780. Winship, T. and Greene, R.: Brit. J. Cancer, *9:*401, 1955.
781. Kenyon, R. and Ackerman, L. V.: Cancer: *8:*964, 1955.
782. Mortensen, J. D., Woolner, L. B. and Bennett, W. A.: Cancer, *9:*306, 1956.
783. Fitzgerald, P. J. and Foote, F. W., Jr.: J. Clin. Endocrinol., *9:*1153, 1949.
784. Fitzgerald, P. J.: Brookhaven Symposia in Biology, No. 7, p. 220, 1954.
785. Fitzgerald, P. J., Foote, F. W., Jr., and Hill, R. F.: Cancer, *3:*86, 1950.
786. Keston, A. S., Ball, R. P., Frantz, V. K. and Palmer, W. W.: Science, *94:*362, 1942.
787. Frantz, V. K., Ball, R., Keston, A. S. and Palmer, W. W.: Ann. Surg., *119:*668, 1944.
788. Robbins, J., Rall, J. E. and Rawson, R. W.: J. Clin. Endocrinol., *15:*1315, 1955.
789. Pochin, E. E., Cunningham, R. M. and Hilton, G.: J. Clin. Endocrinol., *14:*1300, 1954.
790. Robbins, J., Rall, J. E. and Rawson, R. W.: J. Clin. Endocrinol., *13:*852, 1953.
791. Rawson, R. W., Skanse, B. N., Marinelli, L. D. and Fluharty, R. G.: Cancer, *2:*279, 1949.
792. Leiter, L., Seidlin, S. M., Marinelli, L. D. and Baumann, E. J.: J. Clin. Endocrinol., *6:*247, 1946.
793. Seidlin, S. M. and Marinelli, L. D.: Bull. New York Acad. Med., *21:*440, 1945.
794. Cunningham, R. M., Hilton, G. and Pochin, E. E.: Brit. J. Radiol., *28:*252, 1955.
795. Rawson, R. W. and Rall, J. E.: M. Clin. North America, *36:*639, 1952.
796. Rawson, R. W., Marinelli, L. D., Skanse, B. N., Trunnell, J. B. and Fluharty, R. G..: J. Clin. Endocrinol., *10:*826,1948.
797. Trunnell, J. B., Marinelli, L. D., Duffy, B. J., Jr., Hill, R., Peacock, W. and Rawson, R. W.: J. Clin. Endocrinol., *9:*1138, 1949.
798. Seidlin, S. M., Oshry, E. and Yalow, A. A.: J. Clin. Endocrinol., *8:*423, 1948.
799. Seidlin, S. M., Rossmann, I., Oshry, E. and Siegel, E.: J. Clin. Endocrinol., *9:*1122, 1949.
800. Trunnell, J. B., Rawson, R. W., Marinelli, L. D. and Hill, R.: J. Clin. Endocrinol., *8:*598, 1948.
801. Sturgeon, C. T., Davis, F. E., Catz, B., Petit, D. and Starr, P.: J. Clin. Endocrinol., *13:*1391, 1953.
802. Kramer, S., Concannon, J. P., Evans, H. D. and Clark, G. M.: Brit. J. Radiol., *28:*307, 1955.

803. Dobyns, B. M. and Maloof, F.: J. Clin. Endocrinol., *11:*1323, 1951.
804. Rall, J. E., Miller, W. N., Foster, C. G., Peacock, W. C. and Rawson, R. W.: J. Clin. Endocrinol., *11:*1273, 1951.
805. Seidlin, S. M.: M. Clin. North America, *36:*663, 1952.
806. Rawson, R. W. and Rall, J. E.: Treatment of Cancer and Allied Diseases, 2nd ed. New York, Paul B. Hoeber, Inc. (In press.) Chapter on Neoplasms of the Thyroid.
807. Sonenberg, M. and Rall, J. E.: M. Clin. North America, *40:*821, 1956.
808. Shumway, M. and Davis, P. L.: J. Clin. Endocrinol., *14:*742, 1954.
809. Hellwig, C. A. and Wilkinson, P. N.: A.M.A. Arch. Pathol., *62:*23, 1956.
810. Sheets, R. F.: J.A.M.A., *157:*139, 1955.
811. Perloff, W. H.: J. Clin. Endocrinol., *16:*542, 1956.
812. Lasser, H. P.: J.A.M.A., *152:*1133, 1953.
813. Crile, G., Jr.: Ann. Int. Med., *37:*519, 1952.
814. Werner, S. C.: J. Clin. Endocrinol., *13:*1332, 1953.
815. Kahn, J., Spritzler, R. J. and Shector, W. E.: Ann. Int. Med., *39:*1129, 1953.
816. Teitelman, S. L. and Rosenberg, E. F.: Ann. Int. Med., *38:*1062, 1953.
817. Clark, D. E., Nelsen, T. S. and Raiman, R. J.: J.A.M.A., *151:*551, 1953.
818. Cutler, M.: J.A.M.A., *155:*650, 1954.
819. Hunter, R. C., Jr. and Sheehan, D. J.: New England J. Med., *251:*174, 1954.
820. Gelfland, M. L., Little, A. S. and Hoffman, K. F.: Am. J. M. Sc., *229:*69, 1955.
821. Izak, G. and Stein, Y.: Lancet, *270:*225, 1956.
822. Benjamin, Z. H.: Am. J. Med., *18:*677, 1955.
823. McGovern, F. H.: Laryngoscope, *65:*199, 1955.
824. Taylor, L.: Ann. Int. Med., *44:*1082, 1956.
825. Chatton, P., Rochedix, J., Pellisier, M. and Beltrando, L.: J. radiol. et électrol., *35:*560, 1954.
826. King, B. T. and Rossellini, H.: J.A.M.A., *129:*267, 1945.
827. Reveno, W. S. and Rosenbaum, H.: New England J. Med., *245:*364, 1951.
828. Schlicke, C. P.: Arch. Surg., *63:*656, 1951.
829. Fraser, R. and Harrison, R. J.: Lancet, *262:*382, 1952.
830. Altemeier, W. A.: Tr. Am. Goiter A., p. 242, 1951.
831. Hashimoto, H.: Arch. f. klin. Chir., *97:*219, 1912.
832. Riedel, B.: Verhandl. d. deutsch. Ges. f. Chir., *25:*101, 1896.
833. Statland, H., Wasserman, M. M. and Vickery, A. L.: Arch. Int. Med., *88:*659, 1951.
834. Heptinstall, R. H. and Eastcott, H. H. G.: Brit. J. Surg., *41:*471, 1954.
835. Fisher, E. R. and Creed, D. L.: Am. J. Surg., *91:*60, 1956.
836. Marshall, S. F. and Meissner, W. A.: Ann. Surg., *141:*737, 1955.
837. Gribets, D., Talbot, N. B. and Crawford, J. D.: New England J. Med., *250:*555, 1954.
838. Davis, H. C. and Hanske, E. A.: A.M.A. Am. J. Dis. Child., *90:*173, 1955.
839. Dailey, M. E., Lindsay, S. and Skahen, R.: A.M.A. Arch. Surg., *70:*291, 1955.
840. Glass, H. G., Waldron, G. W. and Brown, W. G.: Cancer, *9:*310, 1956.
841. Lindsay, S. and Dailey, M. E.: J. Clin. Endocrinol., *15:*1332, 1955.
842. Fromm, G. A., Lascano, E. F. and Goni Moreno, I.: Am. J. Clin. Pathol., *26:*799, 1956.
843. Skirpan, P., Reich, A. and Crile, G., Jr.: Am. J. Clin. Pathol., *25:*1274, 1955.
844. Cooke, R. T. and Luxton, R. W.: Lancet, *268:*968, 1955.
845. Luxton, R. W. and Cooke, R. T.: Lancet, *271:*105, 1956.
846. Shaw, A. F. B. and Smith, R. P.: Brit. J. Surg., *13:*93, 1925.
847. McCarrison, R.: Brit. M. J.: *1:*5, 1929.
848. Clausen, H. J.: Proc. Soc. Exper. Biol. & Med., *83:*835, 1953.
849. Skillern, P. G., Crile, G., Jr., McCullagh, E. P., Hazard, J. B., Lewis, L. A. and Brown, H.: J. Clin. Endocrinol., *16:*35, 1956.
850. Blake, K. W. and Sturgeon, C. T.: Surg. Gynec. & Obst., *97:*312, 1953.
851. Karhausen, L. and Zylberszac, S.: Brit. M. J., *2:*766, 1955.
852. Doniach, D. and Hudson, R. V.: Brit. M. J., *1:*672, 1957.
853. McConahey, W. M. and Keating, F. R.: J. Clin. Endocrinol., *11:*1116, 1951.
854. Furr, W. E., Jr. and Crile, G., Jr.: J. Clin. Endocrinol., *14:*79, 1954.
855. Ewing, J.: Neoplastic Diseases: Treatise on Tumors. 2nd ed. Philadelphia, W. B. Saunders Co., 1922.
856. Graham, A.: West. J. Surg., *39:*681, 1931.
857. McClintock, J. C. and Wright, A. W.: Ann. Surg., *106:*11, 1937.
858. Goetsch, E.: Am. J. Surg., *82:*71, 1951.
859. Goetsch, E. and Kamner, M.: J. Clin. Endocrinol., *15:*1010, 1955.
860. McKnight, R. B. and Thomas, C. G., Jr.: Am. Surgeon, *21:*887, 1955.

CHAPTER 18

By MAX MILLER, M.D., AND JOSEPH M. HAYMAN, JR., M.D.

Diseases of the Kidney

INTRODUCTION

Proper understanding of the various forms of renal disease can be based only on a knowledge of the structure of the kidney and the function of its component parts and the alterations produced therein by disease.

Each human kidney is composed of approximately 1,250,000 units or nephrons, each consisting of a vascular tuft or glomerulus which is invaginated into the expanded closed end of a long tubule (Fig. 1). The tubule presents a different structure in its different segments. The tubules in turn empty through collecting tubules into the pelvis of the kidney and thence through the ureter into the bladder. In the glomerular capillaries only a thin capillary wall, a basement membrane and the visceral layer of Bowman's capsule, with a combined thickness of about 1 micron, separate the blood from the glomerular space. Studies with the electron microscope, however, have shown that the finer details of these structures is exceedingly complex.[1] The basement membrane of the tubule is expanded over the glomerulus as Bowman's capsule, and is then reflected onto the capillary endothelium as a continuous structure. On the outer side of this basement membrane are epithelial cells continuous with those lining Bowman's capsule, but which have been called podocytes because of their peculiar foot processes. These cells have long, thick trabeculae which end in foot processes that lie on the extracapillary surface of the basement membrane to interdigitate with the foot processes of the same or other podocytes. The glomerular endothelium is a thin layer of protoplasm lying just inside the basement membrane. The cell bodies are syncytial, and form a stalk around which the capillary rete courses into and out of the glomerulus. This endothelial stalk constitutes what has been called the intercapillary space, the glomerular stalk or mesangium. The nephric tubule consists of a single layer of epithelial cells delimited externally by a well defined basement membrane. Conventionally the tubule is divided into a proximal convoluted portion, loop of Henle and distal convolutions, which unite with a collecting duct. Because of the paucity of our knowledge of the functional significance of every cytologic transition, it might be better to think of a proximal segment including the descending limb of Henle's loop, a thin segment and a distal segment.[2] The length of these segments varies considerably in different nephrons. The blood supply of the kidneys is huge, being in the range of 1200 ml. per minute, or about one fifth of the cardiac output. The renal artery, branching directly from the abdominal aorta, is short and has a large diameter. After subdividing in the kidney, finer branches (afferent arterioles, vessels of a diameter of about 50 microns containing muscle fibers) enter the glomerulus and break up into a number of capillary loops which make up the glomerular tuft. These capillaries unite

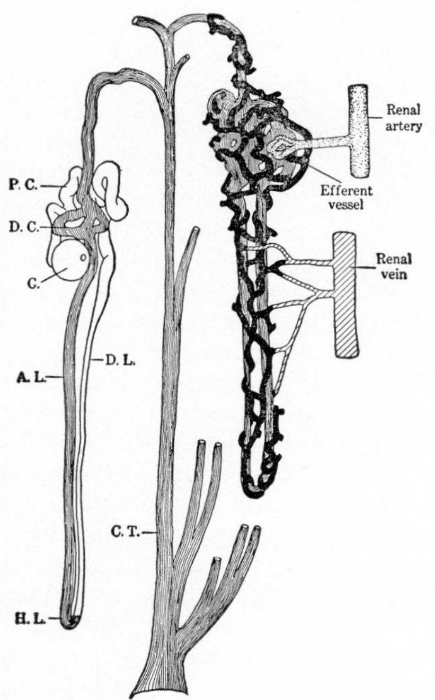

FIG. 1. On the right the tubule is drawn after a diagram of G. C. Hubers. The tubule is outlined from the capsule to the loop of Henle, and is shaded from that point to the end of the collecting tubule. On the left a diagram of the circulation is added: G., glomerulus; P.C., proximal convoluted tubule; D.L., descending limb; H.L., loop of Henle; A.L., ascending limb; D.C., distal convoluted tubule; C.T., collecting tubule. (From A. R. Cushny, The Secretion of the Urine, Longmans, Green and Co., Ltd., London.)

to form the efferent arteriole, which leaves the glomerular tuft close to the point of entrance of the afferent vessel. In the nephrons in the outer two thirds of the cortex the diameter of the efferent arteriole is about one half that of the afferent, and it almost immediately breaks up into a second network of capillaries supplying the adjacent tubule. In the nephrons in the inner third of the cortex (juxtamedullary) the caliber of the efferent vessel is almost as large as, or even larger than, that of the afferent arteriole, and it proceeds directly as a single large trunk into the medulla where it divides into a group of straight parallel vessels (vasa recta) which descend farther into the medulla before turning sharply toward the cortex to drain into the venous system.[3] Because of these anatomic differences in the cortical and deeper glomeruli, the latter offer less resistance to blood flow, and under conditions of low blood pressure or reduced blood flow may be the only ones perfused.[4] It is significant that in mammals the tubules are not supplied by blood from any direct major arterial vessels; most of the blood, consequently, has first passed through a glomerulus. Obliterative lesions of the glomerulus involving the vessels, then, should result in obstruction of the tubular circulation. Exceptionally, however, small twigs (Ludwig's artery) branching from the afferent arteriole may circumvent the glomerulus and supply the tubules. These are usually of no functional significance, but in chronic renal disease involving glomerular circulation they may maintain some tubular blood supply. It has not been shown, however, that such "aglomerular tubules" are functional in man. Recent evidence indicates that "plasma skimming" may occur in the renal circulation to a greater extent than in other organs, so that afferent arterioles branching from the proximal portion of the lobular arteries receive blood with a relatively low hematocrit, while those arising more distally receive blood with a relatively high hematocrit.[5] This implies that there must be short cut postglomerular capillaries by which corpuscles can pass directly to the venous system without following the circuitous route of the peritubular capillaries. Such bypasses, however, have not been demonstrated anatomically. The kidney has an abundant sympathetic nerve supply arising from the sixth thoracic to the third lumbar segment and includes both vasoconstrictor and afferent fibers. In spite of descriptions of parasympathetic fibers from the vagus reaching the kidney, no direct vagal branches have been found and vasodilator fibers have not been demonstrated. Nerve endings have also been described between the cells of the tubules and of Bowman's capsule. Complete denervation of the kidney does not result in any change in the composition of the urine. Any effect on urine formation caused by section or stimulation of any of the renal nerves can be explained by the effect on the vascular system of the kidney.

It is apparent from the unique structure of the glomerulus that it is admirably fitted to act as a filter. The classic experiments of Richards, Walker and their collaborators[6,7] showed that fluid collected by micro pipettes from Bowman's space in the frog, Necturus, snake, guinea pig and rat was normally protein-free within the limit of the analytic method (about 30 mg./100 ml.) and had the composition to be expected of a simple ultrafiltrate. Hayman[8] and White[9] showed by direct measurement in the frog and in Necturus that there was sufficient pressure for filtration to occur. In the frog the average mean value of the diastolic pressure in the glomerular capillaries was 54 per cent of the systolic aortic pressure. If these results can be transferred to the human kidney, the following relationships occur:

$$P_b^{(60)} - P_o^{(25)} - P_c^{(5)} = P_f^{(30)}$$

where P_b = capillary blood pressure in millimeters of mercury, P_o = osmotic pressure of proteins, P_c = intracapsular pressure, and P_f = effective filtration pressure. That these concepts have clinical significance is supported by the observations that a fall in systemic blood pressure to 75 mm. of mercury or less usually results in cessation of urine flow, and that when ureteral pressure is raised to about 30 mm. above atmospheric pressure urine formation ceases, indicating that ureteral pressure, transmitted back through the tubules, neutralizes the filtration pressure in the glomeruli. The volume of glomerular filtrate in the *normal* kidney (inulin clearance) is about 125 ml. per minute, or 180 liters per day.[10] Since the normal urine volume is 1 to 2 liters, 99 per cent of the glomerular filtrate must be reabsorbed by the tubules, of which about two thirds is reabsorbed in the proximal tubule.

On the basis of available evidence, it is believed that the reabsorption of glucose, phosphate, uric acid, potassium, some of the sodium and chloride takes place in the proximal tubule by an iso-osmotic process, so that the fluid delivered to the distal tubule is still iso-osmotic with the glomerular filtrate but considerably changed in its composition.[11,12] The capacities of the transport mechanisms involved in reabsorption are limited. Thus, when the load of glucose, for instance, delivered to the tubules in the glomerular filtrate exceeds the reabsorptive capacity of the tubules, sugar appears in the urine. A considerable fraction (40 to 60 per cent) of the filtered urea is reabsorbed by passive diffusion as the tubular urine is progressively concentrated by the reabsorption of water. This is not surprising since urea is one of the most diffusible organic compounds known and is distributed throughout the body water. Rather, it is remarkable that the tubules can concentrate it to the extent they do. In the distal tubule a variable proportion of the remaining water and salts is reabsorbed, yielding a hypotonic or hypertonic urine. In this segment also the urine is acidified by an ion exchange mechanism, H^+ and K^+ from the tubule cells being exchanged for Na^+ in the tubular urine.[13] This exchange is facilitated by the enzyme carbonic anhydrase. Substances such as sulfanilamide and Diamox, which inhibit the enzyme, lead to diuresis and increased excretion of base, chiefly as bicarbonate. Conservation of base is also accomplished by the secretion of ammonia by the cells of the distal tubule.[14] Ammonia is formed by deamination of amino acids, chiefly glutamine, by the enzyme glutaminase, which is present in the renal tubule cells. Other enzymes, amino acid oxidases, form ammonia and keto acids from the oxidative deamination of amino acids. Normally from 30 to 50 mEq. of excess acid are neutralized by ammonia, but under conditions of stress, as in the excretion of the large quantities of the ketone acids produced in diabetic acidosis, ten times as much (300 to 500 mEq.) ammonia may be produced.

In chronic renal disease the capacity of the kidney to form ammonia may be markedly reduced, with only 0.5 to 15 mEq. of excess acid being neutralized daily by this mechanism. When to this is added the decrease in excretion of titrable acid, it is apparent that the body stores of available base can be rapidly exhausted. The kidney plays a fundamentally important role in the regulation of acid-base balance, and renal failure from whatever cause is accompanied by acidosis.

Nonexcretory functions of the kidney include the synthesis of hippuric acid from benzoic acid and glycine,[15] the oxidation of the keto acids, B-hydroxybutyric and acetoacetic acid, the conversion of succinate to malate,[16] the synthesis of glycocyamine from arginine and glycine,[17] and the secretion of renin which may be a factor in certain types of hypertension.[18]

Since the glomerular filtrate is iso-osmotic with the plasma, the excretion of a hypertonic urine means that water has been reabsorbed to a greater degree than solutes or that substances have been added to the tubular fluid by secretion. Similarly, the excretion of a hypotonic urine means that solutes have been reabsorbed to a greater degree than water. The volume of urine which would contain the osmotically active constituents in an iso-osmotic solution has been called the osmolar clearance. In a hypertonic urine the "free water" clearance would have a negative value.

Changes in "facultative" water reabsorption in diuresis or antidiuresis are mediated by the antidiuretic hormone from the supraopticohypophyseal system. The classic studies of Verney[19] have indicated that the secretion of antidiuretic hormone is mediated through *osmoreceptors* in the hypothalamus, osmotic dilution of the plasma inhibiting secretion and osmotic concentration stimulating it. Thus, variations in excretion of antidiuretic hormone operate to maintain water balance. The reabsorption of sodium and the excretion of potassium are under the control of the hormones secreted by the adrenal glands. Several of these, desoxycorticosterone, cortisone, hydrocortisone and aldosterone, have an effect on sodium secretion. Aldosterone differs from the others in that it does not seem to be dependent on ACTH secretion by the anterior pituitary. It has been postulated that the excretion of sodium, and hence the extracellular volume, is controlled by "volume receptors" located somewhere in the body; but where, or whether activated by changes in blood volume, plasma colloid osmotic pressure, interstitial fluid volume, or some other factor, is unknown.

TESTS OF RENAL FUNCTION

Since the kidney is made up of essentially similar units, the nephrons, each composed of a glomerulus, its tubule and vascular supply, tests for renal function should be designed to evaluate the integrity of each of the component parts. From a clinical point of view, however, it must be evident that disease processes seldom affect one subdivision without involving the others to a greater or less degree. For example, a sclerosing or necrotizing process in the afferent arterioles of the glomeruli, as in nephrosclerosis, may result in (1) decreased blood flow to the nephron, (2) decreased filtration in the glomerulus, (3) alteration in glomerular permeability (from anoxia) with consequent leakage of protein and cellular elements, (4) impairment of tubular function because of (a) reduction in blood supply and anoxia since the tubular blood supply is a continuation of the glomerular or (b) disuse tubular atrophy from obliteration of the glomerular function.[20] Similarly, glomerular disease, as in glomerulonephritis, will affect also the blood supply of the nephron and the function of the tubule. Disease of the tubule with obstruction from casts, as in multiple myeloma, or from interstitial exudate, as in pyelonephritis, may bring about atrophy of the entire nephron, including its glomerulus. Most renal function tests have a variation of at least 5 to 10 per cent; with 2,500,000 nephrons, the disappearance of even significantly large numbers—100,000 to 200,000—could not be accurately determined. Consequently, disease processes of the kidney that are not extensive can be quantitatively assayed only with difficulty. Moreover, the reaction of the glomerular tuft to injurious agents, chemical, bacterial or degenerative, is essentially similar, resulting either in obstruction or increased permeability. In like manner, chemical agents (mercury, carbon tetrachloride, sulfonamides) that poison the tubules, or damage from anoxia will produce similar functional changes, indistinguishable by tests available at present. With certain exceptions that will be pointed out later, the clinical history and course is of much more value in evaluating the pathogenic factors in renal disease than are function tests.

Attempts have been made to correlate renal function tests with kidney mass. Except for kidneys markedly reduced in size by disease, the correlation was frequently grossly inexact because of the complete disappearance of glomeruli and replacement by scar tissue. In patients with primarily glomerular disease, Hayman et al.[21] were able to correlate the magnitude of the urea and creatinine clearance tests and maximum specific gravity of the urine (concentration test) with the actual number of glomeruli, as estimated after postmortem perfusion. While both clearances fall progressively with reduction in the number of glomeruli, maximum specific gravity levels off at approximately 1.010 when the glomerular count falls to 700,000 per kidney, corresponding to a urea or creatinine clearance value of 35 per cent of normal. It is at this point, also, that retention of urea and other nitrogenous substances begins. No correlation between clearance values and number of glomeruli could be obtained in patients with primarily tubular damage.

Smith and his co-workers[10] have developed a series of renal function tests designed to test the separate functions of the kidney. Inulin and mannitol clearances have been used as a measure of the volume of glomerular filtrate, Diodrast and p-aminohippuric acid as a measure of renal blood flow. In addition, the maximal capacity of the tubules to reabsorb glucose, vitamin C, etc., and to secrete Diodrast, phenol red, penicillin, etc., has been said to "afford absolute measurements of the mass of functioning tissue." There is sufficient evidence now at hand to indicate that the volume of glomerular filtrate and renal blood flow can be approximately determined in normal man by these methods, but their validity in cases of tubular disease is doubtful. Bobey et al.[22] have shown in dogs that in uranium poisoning extraction ratios of Diodrast bear no relationship to blood flow directly determined. Similarly, inulin and creatinine clearances were decreased markedly, the latter to a greater degree, so that inulin/creatinine ratios were as high as 1.4 instead of unity as in the normal dog. In view of the fact that glomerular damage is not conspicuous in uranium poisoning and that the actual blood flow is normal, it seemed probable that the reduced clearances were due to back diffusion of the inulin and creatinine through the damaged tubular cells, rather than to decrease in volume of glomerular filtrate. Selkurt[23] has found in dogs with hemorrhagic shock and in renal ischemia with resulting tubular damage that there were large disparities between blood flow based on the p-aminohippuric clearance and the direct renal blood flow measurements, and that creatinine clearance lost its value as a measure of glomerular filtration. It is for these reasons, therefore, that the tremendous amount of data collected in patients with renal tubular disease using these newer clearance techniques may not have the physiologic or clinical significance ascribed to them by their authors.

The use of venous catheterization has permitted direct sampling of renal venous blood in human subjects and determination of the renal extraction of various substances. The extraction of p-aminohippurate may then be used as a true measure of renal blood flow.

Valuable information about the changes in various diseases of the kidney has been gathered by Bradley.[24] This method is not applicable for general clinical use.

Despite the reservations set forth in the preceding paragraphs, the physician has available a battery of tests which will tell him in most cases whether the glomerulus or tubule is predominantly involved and which will furnish him a rough quantitative estimate of the amount of impairment or destruction. Five procedures will usually suffice: (1) measurement of proteinuria, (2) examination of the urinary sediment, (3) determinations of urinary concentrating power, (4) urea clearance tests and (5) analysis of blood for nonprotein nitrogen (blood urea nitrogen or serum creatinine may be substituted for NPN) and, if nitrogen retention is present, determination of acid-base balance by means of carbon dioxide content or combining power and serum Na, K and Cl. Procedures 4 and 5 are not indicated in most instances, except where there is serious impairment of function.

1. The presence of protein in the urine by clinical tests is the commonest sign of kidney disease. Up to 100 mg. of protein may be present in the twenty-four-hour urine from normal persons, but this can be detected only by special methods. Considerably more protein probably leaks through even normal glomeruli in very low concentration in the course of a day, the bulk of which is reabsorbed by the tubules, presumably through a process akin to phagocytosis which has been called athrocytosis.[25] Clinical proteinuria results from more protein in the glomerular filtrate than can be reabsorbed by the tubules. Many young people will show proteinuria when erect, especially if standing with some lordosis. This orthostatic proteinuria is best explained as due to increased venous pressure from compression of the inferior cava by a downward rotation of the liver.[26] Urinary protein consists almost entirely of serum albumin and globulin, the former usually in greater quantity because of its smaller molecular size. A daily excretion of more than 3 to 5 gm. of protein, if persistent, will usually result in depletion of plasma proteins with consequent edema.

2. Microscopic examination of the sediment in parenchymal disease of the kidney may yield important information regarding the nature of the involvement. An excess number of red blood cells can be considered as being glomerular in origin, the erythrocytes escaping from ruptured glomerular capillaries. Although hematuria in varying degree is characteristic of glomerulonephritis, red cells may be found in the urine in embolic glomerulonephritis (thrombosis of capillaries with rupture) and in severe essential or malignant hypertension (thrombosis of arterioles) or focal glomerulitis. Excess white blood cells and epithelial cells are more characteristic of pyelonephritis. The Addis method of counting the total number of erythrocytes, leukocytes and casts in a twelve-hour specimen,[27] if done carefully, eliminates the variation in concentration due to fluctuations in water excretion, and, by comparison with other counts, indicates the direction and rate of progress of the renal damage. Upper limits of normal, according to Addis, are 500,000 erythrocytes, 1,000,000 leukocytes and epithelial cells, and 5000 casts in twelve hours. Other observers have extended these limits to twice these values.

3. The specific gravity or concentration test is probably the simplest, most generally useful test of renal function. With restriction of fluid the normal kidney can excrete a urine of specific gravity of 1.025 or above; in tubular disease or with reduction in kidney mass, the specific gravity falls proportionately and finally becomes fixed at approximately 1.010.* The specific gravity is a measure of the concentration of the dissolved constituents, since it is an additive function of the specific gravity

* Specific gravity is referred to here as nonprotein specific gravity. A protein concentration of 1 gm. per 100 ml. of urine elevates the gravity 0.003. If proteinuria is considerable, the specific gravity should be corrected accordingly.

contributions of each of the individual components of the urine.[28] In a person with normal kidneys and eating the usual American diet, urea makes up from 15 to 25 per cent, chloride 21 to 36 per cent, sulfate 7 to 12 per cent, phosphate 8 to 17 per cent, bicarbonate up to 6 per cent, and creatinine 1 to 2 per cent of the total specific gravity of the urine. Urines of low specific gravity from normal kidneys are simply the result of dilution, the relative composition remaining the same.[29] In advanced renal disease, the specific gravity of the urine becomes fixed, but here again the relative composition is not altered from the normal.[30] This loss of ability to excrete a concentrated urine when fluid is restricted is to be interpreted clinically as an indication of tubular damage or reduction in renal mass.[31]

4. Since the level of blood urea does not rise significantly until over 50 per cent of the nephrons are not functioning, and since the rate of urinary urea excretion is controlled by other factors than renal mass (e.g., blood levels, urine flow), these determinations separately have clinically not been of too great value in many cases. Introduced by Van Slyke,[32] the urea clearance test has become a useful procedure in the evaluation of disturbed renal function. Urea clearance depends on two processes, glomerular filtration and tubular reabsorption, 40 to 50 per cent of the filtered urea being absorbed. In general, it may be said that in renal disease reduction of urea clearance parallels the fall in inulin and creatinine clearances, and hence yields the same information as these more technically complicated clearances. Nevertheless, there are circumstances in which fall in urea clearance does not necessarily indicate intrinsic renal involvement. Decrease in protein intake may result in a 25 per cent fall in urea clearance in normals,[33] presumably because of reduction in renal blood flow and glomerular filtration. In cardiac failure with similar alterations in renal hemodynamics urea clearances may be as low as 35 per cent of normal.[34] In temporary hypotensive states, as in surgical shock, reduced filtration may result in abnormally low clearance values. In all these cases, however, the ability to form a urine of high specific gravity is not lost, indicating the extrarenal origin of the reduced clearances. The combined measurement of urea clearance and concentrating ability is of great importance in evaluating the renal factors in impairment of function.

5. Analysis of blood for retention of nitrogenous substances is of little value when renal disease is not extensive. Correlation of blood urea and nonprotein nitrogen levels with urea clearance and number of glomeruli in glomerulonephritis and nephrosclerosis shows that retention does not consistently occur until urea clearance has fallen to levels of 30 to 35 per cent of normal[21] and when the number of glomeruli have been reduced to below 700,000 per kidney. With greater involvement, however, the nitrogen levels progressively rise and can be regarded as being proportional to the degree of renal decompensation. For practical purposes, measurement of nonprotein nitrogen, urea nitrogen or creatinine is of equal value, since all three rise at about the same rate. Determinations of acid-base balance are not usually indicated until the stage of nitrogen retention is reached, except when extrarenal factors affecting electrolyte balance are present. Salt wastage and failure of ammonia production occur in renal failure, but the degree is so variable that laboratory assistance is essential if therapeutic corrective measures are to be instituted. Correction of salt depletion, acidosis and dehydration may bring about striking improvement, chiefly the result of increased renal blood flow and glomerular filtration.

CLASSIFICATION OF DISEASES OF THE KIDNEY

Classification of the diseases of the kidney has always been confusing, partly because of the tendency noted by Addis[35] that "Every student of Bright's disease constructs his own classification to meet his own individual needs and interests." Although some diseases involve chiefly the glomeruli and others the tubules or interstitial tissue, the kidney becomes diseased as a whole. Rarely, if ever, are pathologic processes confined entirely to one structure. Moreover, similar pathologic changes may result from diverse etiologic factors. Although early in the course of a disease the principal defect may be in glomeruli, tubules or blood vessels, in the later and terminal stages of renal insufficiency not only is the etiology difficult to determine in the clinic, but the histologic picture is often confusing to the pathologist.

The following group is modified from that of Bell[36] and appears to accord best with the known facts of pathologic anatomy and physiology.

1. Glomerular diseases
   - Diffuse proliferative glomerulonephritis
   - Membranous glomerulonephritis
2. Tubular diseases
   - Degenerative tubular disease
   - Obstructive tubular disease
   - Metabolic tubular disease
3. Diseases of the interstitial tissue (pyelonephritis)
4. Diseases of the vascular system
   - Arteriosclerosis of the kidneys
   - Collagen diseases of the kidneys

GLOMERULONEPHRITIS

Although the exact pathogenesis of acute diffuse glomerulonephritis is still to be elucidated, its association with acute infections, particularly those of the upper respiratory tract due to hemolytic streptococci (Group A of Lancefield) is well established. Longcope[37] reported preceding streptococcal infections in 85 per cent of the patients with acute nephritis in his series, and Fishberg states that at least 90 per cent of glomerulonephritis follows sore throat. The studies of Rammelkamp, Weaver and Dingle[38] have gone far in clearing up many questions of this relationship of streptococcal infection and glomerulonephritis. Rammelkamp pointed out that, although both acute glomerulonephritis and acute rheumatic fever are considered to be complications of streptococcal infections, there are a number of differences in the natural history of the two conditions. Rheumatic fever develops in approximately 3 per cent of all persons infected with Group A streptococci, irrespective of the particular type of organism in Group A. Acute nephritis, on the other hand, follows infection with certain nephritic strains only, of which Type 12 is the most common. Thus, in contrast to rheumatic fever, the type of infecting organism seems to be of primary importance. A streptococcal infection of the upper respiratory tract is the most common preceding infection, but about 10 per cent of cases of acute nephritis follow skin and wound infections. Other cases are apparently associated with pneumococcal or gram-negative coccal infections.

The association of chronic glomerulonephritis with infection is much less clear, although exacerbations of the disease with streptococcal infections are well recognized. The majority of students at the present time believe that all cases of chronic glomerulonephritis have originated as acute glomerulonephritis, which has then progressed steadily or through a latent period into the chronic phase. The proportion of cases of recognized acute nephritis which become chronic differs considerably in different series, from 42 per cent in Murphy and Rastetter's[39] series to 4 per cent reported by Leavell.[40] Since the severity and course of acute nephritis are entirely independent of the severity of the preceding infection, and since in chronic glomerulonephritis the clinical course and pathologic changes are indistinguishable in cases in which a preceding acute phase has been recognized and in which it has not, it seems highly probable that all have a common pathogenesis. Many cases of acute nephritis are mild, recognized only by careful search and, if edema has been inconspicuous, those afflicted are unlikely to have sought medical attention.

Many attempts to produce the disease picture of acute or chronic glomerulonephritis in animals as it occurs in humans have been made without success.

The most suggestive and promising line of investigation was started by Masugi.[41] He demonstrated that an antikidney serum, produced by the injection of emulsion of rabbit kidneys into ducks, when injected into rabbits, was followed after an interval of several days by oliguria, albuminuria and hematuria. These observations have been confirmed and extended by others.[42,43] After the injection of nephrotoxic serum, the animal remains well for several days, and urine shows no abnormalities. Then albumin, casts and erythrocytes appear in the urine, often preceded by a short period of oliguria and some rise in blood pressure. Blood urea retention is usually present, and in some animals ascites and edema of the extremities develop. Animals may die in uremia within a few days. Usually if the animal survives the first twenty days, recovery follows. In some animals, however, a chronic progressive nephritis has followed a single injection of nephrotoxic serum, which in the course of many months becomes associated with edema, hypertension, nitrogen retention and depression of renal function. The pathologic lesions in these animals bear a close resemblance to chronic glomerulonephritis in man. These observations are of particular importance because they demonstrate that a single insult to previously normal kidneys may initiate a chronic progressive disease. If these observations are applicable to man, it can be hypothesized that an infectious agent, such as the hemolytic streptococcus, can produce nephrotoxic immune bodies within susceptible individuals. These may then produce an acute nephritis which, in some individuals, fails to heal and which, once started, goes on to the production of chronic kidney disease. Such a hypothesis offers a possible explanation for those cases of chronic glomerulonephritis in which the most careful search fails to demonstrate any persisting infection.

Lange[44] has reported high titers of antibody to human kidney in both acute and chronic glomerulonephritis. Fischel and Gajchisek[45] and others have found that serum complement is abnormally low during the first ten days of acute nephritis. Thus, although the picture is not entirely clear, the evidence all points to the concept that the development of acute glomerulonephritis depends on the development of some sort of antibodies in certain persons who have suffered an infection with particular strains of beta hemolytic streptococci.

The cardinal symptoms of acute glomerular nephritis are hematuria, hypertension and edema. They are not all demonstrably present in every case and, as Murphy and Rastetter[39] point out, if the presence of all three is required for a diagnosis many mild cases will be overlooked, and not until years later when chronic nephritis is obvious will the significance of the mild early episode be apparent. The diagnosis of acute diffuse glomerulonephritis, except in the presence of anuria, is untenable without the excretion of albumin and red cells. In addition to the urinary findings, hypertension was present in 70 per cent of Hayman and Martin's[46] series, and edema in 59 per cent. Albumin and erythrocytes in the urine are manifestations of glomerular damage. But the degree of urinary abnormality is not necessarily related to the severity of the nephritis; for, as Bell pointed out, the blood flow through a severely damaged glomerulus may be greatly reduced or completely obstructed so that little or no filtration takes place. As the inflammatory process subsides, blood flow through severely damaged glomeruli returns, and the excretion of albumin and red cells may even increase temporarily.

The edema of acute nephritis, which may come on very suddenly and be accompanied by a normal concentration of plasma proteins, has been regarded as a manifestation of a generalized increase in capillary permeability occurring in this disease. More recent measurements of the protein content of the edema fluid in acute glomerulonephritis have shown it to be of the same order as that found in cardiac edema. The most important factor in the edema formation appears to be retention of salt and water consequent to a reduced volume of glomerular filtrate.

As long ago as 1879, Goodhart[47] called attention to the occurrence of cardiac failure in the early stages of acute nephritis. At first regarded as a rarity, the incidence of demonstrable cardiac involvement has been found frequently with more careful studies. Whitehill, Longcope and Williams[48] found some degree of cardiac failure as shown by dilatation of the ventricles in 17 per cent of mild cases of acute nephritis and in 90 per cent of severe cases. In these there was dyspnea, orthopnea and elevated venous pressure, and the nephritis might readily be overlooked as the basic cause. The cause of these evidences of heart failure is not clear. That the hypertension is not the sole cause is evidenced by the lack of correlation between blood pressure and cardiac enlargement and its occurrence in the absence of significant hypertension (Levy[49]) or even of any hypertension at all. Whitehill, Longcope and Williams believed that the cardiac damage is intimately associated with the pathogenesis of acute nephritis and is an expression of widespread capillary damage. Moreover, the electrocardiographic changes reported by Levy,[49] Master, Jaffe and Dack,[50] Langendorf and Pick[51] and others are indicative of myocardial damage rather than mechanical factors.

The mechanism of the elevated blood pressure in acute glomerulonephritis is also far from clear. In some cases the pressure never exceeds normal limits during the entire course of the disease; in others, it manifests wide fluctuations. Marked elevation may occur early or may develop some time after the onset. The height of the blood pressure is of little value in prognosis as shown by the observation that cases with systolic pressure of 180 to 200 mm. of mercury may show rapid improvement with a return of pressure to normal levels, while others with only questionable elevation may progress to a chronic disease. The conditions seem to be present to account for the hypertension on the basis of the Goldblatt mechanism of renal ischemia. Obstruction to blood flow through the glomerular capillary loops is apparent in histologic sections as a result of swelling of the capillary endothelium, and Hayman[52] found that resistance to perfusion was increased in kidneys from patients dying of acute glomerulonephritis. Dexter and Haynes[53] and Braun-Menéndez et al.[54] have reported the detection of renin in the systemic blood of patients with acute glomerulonephritis. Earle, Taggart and Shannon,[55] on the other hand, by clearance methods found normal renal blood flows but low glomerular filtration rates in four cases of acute nephritis, and they believe that there may actually be a renal hyperemia, indicated by a high PF/Tm ratio. They could not specifically relate hypertension to any measured kidney function.

Whatever the mechanism of the hypertension, it does seem to be related to the cerebral manifestations of the disease. When the pressure rises rapidly there may develop severe headache, nausea, vomiting, somnambulance and mental confusion. Generalized clonic convulsions may occur. These are much more common in children than in adults. The convulsions are not related to nitrogen retention, but are probably associated with arteriolar spasm and with cerebral edema. Retinal changes are rare in acute glomerulonephritis, but patients with cerebral symptoms usually complain of some blurring of vision, and examination shows narrowing of arteries and occasionally hemorrhages and papilledema. Exudate is rare.

Other symptoms in glomerulonephritis include fever, pain in the lumbar region, abdominal pain (often with persistent nausea and vomiting) and cough. There is usually no anemia, but a moderate leukocytosis is not uncommon.

The urine volume in acute nephritis may be normal, but it is usually somewhat reduced, at least early in the disease. Marked oliguria, with passage of less than 100 ml. daily, or complete anuria occurs in the more severe case. In most instances the specific gravity of the urine is normal or high, 1.020 to 1.030, indicating that as a rule tubular function is well preserved. Occasionally, however, a patient will excrete only a small volume of dilute urine. These cases represent a more widespread renal damage with impairment of tubule cells. The prognosis in such instances is grave. A low specific gravity alone does not carry such a grave prognosis unless the volume is also low, for many mild cases are experiencing a spontaneous diuresis when they first come under observation. The amount of albumin and blood varies tremendously and does not bear any relation to the ultimate outcome. Usually the albumin does not exceed 0.2 to 0.4 per cent and is the last abnormality to disappear.

Renal function, as measured by clearance methods, is normal in about half the cases. Others show a moderate reduction in inulin and urea clearances with moderate nitrogen retention. In severe cases, with impairment of tubular function, nitrogen retention is marked, and all clearances are reduced to low levels. In such cases the interpretation of inulin and Diodrast clearances is uncertain, because in the presence of severe tubular damage these clearances cease to be reliable measures of the volume of glomerular filtrate and of renal plasma flow.

Only a very small proportion of patients with acute nephritis die during the acute attack, although the mortality in reported series from hospital practice varies from 5 to 9 per cent. But such series do not include the many mild cases which are either completely overlooked or not admitted to hospital. In fatal cases death results from hypertensive encephalopathy associated with convulsions, heart failure, uremia or secondary sepsis. In carefully studied series, 42 to 80 per cent of patients recover completely, on the basis of freedom from edema, normal blood pressure and completely normal urine and kidney function. The majority of patients who recover from acute nephritis do so in six months or less. Addis[35] says that healing occurs in the first year in 75 per cent of those who recover, and that there is no record of healing after five years. Once healed, a recurrence of acute nephritis is apparently no more likely to occur than in persons who have never had the disease. A recurrence would be likely only after another infection with a nephrotoxic type of streptococcus; infections with other types of hemolytic streptococci would not be followed by a second attack of nephritis. A certain proportion of patients with acute nephritis continue to show albumin and red cells in the urine and progress under observation into typical chronic glomerulonephritis. The number of these has varied from 4 to 42 per cent in different series. The course of nephritis, from the acute attack, can be illustrated in diagram [A] below, modified slightly from Addis.[35]

Patients in the latent stage are symptom-free but continue to excrete abnormally large amounts of albumin or numbers of red cells, as measured by an Addis count, without detectable impairment of renal function. They are not out of danger but are subject to exacerbations of nephritis with recurrent infections. The active stage may develop directly from an acute glo-

[A]

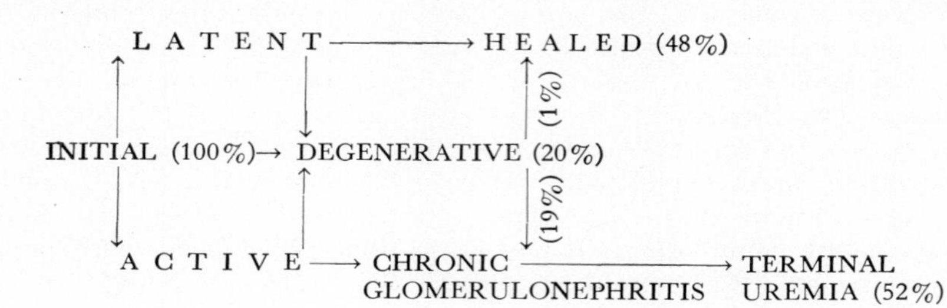

merulonephritis or after a period of latency. The active stage may also be called subacute. It may be considered to be present when urinary abnormalities have lasted for three months or longer. Some cases during this period show a continuous excretion of abnormal amounts of protein and numbers of erythrocytes, persistent edema and a gradually rising blood pressure, but with kidney function still well preserved and no nitrogen retention. When the destructive process in the kidney has progressed to a point where nitrogen retention is evident, or progressive decrease in kidney function is measurable, the patient may be thought of as having passed into the stage of irreversible, chronic glomerulonephritis which will end in uremic death unless life is cut short by some other intercurrent affliction. Apparently some patients in the active stage may cease to excrete appreciable numbers of red cells but continue to put out sufficient protein in the urine so that their plasma proteins are gradually reduced and the so-called nephrotic syndrome develops, which is characterized by edema, massive albuminuria, low plasma proteins, elevated blood cholesterol, normal blood pressure and normal or nearly normal kidney function as measured by clearance tests.

Chronic glomerulonephritis may present an even more variegated picture than acute nephritis. Patients usually consult a physician because of persistent, usually dependent, edema, or recurrent headaches, usually associated with hypertension, or exertional dyspnea, or because albumin and red cells have been found in the urine in the course of a routine examination for employment or insurance. Although there are many cases of chronic glomerulonephritis in which the evolution from an acute phase has taken place under observation, there are many in which no history of the acute attack can be obtained. In such cases it is probable that the initial acute attack was so mild that it passed unnoticed by the patient. Chronic glomerulonephritis occurs at all ages, but like acute nephritis, it is more common in the younger age groups, about half the cases terminating in the second and third decades.

The fundamental pathologic change in chronic glomerulonephritis is the destruction of more and more nephrons. The kidneys in chronic nephritis are characteristically reduced in size, but not always; even at death the kidneys may be of almost normal size. Gross kidney weight does not parallel the number of remaining nephrons, because of variations in the hypertrophy of those remaining and the amount of fat or fibrous tissue replacement. Nor can the extent of nephron destruction be judged by the number of hyalinized glomeruli seen in histologic sections; Moritz and Hayman[56] showed that such scars disappear in time without leaving a detectable trace. The number seen in an ordinary histologic section is an indication of the activity of the process, rather than of its extent. By actually counting the number of remaining nephrons in cases of chronic glomerulonephritis, Hayman, Martin and Miller,[57] showed a definite correlation with the degree of renal functional impairment as measured by the urea clearance and concentration tests (Fig. 2). Oliver,[58] by maceration and isolation of individual nephrons, has vividly pictured the distortion in architecture which takes place in chronic nephritis. Some nephrons are atrophic, while others are definitely hypertrophic, the hypertrophy affecting particularly the proximal convoluted tubule. Some tubules whose glomerulus has been destroyed persist as aglomerular tubules. Smith[59] has suggested that these aglomerular tubules persisting in the nephritic kidney may acquire new capacities, particularly excretion of water, and may become comparable in function to the aglomerular tubules of certain fish. There is no evidence for this hypothesis, however, at least as far as excretion of urea or creatinine is concerned.

The clinical picture of chronic glomerulonephritis varies greatly, depending upon the stage and tempo of the dis-

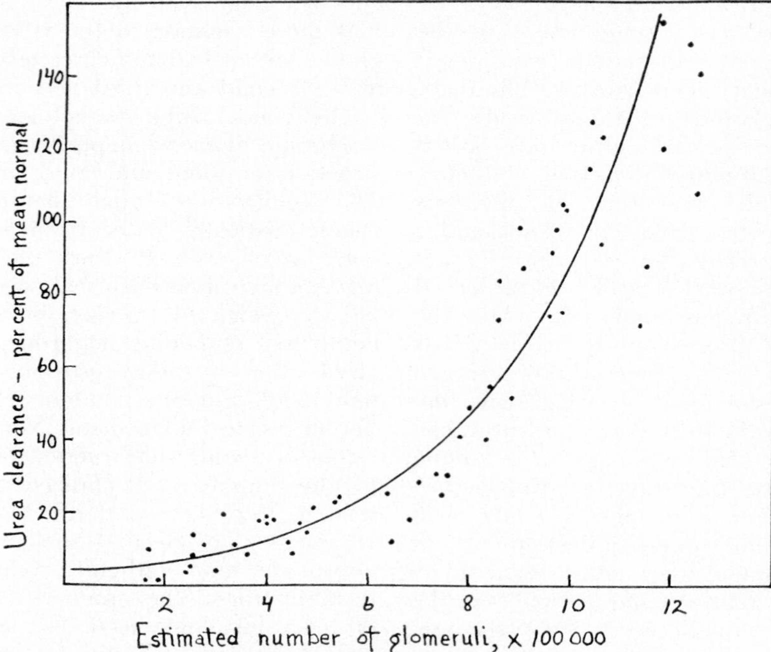

FIG. 2. Relation between urea clearance and the estimated number of glomeruli per kidney in patients without evidence of renal disease and patients with chronic Bright's disease.[57]

ease. Some cases evolve rapidly from the acute stage, with persistent albuminuria, hematuria and edema, with increasing hypertension and diminishing renal function, and death in uremia occurs within three to six months of the onset. In others, after the initial stage, blood pressure returns to normal and red cells disappear from the urine, although massive albuminuria persists and edema becomes pronounced. This so-called nephrotic stage of glomerulonephritis may persist for months or years. Eventually the albuminuria decreases and edema disappears, but hypertension becomes manifest and a progressive decrease in renal function can be detected. Other patients continue to show slight or moderate elevation of blood pressure after an acute attack, with only a slight albuminuria. For a long time, even many years, the clinical course of this group closely resembles that of primary or essential hypertension. However, if a careful examination of the urinary sediment is made during this period by Addis's technique, an abnormal excretion of erythrocytes can usually be demonstrated. These persons may have few symptoms in spite of hypertension, although some nocturia is usually present. Finally, impairment of renal function appears, and the progress of the disease is then usually rapid. Occasionally cardiac failure or cerebral hemorrhage terminates the picture while renal function is still fairly well preserved. In such cases, particularly, if a history of an initial attack is not obtained, differentiation from essential hypertension (arteriolar nephrosclerosis) may be impossible. Other cases first come under observation during an exacerbation, when the history of a recent tonsillitis or other infection and the urinary findings seem typical of an acute nephritis; only the presence of the combination of cardiac hypertrophy, anemia, retinal changes and unexpectedly low renal function points to the existence of long standing disease.

Many cases of chronic glomerulonephritis are free from edema. When edema is present, it may be either of the nephrotic type, associated with lowered plasma proteins, or cardiac in origin. Treatment of the cardiac failure will often lead to a striking reduction in the edema. Practically all cases of chronic nephritis have some degree of hypertension, except during the nephrotic stage or in the presence of advanced tuberculosis or other cachectic state. The blood pressure is usually not elevated to the degrees seen in arteriolar nephrosclerosis, and does not show the fluctuations which are characteristic of the early stages of the latter disease. Although systolic pressures of 250 and diastolic pressures of 150 or more do occur in chronic nephritis, the more usual range is 160 to 180 systolic and 100 to 120 diastolic. There is so much overlap, however, in the range of blood pressures in chronic nephritis and arteriolar nephrosclerosis that the degree of hypertension is not a useful point in differential diagnosis. Cardiac failure, nocturnal dyspnea and edema do occur in chronic nephritis, but they are not nearly so frequent as in arteriolar nephrosclerosis: the typical ending is uremia. Retinal lesions with hemorrhage, exudate and papilledema also occur, but again all are more characteristic of primary vascular disease.

Gastrointestinal symptoms, anorexia, nausea and vomiting are manifestations of chronic nitrogen retention and uremia. The same is true of the characteristic anemia which tends to parallel the degree of impaired renal function. It is usually normoblastic in type, and counts of 2,000,000 red cells and 40 per cent hemoglobin are not uncommon. Reticulocytes are scarce. The bone marrow is either normal or hyperplastic. The mechanism of the anemia is obscure, but it is probably due to depression of the bone marrow by retained metabolites. At times there may be a definitely hemolytic component. It is not improved by liver or iron therapy. In many cases misguided restriction of diet over prolonged periods has been a contributing factor.

The urine in chronic glomerulonephritis is usually increased in volume, amounting to 2 to 3 liters per day. The specific gravity is low, and the patient cannot elaborate a concentrated urine during a concentration test. In severe impairment, the specific gravity becomes fixed within a point or two of 0.010. The reason for the polyuria has been puzzling. Since the major pathologic change in chronic nephritis is a reduction in the number of nephrons, if the remaining tubules functioned in a normal manner, it might be expected that such a kidney would excrete a small volume of urine of a normal specific gravity. That it does not has been correlated with the hypertrophy and changes in histologic appearance described by Oliver and others as evidence that even the remaining tubules are physiologically damaged. But Hayman[31] and collaborators showed that in dogs hyposthenuria and polyuria were the result of simple surgical reduction in kidney mass, and that in these animals a urine of high specific gravity was excreted when the blood pressure was lowered or the concentration of plasma proteins increased. On the other hand, in animals in which the tubules had been specifically damaged by uranium or ureteral obstruction, these maneuvers were without effect on the urinary specific gravity; furthermore, patients with chronic nephritis, who have shown a low fixed specific gravity on concentration tests not infrequently excrete a considerably more concentrated urine if the blood pressure drops to the neighborhood of 100 mm. of mercury systolic. It seems reasonable to assume, therefore, that both the reduction in the number of nephrons and some loss of concentrating power on the part of those remaining are factors in the production of the polyuria and hyposthenuria of chronic nephritis.

Kidney function tests do not show a decrease in function corresponding to the degree of reduction of kidney mass. But the mass of a kidney is no indication of the number of nephrons it contains. When the urea clearance test, for instance, is plotted against the number of remaining nephrons, obtained by count after death, a decrease in clearance with a reduction in the number of nephrons is apparent.[57] The relation, however, is not linear, clearance being reduced more rapidly than the number of nephrons (Fig. 2). This, of course, can be attributed to the fact that many of the remaining glomeruli are not normal, their filtering surface presumably having been reduced. When the maximum specific gravity is similarly plotted against the number of glomeruli, the shape of the curve is different from that afforded by a correlation of clearance value and number of glomeruli. The curve descends approximately in a straight line from the normal range to the point representing about 700,000 or 800,000 remaining nephrons and a maximum specific gravity of 1.010, and then is horizontal in spite of further reduction in nephrons. The point of apparent discontinuity corresponds to about 35 per cent of normal urea or creatinine clearance. The reason for this distribution invites speculation. Van Slyke[60] and his associates found that the urea clearance was reduced to 40 per cent of the mean normal before there was any retention of urea. In the data of Hayman and collaborators there were only four patients with glomerular counts above 800,000 in whom the urea nitrogen content of the blood was above 20 mg. per 100 ml.; only two with glomerular counts below this figure showed a blood urea nitrogen below 20, and in only four was it below 30 mg. per 100 ml. Thus, the concentration test is a satisfactory indication of kidney function and reduction in the number of nephrons until the gravity becomes fixed at 1.010. At that point this test gives no indication whether sufficient nephrons remain to maintain function for several years, or whether they have been reduced to a point where uremia is imminent. Under this condition, further information must be sought by clearance tests.

Treatment of Glomerulonephritis

In the patient exhibiting mild acute glomerulonephritis without hypertension, edema or nitrogen retention, probably no specific therapy is indicated. In the presence of any symptoms other than minimal albuminuria and microscopic hematuria, the patient should be put to bed. The question is: How long should he be kept there? Certainly until blood pressure is normal, all edema has disappeared and the urine is improving. Since proteinuria and hematuria are increased in the erect posture, it would be desirable to prescribe bed rest until the urine is normal, but this is not always feasible. It is probably proper to allow the patient to get up gradually when his twenty-four-hour protein excretion is below 0.2 gm. and the red cells under 10 million. If there is a marked increase in proteinuria when he is ambulatory, further bed rest is indicated. In children, bed rest should be continued for four to six months if necessary. It is often impossible to keep an adult, especially the breadwinner, confined so long. Even adults should be kept in bed until two weeks after the urine has stopped showing progressive improvement.

There is some difference of opinion on diet. On the principle that a damaged part should be rested, and because rats given high protein diets showed greater renal hypertrophy than controls, and because some strains of rats with nephrotoxic nephritis did better on low protein diets, Addis believed that dietary protein should be reduced to about 0.2 gm. per kg. for the first week or ten days, and adequate calories provided with carbohydrate, cream, butter and olive oil. He continued protein restriction at 0.75 gm. per kg. or 40 to 50 gm. for an adult as long as there was any evidence of a renal lesion. On the other hand, in a controlled study Mortensen[61] found that patients with postscarlatinal nephritis recovered just as promptly and, in fact, showed a more rapid subsidence of proteinuria on a relatively high protein diet. Naeraa[62] studied ten patients on a 40 gm. and 125 gm. protein diet; aside from a transient increase in hematuria when first taking the high diet, they showed no other ill effects and felt better. A middle course is probably best, giving only fruit juice or tea for the first twenty-four hours, and then limiting protein to 20 to 30 gm. for the first week, gradually increasing protein until at the end of ten days or two weeks the patient is back on a normal protein intake. In the presence of marked oliguria or anuria, the Borst[63] diet of sugar, butter and orange juice is useful.

Salt should be restricted in the presence of edema, and it is obvious that other sodium compounds such as sodium bicarbonate, the sodium glutamate used as flavoring agent and most salt substitutes should be eliminated. The volume of fluid permissible varies with the urine volume. If ingested fluid is not excreted, it can only accumulate, leading to increased blood volume, edema, pulmonary congestion and circulatory failure. Diuretics have no place in treatment. Nothing can increase urine volume until the swelling of the glomerular capillary endothelium subsides, and no known drugs influence this. Fluid intake should be restricted to enough to make up for water loss in urine, expired air and insensible perspiration. A good rule is to give 500 to 1000 ml. more than the previous day's urine volume, the larger quantity in hot weather or in the presence of fever.

Since glomerulonephritis results from streptococcal infection, and since the relation of persistence of organisms to the course of the renal lesion, if any, is unknown, it is logical to attempt to eradicate the streptococci. Longcope used sulfonamides routinely in his patients, reporting conservatively that it did not seem to do them any harm, and that he thought the drug was beneficial. Rigdon,[64] however, pointed out the similarity of the lesions in acute nephritis and in sulfonamide sensitivity; he believes that sulfonamides should not be used. Since early penicillin treatment of Type 12 streptococcal infections apparently definitely reduces the incidence of acute nephritis,[65] it seems reasonable to give a course of 300,000 units daily for five to ten days even if the renal lesion is present when the patient is first seen. There is no evidence that the routine use of antibiotics is of any value after the initial stage. There is no evidence that tonsillectomy affects the course of the disease. Obvious foci which do not respond to antibiotics should be treated surgically as they would be in the absence of nephritis. On the hypothesis that acute nephritis is a manifestation of hypersensitivity, Craig[66] tried antihistamine drugs and reported a rapid disappearance of albumin. We have been completely unable to confirm this or to see any effect of these drugs on any of the symptoms or signs of the disease. Farnsworth[67] treated three patients with ACTH and concluded that the hematuria, azotemia and hypertension of acute nephritis can be favorably modified by activation of the adrenal cortex by ACTH. Thorn,[68] and Mitchell and Valk, however, were unable to confirm this. In some patients hematuria was increased. We have not detected any benefit from ACTH or cortisone in the acute stage, although at least temporary benefit is obtained in the nephrotic phase. Nor does ascorbic acid, even in large doses, have any effect on the hematuria, although its use has been recommended.

Treatment in acute nephritis is directed toward the control of specific symptoms. Digitalis should be given for signs of congestive failure. There is no objection to the use of mild sedatives if they are indicated. During the period of dietary restriction vitamin supplements may be given, although their necessity during the short period of low intake is theoretical. Intravenous or intramuscular magnesium sulfate is the best means of controlling convulsions if they occur. The effect is due to the depression of nervous tissue by the magnesium ion and not to any dehydrating action. It may be given slowly intravenously as a 0.5 to 2.0 per cent solution until convulsions stop or to a total of 10 gm. for an adult. Respiratory depression is the danger. The disappearance of knee jerks is a good guide for caution. Respiratory depression, if it does occur, can be promptly overcome by intravenous injection of a calcium salt.

Since the renal lesion in acute nephritis is usually reversible, at least to some degree, the use of an artificial kidney is logical in patients with anuria and acute uremia. The object is simply to restore electrolyte balance and reduce nitrogen retention, thus giving a little more time for subsidence of the swelling of capillary endothelium. The use of the artificial kidney is not a minor procedure, but we have had a few patients whose lives were probably saved by it.

The treatment of uremia is disappointing, but occasionally striking temporary improvement can be obtained. This is not due to any improvement in the kidneys themselves, but largely to the correction of "extrarenal" factors, such as dehydration or disturbance in acid-base balance which have resulted from loss of the ability of the kidney to play its normal role in the regulation of the internal milieu. An understanding of the disturbances in body economy suggests appropriate measures. If, as is often the case, the patient is dehydrated, the intravenous infusion of 1500 ml. of normal saline is indicated. Careful watch must be kept, however, that the heart is not overloaded, and, if there is any increase in venous pressure, the fluid should be given subcutaneously. Administration of salt solution should be continued until there is a definite increase in urine volume and decrease in nitrogen retention, or until the development of edema shows that the capacity of the kidneys to excrete water has been exceeded. The distressing dyspnea of acidosis, resulting from retention of phosphates and sulfates and consequent reduction of bicarbonate, may be relieved by 10 to 20 gm. of sodium bicarbonate by mouth in divided doses, or 200 to 300 ml. of a 5 per cent solution intravenously. Tetany may require infusion of calcium chloride or gluconate solution. The retention of potassium and its slow rate of excretion[69] are probably rarely sufficient to be harmful in themselves, but potassium salts should certainly be administered with great caution. On the other hand, Brown and co-workers[70] describe two cases of chronic nephritis suffering attacks resembling those of familial periodic paralysis which were relieved by administration of potassium.

Anorexia is usually such a prominent symptom of uremia that the dietary problem resolves itself into allowing anything which the patient will eat. Protein restriction is usually ineffective, even if desirable, since it is generally impossible to provide sufficient calories on a protein-restricted diet to prevent wasting of tissue protein. Salt restriction is not indicated in the absence of edema and, if rigidly enforced, may even lead to decrease in kidney function and deepening uremia. Palliative blood transfusion is the only reliable method of increasing the blood count. Headache may be relieved by phenacetin, acetylsalicylic acid or codeine. If persistent and accompanied by marked hypertension or papilledema, intravenous injection of hypertonic sugars may afford relief for several days. Convulsions may at times be controlled by the use of magnesium sulfate, as described in the treatment of acute nephritis.

INTERCAPILLARY GLOMERULOSCLEROSIS

Although the presence in some diabetic patients of a syndrome characterized by massive proteinuria and edema was described by Naunyn[71] in 1910, and renal glomerular changes consisting of sharply defined, mostly roundish, homogeneous formations were observed by Fahr[72] in 1924, it remained for Kimmelstiel and Wilson[73] twelve years later to correlate a distinctive lesion of the renal glomerulus with a clinical syndrome of diabetes, hypertension and a nephrotic syndrome. The work was soon confirmed by other investigators,[74,75] and the fully developed "nodular" form, consisting of one or more hyaline spherical masses, usually situated in the central part of the glomerular lobule and appearing to be located between the capillaries, has come to be regarded as being almost specific for diabetes.[76,77,78] In only very rare instances has it been found in patients not known to have diabetes. More recently, another lesion in the glomerulus associated specifically with diabetes was described, first by Laipply[79] as "focal fibrosis"; this description has been greatly extended and clarified by Bell.[77] who uses the term "diffuse type" for a diffuse thickening and hyalinization of the intercapillary septa. The diffuse lesion is frequently associated with the nodular form. The Kimmelstiel-Wilson clinical syndrome may develop in cases with diffuse lesions, in which nodules are minimal or entirely absent. Most other authors have not agreed with this concept of specificity for the "diffuse" type, but Bell[77] maintains that in diabetes there is invariably more or less hyaline in the afferent arteriole in association with an intercapillary lesion, and this combination is rarely seen in any other type of nondiabetic renal disease. There is still much dispute regarding the histogenesis of the hyaline deposit, whether it originates in the intercapillary connective tissue,[76] from thickening and splitting of the inner capillary basement membranes,[77,80] or by deposition in the intercapillary spaces beneath intact basement membranes.[81,82] The lesions take the periodic acid-Schiff stain, suggesting that they contain a polysaccharide, but otherwise very little is known for certain of the histochemical aspects. At necropsy the nodular lesions are found in from 14 to 30 per cent (average: 18.5 per cent of 2143 cases) of all diabetic patients in various series reported since 1951.[77,83,84,85,86,87,88] Taft[89] found a comparable prevalence in twenty cases examined by needle biopsy during life. The diffuse lesion is found in addition or alone in an equal number of instances, but data concerning this is more limited.[77] The longer the duration of the diabetes, the more frequently do the lesions occur, and the greater is the degree of involvement. The clinical manifestations of the disease in cases *with the advanced lesion*[76] include proteinuria, impairment of renal function (50 to 75 per cent), uremia (20 per cent), edema of the nephrotic type (10 per cent) and hypertension (60 per cent). Associated retinopathy occurs frequently (86 per cent). In the early stages even proteinuria may be absent or minimal, and the frequent occurrence of other renal diseases in patients with diabetes, such as pyelonephritis and nephrosclerosis, may make the clinical diagnosis difficult. Renal function studies, as in other types of renal disease, are not helpful in establishing the diagnosis, but when done serially will aid in determining the rate of progression and the prognosis. The life of the patient with diabetes has been prolonged by the judicious use of insulin to prevent acidosis, and the advent of antibiotics has reduced the number of deaths from infection, with the result that diabetics today are living on into the period when death from renal failure assumes more and more importance. Of 1072 diabetic patients of the Joslin Clinic reported by White[90] in 1956 who had been juvenile diabetics and who had had their diabetes at least twenty years, renal disease alone accounted for one half of all the deaths.

THE NEPHROTIC SYNDROME

The term nephrosis, which has caused so much confusion in the literature, was introduced in 1905 by Friedrich Mueller to describe certain degenerative lesions in the kidneys which he believed could not properly be called nephritic, i.e., inflammatory. The striking histologic change consisted of various degrees of tubular degeneration, as seen in mercurial poisoning, chronic jaundice, hydronephrosis, and in the deposition of lipids in the tubule cells. This last was found particularly in cases associated with massive albuminuria and edema, so that the condition was spoken of as "lipoid nephrosis," and yet the overwhelming weight of evidence indicates that albuminuria occurs from an increased permeability of the glomerular membrane. By the use of the Mallory Heidenhain stain, Bell[91] has repeatedly shown marked thickening of the basement membrane in cases of lipoid nephrosis and classifies the condition as membranous glomerulonephritis. He believes that whether a glomerulonephritis is of the azotemic or hydropic type depends on the nature of the glomerular lesion. If endothelial hyperplasia leads to obstruction of the glomerular capillaries, there is associated nitrogen retention and hypertension; if the capillaries remain permeable to blood, but a large amount of protein escapes in the urine, the nephrotic syndrome develops. In this syndrome the urine is usually of a normally high specific gravity, so that, in spite of the histologic appearance of the tubule cells, there is little functional impairment.

The clinical state characterized by the presence of edema, albuminuria and decreased serum albumin can be defined as the "nephrotic syndrome." As such, it may occur (1) as a result of primary systemic amyloidosis or secondary amyloidosis, where the kidneys are involved in the disease process; (2) as a rare manifestation of secondary syphilis; (3) in diabetes of long duration with the development of intercapillary glomerulosclerosis; (4) in disseminated lupus erythematosus; (5) following bilateral renal vein thrombosis;[92] (6) as a result of drug toxicity, such as tridione,[93] gold salts,[94] or following poison oak dermatitis[95] or bee stings;[96] (7) in toxemia of pregnancy; (8) as a stage in the course of some cases of chronic glomerulonephritis. Whether "genuine lipoid nephrosis" also occurs as a distinct entity is a subject of controversy. Those who believe that it does point to the frequent absence of any preceding infection, the absence of hypertension, cardiac enlargement, hematuria or functional renal impairment, the deficient plasma protein regeneration, even when a positive nitrogen balance is attained, and the fact that some patients, particularly children, recover completely for reasons as obscure as those causing the condition. Those who hold the opposite view point out that the vast majority of patients showing the nephrotic syndrome (aside from amyloid disease) either have had a known preceding acute nephritis or—if followed long enough, provided they do not die of intercurrent infection—lose the edema, develop hypertension and hematuria and present the characteristic picture of chronic glomerulonephritis. Histologically, all gradations can be recognized between the typical picture of nephritis and those in whom no glomerular lesion can be recognized, although, because of the albuminuria, the glomeruli cannot be considered to have been physiologically normal. All agree that cases fulfilling all the criteria of "genuine lipoid nephrosis" are extremely rare, many experienced clinicians never having seen a case. Certainly borderline cases occur, and apparently pure cases of nephrosis may progress to a "mixed" form. One, therefore, has to assume either that the two conditions are fundamentally related or that the patient has two distinct diseases. The problem is not an easy one. Qualitative abnormalities in the serum proteins in the nephrotic syndrome have been described by a number of workers using different methods, such as electrophoresis, precipitin reactions to immune sera and quantitation of the amino acid content. But the view that nephrosis is a general metabolic disorder, with secondary involvement of the kidneys, is not supported by satisfactory evidence. In spite of the marked increase in blood lipids, there is no satisfactory evidence to warrant inclusion of lipid nephrosis among the primary disturbances of lipid metabolism. The accepted diseases of lipid metabolism are not associated with significant lipid infection of the kidneys, and clinically bear no resemblance to lipoid nephrosis.

Clinically, the nephrotic syndrome, whatever its cause, is characterized by massive albuminuria, edema and reduced plasma protein concentration, and usually is accompanied by an increase in plasma lipids and a low basal metabolic rate. In the "pure" form, hematuria, hypertension and nitrogen retention are lacking, although the vast majority of cases show one or more of these signs at some time during their course. The onset is usually insidious; the patient feels weak and tires easily over a period of weeks or months, but usually does not consult a physician until the edema becomes obvious. To the patient, the edema is the disease. It is usually dependent at first, then generalized, and often associated with ascites and hydrothorax. It is a peculiarly soft edema, pitting easily on pressure, and is entirely extracellular. The protein content is extremely low, usually less than 0.1 mg. per 100 ml. The amount of edema varies inexplicably at times and cannot be correlated with changes in the concentration of plasma proteins or the amount of protein excreted in the urine. Physical examination is negative except for the massive edema.

The amount of protein in the urine varies from 4 to 30 gm. per day. It is almost entirely albumin. The urine volume is reduced and the specific gravity normally high. The sediment contains many white cells and not infrequently large numbers of casts. Red cells must be either absent or present in only normal numbers if the possibility of a "pure" nephrosis is to be considered. Chemical examination of the blood shows a reduction of serum proteins from the normal 7 per cent to less than 4 per cent in most cases. The reduction is due principally to loss of the smaller and therefore osmotically more active albumin, so that the normal albumin-globulin ratio of 1.5 to 2.5 is reduced to 1 or less. The resulting decrease in colloid osmotic pressure of the blood is of fundamental importance in the production of the edema. This clinical application of the Starling hypothesis was first made by Epstein in 1917, who pointed out that the reduction in plasma colloid osmotic pressure would disturb the normal relationship between intracapillary pressure, tending to force fluid out of the capillaries, and the colloid osmotic pressure, tending to hold it in.

Whether renal handling of sodium and water is also important in the accumulation or disappearance of edema in the nephrotic syndrome has been the subject of many investigations, but not until recently has any significant evidence been advanced in support of these concepts. Wilson[97] has observed increased levels of Pitressin-like substances in the tissue fluids in nephrosis, and Luetscher[98] has isolated the potent, sodium-retaining adrenal cortical hormone, aldosterone, from the urine of edematous patients with nephrosis in quantities at least ten times that obtained from urine of normal men. Both of these substances must exert their effect on the kidney. Aldosterone excretion in the urine in nephrosis seems to be inversely correlated with the output of sodium. When therapy with steroids or intravenous albumin results in the elimination of edema, the output of aldosterone diminishes as diuresis increases. When treatment fails to reduce aldosterone output, sodium excretion does not increase. However, the whole problem of aldosterone metabolism in edematous states, and in the nephrotic syndrome in particular, needs further elucidation.

The endogenous origin of the hyperlipemia in the nephrotic syndrome is shown by the fact that it is not affected by exogenous lipids, nor is it due to disturbance in the oxidation of fat. The two hypotheses which have been advanced to account for the lipemia, namely, as an attempt at compensation for the low plasma proteins and as a primary disturbance of lipid metabolism, are insufficiently supported by experimental or clinical evidence. Heymann and Clark,[99] on the basis of extensive animal experiments and observations on nephrotic children, believe that the hyperlipemia is of renal origin and that the kidneys normally exert some influence on blood lipid concentration which is disturbed in the nephrotic syndrome. There is an increase in both fats and lipids, but for practical purposes an estimation of the blood cholesterol is the most satisfactory clinical test. In most cases the plasma cholesterol is above 300 mg. per 100 ml. and may exceed 1000. In general, higher values are found in association with marked edema and hypoproteinemia, but this is not always so. In those cases which pass into the picture of chronic glomerulonephritis, the concentration of plasma lipids falls as nitrogen retention develops. Both cholesterol and lipid phosphorus also fall if the renal disease improves.[100]

The cause of the low basal metabolic rate frequently seen in the nephrotic syndrome is not clear. Part of it is artefact, the calculation having been based on the edematous weight and not on the normal edema-free weight. But even when correction is made for edema, the rates are usually below the normal range. There is no clinical evidence of thyroid dysfunction. Such patients can take large quantities of thyroid extract with little effect on the disease or on the basal metabolic rate itself.

Kidney function, as measured by concentration and clearance tests, is usually normal. Emerson and Dole[101] report not only abnormally high urea clearances in nephrotic children, but increased inulin and Diodrast clearances as well. The urea clearances were 128 to 192 per cent of normal per square meter of body surface, the inulin 140 to 220, and the Diodrast clearance 95 to 185 per cent as great as the mean normal values. If the increase in Diodrast clearance is taken to indicate an increase in renal blood flow, it is difficult to correlate with the decrease in blood volume found by Gibson and Harris.[102] Errors in calculation of the amount of Diodrast bound to protein might give erroneously high Diodrast clearances, but this would not account for the high inulin clearance.

The concentration of serum calcium is low in nephrosis,[103] paralleling the decrease in protein concentration. The decrease is all due to calcium bound to protein; for the diffusible calcium is normal[104] and tetany therefore never occurs, even when the total calcium falls to "tetanic" levels. Emerson and Beckman,[105] however, have noticed that there is a distinct abnormality in the calcium metabolism of nephrotic children, characterized by generalized rarefaction of diaphyseal bone and relatively good calcification in the region of epiphyseal growth. An abnormally great percentage of ingested calcium is excreted in the stools, and virtually none in the urine.

The diagnosis of the nephrotic syndrome is relatively simple. Diagnosis of "genuine" or "pure" lipoid nephrosis, if it exists as a distinct entity, is extremely difficult. It must be distinguished from the nephrotic syndrome occurring in the other diseases listed earlier. Primary systemic amyloidosis should be suspected if cardiac failure or abnormal rhythms are encountered in the absence of hypertension and renal failure, if macroglossia with dysarthria and dysphagia are present, and if skin or mucous membrane lesions due to infiltration with amyloid and local hemorrhages occur. The Congo red test is seldom positive, and diagnosis premortem can be made with certainty only by biopsy of accessible lesions. Secondary amyloidosis should be kept in mind when the primary disease complexes are present and associated with extensive tissue destruction and infection. History of syphilis, a positive serologic test and dramatic disappearance of the nephrotic syndrome with antisyphilitic therapy will establish syphilis as the cause. Bilateral renal vein thrombosis is suggested when signs of inferior vena cava obstruction are present, when rapid changes in kidney size with hematuria and pain point to infarction, and, in addition, when recurrent pulmonary infarctions occur. Intercapillary glomerulosclerosis seldom presents any diagnostic challenge, since diabetes has usually been present for a long period, and diabetic retinitis can be found almost 90 per cent of the time. Lupus erythematosus may not be obvious in the early stages, but a positive L.E. test, if present, will help to point to this possibility. In late stages when fever, arthralgia, cardiac murmurs, skin rash, serous effusions and other manifestations of disseminated disease are found, the diagnosis is readily made. A careful history will rule out obvious drug toxicity or the other specific events, such as bee sting or poison oak, as a cause, and toxemia of pregnancy rarely poses any diagnostic problem. A history of onset with acute glomerulonephritis, or the presence of hypertension, hematuria or impaired renal function decides in favor of glomerulonephritis. On the other hand, many cases of glomerulonephritis have an insidious onset and may show the characteristic picture of nephrosis. Before a case can be accepted as representing the entity of "chronic nephrosis" it must not only present the clinical and biochemical characteristics, but observations must be available that there was no hypertension or hematuria at the onset of the albuminuria, and the patient must be followed to autopsy or must be observed for at least ten years.

Treatment of the Nephrotic Syndrome

Treatment of the nephrotic syndrome is essentially treatment of the major symptom, edema. The value of bed rest is a decision to be made in each case depending on the amount of edema, the general condition of the patient and the effect of activity on the retention of water. The principal weapons in management are restriction of sodium, both chloride and bicarbonate, and a liberal protein diet. Although in some patients whose salt intake has actually been reduced to 1 gm. a day, a more liberal intake of distilled water is not followed by its retention, such a low intake of salt is difficult to secure; this is simplified by administering a cation exchange resin. Because of the continued loss of protein in the urine and the low plasma protein, a liberal protein intake is rational. However, it is extremely difficult to secure any increase in plasma protein even with relatively high protein diets. Plasma proteins are not fixed but are apparently in a dynamic equilibrium with the protein stores in the body. It seems that the level of plasma protein does not fall until these stores are pretty well exhausted and that they do not increase until such stores have been replenished. High protein feeding is followed by an increased nitrogen excretion but, even when a positive nitrogen balance is attained, the plasma protein concentration usually shows no change. Injection of testosterone propionate[106] is followed by a definite increase in nitrogen retention, but the accompanying retention of water makes its use impractical. From experiments on dogs kept on protein-deficient diets[107] and then fed protein, it can be estimated that in man an increase of 1 gm. per 100 ml. in the concentration of serum albumin or a total increase of 30 gm. in plasma albumin on the basis of a plasma volume of 3000 ml. may require the retention in the entire body of 750 gm. of protein[108] This concept also helps to explain why it is impossible to secure an increase in plasma albumin by the intravenous injection of any reasonable quantities of the recently introduced protein digests. Practically, a diet containing 100 to 120 gm. of protein is usually about all that patients can take.

Many attempts have been made to increase the plasma colloid osmotic pressure by infusion of acacia, plasma, dextran or serum albumin. The last two may lead to effective removal of edema in about one half of patients with the nephrotic syndrome. Administration of acacia was introduced by Hartman in 1933,[109] but favorable reports have been few and evidence that acacia accumulates in the viscera, especially in the liver, has discouraged its use. Whole plasma may be beneficial, but it has the disadvantage of the quantity of salt present. Part of any injected protein is promptly lost in an increased proteinuria and part apparently goes into tissue stores. The failure to detect an increase in plasma concentration may be masked by an increase in plasma volume. It has been estimated that for every gram of protein added to plasma, 25 ml. or more of interstitial fluid is drawn into the plasma by osmotic forces. Injection of relatively large amounts of plasma, of the order of 500 ml. daily for five to seven days, is at times followed by a considerable diuresis, loss of weight and temporary improvement. Concentrated human serum albumin in a salt-poor solution, given intravenously in doses of 25 gm. twice daily for four to five days is more effective[110] but has the disadvantage of high cost. Similar results can be obtained after the use of dextran, but this does not add to the protein stores in the body.

When the edema is marked, the use of various diuretics may be of some help. Among these may be mentioned (1) the cation exchange resins (ammonium and potassium cycle) in doses of 15 gm. after each meal to reduce sodium absorption from the gastrointestinal tract, (2) intramuscular mercurial diuretics, usually in combination with a preparatory course of ammonium chloride in doses of 6 to 10 gms. daily for two or three days before, but not if renal insufficiency is present, (3) urea intermittently for three or four days at a time, in doses of 5 to 20 gm. three times daily after meals, but this is also contraindicated in renal failure, (4) aminometramide (Mictine) and the carbonic anhydrase inhibitor acetazoleamide (Diamox) may also be of value, (5) the new drug chlorothiazide (Diuril) seems to have great promise as a diuretic agent, with successful results when other diuretics have failed.

Since infection may be a major hazard in patients with the nephrotic syndrome, the prompt treatment of intercurrent infections with a specific antibiotic, or with a broad-spectrum agent if the organism has not been identified, has helped greatly to reduce morbidity and immediate fatality rate. The prophylactic use of antibiotics has not been favored because of the known hazard of producing antibiotic-resistant strains of bacteria. Contacts with persons harboring known infections should be avoided or reduced to a minimum.

The use of nitrogen mustard intravenously for one to three days in a total dose of 0.3 to 0.4 mg./kg. has been attended with favorable results in some patients,[111] but the side effects of nausea and vomiting may be conspicuous; this mode of therapy has not received wide acceptance. With the advent of hormone therapy in 1952 (ACTH, cortisone and derivatives related to cortisone), a new era in the management of the nephrotic syndrome has emerged. Initially these hormones were used for short periods of time, and striking elimination of edema was the most important result noted. Adequate dosage by today's standards are as follows: lyophilized ACTH, 25 mg. every six hours, or purified ACTH gel, 40 units every 12 hours intramuscularly; 20 to 30 mg. of ACTH in a 5 or 10 per cent glucose solution, given intravenously in a slow constant drip over an 8 to 10 hour period daily for 7 to 10 days; cortisone or hydrocortisone acetate, 100 mg. by mouth every 6 hours, or prednisone or prednisolone acetate, 20 to 25 mg. by mouth every 6 hours. With these dose regimens given over periods from 10 days to two weeks, complete disappearance of edema can be expected in about two thirds of cases, either during the course of therapy or within three to seven days following the abrupt cessation of hormone therapy. Some of the patients treated in this manner not only show this improvement in fluid balance, but also have marked diminution of proteinuria, or even complete disappearance (in one of five cases) and correction of the other biochemical changes found in nephrosis. Since relapse following discontinuance of therapy occurred in the first few months, the use of maintenance therapy, either according to the plan of intermittent heavy dosage suggested by Lange[112] or the continuous administration as devised by Merrill[113] has been gaining wider acceptance. With long-term treatment a greater number of sustained remissions will occur, and evidence has now been advanced of an increased survival rate as compared with patients who received only short courses of treatment.[114] Galan[115] reports complete clinical-biochemical remissions in 81 per cent of children treated with large doses of prednisone orally, given for an average of 73 days. In twelve adult cases treated in our clinic, three have shown complete remissions lasting from one to three years, and two others have only slight to moderate albuminuria without edema. Baxter[116] and Luetscher[117] report similar results in adults. The mechanism of action of these agents is not clear, but the practical results of improved filtration rate, reduction of abnormal glomerular permeability, decreased output of aldosterone, diuresis normally leading to complete elimination of edema, and reduction or abolition of proteinuria in a significant number of cases have made secure the use of steroid hormones as the treatment of choice in the nephrotic syndrome. The hazards of long-term steroid therapy, under strict clinical and laboratory control, are not as serious as the long-term outcome of the nephrotic syndrome.

GOUT

There is only one lesion that is characteristic of the "gouty kidney," the deposition of urates in the medulla.[118] The problem is the frequency of this lesion and whether it is the cause or result of renal insufficiency. Since sodium urate is soluble in water, the presence of deposits may easily be missed unless the tissue has been fixed in absolute alcohol. The deposits are sodium urate, and there is a reactive inflammation or necrotic foci about them. Pathologists are not agreed as to whether the deposits occur first in the tubule cells, which then desquamate, or whether the urates are first precipitated in the lumen of the distal tubules. These deposits then cause an inflammatory reaction with necrosis and desquamation of the adjacent tubule cells. Whichever mechanism is the more important, it is quite believable that such blocking of tubules would predispose to the development of the areas of pyelonephritis so commonly seen in the gouty kidney.

There is some old experimental evidence suggesting that sodium urate is nephrotoxic. Folin, Berglund and Derick[119] found that after intravenous injection in dogs uric acid accumulated in the kidney, but not in any other tissue, and that the accumulated urate was followed by a temporary rise in nonprotein nitrogen and a decrease in renal function. Dunn and Polson[120] found that intravenous injection of large doses of lithium urate in rabbits caused necrosis of the ascending limb of Henle's loop and collecting tubules, while smaller doses for 18 to 25 days led to dilation and flattening of the epithelium without necrosis.

A possible explanation of the pathogenesis of these lesions may be found in the mechanism of urate excretion. The urate clearance is normally only 6 to 12 ml. per minute, or 5 to 10 per cent of the glomerular filtration rate.[121] This is not due to plasma binding or nonfilterable aggregates, as Berliner[122] found the urate of both normal and gouty plasma completely filterable, and Bordley and Richards[123] showed that the concentration of urate in the glomerular fluid of snakes and frogs was the same as in plasma. The low urate clearance must therefore be due to reabsorption in the tubules. This is an active process, and not a passive back diffusion as with urea. The evidence for this is that injection of urate increases the clearance up to 40 per cent or more of the inulin clearance with a Tm of about 15 mg. per minute, that with diuresis the urine concentration may be lower than in plasma, and that drugs such as cinchophen, Salyrgan and probenecid (benemid), which interfere with the absorptive power of the tubule cells, increase urate clearance without affecting glomerular filtration rate or urea clearance. The reabsorption of urate differs from that of glucose, however, for although the capacity of the tubules to reabsorb urate is so great that it is never saturated under physiologic conditions, some urate continues to be excreted. The excretion of urate is apparently determined by both the total transport capacity of the tubule cells and the affinity of the transporting system for urate. Thus, young gouty patients excrete a greater amount of urate than normal people both on an average and on a low purine diet, but not as much as a normal person whose plasma level has been raised.

In the gouty patient the concentration of urate in plasma, and therefore in glomerular filtrate, is high. Since the same percentage is excreted, the concentration of urate in the reabsorbed fluid is also elevated. Could this long exposure to slightly increased amounts of a substance which is nephrotoxic in large quantities produce tubular damage? Talbott has suggested a similar mechanism, but would make the initial step the precipitation of sodium urate in the lumen of the tubules, which then promotes chronic degenerative changes. If this hypothesis is correct, we would expect the renal lesion in gout to be one of slow development, and this is usually so. Young gouty patients have normal kidney function, even by clearance tests. The first evidence of renal damage is usually some loss of concentrating power and decreased PSP excretion. But since the urine is normal on routine examination, or at most contains only a trace of albumin, these tests are not often carried out.

Progressive renal damage in both gouty and nongouty patients is associated with an increase rather than decrease in urate excretion relative to glomerular filtration rate. Only when filtration is reduced to a negligible amount does retention of urate from failure of renal excretion assume pathologic significance. The urine may show a trace of albumin, but the sediment remains normal and there is no elevation of blood pressure unless there is a complicating pyelonephritis or nephrosclerosis. The progress of the renal lesion is slow; it may be years before azotemia develops, and even a stage of chronic uremia may persist for several years before death. Renal insufficiency is the commonest cause of death in gout, especially before the age of 50. In a series of 77 autopsied cases Gudzent[124] found only four which showed no evidence of kidney disease.

The beneficial effect of probenecid is due to increased excretion of urates. Probenecid interferes with or blocks the transport mechanism involved in the reabsorption of urates, so that a greater fraction of that contained in the glomerular filtrate is excreted.[125] Prolonged administration of probenecid not only has prevented acute attacks of gouty arthritis, but has been accompanied by decrease in the size of tophi. There appears to be no reason why the renal lesions should not share, at least to some extent, in this mobilization of urate deposits.

NEPHROCALCINOSIS

The term nephrocalcinosis is used to describe deposits of calcium in the kidney which may or may not be visible by x-ray. It occurs in a number of conditions which have widely different etiologies.[126] The deposits of calcium may be in the pyramids alone, in the cortex, or in both. Some are associated with nephrolithiasis and some are not. The pathologic physiology is not clear in many cases, and the classification of cases of nephrocalcinosis is therefore somewhat arbitrary. For the purpose of description they may be divided into: (1) dystrophic or secondary calcification in a previously damaged kidney, (2) nephrocalcinosis with hypercalcemia, and (3) nephrocalcinosis from a primary defect in the way the kidney handles calcium.

Dystrophic calcification is a common occurrence in necrotic cells anywhere in the body. Possibly the most important factor leading to the deposition of calcium is an elevation of intracellular *p*H and the consequent decrease in solubility of the calcium-phosphate of the plasma. Such dystrophic calcification is seen best in the tuberculous tubule, but it is seen also in mercurial nephrosis, sulfonamide poisoning, as pointed out by Engel,[127] chronic pyelonephritis and occasionally in chronic glomerulonephritis (especially when there has been a high calcium ingestion). In this group the presence and nature of the pre-existing renal disease is usually apparent, and it is problematic how much, if at all, the calcinosis contributes to the development of renal failure.

In the second group the problem becomes more complicated. The mechanism by which a disturbance in calcium metabolism, usually accompanied by hypercalcemia, leads to renal failure is obscure. If we knew more about the way in which calcium is excreted, it would be helpful. Study of calcium excretion is handicapped by the fact that we do not know how much of the calcium in plasma is filterable. Part is combined with protein and is therefore nonfilterable. Of the remainder, an unknown fraction is presumed to be present in some colloidal complex which is presumably nonfilterable. If we assume a normal plasma calcium of 10 mg. per 100 ml. and further assume that 25 per cent is filterable, there would be some 4.05 gm. filtered per day, of which about 200 mg. might be excreted and 3.8 gm. reabsorbed. The question is, whether with hypercalcemia and a high concentration of calcium in the glomerular filtrate, the tubule cells are damaged by a high concentration of calcium within them as a consequence of increased reabsorption, or whether they are damaged mechanically by the precipitation of calcium salts in the lumen of the tubules. There does not seem to be any evidence on which to decide; it may well be that both mechanisms are operative.

In these disturbances of calcium metabolism with hypercalcemia and hypercalcuria, there are polyuria, low specific gravity, decreased PSP excretion and nitrogen retention. Albuminuria, abnormal sediment and hypertension are absent. A similar picture is seen in hyperparathyroidism, vitamin D poisoning, excessive ingestion of milk and alkali,[126] metastatic bone disease, multiple myeloma, sarcoidosis and prolonged immobilization.[129] There may or may not be nephrocalcinosis demonstrable by x-ray.

Unless the underlying process has persisted for a long time, kidney function returns to normal with correction of the underlying cause, whether this is by removal of a parathyroid tumor, stopping excessive vitamin D or milk and alkali, or allowing a child to move around.

The third group, in which the primary fault appears to be in the kidney, includes three interesting conditions.

The first of these has been called "renal tubular acidosis" by Albright.[130] The kidney, for some reason, seems unable to form a normal amount of ammonia or to exchange hydrogen for sodium. Calcium is therefore excreted as a basic cation. There are a high serum chloride, low CO_2, and normal calcium and phosphorus. The urine is dilute and contains excessive quantities of calcium. Albuminuria or an abnormal sediment is unusual. Nephrocalcinosis and nephrolithiasis are common. Support for this theory of pathogenesis is that renal function improves, calcium excretion decreases, and the size and number of stones may diminish when extra alkali is supplied, preferably in the form of sodium citrate mixture, to compensate for the renal defect. It should be pointed out that the amount of calcium visible in x-rays varies greatly, and does not seem to bear any relation to the degree of renal impairment.

The second condition in this group is the Fanconi syndrome.[131] This is hereditary and is characterized by impaired growth, rickets, albuminuria, renal glycosuria, persistently alkaline urine and increased excretion of amino acids, calcium and phosphorus. These cases differ from the first group in that the acidosis (increased excretion of base) is secondary to the increased excretion of organic acids rather than to a diminished ability of the kidney to make ammonia. The essential defect would appear to be an inability of the tubular epithelium to reabsorb amino acids.

Finally, there is a considerable number of cases in which the only apparent defect seems to be an inability of the tubule cells to reabsorb calcium, or, to put it another way, "a propensity of the kidney to excrete an increased amount of calcium for any given level of calcium in the serum." This results in hypercalciuria without hypercalcemia.

TABLE 1. SERUM AND URINE IN NEPHROCALCINOSIS WITHOUT HYPERCALCEMIA

	SERUM			URINE			
	Ca	CO_2	Cl	Ca	NH_4	Organic Acids	Sugar
Tubular acidosis	N-L	L	H	H	L	L	0
Fanconi syndrome	N-L	L	N	H	H	H	+
Idiopathic hypercalciuria	N-L	N	N	H	N	N	0

H = high N = normal L = low

Most of these cases come under observation because of stone. Nephrocalcinosis demonstrable by x-ray is not common. Renal function, except for the hypercalciuria, may be well preserved for a long period. But because of obstruction, from either a calculus or deposits of calcium in the lumen of the tubules, pyelonephritis is common. The correct diagnosis can be made only by demonstrating a high urinary calcium excretion on a low calcium diet and a normal or low serum calcium. In contrast to the cases of "renal acidosis," the calcium excretion is not diminished by alkali therapy.

Table 1 contrasts the pertinent findings in the serum and urine from patients with nephrocalcinosis without hypercalcemia in the three syndromes of tubular acidosis, Fanconi syndrome and idiopathic hypercalciuria.

SARCOIDOSIS

Since the recognition of sarcoidosis as a generalized disease which may involve any organ, reports of abnormalities in the urine, usually a transient albuminuria and cylindruria in the acute stage, are not uncommon. In a smaller number of cases the urinary findings and disturbance of renal function are sufficiently marked to suggest serious disease of the kidney. These cases are usually associated with hypercalcemia and hypercalciuria.

Descriptions of the renal lesion in sarcoidosis are varied. Apparently three distinct changes may occur. Teilum[132] has described thickening and hyaline changes in the basement membrane of the glomerular tuft, without granuloma. He suggests that hyalinosis of the vascular membranes may be the characteristic change in sarcoidosis, in common with other "hyperglobinotic" diseases such as disseminated lupus. Secondly, there may be typical sarcoid granuloma in the capsule, cortex and medulla. These vary from a few scattered lesions to massive infiltration. Finally, the great majority of cases with renal insufficiency or marked impairment of kidney function have shown the pathologic picture associated with hypercalcemia and hypercalciuria: calcification around and within the tubules of the medulla and portions of the cortex, distortion of the tubules and calcium casts. Sarcoid granulomata themselves rarely, if ever, are the cause of renal functional impairment, since massive infiltration may exist with normal function, and renal failure occurs without granulomata. A few authors believe that occasionally the granulomatous lesions may be extensive enough to reduce kidney function. It is interesting that in Berger and Relman's case,[133] in addition to sarcoid granulomata, renal biopsies showed thickening of the capsular basement membrane and irregular thickening and hyaline appearance of the basement membrane in the glomerular tufts, whose epithelium was unusually prominent. The incidence of granulomatous lesions in the kidneys at autopsy was 8 in 117 cases (6.5 per cent) in Branson and Park's[134] series and 17 in 92 (19 per cent) reported by Longcope and Freiman.[135]

Hypercalcemia in sarcoid was first

recognized by Harrell and Fisher,[136] who pointed out that the serum phosphorus was not reduced as it is in uncomplicated hyperparathyroidism. The increased plasma globulin and total protein were not sufficient to account for the increase in serum calcium, which might be as high as 15 mg. per 100 ml. The mechanism of the hypercalcemia in sarcoidosis is not clear. Probably the most popular explanation is to attribute it to increased osteolysis from sarcoid infiltration of the bones. Schaumann[137] has pointed out that diffuse invasion of the bones may give simply the appearance of osteoporosis in roentgenograms without localized lesions. Albright's metabolic studies suggested that the hypercalcemia of sarcoidosis was associated with a primary abnormality in calcium metabolism rather than with bone involvement. This is supported by the experiments of Henneman, Carroll and Dempsey,[138] who in balance studies found an excessive absorption of calcium from the intestinal tract, and consequent hypercalcemia, as though sarcoid caused the excessive endogenous production of a vitamin D-like substance. The reason or mechanism of this, if it occurs, is obscure.

Many of the usual concomitants of chronic nephritis, e.g., retinal exudates and hemorrhages, cardiac enlargement and edema, are absent or very inconspicuous. A marked grade of renal insufficiency may exist without elevation of blood pressure. The urinary sediment is unusual in that the excretion of red cells, casts and albumin seems low in proportion to the degree of functional failure present. Polyuria, nocturia and polydypsia occur with striking frequency. Although no one of these features suggests a differential point, the combination is sufficiently bizarre to suggest that one is not dealing with one of the more common types of chronic renal failure.

The hypercalciuria and hypercalcemia regress with clinical improvement of the sarcoidosis. This is accompanied by improvement in concentrating power, PSP excretion and urea clearance. Cortisone and ACTH produce a rapid fall in serum calcium and improvement in renal function which may occur with no detectable change in the granulomata in the kidneys.

COLLAGEN DISEASES

The term collagen disease is used with varying connotation. Some would include rheumatic fever, rheumatoid arthritis, acute glomerulonephritis and any condition in which connective tissue is involved. For the purpose of this discussion it will be limited to disseminated lupus erythematosus, polyarteritis nodosa and scleroderma. Renal involvement may occur in all, but the incidence, characteristics and pathologic changes are quite different, although in some cases, as with other types of renal disease, a definitive diagnosis may be very difficult on the basis of pathologic histology alone.

Lupus Erythematosus

Klemperer[139] has emphasized a characteristic change in the basement membrane of the glomerular capillaries, characterized by a focal, acidophilic, homogenous, generally nongranular thickening of one or more segments, suggesting a wire loop. Such lesions are found in from 50 to 80 per cent of patients dying of disseminated lupus. Arteritis simulating polyarteritis or other types of arteritis is uncommon, and the tubules show little change.

Albuminuria and hematuria occur at some time in about one half the cases of disseminated lupus, and once present usually persist. Hypertension occurs in only about 25 per cent, and about the same number or less die in uremia. Krupp[140] has made an interesting observation on the difference in the urinary sediment in lupus and in glomerulonephritis. In the latter, the sediment is usually characteristic of the stage of the disease, while in the former the sediment is as though all stages were telescoped together, showing red cells, red cell casts, degenerated tubular cells and broad casts in the same field. Occasion-

TABLE 2. CHARACTERISTIC CHANGES IN THE "COLLAGEN DISEASES"

	GLOMERULI	ARTERIES	THROMBOSIS	ALBUMINURIA, HEMATURIA	EYEGROUNDS	ELEVATED B.P.
Disseminated lupus	"Wire loop" (60%)	"Fibrinoid degeneration"	Occasional	Common (70%)	Exudate	20%
Polyarteritis nodosa	Local fibrinoid necrosis	Aneurysms Perivascular infiltration	Common	Intermittent (80%)	Hemorrhages Vascular lesions	50%
Scleroderma	Normal	Intimal "basophilic mucoid"	No	Terminal	Normal	Rare

ally patients with disseminated lupus develop a typical nephrotic syndrome.

Polyarteritis Nodosa

The characteristic renal lesions in polyarteritis nodosa are in the arteries and consist of localized disruption of the internal elastic lamina and perivascular cellular infiltration, often with small aneurysms. These lead to thrombosis and infarction, which occurs in about half of the cases and is the only lesion to suggest the diagnosis grossly. The arterial lesions are characteristically in the small arteries, the afferent glomerular vessesl not being commonly involved, in contrast to glomerulonephritis and nephrosclerosis.

The incidence of renal involvement in polyarteritis is 75 or 80 per cent of autopsied cases.[141] Only about half the patients, including those with abnormal urine, develop hypertension, and of these about one third develop renal insufficiency. In contrast to disseminated lupus, evidence of renal involvement does not particularly alter the prognosis, for after persisting for some weeks evidence of kidney involvement may completely disappear. The occurrence of albuminuria in any febrile disease with multiple symptoms, negative blood cultures and normal blood pressure may first arouse suspicion of polyarteritis. Albuminuria may be the only symptom of renal involvement, and renal function may be well preserved. When, however, albuminuria is followed by hematuria, hypertension and decreasing kidney function, the prognosis is gravely altered with death in uremia likely. The eyegrounds may show more extensive lesions than the exudate and flame-shaped hemorrhages of lupus, including involvement of retinal arterioles, arterial occlusion, aneurysms and retinal detachment.

Scleroderma

Renal involvement is relatively uncommon in scleroderma. Kidney lesions when present have frequently been described as those of arteriolar nephrosclerosis or pyelonephritis. Moore and Sheehan[142] believe that if it is sought there is usually a characteristic lesion, consisting of intimal thickening with a basophilic mucoid appearance in the *intralobular* arteries. The media appears normal, but stretched, so that the overall diameter of the vessel is increased although the lumen is diminished. The parenchyma supplied by involved vessels shows shrunken glomeruli and atrophic tubules or infarction.

Clinical evidence of renal involvement in scleroderma is unusual. There is no mention of it by O'Leary and Nomland[143] in their review of 103 cases, and Burman[144] believes that any association is coincidental. But renal insufficiency is present in practically all fatal cases. Albuminuria and decreased renal function are late manifestations, and when they occur they indicate a grave prognosis. In one case reported from Barnes Hospital urine and renal function were entirely normal a month before death in uremia, with fixed specific gravity, albuminuria and hematuria.

Table 2 compares the changes in the kidneys, in the eyegrounds and in blood pressure in disseminate lupus, polyarteritis nodosa and scleroderma.

POTASSIUM AND KIDNEY FUNCTION

Impaired renal function is found with both hyperkalemia and hypokalemia and with the excretion of either diminished quantities or excessive amounts of potassium.

An understanding of the relation of potassium metabolism and renal function is made difficult by the complicated process of potassium excretion. Potassium is freely filterable, and the amount excreted is usually less than that calculated to be in the glomerular filtrate. But after potassium loading in both animals and man the amount excreted may be greater than that calculated to be in the glomerular filtrate, so that the tubule cells have the capacity to secrete potassium. Wirz and Bott[145] have found that in the rat the fluid in the lower proximal tubule is practically potassium-free, indicating that normally filtered potassium is completely reabsorbed, and that the excreted represents secretion by the distal tubule. There is good evidence that this is due to an ion exchange mechanism by which potassium in the renal tubule cell is exchanged for sodium in the glomerular filtrate. Increased potassium excretion may thus be due to diminished reabsorption from glomerular filtrate or to increased secretion, and diminished excretion to increased reabsorption or impaired tubular secretion. The normal kidney has a tremendous capacity to excrete potassium, handling even 20 to 40 gm. (1000 mEq.) per day without difficulty. After ingestion of 3 to 5 mEq./kg. there may, however, be a transient increase of 1 to 2 mEq. per liter in serum potassium. Continued administration enhances the ability of the kidney to excrete potassium.

Much attention has been paid to potassium intoxication in renal disease. Except in acute renal failure, the importance of potassium retention has probably been overstressed. In chronic kidney disease the elevation of serum potassium is usually only moderate except terminally. Elevation of serum potassium to 5.5 mEq. occurs in approximately half the patients with a blood urea nitrogen over 100 mg. per 100 ml., but elevations above 6.5 mEq. are uncommon and usually occur only with severe oliguria. Although potassium intoxication may be the immediate cause of death, it is not a limiting factor in the patient's survival as, for example, sodium depletion may be. The recognition and treatment of a salt-wasting disorder often result in prolonged survival, but this is rarely true in the case of hyperkalemia. In most instances it appears that hyperkalemia of a sufficient degree to cause death occurs only in association with a general deterioration of renal function at the terminal phase of renal insufficiency.

The disturbance in renal function and the pathologic changes in the kidney associated with potassium depletion in man have only recently been recognized. It has been well known that experimental depletion of potassium produces renal tubular lesions in rats characterized particularly by extensive vacuolization. Perkins, Petersen and Riley[146] were the first to attribute clearly a renal tubular lesion in man to potassium deficiency. The subject is well reviewed by Relman and Schwartz.[147]

Potassium depletion is most commonly associated with protracted diarrhea, including the prolonged use of cathartics, but it may also occur with cortisone treatment, primary aldosteronism and versene poisoning. The clinical manifestations of abnormal renal function have probably been overlooked because they are neither striking nor particularly specific. There is loss of concentration power, reduction of phenol red excretion and some reduction in the clearance of urea, creatinine and inulin, but no significant elevation of blood nonprotein nitrogen. Routine urinalysis is normal or shows only minimal albuminuria and cylindruria. Renal biopsies and postmortem examinations have shown hydropic and degenerative changes confined chiefly to the convoluted tubules without significant glomerular or vascular disease. Restoration of potassium balance usually leads to a return of kidney function to or toward normal and total healing or marked improvement in the tubular lesion as seen in repeated renal biopsies.[148]

It seems that the nephropathy of potassium depletion may be a relatively common clinical and pathologic entity that may complicate a variety of situations. Potassium depletion should be added to the list of causes of reversible renal diseases.

ARTERIOSCLEROSIS

Arteriosclerosis of the larger branches of the renal arteries usually has very little clinical significance except when the main renal artery is narrowed sufficiently to produce hypertension in a manner analogous to that found in animals after experimental narrowing of the main renal artery. Although well substantiated cases of this sort have been described,[149] their numbers are comparatively few. In such cases, cure of the hypertension may be effected by nephrectomy[150] or arterial graft.[151] If occlusion of large branches of the renal arteries occurs, wedge-shaped areas of atrophy may be present with resulting superficial depressions, but these are seldom extensive enough to cause any functional disturbance.

ARTERIOSCLEROSIS AND PRIMARY HYPERTENSION (ARTERIOLAR NEPHROSCLEROSIS)

"The question whether essential hypertension in both the benign and malignant forms is primarily of renal origin is still the main point in dispute among investigators in this field."[152] Some twenty-five years ago Goldblatt[153] produced hypertension in animals by partial constriction of the main renal arteries by means of an adjustable clamp. Depending upon the degree of constriction, the animals developed a condition which was indistinguishable from benign essential hypertension in human beings (rise in both systolic and diastolic blood pressures with no detectable change in renal excretory function) or a malignant hypertension, with renal excretory failure, uremia and necrotizing arteriolitis at autopsy.

Moritz and Oldt[154] compared the occurrence of arteriolar sclerosis in the various organs of one hundred nonhypertensive subjects and an equal number with hypertension. In the hypertensive group 97 per cent showed arteriosclerosis of the small renal arteries, compared with only 12 per cent in patients with normal blood pressure. The difference in the incidence and degree of sclerosis was much greater in the kidneys than in the other organs of the two groups. This finding and the results of Goldblatt's experiments led to the search for a chemical agent of renal origin as the cause of hypertension. Tigerstedt and Bergman[155] in 1898 had made a crude extract of kidneys which was capable of inducing a pressor response when injected intravenously, and which they called renin. Wakerlin[156] found that heterologous renin was antigenic and would produce antirenin which was capable of lowering the blood pressure of animals with experimental hypertension. Renin, however, is not directly pressor, but as an enzyme reacts with its substrate, an α_2 globulin present in systemic blood, to produce a pressor polypeptide, called hypertensin by the South American investigators[157] and angiotonin by Page and co-workers.[158] In order to confirm the theory of the renal origin of hypertension and the renin-hypertensin mechanism, it was necessary to demonstrate the presence of hypertensin in the blood of experimental animals and man with this elevated blood pressure.

Since attempts to demonstrate hypertensin in arterial blood were unsuccessful, many investigators abandoned the renin-hypertensin theory and sought for other pressor substances by which persistent hypertension might be mediated. Grollman[159] believed that hypertension resulted from a deficiency of an antipressor substance elaborated by the kidneys. Shorr[160] described a derangement in the hepatorenal vasoactive principles, vasoexcitor material (VEM) and vasodepressor material (VDM). Heymans and Bouckaert[161] claimed to have produced experimental hypertension by carotid sinus denervation which could be reduced by sympathectomy.

In 1948 Goldblatt[162] showed that hypertensin was present in the blood of dogs with experimental hypertension. Using more refined methods, Kahn and Skeggs[163] and their co-workers not only confirmed this, but showed the presence of large amounts of hypertensin in the blood of patients with malignant hypertension. Much smaller but still significant amounts were found in the blood of patients with the benign form of the disease. Further purification of hypertensin showed that it exists in two forms.[164] The first, which has been called hypertensin I, is the initial product of the reaction of renin on its substrate and is nonpressor. It is converted to hypertensin II by the action of an enzyme present in plasma which requires chloride for its activation. Hypertensin II is an intense vasoconstrictor, being at least four times as powerful as norepinephrine on a weight for weight basis. Qualitative analysis showed that hypertensin I consists of 8 amino acids in approximately unimolar proportion (aspartic, proline, valine, isoleucine, leucine, tyrosine, phenylalanine, arginine) and two moles of histidine.[165] Hypertensin II lacks leucine and one mole of histidine, and the amino acids are arranged in the following order: asp—arg—val—tyr—iso—hist—pro—phe.[166] It is intensely vasoconstrictor, and this action is completely destroyed by the removal of phenylalanine from the end of the chain.

Thus an impressive body of evidence supports the conclusion that the rise in blood pressure in essential hypertension is caused by the renin-hypertensin mechanism, initiated by a relative renal ischemia.

The structural changes in the renal arterioles in arteriolar nephrosclerosis consist, first, in a subintimal deposit of a hyaline material. As this increases in amount, the lumen becomes narrowed and atrophy of the muscular layer appears. The glomeruli and tubules supplied by these arterioles become so ischemic that they are rendered functionally incompetent. The glomeruli become shrunken or fibrosed or converted to hyaline balls, and the corresponding tubules undergo atrophy, partly from ischemia and partly from disuse. In many cases thrombosis of the arterioles, with or without necrosis of the arteriolar wall, may be present. In hypertension with renal insufficiency Bell[167] describes the frequent occurrence of focal glomerulitis, an exudative and proliferative lesion in the glomerular capillaries.

Death from renal insufficiency in hypertensive disease occurs in only 8 to 10 per cent of cases. The major causes of death are congestive heart failure, coronary thrombosis and cerebral vascular accident. When renal failure supervenes in hypertensive disease, it may appear slowly over a period of years or rapidly over a period of weeks or months. In the first instance, usually encountered in the older age group, postmortem examination of the kidney reveals only widespread arteriolosclerotic foci of atrophy. In the other group, when the progress of the disease is rapid, the diffuse necrotizing arteriolar lesions characteristic of the "malignant" phase are present. As a rule, these latter cases occur most frequently in younger persons (in the thirties or forties) and are often associated with neuroretinopathy and hematuria.

Arteriolar nephrosclerosis occurs more commonly in females. Probably the role of toxemia of pregnancy in initiating permanent vascular disease is a factor in this greater incidence. There seems to be a strong familial tendency to the disease, as illustrated by Ayman's[168] studies. In families where both parents had hypertension, 46 per cent of the children had high blood pressure, as compared with a 28 per cent incidence when one parent had hypertension, and only 3 per cent when both parents had normal blood pressure. Draper[169] has emphasized the "sthenic" type (short, stocky, heavy skeletal frame, broad deep chest and marked tendency to obesity)

TABLE 3. RENAL FUNCTION TESTS IN HYPERTENSIVE RENAL DISEASE

URINE	STAGE I. NO PROTEINURIA SEDIMENT NORMAL	STAGE II. PROTEINURIA PRESENT	STAGE III. PROTEINURIA PRESENT HEMATURIA IN 50–70%
Maximal concentrating power	Normal	Normal or slightly decreased	Lost (1.010)
Urea and inulin clearance	Normal	Normal or slightly decreased	Markedly reduced
Diodrast or PAH clearance	Reduced	Reduced	Markedly reduced
Inulin clearance / Diodrast clearance ("filtration fraction")	Increased	Increased	Increased?
Maximal tubular excretory capacity (Diodrast Tm)	Reduced	Reduced	Markedly reduced
Maximal tubular reabsorptive capacity (Glucose Tm)	Normal	Normal or slightly decreased	Markedly reduced

as being particularly susceptible toward hypertensive vascular disease.

The clinical picture of arteriolar nephrosclerosis is determined naturally by the various manifestations of hypertension. For long periods of time the urine may show no changes. If death from cerebral or cardiac complications does not occur, proteinuria and cylindruria appear. In "benign" hypertension renal function decreases slowly, but only rarely does renal failure appear. "Malignant" hypertension is characterized by the abrupt acceleration of the course of hypertension, leading to renal failure as the principal cause of death. The change in rate of evolution of the disease is usually marked by an increase in proteinuria and the appearance of gross painless hematuria in 20 per cent of patients and of intermittent microscopic hematuria in 50 to 70 per cent. Neuroretinopathy with papilledema, hemorrhages and exudate, and arteriolar constriction, causing blurring of vision, are present in a majority of these cases. The blood pressure is almost invariably markedly elevated, pressures above 230 mm. Hg systolic and 120 diastolic being found in over four fifths of this group. Cardiac failure, the result of hypertensive heart disease or coronary sclerosis, may be present to complicate the picture, adding to the renal burden. At this stage may appear hypertensive encephalopathy as indicated by convulsions or episodes of transient paralysis or aphasia. In a few cases paroxysmal abdominal pain may simulate peptic ulcer or cholelithiasis. The widespread necrotizing arteriolitis may rarely produce bizarre manifestations, such as hemoptysis, gastrointestinal hemorrhage, or mesenteric thrombosis. Renal function tests during the various stages of hypertensive renal disease have been characterized in Table 3, adapted from Goldring and Chasis. Stage I: "Essential" hypertension, without abnormalities in urine; Stage II: Long-standing hypertension, with beginning renal involvement; Stage III: Terminal phase ("malignant"), with renal insufficiency.

The diagnosis of arteriolar nephrosclerosis must be considered when hypertension develops in a person who is usually in the middle age or older age group, followed by the appearance of proteinuria and cylindruria, finally terminating in renal insufficiency. The greatest difficulty in diagnosis lies in those cases in which an adequate history is not available or in which the whole course of the disease has not been observed. The end stage of chronic glomerulonephritis may be indistinguishable from that of arteriolar nephrosclerosis. Factors which may help differentiate between the two may be summarized as follows: (1) If hypertension has been present before the appearance of proteinuria, the diagnosis of nephrosclerosis is certain; in glomerulonephritis albuminuria appears coincident with or prior to the hypertension. (2) Nephrosclerosis is more common in the middle or older age group; glomerulonephritis occurs predominantly in the young. (3) Hypertension is, on the average, much higher in nephrosclerosis as indicated by the fact that systolic pressures over 230 mm. of mercury are present in three fourths of cases of nephrosclerosis, as compared with only one fourth of cases in glomerulonephritis. (4) Hematuria is present ordinarily only in the terminal stages of nephrosclerosis and then intermittently in most cases, whereas constant microscopic hematuria is characteristic of glomerulonephritis. (5) Anemia, although present in the end stages of both nephrosclerosis and glomerulonephritis, tends to occur with less severity and frequency in the former.

Arteriolar nephrosclerosis may be associated with lead poisoning or may develop as a sequela of toxemia of pregnancy. It must be kept in mind that the syndrome of "malignant hypertension" may occur in association with a number of diseases in which hypertension is present, such as pyelonephritis and Cushing's syndrome.[170]

The prognosis of arteriolar nephrosclerosis is variable, as is evident from the previous discussion. In the older age group the renal disease may progress so slowly that death will occur from cardiac or cerebral complications. When renal function is significantly reduced, and when neuroretinopathy is present, the disease usually runs its course within a few months. The benign form may at any time develop the features of the "malignant" type, making serial observations essential for an accurate prognosis. Although extreme elevations of blood pressure are indicative usually of a poor outcome, there exists so much variability that the duration of the disease cannot be predicted in the absence of indications of widespread vascular disease. Thus, patients with blood pressures of 230 mm. Hg systolic and 120 diastolic or over with normal renal function and without neuroretinopathy may have many years of moderate activity with few, if any, symptoms.

At present there is no specific treatment for arteriolar nephrosclerosis. Treatment, therefore, involves the problem of the management of hypertension and chronic nephritis. The latter has already been discussed; the former is concerned with the care of the various manifestations of hypertension, involving a recognition of the psychic factors in the disease, the control of cardiac failure and angina and a sufficient knowledge of the countless procedures suggested for the treatment of hypertension to protect the patient from unnecessary and possibly harmful treatment.

PYELONEPHRITIS

The importance of pyelonephritis as the cause of chronic renal disease is becoming recognized. Although acute pyelonephritis (improperly called pyelitis) has long been recognized, a chronic form is not even mentioned in the twelfth edition of Osler's text published in 1935. The importance of chronic pyelonephritis was pointed out in the papers of Longcope and Winkenwerder[171] and of Weiss and Parker.[172] Now Allen[173] says that pyelonephritis is the most common renal lesion seen at autopsy, and McManus[174] states that all or nearly all adults show microscopic foci of chronic pyelonephritis and that in many the disease is marked.

Pyelonephritis differs from other types of chronic kidney disease in that it results from the actual presence of organisms in the kidney. The organisms commonly associated with pyelonephritis are those found in the normal flora of the intestinal tract, coliform bacilli in about 80 per cent, enterococci, staphylococci and less frequently, Proteus and Pseudomonas. Pyelonephritis is primarily an infection of the interstitial tissues. It presents certain peculiarities as an infectious process. Although most of the causative bacteria are susceptible to one or more chemotherapeutic agents, the results of drug therapy are surprisingly poor. Instead of the purulent exudate usually produced by the organisms, they seem capable in the kidney of establishing an infection of extraordinary chronicity, characterized by some cellular infiltrate, some scarring and great difficulty in demonstrating organisms.

The question of the route by which organisms reach the kidney is unsettled. There is little support for the theory that bacteria travel directly from the intestine to the kidney via lymphatic vessels, or that they are carried from the lower urinary tract in periureteral lymphatics.[175] Ascending infection via the urinary passages appears to be the route in some cases, probably mediated through vesico-ureteral reflex and reverse ureteral peristalsis. The hematogenous route also undoubtedly occurs, not only in recognized septicemia, but after instrumentation of the urethra, after which bacteremia has been found in a significant proportion of cases. It seems reasonable to assume that instrumentation may not be required, but that bacteremia may occur in the presence of a lower urinary tract infection as a result of normal lymphatic drainage, perhaps augmented by an overdistended bladder, micturition or straining at stool.

Pyelonephritis is most common in the presence of some obstructive lesion in the lower urinary tract, pregnancy, diabetes mellitus and as a complication of pre-existing renal disease. Ehrström[176] has reported 80 cases of pyelonephritis after tonsillitis in 300 children, the majority occurring after a two-week interval. He also described 10 cases of typical acute glomerulonephritis after tonsillitis in which there were colon bacilli in the urine. Experimentally, intravenous injection of bacteria produces pyelonephritis only if the ureter is obstructed[177] or if the kidney is injured as by massage.[178] These observations raise the question whether pyelonephritis is a primary disease or whether it is simply an infection in a *locus minoris resistentiae*. Dubos[179] has pointed out the difference in bacterial growth in vitro and in vivo. In the animal, changes in the local intracellular or interstitial environment may favor or inhibit bacterial growth. In the conditions in which pyelonephritis is common there would seem to be abnormal conditions in the kidney; certainly this is true in glomerulonephritis. In diabetes there are undoubtedly abnormal concentrations of glucose and keto acids and a low glycolytic metabolism. Even partial ureteral obstruction leads to changes in renal blood flow and to some cellular change as shown by the decrease in tubular function which accompanies all types of obstruction. In pregnancy there is certainly a change in hormonal content. Such a hypothesis would help to explain the frequent recurrence of attacks of pyelonephritis after apparent cure and the recovery of different organisms in different attacks. It also implies that treating any bacterial infection present can be of only limited value; it is treating a symptom, not a cause. It is far more important to correct the underlying abnormality that has made the infection possible.

Pyelonephritis may be either unilateral or bilateral, the latter being much more common in the chronic stage. Weiss and Parker[172] divided pyelonephritis into four types: acute, chronic, healed and healed with acute exacerbations.

Acute pyelonephritis is characterized by sudden onset with chill, fever, headache, prostration, pain in the loin, frequency and burning on micturition. There is usually a moderate leukocytosis. The urine contains large numbers of pus cells and usually some albumin. In some instances symptoms are minimal, and only the urinary abnormalities establish the diagnosis. Elevation of arterial pressure does not occur, and kidney function is usually not significantly impaired. Pathologically there is an acute inflammation of the pelvic wall. The extent of involvement in the renal parenchyma varies considerably. In more severe cases yellow streaks extending from the pelvis to the cortex are evident. The tubules contain pus, and there is an infiltration of leukocytes in the intertubular connective tissue, periglomerular lymphatics, and even in the glomeruli.

The symptoms and pathologic changes of chronic pyelonephritis are much less constant. Weiss and Parker set down four criteria which they believed permitted a reasonably accurate pathologic diagnosis. These are: the presence of so-called colloid casts, infiltration of the interstitial tissues with lymphocytes and plasma cells, pericapsular fibrosis and inflammation of the renal pelvis. Unfortunately these criteria are not always all present and their significance is not accepted by all pathologists. Many believe that colloid casts may occur in other types of kidney disease. Boyd[180] holds that when the original inflammation has been more diffuse than focal the picture may be indistinguishable from primary vascular disease. Periglomerular fibrosis is seen in other types of chronic kidney disease. These points are emphasized only to show that the difficulty in the diagnosis of chronic pyelonephritis is not limited to the clinic; even at the autopsy table it is frequently not a clear-cut entity.

Chronic pyelonephritis differs from other types of chronic kidney disease in the variability of the degree of renal insufficiency. In glomerulonephritis, nephrosclerosis and many cases of polycystic disease, the progress is relentless and irreversibly downhill, corresponding to the destruction of the nephrons. In pyelonephritis, however, a severe renal insufficiency may show considerable functional improvement. In the other types of chronic renal disease the remaining nephrons are more or less normal; in pyelonephritis, in addition to destruction of nephrons, there is a definite element of tubular damage. This latter is a reversible process so that with relief of obstruction, temporary control of infection or correction of metabolic fault, there may be a considerable improvement in renal function.

The relation of pyelonephritis to hypertension is another problem. Some cases are associated with marked hypertension. This is perhaps best demonstrated by those cases of unilateral pyelonephritis in which the hypertension is cured by nephrectomy. The question of the incidence of hypertension in pyelonephritis and of pyelonephritis in malignant hypertension remains a moot one. Crabtree and Prien[181] found that only 7 and 20 per cent, respectively, of patients with pyelonephritis of pregnancy were hypertensive 10 to 18 years later. On the other hand, Saphir and Taylor,[182] in a study of 50 cases of malignant hypertension with renal insufficiency and an equal number of benign hypertensives, concluded that 86 per cent of the former were caused by pyelonephritis. Nevertheless, there was no evidence of active infection in these patients and the observers suggested the name pyelonephritis lenta for them.

Arterial disease in pyelonephritis differs from that in benign nephrosclerosis since the lesions tend to be confined to the kidney. Involvement of retinal, cerebral and coronary vessels is less common, although it may be present in long-standing cases. The mechanism of the hypertension is best explained by the Goldblatt hypothesis—an increased output of renin from ischemic renal tissue. It is assumed that man is more like the rat than the dog in that a unilateral lesion may cause hypertension. The beneficial effect of unilateral nephrectomy is hard to explain on any but a humoral mechanism. The absence of hypertension in some cases could be explained by assuming that the involvement was patchy, the involved areas converted to more or less avascular scars and the blood flow through the remaining "renal" tissue was normal.

The clinical picture of chronic pyelonephritis is variable, and frequently the symptoms are so mild that the disease escapes recognition until the terminal stage. A history of an acute attack followed by persistent or intermittent pyuria should arouse suspicion. Persistent albuminuria may be more striking than the pyuria. Urine cultures are frequently sterile, and the significance of small numbers of organisms is doubtful. It is probable that up to 10^5 organisms may be found per ml. in normal urine, because of unavoidable contamination from the surface of the urethra during urination or catheterization. If bacteria cannot be demonstrated in a stained smear of the urinary sediment, a positive culture is in all probability the result of contamination. Pyelograms may show deformities of the pelvis, calyces or ureters, but are frequently normal. As the disease progresses, renal function becomes impaired, with excretion of an increased volume of dilute urine, loss of concentrating power, reduced clearances and nitrogen retention. The cause of death is usually renal failure with uremia; cardiac failure or cerebral hemorrhage is rare.

Acute pyelonephritis with fever should be treated by bed rest, a soft diet and liberal amounts of fluid, 3000 to 4000 ml. daily. If the urine is highly acid, the intense urgency and frequency can often be relieved by making the urine alkaline. Cultures of the urine should be obtained, and the sensitivity of the organism to sulfonamides and the various antibiotic drugs determined. The efficacy of the new antibiotics has rendered obsolete the use of the older urinary antiseptics, such as methenamine, pyridium and mandelic acid.

The value of the sulfonamides in the treatment of urinary tract infection is well established. The substituted sulfonamides were introduced in order to broaden the effective action against more strains of such organisms as pneumococci, staphylococci, Proteus and Pseudomonas groups. Any of the sulfonamides are quite effective against most strains of *E. coli*. There is really relatively little to choose between the various sulfonamides. It is much better to choose one of the commonly used compounds with a proved history of clinical effectiveness and to learn to use it well, than to change from one to another without good evidence. With the development of the antibiotics, interest has been transferred to these agents. Penicillin is most commonly used; it is effective against enterococci, some strains of staphylococci and strains of Proteus that do not produce indole. Streptomycin is effective against *E. coli*, *A. aerogenes* and some strains of staphylococci. It is more effective in an alkaline urine, so that alkalies should be given routinely with it. Resistant strains develop rapidly. Polymyxin B is effective against *E. coli*, *A. aerogenes* and *Ps. aeruginosa*, but because of the high incidence of renal and neurologic toxicity its use should be reserved for infections resistant to other forms of therapy. There is a close correlation between in vitro sensitivity and the effectiveness of chlortetracycline, oxytetracycline and tetracycline, but failures frequently occur because of reinfection with different organisms.[183]

Because of the importance of obstruction in favoring the localization of infection in the urinary tract, any patient having recurrent attacks of pyelonephritis or in whom the urine does not become completely normal in a few weeks should be subjected to careful and thorough urologic study.

MULTIPLE MYELOMA

Multiple myeloma is another cause of renal insufficiency that is frequently overlooked. The patients, 40 years of age or over, with fixed specific gravity of the urine, albuminuria, moderate cellular excretion, nitrogen retention and a normal blood pressure, are frequently carried erroneously as chronic nephritics for years before the correct diagnosis is established. In any patient past 40, particularly a male, who presents with albuminuria, impairment of renal function and a normal blood pressure, multiple myeloma must be considered. It should be emphasized that renal insufficiency with a "myeloma kidney" may occur in the absence of bone pain, bone lesions, increase in serum globulin or plasma cells in the peripheral blood.

Severe impairment of renal function is common in multiple myeloma, occurring in 86 per cent of the cases reported by Geschickter and Copeland.[184] In Bell's series[185] of 41 autopsied cases, 13 showed characteristic changes in the kidney (myeloma kidney) of which 9 had died in uremia, only one having a blood pressure over 150 mm. Hg systolic and 90 diastolic. But by no means do all cases show renal involvement. The excretion of Bence Jones protein is characteristic of myeloma, but not all cases show this abnormal protein. These valid but isolated observations are brought into order by the correlation that only those cases showing Bence Jones proteinuria develop renal insufficiency. Moreover, Bence Jones proteinuria is common in cases with low serum globulin rather than with high.[186]

The myeloma kidney is usually of normal size, smooth and pale. Grossly it does not look too abnormal. Microscopically, there is an interstitial infiltration with mononuclear cells and dense acidophilic casts plugging the tubules and surrounded by foreign body grant cells. Oliver[187] has pointed out that, in contrast to most other types of renal disease, these casts are not only more numerous but may extend even up to the proximal tubule. These casts do not take the stain for amyloid, and are probably precipitated Bence Jones protein. Ehrlich and Bell feel that the renal damage is caused by these obstructing casts which, acting as foreign bodies, lead to tubular atrophy. Because of the number of such casts there may be more basis for believing in such an obstructive mechanism here than in most other conditions, but the mechanism is probably not so simple. Even in multiple myeloma all the tubules are not obstructed. It is probable that the hyaline droplets in the tubule cells represent filtered Bence Jones protein which is in the process of reabsorption. Although the reabsorption of normal plasma protein may give very sick-looking tubule cells, as in the nephrotic syndrome, these proteins are apparently nontoxic to the cells and tubular function remains good. It does not follow that Bence Jones protein is equally harmless. Blackman[188] believes that although albumin is harmless, beta globulin and Bence Jones protein are not. The hypercalcemia and hypercalciuria commonly found in multiple myeloma, probably associated with rapid demineralization of bone in advanced or rapidly spreading disease, may well be another factor. The relative importance of these three factors—tubular obstruction, toxic damage from reabsorbed Bence Jones protein and hypercalciuria—cannot be determined. Attempts to explore the nature of the renal lesion by studies with the clearance techniques have not yielded consistent results. In 15 cases without severe renal insufficiency, Armstrong[189] found the glomerular filtration rate reduced to a greater extent than tubular excretory capacity. In the patients studied by Goldman, Adams and Luchsinger[190] there was a parallel reduction in estimated renal plasma flow, glomerular filtration and tubular excretory capacity. Such studies serve chiefly to point up the difficulty in interpreting clearances in physiologic terms in the presence of possible tubular damage unless extraction ratios are determined.

From the practical standpoint, multiple myeloma must be considered in any patient over 40, particularly a man, with nonhypertensive renal insufficiency or albuminuria. This is nearly always associated with the presence of Bence Jones protein. If this protein is not present, multiple myeloma can probably be excluded as the cause of the renal disease.

LOWER NEPHRON NEPHROSIS

During World War II attention was directed to a large number of patients who developed oliguria, anuria and renal failure following crushing injury to muscle in air raids,[191] and after severe battle wounds. The syndrome had been described in the German literature after the First World War.[192] The clinical picture and the renal changes, however, are not limited to the crush syndrome. Similar or identical lesions have been found after severe burns, transfusions with incompatible blood, heat stroke, blackwater fever, some toxemias of pregnancy, sulfonamide poisoning and poisoning with mercury, arsenic, carbon tetrachloride or some other chemical agents. Except for the poisoning group, these conditions all have features in common. In each, there has been destruction of tissue or of blood, and there has usually been a period of shock with low blood pressure.

The development of renal insufficiency is essentially the same in all. The first urine passed after injury may be of normal specific gravity, but may contain albumin, hemoglobin or myoglobin. Oliguria develops rapidly, the small volume of urine having a low specific gravity approximating 1.010. This small volume of dilute urine is characteristic of tubular damage. Uremia with marked nitrogen and creatinine retention develops rapidly. Disturbances in the plasma electrolytes are accentuated in the presence of vomiting or dehydration. In some patients the cardiac irregularities and electrocardiographic changes associated with potassium retention develop. There is usually little hypertension, and edema, if present, is due to excessive administration of fluids. In favorable cases the urine volume increases after four or five days, followed by a polyuria of dilute urine and decrease in blood nitrogen. Recovery of concentrating power, however, may require several weeks or months. In those patients who recover there is little or no residual renal impairment. The fatality rate in patients who developed anuria has been very high, probably in the neighborhood of 90 per cent, the majority dying within eight days.

The pathologic changes have been summarized by Lucké.[193] The kidneys are swollen, pale and soft. Microscopically there is focal degeneration and necrosis of the epithelial cells of the distal convoluted tubule and ascending limb of Henle's loop, associated with edema and cellular reaction around the more severely damaged portions of the tubules. There is frequently thrombosis of the adjacent veins. It is this localization of the pathologic lesions to the distal tubule that led to the name lower nephron nephrosis. In cases of poisoning with mercury and most other renal poisons the damage is principally in the proximal tubule, although the clinical picture is the same.

The pathogenesis of these lesions has not yet been established. It is probable that several factors are concerned, their combination depending upon the precipitating condition. Among etiologic factors which have been considered are possible injury to the kidney produced by the excretion of hemoglobin, myoglobin or their degradation products, nephrotoxic substances such as adenosine triphosphate arising from injured tissue, and the injurious effect of renal anoxia.[194] For a discussion of opposing views on the mechanism of injury from hemoglobinuria the papers of Yuile,[195] Bott and Richards,[196] and Foy, Altmann, Barnes and Kondi[197] should be consulted. Evidence is accumulating that the most important factor is damage to tubule cells resulting from anoxia. The deleterious effect of inadequate circulation upon the kidneys has been extensively studied in relation to shock, and a large proportion of patients developing lower nephron nephrosis have been in shock from their primary injury. Renal ischemia may result from low systemic blood pressure, diminished blood volume or local renal vasoconstriction. The duration of ischemia is important in determining the degree of renal injury; if sufficiently prolonged there is irreversible damage to tubule cells.[198] Trueta[3] and his associates believe that ischemia of the renal cortex may result from diversion or shunting of the renal blood flow through the deeper juxtamedullary glomeruli. While these are preferentially perfused under conditions of low blood pressure in the rabbit,[4] there is no convincing evidence of any diversion of blood through juxtamedullary paths either in this animal, dog or man.[199] All the data indicate that in the oliguria of traumatic or toxic origin renal blood flow is consistently reduced, renal A-V oxygen difference is increased rather than decreased and the extraction of PAH recovers ahead of the PAH clearance, which would not be the case if there were an increase in blood flow through juxtamedullary tissue.

Three principal hypotheses have been advanced to account for the oliguria and anuria. Inadequate renal circulation is undoubtedly the chief factor during shock, but cannot account for persistent anuria after re-establishment of the circulation. Mechanical blockage of tubules with debris and heme masses has been suggested, but seems inadequate, for histologically all tubules are not obstructed and in many cases heme casts are scanty or may even be absent. Nor is there the dilatation of glomerular spaces and upper segments to be expected when obstruction is complete. The most plausible hypothesis is that when the tubules become injured beyond a certain degree their permeability is altered and reabsorption becomes unselective. After poisoning frogs with mercuric chloride, and then examining the exposed kidneys of the living animals, Richards[200] found that the glomerular circulation and the volume and composition of the filtrate were approximately normal, but that no urine issued from the ureters. The only possible explanation was that because of loss of selective permeability of the dead tubule cells the osmotic pressure of the blood in the peritubular capillaries was able to draw back all or nearly all of the glomerular filtrate. It seems that the results are the same whether the damaged tubule segments are in the proximal or distal portion of the tubule.

Treatment of Lower Nephron Nephrosis

Unless the tubular damage has been too severe, it is a reversible process and recovery can take place. The problem then is to attempt to prevent death in uremia before this has occurred. In the past, many patients have been killed with pulmonary edema by the overenthusiastic administration of fluids in an effort to establish urine flow. There is no known means of establishing urine secretion until there has been some recovery of the tubule cells. With little or no urine secretion, fluid intake should, therefore, be limited to 500 to 1000 ml. (enough to take care of extrarenal loss) more than the previous day's urine volume. As urine volume increases with recovery, fluid intake should be increased. Satisfactory conditions are established when urine volume and fluid intake are at a level which is accompanied by a falling blood nitrogen, whether this be 3000 or 5000 ml. daily. Since the sodium and chloride concentration in the urine usually ranges between 25 and 50 mEq./liter, sodium chloride should not be given during the oliguric phase except to correct salt depletion from extrarenal losses (vomiting, diarrhea, etc.). During the period of diuresis, however, when the large volume of urine carries away corresponding amounts of sodium, salt replacememt may become a necessity. Measurement of the excretion of these ions in the urine is essential if the amounts for administration are to be selected accurately. Potassium should be rigidly excluded from the intake during the oliguric phase. If nausea, vomiting or diarrhea is present, all oral intake should be stopped and fluids should be given parenterally in amounts sufficient to prevent dehydration. When tolerated, the diet should be low in protein and high in carbohydrate and fat, in order that protein catabolism be kept at a minimum.

Much interest has been aroused by attempts to prevent uremic death by the use of artificial dialysing devices. Although peritoneal lavage and intestinal perfusion are capable of removing large amounts of nitrogen, there is considerable difficulty in maintaining fluid and electrolyte balance. Peritonitis may occur after repeated peritoneal lavage in spite of antibiotics. For these reasons,

TABLE 4. THE EFFECT OF TREATMENT WITH THE ARTIFICIAL KIDNEY (SKEGGS-LEONARDS) ON THE CHEMICAL COMPOSITION OF PLASMA

	BEFORE TREATMENT	AFTER TREATMENT
Blood urea N, mg. per 100 ml.	113	30
Creatinine, mg. per 100 ml.	16	5
CO_2, volumes per 100 ml.	33	58
Chloride, mEq. per liter	79	101
Phosphorus, mg. per 100 ml.	11.1	3.8
Sodium, mEq. per liter	122	135
Potassium, mEq. per liter	6.0	5.4

ARTIFICIAL KIDNEY DATA

Number of units	12
Cellophane area	20,000 sq. cm.
Volume of blood in "kidney"	600 ml.
Time of dialysis	6 hrs.
Blood flow through "kidney"	200 ml./min.
Average urea clearance	155 ml./min.
Total urea removed	66 gm.
Hemolysis	None

This patient was oliguric as a result of carbon tetrachloride poisoning.

both of the methods have been supplanted by the "artificial kidney." After heparinizing the patient, blood is taken from an artery or large vein, circulated through cellophane tubing in contact with dialysing fluid and returned to the patient by way of another vein. The ideal dialysing fluid should contain electrolytes in the same concentration as that present in normal extracellular fluid. There are several models of the "artificial kidney" in use which are mechanically capable of efficient and rapid dialysis.[201,202] The revolutionary model of Skeggs, Leonards and Heisler[203] appears to be the most compact and efficient. With it urea clearances as high as 180 ml. per minute have been obtained, and the blood urea level reduced more than half in less than five or six hours. Table 4 shows the changes in chemical composition of the plasma in a patient treated with the Skeggs-Leonards model. The reduction in azotemia and the restoration of acid-base and electrolyte balance within a few hours was accompanied by striking clinical improvement. These artificial kidneys still require highly trained teams, familiar with the mechanical complexities of the models and expert in the problems of fluid and electrolyte management.

References

1. Mueller, C. B., Mason, A. D. and Stout, D. G.: Am. J. Med., *18:*267, 1955.
2. Smith, H. W.: Principles of Renal Physiology. New York, Oxford University Press, 1956.
3. Trueta, J., Barclay, A. E., Daniel, P. M., Franklin, K. J. and Prichard, M. M. L.: Studies of the Renal Circulation, Springfield, Ill., C. C Thomas, 1947.
4. Insull, W., Jr., Tillotson, I. G., and Hay-676, 1950.
5. Pappenheimer, J. R., and Kinter, W. B.: Am. J. Physiol., *185:*377, 1956.
6. Richards, A. N.: Proc. Roy. Soc. London (B), *126:*398, 1938.
7. Walker, A. M., Bott, P. A., Oliver, J. and MacDowell, M. C.: Am. J. Physiol., *134:*580, 1941.
8. Hayman, J. M., Jr.: Am. J. Physiol., *79:*389–409, 1927.
9. White, H. L.: Am. J. Physiol., *90:*689, 1929.
10. Smith, H. W.: The Kidney. New York, Oxford University Press, 1951.
11. Taggart, J. V.: Am. J. Med., *9:*678, 1956.
12. Cohen, J. J., Berglund, F. and Lotspeich, W. D.: Am. J. Physiol.: *179:*627, 1954.
13. Pitts, R. F., Ayer, J. L. and Schiess, W. A.: J. Clin. Invest., *28:*35, 1949.
14. Pitts, R. F.: Arch. Int. Med., *89:*864, 1952.
15. Bunge, G. and Schmiedeberg, O.: Arch. exp. Path. u. Pharmakol., *6:*233, 1876.
16. Craig, J. W., Miller, M., Drucker, W. R., Woodward, H., Brofman, B. L. and Pritchard, W. H.: J. Clin. Invest., *30:*634, 1951.
17. Borsook, H., Dubnoff, J. W., Lilly, J. C. and Marriott, W.: J. Biol. Chem., *138:*405, 1941.
18. Goldblatt, H.: Physiol. Rev., *27:*120, 1947.
19. Verney, E. B.: Proc. Roy. Soc. London (B), *135:*25, 1947.
20. Bell, E. T.: Renal Diseases. Philadelphia, Lea & Febiger, 1946.

21. Hayman, J. M., Jr., Martin, J. W., Jr. and Miller, M.: Arch. Int. Med., *64:* 69–83, 1939.
22. Bobey, M. E., Longley, L. P., Dickes, R., Price, J. W. and Hayman, J. M., Jr.: Am. J. Physiol., *139:*155, 1943.
23. Selkurt, E. E.: Am. J. Physiol., *145:*699, 1946.
24. Bradley, S. E., Bradley, G. P., Tyson, C. J., Curry, J. J. and Blake, W. D.: Am. J. Med., *9:*766, 1950.
25. Rather, L. J.: Stanford M. Bull., *6:*117, 1948.
26. Bull, G. M.: Clin. Sc., *7:*77, 1949.
27. Addis, T.: J. Clin. Invest., *2:*409, 1926.
28. Price, J. W., Miller, M. and Hayman, J. M., Jr.: J. Clin. Invest., *19:*537, 1940.
29. Miller, M., Price, J. W. and Longley, L. P.: J. Clin. Invest., *20:*31, 1941.
30. Miller, M., Price, J. W. and Hayman, J. M., Jr.: Unpublished studies.
31. Hayman, J. M., Jr., Shumway, N. P., Dumke, P. and Miller, M.: J. Clin. Invest., *18:*195, 1939.
32. Möller, E., McIntosh, J. F. and Van Slyke, D. D.: J. Clin. Invest., *6:*427, 1928; *6:*485, 1928.
33. Longley, L. P. and Miller, M.: Am. J. M. Sc., *203:*253, 1942.
34. Seymour, W. B., Pritchard, W. H., Longley, L. P. and Hayman, J. M., Jr.: J. Clin. Invest., *21:*229, 1942.
35. Addis, T.: Glomerular Nephritis. New York, The Macmillan Co., 1948.
36. Bell, E. T.: Renal Diseases. Philadelphia, Lea & Febiger, 1946.
37. Longcope, W. T.: Bull. Johns Hopkins Hosp., *45:*335, 1929.
38. Rammelkamp, C. H., Weaver, R. F. and Dingle, J. H.: Tr. A. Am. Physicians, *65:*168, 1952.
39. Murphy, F. D. and Rastetter, J. W.: J.A.M.A., *111:*668, 1938.
40. Leavell, B. C., Becksmith, J. R. and Wood, J. E., Jr.: Virginia M. Monthly, *66:*326, 1939.
41. Masugi, M.: Beitrz. path. Anat. u. z. allg. Path., *92:*429, 1934.
42. Smadel, J. E. and Farr, L. E.: J. Exper. Med., *65:*527, 1937.
43. Kay, C. F.: J. Exper. Med., *72:*559, 1940.
44. Lange, K., Grag, F., Oberman, J., Slobody, L., Ogin, G. and Lo Casto, F.: Arch. Int. Med., *88:*433, 1951.
45. Fischel, E. E. and Gajchisek, D. C.: Am. J. Med., *12:*190, 1952.
46. Hayman, J. M., Jr. and Martin, J. W., Jr.: Am. J. M. Sc., *200:*505, 1940.
47. Goodhart, J. F.: Guy's Hosp. Rep., *24:* 153, 1879.
48. Whitehill, R. M., Longcope, W. T. and Williams, R.: Bull. Johns Hopkins Hosp., *64:*83, 1939.
49. Levy, I. J.: Am. Heart J., *5:*277, 1930.
50. Master, A. M., Jaffe, N. L. and Dack, S.: Arch. Int. Med., *60:*1016, 1937.
51. Langendorf, R. and Pick, A.: Acta. med. scandinav., *94:*1, 1938.
52. Hayman, J. M., Jr.: J. Clin. Invest., *8:*89, 1929.
53. Dexter, L. and Haynes, F. W.: Proc. Soc. Exper. Biol. & Med., *55:*288, 1944.
54. Braun-Menéndez, E., Fasciolo, J. C., Leloir, L. F., Munoz, J. M. and Taquini, A. C.: Renal Hypertension. Springfield, Ill., C. C Thomas, 1946.
55. Earle, D. P., Taggart, J. V. and Shannon, J. A.: J. Clin. Invest., *23:*119, 1944.
56. Moritz, A. R. and Hayman, J. M., Jr.: Am. J. Path., *10:*505, 1934.
57. Hayman, J. M., Jr., Martin, J. W., Jr. and Miller, M.: Arch. Int. Med., *64:* 69, 1939.
58. Oliver J.: Harvey Lectures, Series 40, New York, 1944.
59. Smith, H. W.: J. Mt. Sinai Hosp., *10:*41, 1943.
60. Van Slyke, D. D., McIntosh, J. F., Möller, E., Harmon, R. R. and Johnston, C.: J. Clin. Invest., *8:*357, 1930.
61. Mortensen, V.: Acta med. scandinav., *129:*321, 1947.
62. Naeraa, A.: Act med. scandinav., *95:*359, 1938.
63. Borst, J. G.: Lancet, *1:*824, 1948.
64. Rigdon, R. H., Siddon, W. H. and Fletcher, D. E.: Am. J. Med., *6:*177, 1949.
65. Stetson, C. A., Rammelkamp, C. H., Jr., Krause, R. M., Kohen, R. J. and Perry, W. D.: Medicine, *34:*431, 1955.
66. Craig, J., Clark, N. S. and Chalmers, J. D.: Brit. M. J., *1:*6, 1949.
67. Farnsworth, E. B.: Proc. Soc. Exper. Biol. & Med., *74:*57, 1950.
68. Thorn, G. W., Merrill, J. P., Smith, S., Roche, M. and Frawley, T. F.: Arch. Int. Med., *86:*319, 1950.
69. Keith, N. M., King, H. E. and Osterberg, A. E.: Arch. Int. Med., *17:*675, 1943.
70. Brown, M. R., Currens, J. H. and Marchand, J. F.: J.A.M.A., *124:*545, 1944.
71. Naunyn, B.: Der Diabetes Mellitus. In Nothnagel, H.: Specielle Pathologie und Therapie. Vol. VII. Wien und Leipzig, Alfred Hölder, 1910.
72. Fahr, T.: Virchow's Arch. f. path. Anat., *248:*323, 1924.
73. Kimmelstiel, P. and Wilson, C.: Am. J. Path., *12:*83, 1936.
74. Newburger, R. A. and Peters, J.: Arch. Int. Med., *64:*1252, 1939.
75. Siegal, S. and Allen, A. C.: Am. J. M. Sc., *201:*516, 1941.
76. Kimmelstiel, P. and Porter, W. B.: New England J. Med., *238:*876, 908, 1948.
77. Bell, E. T.: Diabetes, *2:*376, 1953.
78. Lambie, A. T. and Macfarlane, A.: Quart. J. Med., *24:*125, 1955.
79. Laipply, T. C., Eitzen, O. and Dutra, F. R.: Arch. Int. Med., *74:*354, 1944.

80. Allen, A. C.: Arch. Path. *32:*22, 1941.
81. McManus, J. F. A.: Medical Diseases of the Kidney. Philadelphia, Lea & Febiger, 1950, pp. 57 and 149.
82. Churg, J. and Grishman, E.: Am. J. Path., *29:*199, 1953.
83. Gilliland, I.: Brit. M. J., *1:*916, 1951.
84. Aarseth, S.: Acta med. scandinav., supplement 281, 1953.
85. Smith, J. F., Bolton, J. R. and Turnbull, A. L.: J. Path. & Bact., *70:*475, 1953.
86. Anderson, G. S.: J. Path. & Bact., *67:*241, 1954.
87. Dana, G. W. and Zubrod, C. G.: Bull. Johns Hopkins Hosp., *95:*338, 1954.
88. Epstein, F. H. and Zupa, V. J., New England J. Med., *254:*896, 1956.
89. Taft, H. P., Finck, E. S. and Joske, R. A.: Australasian Ann. Med., *3:*189, 1954.
90. White, P.: Diabetes, *5:*445, 1956.
91. Bell, E. T.: Renal Diseases. Philadelphia, Lea & Febiger, 1946.
92. Blainey, J. D., Hardwicke, J. and Whitfield, A. G. W.: Lancet, *2:*1208, 1954.
93. Barnett, H. L., Simons, D. J. and Wells, R. E., Jr.: Am. J. Med., *4:*760, 1948.
94. Valley-Radot, P., Mauric, G., Wolfromm, R. and Guiot, G.: Bull. et Mém. Soc. med. Hôp., Paris, *58:*96, 1942.
95. Rytand, O. A.: Am. J. Med., *5:*548, 1948.
96. Rytand, O. A.: Stanford M. Bull., *13:*224, 1955.
97. Wilson, H. E. C. and Muirhead, A.: Acta paediat., *45:*77, 1956.
98. Luetscher, J. A., Jr., Dowdy, A., Harvey, J., Neher, R. and Wettstein, A.: J. Biol. Chem., *217:*505, 1955.
99. Heymann, W. and Clark, S. C.: Am. J. Dis. Child., *70:*74, 1945.
100. Peters, J. P. and Man, E. B.: J. Clin. Invest., *22:*721, 1943.
101. Emerson, K., Jr. and Dole, V. P.: J. Clin. Invest., *22:*447, 1943.
102. Gibson, J. G. and Harris, A. W.: J. Clin. Invest., *18:*483, 1939.
103. Salvesen, H. A. and Linder, G. C.: J. Biol. Chem., *58:*617, 1923.
104. Liu, S. H.: Proc. Soc. Exper. Biol. & Med., *24:*817, 1926.
105. Emerson, K., Jr. and Beckman, W. W.: J. Clin. Invest., *24:*564, 1945.
106. Bassett, S. H., Keutman, E. H. and Kochakian, C. D.: J. Clin. Endocrinol., *3:*400, 1943.
107. Elman, R., Brown, F. A. and Wolf, H.: J. Exper. Med., *75:*461, 1942.
108. Thorn, G. W.: New England M. J., *229:* 33, 1943.
109. Hartman, A. F., Senn, M. J. E., Nelson, M. V. and Perley, A. M.: J.A.M.A., *100:*251, 1933.
110. Luetscher, J. A., Jr., Hall, A. O. and Kremer, V. L.: J. Clin. Invest., *28:*700, 1949 and *29:*896, 1950.
111. Taylor, R. D., Corcoran, A. C. and Page, I. H.: J. Lab. & Clin. Med., *36:*996, 1950.
112. Lange, K., Slobody, L. and Strong, R.: Pediatrics, *15:*156, 1955.
113. Merrill, A. J., Wilson, J. and Timberlake, L. F.: Arch. Int. Med., *94:*925, 1954.
114. Riley, C. M. and Davis, R. A.: Am. J. Dis. Child., *90:*534, 1955.
115. Galan, E. and Maso, C.: Pediatrics, *20:* 610, 1957.
116. Baxter, J. H., Goodman, H. C. and Orloff, J.: J. Clin. Invest., *35:*689, 1956.
117. Luetscher, J. A., Jr. and Mulrow, P. J.: Disease-a-Month Series, August, 1956. Chicago, The Year Book Publishers.
118. Modern, F. W. S. and Meister, L.: M. Clin. North America, July, 1952.
119. Folin, O., Berglund, H. and Derick, C.: J. Biol. Chem., *60:*361, 1924.
120. Dunn, J. S. and Polson, C. J.: J. Path. & Bact., *29:*337, 1926.
121. Coombs, F. S., Pecora, L. J., Thorogood, E., Consolazio, W. V. and Talbot, J. H.: J. Clin. Invest., *19:*525, 1940.
122. Berliner, R. W., Hilton, J. G., Yü, T. F. and Kennedy, T. J., Jr.: J. Clin. Invest., *29:*396, 1950.
123. Bordley, J. and Richards, A. N.: J. Biol. Chem., *101:*193, 1933.
124. Gudzent, F.: Gicht und Rheumatismus. Berlin, Springer, 1928.
125. Sirota, J. H., Yü, T. F. and Gutman, A. B.: J. Clin. Invest., *31:*692, 1952.
126. Mortensen, S. D. and Emmett, J. L.: J. Urol., *71:*398, 1954.
127. Engel, W. J.: J.A.M.A., *145:*288, 1951.
128. Kessler, E.: Ann. Int. Med., *42:*324, 1955.
129. Halvorsen, S.: Acta. med. scandinav., *149:*401, 1954.
130. Albright, F. and Reifenstein, E. C.: The Parathyroid Glands and Metabolic Bone Disease. Baltimore, Williams and Wilkins Co., 1948.
131. McCune, D. J., Mason, H. H. and Clarke, H. T.: Am. J. Dis. Child., *65:*81, 1943.
132. Teilum, G.: Acta path. microbiol. scandinav., *28:*294, 1951.
133. Berger, K. W. and Relman, A. S.: New England J. M., *252:*44, 1955.
134. Branson, J. H. and Park, J. H.: Ann. Int. Med., *40:*111, 1954.
135. Longcope, W. T. and Freiman, D. G.: Medicine, *31:*1, 1952.
136. Harrell, G. T. and Fisher, S.: J. Clin. Invest., *18:*687, 1939.
137. Schaumann, J.: Acta radiol., *7:*358, 1926.
138. Henneman, P. H., Carroll, E. L. and Dempsey, E. F.: J. Clin. Invest., *33:* 941, 1954.
139. Klemperer, P.: Ann. Int. Med., *28:*1, 1948.
140. Krupp, M. A.: Arch. Int. Med., *71:*54, 1943.

141. Dawson, J., Ball, J. and Platt, R.: Quart. J. Med., *41:*175, 1948.
142. Moore, H. C. and Sheehan, H. L.: Lancet, *1:*68, 1952.
143. O'Leary, P. A., and Nomland, R.: Am. J. M. Sc., *180:*95, 1930.
144. Burman, H.: Am. J. M. Sc., *216:*458, 1948.
145. Wirz, H. and Bott, P. A.: Proc. Soc. Exper. Biol. & Med., *87:*405, 1954.
146. Perkins, J. G., Petersen, A. B. and Riley, J. A.: Am. J. Med., *8:*115, 1950.
147. Relman, A. S. and Schwartz, W. B.: New England J. Med., *255:*195, 1956.
148. Schwartz, W. B. and Relman, A. S.: J. Clin. Invest., *32:*258, 1953.
149. Yuile, C. L.: Am. J. M. Sc., *207:*394, 1944.
150. Howard, J. E., Berthrong, M., Gould, D. M. and Yendt, E. R.: Bull. Johns Hopkins Hosp., *94:*51, 1954.
151. Pontasse, E. F., Humphries, A. W., McCormack, L. J. and Corcoran, A. C.: J.A.M.A., *161:*419, 1956.
152. Kahn, J. R.: Am. J. Clin. Path., *26:*521, 1956.
153. Goldblatt, H., Lynch, J., Hanzal, R. F. and Summerville, W. W.: J. Exper. Med., *59:*347, 1934.
154. Moritz, A. R. and Oldt, M. R.: Am. J. Path., *13:*679, 1937.
155. Tigerstedt, R. and Bergman, P. G.: Skand. Arch. Physiol., *8:*223, 1898.
156. Wakerlin, G. E. and Johnson, C. A.: Proc. Soc. Exper. Biol. & Med., *46:*104, 1941.
157. Braun-Menéndez, E., Fasciolo, J. C., Leloir, L. F. and Munoz, J. M.: J. Physiol., *98:*283, 1940.
158. Kohlstaedt, K. G., Page, I. H. and Helmer, O. M.: Am. Heart J., *19:*92, 1940.
159. Grollman, A., Harrison, T. B. and Williams, J. R., Jr.: Blood, Heart and Circulation Symposium. Washington, D.C., Am. A. Adv. Sc., 1940, pp. 274.
160. Shorr, E., Zweifach, B. W., Furchott, R. F. and Baez, S.: Fed. Proc., *7:*115, 1948.
161. Heymans, C. and Bouckaert, J. J.: Proc. Soc. Exper. Biol. & Med., *39:*94, 1938.
162. Gollan, F., Richardson, E. and Goldblatt, H.: J. Exper. Med., *88:*389, 1948.
163. Kahn, J. R., Skeggs, L. T., Jr., Shumway, N. P. and Wisenbaugh, P. E.: J. Exper. Med., *95:*523, 1952.
164. Skeggs, L. T., Jr., Marsh, W. H., Kahn, J. R. and Shumway, N. P.: J. Exper. Med., *99:*275, 1954.
165. Skeggs, L. T., Jr., Marsh, W. H., Kahn, J. R. and Shumway, N. P.: J. Exper. Med., *102:*435, 1955.
166. Skeggs, L. T., Jr., Lentz, K. E., Kahn, J. R., Shumway, N. P. and Woods, K. R.: J. Exper. Med., *104:*193, 1956.
167. Bell, E. T.: Renal Disease. 2nd. ed. Philadelphia, Lea & Febiger, 1950.
168. Ayman, D.: Arch. Int. Med., *53:*792, 1934.
169. Draper, G.: Human Constitution. Philadelphia, W. B. Saunders Co., 1924.
170. Derow, H. A. and Altschule, M. D.: Ann. Int. Med., *14:*1768, 1941.
171. Longcope, W. T. and Winkenwerder, W. L.: Bull. Johns Hopkins Hosp., *53:*255, 1933.
172. Weiss, S. and Parker, F., Jr.: Medicine, *18:*221, 1939.
173. Allen, A. C.: The Kidney, Medical and Surgical Diseases. New York, Grune and Stratton, 1951.
174. McManus, J. F. S.: Medical Diseases of the Kidney. Philadelphia, Lea & Febiger, 1950.
175. Beeson, P. B.: Yale J. Biol. & Med., *28:*81, 1955.
176. Ehrström, M. C.: Acta med. scandinav., *119:*122, 1944.
177. Mallory, G. K., Crane, A. R. and Edwards, J. E.: Arch. Path., *30:*330, 1940.
178. Brande, A. I., Shapiro, A. P. and Siemienski, J.: J. Clin. Invest., *34:*1489, 1955.
179. Dubos, R. J.: Biochemical Determinants of Microbial Disease. Cambridge, Mass., Harvard University Press, 1954.
180. Boyd, W.: Canad. M.A.J., *47:*128, 1942.
181. Crabtree, E. G. and Prien, E. L.: J. Urol., *42:*982, 1939.
182. Saphir, O. and Taylor, B.: Ann. Int. Med., *36:*1017, 1952.
183. Kass, E. H.: Am. J. Med., *18:*764, 1955.
184. Geschickter, C. F. and Copeland, N. M.: Arch. Surg., *16:*807, 1928.
195. Yuile, C. L.: Physiol. Rev., *22:*19, 1942.
186. Snapper, I., Turner, L. B. and Moscovitz, H. L.: Multiple Myeloma. New York, Grune and Stratton, 1953.
187. Oliver, J.: Harvey Lectures, *40:*102, 1944.
188. Blackman, C., Barker, W., Buell, M. and Davis, B.: J. Clin. Invest., *23:*163, 1944.
189. Armstrong, J. B.: Am. J. Med. Sc., *219:*488, 1950.
190. Goldman, R., Adams, W. S. and Luchsinger, E.: J. Lab. & Clin. Med., *40:*519, 1952.
191. Bywaters, E. G. L. and Beall, D.: Brit. M. J., *1:*427, 1941.
192. Minami, S.: Arch. f. path. Anat., *245:*247, 1923.
193. Lucké, B.: Mil. Surg. *99:*371, 1946.
194. Oliver, J., MacDowell, M. and Tracy, A.: J. Clin. Invest., *30:*1307, 1951.
195. Yuile, C. L.: Physiol. Rev., *22:*19, 1942.
196. Bott, P. A., and Richards, A. N.: J. Biol. Chem., *141:*291, 1941.
197. Foy, H., Altmann, A., Barnes, H. D. and Kondi, A.: Tr. Roy. Soc. Trop. Med. and Hyg., *36:*197, 1943.

198. Van Slyke, D. D.: Ann. Int. Med., *28:* 701, 1948.
199. Maxwell, M. H., Breed, E. S. and Smith, H. W.: Amer. J. Med., *9:*216, 1950.
200. Richards, A. N.: Tr. A. Am. Physicians, *44:*64, 1929.
201. Merrill, J. P., Thorn, G. W., Walter, C. W., Callahan, E. J., 3rd and Smith, L. H., Jr.: J. Clin. Invest., *29:*412, 1950.
202. Murray, G., Delorme, E. and Thomas, N.: Brit. M. J., *2:*887, 1949.
203. Skeggs, L. T., Jr., Leonards, J. R. and Heisler, C. R.: Proc. Soc. Exper. Biol. & Med., *72:*539, 1949.

Appendix

By GARFIELD G. DUNCAN, M.D.

Composition of Foods. With the general adoption of the Food Exchange System (p. 819), it appears superfluous to include the percentage value of protein, fat and carbohydrate of the common foods. However, for those who may use such data, attention is drawn to the revised brochure—Composition of Foods, U.S. Dept. of Agriculture, Agriculture Handbook No. 8, June, 1950.

Determination of Basal Energy Requirements*

The DuBois Normal Standards† as Modified by Boothby and Sandiford (from the Mayo Clinic), Am. J. Physiol., 90: 291, 1929

Calories per Square Meter per Day

AGE	MALES	FEMALES	AGE	MALES	FEMALES
5	1272	1238	20–24	984	886
6	1265	1217	25–29	967	878
7	1248	1162	30–34	955	869
8	1229	1154	35–39	931	859
9	1210	1126	40–44	919	847
10	1188	1099	45–49	907	840
11	1166	1070	50–54	893	828
12	1147	1042	55–59	878	818
13	1130	1028	60–64	864	811
14	1109	984	65–69	847	802
15	1087	950	70–74	(835)	(787)
16	1073	924	75–79	(820)	(775)
17	1049	898			
18	1030	895			
19	1010	892			

* From Frances Stern: Applied Dietetics, Williams and Wilkins, Baltimore, 1936, p. 105.

† For convenience the calories for the day have been used, rather than calories per hour, as in the original table.

Heights and Weights of 221,819 Men Fifteen or More Years of Age (with Clothes*)

AGE	GRADED AVERAGE WEIGHT IN POUNDS WITH CLOTHES																	
	Feet and Inches with Shoes																	
	5–0	5–1	5–2	5–3	5–4	5–5	5–6	5–7	5–8	5–9	5–10	5–11	6–0	6–1	6–2	6–3	6–4	6–5
15	107	109	112	115	118	122	126	130	134	138	142	147	152	157	162	167	172	177
16	109	111	114	117	120	124	128	132	136	140	144	149	154	159	164	169	174	179
17	111	113	116	119	122	126	130	134	138	142	146	151	156	161	166	171	176	181
18	113	115	118	121	124	128	132	136	140	144	148	153	158	163	168	173	178	183
19	115	117	120	123	126	130	134	138	142	146	150	155	160	165	170	175	180	185
20	117	119	122	125	128	132	136	140	144	148	152	156	161	166	171	176	181	186
21	118	120	123	126	130	134	138	141	145	149	153	157	162	167	172	177	182	187
22	119	121	124	127	131	135	139	142	146	150	154	158	163	168	173	178	183	188
23	120	122	125	128	132	136	140	143	147	151	155	159	164	169	175	180	185	190
24	121	123	126	129	133	137	141	144	148	152	156	160	165	171	177	182	187	192
25	122	124	126	129	133	137	141	145	149	153	157	162	167	173	179	184	189	194
26	123	125	127	130	134	138	142	146	150	154	158	163	168	174	180	186	191	196
27	124	126	128	131	134	138	142	146	150	154	158	163	169	175	181	187	192	197
28	125	127	129	132	135	139	143	147	151	155	159	164	170	176	182	188	193	198
29	126	128	130	133	136	140	144	148	152	156	160	165	171	177	183	189	194	199
30	126	128	130	133	136	140	144	148	152	156	161	166	172	178	184	190	196	201
31	127	129	131	134	137	141	145	149	153	157	162	167	173	179	185	191	197	202
32	127	129	131	134	137	141	145	149	154	158	163	168	174	180	186	192	198	203
33	127	129	131	134	137	141	145	149	154	159	164	169	175	181	187	193	199	204
34	128	130	132	135	138	142	146	150	155	160	165	170	176	182	188	194	200	206
35	128	130	132	135	138	142	146	150	155	160	165	170	176	182	189	195	201	207
36	129	131	133	136	139	143	147	151	156	161	166	171	177	183	190	196	202	208
37	129	131	133	136	140	144	148	152	157	162	167	172	178	184	191	197	203	209
38	130	132	134	137	140	144	148	152	157	162	167	173	179	185	192	198	204	210
39	130	132	134	137	140	144	148	152	157	162	167	173	179	185	192	199	205	211
40	131	133	135	138	141	145	149	153	158	163	168	174	180	186	193	200	206	212
41	131	133	135	138	141	145	149	153	158	163	168	174	180	186	193	200	207	213
42	132	134	136	139	142	146	150	154	159	164	169	175	181	187	194	201	208	214
43	132	134	136	139	142	146	150	154	159	164	169	175	181	187	194	201	208	214
44	133	135	137	140	143	147	151	155	160	165	170	176	182	188	195	202	209	215
45	133	135	137	140	143	147	151	155	160	165	170	176	182	188	195	202	209	215
46	134	136	138	141	144	148	152	156	161	166	171	177	183	189	196	203	210	216
47	134	136	138	141	144	148	152	156	161	167	171	177	183	190	197	204	211	217
48	134	136	138	141	144	148	152	156	161	166	171	177	183	190	197	204	211	217
49	134	136	138	141	144	148	152	156	161	166	171	177	183	190	197	204	211	217
50	134	136	138	141	144	148	152	156	161	166	171	177	183	190	197	204	211	217
51	135	137	139	142	145	149	153	157	162	167	172	178	184	191	198	205	212	218
52	135	137	139	142	145	149	153	157	162	167	172	178	184	191	198	205	212	218
53	135	137	139	142	145	149	153	157	162	167	172	178	184	191	198	205	212	218
54	125	137	139	142	145	149	153	158	163	168	173	178	184	191	198	205	212	219
55	135	137	139	142	145	149	153	158	163	168	173	178	184	191	198	205	212	219

* Association of Life Insurance Directors and Actuarial Society of America, New York, 1912, p. 38. Published by a committee. Allow 1 inch for shoes and 10 pounds for clothes.

Heights and Weights of 136,504 Women Fifteen or More Years of Age (with Clothes)

AGE	GRADED AVERAGE WEIGHT IN POUNDS WITH CLOTHES																
	Feet and Inches with Shoes																
	4–8	4–9	4–10	4–11	5–0	5–1	5–2	5–3	5–4	5–5	5–6	5–7	5–8	5–9	5–10	5–11	6–0
15	101	103	105	106	107	109	112	115	118	122	126	130	134	138	142	147	152
16	102	104	106	108	109	111	114	117	120	124	128	132	136	139	143	148	153
17	103	105	107	109	111	113	116	119	122	125	129	133	137	140	144	149	154
18	104	106	108	110	112	114	117	120	123	126	130	134	138	141	145	150	155
19	105	107	109	111	113	115	118	121	124	127	131	135	139	142	146	151	155
20	106	108	110	112	114	116	119	122	125	128	132	136	140	143	147	151	156
21	107	109	111	113	115	117	120	123	126	129	133	137	141	144	148	152	156
22	107	109	111	113	115	117	120	123	126	129	133	137	141	145	149	153	157
23	108	110	112	114	116	118	121	124	127	130	134	138	142	146	150	153	157
24	109	111	113	115	117	119	121	124	127	130	134	138	142	146	150	154	158
25	109	111	113	115	117	119	121	124	128	131	135	139	143	147	151	154	158
26	110	112	114	116	118	120	122	125	128	131	135	139	143	147	151	155	159
27	110	112	114	116	118	120	122	125	129	132	136	140	144	148	152	155	159
28	111	113	115	117	119	121	123	126	130	133	137	141	145	149	153	156	160
29	111	113	115	117	119	121	123	126	130	133	137	141	145	149	153	156	160
30	112	114	116	118	120	122	124	127	131	134	138	142	146	150	154	157	161
31	113	115	117	119	121	123	125	128	132	135	139	143	147	151	154	157	161
32	113	115	117	119	121	123	125	128	132	136	140	144	148	152	155	158	162
33	114	116	118	120	122	124	126	129	133	137	141	145	149	153	156	159	162
34	115	117	119	121	123	125	127	130	134	138	142	146	150	154	157	160	163
35	115	117	119	121	123	125	127	130	134	138	142	146	150	154	157	160	163
36	116	118	120	122	124	126	128	131	135	139	143	147	151	155	158	161	164
37	116	118	120	122	124	126	129	132	136	140	144	148	152	156	159	162	165
38	117	119	121	123	125	127	130	133	137	141	145	149	153	157	160	163	166
39	118	120	122	124	126	128	131	134	138	142	146	150	154	158	161	164	167
40	119	121	123	125	127	129	132	135	138	142	146	150	154	158	161	164	167
41	120	122	124	126	128	130	133	136	139	143	147	151	155	159	162	165	168
42	120	122	124	126	128	130	133	136	139	143	147	151	155	159	162	166	169
43	121	122	125	127	129	131	134	137	140	144	148	152	156	160	163	167	170
44	122	124	126	128	130	132	135	138	141	145	149	153	157	161	164	168	171
45	122	124	126	128	130	132	135	138	141	145	149	153	157	161	164	168	171
46	123	125	127	129	131	133	136	139	142	146	150	154	158	162	165	169	172
47	123	125	127	129	131	133	136	139	142	146	151	155	159	163	166	170	173
48	124	126	128	130	132	134	137	140	143	147	152	156	160	164	167	171	174
49	124	126	128	130	132	134	137	140	143	147	152	156	161	165	168	172	175
50	125	127	129	131	133	135	138	141	144	148	152	156	161	165	169	173	176
51	125	127	129	131	133	135	138	141	144	148	152	157	162	166	170	174	177
52	125	127	129	131	133	135	138	141	144	148	152	157	162	166	170	174	177
53	125	127	129	131	133	135	138	141	144	148	152	157	162	166	170	174	177
54	125	127	129	131	133	135	138	141	144	148	153	158	163	167	172	174	177
55	125	127	129	131	133	135	138	141	144	148	153	158	163	167	171	174	177

* Association of Life Insurance Directors and Actuarial Society of America, New York, 1912, p. 67. Published by a committee. Allow $1\frac{1}{2}$ inches for shoes and 6 pounds for clothes

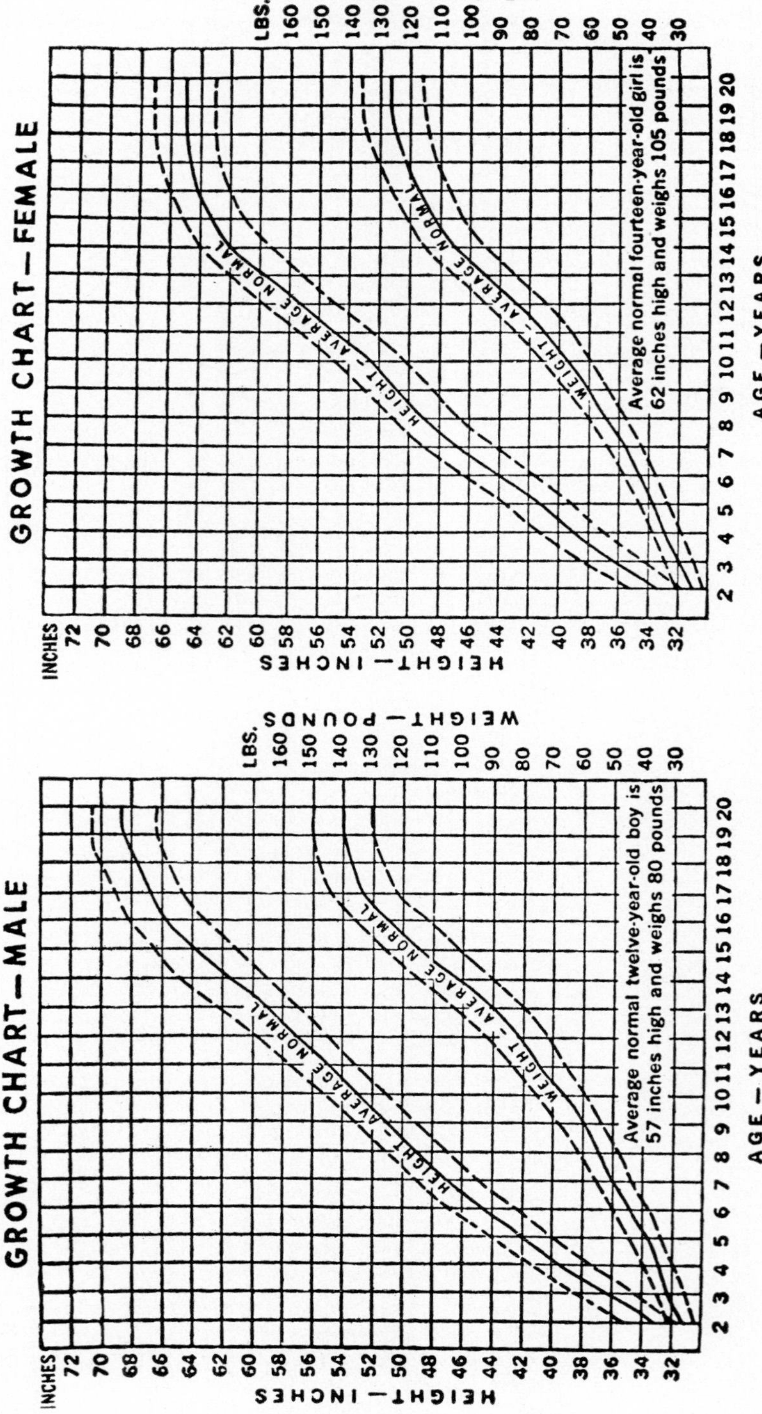

Fig. 1. Normal growth patterns. Solid lines indicate average normals; broken lines, 10 per cent above or below ideal normals. (Presented through the courtesy of Dr. J. H. Barach.)

Heights and Weights of Children between One and Four Years of Age (without Clothes) *

5602 BOYS		AGE, MONTHS	4821 GIRLS	
Height, Inches	Weight, Pounds		Height, Inches	Weight, Pounds
26.5	18.0	6	25.9	16.8
27.3	19.1	7	26.5	17.4
27.6	19.8	8	27.0	18.3
28.1	20.4	9	27.6	19.1
28.5	20.9	10	27.9	19.5
29.0	21.4	11	28.4	20.1
29.4	21.9	12	28.9	20.8
29.9	22.9	13	29.4	21.0
30.3	23.0	14	29.5	21.6
30.8	23.6	15	30.1	21.9
31.1	24.1	16	30.5	22.6
31.4	24.5	17	30.8	22.9
31.8	24.6	18	31.1	23.4
32.3	25.5	19	31.5	23.8
32.6	25.8	20	32.0	24.1
32.9	25.8	21	32.3	24.8
33.3	26.9	22	32.6	25.3
33.6	27.0	23	32.9	25.6
33.8	27.1	24	33.4	26.4
34.0	27.9	25	33.8	26.9
34.1	28.3	26	33.9	27.3
34.8	29.0	27	33.9	27.3
35.1	29.1	28	34.6	27.8
35.4	29.3	29	34.8	27.8
35.4	29.5	30	34.9	28.3
35.5	30.5	31	35.1	28.8
36.0	30.6	32	35.4	29.0
36.1	30.6	33	35.6	29.1
36.5	31.1	34	36.5	30.1
36.8	31.9	35	36.5	30.3
37.1	32.3	36	36.8	30.5
37.4	32.3	37	36.8	30.8
37.5	32.4	38	37.0	31.0
37.9	33.1	39	37.3	31.6
38.4	33.5	40	37.5	32.0
38.6	33.6	41	37.8	32.3
38.6	33.8	42	38.0	32.5
38.8	33.8	43	38.3	32.8
38.9	34.3	44	38.5	33.0
39.0	34.5	45	38.5	33.5
39.0	34.8	46	38.8	33.5
39.3	35.8	47	38.9	33.5
39.5	35.9	48	39.0	33.8

* Crum, F. S.: Quarterly Publication of the American Statistical Association, Boston, September, 1916, N.S., No. 115, 15, 332.

Height—Weight—Age Table (Boys)

HEIGHT, INCHES	5 YRS.	6 YRS.	7 YRS.	8 YRS.	9 YRS.	10 YRS.	11 YRS.	12 YRS.	13 YRS.	14 YRS.	15 YRS.	16 YRS.	17 YRS.	18 YRS.	19 YRS.
38	34	34													
39	35	35													
40	36	36													
41	38	38	38												
42	39	39	39	39											
43	41	41	41	41											
44	44	44	44	44											
45	46	46	46	46	46										
46	47	48	48	48	48										
47	49	50	50	50	50	50									
48		52	53	53	53	53									
49		55	55	55	55	55	55								
50		57	58	58	58	58	58	58							
51			61	61	61	61	61	61							
52			63	64	64	64	64	64	64						
53			66	67	67	67	67	68	68						
54				70	70	70	70	71	71	72					
55				72	72	73	73	74	74	74					
56				75	76	77	77	77	78	78	80				
57					79	80	81	81	82	83	83				
58					83	84	84	85	85	86	87				
59						87	88	89	89	90	90	90			
60						91	92	92	93	94	95	96			
61							95	96	97	99	100	103	106		
62							100	101	102	103	104	107	111	116	
63							105	106	107	108	110	113	118	123	127
64								109	111	113	115	117	121	126	130
65								114	117	118	120	122	127	131	134
66									119	122	125	128	132	136	139
67									124	128	130	134	136	139	142
68										134	134	137	141	143	147
69										137	139	143	146	149	152
70										143	144	145	148	151	155
71										148	150	151	152	154	159
72											153	155	156	158	163
73											157	160	162	164	167
74											160	164	168	170	171

Prepared by Bird T. Baldwin, Ph.D., and Thomas D. Wood, M. D.

Height—Weight—Age Table (Girls)

HEIGHT, INCHES	5 YRS.	6 YRS.	7 YRS.	8 YRS.	9 YRS.	10 YRS.	11 YRS.	12 YRS.	13 YRS.	14 YRS.	15 YRS.	16 YRS.	17 YRS.	18 YRS.
38	33	33												
39	34	34												
40	36	36	36											
41	37	37	37											
42	39	39	39											
43	41	41	41	41										
44	42	42	42	42										
45	45	45	45	45	45									
46	47	47	47	48	48									
47	49	50	50	50	50	50								
48		52	52	52	52	53	53							
49		54	54	55	55	56	56							
50		56	56	57	58	59	61	62						
51			59	60	61	61	63	65						
52			63	64	64	64	65	67						
53			66	67	67	68	68	69	71					
54				69	70	70	71	71	73					
55				72	74	74	74	75	77	78				
56					76	78	78	79	81	83				
57					80	82	82	82	84	88	92			
58						84	86	86	88	93	96	101		
59						87	90	90	92	96	100	103	104	
60						91	95	95	97	101	105	108	109	111
61							99	100	101	105	108	112	113	116
62							104	105	106	109	113	115	117	118
63								110	110	112	116	117	119	120
64								114	115	117	119	120	122	123
65								188	120	121	122	123	125	126
66									124	124	125	128	129	130
67									128	130	131	133	133	135
68									131	133	135	136	138	138
69										135	137	138	140	142
70										136	138	140	142	144
71										138	140	142	144	145

Prepared by Bird T. Baldwin, Ph.D., and Thomas D. Wood, M. D.

Index